D1609512

EXPERTddx

HEAD AND NECK

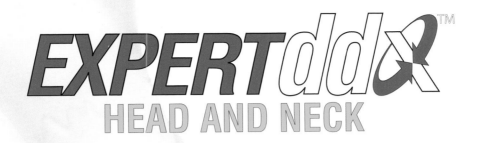

EXPERTddx™
HEAD AND NECK

H. Ric Harnsberger, MD
Professor of Radiology and Otolaryngology
R.C. Willey Chair in Neuroradiology
University of Utah School of Medicine
Salt Lake City, Utah

Michelle A. Michel, MD
Professor of Radiology and Otolaryngology
Chief, Head and Neck Neuroradiology
Medical College of Milwaukee
Milwaukee, Wisconsin

C. Douglas Phillips, MD, FACR
Professor of Radiology
Director of Head and Neck Imaging
Weill-Cornell Medical College
New York-Presbyterian Hospital
New York, New York

Patricia A. Hudgins, MD
Professor of Radiology and Otolaryngology
Head and Neck Radiology
Emory University School of Medicine
Atlanta, Georgia

Richard H. Wiggins, III, MD
Associate Professor of Radiology, Otolaryngology, Head and
Neck Surgery, and Biomedical Informatics
University of Utah School of Medicine
Salt Lake City, Utah

Christine M. Glastonbury, MBBS
Associate Professor of Clinical Radiology, Otolaryngology, and
Radiation Oncology
University of California, San Francisco
San Francisco, California

Bernadette L. Koch, MD
Associate Professor of Radiology and Pediatrics
Cincinnati Children's Hospital Medical Center
Cincinnati, Ohio

Kristine M. Mosier, DMD, PhD
Associate Professor of Radiology
Chief, Head and Neck Imaging
Department of Radiology
Section of Neuroradiology
Indiana University School of Medicine
Indianapolis, Indiana

H. Christian Davidson, MD
Associate Professor of Radiology
University of Utah School of Medicine
Salt Lake City, Utah

Joel K. Curé, MD
Associate Professor of Radiology and Neurology
University of Alabama Medical Center
Birmingham, Alabama

AMIRSYS®
Names you know. Content you trust.®

AMIRSYS®

Names you know. Content you trust.®

First Edition

Composition by Amirsys, Inc., Salt Lake City, Utah

Printed in Canada by Friesens, Altona, Manitoba, Canada

ISBN: 978-1-931884-11-2

Notice and Disclaimer

Library of Congress Cataloging-in-Publication Data

Expertddx. Head and neck / [edited by] H. Ric Harnsberger. -- 1st ed.
   p. ; cm.
 Includes index.
 ISBN 978-1-931884-11-2
 1. Head--Diseases--Diagnosis--Atlases. 2. Neck--Diseases--Diagnosis--Atlases. 3. Diagnosis, Differential--Atlases. I. Harnsberger, H. Ric. II. Title: Head and neck.
 [DNLM: 1. Head--physiopathology--Handbooks. 2. Neck--physiopathology--Handbooks. 3. Diagnosis, Differential--Handbooks. 4. Diagnostic Imaging--Handbooks. WE 39 E955 2009]

 RC936.E97 2009
 617.5'3--dc22

                        2009004041

To our families and loved ones whose wholehearted support helped us sustain our efforts during the long hours of creating this unique book. Thank you all for that!

The <u>EXPERTddx: Head and Neck</u> author team

Norm's doing good. 74?

Ric

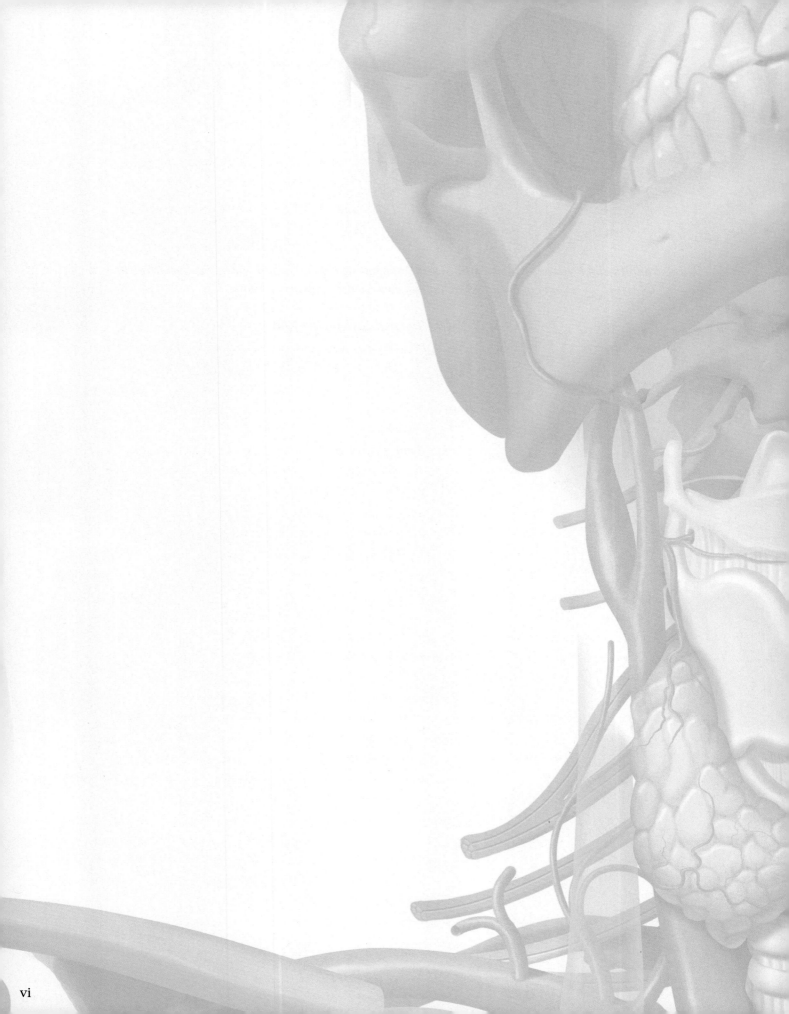

CONTRIBUTORS

Below are listed the stalwart group of physicians who took the time
to help find the case material necessary to fill the extensive image
galleries of *EXPERTddx: Head and Neck*. Without their
willingness to "share the wealth," this book would have been far
less rich an offering. Thanks to you all.
No book of this nature could have been done alone!

H. Ric Harnsberger, MD

Anil T. Ahuja, MD; Hong Kong, China
Susan I. Blaser, MD; Toronto, Canada
Barton F. Branstetter, MD; Pittsburgh, PA
Philip Chapman, MD; Huntsville, AL
Rebecca Cornelius, MD; Cincinnati, OH
Joel K. Curé, MD; Birmingham, AL
H. Christian Davidson, MD; Salt Lake City, UT
Nancy J. Fischbein, MD; Stanford, CA
Lindell R. Gentry, MD; Madison, WI
Lawrence E. Ginsberg, MD; Houston, TX
Christine M. Glastonbury, MBBS; San Francisco, CA
Gary L. Hedlund, DO; Salt Lake City, UT
Peter Hildenbrand, MD; Burlington, MA
Patricia A. Hudgins, MD; Atlanta, GA
Bernadette Koch, MD; Cincinnati, OH
Timothy S. Larson, MD; Charlotte, NC
Laurie A. Loevner, MD; Philadelphia, PA
André Macdonald, MBChB; Asheville, NC
Michelle M. Michel, MD; Milwaukee, WI
Kevin R. Moore, MD; Salt Lake City, UT
Kristine M. Mosier, MD; Indianapolis, IN
C. Douglas Phillips, MD; New York, NY
Edward Quigley, MD; Salt Lake City, UT
Charles Schatz, MD; Beverly Hills, CA
Anthony J. Scuderi, MD; Johnstown, PA
Lubdha M. Shah, MD; Salt Lake City, UT
Deborah R. Shatzkes, MD; New York, NY
Hilda Stambuk, MD; New York, NY
Brian M. Steele, DO; Denver, CO
Robert Wallace, MD; Phoenix, AZ
Richard H. Wiggins, III, MD; Salt Lake City, UT

Special thanks to Larry Ginsberg, Phil Chapman, and Peter Hildenbrand who contributed
above and beyond any possible expectation for their generosity with their case material.

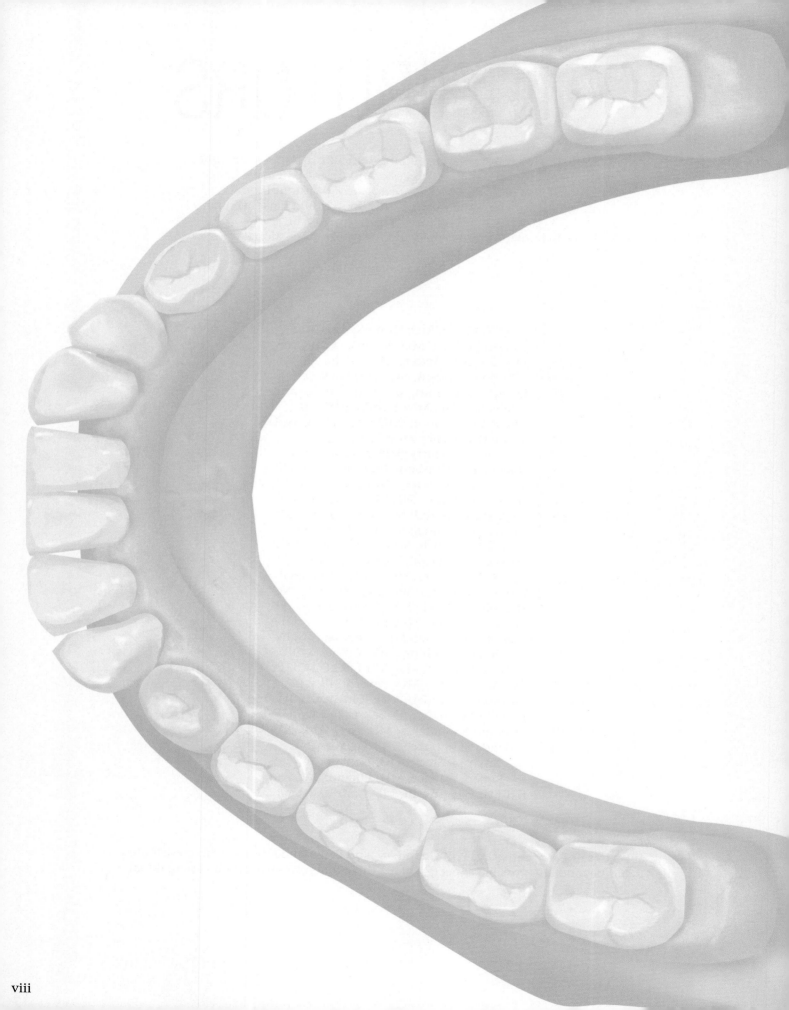

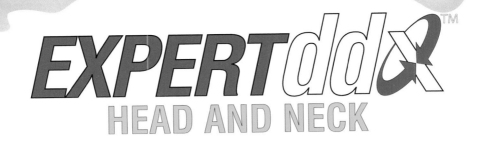

Once the appropriate technical protocols have been delineated, the best quality images obtained, and the cases queued up on PACS, the diagnostic responsibility reaches the radiology reading room. The radiologist must do more than simply "lay words on" but reach a real conclusion. If we cannot reach a definitive diagnosis, we must offer a reasonable differential diagnosis. A list that's too long is useless; a list that's too short may be misleading. To be useful, a differential must be more than a rote recitation from some dusty book or a mnemonic from a lecture way back when. Instead, we must take into account key imaging findings and relevant clinical information.

With these considerations in mind, we at Amirsys designed our Expert Differential Diagnoses series— EXPERTddx for short. Leading experts in every subspecialty of radiology identified the top differential diagnoses in their respective fields, encompassing specific anatomic locations, generic imaging findings, modality-specific findings, and clinically based indications. Our experts gathered multiple images, both typical and variant, for each EXPERTddx. Each features at least eight beautiful images that illustrate the possible diagnoses, accompanied by captions that highlight the pertinent imaging findings. Hundreds more are available in the eBook feature that accompanies every book. In classic Amirsys fashion, each EXPERTddx includes bulleted text that distills the available information to the essentials. You'll find helpful clues for diagnoses, ranked by prevalence as Common, Less Common, and Rare but Important.

Our EXPERTddx series is designed to help radiologists reach reliable—indeed, expert—conclusions. Whether you are a practicing radiologist or a resident/fellow in training, we think the EXPERTddx series will quickly become your practical "go-to" reference.

Anne G. Osborn, MD
Executive Vice President and Editor-in-Chief, Amirsys Inc.

Paula J. Woodward, MD
Executive Vice President and Medical Director, Amirsys Inc.

H. Ric Harnsberger, MD
CEO, Amirsys Inc.

PREFACE

When we wrote our first book, *Diagnostic Imaging: Head and Neck*, we were determined to create a comprehensive, diagnosis-based resource for radiologists seeking knowledge in the head and neck area. *Diagnostic and Surgical Imaging Anatomy: Brain, Head and Neck, Spine* followed with a goal to tackle the challenging anatomic substrate of the head and neck. Both these books have found a real audience in the imaging community (many thanks for that!). So why another book? Now that the radiologist can review the details of a specific diagnosis and feels comfortable with the underlying anatomy, one final question remains unanswered: "What is the differential diagnosis for that finding on my scan?" *EXPERTddx: Head and Neck* is designed to answer that question. It is aimed at busy radiologists who discover a finding on their head and neck study and want a statistically driven differential diagnosis list to activate their thought processes.

This one-of-a-kind book contains over 160 expert differential diagnoses, representing an exhaustive spectrum of head and neck imaging challenges. The book is organized first by anatomic area, then divided into the four classic differential diagnosis types: 1) anatomy-based, 2) general imaging finding–based, 3) modality-based, and 4) clinically based. Each differential diagnosis chapter has key facts, imaging findings, and image(s) for every diagnosis in the list. Thousands of images were chosen from a comprehensive library created by the authors and an intrepid case team. Never before has a book been published with such a wide variety of images of head and neck lesions. The eBook companion contains hundreds more images, adding to the richness of the final product.

If you have comments or suggestions for other "must have" differentials, we would be happy to hear from you at feedback@amirsys.com.

We hope this book becomes a critical part of your daily practice or a useful study guide if you are just entering our specialty. As the third and final component of the Amirsys Head and Neck trilogy, *EXPERTddx: Head and Neck* represents the culmination of a decade-long quest to create a distilled but comprehensive textbook series that demystifies the field of head and neck imaging. *Enjoy!*

H. Ric Harnsberger, MD
Professor of Radiology and Otolaryngology
R.C. Willey Chair in Neuroradiology
University of Utah School of Medicine
Salt Lake City, Utah

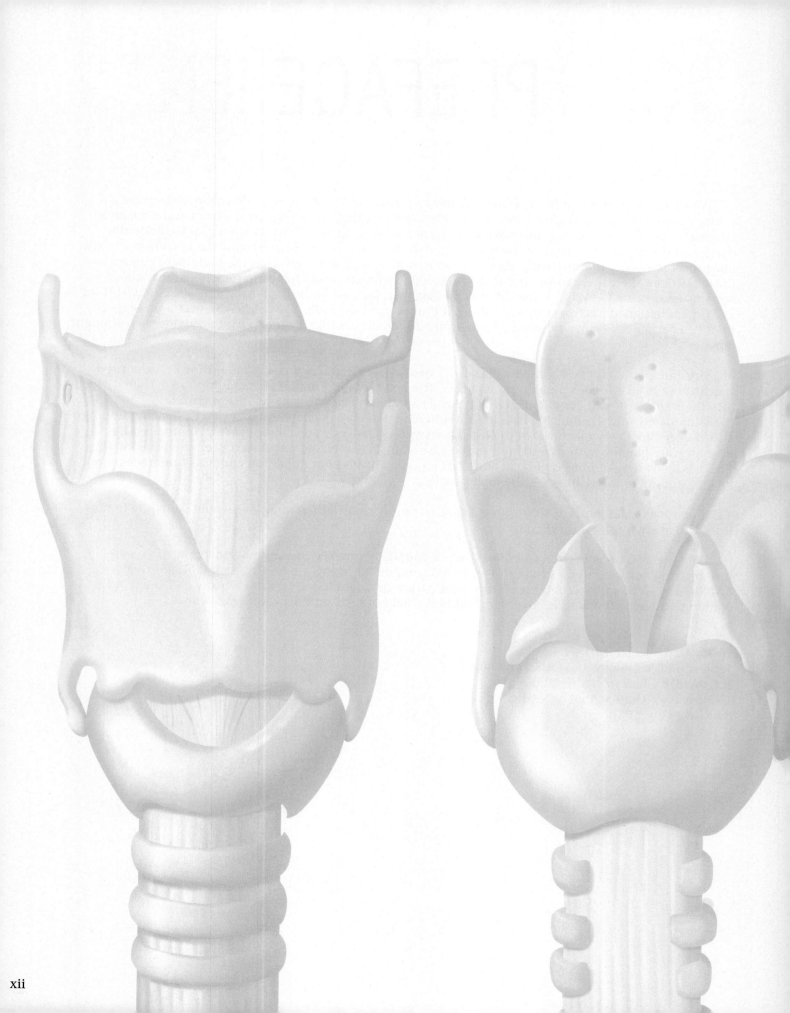

ACKNOWLEDGMENTS

Text Editing

Ashley R. Renlund, MA

Kellie J. Heap

Arthur G. Gelsinger, MA

Image Editing

Jeffrey J. Marmorstone

Christopher Odekirk

Medical Text Editing

Logan A. McLean, MD

Art Direction and Design

Lane R. Bennion, MS

Richard Coombs, MS

Production Lead

Melissa A. Hoopes

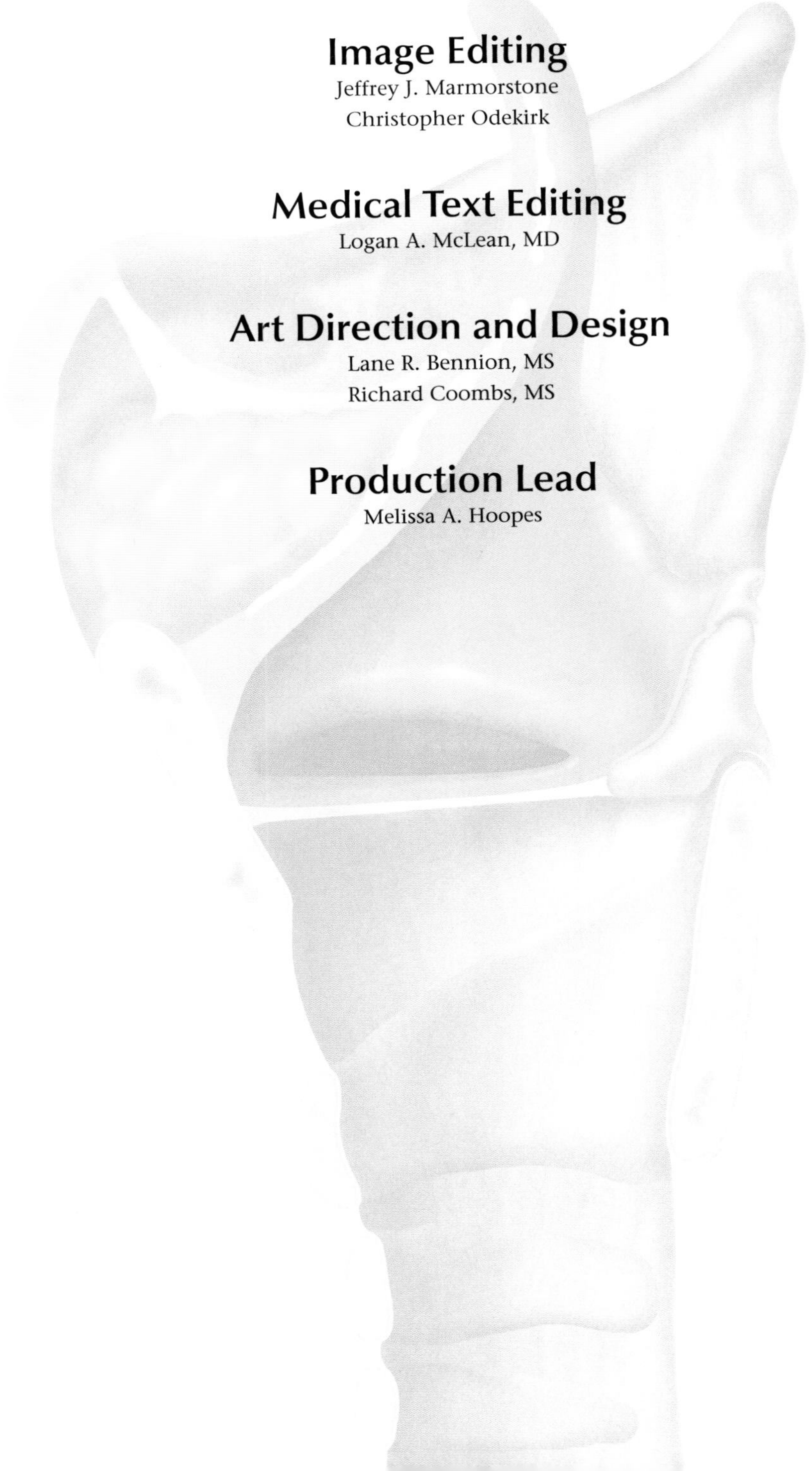

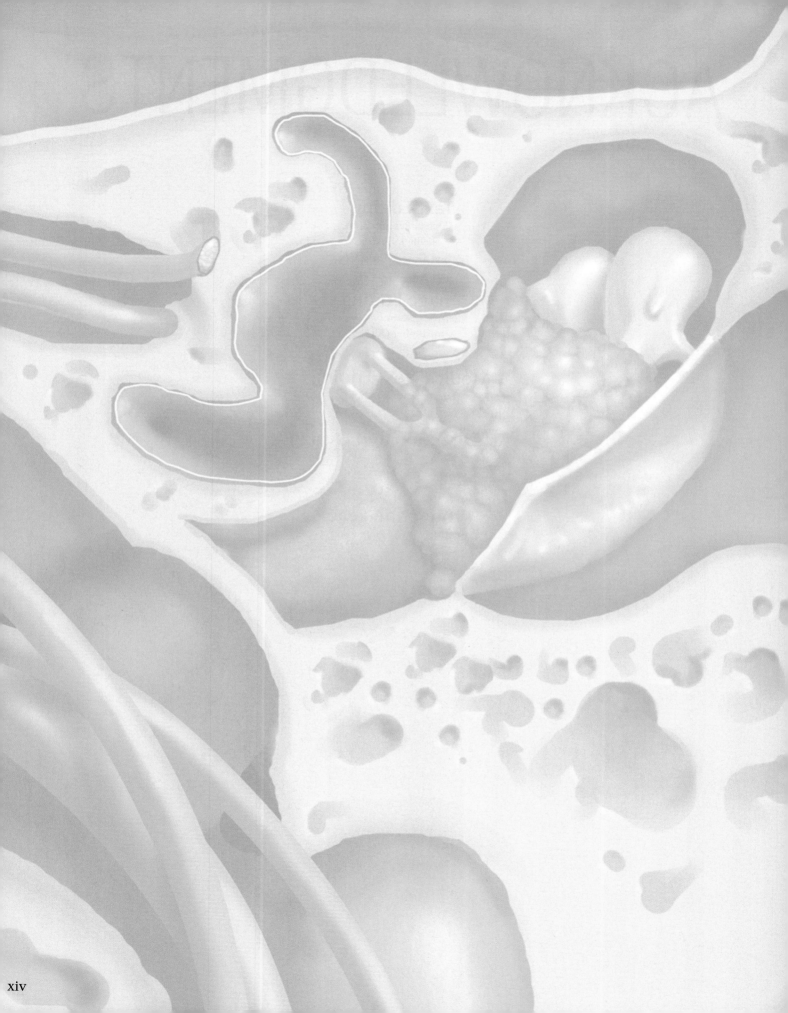

SECTIONS

Suprahyoid & Infrahyoid

Oral Cavity, Mandible & Maxilla

Hypopharynx & Larynx

Lymph Nodes

Trans-spatial, Multi-spatial in Head and Neck

Sinus & Nose

Orbit

Temporal Bone

Skull Base

CPA-IAC & Posterior Fossa

Cranial Nerve & Brainstem

TABLE OF CONTENTS

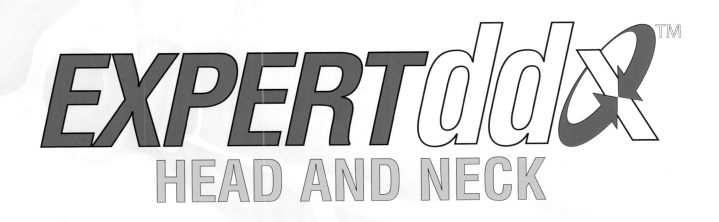

SECTION 1
Suprahyoid & Infrahyoid

Anatomically Based Differentials

Generic Imaging Patterns

Clinically Based Differentials

PARAPHARYNGEAL SPACE LESION

DIFFERENTIAL DIAGNOSIS

Common
- Direct Extension into PPS from Neoplasm from Adjacent Space
  - Pharyngeal Mucosal Space/Surface (PMS) ⇒ PPS
    - Nasopharyngeal Carcinoma
    - SCCa, Palatine Tonsil
    - Non-Hodgkin Lymphoma, PMS
  - Masticator Space (MS) ⇒ PPS
    - Sarcoma, MS
    - Rhabdomyosarcoma, MS
  - Parotid Space (PS) ⇒ PPS
    - Benign Mixed Tumor, PS
    - Adenoid Cystic Carcinoma, PS
    - Mucoepidermoid Carcinoma, PS
- Direct Extension into PPS from Abscess from Adjacent Space
  - Abscess, MS
  - Tonsillar Abscess, PMS
  - Parotiditis, Acute, PS

Less Common
- Primary PPS Lesion
  - Pterygoid Venous Plexus Asymmetry
  - Venolymphatic Malformation
  - Lipoma

Rare but Important
- Benign Mixed Tumor, PPS
- 2nd Branchial Cleft Cyst, Variant
- Ranula, Diving

ESSENTIAL INFORMATION

Key Differential Diagnosis Issues
- Parapharyngeal space lesion (PPS) is suprahyoid only
- PPS most commonly affected secondarily by local malignancy or infection, as primary PPS lesions are rare
  - Most deep lobe parotid tumors have mass effect on lateral aspect of PPS
  - When tumor is large, may be difficult to determine if site of origin is parotid gland or primary PPS
  - Nasopharyngeal & oropharyngeal malignancy flatten medial aspect of PPS

Helpful Clues for Common Diagnoses
- **Pharyngeal Mucosal Space/Surface (PMS) ⇒ PPS**
  - Medial wall PPS bulges laterally when lesion located in PMS
  - **Nasopharyngeal Carcinoma**
    - CT/MR: Lateral pharyngeal recess tumor bulges into medial PPS
    - Direct invasion of carotid space or bony skull base possible
  - **SCCa, Palatine Tonsil**
    - Tumor staged as T4 if PPS invaded
    - CT/MR: Tumor arises in tonsillar fossa, extends laterally with either mass effect or direct invasion of PPS
    - Induration of PPS fat and irregular margin between fat and tumor are key findings
  - **Non-Hodgkin Lymphoma, PMS**
    - CT/MR: Bulky PMS tumor bulges medial wall of PPS, without direct invasion
- **Masticator Space (MS) ⇒ PPS**
  - Lateral wall PPS bulges medially when lesion located in MS
  - **Sarcoma, MS**
    - CT/MR: Aggressive MS tumor ± calcific matrix
  - **Rhabdomyosarcoma, MS**
    - CT/MR: Aggressive noncalcified MS tumor in child
- **Parotid Space (PS) ⇒ PPS**
  - **Benign Mixed Tumor, PS**
    - Benign deep lobe tumor often asymptomatic until large
    - May be hard to determine if tumor is from parotid or primary PPS
    - CT/MR: Large well-circumscribed mass flattening lateral aspect of PPS
  - **Adenoid Cystic Carcinoma, PS**
    - CT/MR: Invasive parotid mass with propensity for perineural spread (CN7)
  - **Mucoepidermoid Carcinoma, PS**
    - CT/MR: Invasive parotid mass; enhances, "feathery" margins
- **Direct Extension into PPS from Abscess from Adjacent Space**
  - **Abscess, MS**
    - Odontogenic origins; recent tooth extraction or lucency around molar
    - CT/MR: Pus pocket in MS; edematous muscles; induration of PPS from lateral aspect
  - **Tonsillar Abscess, PMS**

PARAPHARYNGEAL SPACE LESION

- CT/MR: Palatine tonsil pus with surrounding edema & induration; mass effect on medial wall of PPS
  - **Parotiditis, Acute, PS**
    - CT/MR: Edematous parotid gland with possible stone in duct; swollen deep lobe causes mass effect on lateral wall of PPS

Helpful Clues for Less Common Diagnoses
- **Pterygoid Venous Plexus Asymmetry**
  - Prominent venous plexus at pterygoid plates involves PPS & MS
    - May simulate venous malformation
  - CECT: Asymmetric prominent venous enhancement in MS & anterior PPS near pterygoid plates
- **Venolymphatic Malformation**
  - Common congenital suprahyoid trans-spatial lesion usually presents in childhood
  - CT/MR: Involves multiple contiguous spaces, including PPS
    - Appearance determined by whether lesion is primarily venous, lymphatic, or mixed in composition
    - Venous components enhance, but both venous & lymphatic portions are T2 bright
- **Lipoma**
  - Benign fatty tumor almost always incidental finding
  - CT/MR: Enlarged but otherwise normal-appearing PPS

- Should have no soft tissue component and no enhancement

Helpful Clues for Rare Diagnoses
- **Benign Mixed Tumor, PPS**
  - Arises in PPS from ectopic salivary gland rests
    - Primary PPS benign mixed tumor has no connection to deep lobe of parotid gland
    - Tumor often large when diagnosed
    - PPS lesions "silent" and asymptomatic
  - CT/MR: Variable enhancement
    - Ovoid mass typically T1 low, T2 high on MR
    - If part of mass appears more aggressive or irregular, think of malignancy arising in BMT, "carcinoma ex pleomorphic adenoma"
- **2nd Branchial Cleft Cyst, Variant**
  - Primary cyst in PPS most likely branchial in origin
  - CT/MR: Benign nonenhancing cyst
    - May point or be connected to palatine tonsil area
- **Ranula, Diving**
  - Sublingual gland retention cyst ruptures into submandibular (SMS) & parapharyngeal spaces
  - CT/MR: "Tail" sign in sublingual space leads to SMS & PPS cystic components
    - PPS component rarest area for pseudocyst to spread

Nasopharyngeal Carcinoma

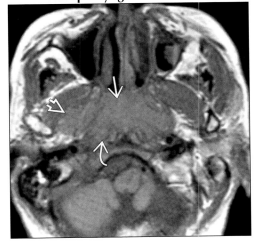

Axial T1WI MR shows a nonkeratinizing EBV-positive nasopharyngeal carcinoma filling the pharyngeal mucosal space ➡. The parapharyngeal space ➡ and prevertebral muscles ➡ are invaded by the tumor.

Nasopharyngeal Carcinoma

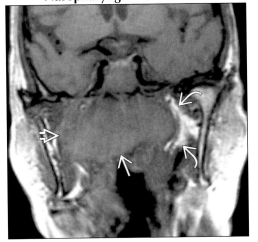

Coronal T1WI MR in the same patient reveals carcinoma ➡ in the nasopharyngeal mucosal space invading laterally into the right parapharyngeal space ➡. Note the normal left parapharyngeal space ➡.

PARAPHARYNGEAL SPACE LESION

(Left) Axial CECT shows a large palatine tonsil SCCa invading posterolaterally into the parapharyngeal space ➡. Note the fatty triangle of the normal contralateral parapharyngeal space ➡.
(Right) Axial CECT in the same patient demonstrates the palatine tonsillar SCCa invading the sublingual space ➡ and lateral parapharyngeal space ➡. Bilateral malignant level II nodes ➡ are visible.

SCCa, Palatine Tonsil

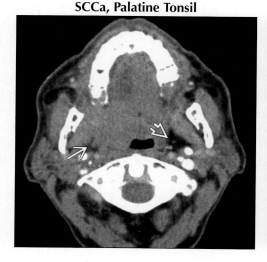

SCCa, Palatine Tonsil

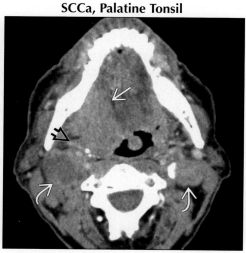

(Left) Axial CECT demonstrates a bulky bilateral nasopharyngeal non-Hodgkin lymphoma bulging into both parapharyngeal spaces ➡. The feathery appearance ➡ on the left suggests invasion of the parapharyngeal space.
(Right) Axial CECT in the same patient shows a mass nearly obliterating the left parapharyngeal space ➡.

Non-Hodgkin Lymphoma, PMS

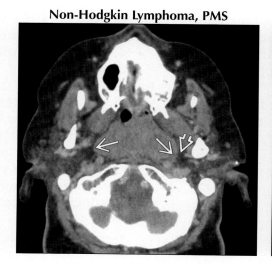

Non-Hodgkin Lymphoma, PMS

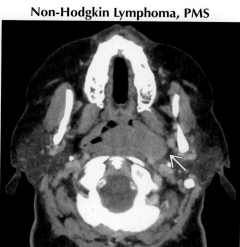

(Left) Axial CECT shows a masticator space osteosarcoma with destruction of the mandible and extension through the maxillary sinus wall ➡. Note the mass effect on the parapharyngeal space ➡.
(Right) Axial bone CT in the same patient demonstrates "sunburst" malignant periosteal changes ➡ of osteosarcoma. Parapharyngeal space compression ➡, from lateral to medial, is characteristic of a masticator space tumor.

Sarcoma, MS

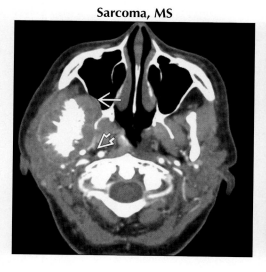

Sarcoma, MS

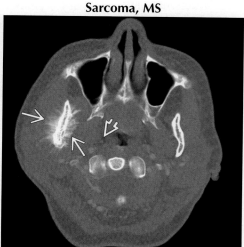

PARAPHARYNGEAL SPACE LESION

Rhabdomyosarcoma, MS

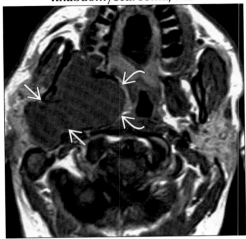

Rhabdomyosarcoma, MS

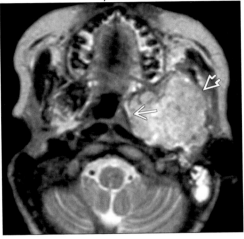

(Left) Axial T1WI MR shows a bulky mass arising in the right masticator space, extending through the stylomandibular tunnel laterally ➡, and bulging into the parapharyngeal space ➡. A smooth interface with PPS fat suggests there is no direct invasion through fascia. (Right) Axial T2WI MR reveals a large rhabdomyosarcoma in the medial masticator space, destroying the mandible ➡ and invading the parapharyngeal space ➡.

Benign Mixed Tumor, PS

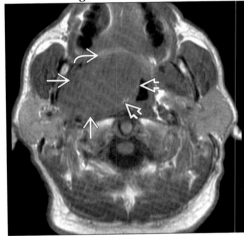

Benign Mixed Tumor, PS

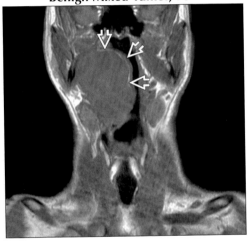

(Left) Axial T1WI MR shows a large deep parotid tumor ➡ with effacement of the pterygoid muscles, airway compromise, and a mass effect on the soft palate ➡. The parapharyngeal space ➡ is markedly flattened but not invaded. (Right) Coronal T1WI MR in the same patient confirms that the parapharyngeal space ➡ is stretched over the mass but not invaded.

Adenoid Cystic Carcinoma, PS

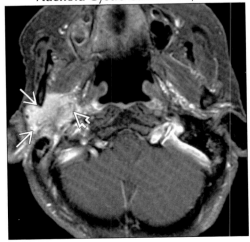

Adenoid Cystic Carcinoma, PS

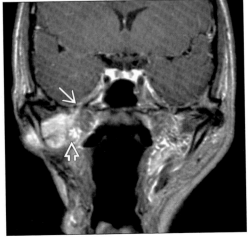

(Left) Axial T1 C+ FS MR shows an enhancing invasive recurrent tumor in the parotid gland ➡ with extension into the parapharyngeal space ➡ in a patient previously treated for parotid adenoid cystic carcinoma. Parapharyngeal fat has been replaced by tumor. (Right) Coronal T1 C+ FS MR in the same patient demonstrates a deep lobe tumor extending into the parapharyngeal space ➡ & a perineural tumor ➡ on the CN5/V3 division at the foramen ovale.

1

PARAPHARYNGEAL SPACE LESION

(Left) Axial CECT shows a mass in the superficial ➡ and deep lobes ➡ of the parotid gland, effacing the lateral PPS ➡. The feathery periphery of the mass is characteristic of parotid malignancy. *(Right)* Axial CECT shows a multilocular masticator space abscess with pus around the mandible ➡ and within the lateral pterygoid muscle ➡. The parapharyngeal space ➡ is effaced by the adjacent infection.

Mucoepidermoid Carcinoma, PS

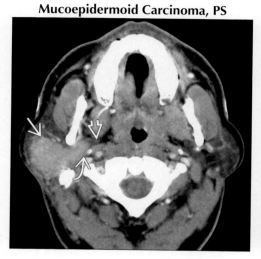

Abscess, MS

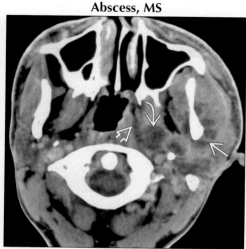

(Left) Axial CECT in a patient with a 2 week history of tonsillitis shows pus in the parapharyngeal space ➡ with a large inflamed palatine tonsil ➡ and masticator space phlegmon ➡. *(Right)* Axial CECT in the same patient reveals an inferior palatine tonsil abscess ➡ causing extensive submandibular space cellulitis ➡ and parapharyngeal & masticator space abscess (not shown).

Tonsillar Abscess, PMS

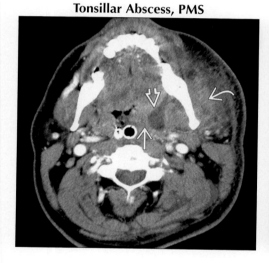

Tonsillar Abscess, PMS

(Left) Axial CECT reveals a diffusely enlarged left parotid gland with inhomogeneous enhancement, secondary to acute acalculous parotiditis. The deep lobe is swollen ➡. Note the induration of the parapharyngeal space fat ➡. *(Right)* Axial CECT demonstrates a prominent asymmetric left pterygoid venous plexus as racemose enhancement in the deep masticator ➡ and anterior parapharyngeal ➡ space.

Parotiditis, Acute, PS

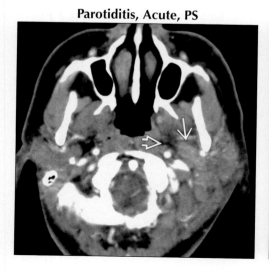

Pterygoid Venous Plexus Asymmetry

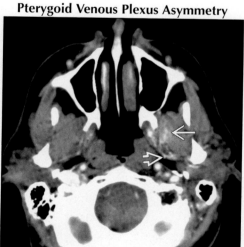

1

PARAPHARYNGEAL SPACE LESION

Venolymphatic Malformation

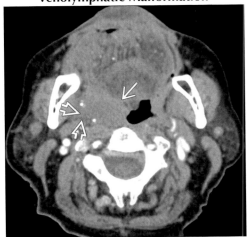

Venolymphatic Malformation

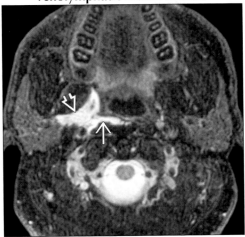

(Left) Axial CECT in a patient with violaceous oropharyngeal mucosa shows a tissue density venous malformation with phleboliths, involving the pharyngeal mucosal ➡ and parapharyngeal ➡ space. (Right) Axial T2WI FS MR reveals a high signal venolymphatic malformation that fills the parapharyngeal space ➡ and ipsilateral retropharyngeal space ➡. The trans-spatial nature, fluid signal, and shape all suggest venolymphatic malformation.

Lipoma

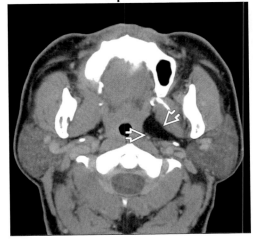

Benign Mixed Tumor, PPS

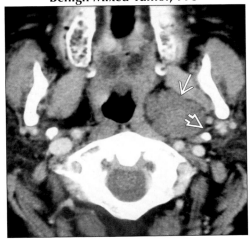

(Left) Axial CECT demonstrates a lipoma in the parapharyngeal space ➡. This lipoma extended inferiorly and involved the submandibular space (not shown). (Right) Axial CECT shows an ovoid benign mixed tumor ➡ centered in the parapharyngeal space. Note the sharp delineation ➡ between the deep lobe of the parotid gland and the tumor, indicating that the lesion arose in the parapharyngeal space and not in the deep lobe of the parotid gland.

2nd Branchial Cleft Cyst, Variant

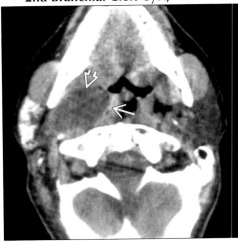

Ranula, Diving

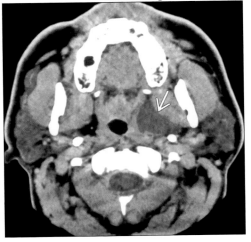

(Left) Axial NECT reveals an ovoid low-density cyst in the right parapharyngeal space ➡, deep to the palatine tonsil ➡. This is a rare example of a 2nd branchial cleft cyst projecting superiorly into the parapharyngeal space. (Right) Axial CECT reveals a fluid density lesion ➡ in the left parapharyngeal space. This superior extension of a diving ranula is confirmed on inferior images, defining the ranular sublingual space origin (not shown).

PHARYNGEAL MUCOSAL SPACE LESION, NASOPHARYNX

DIFFERENTIAL DIAGNOSIS

Common
- Adenoid Tissue, Prominent/Asymmetric
- Adenoid Inflammation
- Tornwaldt Cyst
- Retention Cyst, PMS
- Nasopharyngeal Carcinoma
- Non-Hodgkin Lymphoma, PMS

Less Common
- Post-Radiation Mucositis, PMS
- Benign Mixed Tumor, PMS

Rare but Important
- Minor Salivary Gland Malignancy, PMS
- Rhabdomyosarcoma
- Extraosseous Chordoma, PMS

ESSENTIAL INFORMATION

Key Differential Diagnosis Issues
- Remember, referring clinician can visualize mucosal surface
  - Carcinoma usually has mucosal ulceration
  - Lymphoma & other malignancies are submucosal
  - Caveat: Don't read CT or MR of pharyngeal mucosal space (PMS) without knowing what clinician sees!
- Big 3 tumors of this area are nasopharyngeal carcinoma, non-Hodgkin lymphoma, & minor salivary gland malignancy
  - Arise from principal normal PMS structures: Mucosal surface, lymphatic ring, & minor salivary glands
  - Close proximity to skull base explains why intracranial and cavernous sinus invasion are common with malignant lesions
    - Both CT (bone window) and MR are always indicated when PMS lesion involves skull base
- Nasopharyngeal mucosal space masses invade parapharyngeal space from medial to lateral

Helpful Clues for Common Diagnoses
- **Adenoid Tissue, Prominent/Asymmetric**
  - Key facts: Adenoids involute by 40 years
    - May be prominent if adult had tonsillectomy

- HIV and other immune-stimulating exposures can result in prominent adenoidal tissue
  - Imaging
    - Midline nasopharyngeal soft tissue
    - No extension through deep fascia or laterally into parapharyngeal space (PPS)
- **Adenoid Inflammation**
  - Key facts: Presents as acute pharyngitis
  - Imaging: Adenoidal ± lingual ± palatine tonsil enlargement
    - Peritonsillar soft tissue edema
    - Intratonsillar enhancing septa common
- **Tornwaldt Cyst**
  - Key facts: Common, clinically incidental
    - Midline cystic lesion present on 5% of all brain MR
    - Cyst of notochordal remnant
  - Imaging
    - Nonenhancing cyst between prevertebral muscles
    - May be high T1 signal if proteinaceous
- **Retention Cyst, PMS**
  - Key facts
    - Common, incidental, and asymptomatic
    - Submucosal cyst located either laterally or in midline
  - Imaging
    - Nonenhancing single or multiple smooth cysts
    - Pear-shaped if located in lateral pharyngeal recess
- **Nasopharyngeal Carcinoma**
  - Key facts
    - SCCa with 3 distinct subtypes & strong relationship with Epstein-Barr virus
    - Very common in Chinese population, including those who relocate to USA
    - 90% have nodal metastases at diagnosis, ± retropharyngeal nodal chain
  - Imaging
    - Mass centered in lateral nasopharynx (NP) with invasion
    - Typical patterns of invasion from NP into nasal cavity, soft palate, parapharyngeal space, prevertebral muscles, or directly into clivus or sphenoid sinus
- **Non-Hodgkin Lymphoma, PMS**
  - Key facts

- Non-nodal lymphoma originates in nasopharyngeal component of Waldeyer lymphatic ring (adenoidal component)
  - Imaging
    - Bulky homogeneous mass with variable enhancement and low T2 signal
    - Mass may be located only in mucosal space or extend beyond fascia into PPS, retropharyngeal space, or skull base

Helpful Clues for Less Common Diagnoses
- **Post-Radiation Mucositis, PMS**
  - Key facts
    - History critical as patient will have received radiation therapy (XRT) for head and neck malignancy
    - Enhancing mucosa usually within 1st year after XRT; then gradual decrease in degree of enhancement
  - Imaging
    - Thin, non-mass-like, and symmetric enhancement of entire mucosal surface that was included in XRT field
- **Benign Mixed Tumor, PMS**
  - Key facts
    - Salivary gland rests scattered throughout mucosa of PMS
    - Benign mixed tumor develops from minor salivary gland rests
    - Presents as painless submucosal mass
    - Patient may report ear "fullness" or ↓ hearing if eustachian tube affected

- Compared with nasopharyngeal carcinoma, minor salivary gland tumors are submucosal & have high T2 signal
  - Imaging
    - Smooth enhancing submucosal mass with high T2 MR signal
    - Fluid in mastoids & middle ear cavity when there is mass effect on eustachian tube in nasopharynx

Helpful Clues for Rare Diagnoses
- **Minor Salivary Gland Malignancy, PMS**
  - Key facts: Develops from salivary rests in mucosa of PMS
    - Perineural extension makes pain common
  - Imaging: Submucosal but deeply invasive
    - Higher in T2 signal than SCCa
- **Rhabdomyosarcoma**
  - Key facts: Nasopharynx is 2nd most common H&N site after orbit
    - Pediatric or young adult patients
  - Imaging: Invasive nasopharynx mass
    - Skull base & intracranial extension common
- **Extraosseous Chordoma, PMS**
  - Key facts: Primary malignant tumor of notochord origin
    - Rarely extraosseous
  - Imaging: Very hyperintense on T2
    - Heterogeneous enhancement
    - May have anterior clival tract

Adenoid Tissue, Prominent/Asymmetric

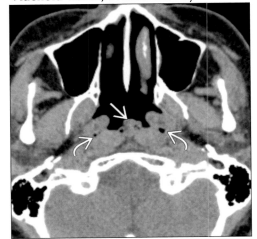

Axial NECT shows prominent midline soft tissue ➡ on mucosal surface in a patient years after adenoidectomy. In contrast, nasopharyngeal carcinoma arises laterally, in the fossa of Rosenmüller ➡.

Adenoid Inflammation

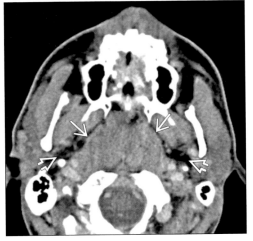

Axial CECT shows large edematous adenoidal tonsils ➡ without intratonsillar or peritonsillar abscess. The lateral fatty parapharyngeal spaces ➡ are easily seen and uninvolved.

PHARYNGEAL MUCOSAL SPACE LESION, NASOPHARYNX

Tornwaldt Cyst

Tornwaldt Cyst

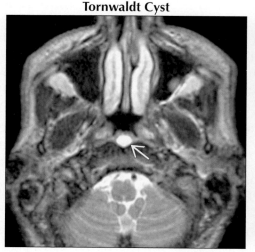 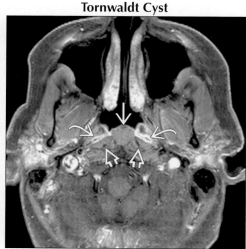

(Left) Axial T2WI MR demonstrates an ovoid, well-circumscribed, high signal intensity, midline benign cyst ➡ between the prevertebral muscles. *(Right)* Axial T1 C+ FS MR demonstrates a nonenhancing Tornwaldt cyst ➡ between the prevertebral muscles ⮕. Note the normal enhancing mucosa of the lateral pharyngeal recess ➡.

Retention Cyst, PMS

Retention Cyst, PMS

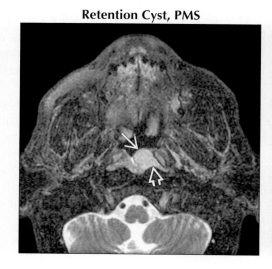 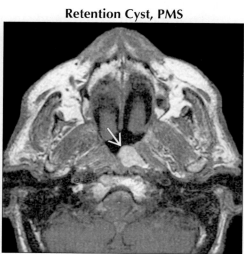

(Left) Axial T2WI FS MR shows a high signal, well-circumscribed cyst ➡ in the lateral nasopharynx. Note smooth interface with the prevertebral muscles ⮕, as the cyst does not extend through the fascia. *(Right)* Axial T1WI MR in the same patient reveals that the cyst ➡ is relatively high signal, consistent with proteinaceous contents. Some complex cysts may even be low signal on T2 sequences. Lack of local invasion helps determine that this is a benign lesion.

Nasopharyngeal Carcinoma

Nasopharyngeal Carcinoma

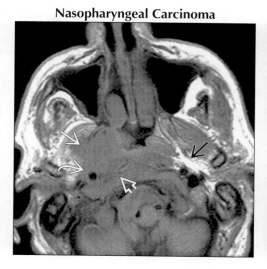 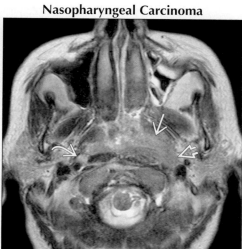

(Left) Axial T1WI MR demonstrates a large mass invading into the right parapharyngeal space ➡, carotid space ⮕, & the prevertebral muscles ➡. Note the normal left parapharyngeal space ➡. *(Right)* Axial T2WI MR in another patient shows a low signal mass ➡ arising on the left side and extending to the right. Note the deep lateral invasion ➡ into surrounding spaces on the left. Retropharyngeal adenopathy ➡ is common in nasopharyngeal carcinoma.

PHARYNGEAL MUCOSAL SPACE LESION, NASOPHARYNX

Non-Hodgkin Lymphoma, PMS

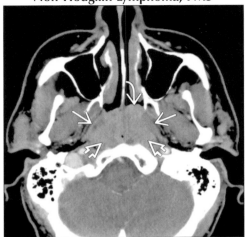

Post-Radiation Mucositis, PMS

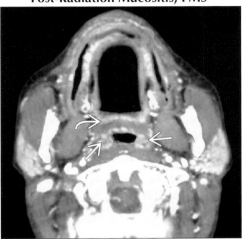

(Left) Axial CECT shows a nonenhancing bulky PMS mass ➡. Note anterior extension into the posterior nasal cavity ➡. The mass is inseparable from the prevertebral muscles ➡, suggesting that invasion has occurred. *(Right)* Axial CECT shows symmetric marked enhancement on all mucosal surfaces, including nasopharyngeal ➡. Note similar enhancement of soft palate ➡. Symmetry and direct visualization of inflamed mucosa exclude recurrent mucosal SCCa.

Benign Mixed Tumor, PMS

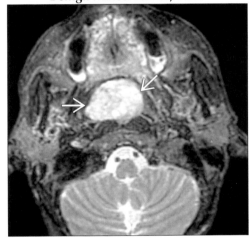

Minor Salivary Gland Malignancy, PMS

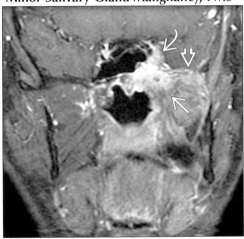

(Left) Axial T2WI FS MR shows a smooth hyperintense benign mixed tumor ➡ obliterating the nasopharyngeal airway. Note the absence of invasion into the adjacent tissues. *(Right)* Coronal T1 C+ FS MR shows an enhancing mass originating in the lateral nasopharynx, deeply invasive into the masticator space ➡. Note the intracranial extension along the floor of the middle cranial fossa ➡ and cavernous sinus ➡.

Rhabdomyosarcoma

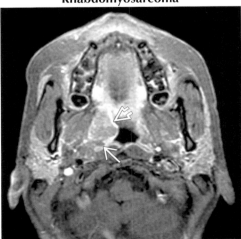

Extraosseous Chordoma, PMS

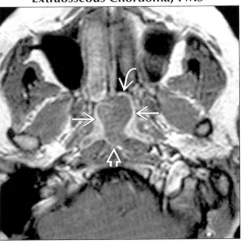

(Left) Axial T1 C+ FS MR reveals a minimally enhancing mass in the pharyngeal mucosal space ➡. On this image there are no invasive features, and biopsy is critical to make the diagnosis. Note mass effect on torus tubarius ➡, which explains why this patient presented with serous otitis and hearing loss. *(Right)* Axial T1 C+ MR demonstrates a midline mass ➡ extending from the posterior midline mucosa of the nasopharynx ➡ into the posterior nasal cavity ➡.

1

PHARYNGEAL MUCOSAL SPACE LESION, OROPHARYNX

DIFFERENTIAL DIAGNOSIS

Common
- Tonsillar Tissue, Prominent/Asymmetric
- Palatine Tonsil Abscess
- Tonsillar Inflammation
- Retention Cyst, PMS, Oropharynx
- Lingual Tonsil SCCa
- Palatine Tonsil SCCa
- Non-Hodgkin Lymphoma

Less Common
- Post-Radiation Mucositis
- Benign Mixed Tumor, PMS
- Vallecular Cyst
- Thyroglossal Duct Cyst

Rare but Important
- Minor Salivary Gland Malignancy, PMS
- Rhabdomyosarcoma

ESSENTIAL INFORMATION

Key Differential Diagnosis Issues
- Oropharyngeal mucosal space/surface (PMS) location includes all mucosa between soft palate and tip of epiglottis
  - Medial parapharyngeal space (PPS) effaced or displaced by PMS lesion
- Most common malignant tumors (SCCa, NHL, minor salivary gland malignancy) frequently indistinguishable on CT/MR
  - SCCa typically presents with mucosal ulceration seen on direct examination

Helpful Clues for Common Diagnoses
- **Tonsillar Tissue, Prominent/Asymmetric**
  - Key facts: Benign tonsillar hyperplasia usually incidental finding or secondary to recurrent infections
  - Imaging: Enlarged tonsil without discrete mass or local invasion
- **Palatine Tonsil Abscess**
  - Key facts: Progression of tonsillar inflammation and edema → phlegmon → discrete abscess
    - Abscess treated with incision & drainage
    - May be complicated by peritonsillar abscess if extension to surrounding PPS, submandibular space (SMS), or masticator space (MS)

- Imaging: Enlarged tonsil with central low density surrounded by peripheral enhancement on CECT
    - Frequent bulky reactive bilateral cervical adenopathy
- **Tonsillar Inflammation**
  - Key facts: Presents as acute pharyngitis, usually bilateral, involving both palatine tonsils
    - No central low density collection; helps differentiate inflammation (treated with antibiotics) from abscess (may be treated surgically)
  - Imaging: Bilateral palatine ± lingual ± adenoid tonsil enlargement with edema of peritonsillar soft tissues
    - Enlarged heterogeneously enhancing tonsils with characteristic internal enhancing septa
- **Retention Cyst, PMS, Oropharynx**
  - Key facts: Benign, postinflammatory, asymptomatic, & epithelial-lined mucosal cyst in PMS
  - Imaging: Low-density homogeneous cyst without enhancement on CECT
    - MR: Isointense or hyperintense on T1 (depending on proteinaceous contents); hyperintense on T2
- **Lingual Tonsil SCCa**
  - Key facts: Invasive or exophytic mass at base of tongue with mucosal ulceration seen on physical examination
    - SCCa of lingual & palatine tonsil are common
    - Associated with smoking & human papilloma virus
    - Treated with chemoradiation
    - Adenopathy in levels II and III common at presentation
  - Imaging: Small SCCa may appear as subtle mucosal asymmetry
    - Isointense on T1 & isointense or slightly hyperintense to muscle on T2
    - Enhancement on T1 C+ MR aids in delineation of interface between tumor & muscle
- **Palatine Tonsil SCCa**
  - Key facts: Etiology and behavior similar to SCCa at base of tongue (lingual tonsil)
  - Imaging: Enhancing mass centered in palatine tonsil with invasive deep margins

- T1 FS C+ MR most helpful to assess extent of tumor
- **Non-Hodgkin Lymphoma**
  - Key facts: Extranodal lymphoma involving either lingual lymphoid tissue or palatine tonsils
    - Associated with bulky cervical adenopathy > 50% of cases
  - Imaging: Poorly circumscribed, diffusely infiltrative mass, more often bilateral than SCCa
    - Homogeneous mass, isodense on CECT, most commonly hyperintense on T2
    - Diffuse enhancement without presence of internal enhancing tonsillar septa

Helpful Clues for Less Common Diagnoses
- **Post-Radiation Mucositis**
  - Key facts: History of radiation therapy & diffuse mucosal enhancement helps differentiate mucositis from recurrent mucosal neoplasm
  - Imaging: Acute phase shows diffuse thickening & mucosal edema with ill-defined soft tissue planes
    - Diffuse T2 hyperintensity may persist for several years post-therapy
    - Focal nodularity or enhancement deep to mucosa suggests recurrent tumor, especially if patient reports pain
- **Benign Mixed Tumor, PMS**
  - Key facts: Slow-growing submucosal painless tumor originating in minor salivary glands

- Imaging: Variably enhancing, well-circumscribed mass on CECT/MR
  - May contain calcifications & cystic areas
  - Most commonly T2 hyperintense with T1 C+ homogeneous enhancement
- **Vallecular Cyst**
  - Key facts: Unilocular benign cystic mass located in vallecula
  - Imaging: Hypodense nonenhancing cyst with preservation of soft tissue planes on CECT
    - T2 hyperintense lesion with variable T1 characteristics due to proteinaceous contents
- **Thyroglossal Duct Cyst**
  - Key facts: May occur anywhere between foramen cecum of tongue & thyroid
  - Imaging: Midline nonenhancing lingual tonsil cyst at location of foramen cecum
  - Be sure to look along entire course of duct for ectopic thyroid tissue

Helpful Clues for Rare Diagnoses
- **Minor Salivary Gland Malignancy, PMS**
  - Enhancing infiltrating mass with propensity for perineural & perivascular spread, especially CNV2 & CNV3
- **Rhabdomyosarcoma**
  - Large heterogeneous enhancing trans-spatial mass usually hyperintense on T2 MR

Tonsillar Tissue, Prominent/Asymmetric

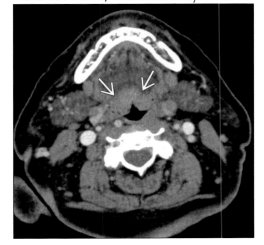

Axial CECT demonstrates prominent tissue ➡ mimicking a mass at the base of the tongue. The lack of deep invasion suggests benign hypertrophy, but normal mucosal examination is needed to confirm.

Palatine Tonsil Abscess

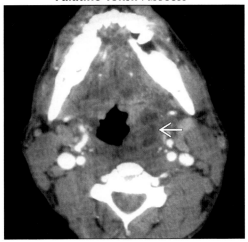

Axial CECT shows an abscess ➡ of the left palatine tonsil. Note the central low density, consistent with necrotic debris, surrounded by an enhancing rim.

PHARYNGEAL MUCOSAL SPACE LESION, OROPHARYNX

(Left) Axial CECT shows bilateral large palatine tonsillar abscesses ➡. Both are contained within the tonsil, with no peritonsillar component. Note the marked narrowing of the oropharyngeal airway ➡. *(Right)* Axial CECT shows large bilateral palatine tonsils ➡. The lack of central necrosis and striated enhancement pattern is typical for inflammation without abscess.

Palatine Tonsil Abscess

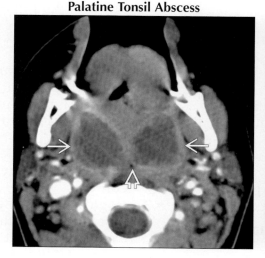

Tonsillar Inflammation

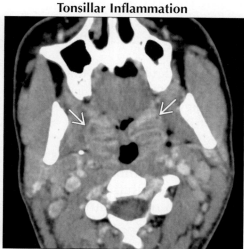

(Left) Axial CECT reveals a large primarily low-density submucosal cystic lesion ➡ in the superior oropharynx with a fluid-fluid level ➡ indicating previous hemorrhage. Note lack of deep extension into PPS ➡. *(Right)* Axial CECT shows an enhancing invasive right base of tongue mass ➡ that crosses midline. The lesion is apparent because of excellent contrast technique. Note the prior nodal neck dissection ➡ with loss of fat around the carotid artery.

Retention Cyst, PMS, Oropharynx

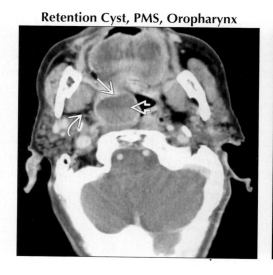

Lingual Tonsil SCCa

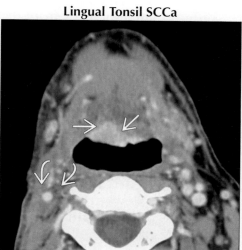

(Left) Axial T1 C+ FS MR demonstrates a large avidly enhancing tonsillar mass ➡ with extension to the oral cavity ➡ and carotid space ➡. An enhancing pathologic lymph node ➡ is seen in the left retropharyngeal space. *(Right)* Axial CECT depicts a large exophytic homogeneous mass centered in the right palatine tonsil ➡. The left tonsil is prominent ➡ but normal. Mucosa is usually intact in patients with oropharyngeal lymphoma.

Palatine Tonsil SCCa

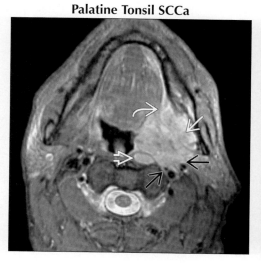

Non-Hodgkin Lymphoma

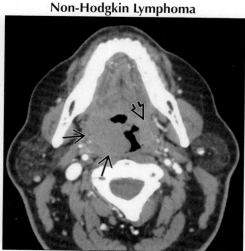

Post-Radiation Mucositis

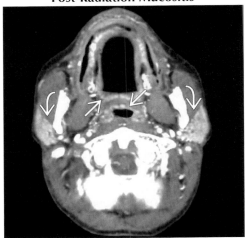

Benign Mixed Tumor, PMS

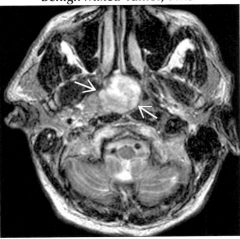

(Left) Axial CECT shows diffuse superficial mucosal enhancement, including the soft palate ➡. Marked parotid enhancement ➡ may also be present after radiation therapy to head and neck. *(Right)* Axial T2WI MR shows a large mass ➡ involving the right pharyngeal mucosal space with significant narrowing of the airway. Note the heterogeneous but mostly high T2 signal. The tumor is well circumscribed with no deep invasion.

Vallecular Cyst

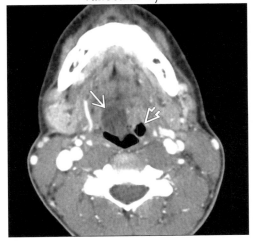

Thyroglossal Duct Cyst

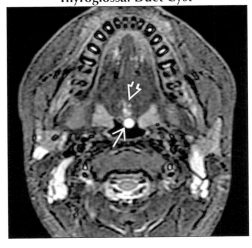

(Left) Axial CECT shows a paramedian nonenhancing mucoid density cyst ➡ projecting from the lingual tonsil into the vallecula. Note the normal opposite vallecula ➡. *(Right)* Axial T2WI FS MR reveals a thyroglossal duct cyst ➡ located at the midline base of the tongue. Note the linear high signal ➡ at the foramen cecum from the persistent thyroglossal duct remnant.

Minor Salivary Gland Malignancy, PMS

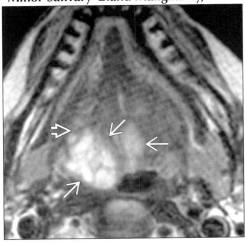

Rhabdomyosarcoma

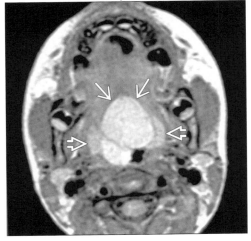

(Left) Axial T2WI MR shows an adenoid cystic carcinoma ➡ of the tonsil invading the oral cavity sublingual space ➡. High T2 signal is characteristic of minor salivary gland malignancy; SCCa is usually lower in signal. *(Right)* Axial T1 C+ MR in a child reveals a rhabdomyosarcoma arising from the lingual tonsil ➡. The bilobed enhancing mass results in marked airway compromise. Note different enhancement pattern between the mass and the palatine tonsils ➡.

MASTICATOR SPACE LESION

DIFFERENTIAL DIAGNOSIS

Common
- Fracture, Mandible
- Abscess, Masticator Space
- Benign Masticator Muscle Hypertrophy
- Motor Denervation CN5
- Pterygoid Venous Plexus Asymmetry
- Metastasis, Mandible-Maxilla
- Sarcoma, Other, Masticator Space
- Osteosarcoma, Mandible-Maxilla

Less Common
- Chondrosarcoma, Masticator Space
- Perineural Tumor, CNV3, MS
- Schwannoma, CNV3, MS
- Ameloblastoma
- Osteoradionecrosis, Mandible-Maxilla
- Odontogenic Keratocyst

Rare but Important
- Synovitis, Pigmented Villonodular, TMJ
- Chondromatosis, Synovial, TMJ
- Cyst, Dentigerous (Follicular)
- Cherubism, Mandible-Maxilla

ESSENTIAL INFORMATION

Key Differential Diagnosis Issues
- Masticator space (MS) has wide differential
- Most pathology related to mandible, teeth, or temporomandibular joint (TMJ)
- Imaging strategy
  - CT 1st line imaging tool
    - Review on both soft tissue and bone algorithm and windows
  - CECT important for evaluation of infectious process or masses
    - Abscesses can be subtle
    - Look for focal areas of low density
  - Bone CT
    - Look for fracture
    - If mandible lesion: Determine relationship to teeth
    - If infection: Look for empty tooth socket from recent extraction
    - If MS mass: Look for bone erosion & check for skull base involvement
  - MR with contrast complementary
    - Characterization of noninfectious masses
    - Perineural tumor to foramen ovale (CNV3)
    - Evaluation of skull base involvement &/or intracranial extension

Helpful Clues for Common Diagnoses
- **Fracture, Mandible**
  - Key facts
    - Mandible simulates ring so usually find 2nd fracture &/or TMJ dislocation
    - 15% have facial fractures
  - Imaging
    - CT: Linear lucency ± displacement
- **Abscess, Masticator Space**
  - Key facts: Most common MS mass
    - Usually dental source of infection
  - Imaging
    - CECT: Swelling of masticator muscles
    - Pus often subtle, ill-defined low density
    - Bone CT: Recently extracted tooth
- **Benign Masticator Muscle Hypertrophy**
  - Key facts
    - Uni- or bilateral muscle enlargement
  - Imaging: Muscles have normal density/intensity & enhancement
- **Motor Denervation CN5**
  - Key facts
    - Altered appearance of masticator muscles from loss of CNV3 innervation
  - Imaging
    - Acute/subacute: Swelling of muscles with edema, enhancing muscles
    - Late subacute: ↓ swelling & enhancement
    - Chronic: Fatty atrophy, no enhancement
- **Pterygoid Venous Plexus Asymmetry**
  - Key facts
    - Unilateral prominence usually incidental
  - Imaging
    - CT/MR: Enhancing tubular structures in medial MS or parapharyngeal space
- **Metastasis, Mandible-Maxilla**
  - Key facts
    - Uncommon; mimics dental disease
    - Most often: Breast, thyroid, kidney, lung
  - Imaging
    - Single/multiple, lytic/sclerotic lesions
- **Sarcoma, Other, Masticator Space**
  - Key facts: Rhabdomyosarcoma, leiomyosarcoma, liposarcoma, Ewing, & synovial sarcoma
  - Imaging: Aggressive, poorly defined mass
- **Osteosarcoma, Mandible-Maxilla**
  - Key facts
    - Malignant tumor with osteoid matrix

- Imaging
  - Ill-defined expansile mandibular mass
  - CT: Often tumoral calcification ± aggressive periosteal reaction

Helpful Clues for Less Common Diagnoses
- **Chondrosarcoma, Masticator Space**
  - Key facts
    - Malignant cartilage origin tumor
    - Arises in masticator space or TMJ
  - Imaging
    - CT: Focal calcifications or chondroid matrix, less so in higher grade tumor
    - MR: Typically T2 hyperintense, variable enhancement
- **Perineural Tumor, CNV3, MS**
  - Key facts
    - Spread of tumor along mandibular nerve
  - Imaging
    - CT: Widened inferior alveolar canal &/or foramen ovale
    - MR: Thickening and enhancement along CNV3 to foramen ovale
- **Schwannoma, CNV3, MS**
  - Key facts
    - Benign peripheral nerve sheath tumor
  - Imaging
    - Ovoid enhancement along CNV3 course
- **Ameloblastoma**
  - Key facts
    - Benign, locally aggressive odontogenic epithelial tumor
  - Imaging
    - Expansile mass; solid, cystic, or mixed

- **Osteoradionecrosis, Mandible-Maxilla**
  - Key facts
    - Loss of bone vitality after radiation
  - Imaging
    - CT: Lytic permeative change, cortical loss
    - MR: Marrow bright on T2, dark on T1
- **Odontogenic Keratocyst**
  - Key facts: Typically posterior mandible
  - Imaging
    - CT/MR: Expansile mass with cortical thinning, no enhancement

Helpful Clues for Rare Diagnoses
- **Synovitis, Pigmented Villonodular, TMJ**
  - Key facts
    - Monoarticular inflammatory arthropathy
  - Imaging
    - Bone CT: Articular erosions, cysts
    - MR: Heterogeneous mass, dark T2 signal
- **Chondromatosis, Synovial, TMJ**
  - Key facts
    - Benign calcifying synovial metaplasia
  - Imaging
    - CT: Calcified loose bodies in TMJ
    - MR: T1 & T2 focal signal loss
- **Cyst, Dentigerous (Follicular)**
  - Key facts: Also known as follicular cyst
  - Imaging
    - Well-defined expansile cyst surrounding impacted/unerupted tooth crown
- **Cherubism, Mandible-Maxilla**
  - Key facts: Bony dysplasia confined to jaw
  - Imaging: Expansile symmetric jaw remodeling

Fracture, Mandible

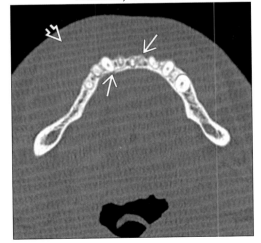

Axial bone CT demonstrates subtle swelling of the soft tissues of the right chin ⬦. Careful review of bone CT reveals an even more subtle fracture line ➡ through the cortex of the alveolar portion of mandible.

Fracture, Mandible

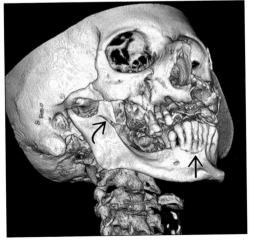

3D reformat from same patient shows a fracture of the right mandibular alveolar ridge ➡ from the central incisor to the 2nd premolar. Note ipsilateral coronoid process fracture with displacement ➘.

MASTICATOR SPACE LESION

(Left) Axial CECT reveals marked left cheek swelling with heterogeneous density of medial pterygoid and masseter muscles containing focal areas of low density ➥ indicative of pus in the masticator space. *(Right)* Axial bone CT in the same patient reveals source of collections to be infected tooth socket after recent extraction ➡. This is the most common cause of masticator space infection & should be carefully sought whenever masticator space infection is suspected.

Abscess, Masticator Space

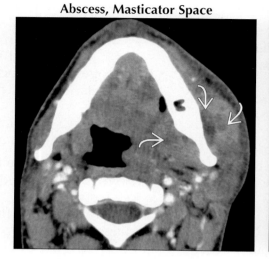

Abscess, Masticator Space

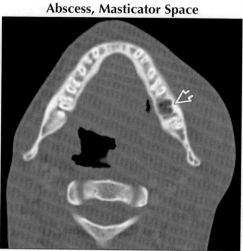

(Left) Axial CECT demonstrates bilateral, although asymmetric, enlargement of masticator muscles. Note greater enlargement of left medial pterygoid ➡ and masseter ➡ muscles relative to right but symmetric density and no abnormal enhancement. *(Right)* Axial NECT in a patient with squamous cell carcinoma of the face and a perineural tumor involving the 5th cranial nerve reveals denervation atrophy of the right masseter ➡ and medial pterygoid ➡ muscles.

Benign Masticator Muscle Hypertrophy

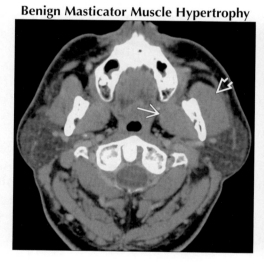

Motor Denervation CN5

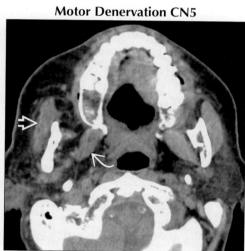

(Left) Axial CECT reveals a mass-like appearance of the left pterygoid venus plexus ➡ relative to the right ➡ at the deep aspect of lateral pterygoid muscle. This can be an incidental benign finding or associated with carotico-cavernous fistula. *(Right)* Axial bone CT in a patient with jaw pain reveals a lytic destructive process centered in posterior body of mandible with cortical erosion ➡. This was the only metastasis from previously unsuspected lung cancer.

Pterygoid Venous Plexus Asymmetry

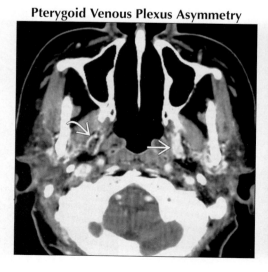

Metastasis, Mandible-Maxilla

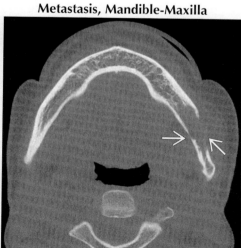

MASTICATOR SPACE LESION

Sarcoma, Other, Masticator Space

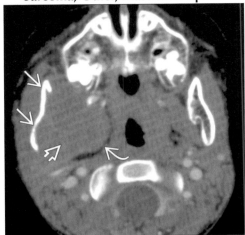

Sarcoma, Other, Masticator Space

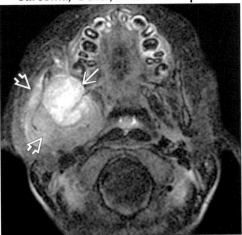

(Left) Axial CECT in a young child reveals a large mass in right deep face ➡, isodense to muscle. Destruction of medial mandible ➡ and posteromedial displacement of parapharyngeal fat ➡ indicate this aggressive process arises in masticator space. *(Right)* Axial T2WI FS MR in the same patient shows this rhabdomyosarcoma ➡ to be more heterogeneous. Area of intrinsic T2 hyperintensity ➡ was nonenhancing and necrotic on post-gadolinium images.

Osteosarcoma, Mandible-Maxilla

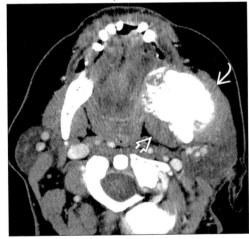

Osteosarcoma, Mandible-Maxilla

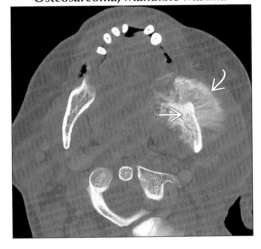

(Left) Axial CECT shows a large, markedly dense mass centered in the left masticator space and involving or displacing the masseter ➡ and medial pterygoid ➡ muscles. *(Right)* Axial bone CT in the same patient reveals the hyperdensity to be bone formation in mass centered at left mandibular angle. Lesion has features of osteosarcoma with classic sunburst pattern periosteal reaction ➡. Note that involved mandibular marrow is sclerotic ➡.

Chondrosarcoma, Masticator Space

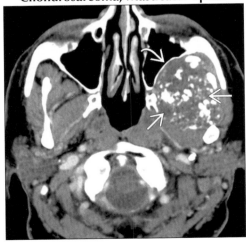

Chondrosarcoma, Masticator Space

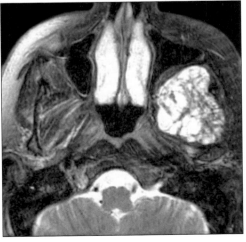

(Left) Axial CECT shows a low-density mass ➡ with intrinsic calcifications filling the left infratemporal fossa. The mass is surprisingly large without cheek expansion, although it deforms the posterior wall of the left maxillary sinus ➡. *(Right)* Axial T2WI FS MR in the same patient reveals a well-defined mass filling the infratemporal fossa. The mass is heterogeneous but predominantly hyperintense, which is typical of chondroid tumors.

1

MASTICATOR SPACE LESION

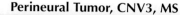

(Left) Axial T1 C+ FS MR shows a patient with facial deformity ➡ from prior left segmental mandibulectomy for adenoid cystic carcinoma, with very subtle asymmetric enhancement of muscles of mastication ➡. Note also the abnormal enhancement at the mandibular foramen ➡. *(Right)* Coronal T1 C+ FS MR in the same patient reveals a thick enhancing perineural tumor tracking through masticator space to foramen ovale ➡ along mandibular nerve ➡.

Perineural Tumor, CNV3, MS

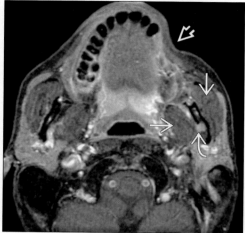

Perineural Tumor, CNV3, MS

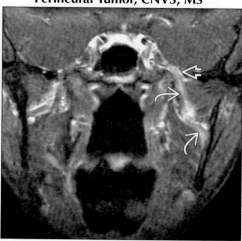

(Left) Coronal T1WI FS MR demonstrates a large, well-defined, homogeneously enhancing, solid mass ➡ in the right masticator space extending through the central skull base to the middle cranial fossa. *(Right)* Coronal T1 C+ FS MR in a young patient with a diagnosis of neurofibromatosis type 2 shows similar spread of a mandibular nerve (V3) schwannoma ➡ through the enlarged foramen ovale ➡ to the right Meckel cave.

Schwannoma, CNV3, MS

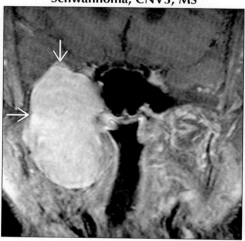

Schwannoma, CNV3, MS

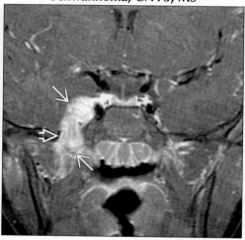

(Left) Axial bone CT shows an expanded body of the right mandible associated with unerupted & malpositioned 3rd molar tooth ➡. Lesion has benign character with expansion and marked thinning of buccal & lingual cortex with focal cortical dehiscence ➡. *(Right)* Axial bone CT demonstrates heterogeneous "moth-eaten" destruction of the right hemimandible with focal areas of intraosseous gas ➡. Evolving intraosseous bone sequestrum is also noted ➡.

Ameloblastoma

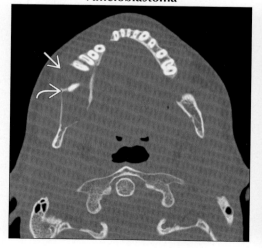

Osteoradionecrosis, Mandible-Maxilla

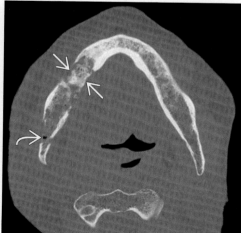

MASTICATOR SPACE LESION

Odontogenic Keratocyst

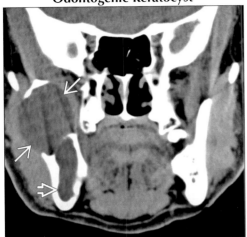

Odontogenic Keratocyst

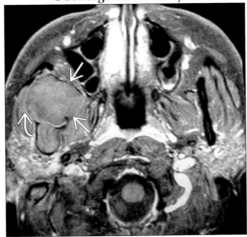

(Left) Coronal NECT reveals an expansile unilocular cystic lesion arising in the right mandibular ramus ➡ and expanding cephalad into the masticator space. Note the marked thinning of the cortex in some areas ➡. (Right) Axial T1 C+ FS MR in the same patient shows an expansile lesion ➡ without appreciable enhancement, indicating a truly cystic nature. The keratocyst extends laterally into the masseter muscle ➡.

Synovitis, Pigmented Villonodular, TMJ

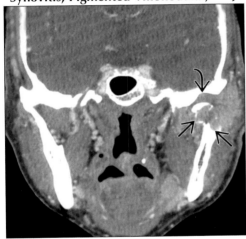

Chondromatosis, Synovial, TMJ

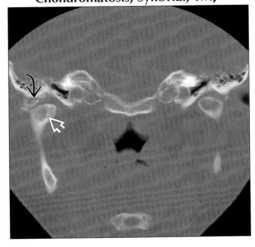

(Left) Coronal CECT demonstrates a moderately enhancing soft tissue mass centered around the left TMJ associated with erosion of the mandibular condyle ➡ and glenoid fossa ➡. There is no evidence of new bone formation or calcifications. (Right) Coronal bone CT shows subtly sclerotic right mandibular condyle ➡. The articular surface is slightly irregular, suggesting degenerative change, but small calcified bodies ➡ are also evident in the joint.

Cyst, Dentigerous (Follicular)

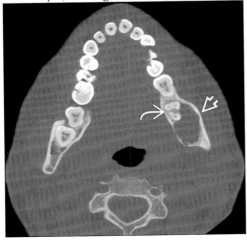

Cherubism, Mandible-Maxilla

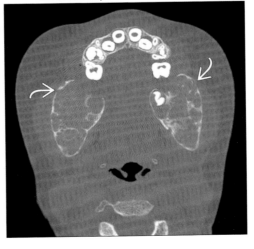

(Left) Axial bone CT demonstrates smooth-walled cystic expansion of left hemimandible ➡, abutting an impacted left 3rd mandibular molar ➡. There is no abnormal calcification, periosteal reaction, or associated soft tissue mass. (Right) Axial bone CT in a child shows symmetric expansion of angles of mandible with multiloculated appearance. No cortical destruction evident though remaining cortex is markedly thinned and focally dehiscent in places ➡.

BUCCAL SPACE LESION

DIFFERENTIAL DIAGNOSIS

Common
- Accessory Parotid Gland
- SCCa, Nodes
- SCCa, Buccal Mucosa
- Minor Salivary Gland Malignancy, Oral
- Fungal Sinusitis, Invasive

Less Common
- Juvenile Angiofibroma
- Venous Malformation, Buccal Space
- Abscess, Masticator Space
- Perineural Tumor, CNV2
- SCCa, Sinonasal
- Non-Hodgkin Lymphoma

Rare but Important
- Sarcoma, Other, Masticator Space
- Lipoma, Buccal Space

ESSENTIAL INFORMATION

Key Differential Diagnosis Issues
- Buccal space (BS) is pyramidal fat-filled space of midface; forms padding of cheeks
- No defined fascial boundaries
  - Medial border: Buccinator muscle
  - Lateral border: Muscles of facial expression
  - Posterior border: Masseter, mandible, pterygoid muscles, parotid gland
  - Superior extent: Retromaxillary fat pad
- BS predominantly fat & small nodes
  - Parotid duct traverses BS; pierces buccinator at level of upper 2nd molar
  - Accessory parotid gland found in ≈ 20%
- Majority of BS pathology is nodal disease or extension of pathology from adjacent structures & spaces
  - Oral cavity and specifically buccal mucosa
  - Maxillary sinus infection or tumor
  - Masticator & parotid infection or tumor
- Imaging strategies
  - Either CT or MR useful for evaluation of BS
  - Buccal masses, especially adjacent to mandible/maxilla, often subtle on imaging
    - Look for asymmetry of fat density (CT) or signal intensity (T1 MR)
    - Caveat: Dental amalgam obscures BS disease on CT or MR

Helpful Clues for Common Diagnoses
- **Accessory Parotid Gland**

- Key facts: "Extra" parotid tissue (20%)
  - Subject to same inflammatory & neoplastic processes as parotids
  - Imaging: Anterior aspect of masseter surface separate from remaining parotid
    - Texture and CT density/MR intensity & C+ same as parotids
- **SCCa, Nodes**
  - Key facts: Facial lymph node group
    - Primary lesion from buccal mucosa, maxillary sinus, or skin tumor
  - Imaging: Rounded mass typically lateral to facial vein & artery
    - Necrosis/cystic change may be evident
- **SCCa, Buccal Mucosa**
  - Key facts: Lesion clinically evident; can be subtle on imaging
  - Imaging: Look for asymmetry of thickness of buccinator & infiltration of buccal fat
    - Noncontrast CT or T1 MR shows fat infiltration well
    - Coronal imaging often most helpful for extent of lesion & buccinator involvement
    - Nodal drainage to level I and II
- **Minor Salivary Gland Malignancy, Oral**
  - Key facts: Clinically evident lesion
  - Imaging: Performed to evaluate for soft tissue extent, bone invasion, & adenopathy
    - CT or T1 MR: Look for infiltration of fat
- **Fungal Sinusitis, Invasive**
  - Key facts: Aggressive, often rapidly progressive infection
    - May not be clinically suspected
    - Maintain high index of suspicion for immunosuppressed patient (steroid use, diabetes, malignancy, chemotherapy, chronic renal disease)
  - Imaging: CT 1st line study for sinusitis
    - Look for infiltration of buccal fat around maxillary sinus
    - Bone destruction NOT feature until late in process
    - MR: Best modality, especially T2 fat saturated, for full extent of infection

Helpful Clues for Less Common Diagnoses
- **Juvenile Angiofibroma**
  - Key facts: Male teenagers
    - Most often present with epistaxis

BUCCAL SPACE LESION

- Imaging: Hypervascular benign tumor of nose that originates near sphenopalatine foramen margin
- Multiple directions of spread possible
  - Medial: Fills nasal cavity & nasopharynx
  - Superior: Anterior cranial fossa
  - Posterior: Sphenoid bone & sinus
  - Lateral: Through pterygomaxillary fissure to masticator space & retromaxillary fat of buccal space

- **Venous Malformation, Buccal Space**
  - Key facts: Vascular nonneoplastic lesion found in any spaces of head & neck
  - Imaging: Mixed enhancing lobulated mass with hyperdense phleboliths (CT)
    - Presence of phleboliths (on any imaging modality) virtually diagnostic
    - MR: T2 hyperintense & hypointense phleboliths; mixed enhancement

- **Abscess, Masticator Space**
  - Key facts: Abscess from dental disease
    - Either maxillary or mandibular infection can involve adjacent buccal space
  - Imaging: Loss of clarity of buccal fat ± rim-enhancing low-density collection (CT)
    - Bone windows to identify infected tooth
    - Note that facial pus often does NOT form well-defined collection
    - MR: Infiltration of fat best seen on T2; focal collection best seen on T1 C+ FS

- **Perineural Tumor, CNV2**
  - Key facts: Infraorbital nerve traverses portion of retromaxillary fat of BS
    - Primary tumor: Cheek melanoma, SCCa

- Imaging: MR more sensitive than CT, especially T1 C+ FS
  - CT or MR: Thickening & C+ CNV2
  - Carefully review nerve course: Infraorbital canal → pterygopalatine fossa
- **SCCa, Sinonasal**
  - Key facts: Any maxillary sinus malignancy may invade through anterolateral or posterolateral wall to BS
    - Primary mass is destructive
    - SCCa heterogeneous & necrotic
  - Imaging: Asymmetry of buccal fat, bone destruction (CT)
    - MR: Infiltration of BS, orbit
- **Non-Hodgkin Lymphoma**
  - Key facts: BS secondarily involved by adjacent facial primary NHL
  - Imaging: Mass infiltrates masticator & parotid spaces and maxillary sinus
    - NHL in BS facial lymph node

Helpful Clues for Rare Diagnoses
- **Sarcoma, Other, Masticator Space**
  - Key facts: Fibro-, synovial, undifferentiated sarcoma
  - Imaging: Invasive mass involves BS
- **Lipoma, Buccal Space**
  - Key facts: Lipoma can involve any space(s)
  - Imaging: Low density (CT) and high T1 (MR) signal mass
    - Fat-saturation sequences decrease fat signal

Accessory Parotid Gland

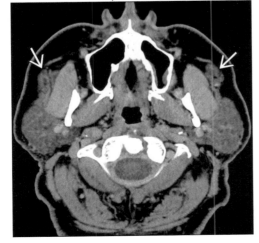

Axial CECT reveals bilateral soft tissue masses ➡ overlying the masseter muscles. Their density, texture, and enhancement characteristics appear almost identical to those of normal parotid glands.

Accessory Parotid Gland

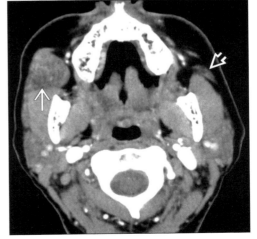

Axial CECT shows large round mass ➡ immediately anterior to right masseter muscle. This proved to be a benign mixed tumor arising in the accessory parotid. Note the contralateral accessory parotid ➡.

BUCCAL SPACE LESION

(Left) Axial CECT demonstrates a cystic/necrotic mass ➡ in the left buccal space, abutting the anterior margin of the masseter muscle and adjacent to the facial vein and distal parotid duct ➡.
(Right) Axial T1WI MR reveals a soft tissue mass ➡ isointense to the muscle but with an ill-defined anterior margin infiltrating right buccal fat. This asymmetry of fat may seem obvious but can be a "blind spot" on imaging.

SCCa, Nodes

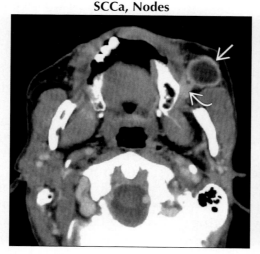

SCCa, Buccal Mucosa

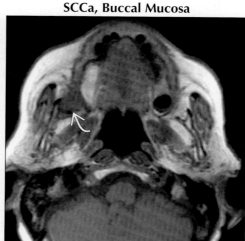

(Left) Axial T1 C+ FS MR shows an irregular rim-enhancing cystic mass ➡ with solid enhancement at buccal mucosa ➡. FNA of cheek mass suggested salivary tissue; final pathology showed poorly differentiated carcinoma.
(Right) Axial NECT reveals partial opacification of left maxillary sinus in a patient with a history of lymphoma. More significant, there is marked infiltration of buccal space fat ➡. This was proven to be aspergillus infection.

Minor Salivary Gland Malignancy, Oral

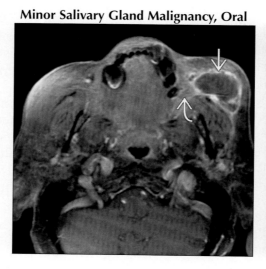

Fungal Sinusitis, Invasive

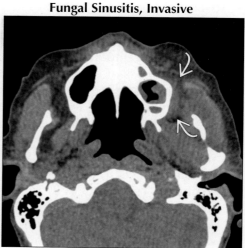

(Left) Axial CECT reveals a large angiofibroma ➡ that has herniated into the buccal space from the pterygopalatine fossa, displacing facial vein ➡ anteriorly and distending left cheek. *(Right)* Axial STIR MR shows a complex mostly T2 hyperintense cheek mass predominantly in buccal space ➡ but extending deep into oral cavity ➡. Rounded areas of low signal intensity representing phleboliths ➡ are a key finding to make this diagnosis.

Juvenile Angiofibroma

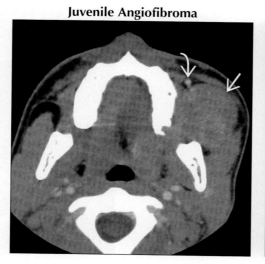

Venous Malformation, Buccal Space

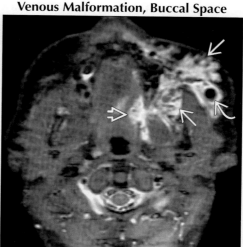

1

BUCCAL SPACE LESION

Abscess, Masticator Space

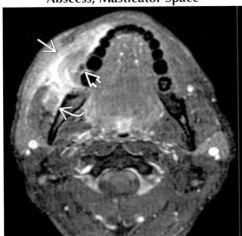

Perineural Tumor, CNV2

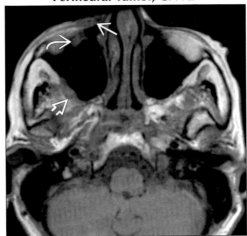

(Left) Axial T1 C+ FS MR shows extensive inflammation and enhancement of right buccal space ➡ and anterior masseter muscle ➡. Focal peripherally enhancing fluid collection ➡ adjacent to mandible is also evident in this infection of dental origin. *(Right)* Axial T1WI MR shows a patient with prior resection of facial skin SCCa ➡. Recurrence is seen as perineural tumor along infraorbital nerve ➡ through retromaxillary fat ➡ to pterygopalatine fossa.

SCCa, Sinonasal

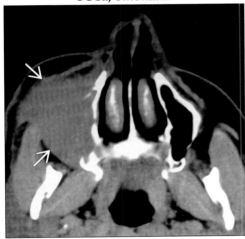

Non-Hodgkin Lymphoma

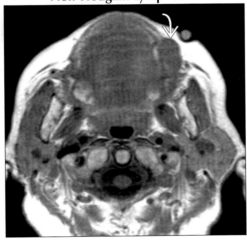

(Left) Axial NECT demonstrates a large soft tissue mass filling the right maxillary sinus with extensive sinus wall bone destruction. There is direct extension into the buccal space ➡ with pre- and retro-maxillary fat involvement. *(Right)* Axial T1WI MR reveals a soft tissue mass in the left buccal space ➡. Clinically this was a palpable submucosal mass rather than a buccal mucosal lesion. Pathological examination found a B-cell lymphoma.

Sarcoma, Other, Masticator Space

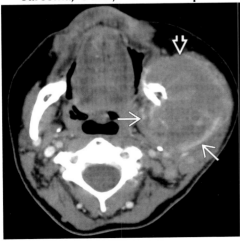

Lipoma, Buccal Space

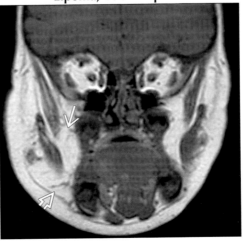

(Left) Axial CECT shows a large heterogeneous mass ➡ that arises in masticator space, surrounding mandible and engulfing pterygoid & masseter muscles. The mass invades buccal space ➡. This tumor was found to be undifferentiated pleomorphic sarcoma. *(Right)* Coronal T1WI MR shows buccal space lipoma presenting as facial asymmetry in a child. Right buccal fat is enlarged ➡ compared to left side with contiguous enlargement of inferior submandibular fat ➡.

DIFFERENTIAL DIAGNOSIS

Common
- Benign Mixed Tumor, Parotid
- Warthin Tumor
- Metastatic Disease, Nodal, Parotid

Less Common
- Salivary Gland Malignancies
  - Mucoepidermoid Carcinoma, Parotid
  - Adenoid Cystic Carcinoma, Parotid
  - Malignant Mixed Tumor, Parotid
  - Acinic Cell Carcinoma, Parotid
  - Adenocarcinoma, Parotid
  - Ductal Carcinoma, Parotid
  - Squamous Cell Carcinoma, Parotid
- Non-Hodgkin Lymphoma, Parotid
- Schwannoma, Parotid
- Infantile Hemangioma
- Lipoma

Rare but Important
- Oncocytoma, Parotid
- Venous Malformation
- Lymphatic Malformation
- 1st Branchial Cleft Cyst
- Neurofibromatosis Type 1
- Rhabdomyosarcoma

ESSENTIAL INFORMATION

Key Differential Diagnosis Issues
- Overlapping features of parotid space (PS) masses can make imaging diagnosis difficult
  - Different malignant cell types are radiologically indistinguishable
- Many lesions require FNA/resection for diagnosis, but imaging can localize & guide surgeon to likely diagnosis
  - Caveat: Beware of FNA pitfalls in parotid!
- Small well-defined lesion of PS
  - Almost impossible to distinguish node from benign or low-grade neoplasm
- Larger lesions of PS
  - Any loss of margin definition raises concern for malignancy
- Imaging strategies
  - CT can localize, enumerate, determine cystic vs. solid, assess for neck nodes
  - US guides FNA of superficial lobe lesion
  - MR best characterizes lesions
    - T1: Evaluate lesion margins & extent

- T1 C+ FS: Clarify solid or cystic, evaluate CN7 for perineural tumor
  - MR T2 FS: Solid lesion's signal intensity can suggest benign or malignant
    - High T2 signal in solid lesion suggests benign (BMT) or low-grade malignancy
    - Low T2 signal seen with higher grade solid tumors
- FDG PET of little use in characterization of parotid masses
  - High SUV may be seen with BMT, malignancy, inflammation
  - Low SUV may be seen with malignant tumors such as adenoid cystic carcinoma

Helpful Clues for Common Diagnoses
- **Benign Mixed Tumor, Parotid**
  - Key facts: a.k.a., pleomorphic adenoma
    - 80% of parotid tumors
  - Imaging: Sharp margins
    - T2 MR: Solid, mostly hypertense
    - T1 C+ MR: Heterogeneous if large
- **Warthin Tumor**
  - Key facts: Tobacco-linked benign tumor
  - Imaging: Typically at tail of parotid
    - May be multiple, solid, or cystic
    - T2 MR: Bright if cystic or solid
- **Metastatic Disease, Nodal, Parotid**
  - Key facts: Scalp, EAC, or cheek skin SCCa or melanoma
    - Systemic metastases rarely occur in PS
  - Imaging: ≤ 1.5 cm superficial mass(es)
    - Other periparotid, occipital, or level II or VA nodes often found

Helpful Clues for Less Common Diagnoses
- **Salivary Gland Malignancies**
  - Multiple less common lesions included
  - Typically no imaging features distinguish these carcinomas
  - When small or low grade, these may appear well defined and mimic node or BMT
    - Look for ill-defined margin as clue to malignancy
    - Look for low T2 signal in solid mass as clue to malignancy
    - Always look for perineural tumor spread along CN7 in temporal bone!
  - **Malignant Mixed Tumor, Parotid**
    - Key facts: Most often arises in longstanding benign mixed tumor

- Imaging: Indistinguishable from other high-grade malignancies
  - **Squamous Cell Carcinoma, Parotid**
    - Key facts: De novo or extranodal spread of metastatic parotid nodal disease
    - Imaging: If de novo, mimics other high-grade parotid neoplasms; if in parotid nodes, typically multiple coalescent nodules
- **Non-Hodgkin Lymphoma, Parotid**
  - Key facts: With parotid nodes or gland
  - Imaging: If in parotid nodes, mimics other metastatic nodal disease
    - Primary parotid lymphoma mimics other salivary malignancies
- **Schwannoma, Parotid**
  - Key facts: Often arises from small nerves, not from facial nerve itself
  - Imaging: Well-defined oval mass in superficial lobe
    - MR: Target appearance with peripheral lower T2 signal, T1 C+ enhancement
- **Infantile Hemangioma**
  - Key facts: Clinical history is key
    - Rapidly enlarging mass in 1st year of life
  - Imaging: Diffusely enlarged gland with marked contrast enhancement
- **Lipoma**
  - Imaging: Markedly low density (CT)
    - MR: T1 hyperintense, but dark with any fat-saturation sequence

Helpful Clues for Rare Diagnoses
- **Oncocytoma, Parotid**

- Key facts: Benign lesion
  - Associated with prior radiation
  - Imaging: Small, well defined; mimics node
- **Venous Malformation**
  - Key facts: Often trans-spatial
    - Multilobulated, loculations ± fluid levels
  - CT/MR: Diffusely enhancing; phleboliths
    - MR: T2 hyperintense with diffuse C+
- **Lymphatic Malformation**
  - Key facts: Often trans-spatial
    - Multilobulated, cystic, ± fluid levels
  - CT/MR: Cystic, lobulated without C+
    - MR: T2 bright, ± blood-fluid levels
- **1st Branchial Cleft Cyst**
  - Key facts: 2 cyst types
    - Type 1: Preauricular or intraparotid; ± sinus tract to middle ear or medial EAC
    - Type 2: Posterior or inferior to angle of mandible; ± sinus tract to lateral EAC
- **Neurofibromatosis Type 1**
  - Key facts: Plexiform lesion seen with NF1
  - Imaging: Lobulated, infiltrating lesion
- **Rhabdomyosarcoma**
  - Key facts: Enlarging PS mass in child
  - Imaging: Infiltrating, patchy C+ mass

SELECTED REFERENCES

1. Wong KT et al: Vascular lesions of parotid gland in adult patients: diagnosis with high-resolution ultrasound and MRI. Br J Radiol. 77(919):600-6, 2004
2. Tart RP et al: CT and MR imaging of the buccal space and buccal space masses. Radiographics. 15(3):531-50, 1995
3. Freling NJ et al: Malignant parotid tumors: clinical use of MR imaging and histologic correlation. Radiology. 185(3):691-6, 1992

Benign Mixed Tumor, Parotid

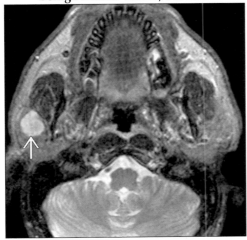

Axial T1WI FS MR shows a solitary sharply defined T2 hyperintense mass ➡ in the superficial lobe of the right parotid gland. Fat saturation accentuates the intrinsic high signal in this lesion.

Benign Mixed Tumor, Parotid

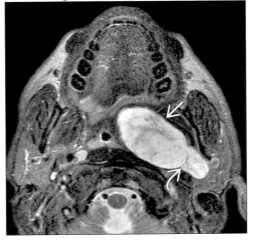

Axial T2WI FS MR reveals a large but well-defined hyperintense mass ➡ in the deep face. The mass extends to the superficial lobe of the parotid through the stylomandibular notch ➡.

PAROTID SPACE MASS

Warthin Tumor

Warthin Tumor

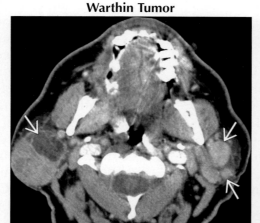
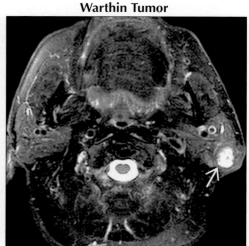

(Left) Axial CECT reveals multiple bilateral cystic and solid masses ➡ at the angle of the mandible. Subtle peripheral parotid tissue indicates tumors are within parotid. *(Right)* Axial T2WI FS MR shows a solitary diffusely hyperintense mass ➡ in the superficial lobe of the left parotid gland, lateral to the expected course of the intraparotid facial nerve. Post-contrast enhancement showed this mass to be predominantly solid.

Metastatic Disease, Nodal, Parotid

Metastatic Disease, Nodal, Parotid

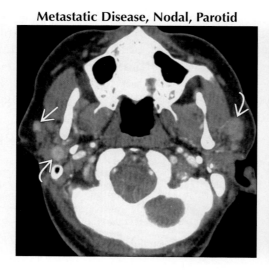
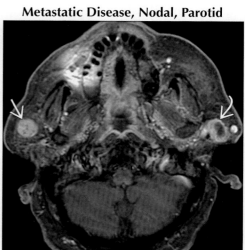

(Left) Axial CECT shows bilateral lesions within the parotids ➡, with the right lesion showing greater enhancement. An additional smaller lesion on the right ➡ may represent a further metastasis or a benign node. *(Right)* Axial T1 C+ FS MR reveals a solid mass ➡ in the superficial lobe of the right parotid and a partially necrotic or cystic mass ➡ in the superficial lobe of the left parotid.

Mucoepidermoid Carcinoma, Parotid

Mucoepidermoid Carcinoma, Parotid

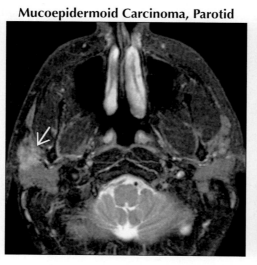
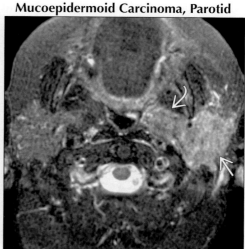

(Left) Axial T2WI FS MR shows a small lesion in the superficial lobe of the right parotid gland ➡. While not a large lesion, its ill-defined contours and intermediate signal intensity favor malignancy. *(Right)* Axial T2WI MR shows a large mass with ill-defined margins infiltrating much of the left parotid superficial ➡ and deep ➡ lobes. The mixed signal, only slightly higher than contralateral normal parotid gland, is consistent with a high-grade tumor.

PAROTID SPACE MASS

Adenoid Cystic Carcinoma, Parotid

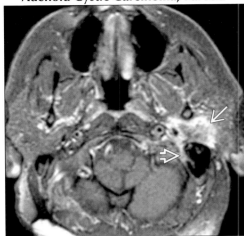

Malignant Mixed Tumor, Parotid

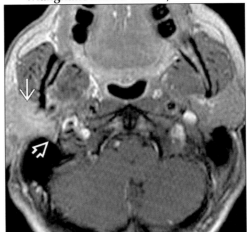

(Left) Axial T1 C+ FS MR shows a poorly marginated mass straddling superficial and deep lobes of the left parotid ➡. The heterogeneously enhancing tumor extends to the stylomastoid foramen ➡ of the facial nerve. *(Right)* Axial T1 C+ FS MR demonstrates diffuse right parotid enhancement ➡ from an infiltrative tumor, which extends posteromedially to the stylomastoid foramen ➡. A tumor involving the facial nerve was found at surgery.

Acinic Cell Carcinoma, Parotid

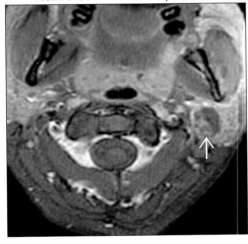

Adenocarcinoma, Parotid

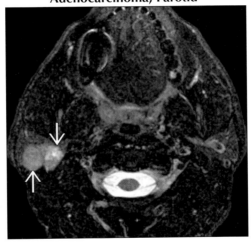

(Left) Axial T1 C+ FS MR shows a heterogeneous cystic & solid mass ➡ in the superficial left parotid lobe in a 19 year old woman. Metastatic neck adenopathy was also present at the time of tumor resection. *(Right)* Axial T2WI FS MR shows a heterogeneous, but predominantly intermediate, signal intensity mass ➡ in the right parotid. FNA had suggested benign mixed tumor vs. adenoid cystic carcinoma, but final pathology was adenocarcinoma NOS.

Ductal Carcinoma, Parotid

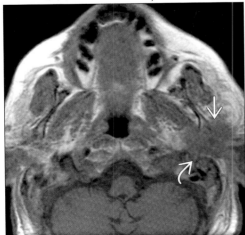

Squamous Cell Carcinoma, Parotid

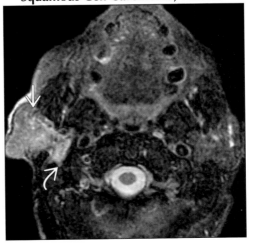

(Left) Axial T1WI MR shows an aggressive-appearing mass ➡ infiltrating the superficial and deep lobes of the left parotid and extending to the left stylomastoid foramen ➡. *(Right)* Axial T2WI FS MR shows an infiltrating mass ➡ involving the entire right parotid gland and extending toward the right stylomastoid foramen ➡. The lesion is hyperintense to normal parotid but generally of intermediate signal intensity.

PAROTID SPACE MASS

(Left) Axial CECT shows a large moderately enhancing mass ➡ involving the left parotid. The margins appear relatively well defined, mimicking a low- to intermediate-grade primary parotid tumor. A separate nodal mass ➡ is also noted. **(Right)** Axial CECT shows a well-defined nodule ➡ within the right parotid tail, but also bilateral neck adenopathy ➡. Multiple right parotid nodules were found.

Non-Hodgkin Lymphoma, Parotid

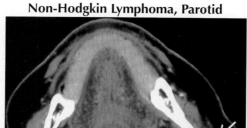

Non-Hodgkin Lymphoma, Parotid

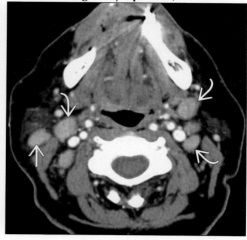

(Left) Axial T2WI FS MR shows a solitary well-defined hyperintense mass in the left parotid ➡ with a peripheral intermediate intensity rim ➡, which can be described as target-like. Despite the central high signal, this was a solid mass on T1 MR (not shown). **(Right)** Axial CECT shows a diffusely enlarged, intensely enhancing left parotid gland ➡ in an infant. The clinical history of a rapidly enlarging facial mass is key.

Schwannoma, Parotid

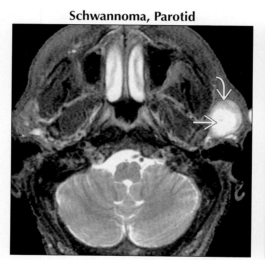

Infantile Hemangioma

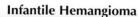
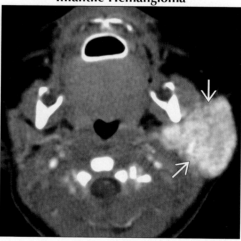

(Left) Axial NECT shows a well-defined, markedly hypodense mass ➡ in the superficial lobe of the right parotid. The fat density on CT is key for the diagnosis. **(Right)** Axial CECT shows a small well-defined mass ➡ in the left superficial lobe with a slightly lobulated contour. There are no specific imaging features to distinguish this lesion from a parotid lymph node.

Lipoma

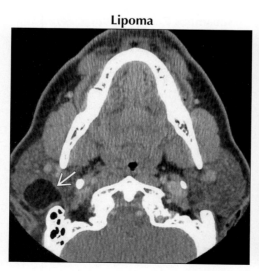

Oncocytoma, Parotid

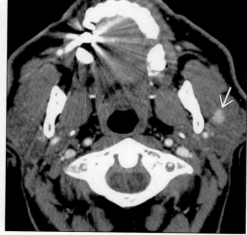

PAROTID SPACE MASS

Venous Malformation

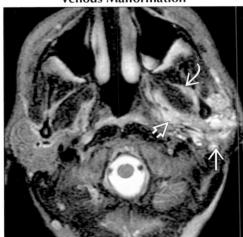

Lymphatic Malformation

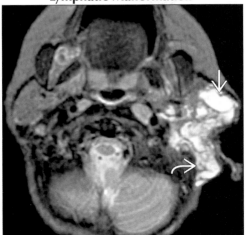

(Left) Axial T2WI MR shows diffuse infiltration of the superficial ➡ and deep ➡ lobes of the left parotid gland and the masticator space ➡. This trans-spatial, but otherwise nonaggressive appearance, favors a congenital lesion. *(Right)* Axial T2WI FS MR reveals a hyperintense mass with large ➡ and smaller ➡ "pools" replacing the left parotid gland. The lack of enhancement favors lymphatic malformation rather than venolymphatic malformation.

1st Branchial Cleft Cyst

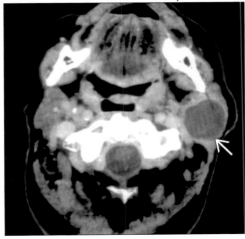

1st Branchial Cleft Cyst

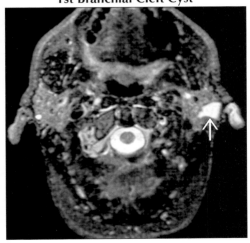

(Left) Axial CECT shows a well-defined intraparotid cyst with a smooth but enhancing periphery ➡, suggesting prior superimposed infection. *(Right)* Axial T2WI FS MR demonstrates a hyperintense cystic mass ➡ within the left parotid gland, extending toward the left external auditory canal.

Neurofibromatosis Type 1

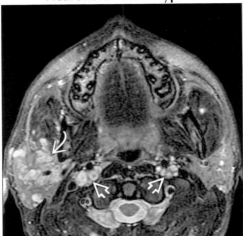

Rhabdomyosarcoma

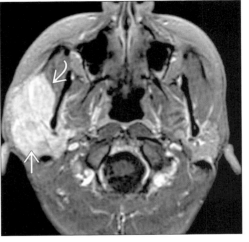

(Left) Axial T2WI FS MR shows an irregular lobulated mass in the right parotid and also involving the masseter muscle ➡. Separate bilateral carotid space nerve sheath lesions ➡ are also noted in this patient with neurofibromatosis type 1. *(Right)* Axial T1 C+ FS MR reveals a homogeneously enhancing mass ➡ diffusely infiltrating the right parotid and the adjacent right masseter muscle ➡.

CAROTID SPACE LESION

DIFFERENTIAL DIAGNOSIS

Common
- Reactive Lymph Nodes
- Atherosclerosis, Carotid Artery, Neck
- Thrombosis, Jugular Vein, Neck
- SCCa, Nodes
- Dissection, Carotid Artery, Neck
- Paraganglioma, Carotid Body
- Schwannoma, Carotid Space

Less Common
- Paraganglioma, Glomus Vagale
- Non-Hodgkin Lymphoma, Lymph Nodes
- Hodgkin Lymphoma, Lymph Nodes
- Neurofibroma, Carotid Space
- Fibromuscular Dysplasia, Carotid, Neck

Rare but Important
- Pseudoaneurysm, Carotid Artery, Neck
- Radiation Changes, Chronic
- Metastases, Systemic, Nodal
- Meningioma, Carotid Space
- Carotidynia, Acute Idiopathic

ESSENTIAL INFORMATION

Key Differential Diagnosis Issues
- Carotid space (CS) anatomic definition
  - Extent: Skull base (jugular foramen/carotid canal) to aortic arch
  - Contents: Suprahyoid CS contains CN9-12, internal carotid artery (ICA), internal jugular vein (IJV)
    - Infrahyoid CS: CN10, common carotid artery (CCA), IJV
    - Internal jugular nodes on CS surface
  - Fascia: All 3 layers of deep cervical fascia make up carotid sheath
- CS lesion definition: On surface of CS, involves carotid sheath or structures of CS
- CS mass displacement pattern depends on level of lesion
  - Nasopharyngeal CS mass: Parapharyngeal space (PPS) displaced anteriorly, styloid process displaced anterolaterally
  - Oropharyngeal CS mass: PPS displaced anteriorly, posterior belly of digastric displaced laterally
  - Infrahyoid neck CS mass: Surrounds CCA
    - May separate CCA from IJV
- Carotid space lesion general comments
  - ICA or CCA may be source of lesion

- Aneurysm, pseudoaneurysm, dissection
  - Finding artery lumen is primary task
- Hypervascular lesions suggested by vascular flow voids (paraganglioma)
- Lymph node diseases display multiple masses lateral to vascular structures
  - Remember internal jugular nodal chain is along surface of CS, not within CS

Helpful Clues for Common Diagnoses
- **Reactive Lymph Nodes**
  - Key facts: Common in younger patients
  - Imaging: Multiple enhancing ovoid lesions
    - When uniformly enlarged, may be difficult to distinguish from lymphoma
- **Atherosclerosis, Carotid Artery, Neck**
  - Key facts: Older patient, associated with cardiovascular & peripheral vascular disease
  - Imaging: Calcific & fibrofatty thickening of carotid artery vessel wall
    - Vessel often tortuous ± modestly dilated
    - Luminal narrowing often present
- **Thrombosis, Jugular Vein, Neck**
  - Key facts: Prior hospitalization with indwelling IJV line
  - Imaging: Nonenhancing jugular vein
    - ± Inflammatory changes around CS
    - ± Retropharyngeal edema
- **SCCa, Nodes**
  - Key facts: Multiple internal jugular chain nodes surround CS
    - History of cancer is significant
  - Imaging: Extranodal spread can invade carotid space directly
- **Dissection, Carotid Artery, Neck**
  - Key facts: Ipsilateral Horner syndrome, history of prior trauma, vasculopathy
  - Imaging: CA lumen compromised; overall cross sectional area of CA increases
    - Begins above bifurcation; terminates at carotid canal of skull base
    - High density/intensity mural thrombus
- **Paraganglioma, Carotid Body**
  - Key facts: Multiple paragangliomas, especially if familial
    - Check for other tumors
  - Imaging: Carotid bifurcation mass
    - "Splays" ICA & ECA
    - CT: Intense enhancement
    - MR: High velocity flow voids within lesion & along lesion margin

CAROTID SPACE LESION

- **Schwannoma, Carotid Space**
  - Imaging: Fusiform CS mass
    - CA displaced anteriorly or anteromedially
    - Intensely enhancing ± intramural cysts

Helpful Clues for Less Common Diagnoses

- **Paraganglioma, Glomus Vagale**
  - Key facts: Arises in vagal nodose ganglion
  - Imaging: Centered ~ 2 cm below skull base
    - Displaces PPS anteriorly
    - CT: Intense enhancement
    - MR: Flow voids ("pepper")
- **Non-Hodgkin Lymphoma, Lymph Nodes**
  - Key facts: Isolated to neck or part of systemic disease
  - Imaging: Bilateral multiple nodal masses
    - Heterogeneous enhancement possible
    - Large nonnecrotic nodes in typical & atypical chains
    - Waldeyer lymphatic ring ± involved
- **Hodgkin Lymphoma, Lymph Nodes**
  - Key facts: Younger patient with diffuse lymphadenopathy; night sweats
  - Imaging: Multiple large, ovoid lesions
    - Often unilateral with homogeneous enhancement
- **Neurofibroma, Carotid Space**
  - Key facts: Solitary or plexiform NF
    - When solitary, often NOT associated with NF1
  - Imaging: Fusiform, well-circumscribed shape (solitary NF)
    - CT: Lower density on NECT

- MR: Characteristic "target" sign appearance on T2 images
- If plexiform NF, mass poorly circumscribed, "invasive appearing"
- **Fibromuscular Dysplasia, Carotid, Neck**
  - Key facts: Medium to large artery wall dysplasia in younger women
  - Imaging: 3 appearances
    - Multifocal stenosis, long tubular stenosis, and single arterial wall outpouching

Helpful Clues for Rare Diagnoses

- **Pseudoaneurysm, Carotid Artery, Neck**
  - Key facts: Trauma or CA dissection history
  - Imaging: Focal dilatation of carotid artery
    - CT: Rings of Ca++ & thrombus
    - MR: Vascular flow phenomena ± complex wall signal
    - CTA, MRA, or angio correlation key
- **Radiation Changes, Chronic**
  - Key facts: Prior H&N tumor history
  - Imaging: Skin thickening, fascial thickening, fatty involution
    - "Blurring" of vasculature within CS
    - Carotid wall thickening ± aneurysm
- **Metastases, Systemic, Nodal**
  - Key fact: Chest or abdomen cancer
  - Imaging: Supraclavicular pathologic nodes
- **Meningioma, Carotid Space**
  - Key facts: Arises from jugular foramen
  - Imaging: Bilobed-enhancing mass
- **Carotidynia, Acute Idiopathic**
  - Key facts: Local pain important clue
  - Imaging: "Blurring" of CS tissue planes

Reactive Lymph Nodes

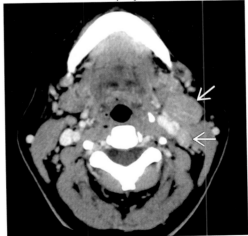

Axial CECT shows reactive adenopathy with minimal nodal enhancement. Multiple rounded masses ➡ along the surface of the carotid space are seen anterior and posterior to the carotid artery and jugular vein.

Atherosclerosis, Carotid Artery, Neck

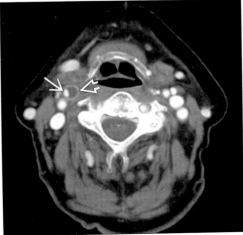

Axial CECT demonstrates significant narrowing of the ICA lumen ➡ by a soft atherosclerotic plaque ➡. US, CTA, MRA, or angiography can be used to further assess such a lesion.

CAROTID SPACE LESION

(Left) Axial CECT shows that the left internal jugular vein is thrombosed ➡. Note the loss of soft tissue planes, mild peripheral enhancement of the vein, and uniform low-density thrombus within the lumen.
(Right) Axial T2WI FS MR reveals a hyperintense left jugulodigastric malignant lymph node ➡ situated just anterior to the carotid bifurcation ⮞ and internal jugular vein ⮞ of the carotid space proper.

Thrombosis, Jugular Vein, Neck

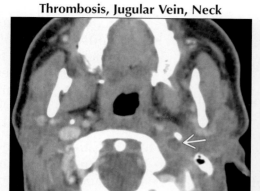

SCCa, Nodes

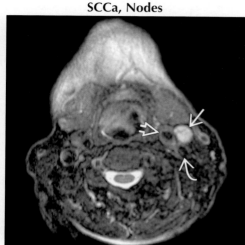

(Left) Axial T1WI MR demonstrates a hyperintense subintimal hematoma ➡ enlarging the right internal carotid artery cross section. The low signal arterial lumen is only minimally narrowed.
(Right) Axial CECT reveals the typical appearance of a homogeneously enhancing carotid body paraganglioma ➡. The external carotid ⮞ and internal carotid ⮞ arteries are splayed, and there are many prominent vessels along the anterior margin of the tumor.

Dissection, Carotid Artery, Neck

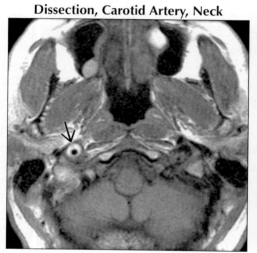

Paraganglioma, Carotid Body

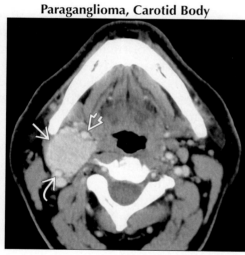

(Left) Axial T1 C+ FS MR shows an enhancing carotid space schwannoma ➡ with multiple intramural cysts ➡. The absence of flow voids and the presence of intramural cysts make a schwannoma the most likely diagnosis. **(Right)** Axial T1 C+ MR reveals an ovoid mass ➡ centered approximately 2 cm below the skull base in the carotid space. Note the heterogeneous enhancement with central low signal flow voids.

Schwannoma, Carotid Space

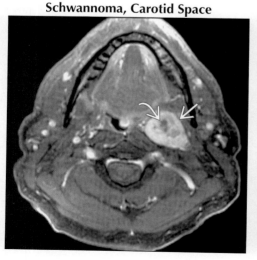

Paraganglioma, Glomus Vagale

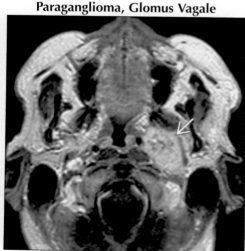

CAROTID SPACE LESION

Non-Hodgkin Lymphoma, Lymph Nodes

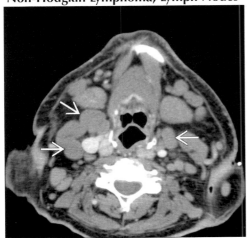

Hodgkin Lymphoma, Lymph Nodes

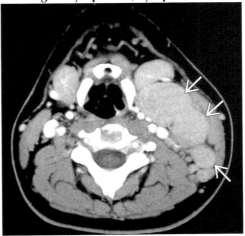

(Left) Axial CECT demonstrates multiple, rounded, uniform density masses adjacent to the carotid space ➡. Internal jugular chain lymph nodes are closely associated with the carotid space but not within the space itself. (Right) Axial CECT shows moderately enhancing, unilateral, bulky Hodgkin lymphoma lymph nodes ➡. The internal jugular nodes are found in the superficial carotid space fascia.

Neurofibroma, Carotid Space

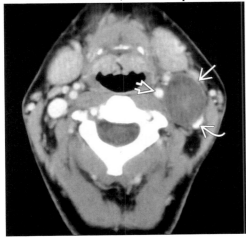

Fibromuscular Dysplasia, Carotid, Neck

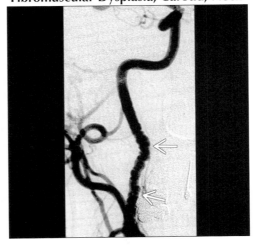

(Left) Axial CECT demonstrates a low-density isolated neurofibroma ➡ in the carotid space, which displaces the internal carotid artery ➡ anteromedially and the internal jugular vein ➡ posterolaterally. Note the density is between the muscle and fat. (Right) Anteroposterior internal carotid artery angiogram shows the typical "string of beads" appearance ➡ of fibromuscular dysplasia in this younger female patient with transient ischemic attacks.

Pseudoaneurysm, Carotid Artery, Neck

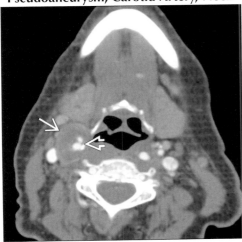

Radiation Changes, Chronic

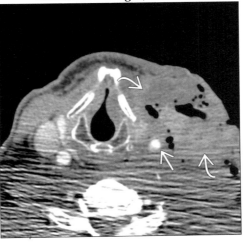

(Left) Axial CECT shows a large, clot-filled carotid artery pseudoaneurysm ➡ surrounding the carotid bifurcation ➡. (Right) Axial CECT reveals a persistent massive extranodal tumor that has injured the common carotid artery wall. Extensive extranodal tumor ➡ extends to the overlying skin and infiltrates through the carotid space, encasing the common carotid ➡.

CAROTID ARTERY LESION

DIFFERENTIAL DIAGNOSIS

Common
- Atherosclerosis, Carotid Artery, Neck
- Carotid Artery, Tortuous, Neck
- Fibromuscular Dysplasia, Carotid, Neck
- Dissection, Carotid Artery, Neck

Less Common
- Carotidynia, Acute Idiopathic
- Pseudoaneurysm, Carotid Artery, Neck

Rare but Important
- Aneurysm, Carotid Artery, Neck
- Takayasu Arteritis, Carotid Artery, Neck
- Carotid Artery, SCCa Nodal Involvement
- Radiation Changes, Acute, Carotid Artery
- Radiation Changes, Chronic, Carotid Artery

ESSENTIAL INFORMATION

Key Differential Diagnosis Issues
- DDx describes primary lesions of carotid artery lumen or perivascular soft tissues
  - Primary disease in this location often accompanied by thromboembolic phenomena; i.e., TIA or cerebral infarction
  - Perivascular disease will most commonly be inflammatory in nature
  - Review of any lesion contiguous with carotid artery should include assessment of carotid lumen
- Adequate depiction of carotid artery lumen is critical imaging element
  - CT is best performed with adequate arterial opacification; MRA is more reliable than other MR sequences to evaluate status of vascular lumen
    - Reconstructions may be necessary to evaluate vessel lumen to advantage
    - Maximum-intensity projection, volume-rendered and curvilinear MPR, or volume depiction techniques may be used
- Stack review of vascular structures of neck with occasional reconstructed images is optimal

Helpful Clues for Common Diagnoses
- **Atherosclerosis, Carotid Artery, Neck**
  - Key facts: May be asymptomatic; should be evaluated on all studies of H&N

- CT: Calcific & fibrofatty disease of vessel wall with accompanying luminal narrowing is most common appearance
- **Carotid Artery, Tortuous, Neck**
  - Key facts
    - Tortuosity of cervical carotid artery can be evaluated with careful tracing of vessel on contiguous stack images
    - Unusual tortuosity of cervical ICA may result in prominent submucosal "mass"
  - Imaging
    - Tortuous ectatic carotid arteries may loop into retropharyngeal space
- **Fibromuscular Dysplasia, Carotid, Neck**
  - Key facts: Medium to large artery wall dysplasia in young to middle-aged women
  - Imaging: 3 appearances
    - Multifocal stenosis ("string of beads")
    - Long tubular stenosis
    - Single outpouching from arterial wall
    - CTA, MRA, or angiography key
    - Caveat: Difficult diagnosis with axial CECT
- **Dissection, Carotid Artery, Neck**
  - Key facts
    - Classic clinical symptom complex: Horner syndrome, neck pain, & TIA-CVA
    - History of trauma (penetrating or blunt) may help make dissection diagnosis
    - Dissection may be etiology of cerebral infarction in young patient
    - Associations of carotid dissection: Blunt neck trauma (seat belt injury), iatrogenic causes, collagen vascular diseases, fibromuscular dysplasia, chiropractic manipulation or vigorous neck torsion, & occasional idiopathic etiology
  - Imaging: Carotid dissection results in 2 typical imaging manifestations
    - Intimal rupture & hematoma dissecting through media results in enlargement of vessel cross-section
    - Same phenomenon results in arterial lumen narrowing or occlusion
    - Smooth tapering occlusion of ICA beyond bifurcation is often seen when patients are studied at symptom onset

Helpful Clues for Less Common Diagnoses
- **Carotidynia, Acute Idiopathic**
  - Key facts: Presents with localized pain & inflammatory change

CAROTID ARTERY LESION

- Typically accompanied by significant pain over bifurcation
  - Imaging: Localized carotid space (CS) inflammatory findings
    - Blurring of tissue planes in & around CS
    - Exaggerated perivascular enhancement without discrete mass
- **Pseudoaneurysm, Carotid Artery, Neck**
  - Key facts
    - Pseudoaneurysm of carotid artery at skull base is strongly suggestive of prior carotid dissection
    - Carotid blow out is unique form of carotid artery pseudoaneurysm associated with contiguous tumor involvement of vessel wall
    - Blow out typically follows multimodality therapy for cancer; surgery, chemotherapy, & radiation therapy
  - Imaging
    - Aneurysm sac made up of < 3 walls; hence term pseudoaneurysm
    - "Onion skin" or lamellated layers of thrombotic material in wall not uncommon

Helpful Clues for Rare Diagnoses

- **Aneurysm, Carotid Artery, Neck**
  - Key facts: Atherosclerotic disease or collagen vascular disease may predispose
    - Pulsatility is not useful clinical sign for carotid artery aneurysms
    - Any lesion contiguous with carotid may transmit pulsations

- Imaging: Fusiform dilatation of common or internal carotid artery
- **Takayasu Arteritis, Carotid Artery, Neck**
  - Key facts: Proximal vessel involvement; originate from arch, extends into inferior cervical neck arterial walls
    - Diagnosis of exclusion in young adults with CVA
  - Imaging: Smooth tapering stenoses or occlusions, wall thickening
- **Carotid Artery, SCCa Nodal Involvement**
  - Key facts: Can limit surgical dissection or require grafting
    - Predisposes to carotid blow out
  - Imaging
    - Extranodal tumor visible
    - Obliteration of fat planes in circumferential fashion around carotid
- **Radiation Changes, Acute, Carotid Artery**
  - Key facts: Inflammatory change of vessel during radiation therapy
    - Carotid radiation changes occur with significant radiation changes to overlying skin & soft tissues
  - Imaging: Thickened vessel wall, edema, perivascular inflammatory change
- **Radiation Changes, Chronic, Carotid Artery**
  - Key facts: Findings resemble accelerated atherosclerosis
  - Imaging: Wall thickening, calcifications, vessel stenoses, & occlusions

Atherosclerosis, Carotid Artery, Neck

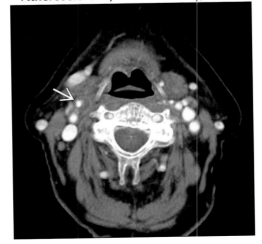

Axial CECT reveals high-grade stenosis of the proximal internal carotid artery ➡ due to atherosclerotic plaque. Plaque in this case is largely fibrofatty and eccentric.

Atherosclerosis, Carotid Artery, Neck

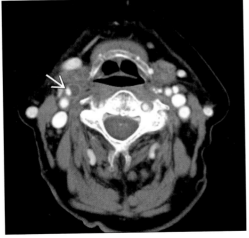

Axial CECT shows a typical CECT appearance of high-grade stenosis of the proximal internal carotid artery due to atherosclerotic plaque. Note hemodynamically significant luminal compromise ➡.

CAROTID ARTERY LESION

(Left) Axial CECT demonstrates bilateral tortuous internal carotid arteries ➡. Distortion of the posterior wall of the hypopharynx may be associated. Pulsatile masses may be mistaken for vascular tumors. (Right) Axial CECT reveals short segment bilateral tortuous carotid arteries ➡. The left ICA is horizontal within this section. Following the vessel on stacked images allows the diagnosis.

Carotid Artery, Tortuous, Neck

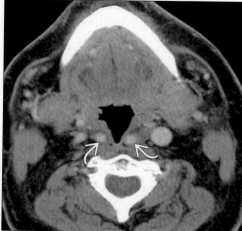

Carotid Artery, Tortuous, Neck

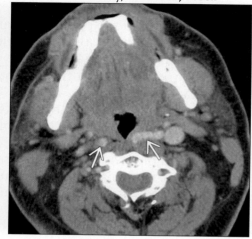

(Left) MRA of suprahyoid neck reveals internal carotid artery findings typical of fibromuscular dysplasia. Note the "string of beads" appearance ➡ created by alternating web-like narrowing and modest dilatation of the internal carotid artery. (Right) MRA demonstrates the most common imaging manifestation of fibromuscular dysplasia, the "string of beads" ➡. Patients with FMD are predisposed to carotid artery dissection.

Fibromuscular Dysplasia, Carotid, Neck

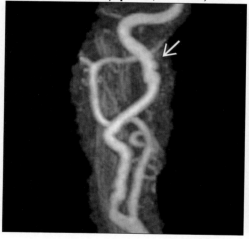

Fibromuscular Dysplasia, Carotid, Neck

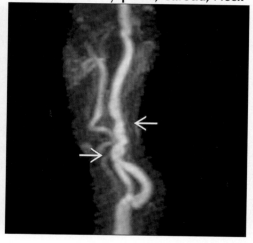

(Left) Axial T1WI MR shows right ICA dissection with the mural hematoma evident as crescentic high signal intensity ➡ with an enlarged cross section of the vessel and narrow low signal lumen ➡. (Right) Oblique sagittal MRA shows an internal carotid artery dissection. The high signal of the mural hematoma ➡ parallels the true lumen, which is even higher signal ➡.

Dissection, Carotid Artery, Neck

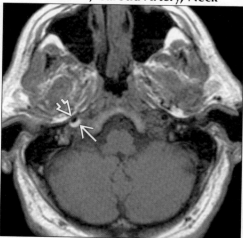

Dissection, Carotid Artery, Neck

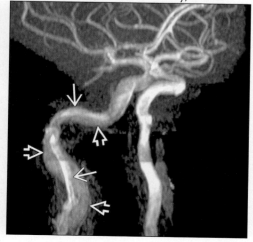

CAROTID ARTERY LESION

Pseudoaneurysm, Carotid Artery, Neck

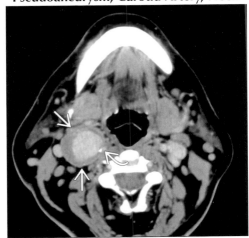

Pseudoaneurysm, Carotid Artery, Neck

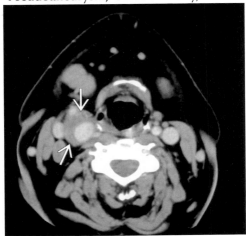

(Left) Axial CECT reveals a carotid artery pseudoaneurysm as displaced calcifications ➡ and "onion skin" layers of thrombosis of the wall ➡. *(Right)* Axial CECT shows the classic CT features of a carotid artery pseudoaneurysm (CAPA). The thrombosis ➡ is largely lateral to residual lumen.

Takayasu Arteritis, Carotid Artery, Neck

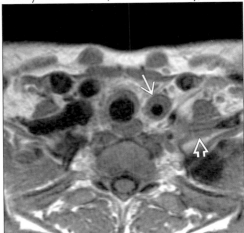

Takayasu Arteritis, Carotid Artery, Neck

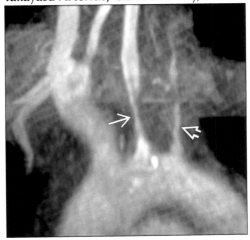

(Left) Axial T1WI MR shows a typical appearance of Takayasu arteritis. Note the eccentric wall thickening and narrowing of the left common carotid artery ➡ and left subclavian artery ➡. *(Right)* MRA shows typical findings of Takayasu arteritis. Maximum-intensity projection reformations demonstrate narrowing of the left common carotid artery ➡ and subclavian artery ➡.

Carotid Artery, SCCa Nodal Involvement

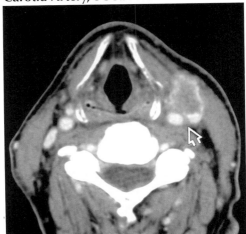

Carotid Artery, SCCa Nodal Involvement

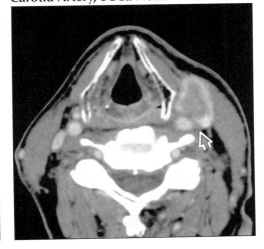

(Left) Axial CECT shows a recurrent nodal-extranodal squamous cell carcinoma invading carotid space, seen as enhancing tissue between the carotid artery and the internal jugular vein ➡. *(Right)* Axial CECT shows a recurrent nodal-extranodal squamous cell carcinoma invading the carotid space, with blurred fat planes ➡ but normal carotid lumen.

PERIVERTEBRAL SPACE LESION

DIFFERENTIAL DIAGNOSIS

Common
- Metastasis, Vertebral Body, PVS
- Infection, Perivertebral Space
- Schwannoma, Brachial Plexus, PVS
- Longus Colli Tendinitis

Less Common
- Chordoma, PVS
- Venous Malformation, PVS
- Neurofibromatosis Type 1
- Lipoma, PVS
- Non-Hodgkin Lymphoma, PVS

Rare but Important
- Lymphatic Malformation, PVS
- Hypertrophy, Levator Scapulae Muscle
- Fibromatosis, PVS
- Hemangiopericytoma, PVS

ESSENTIAL INFORMATION

Key Differential Diagnosis Issues
- Perivertebral space (PVS) has 2 components
  - Prevertebral: Vertebral body, prevertebral & scalene muscles, brachial plexus
  - Paraspinal: Paraspinal muscles, posterior spinal elements
- Most PVS lesions arise from vertebral body: Metastases, infection
- Deep layer of deep cervical fascia surrounds PVS
  - Confines lesions; "directs" them to spread into epidural area

Helpful Clues for Common Diagnoses
- **Metastasis, Vertebral Body, PVS**
  - Key facts
    - Diagnosis of neoplasm may not be known
    - Perivertebral space involvement secondary to vertebral body disease
  - Imaging
    - Replacement of normal marrow signal intensity of involved vertebra on MR
    - CECT: Lytic or sclerotic vertebral body lesion with contiguous soft tissue abnormality in PVS
- **Infection, Perivertebral Space**
  - Key facts
    - Elevated white count, fever, and local pain and tenderness
    - Epidural involvement may result in cord compression or radicular symptoms
  - Imaging
    - Disease in disc space or vertebral body osteomyelitis with contiguous inflammatory mass
    - CECT: Abscess formation will lead to peripheral enhancement of fluid collection
- **Schwannoma, Brachial Plexus, PVS**
  - Key facts
    - Often asymptomatic PVS mass
  - Imaging
    - May appear embedded in scalene muscles
    - CECT: Lesion often extends to spinal canal; smoothly enlarges neural foramen
    - MR: High signal on T2; enhances heterogeneously when larger, with intratumoral cyst formation
- **Longus Colli Tendinitis**
  - Key facts
    - Crystal deposition disease with involvement of skull base musculature
    - Infectious etiology may be suspected
  - Imaging
    - CT: Calcifications anterior to C2
    - CT/MR: May present with retropharyngeal effusion

Helpful Clues for Less Common Diagnoses
- **Chordoma, PVS**
  - Key facts
    - Unusual lesion of cervical vertebral body with PVS mass
  - Imaging
    - CT: Irregular bone destruction of involved vertebral body
    - CT/MR: Enhances avidly following contrast administration
    - MR: May show characteristic high signal intensity on T2
- **Venous Malformation, PVS**
  - Key facts
    - Rarely symptomatic
    - May be palpable as soft ill-defined mass
  - Imaging
    - CT: Lobulated soft tissue mass with phleboliths
    - MR: Variable appearance based on size of venous channels

- CT/MR: May also exhibit regional fat hypertrophy
- **Neurofibromatosis Type 1**
  - Key facts
    - Multilevel spinal nerve root tumors, often in PVS in patient with NF1
    - May involve multiple nerve roots, and described as "plexiform"
  - Imaging
    - CT: Isodense to spinal cord, near fluid density, often follows brachial plexus roots
    - MR: Near isointense to spinal roots or cord, variable enhancement
    - MR: "Target sign" is very suggestive; high T2 signal intensity periphery & low signal intensity centrally
- **Lipoma, PVS**
  - Key facts
    - Often soft and compressible mass
  - Imaging
    - CT: Uniform fat density
    - MR: Uniform high T1 signal intensity, intermediate signal on T2
    - CT/MR: Liposarcoma possible when soft tissue is significant component
- **Non-Hodgkin Lymphoma, PVS**
  - Key facts
    - Extranodal, extralymphatic NHL deposit
  - Imaging
    - CT/MR: Infiltrating mass in PVS ± epidural disease

Helpful Clues for Rare Diagnoses
- **Lymphatic Malformation, PVS**
  - Imaging
    - CT/MR: Trans-spatial lesion, multilocular and nonenhancing
    - MR: Low T1, high T2 signal
- **Hypertrophy, Levator Scapulae Muscle**
  - Key facts
    - May follow ipsilateral neck dissection with resection of sternocleidomastoid muscle
    - Pseudomass results from muscle hypertrophy
  - Imaging
    - CT/MR: Muscle is normal in CT density and MR signal intensity
- **Fibromatosis, PVS**
  - Key facts
    - Synonym: Desmoid tumor
    - Benign soft tissue tumor often with aggressive appearance
  - Imaging
    - CT/MR: Poorly defined, trans-spatial, soft tissue mass involving muscle bundle
- **Hemangiopericytoma, PVS**
  - Key facts
    - Rare soft tissue tumor of H&N
    - Propensity to develop in posterior perivertebral soft tissues
  - Imaging
    - Hypervascular mass with prominent arterial feeders on angiography
    - CT/MR: Avid enhancement

Metastasis, Vertebral Body, PVS

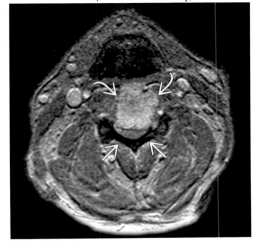

Axial STIR MR shows metastasis to cervical spine, with a tumor in the vertebral body and extension to the perivertebral space ➔ and spinal canal. Note the normal STIR signal of marrow in the lamina ➔.

Metastasis, Vertebral Body, PVS

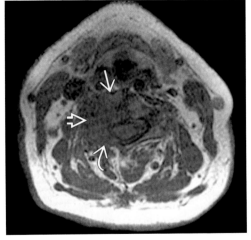

Axial T1WI MR at the C4 level shows a right lateral vertebral body metastasis, including the vertebral body ➔, pedicle ➔, and lamina ➔. Notice that the epidural tumor abuts the spinal cord.

PERIVERTEBRAL SPACE LESION

(Left) *Axial CECT reveals a postoperative paraspinal space abscess, seen as a fluid density collection with minimal marginal enhancement within the paraspinal aspect of the perivertebral space* ➡. **(Right)** *Axial T1 C+ FS MR shows brachial plexus schwannoma* ➡ *as a heterogeneously enhancing rounded mass posterior to and minimally displacing the internal jugular vein* ⮑.

Infection, Perivertebral Space

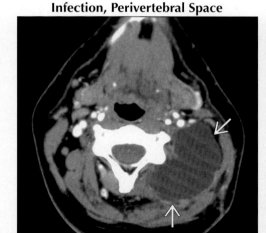

Schwannoma, Brachial Plexus, PVS

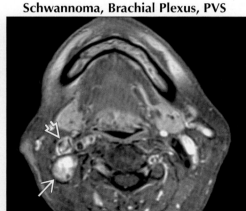

(Left) *Axial CECT demonstrates characteristic calcifications anterior to C1-2* ➡ *located within the longus colli muscle. Retropharyngeal effusion accompanies most cases.* **(Right)** *Axial T2WI MR reveals a cervical chordoma involving the C3 body* ➡ *with extension into the anterior prevertebral part of the perivertebral space. The lesion involves the entirety of the body and extends into the central canal, compressing the cervical cord* ⮑.

Longus Colli Tendinitis

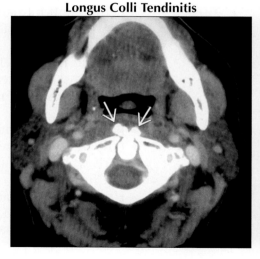

Chordoma, PVS

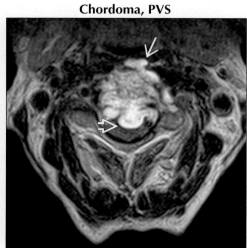

(Left) *Axial T1 C+ FS MR shows a trans-spatial enhancing lesion involving the prevertebral aspect of the perivertebral space* ➡ *and retropharyngeal* ⮑ *and pharyngeal mucosal* ➡ *spaces.* **(Right)** *Axial T2WI MR shows multiple neurofibromas in a child with neurofibromatosis type 1 in the prevertebral* ➡ *and paraspinal* ⮑ *aspects of the perivertebral space.*

Venous Malformation, PVS

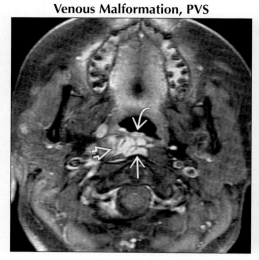

Neurofibromatosis Type 1

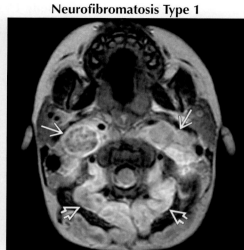

PERIVERTEBRAL SPACE LESION

Lipoma, PVS

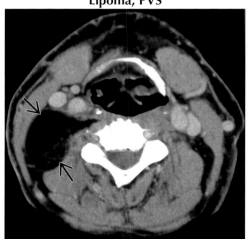

Non-Hodgkin Lymphoma, PVS

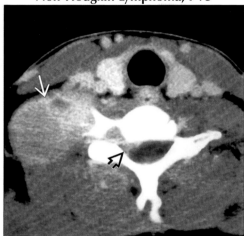

(Left) Axial CECT shows a perivertebral space lipoma with near uniform fat density ➡ and no significant soft tissue mass within the fatty mass. Distortion of the adjacent soft tissues is minimal. *(Right)* Axial CECT reveals a variably enhancing right perivertebral space infiltrating mass ➡ with epidural disease evident ➡. At biopsy, extranodal extralymphatic non-Hodgkin lymphoma was diagnosed.

Lymphatic Malformation, PVS

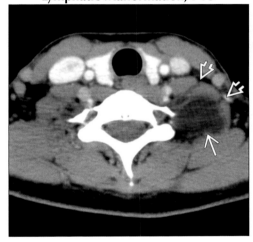

Hypertrophy, Levator Scapulae Muscle

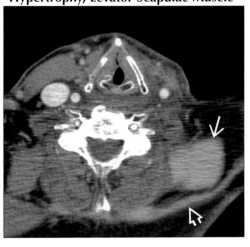

(Left) Axial CECT shows a lobulated, low-attenuation, nonenhancing lymphatic malformation ➡ in the left neck in the deep layer of the deep cervical fascia ➡. Note absence of extension into the neural foramina. *(Right)* Axial CECT shows levator scapulae hypertrophy, with ipsilateral neck dissection (absent internal jugular vein and sternocleidomastoid muscle). The trapezius muscle is atrophic ➡, and the left levator scapulae muscle is hypertrophic ➡.

Fibromatosis, PVS

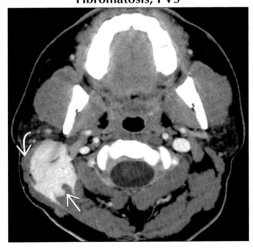

Hemangiopericytoma, PVS

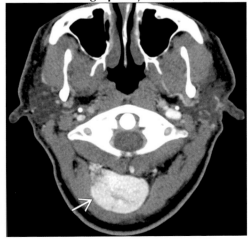

(Left) Axial CECT demonstrates an invasive, enhancing area of fibromatosis involving the right paraspinal ➡ and sternocleidomastoid ➡ muscles. The infiltrating edges of this lesion suggest other malignant conditions. *(Right)* Axial CECT reveals a densely enhancing hemangiopericytoma ➡ in the paraspinal aspect of the perivertebral space. The mass is well marginated, with a small central area of decreased enhancement.

BRACHIAL PLEXUS LESION

DIFFERENTIAL DIAGNOSIS

Common
- Trauma, Brachial Plexus
- Pancoast Tumor
- Metastases, Systemic, Nodal
- Radiation Changes, Subacute
- Radiation Changes, Chronic

Less Common
- Neuroma, Post-Traumatic, Brachial Plexus
- Neurofibromatosis Type 1
- Schwannoma, Brachial Plexus, PVS
- Acute Brachial Plexitis (Parsonage-Turner Syndrome)
- Peripheral Neurolymphomatosis
- Leukemia

Rare but Important
- Brachial Plexus Entrapment (Thoracic Outlet Syndrome)
- Fibromatosis
- Chronic Inflammatory Demyelinating Polyneuropathy (CIDP)
- Hereditary Motor-Sensory Neuropathy

ESSENTIAL INFORMATION

Key Differential Diagnosis Issues
- Brachial plexus innervates arm
  - C5-T1 ventral rami
- Trauma most common cause of plexopathy
  - Stretch injuries → nerve avulsion
- Neoplastic: Metastatic disease > primary
  - Metastatic: Direct tumor spread or nodal
  - Compresses ± invades plexus
- Inflammatory: Acute → chronic plexitis
  - Radiation most common cause
  - Diffuse thickening: Consider hypertrophic polyneuropathies (CIDP, hereditary motor-sensory neuropathy)
- Imaging strategies
  - CT: Allows detection of masses
    - Look for loss of perineural fat
  - MR: Allows detailed evaluation of nerves
    - Enlarged, edematous ± enhancing

Helpful Clues for Common Diagnoses
- **Trauma, Brachial Plexus**
  - Most common cause of brachial plexopathy
    - Stretch injury: Neuropraxia with swollen nerve; most improve

- Nerve avulsion: Pre- or postganglionic
  - Infants: Result of traumatic delivery
    - Erb (C5, 6, ± 7) & Klumpke (C8, T1) palsies
  - Adults: High force, e.g., motorcycle crash
  - Imaging
    - MR typically study of choice
    - Stretch: Enlarged T2 hyperintense nerves
    - Preganglionic avulsion: Root absent ± pseudomeningocele, cord displaced, denervated paraspinous muscles
    - Postganglionic nerve avulsion: Nerve disruption with distal retraction
    - CT myelography shows preganglionic avulsions with absent root
- **Pancoast Tumor**
  - Key facts
    - Apical lung tumor; SCCa most common
  - Imaging
    - CT: Chest wall invasion, loss of fat around subclavian artery
    - MR: Infiltration of lower trunk especially
- **Metastases, Systemic, Nodal**
  - Key facts
    - Most often from breast carcinoma
    - Compresses &/or infiltrates plexus
  - Imaging
    - MR: Enhancing masses compress plexus
    - Nodular or diffuse enhancing tissue
- **Radiation Changes, Subacute**
  - Key facts
    - Uncommon (< 1%); > 6000 cGy
    - Peak at 10-20 months post-radiation
    - Predominantly sensory symptoms
  - Imaging
    - MR: Loss of clarity of plexus
    - T2 hyperintense, variable enhancement
- **Radiation Changes, Chronic**
  - Key facts
    - Fibrosis even > 20 years post-treatment
  - Imaging
    - MR: Loss of clarity of nerves from intermediate T2 scar tissue

Helpful Clues for Less Common Diagnoses
- **Neuroma, Post-Traumatic, Brachial Plexus**
  - Key facts
    - Result of unregulated nerve regeneration
    - ≤ 12 months after injury
  - Imaging
    - MR: Heterogeneously hyperintense & enhancing nodule in plexus

BRACHIAL PLEXUS LESION

- **Neurofibromatosis Type 1**
  - Key facts
    - Plexus neurofibromas rare unless NF1
  - Imaging
    - MR: Symmetrically enlarged, lobulated T2 hyperintense roots
- **Schwannoma, Brachial Plexus, PVS**
  - Key facts
    - Benign Schwann cell neoplasm
  - Imaging
    - T2 hyperintense, ± cystic degeneration
    - Moderate to intense enhancement
- **Acute Brachial Plexitis (Parsonage-Turner Syndrome)**
  - Key facts
    - Idiopathic, viral/postviral, post-vaccination
  - Imaging
    - MR: T2 hyperintense plexus
    - Muscle denervation, then atrophy
- **Peripheral Neurolymphomatosis**
  - Key facts
    - Isolated plexus lymphoma OR with CNS or systemic lymphoma
    - Focal nerve → diffuse infiltration
  - Imaging
    - MR: Smooth thickening, T2 hyperintense enhancing nerve(s)
- **Leukemia**
  - Key facts: Infiltration with leukemic cells
  - Imaging
    - MR: Loss of clarity of plexus elements
    - Smooth thickening, T2 hyperintensity & enhancement

Helpful Clues for Rare Diagnoses

- **Brachial Plexus Entrapment (Thoracic Outlet Syndrome)**
  - Key facts: Nerves compressed or stretched
    - Cervical rib, long C7 transverse process
    - Excessive callus from clavicle/rib fracture
    - Muscle hypertrophy, e.g., anterior scalene
  - Imaging
    - MR may show focal T2 hyperintensity
- **Fibromatosis**
  - Key facts: Spectrum of disease
    - Benign desmoid → aggressive fibromatosis
  - Imaging
    - Variable: Well-defined → infiltrative mass
    - MR: T1 hypo- to isointense to muscle, T2 heterogeneous, enhancing
- **Chronic Inflammatory Demyelinating Polyneuropathy (CIDP)**
  - Key facts: Acquired, immune-mediated
    - Sensory, motor symptoms & areflexia
  - Imaging
    - MR: Diffusely thickened nerve roots
    - Enlarged, moderately enhancing nerves
- **Hereditary Motor-Sensory Neuropathy**
  - Key facts: Many types and subtypes
    - Synonym: Charcot-Marie-Tooth
    - CMT1: Demyelination & remyelination ⇒ "onion bulb" appearance
    - CMT3 = Dejerine-Sottas (infantile form)
  - Imaging
    - Identical appearance to CIDP

Trauma, Brachial Plexus

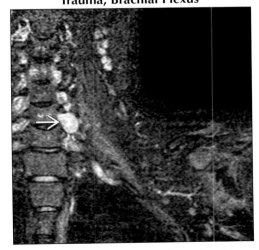

Coronal STIR MR shows a large hyperintense pseudomeningocele ➡ at C6-7, indicating avulsion of the left C7 nerve root. This patient had experienced a prior motorcycle crash.

Trauma, Brachial Plexus

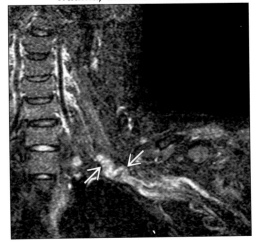

Coronal STIR MR in same patient shows discontinuous, hyperintense, & retracted C7 nerve root ➡, indicating complete avulsion. Injuries to the rest of plexus nerves are also evident.

1

BRACHIAL PLEXUS LESION

Pancoast Tumor

Pancoast Tumor

(Left) Axial CECT reveals a heterogeneous apical lung mass ➡ invading the posterior chest wall. The anterior margin of the tumor nears the posterior margin of the subclavian artery ➡, where trunks of brachial plexus are found. Also note tumor's proximity to the right vertebral artery ➡. *(Right)* Sagittal T1WI MR in the same patient shows a superior sulcal tumor ➡ invading through the chest wall. Anterior limit of tumor ➡ invades fat pad posterior to subclavian artery ➡.

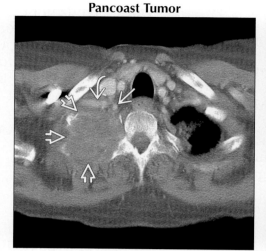
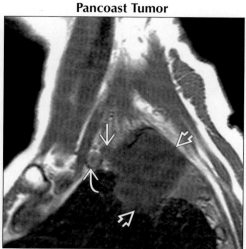

Metastases, Systemic, Nodal

Metastases, Systemic, Nodal

(Left) Axial T1 C+ FS MR in a patient with prior breast cancer demonstrates new supraclavicular mass ➡, the posterior aspect of which abuts the brachial plexus ➡, which is intensely enhancing. Denervation is noted in pectoralis major muscle also ➡. *(Right)* Coronal T1 C+ FS MR in the same patient shows marked enhancement extending proximally along thickened plexus cords ➡ to divisions ➡ and trunks. Both compression and infiltration by tumor are evident.

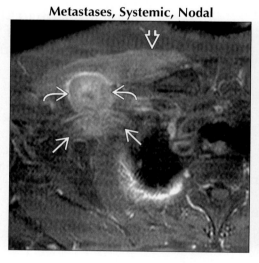
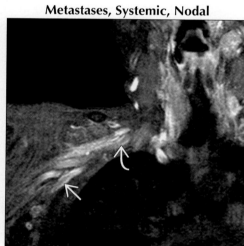

Radiation Changes, Subacute

Radiation Changes, Chronic

(Left) Coronal STIR MR shows diffuse hyperintensity of the plexus relative to muscles and enlargement of roots ➡, trunks ➡, divisions ➡, and proximal cords in a patient with prior radiation for breast cancer and progressive left arm symptoms. *(Right)* Coronal T1WI MR in a different patient shows confluence of roots ➡ and trunks ➡ of the plexus with homogeneous fibrotic tissue. Note the extensive supraclavicular fat stranding ➡.

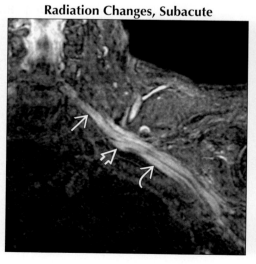
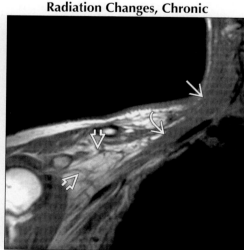

BRACHIAL PLEXUS LESION

Neuroma, Post-Traumatic, Brachial Plexus

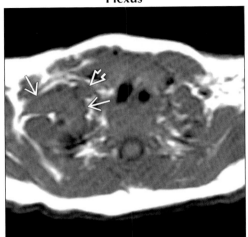

Neuroma, Post-Traumatic, Brachial Plexus

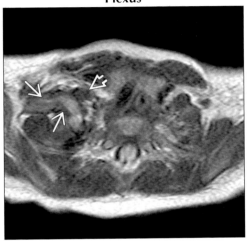

(Left) Axial T1WI MR in an infant demonstrates a tubular mass ⇥ that is isointense to muscle and is located posterior to the anterior scalene muscle ⇥. *(Right)* Axial T2WI MR in the same infant better demonstrates the tubular nature of the hyperintense mass ⇥, which is now more clearly distinguished from the anterior scalene muscle ⇥.

Neurofibromatosis Type 1

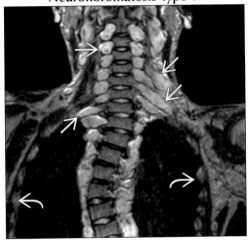

Schwannoma, Brachial Plexus, PVS

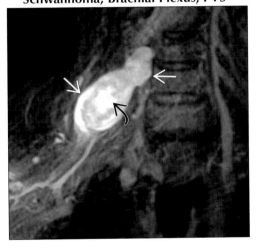

(Left) Coronal T2WI MR in a teenager reveals bilateral lobulated heterogeneous neurofibromas ⇥ involving each cervical and upper thoracic nerve root. This patient had other manifestations of NF1, including intercostal nerve lesions ⇥ and scoliosis. *(Right)* Coronal T2WI FS MR shows a fusiform hyperintense but heterogeneous mass ⇥ oriented along the course of the brachial plexus. Central cystic degeneration ⇗ is typical of a schwannoma.

Acute Brachial Plexitis (Parsonage-Turner Syndrome)

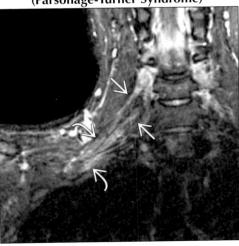

Acute Brachial Plexitis (Parsonage-Turner Syndrome)

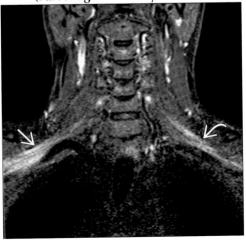

(Left) Coronal STIR MR in a young man with rapid onset of shoulder weakness shows hyperintensity and subtle enlargement of roots ⇥ and trunks ⇥. Symptoms resolved over months with anti-inflammatory treatment, but no cause was determined. *(Right)* Coronal STIR MR in a different patient reveals bilateral asymmetric hyperintensity of the brachial plexus with more marked involvement of right ⇥ than left ⇥. Acute plexitis is bilateral in up to 1/3 of cases.

BRACHIAL PLEXUS LESION

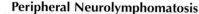

(Left) Coronal STIR MR in a patient with systemic lymphoma and 1 month history of left arm flaccid paralysis demonstrates marked thickening of roots and trunks of left brachial plexus ➡. Tumor involving the left scapula is also apparent ➡. (Right) Coronal T1 C+ FS MR in the same patient shows smooth diffuse enhancement of enlarged left plexus from roots ➡, to divisions ➡ and cords ➡. Intracranial and spinal leptomeningeal recurrence are also found on MR.

Peripheral Neurolymphomatosis

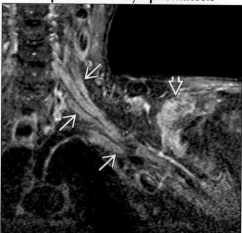

Peripheral Neurolymphomatosis

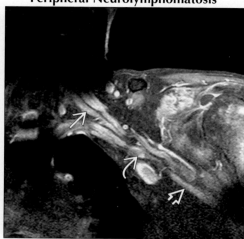

(Left) Coronal STIR MR in a child with previous CNS relapse of ALL, new left shoulder pain, & C8 numbness shows enlargement & hyperintensity of C5 ➡ through C8 ➡. C8 is the largest of affected nerve roots, and the process extended into the trunks. (Right) Axial T1 C+ FS MR in the same child at the cervicothoracic junction level demonstrates asymmetric abnormal enhancement of C8 ➡ and T1 ➡ as they form the lower trunk.

Leukemia

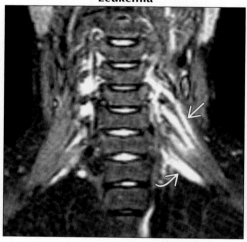

Leukemia

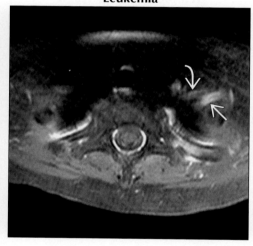

(Left) Coronal STIR MR in a patient with prior snowboarding injury & C8-T1 neuropathy shows an abnormally hyperintense C7 nerve root ➡ directed toward heterogeneous mass of left chest wall ➡. C8 & T1 also extend into mass. (Right) Sagittal STIR MR in the same patient shows a healing rib fracture with hyperintense callus ➡ immediately inferior to the subclavian artery ➡. Note hyperintensity seen in fat ➡ posterior to artery at location of plexus divisions.

Brachial Plexus Entrapment (Thoracic Outlet Syndrome)

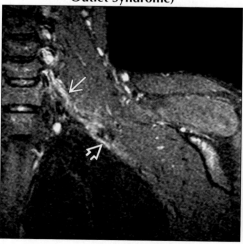

Brachial Plexus Entrapment (Thoracic Outlet Syndrome)

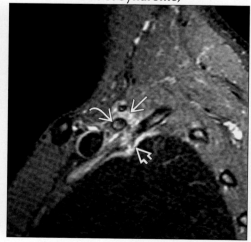

BRACHIAL PLEXUS LESION

Fibromatosis

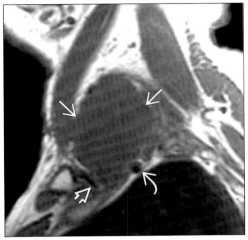

Fibromatosis

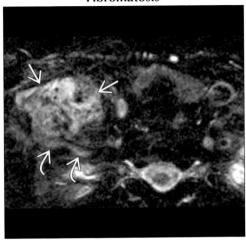

(Left) Sagittal T1WI MR shows a homogeneous mass ➡ in the lower neck that abuts & surrounds subclavian artery ➡ & compresses the vein anteriorly ➡. Brachial plexus divisions are located superior & posterior to the subclavian artery at this level. *(Right)* Axial T2WI FS MR shows marked heterogeneity of a supraclavicular mass ➡ that is rounded with ill-defined margins. The middle trunk of the plexus ➡ is displaced and slightly enlarged.

Chronic Inflammatory Demyelinating Polyneuropathy (CIDP)

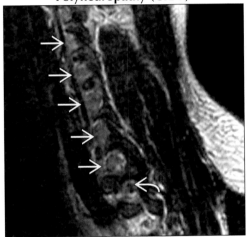

Chronic Inflammatory Demyelinating Polyneuropathy (CIDP)

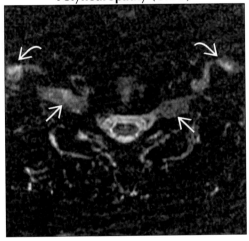

(Left) Sagittal T2WI MR in young man with progressive peripheral numbness, early fatigue, & areflexia shows enlargement & subtle hyperintensity of multiple cervical nerve roots ➡. Note the relatively normal size of the T1 nerve root ➡. Patient also had lumbar abnormalities. *(Right)* Axial T2WI FS MR in the same patient shows enlargement & subtle hyperintensity of exiting ➡ & exited ➡ nerve roots in cervical spine. Electromyography showed demyelination.

Hereditary Motor-Sensory Neuropathy

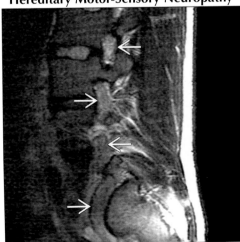

Hereditary Motor-Sensory Neuropathy

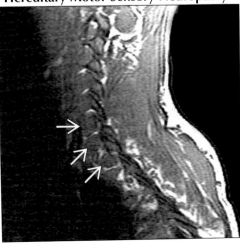

(Left) Sagittal T2WI MR in the same patient demonstrates similar enlargement of slightly hyperintense lumbar nerve roots ➡, filling the neural foramina. (Courtesy L.R. Gentry, MD.) *(Right)* Sagittal T1WI MR in a patient with Charcot-Marie-Tooth demonstrates enlargement of the nerve roots emerging from the cervical foramina ➡. The nerve root enlargement is subtle as nerves are isointense to muscle, but loss of perineural fat is key to diagnosis.

VISCERAL SPACE LESION

DIFFERENTIAL DIAGNOSIS

Common
- Multinodular Goiter
- Colloid Cyst, Thyroid
- Adenoma, Thyroid
- Diverticulum, Esophago-Pharyngeal (Zenker)
- Differentiated Carcinoma, Thyroid
- Differentiated Thyroid Carcinoma, Nodal
- Non-Hodgkin Lymphoma, Thyroid
- Non-Hodgkin Lymphoma, Lymph Nodes

Less Common
- Thyroglossal Duct Cyst
- Anaplastic Carcinoma, Thyroid
- Medullary Carcinoma, Thyroid
- Esophageal Carcinoma, Cervical
- Adenoma, Parathyroid, Visceral Space
- Parathyroid Cyst, Visceral Space
- Thyroiditis, Chronic Lymphocytic (Hashimoto)
- Thymic Remnant, Adult

Rare but Important
- 4th Branchial Anomaly
- Adenoma, Parathyroid, Ectopic
- Paraganglioma, Thyroid

ESSENTIAL INFORMATION

Key Differential Diagnosis Issues
- Visceral space (VS) is defined by middle layer of deep cervical fascia
  - Cylindrical in contour; in anterior midline of infrahyoid neck
- Key contents
  - Thyroid gland, 4 parathyroid glands, cervical trachea, & esophagus
  - Level VI lymph nodal group
- Lesions typically present as masses
- Malignant processes may present with recurrent laryngeal nerve paralysis

Helpful Clues for Common Diagnoses
- **Multinodular Goiter**
  - Key facts: Common visceral space mass
  - Imaging: Heterogeneous, multilobulated thyroid enlargement; 90% calcifications
- **Colloid Cyst, Thyroid**
  - Key facts: Palpable mass or incidental imaging finding
  - Imaging: Cystic well-circumscribed mass
    - Variable CT density & MR intensity

- **Adenoma, Thyroid**
  - Key facts: Benign, often incidental imaging finding
  - Imaging: Circumscribed; usually < 4 cm
    - Heterogeneous enhancement if it's degenerated adenoma
- **Diverticulum, Esophago-Pharyngeal (Zenker)**
  - Key facts: Esophageal pouch forming through Killian dehiscence at C5-6
  - Imaging: Heterogeneous mass posterior, ± left of esophagus
    - Often see fluid-fluid level
- **Differentiated Carcinoma, Thyroid**
  - Key facts: 90% of thyroid malignancies
    - Presents as mass or nodal disease
    - Any neck nodal level, especially level IV
  - Imaging: Well-defined, ill-defined, or invasive thyroid mass ± calcifications
- **Differentiated Thyroid Carcinoma, Nodal**
  - Key facts: Though level VI is frequent site, thyroid tumor may spread to any nodal level including retropharyngeal
  - Imaging: Typically heterogeneous nodes
    - May be solid, cystic, calcified, and variable density/intensity
- **Non-Hodgkin Lymphoma, Thyroid**
  - Key facts: Primary to thyroid gland
    - Presents as rapidly growing mass
  - Imaging: Large homogeneous mass; more compression than invasion
- **Non-Hodgkin Lymphoma, Lymph Nodes**
  - Key facts: When in level VI, often also in mediastinum
  - Imaging: Multiple nodes; may be large without necrosis

Helpful Clues for Less Common Diagnoses
- **Thyroglossal Duct Cyst**
  - Key facts: 25% infrahyoid, usually paramedian
  - Imaging: Cystic mass ± septations; embedded in strap muscles abutting thyroid cartilage
    - Calcification suggests rare carcinoma
- **Anaplastic Carcinoma, Thyroid**
  - Key facts: Undifferentiated carcinoma; rapidly growing, aggressive mass
    - Tends to be more necrotic and frankly invasive than thyroid NHL
  - Imaging: Heterogeneous necrotic thyroid mass invading adjacent structures

1

VISCERAL SPACE LESION

- **Medullary Carcinoma, Thyroid**
  - Key facts: Thyroid neuroendocrine tumor
    - Arises in calcitonin-producing parafollicular C-cells
  - CT: Low-density mass ± fine calcifications
- **Esophageal Carcinoma, Cervical**
  - Key facts: Most often SCCa
  - Imaging: Ill-defined circumferential esophageal thickening
    - When large and infiltrative can be difficult to distinguish from anaplastic thyroid carcinoma
    - Look for cervical and supraclavicular lymph nodes
- **Adenoma, Parathyroid, Visceral Space**
  - Key facts: Presents with hypercalcemia; 20% ectopic especially inferior pair
  - Imaging: Ultrasound & nuclear medicine used more than CT/MR
    - CT: Intense contrast enhancement on early arterial phase imaging
- **Parathyroid Cyst, Visceral Space**
  - Key facts: More common in women; most are nonfunctioning
    - Functioning more common in men; present with hyperparathyroidism
  - Imaging: Cystic lower neck mass; often on left; typically arises from inferior glands
- **Thyroiditis, Chronic Lymphocytic (Hashimoto)**
  - Key facts: Autoimmune disease in which T cells attack thyroid
    - Marked female preponderance

- Imaging: CT shows diffusely enlarged hypodense gland
    - No adenopathy present
- **Thymic Remnant, Adult**
  - Key facts: Residual thymic tissue in lower neck in adult
    - In children, incomplete thymus descent may result in neck mass
  - Imaging: Soft tissue mass(es) in cervicothoracic junction
    - CT density slightly less than muscle

Helpful Clues for Rare Diagnoses
- **4th Branchial Anomaly**
  - Key facts: Different presentations possible
    - Cystic left neck mass, fistula to skin, or recurrent suppurative left thyroiditis
  - Imaging: CT best 1st line for imaging evaluation
    - If suspected, look for connection to pyriform sinus
    - CT with oral barium may reveal pyriform sinus fistula
- **Adenoma, Parathyroid, Ectopic**
  - Key facts: Ectopic location seen in 20%
    - Rare site is intrathyroidal location
  - CT: Arterial phase enhancement with peripheral washout
- **Paraganglioma, Thyroid**
  - Key facts: Rare intrathyroidal location
  - Imaging: Homogeneously enhancing hypervascular masses
    - Look for enlarged feeding arteries

Multinodular Goiter

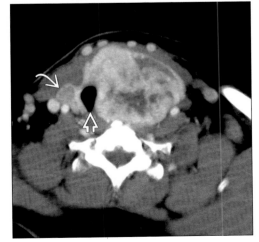

Axial CECT through lower neck reveals asymmetrically enlarged heterogeneous thyroid with markedly enlarged left lobe and smaller but abnormal right ➡ lobe. Trachea is narrowed ➡ and displaced to the right.

Multinodular Goiter

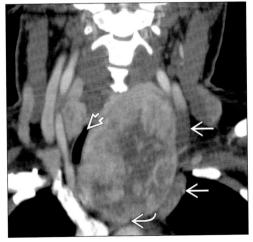

Coronal CECT in the same patient shows inferior extent of heterogeneous enlarged left lobe ➡ and mass effect on trachea ➡. The left lobe distorts the jugular vein ➡, delaying contrast drainage.

1

VISCERAL SPACE LESION

(Left) Axial CECT through lower neck shows a well-defined round cyst ➡ in the right neck, displacing and distorting the larynx. The cyst is heterogeneous with higher density in dependent portion ➡, suggesting recent hemorrhage. *(Right)* Axial T1WI MR demonstrates a large well-defined left neck mass with intrinsic hyperintensity. The presence of thyroid tissue around the periphery ➡ confirms its origin. Aspiration confirmed colloid cyst.

Colloid Cyst, Thyroid

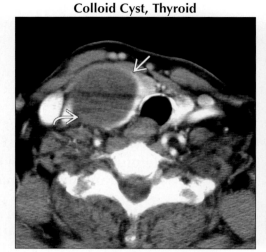

Colloid Cyst, Thyroid

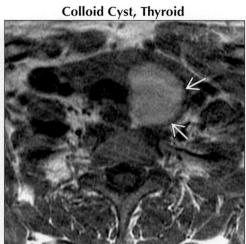

(Left) Axial T1WI MR demonstrates a well-circumscribed nodule replacing much of the right thyroid gland, which is seen along the periphery ➡ of the adenoma. The mass is hypointense with focal areas of T1 hyperintensity ➡, which may be calcification or hemorrhage. *(Right)* Axial CECT at the level of normal right thyroid ➡ gland shows replacement of left lobe by heterogeneous well-defined mass ➡. At resection, lesion was found to be degenerated follicular adenoma.

Adenoma, Thyroid

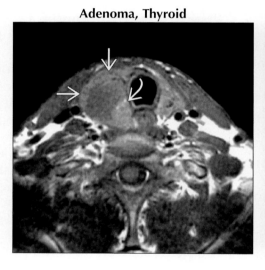

Adenoma, Thyroid

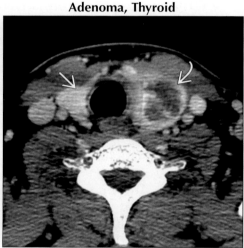

(Left) Axial CECT shows an oval-shaped structure with an air-fluid level ➡ in the midline of the lower neck immediately posterior to the hypopharynx ➡ and anterior to the vertebral body. *(Right)* Axial T2WI MR reveals a large mass anterior to the 1st thoracic vertebra and containing an air-fluid level ➡. The Zenker diverticulum compresses and displaces the esophagus anteriorly ➡.

Diverticulum, Esophago-Pharyngeal (Zenker)

Diverticulum, Esophago-Pharyngeal (Zenker)

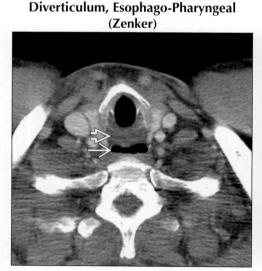

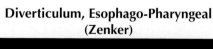

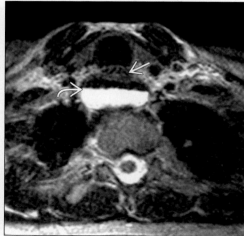

VISCERAL SPACE LESION

Differentiated Carcinoma, Thyroid

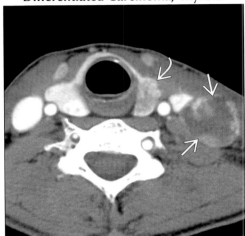

Differentiated Thyroid Carcinoma, Nodal

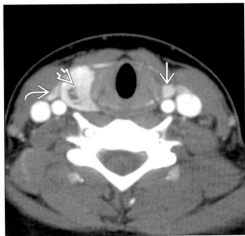

(Left) Axial CECT through the lower neck reveals the heterogeneous appearance of the left thyroid lobe with diffuse low density, suggestive of infiltrating primary tumor ➡. Note the large ipsilateral mostly cystic nodal metastasis ➡. *(Right)* Axial CECT in an 18 year old woman shows a round enhancing node in left neck ➡ with much smaller and less suspicious right neck node ➡. The subtle focal heterogeneous density in right thyroid lobe ➡ is a primary tumor.

Non-Hodgkin Lymphoma, Thyroid

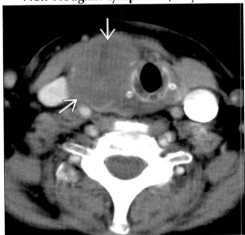

Non-Hodgkin Lymphoma, Thyroid

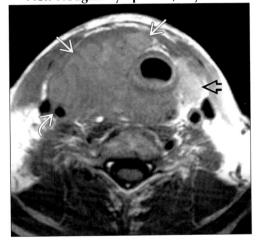

(Left) Axial CECT demonstrates a large circumscribed but hypodense solid right thyroid mass ➡ without necrosis, calcification, or invasion of surrounding structures. *(Right)* Axial T1WI MR reveals a homogeneous solid mass infiltrating the right thyroid lobe ➡. Although circumscribed, the mass infiltrates between the displaced carotid artery and the IJV ➡. The normal bright intensity of the left thyroid is preserved ➡.

Non-Hodgkin Lymphoma, Lymph Nodes

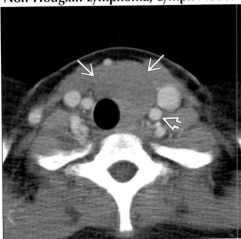

Thyroglossal Duct Cyst

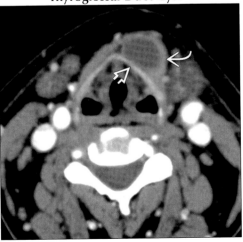

(Left) Axial CECT through the lower neck shows a homogeneous soft tissue mass ➡ abutting the left side of the trachea and displacing the common carotid artery ➡ and jugular vein laterally. *(Right)* Axial CECT shows a well-defined nonenhancing cystic mass immediately lateral to the thyroid cartilage ➡ and deep to the left strap muscles ➡. No soft tissue nodularity or calcifications are evident in this cyst.

VISCERAL SPACE LESION

(Left) Axial CECT in a patient with a rapidly growing mass ➡ reveals a heterogeneous, partially necrotic mass arising from the right thyroid, invading the trachea ➡, and extending into the anterior soft tissues. (Right) Axial CECT through the lower neck reveals a heterogeneously enhancing mass enlarging and distorting the left thyroid lobe ➡. Posteriorly, the mass extends medially, displacing the esophagus ➡ to the right.

Anaplastic Carcinoma, Thyroid

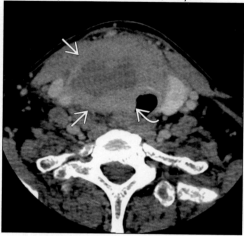

Medullary Carcinoma, Thyroid

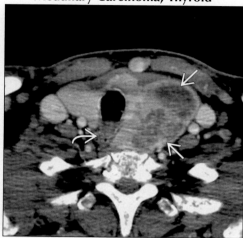

(Left) Axial CECT reveals a solid mass ➡ in the visceral space posterior to the trachea, distorting and displacing the esophageal lumen to the left ➡. The mass extends into lumen and has an indistinct margin with right thyroid lobe. (Right) Axial CECT through the lower neck shows a bulky heterogeneous midline mass ➡ spreading bilaterally through soft tissues of neck, invading the thyroid & right carotid sheath ➡. The tumor also invades the posterior trachea ➡.

Esophageal Carcinoma, Cervical

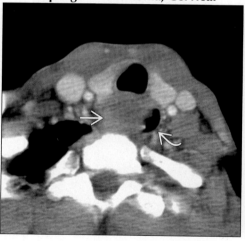

Esophageal Carcinoma, Cervical

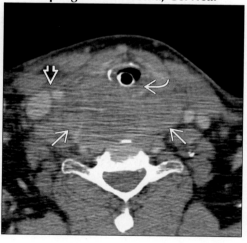

(Left) Axial CECT demonstrates a heterogeneously enhancing well-circumscribed nodule ➡ immediately posterior and medial to the left thyroid lobe but clearly distinct from it. Adenoma is hypodense relative to thyroid tissue. (Right) Axial CECT reveals a well-defined cystic lesion ➡ in the lower right neck immediately posterior to and abutting the right internal carotid artery ➡. This parathyroid cyst has a single septation through the center.

Adenoma, Parathyroid, Visceral Space

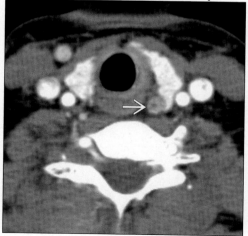

Parathyroid Cyst, Visceral Space

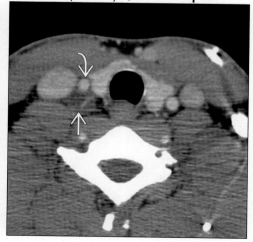

VISCERAL SPACE LESION

Thyroiditis, Chronic Lymphocytic (Hashimoto)

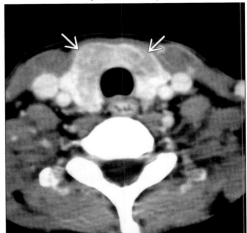

Thymic Remnant, Adult

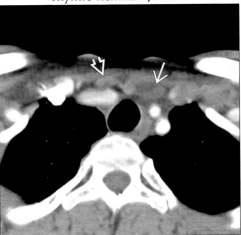

(Left) Axial CECT reveals a diffusely enlarged nodular heterogeneous thyroid gland ➡. The gland is predominantly low in density; there is no evidence of neck adenopathy. *(Right)* Axial CECT shows a well-circumscribed lesion in the left inferior visceral space ➡. A much smaller right-sided lesion is also seen ➡. Both lesions are slightly less dense than muscle on CECT and were shown to be thymic remnants.

4th Branchial Anomaly

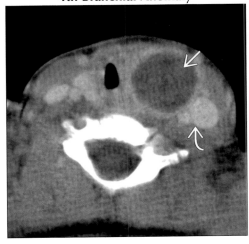

4th Branchial Anomaly

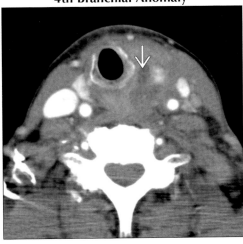

(Left) Axial CECT in a young child shows a well-defined, low-attenuation, nonenhancing left neck mass in the left thyroid lobe ➡, displacing carotid space vessels laterally ➡. *(Right)* Axial CECT in a young adult demonstrates suppurative thyroiditis with left neck inflammation and fluid collection ➡. Left thyroiditis should raise concern for underlying 4th branchial anomaly.

Adenoma, Parathyroid, Ectopic

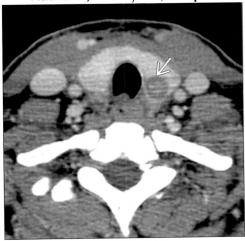

Paraganglioma, Thyroid

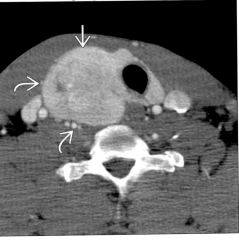

(Left) Axial CECT 3rd pass shows an unusual target-like appearance of the left thyroid nodule ➡. In this phase of enhancement, there is peripheral washout with some residual central enhancement. *(Right)* Axial CECT shows marked enlargement of the right thyroid lobe ➡, which appears well defined but heterogeneously enhancing. Note the enlarged vessels at the periphery of the lesion ➡, indicating that this is a hypervascular mass.

CERVICAL TRACHEAL LESION

DIFFERENTIAL DIAGNOSIS

Common
- Multinodular Goiter
- Differentiated Thyroid Carcinoma, Nodal
- Subglottic-Tracheal Stenosis, Iatrogenic
- Subglottic-Tracheal Stenosis, Congenital

Less Common
- Anaplastic Carcinoma, Thyroid
- Esophageal Carcinoma, Cervical
- Non-Hodgkin Lymphoma, Thyroid
- Amyloidosis
- Wegener Granulomatosis
- Relapsing Polychondritis
- Subglottic-Tracheal Stenosis, Idiopathic

Rare but Important
- Tracheopathia Osteochondroplastica
- SCCa, Trachea
- Adenoid Cystic Carcinoma, Trachea
- Benign Fibrous Histiocytoma
- Mucopolysaccharidoses
- Sarcoidosis, Trachea
- Respiratory Papillomatosis

ESSENTIAL INFORMATION

Key Differential Diagnosis Issues
- Cervical portion of trachea measured from subglottis to manubrium
  - Total trachea length = 11 cm
  - Cervical trachea ≤ 6 cm
  - Normal caliber 2-2.5 cm transverse, 1.5-2 cm anteroposterior; M > F
- Narrowing of tracheal lumen uncommon
- Best imaged using CT ± dynamic expiration

Helpful Clues for Common Diagnoses
- **Multinodular Goiter**
  - Key facts
    - Diffusely enlarged thyroid compresses external trachea
  - Imaging
    - Heterogeneous enlarged thyroid ± calcifications and hemorrhage
    - Low cervical tracheal stenosis from extrinsic compression
- **Differentiated Thyroid Carcinoma, Nodal**
  - Key facts
    - Extrinsic compression by level VI nodes
  - Imaging

- Heterogeneous adenopathy ± calcification
- **Subglottic-Tracheal Stenosis, Iatrogenic**
  - Key facts
    - Airway injury following tracheostomy or prolonged intubation
    - Scarring from pressure injury
  - Imaging
    - Soft tissue thickening with tracheal deformity and stenosis
- **Subglottic-Tracheal Stenosis, Congenital**
  - Key facts
    - Tracheomalacia: Congenital cartilage deficiency resulting in weak tracheal wall
  - Imaging
    - Collapse of lumen during forced expiration
    - Collapse typically > 50%

Helpful Clues for Less Common Diagnoses
- **Anaplastic Carcinoma, Thyroid**
  - Key facts
    - Aggressive primary thyroid tumor
  - Imaging
    - Heterogeneous, often necrotic mass
    - Invasion of trachea & other structures
- **Esophageal Carcinoma, Cervical**
  - Key facts: Usually SCCa
    - Associated with tobacco & alcohol abuse
  - Imaging
    - Concentric or eccentric esophageal thickening
    - Invades posterior trachea
- **Non-Hodgkin Lymphoma, Thyroid**
  - Key facts: B-cell primary lymphoma
    - Rapidly enlarging neck mass
  - Imaging
    - Tumors reasonably homogeneous without necrosis or calcifications
    - Tracheal invasion possible
- **Amyloidosis**
  - Key facts
    - Diffuse or multifocal submucosal infiltrates or large submucosal mass
  - Imaging
    - Luminal narrowing with focal or diffuse thickening of wall ± calcification
- **Wegener Granulomatosis**
  - Key facts: Late manifestation of Wegener
    - Vasculitis with granulomatous inflammation
  - Imaging

- Abnormal tissue within tracheal rings
- **Relapsing Polychondritis**
  - Key facts: Cartilage inflammation + fibrosis
  - Imaging
    - Tracheal thickening and calcification
    - Tracheal collapse with dynamic CT
- **Subglottic-Tracheal Stenosis, Idiopathic**
  - Key facts: Nonspecific inflammatory tissue
  - Imaging
    - Focal or diffuse thickening or mass

Helpful Clues for Rare Diagnoses
- **Tracheopathia Osteochondroplastica**
  - Key facts: Idiopathic progressive disorder
    - Submucosal osteocartilaginous calcified nodules; larynx to main bronchi
  - Imaging
    - Tracheal nodularity ± calcification
    - Posterior membrane spared
- **SCCa, Trachea**
  - Key facts: Most common primary tracheal cancer
    - Aggressive; often presents late
  - Imaging
    - Focal or circumferential invasive mass
- **Adenoid Cystic Carcinoma, Trachea**
  - Key facts: 2nd most common primary tracheal cancer
  - Imaging
    - Homogeneous soft tissue mass
- **Benign Fibrous Histiocytoma**
  - Key facts: Pediatric tumor
    - Benign, recurrent spindle cell tumor
  - Imaging

- Lobulated endoluminal mass
- **Mucopolysaccharidoses**
  - Key facts: Mucopolysaccharide deposits
  - Imaging
    - Tracheal luminal narrowing by soft tissue
- **Sarcoidosis, Trachea**
  - Key facts: ≈ 3% of sarcoidosis patients
    - Submucosal granulomatous lesions
  - Imaging
    - Thickening of tracheal wall
- **Respiratory Papillomatosis**
  - Key facts: Clinical diagnosis
    - HPV-induced laryngeal & tracheal warts
  - Imaging: Usually not obtained

Alternative Differential Approaches
- Also classified by etiology
  - Congenital: Tracheomalacia, hypoplasia
  - Acquired iatrogenic disease
    - Post-tracheostomy scarring
    - Less often trauma or radiation
  - Intrinsic tracheal inflammatory disease
    - Amyloid, Wegener, sarcoid, tracheopathia osteoplastica, relapsing polychondritis, mucopolysaccharidoses
  - Benign tracheal tumors
    - Papillomatosis, fibroma
  - Malignant tracheal tumors
    - SCCa, adenoid cystic carcinoma
  - Extrinsic compression
    - Multinodular goiter, adenopathy
  - Secondary tumor invasion
    - Thyroid or esophageal malignancies

Multinodular Goiter

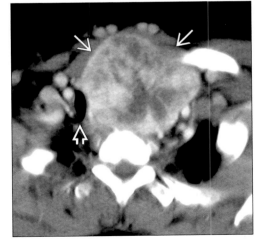

Axial CECT through lower neck reveals markedly compressed & displaced trachea ➡, shifted to the right by enlarged heterogeneous left thyroid lobe ➡. There is no irregularity of tracheal lumen to suggest invasion.

Multinodular Goiter

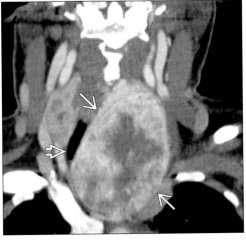

Coronal CECT in the same patient better demonstrates the extent of thyroid enlargement ➡ and cervical tracheal deviation and narrowing ➡. Thyroid goiter extends into the superior mediastinum also.

CERVICAL TRACHEAL LESION

Differentiated Thyroid Carcinoma, Nodal

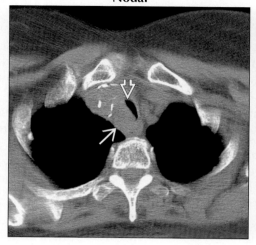

Differentiated Thyroid Carcinoma, Nodal

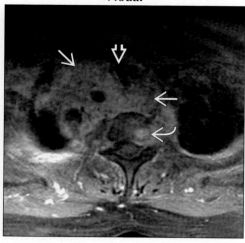

(Left) Axial NECT at level of thoracic inlet demonstrates marked narrowing of the tracheal lumen ⮆ by right paratracheal nodal mass ➡. Extensive mediastinal nodal metastases were also present in this patient with history of papillary thyroid carcinoma. *(Right)* Axial T1 C+ FS MR above sternal notch reveals a heterogeneous soft tissue mass ➡ surrounding and narrowing the trachea ⮆ and encasing the vessels. A C7 vertebral body metastasis ➡ is also evident.

Subglottic-Tracheal Stenosis, Iatrogenic

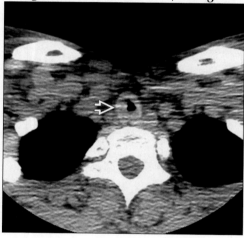

Subglottic-Tracheal Stenosis, Iatrogenic

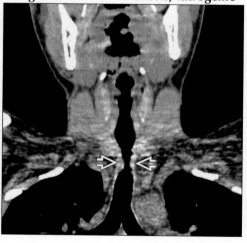

(Left) Axial NECT through the lower neck reveals circumferential irregular tracheal luminal narrowing ⮆ from soft tissue in a patient with a history of prolonged intubation. *(Right)* Coronal NECT reformat in the same patient shows focal short-segment narrowing of trachea ⮆ just above the thoracic inlet and 6 cm from the level of true cords. The outer contour of trachea is preserved with narrowing, secondary to luminal granulomatous tissue.

Subglottic-Tracheal Stenosis, Iatrogenic

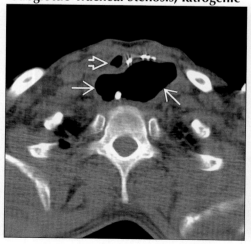

Subglottic-Tracheal Stenosis, Iatrogenic

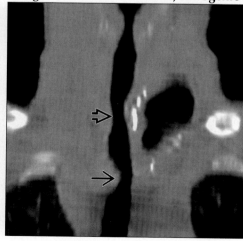

(Left) Axial NECT through the lower neck in a patient with prior esophagectomy and gastric pull-up reveals stomach ➡ in lower neck immediately posterior to narrowed trachea ⮆. Dynamic imaging revealed further collapse in expiration. *(Right)* Coronal NECT in the same patient shows stenosis to be multifocal with narrowing seen at the level of the surgical clips ⮆, approximately 4 cm below the vocal cords, and also at the cervicothoracic junction ➡.

CERVICAL TRACHEAL LESION

Subglottic-Tracheal Stenosis, Congenital

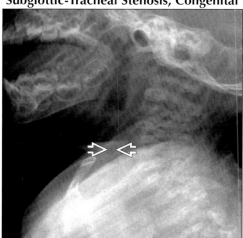

Subglottic-Tracheal Stenosis, Congenital

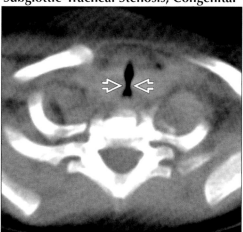

(Left) Lateral radiograph in a 9 month old with stridor reveals narrowing of the anteroposterior caliber of the cervical trachea ➡. Distal trachea has a diameter of 0.62 cm, and diameter at the narrowing is 0.37 cm. (Right) Axial NECT in the same baby reveals a markedly narrowed lower cervical trachea ➡. With dynamic imaging the contour was seen to change from 6 mm in inspiration to 1 mm in expiration. Dynamic CT findings are consistent with tracheomalacia.

Subglottic-Tracheal Stenosis, Congenital

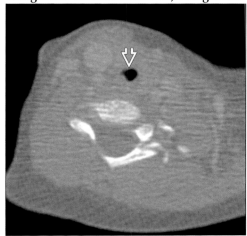

Subglottic-Tracheal Stenosis, Congenital

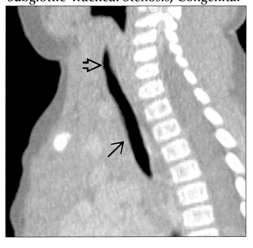

(Left) Axial NECT in an 18 month old with a history of stridor reveals diffusely small caliber trachea ➡ in the lower neck. This also involved the thoracic trachea, although normal branching was evident into the right main stem and left main stem bronchus. No luminal thickening or irregularity is evident. (Right) Sagittal NECT reformat in the same child shows the diffusely small caliber of the cervical trachea ➡ and less affected thoracic trachea ➡, without focal stenosis.

Anaplastic Carcinoma, Thyroid

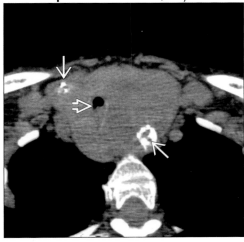

Esophageal Carcinoma, Cervical

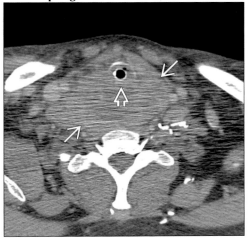

(Left) Axial NECT shows a subtly heterogeneous mass diffusely infiltrating the soft tissues of the neck and encircling, displacing, and narrowing the trachea ➡. Dense calcifications ➡ suggest carcinoma arose within a goiter. (Right) Axial CECT shows a heterogeneous mass ➡ infiltrating neck tissues and the tracheal lumen ➡ of an intubated patient. Mass is centered more midline and in posterior aspect of neck compared to primary thyroid tumors.

Non-Hodgkin Lymphoma, Thyroid

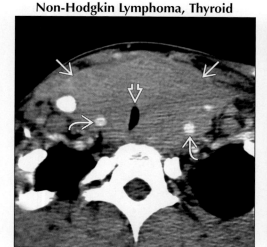

Amyloidosis

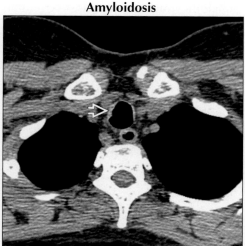

(Left) Axial CECT through cervicothoracic junction shows a large infiltrative homogeneous mass ➔ symmetrically enveloping adjacent structures. There is tracheal compression ➔, encasement, and displacement of great vessels ➔. (Right) Axial NECT reveals subtle eccentric irregularity & thickening of the right anterior tracheal wall ➔, which was also evident throughout the thoracic tracheobronchial tree. Only minimal deformity of tracheal lumen was seen.

Wegener Granulomatosis

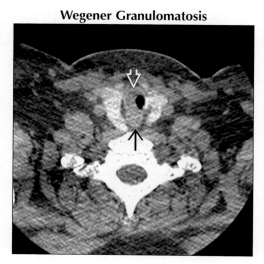

Wegener Granulomatosis

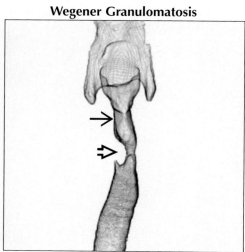

(Left) Axial NECT through the lower neck reveals an eccentric but smooth soft tissue thickening that narrows the tracheal lumen ➔. The soft tissue is slightly less dense than the adjacent esophagus ➔. (Right) 3D reconstructed image of the same study demonstrates an eccentric deformity of the proximal tracheal lumen ➔ below the glottis ➔, secondary to the granulomatous tissue of the tracheal wall.

Relapsing Polychondritis

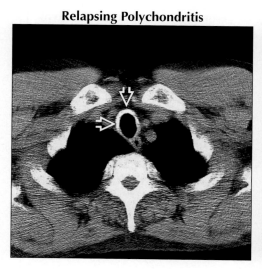

Subglottic-Tracheal Stenosis, Idiopathic

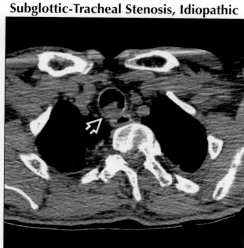

(Left) Axial NECT performed during inspiration shows thickening and smooth calcification ➔ of the tracheal wall, particularly at the right anterior and lateral aspect. The caliber of the tracheal lumen is preserved. (Right) Axial NECT shows a lesion arising from the posterior midline tracheal wall ➔, extending exophytically into the tracheal lumen. No calcifications are evident. Resection revealed florid reactive proliferative tissue that did not recur.

CERVICAL TRACHEAL LESION

Tracheopathia Osteochondroplastica

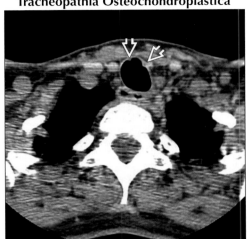

SCCa, Trachea

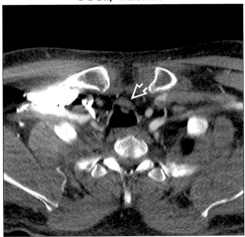

(Left) Axial CECT through the lower neck reveals subtle cervical trachea nodularity with submucosal lesions of the tracheal wall ➡. No significant narrowing of the caliber of the lumen or calcification is evident. *(Right)* Axial CECT through the lower neck in a patient with supraglottic SCCa reveals a soft tissue mass ➡ arising from the anterior and left tracheal wall and appearing to extend both into the lumen and through the contours of the wall.

Adenoid Cystic Carcinoma, Trachea

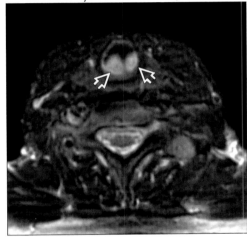

Benign Fibrous Histiocytoma

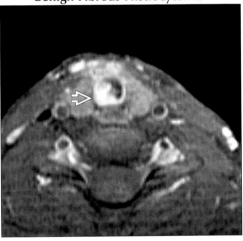

(Left) Axial T2WI FS MR through the neck reveals a bilobed well-defined hyperintense mass ➡ arising from the posterior tracheal wall at the inferior aspect of the cricoid ring. There is no evidence of extension into or through the tracheal wall. *(Right)* Axial T1 C+ FS MR in a 9 year old child reveals an endoluminal mass arising from the right posterolateral tracheal wall ➡. No evidence of invasion through the wall and no neck adenopathy was seen.

Mucopolysaccharidoses

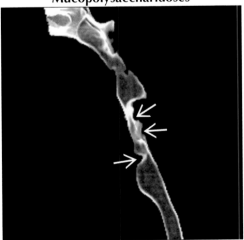

Sarcoidosis, Trachea

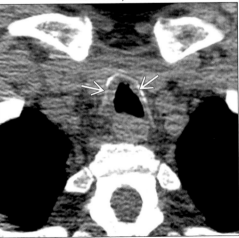

(Left) Lateral 3D reformation shows an irregular subglottis and cervical trachea from the deposition of mucopolysaccharides with multifocal stenoses ➡ in this child with mucopolysaccharidosis type 2 (Hunter syndrome). *(Right)* Axial NECT demonstrates circumferential thickening of the tracheal wall by sarcoid granulomas ➡. This process affected the entire tracheobronchial tree (not shown). (Courtesy P. Boiselle, MD.)

TRACHEOESOPHAGEAL GROOVE LESION

DIFFERENTIAL DIAGNOSIS

Common
- Differentiated Thyroid Carcinoma, Nodal
- Multinodular Goiter
- Adenoma, Thyroid
- Adenoma, Parathyroid, Visceral Space
- Non-Hodgkin Lymphoma, Lymph Nodes
- SCCa, Nodes
- Diverticulum, Esophago-Pharyngeal (Zenker)
- Differentiated Carcinoma, Thyroid

Less Common
- Anaplastic Carcinoma, Thyroid
- Non-Hodgkin Lymphoma, Thyroid
- Medullary Carcinoma, Thyroid
- Schwannoma

Rare but Important
- Esophageal Carcinoma, Cervical
- Thymic Cyst
- Parathyroid Cyst, Visceral Space
- Parathyroid Carcinoma

ESSENTIAL INFORMATION

Key Differential Diagnosis Issues
- Focal mass most often lymph node (level VI), exophytic thyroid mass, or parathyroid lesion
  - Nodes most often thyroid carcinoma
  - Nodal SCCa may be esophageal, laryngeal, or hypopharyngeal primary
  - Exophytic thyroid mass may mimic node or parathyroid adenoma
  - Multinodular goiter may extend cranially along tracheoesophageal (TE) groove
- Infiltrative mass may be neoplasm of thyroid or cervical esophagus
  - Any primary thyroid tumor may extend to TE groove
- TE groove must be carefully reviewed whenever vocal cord paralysis is present
  - Look for malignant lesion invading recurrent laryngeal nerve
  - Rarely from rapid expansion (hemorrhage) of benign lesion

Helpful Clues for Common Diagnoses
- **Differentiated Thyroid Carcinoma, Nodal**
  - Key facts
    - Most common focal mass in TE groove
    - Level IV and VI common sites
  - Imaging
    - Solid, cystic, &/or calcified; often heterogeneous nodes
    - Look for ipsilateral thyroid lesion and additional adenopathy
- **Multinodular Goiter**
  - Key facts
    - Common neck mass; patient usually euthyroid
  - Imaging
    - Heterogeneous, multilobulated gland
    - 90% have calcifications
    - As gland enlarges, often fills TE groove
    - Exophytic component may appear as separate nodule
- **Adenoma, Thyroid**
  - Key facts
    - Common, often incidental lesion
  - Imaging
    - Circumscribed mass, usually < 4 cm
    - When exophytic may mimic focal TE groove mass, such as node
- **Adenoma, Parathyroid, Visceral Space**
  - Key facts
    - Presents with hypercalcemia
    - 20% of glands ectopic
  - Imaging
    - Usually 1-3 cm when detected
    - Mimics enlarged lymph node
    - CECT: Arterial phase enhancement, then washes out
- **Non-Hodgkin Lymphoma, Lymph Nodes**
  - Key facts
    - Level VI nodes may be found as part of neck disease
  - Imaging
    - Homogeneous bulky nodes
    - Uncommonly calcified unless treated
- **SCCa, Nodes**
  - Key facts
    - May arise from primary in cervical esophagus, larynx, or hypopharynx
  - Imaging
    - Small, homogeneous, may be necrotic
- **Diverticulum, Esophago-Pharyngeal (Zenker)**
  - Key facts
    - Pouch created from herniation at Killian dehiscence C5-6 level
  - Imaging

TRACHEOESOPHAGEAL GROOVE LESION

- Heterogeneous mass, most often posterior and left of esophagus
- **Differentiated Carcinoma, Thyroid**
  - Key facts
    - 90% of thyroid malignancies
    - May present as midline mass or with nodal disease
  - Imaging
    - As invasive mass may extend directly into TE groove
    - ± Calcifications

Helpful Clues for Less Common Diagnoses
- **Anaplastic Carcinoma, Thyroid**
  - Key facts
    - Undifferentiated carcinoma; rapidly growing aggressive tumor
  - Imaging
    - Heterogeneous necrotic mass invading perithyroid tissues
- **Non-Hodgkin Lymphoma, Thyroid**
  - Key facts
    - Lymphoma arising in gland
    - Presents as rapidly growing mass
  - Imaging
    - Homogeneous mass; tends to compress rather than invade structures
- **Medullary Carcinoma, Thyroid**
  - Key facts
    - Thyroid neuroendocrine tumor
  - Imaging
    - CECT: Low density mass ± fine calcifications in primary &/or nodes
- **Schwannoma**

- Key facts
  - Painless neck mass; may be incidental
- Imaging
  - Well-defined fusiform mass
  - Larger masses often have intramural cysts

Helpful Clues for Rare Diagnoses
- **Esophageal Carcinoma, Cervical**
  - Key facts
    - Most often SCCa
  - Imaging
    - Ill-defined esophageal thickening; may be eccentric
- **Thymic Cyst**
  - Key facts
    - Embryologic remnant of thymopharyngeal duct
  - Imaging
    - Uni- or multilocular; often in left neck
    - TE groove or lateral to thyroid
- **Parathyroid Cyst, Visceral Space**
  - Key facts
    - Rare cause of hyperparathyroidism
  - Imaging
    - Homogeneous unilocular cyst
- **Parathyroid Carcinoma**
  - Key facts
    - Highly malignant tumor with poor prognosis
  - Imaging
    - Invasive tumor in TE groove
    - Invades thyroid, esophagus, trachea

Differentiated Thyroid Carcinoma, Nodal

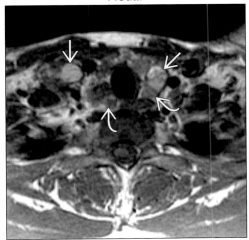

Axial T1WI MR through the lower neck reveals multiple paratracheal nodules ➡ extending into the superior mediastinum. Multiple heterogeneous neck nodes are evident with high T1 signal ➡.

Multinodular Goiter

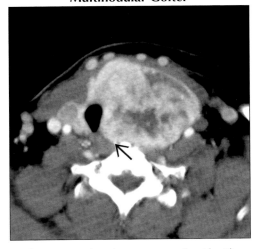

Axial CECT reveals a heterogeneous thyroid with an asymmetrically enlarged left lobe filling the fat plane of the tracheoesophageal groove ➡. The mass is well defined and distinct from the esophagus.

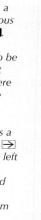

TRACHEOESOPHAGEAL GROOVE LESION

(Left) Axial CECT reveals a well-defined heterogeneous mass in the right lobe ➡. 2nd well-defined lesion posteriorly ➡ appears to be separate from thyroid. At surgery, both nodules were adenomas with the more posterior lesion being exophytic from thyroid. *(Right)* Axial CECT shows a well-circumscribed mass ➡ posterior & medial to the left thyroid lobe ➡. Enhancement has washed out of the adenoma, enhancing distinction from thyroid gland.

Adenoma, Thyroid

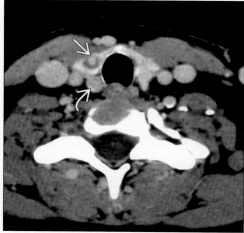

Adenoma, Parathyroid, Visceral Space

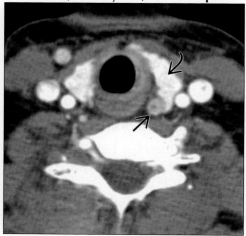

(Left) Axial T1WI MR through the lower neck shows multiple homogeneous masses ➡ bilaterally in the neck with 1 nodal mass in the right tracheoesophageal groove ➡. Nodal masses appear subtly hyperintense to muscle. *(Right)* Axial CECT demonstrates a small, subtle node in the right tracheoesophageal groove ➡, which was found after this patient with esophageal squamous cell carcinoma developed right vocal cord paralysis.

Non-Hodgkin Lymphoma, Lymph Nodes

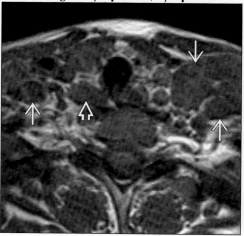

SCCa, Nodes

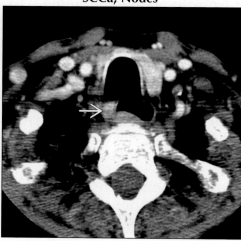

(Left) Axial NECT with oral barium reveals an air-fluid level in a large pouch ➡ situated in the lower right neck. The pouch displaces the esophagus ➡ to the left and pushes carotid sheath to the right ➡. *(Right)* Axial CECT demonstrates an enlarged heterogeneous right neck node ➡ and smaller contralateral node ➡. The right thyroid lobe is enlarged, filing in the fat plane of tracheoesophageal groove ➡. Focal thyroid carcinoma calcifications are also evident.

Diverticulum, Esophago-Pharyngeal (Zenker)

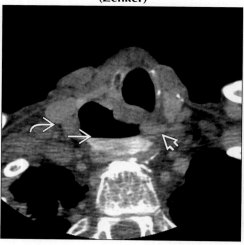

Differentiated Carcinoma, Thyroid

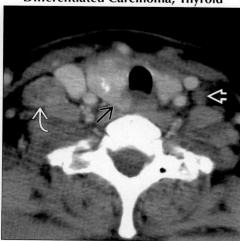

TRACHEOESOPHAGEAL GROOVE LESION

Anaplastic Carcinoma, Thyroid

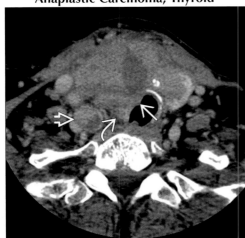

Non-Hodgkin Lymphoma, Thyroid

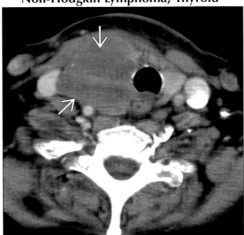

(Left) Axial CECT reveals a large heterogeneous mass replacing the thyroid, invading the trachea ➡ and fat of the tracheoesophageal groove ⮕. Note the ipsilateral level VI node also ⮞. *(Right)* Axial CECT shows a large circumscribed right thyroid mass ➡ without necrosis or calcification. The mass conforms to the tracheal contour and displaces the carotid and jugular vein without clear invasion of the surrounding structures.

Medullary Carcinoma, Thyroid

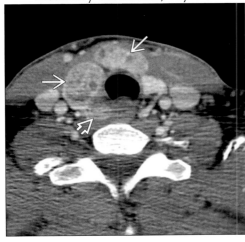

Schwannoma

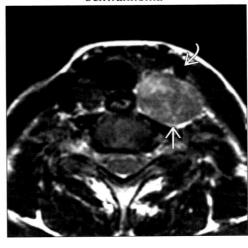

(Left) Axial CECT shows a lobulated and heterogeneous thyroid gland ➡. Additional rounded nodule in the right tracheoesophageal groove ⮕ may represent nodal metastasis or an exophytic lobulated portion of thyroid tumor. *(Right)* Axial T2WI MR demonstrates a heterogeneous mass ➡ in the left tracheoesophageal groove displacing carotid artery ➡ anteriorly. The mass is well defined and clearly separate from the esophagus and thyroid gland.

Esophageal Carcinoma, Cervical

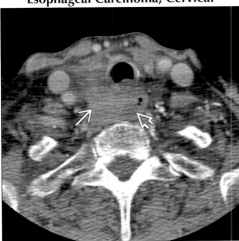

Thymic Cyst

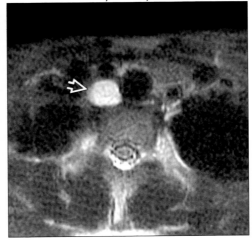

(Left) Axial CECT reveals a soft tissue mass filling the right tracheoesophageal groove ➡ in the lower neck and infiltrating adjacent fat. The mass is inseparable from the enlarged, thickened esophagus ⮕, whose eccentric lumen is a clue to the tumor's origin. *(Right)* Axial T2WI MR demonstrates a variant right-sided thymic cyst in the tracheoesophageal groove ⮕. Most thymic cysts are on the left side of the cervical neck.

POSTERIOR CERVICAL SPACE LESION

DIFFERENTIAL DIAGNOSIS

Common
- Reactive Lymph Nodes
- SCCa, Spinal Accessory Node
- NHL, Spinal Accessory Node
- Differentiated Thyroid Carcinoma, Nodal
- Suppurative Lymph Nodes
- Lymphatic Malformation

Less Common
- Neurofibromatosis Type 1
- Abscess
- Metastases, Systemic, Nodal
- Sarcoidosis, Lymph Nodes
- Tuberculosis, Lymph Nodes
- Lipoma
- Venous Malformation

Rare but Important
- Schwannoma, Posterior Cervical Space
- 3rd Branchial Cleft Cyst
- Liposarcoma
- Sinus Histiocytosis (Rosai-Dorfman)
- Giant Lymph Node Hyperplasia (Castleman)

ESSENTIAL INFORMATION

Key Differential Diagnosis Issues
- Posterior cervical space (PCS) contains fat, nodes, CN11, distal brachial plexus
  - Nodes from spinal accessory & internal jugular chains
  - Internal jugular nodes along posterior margin of internal jugular vein project posterolaterally into PCS when enlarged
- Differential diagnosis therefore includes congenital, fatty, nodal, & neural lesions

Helpful Clues for Common Diagnoses
- **Reactive Lymph Nodes**
  - Key facts: With upper respiratory tract infection
  - Imaging: Ovoid, enhancing multiple nodes
    - Inflammatory septa possible
- **SCCa, Spinal Accessory Node**
  - Key facts: Primary SCCa from nasopharynx or oropharynx
    - Caveat: If "cystic" mass found in adult, look for primary SCCa
  - Imaging: > 1.5 cm nodal masses in PCS
    - Cystic-necrotic appearance common
- **NHL, Spinal Accessory Node**
  - Key facts: Nodal systemic lymphoma
  - Imaging: Large, nonnecrotic nodes in multiple nodal chains
    - Multiple nodal chains involved including retropharyngeal, parotid, spinal accessory, & submandibular
- **Differentiated Thyroid Carcinoma, Nodal**
  - Key facts: Primary tumor may be small & difficult to see on CT or MR
  - Imaging: Nodes may display nodular enhancement or prominent cystic change
    - MR may show distinctive high T1 signal
- **Suppurative Lymph Nodes**
  - Key facts: Defined as "intranodal abscess"
    - Patient often acutely ill with pharyngitis
  - Imaging: Rim-enhancing cystic mass
    - Associated cellulitis common
- **Lymphatic Malformation**
  - Key facts: Lymphatic rest left behind during embryogenesis
    - May be found in any H&N space(s)
  - Imaging: Often trans-spatial lesion
    - Nonenhancing, fluid density (CT)/intensity (MR)

Helpful Clues for Less Common Diagnoses
- **Neurofibromatosis Type 1**
  - Key facts: Any nerve in neck can be affected
    - In PCS, distal brachial plexus root or CN11 most commonly affected
  - Imaging: Neurofibroma or plexiform neurofibroma
    - Neurofibroma: Multi-spatial round to ovoid masses; "target" sign
    - Plexiform: Trans-spatial mass mimics malignancy
- **Abscess**
  - Key facts: Sick patient with tender posterior triangle mass
  - Imaging: Suppurative nodes may precede abscess
    - Trans-spatial rim-enhancing fluid centered on PCS
    - Most commonly affected 2nd space is paraspinal aspect of perivertebral space
- **Metastases, Systemic, Nodal**
  - Key facts: Abdominal or chest malignancy
    - May travel up nodal chains from chest via lymphatic duct or hematogenous route

POSTERIOR CERVICAL SPACE LESION

- Imaging: Nodal or extranodal tumor in supraclavicular neck
  - Internal jugular, spinal accessory, or transverse cervical nodes involved
- **Sarcoidosis, Lymph Nodes**
  - Key facts: Mediastinal nodes commonly associated
    - Nodes usually < 2 cm
  - Imaging: Nonnecrotic lower neck nodes in multiple nodal chains
- **Tuberculosis, Lymph Nodes**
  - Key facts: Scrofula is old term for tuberculosis of neck nodes
  - Imaging: Enhancing necrotic nodes in multiple neck nodal chains
    - May calcify in chronic phase
- **Lipoma**
  - Key facts: Can involve any space(s) in neck
  - Imaging: Fat density/intensity is characteristic
    - If enhancing soft tissue present, consider liposarcoma
- **Venous Malformation**
  - Key facts: Can involve any neck space(s)
  - Imaging: Trans-spatial enhancing mass
    - Phleboliths are characteristic

Helpful Clues for Rare Diagnoses
- **Schwannoma, Posterior Cervical Space**
  - Key facts: CN11 and distal brachial plexus in PCS
  - Imaging: Ovoid or tubular well-circumscribed mass
    - Enhancing ± intramural cysts when large

- **3rd Branchial Cleft Cyst**
  - Key facts: Congenital cyst posterolateral to carotid space
  - Imaging: Ovoid cystic mass in PCS
- **Liposarcoma**
  - Key facts: May arise from preexisting lipoma or as initial lesion
  - Imaging: Invasive mass in PCS
    - May have fat mixed with soft tissue
    - No fatty elements may be visible
- **Sinus Histiocytosis (Rosai-Dorfman)**
  - Key facts: Idiopathic; non-Hodgkin lymphoma mimic
    - Synonym: Massive lymphadenopathy
    - Childhood predilection
  - Imaging: Moderately enhancing, large nonnecrotic nodes in multiple nodal chains in neck
- **Giant Lymph Node Hyperplasia (Castleman)**
  - Key facts: Idiopathic; non-Hodgkin lymphoma mimic
    - 3 types: Hyaline-vascular (≈ 90%), plasma cell, & multicentric type
  - Imaging: Large single or multiple conglomerate nonnecrotic nodes
    - Often avidly enhancing

SELECTED REFERENCES

1. Parker GD et al: Radiologic evaluation of the normal and diseased posterior cervical space. AJR Am J Roentgenol. 157(1):161-5, 1991

Reactive Lymph Nodes

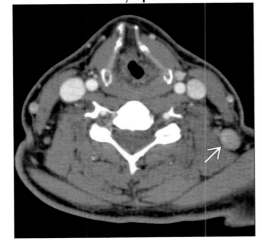

Axial CECT shows a level V spinal accessory reactive node ➜ in the posterior cervical space located just behind the posterior margin of the left sternocleidomastoid muscle.

Reactive Lymph Nodes

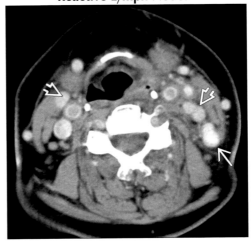

Axial CECT reveals multiple enhancing reactive nodes in the internal jugular ➜ and spinal accessory ➜ nodal chains. The nodes are of varying size and contour, some oval and some more rounded.

POSTERIOR CERVICAL SPACE LESION

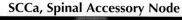

SCCa, Spinal Accessory Node   **SCCa, Spinal Accessory Node**

(Left) Axial T1 C+ FS MR reveals a left lateral nasopharyngeal recess carcinoma ➡ with an associated large retropharyngeal node ⬧.
(Right) Axial T1 C+ FS MR in the same patient shows a large malignant spinal accessory node ➡ in the left posterior cervical space from the nasopharyngeal carcinoma primary. The right neck internal jugular ⬧ and spinal accessory ➡ reactive nodes are also evident.

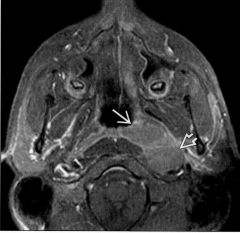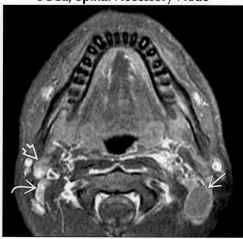

NHL, Spinal Accessory Node   **NHL, Spinal Accessory Node**

(Left) Axial CECT shows multiple spinal accessory lymph nodes ➡ combined with subcutaneous tumor deposits ⬧ in this patient with non-Hodgkin lymphoma. The increase in size and density ➡ of the parotid tail suggests bilateral parotid lymphoma as well.
(Right) Axial CECT demonstrates round nonnecrotic non-Hodgkin lymph nodes in the internal jugular ⬧, submandibular ⬧, and spinal accessory ➡ nodal chains.

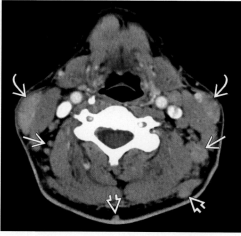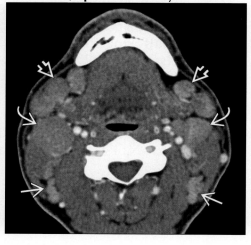

Differentiated Thyroid Carcinoma, Nodal   **Differentiated Thyroid Carcinoma, Nodal**

(Left) Axial CECT shows distinctive cystic ➡ and solid enhancing ⬧ components in this posterior internal jugular node in a patient with differentiated thyroid carcinoma. (Right) Sagittal CECT reformation in the same patient demonstrates the node with cystic ➡ and solid ⬧ components nestled in the cephalad aspect of the posterior cervical space.

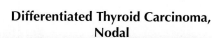

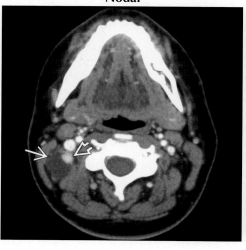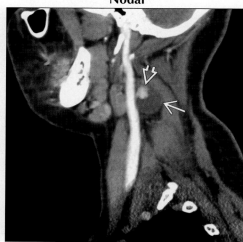

POSTERIOR CERVICAL SPACE LESION

Suppurative Lymph Nodes

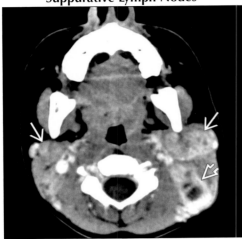

Suppurative Lymph Nodes

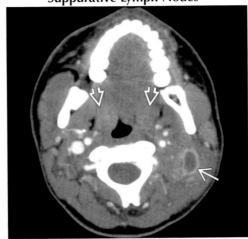

(Left) Axial NECT in a child with sepsis shows bilateral large reactive nodes ➡ accompanied by left spinal accessory suppurative adenopathy ⇨ in the posterior cervical space. *(Right)* Axial CECT in a patient with a sore throat, fever, and a tender left neck mass reveals tonsillitis ➡ with a suppurative node ➡ in the left posterior cervical space. The normal fat planes surrounding the suppurative node are obliterated secondary to associated cellulitis.

Lymphatic Malformation

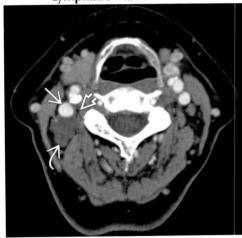

Lymphatic Malformation

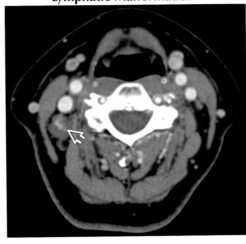

(Left) Axial CECT demonstrates a small lobulated low-attenuation nonenhancing mass in the right posterior cervical space ➡, posterior to the right jugular vein ➡, with minimal extension into the carotid space ⇨. *(Right)* Axial CECT in the same patient shows the inferior end of the lymphatic malformation with small rounded foci of contrast enhancement ⇨ that may represent a venous malformation component.

Neurofibromatosis Type 1

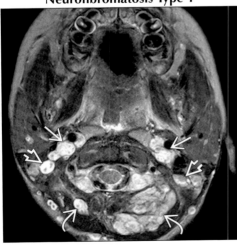

Neurofibromatosis Type 1

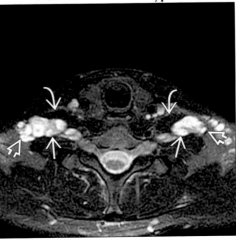

(Left) Axial T2WI MR in a patient with neurofibromatosis type 1 shows multi-spatial neurofibromas affecting the carotid ➡, posterior cervical ⇨, and perivertebral ➡ spaces. *(Right)* Axial T2WI FS MR reveals lobulated hyperintense masses involving the brachial plexus ➡ bilaterally. Note that the lesions are just posterior to the anterior scalene muscles ➡ and extend laterally from the perivertebral space into the posterior cervical space ⇨.

POSTERIOR CERVICAL SPACE LESION

(Left) Axial CECT in a patient with tuberculosis reveals spinal accessory nodes ➡ with a trans-spatial TB abscess involving the posterior cervical ⇨ and perivertebral ➡ spaces. *(Right)* Axial CECT shows a heterogeneously enhancing right inferior neck posterior cervical space systemic metastasis ➡ from lung carcinoma. Note the medially displaced carotid artery ⇨ and compressed internal jugular vein ➡.

Abscess

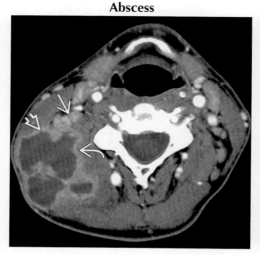

Metastases, Systemic, Nodal

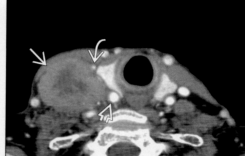

(Left) Axial CECT reveals supraclavicular sarcoidosis nodes in internal jugular ➡ and spinal accessory ➡ chains. Sarcoid nodes usually show no central cystic-necrotic change, looking much like reactive nodes when large. *(Right)* Axial CECT shows nodal ➡ and extranodal ➡ tuberculous disease affecting the posterior cervical space and sternocleidomastoid muscle ➡.

Sarcoidosis, Lymph Nodes

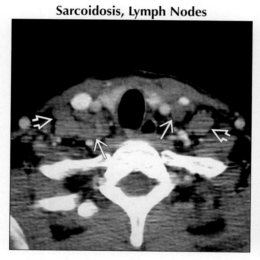

Tuberculosis, Lymph Nodes

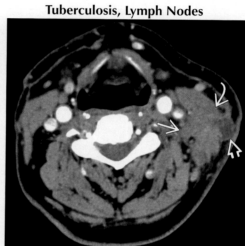

(Left) Axial CECT demonstrates a fat-density mass ➡ in the right posterior cervical space. Absence of soft tissue matrix rules out the possibility of liposarcoma. *(Right)* Axial T1 C+ FS MR depicts a trans-spatial enhancing lesion that involves the retropharyngeal ➡, carotid ➡, posterior cervical ➡, and submandibular ⇨ spaces.

Lipoma

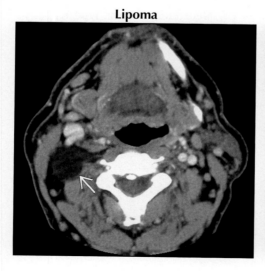

Venous Malformation

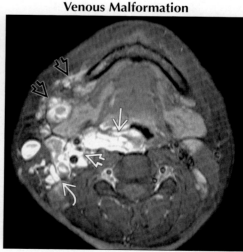

POSTERIOR CERVICAL SPACE LESION

Schwannoma, Posterior Cervical Space

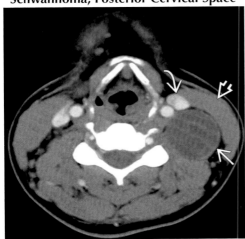

3rd Branchial Cleft Cyst

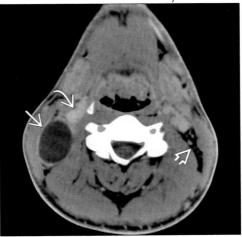

(Left) Axial CECT reveals a well-defined heterogeneous but mostly low-density mass ➡ in the posterior cervical space. The anterior margin of the mass displaces the jugular vein ➡ anteriorly and the sternocleidomastoid muscle ➡ laterally. *(Right)* Axial CECT shows a thin-walled cyst ➡ in the posterior cervical space, deep to the sternocleidomastoid muscle and posterolateral to the carotid sheath ➡. Note the normal left posterior cervical space ➡.

Liposarcoma

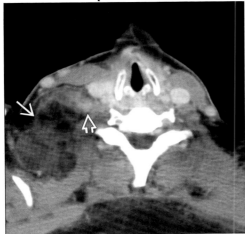

Sinus Histiocytosis (Rosai-Dorfman)

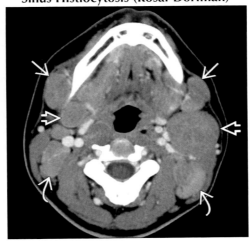

(Left) Axial CECT shows a mixed fat ➡ and enhancing soft tissue ➡ density mass within the right posterior cervical space. *(Right)* Axial CECT demonstrates very large nonnecrotic lymph nodes in the submandibular ➡, internal jugular ➡, and spinal accessory ➡ chains. The initial presumptive diagnosis was non-Hodgkin lymphoma. Tissue diagnosis of sinus histiocytosis is often mimicked by NHL.

Giant Lymph Node Hyperplasia (Castleman)

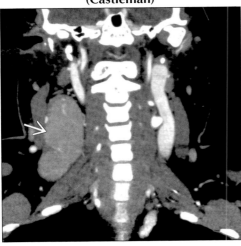

Giant Lymph Node Hyperplasia (Castleman)

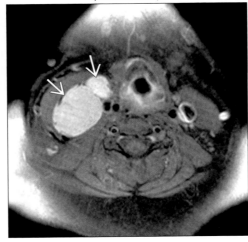

(Left) Coronal CECT shows multiple large, enhancing nonnecrotic lymph nodes ➡ in the right posterior cervical space. Initial diagnosis was non-Hodgkin lymphoma. *(Right)* Axial T1 C+ FS MR in the same patient shows 2 internal jugular chain nodes ➡ with the more lateral node filling the posterior cervical space. Avid uniform enhancement is visible and makes non-Hodgkin lymphoma less likely.

CERVICOTHORACIC JUNCTION LESION

DIFFERENTIAL DIAGNOSIS

Common
- Multinodular Goiter
- Diverticulum, Esophago-Pharyngeal (Zenker)
- SCCa, Nodes
- Differentiated Carcinoma, Thyroid
- Differentiated Thyroid Carcinoma, Nodal
- Metastases, Systemic, Nodal
- Adenoma, Thyroid
- Non-Hodgkin Lymphoma, Lymph Nodes
- Hodgkin Lymphoma, Lymph Nodes
- Pancoast Tumor

Less Common
- Esophageal Carcinoma, Cervical
- Anaplastic Carcinoma, Thyroid
- Non-Hodgkin Lymphoma, Thyroid
- Adenoma, Parathyroid, Visceral Space
- Medullary Carcinoma, Thyroid
- Colloid Cyst, Thyroid
- Thyroiditis, Chronic Lymphocytic
- Schwannoma, Brachial Plexus, PVS
- Metastasis, Vertebral Body, PVS

Rare but Important
- Aneurysm, Subclavian Artery
- Thymic Remnant, Adult
- Thymic Cyst
- Parathyroid Cyst, Visceral Space
- Diverticulum, Lateral Cervical Esophageal
- Diverticulum, Trachea

ESSENTIAL INFORMATION

Helpful Clues for Common Diagnoses
- **Multinodular Goiter**
  - Key facts: Common neck mass
  - Imaging: Heterogeneous, multilobulated, 90% calcifications
    - Must image inferior extent
- **Diverticulum, Esophago-Pharyngeal (Zenker)**
  - Key facts: Zenker diverticulum
    - Herniation between fibers of inferior constrictor muscle at C5-C6
  - Imaging: Heterogeneous mass posterior to and left of esophagus
- **SCCa, Nodes**
  - Key facts: Supraclavicular nodes drain from upper neck nodes
    - If only nodes, think primary lung SCCa
  - Imaging: Rounded supraclavicular mass

- May be necrotic
- **Differentiated Carcinoma, Thyroid**
  - Key facts: 90% of thyroid malignancies
    - Presents as mass or nodal disease
  - Imaging: Well-defined, ill-defined, or invasive mass ± calcifications
- **Differentiated Thyroid Carcinoma, Nodal**
  - Key facts: Level IV & VI common sites for thyroid metastases
  - Imaging: Solid, cystic, ± calcified
    - Ca++ neck node, consider thyroid 1st
    - MR signal variable, including bright T1
- **Metastases, Systemic, Nodal**
  - Key facts: Supraclavicular = Virchow node
    - Melanoma, esophagus, breast, lung, abdominal primaries
  - Imaging: Frequently large when present
- **Adenoma, Thyroid**
  - Key facts: Common, often incidental
  - Imaging: Circumscribed, usually < 4 cm
    - Heterogeneous C+ if degenerated
- **Non-Hodgkin Lymphoma, Lymph Nodes**
  - Key facts: Supraclavicular nodes & levels IV, VB common sites
  - Imaging: Multiple nodes, may be large without necrosis
- **Hodgkin Lymphoma, Lymph Nodes**
  - Key facts: Unilateral supraclavicular & level IV common
  - Imaging: Homogeneous bulky nodes
- **Pancoast Tumor**
  - Key facts: Lung SCCa or adenocarcinoma
    - Frequently present with lower trunk (C8, T1) brachial plexopathy
  - Imaging: Soft tissue mass invading lower neck from lung apex

Helpful Clues for Less Common Diagnoses
- **Esophageal Carcinoma, Cervical**
  - Key facts: Most often SCCa
  - Imaging: Ill-defined circumferential esophageal thickening
- **Anaplastic Carcinoma, Thyroid**
  - Key facts: Undifferentiated carcinoma = rapidly growing, aggressive mass
  - Imaging: Heterogeneous, necrotic thyroid mass invading adjacent structures
- **Non-Hodgkin Lymphoma, Thyroid**
  - Key facts: Primary to thyroid gland
    - Presents as rapidly growing mass
  - Imaging: Large homogeneous thyroid mass, more compression than invasion

CERVICOTHORACIC JUNCTION LESION

- **Adenoma, Parathyroid, Visceral Space**
  - Key facts: Presents with hypercalcemia; 20% ectopic glands, especially inferior pair
  - Imaging: Ultrasound and nuclear medicine used more than CT or MR
- **Medullary Carcinoma, Thyroid**
  - Key facts: Thyroid neuroendocrine tumor
  - Imaging: CT low density mass ± fine Ca++
- **Colloid Cyst, Thyroid**
  - Key facts: Palpable mass or incidental imaging finding
  - Imaging: Cystic well-circumscribed mass
    - Variable CT density & MR intensity
- **Thyroiditis, Chronic Lymphocytic**
  - Key facts: a.k.a., Hashimoto thyroiditis
  - Imaging: Diffusely enlarged low density gland (CT)
- **Schwannoma, Brachial Plexus, PVS**
  - Key facts: Painless lateral neck mass
  - Imaging: Well-circumscribed fusiform mass between anterior & middle scalene muscles
- **Metastasis, Vertebral Body, PVS**
  - Key facts: May present with pain, cord compression
  - Imaging: Destructive solid mass

Helpful Clues for Rare Diagnoses

- **Aneurysm, Subclavian Artery**
  - Key facts: Pulsatile low neck mass
  - Imaging: CT arterial enhancement
    - MR complex signal from flow
- **Thymic Remnant, Adult**
  - Key facts: Residual thymic tissue
  - Imaging: Solid masses in superior mediastinum
    - CT density slightly less than muscle
- **Thymic Cyst**
  - Key facts: Congenital remnant, most commonly in LEFT neck
  - Imaging: Uni- or multilocular lateral mass
- **Parathyroid Cyst, Visceral Space**
  - Key facts: Rare cause of hyperparathyroidism
  - Imaging: Homogeneous unilocular
    - Located posterior to thyroid
- **Diverticulum, Lateral Cervical Esophageal**
  - Key facts: Less common than thoracic lesions
  - Imaging: Lateral outpouching of wall
- **Diverticulum, Trachea**
  - Key facts: Outpouching of tracheal wall
  - Imaging: Posterior & right of trachea
    - Look for tracheal communication

Alternative Differential Approaches

- Extensive DDx list for lesions at cervico-thoracic junction
- Consider lesions by anatomic sites of origin
  - Arising from lower neck: Thyroid, lymph nodes, parathyroid, esophagus, trachea, brachial plexus
  - Arising from chest: Lung apices, great vessels, thymus

Multinodular Goiter

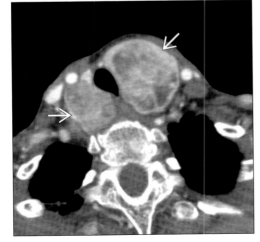

Axial CECT through the cervicothoracic junction demonstrates asymmetrically enlarged heterogeneous thyroid lobes ➡ that displace and distort the trachea as they extend into the superior mediastinum.

Multinodular Goiter

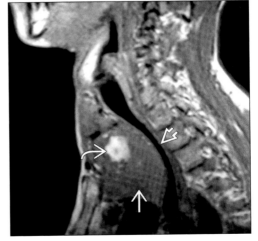

Sagittal T1WI MR shows a large lower neck mass ➡ distorting and compressing trachea ➡ and extending into the superior mediastinum. Focal T1 shortening ➡ may be calcification, hemorrhage, or colloid.

CERVICOTHORACIC JUNCTION LESION

(Left) Axial CECT through the lower neck shows midline air-fluid level ➡ immediately posterior to lowest aspect of hypopharynx ➡ and anterior to vertebral bodies. This is the cranial aspect of the diverticulum, not to be mistaken for abscess. *(Right)* Axial T1 C+ MR through lower neck in a patient with a prior left neck dissection for SCCa of unknown primary shows 2 palpable, heterogeneous recurrent SCCa nodes ➡ compressing the right jugular vein ➡.

Diverticulum, Esophago-Pharyngeal (Zenker)

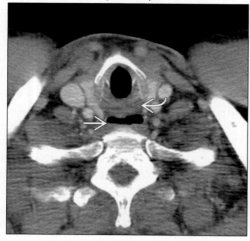

SCCa, Nodes

(Left) Axial CECT shows an enlarged heterogeneous right neck node ➡ abutting the internal jugular vein. A primary tumor was found in the right thyroid lobe ➡, which is heterogeneous and enlarged with several small ill-defined areas of calcification. *(Right)* Axial CECT reveals multiple nodes extending into the superior mediastinum, with a curvilinear rim of calcification seen in 1 ➡ and focal dense calcification in another ➡.

Differentiated Carcinoma, Thyroid

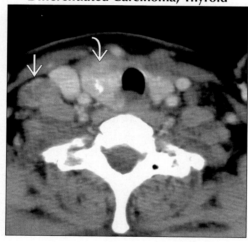

Differentiated Thyroid Carcinoma, Nodal

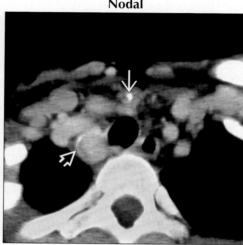

(Left) Axial CECT through the lower neck shows a large heterogeneous supraclavicular mass ➡ displacing & deforming the patent left internal jugular vein ➡. This is a metastatic malignant testicular germ cell tumor. *(Right)* Axial CECT shows a heterogeneous, centrally low-density mass ➡ arising from the left thyroid lobe & extending into the superior mediastinum. This degenerated adenoma appears "necrotic" but is well demarcated from adjacent tissues.

Metastases, Systemic, Nodal

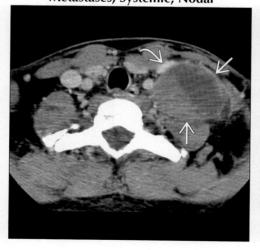

Adenoma, Thyroid

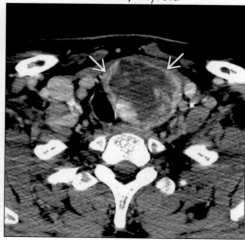

CERVICOTHORACIC JUNCTION LESION

Non-Hodgkin Lymphoma, Lymph Nodes

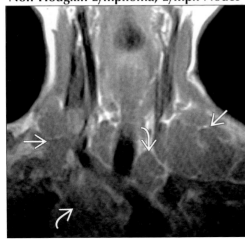

Hodgkin Lymphoma, Lymph Nodes

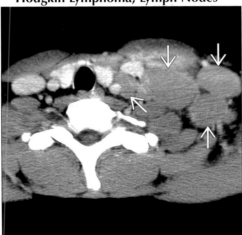

(Left) Coronal T1WI MR shows multiple masses bilaterally in the lower neck ➡ and superior mediastinum ➡ forming nodal conglomerates. The masses appear slightly hyperintense to muscle and displace vascular structures without compressing them. *(Right)* Axial CECT in a patient with Hodgkin lymphoma shows unilateral bulky homogeneous nodes ➡ in the supraclavicular fossa and lower jugular chain. There was no right-sided adenopathy.

Pancoast Tumor

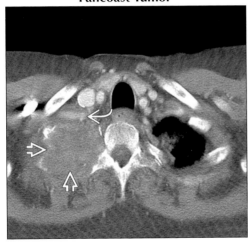

Esophageal Carcinoma, Cervical

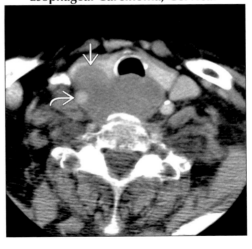

(Left) Axial CECT through the cervicothoracic junction reveals an apical lung mass ➡ destroying the 1st and 2nd ribs and infiltrating the soft tissues posterior to the right subclavian artery ➡, where the brachial plexus is located. *(Right)* Axial CECT shows a bulky homogeneous mass arising from the proximal cervical esophagus and infiltrating the right thyroid ➡. The mass surrounds the right common carotid artery ➡ and invades the trachea.

Anaplastic Carcinoma, Thyroid

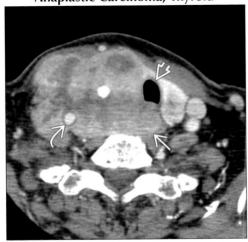

Non-Hodgkin Lymphoma, Thyroid

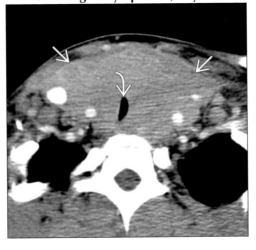

(Left) Axial CECT through the lower neck shows a heterogeneous mass arising from the right thyroid lobe, infiltrating soft tissues of the neck & encircling common carotid artery ➡. The mass cannot be separated from esophagus ➡ or trachea ➡. *(Right)* Axial CECT reveals a mass ➡ infiltrating the lower neck symmetrically and enveloping adjacent tissues. There is compression of the trachea ➡ and bilateral carotid sheath involvement with encasement and displacement of vessels.

CERVICOTHORACIC JUNCTION LESION

(Left) Axial CECT through the neck shows a well-circumscribed but irregularly contoured mass ⇗ immediately posterior to left thyroid lobe. Mass has heterogeneous enhancement and is hypodense, as compared to the thyroid tissue. (Right) Axial CECT through lower neck reveals a heterogeneous mass ⇒ arising from the left thyroid. While not clearly infiltrating the adjacent tissues, the presence of ipsilateral heterogeneous adenopathy ⇒ suggests malignancy.

Adenoma, Parathyroid, Visceral Space

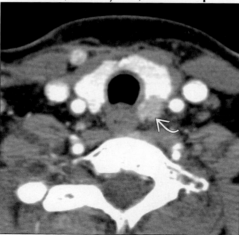

Medullary Carcinoma, Thyroid

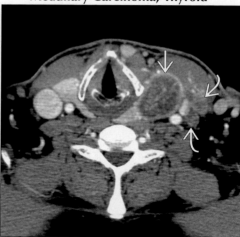

(Left) Axial CECT through the neck shows a well-defined round mass displacing & distorting the larynx. Higher density in dependent portion ⇒ suggests recent hemorrhage. No aggressive features or neck adenopathy is seen. (Right) Axial CECT shows diffuse enlargement of the left and right thyroid lobes and pyramidal lobe. The thyroid gland is diffusely decreased in density and has an almost "infiltrated" appearance. There is no neck adenopathy.

Colloid Cyst, Thyroid

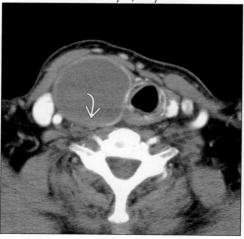

Thyroiditis, Chronic Lymphocytic

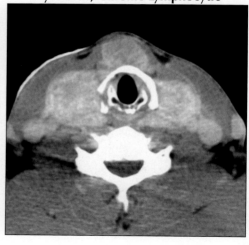

(Left) Axial T2WI MR through the lower neck demonstrates a well-defined hyperintense and heterogeneous round mass adjacent to the anterior ⇒ and middle/posterior ⇒ scalene muscles. (Right) Axial T1 C+ MR reveals a destructive mass centered on the 1st thoracic vertebral body with extensive paravertebral ⇒ & epidural ⇒ tumor and involvement of the adjacent rib ⇒. This was the 1st presentation of renal cell carcinoma.

Schwannoma, Brachial Plexus, PVS

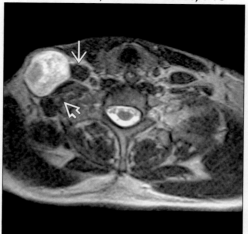

Metastasis, Vertebral Body, PVS

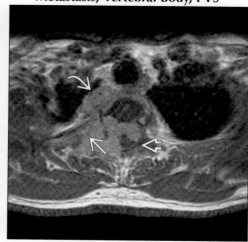

CERVICOTHORACIC JUNCTION LESION

Aneurysm, Subclavian Artery

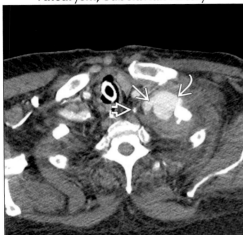

Thymic Remnant, Adult

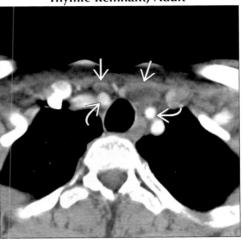

(Left) Axial CECT shows arterial enhancement of the central aspect of a left lower neck mass ➡ arising from the subclavian artery ➡, distal to origin of left vertebral artery ➡. *(Right)* Axial CECT demonstrates 2 well-circumscribed lesions in the lower neck ➡, immediately posterior to the strap muscles and anterior to the common carotid arteries ➡. Both lesions are slightly less dense than muscle. The right lesion is oval, and the left lesion conforms to adjacent tissues.

Thymic Cyst

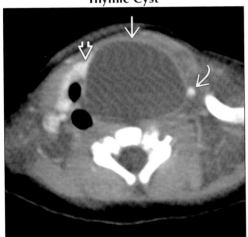

Parathyroid Cyst, Visceral Space

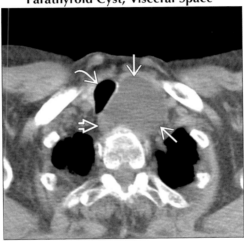

(Left) Axial CECT in a toddler shows a large, low-density, nonenhancing mass ➡ in the lower neck, displacing the left carotid artery ➡ laterally and the visceral space structures to the right of midline. Within the visceral space, the cyst is most intimately related to left thyroid lobe ➡. *(Right)* Axial CECT in an adult shows a low-density mass ➡ at the cervicothoracic junction that appears inseparable from the esophagus ➡ and trachea ➡, both of which are displaced to the right side.

Diverticulum, Lateral Cervical Esophageal

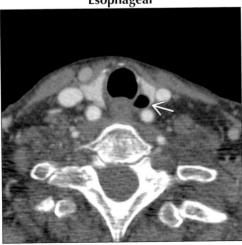

Diverticulum, Trachea

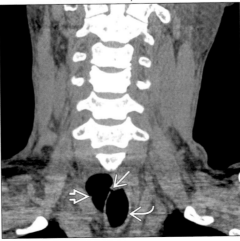

(Left) Axial CECT through the lower neck demonstrates an air-filled structure ➡ immediately lateral to the cervical esophagus in the left tracheoesophageal groove. The medial aspect of the lesion "points" toward the esophagus rather than the trachea. *(Right)* Coronal NECT through the neck was performed following trauma and revealed an incidental small air-filled lesion ➡ to the right of the cervical trachea ➡, with a small track ➡ connecting the 2 structures.

TMJ MASS LESIONS

DIFFERENTIAL DIAGNOSIS

Common
- Trauma/Dislocation, TMJ
- Simple Bone Cyst (Traumatic)
- Fibrous Dysplasia, Mandible-Maxilla
- Calcium Pyrophosphate Dihydrate Deposition Disease, TMJ
- Synovial Chondromatosis, TMJ
- Necrotizing External Otitis
- SCCa, EAC
- Pigmented Villonodular Synovitis, TMJ

Less Common
- Metastasis, Mandible-Maxilla
- Parotid Malignant Neoplasm
- Rhabdomyosarcoma
- Osteosarcoma, Mandible-Maxilla
- Giant Cell Tumor, Skull Base

Rare but Important
- Chondroblastoma, Skull Base
- Chondrosarcoma
- Venous Malformation, TMJ
- Cholesteatoma, EAC
- Interpositional Graft, TMJ
- Abscess, TMJ

ESSENTIAL INFORMATION

Key Differential Diagnosis Issues
- Temporomandibular joint (TMJ) masses can be identified by source
  - Primary joint pathology
  - Mandible or skull base bone pathology
  - Adjacent soft tissue pathology
    - Parotid, masticator space (MS), external auditory canal (EAC)
    - TMJ lesion may present as parotid mass
    - Parotid, MS, or EAC mass may present with TMJ symptoms ± destruction
- Imaging strategy
  - Either CT or MR useful to localize lesion
  - CT best demonstrates bone changes
  - MR may allow better characterization
  - MR evaluates middle cranial fossa

Helpful Clues for Common Diagnoses
- **Trauma/Dislocation, TMJ**
  - Key facts
    - May be acute or chronic presentation
  - Imaging
    - CT: Deformed displaced condyle
    - Look for other mandible fractures
- **Simple Bone Cyst (Traumatic)**
  - Key facts
    - Synonym: Traumatic bone cavity
    - Fluid-filled intraosseous pseudocyst
  - Imaging
    - CT: Thin irregular well-corticated bone
    - MR: T2 hyperintense focal lesion
- **Fibrous Dysplasia, Mandible-Maxilla**
  - Key facts
    - Developmental bone anomaly
  - Imaging
    - CT: Expansile "ground-glass" bone lesion
    - MR: Often heterogeneous, predominantly low signal
- **Calcium Pyrophosphate Dihydrate Deposition Disease, TMJ**
  - Key facts
    - Crystal-induced arthropathy
    - Acute arthropathy = pseudogout
    - TMJ CPPD: Chronic "tophaceous" form
  - Imaging
    - CT: Bone erosion, joint calcification
    - MR: "Tophaceous" deposits hypointense
- **Synovial Chondromatosis, TMJ**
  - Key facts
    - Synovial membrane proliferation and metaplasia → hyaline cartilage nodules
  - Imaging
    - Early: Wide joint space, filling defects
    - Late: Nodules calcify, MR hypointense
- **Necrotizing External Otitis**
  - Key facts
    - Synonym: Malignant otitis externa
    - *Pseudomonas* EAC infection in diabetics
  - Imaging
    - Aggressive enhancing EAC mass
- **SCCa, EAC**
  - Key facts
    - Associated with prior neck radiation
  - Imaging
    - Enhancing destructive EAC mass
    - Intraparotid and level VA nodes
- **Pigmented Villonodular Synovitis, TMJ**
  - Key facts
    - Idiopathic benign synovial proliferation
    - Characteristic hemosiderin deposition
  - Imaging
    - CT: Scalloped condyle & condylar fossa
    - MR: Cystic and solid; variable intensity
    - T2 & GRE: Peripheral low intensity rim

TMJ MASS LESIONS

Helpful Clues for Less Common Diagnoses
- **Metastasis, Mandible-Maxilla**
  - Key facts
    - Lung and breast carcinoma most often
  - Imaging
    - Enhancing destructive mass
    - More often lytic than sclerotic
- **Parotid Malignant Neoplasm**
  - Key facts
    - Wide range of histologies
  - Imaging
    - Invasive enhancing parotid mass
    - Superficial lobe > > deep lobe
- **Rhabdomyosarcoma**
  - Key facts
    - Most common pediatric sarcoma
    - Most often "embryonal" form in H&N
  - Imaging
    - Destructive enhancing masticator mass
- **Osteosarcoma, Mandible-Maxilla**
  - Key facts
    - < 10% osteosarcomas occur here
  - Imaging
    - Aggressive destructive mass
    - "Sunburst" periosteal reaction classic
- **Giant Cell Tumor, Skull Base**
  - Key facts
    - Rare locally aggressive benign tumor
  - Imaging
    - CT: Thin sclerotic cortical shell
    - MR: Low signal on T2

Helpful Clues for Rare Diagnoses
- **Chondroblastoma, Skull Base**

  - Key facts
    - Rare benign cartilage tumor
  - Imaging
    - CT: Multilobulated mixed density mass
    - MR: T2 heterogeneity ± fluid levels
- **Chondrosarcoma**
  - Key facts
    - Rare; most patients in 4th-7th decades
  - Imaging
    - CT: Calcified enhancing mass
    - MR: T2 hyperintense, enhancing mass
- **Venous Malformation, TMJ**
  - Key facts
    - Congenital low-flow malformation
  - Imaging
    - CT: Enhancing mass with phleboliths
    - MR: T2 hyperintense, enhancing mass
- **Cholesteatoma, EAC**
  - Key facts
    - Submucosal EAC mass; mimics SCCa
  - Imaging
    - EAC mass with bone erosions
- **Interpositional Graft, TMJ**
  - Key facts
    - Disc replacement after discectomy
  - Imaging
    - Fat mass within deformed joint
    - May mature into soft tissue
- **Abscess, TMJ**
  - Key facts
    - Usually infected from EAC/mastoid
  - Imaging
    - Distended TMJ, bone destruction
    - Auricular & periauricular swelling

Trauma/Dislocation, TMJ

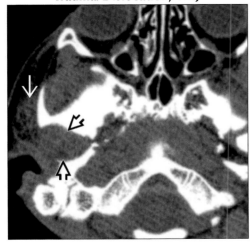

Axial NECT through skull base shows right periauricular swelling ➡ & "empty" TMJ ➡, which appears filled with soft tissue density blood. This scan was performed following a child's fall from a bicycle.

Trauma/Dislocation, TMJ

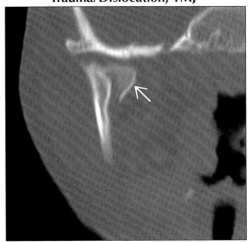

Coronal bone CT in the same child shows intraarticular fracture of right mandibular condyle with medial & anterior displacement of fragment ➡, resulting in subluxation of right temporomandibular joint.

TMJ MASS LESIONS

(Left) Axial bone CT shows mass-like appearance of the left condyle ➡, which is enlarged, deformed, and sclerotic. This is an old healed condylar fracture/subluxation with early secondary degenerative changes. (Right) Coronal CECT demonstrates a sharply defined mildly expansile lucent lesion ➡ in the right mandibular condyle & subcondylar neck. Overlying cortex is thinned but intact, & there are no abnormal matrix calcifications or extraosseous soft tissue.

Trauma/Dislocation, TMJ
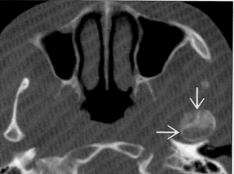

Simple Bone Cyst (Traumatic)
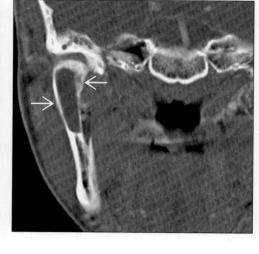

(Left) Coronal T1WI MR shows a soft tissue intensity mass of the left deep face, which appears to arise within expanded left TMJ condyle ➡. Note marked low signal intensity of bone of the expanded condylar fossa ➡ and adjacent pterygoid plates ➡. (Right) Coronal bone CT in the same patient reveals mass is hemifacial fibrous dysplasia. Condyle ➡ is heterogeneous and expanded with deformed mandibular ramus. Note the typical "ground-glass" appearance of sphenoid ➡.

Fibrous Dysplasia, Mandible-Maxilla
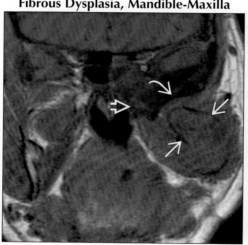

Fibrous Dysplasia, Mandible-Maxilla
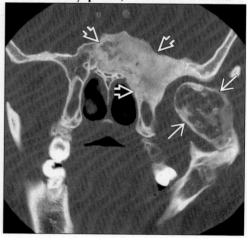

(Left) Axial bone CT through the skull base reveals an extensive mass of calcific density ➡ surrounding the condyle and neck of right hemimandible. There is also erosion of the condylar fossa, which is widening the joint space ➡. (Right) Axial T2WI FS MR shows typical features of TMJ synovial chondromatosis: Distension of the right TMJ joint with hyperintense fluid ➡, which also surrounds hypointense calcified loose bodies ➡.

Calcium Pyrophosphate Dihydrate Deposition Disease, TMJ
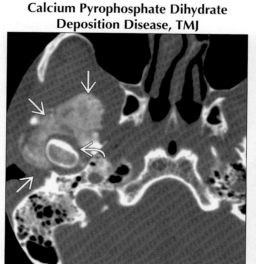

Synovial Chondromatosis, TMJ
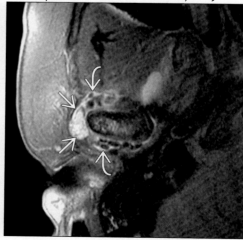

TMJ MASS LESIONS

Necrotizing External Otitis

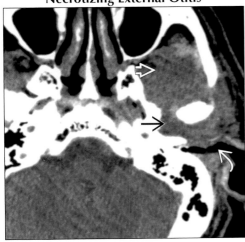

SCCa, EAC

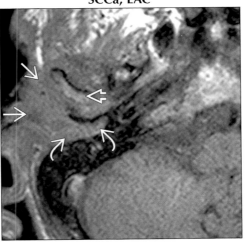

(Left) Axial NECT in a patient with diabetes reveals a markedly narrowed left EAC ➡ from swollen soft tissues. This heterogeneous tissue extends into the left TMJ ➡ and also further anteriorly, with phlegmon in the masticator space ➡. *(Right)* Axial T1WI MR reveals an infiltrating aggressive process filling the EAC ➡ and invading the right temporomandibular joint ➡ and adjacent parotid tissue. Condylar marrow signal ➡ is relatively preserved.

Pigmented Villonodular Synovitis, TMJ

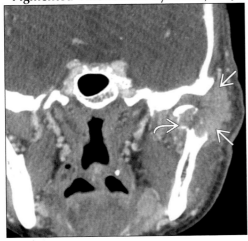

Pigmented Villonodular Synovitis, TMJ

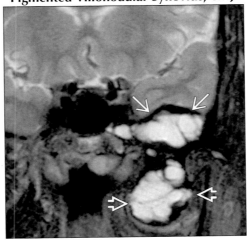

(Left) Coronal CECT demonstrates an enhancing soft tissue mass ➡ centered at left TMJ. There is marked erosion of the mandibular condyle ➡. Surprisingly, patients with PVNS often present with a "parotid mass" rather than TMJ pain. *(Right)* Coronal T2WI FS MR shows a predominantly hyperintense lobulated mass centered on the joint but with both deep face ➡ and intracranial ➡ components. The markedly low signal periphery is characteristic of these lesions.

Metastasis, Mandible-Maxilla

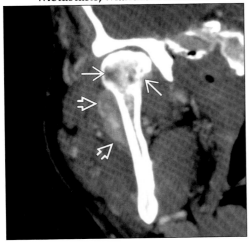

Metastasis, Mandible-Maxilla

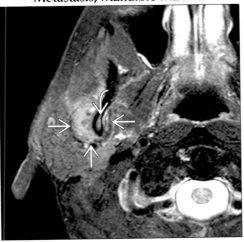

(Left) Coronal CECT demonstrates heterogeneous predominantly lytic right condyle ➡ & neck with an adjacent mass along lateral cortical surface of ramus ➡. This is clearly a mandible origin lesion, & TMJ shows only minimal degenerative changes. *(Right)* Axial T2WI FS MR reveals a heterogeneous mass ➡ surrounding right mandibular ramus & subcondylar neck with intrinsic hyperintensity within mandible ➡. This later proved to be metastatic hepatocellular carcinoma.

TMJ MASS LESIONS

(Left) Axial T1 C+ FS MR demonstrates a poorly marginated enhancing mass ➡ centered in the superficial lobe of the left parotid but infiltrating the right temporomandibular joint and abutting the condylar cortex ➡. *(Right)* Coronal T1WI MR shows a poorly defined infiltrative mass ➡ of the left parotid gland, which engulfs the left TMJ, widens the joint space ➡, & focally destroys the lateral aspect of condyle ➡. This was proven to be squamous cell carcinoma.

Parotid Malignant Neoplasm

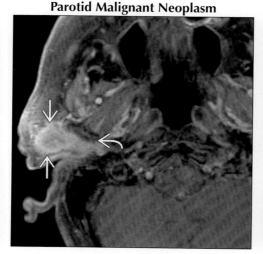

Parotid Malignant Neoplasm

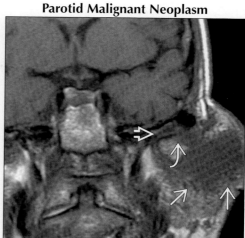

(Left) Coronal T1WI MR shows a large mass ➡ of right deep face destroying much of the right mandible. Only a small portion of condyle remains ➡, and the TMJ appears relatively preserved. The mass extends through foramen ovale ➡. *(Right)* Coronal bone CT reveals an aggressive mandibular ramus process with a soft tissue mass deforming the face ➡. Hyperdense "sunburst" periosteal reaction ➡ and formation of osteoid matrix suggest the diagnosis.

Rhabdomyosarcoma

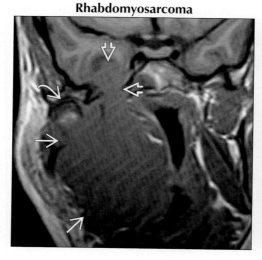

Osteosarcoma, Mandible-Maxilla

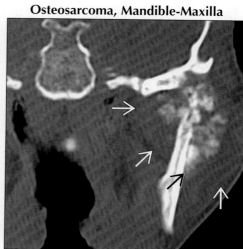

(Left) Coronal bone CT shows a lytic expansile mass ➡ arising from the temporal bone, deforming the floor & lateral wall of the left middle cranial fossa. The mass erodes through to condylar fossa ➡ of TMJ. *(Right)* Coronal bone CT demonstrates predominantly lytic, though partially calcified ➡, mass involving right condylar fossa. Condyle ➡ is intact, indicating that the mass originates from the squamous temporal bone above. *(Courtesy R. Kurokawa, MD.)*

Giant Cell Tumor, Skull Base

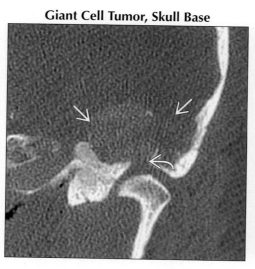

Chondroblastoma, Skull Base

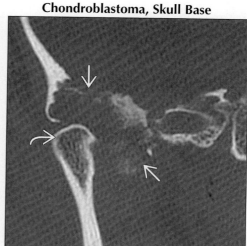

TMJ MASS LESIONS

Chondrosarcoma

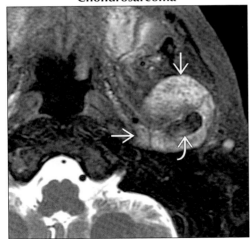

Chondrosarcoma

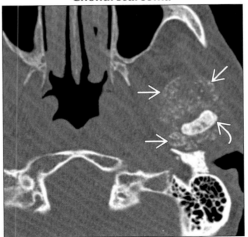

(Left) Axial T2WI FS MR reveals a large soft tissue mass ➡ surrounding the condyle of left TMJ ➡. The mass is heterogeneous but high T2 signal intensity, which is typical of chondroid tumors. The stippled low signal intensity foci are from multiple tumoral calcifications. (Right) Axial bone CT reveals multiple tumoral calcifications ➡. This is reminiscent of synovial chondromatosis, though more irregularly shaped. Note sclerotic appearance of condyle ➡.

Venous Malformation, TMJ

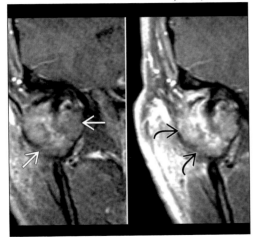

Cholesteatoma, EAC

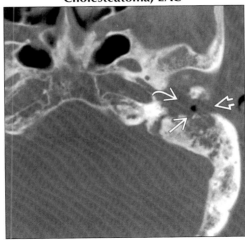

(Left) Coronal T1 C+ FS MR with early ➡ and late ➡ dynamic GD-DTPA injection shows progressive enhancement of a soft tissue mass surrounding the condyle. This is typical of venous malformations. Phleboliths, not evident in this patient, are a sensitive CT or MR finding. (Right) Axial bone CT shows a soft tissue density within the left EAC ➡. Note the osseous destructive changes of the posterior EAC wall ➡ and anterior wall ➡.

Interpositional Graft, TMJ

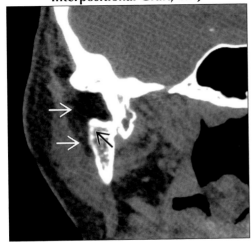

Abscess, TMJ

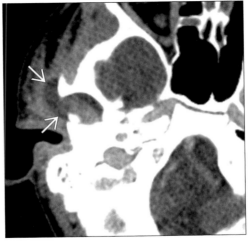

(Left) Coronal NECT shows a fat-density mass ➡ lateral to the foreshortened right mandibular neck ➡. This is autologous fat surgically grafted to reduce the risk of ankylosis at the surgical site. (Right) Axial CECT reveals an abscess ➡ within distended temporomandibular joint in a child with acute suppurative otomastoiditis. TMJ septic arthritis comes more often from adjacent sites rather than hematogenous spread of infection.

CALCIFIED TMJ LESIONS

DIFFERENTIAL DIAGNOSIS

Common
- Degenerative Disease, TMJ
- Chondromatosis, Synovial, TMJ
- Osteochondritis Dissecans, TMJ

Less Common
- Calcium Pyrophosphate Dehydrate Deposition Disease, TMJ
- Ankylosis, TMJ

Rare but Important
- Foreign Body Giant Cell Reaction (Proplast Implant)
- Chondroblastoma, TMJ
- Osteosarcoma, TMJ
- Chondrosarcoma, TMJ
- Osteochondroma, TMJ
- Synovitis, Pigmented Villonodular, TMJ
- Gout, TMJ

ESSENTIAL INFORMATION

Key Differential Diagnosis Issues
- Masses of condyle or joint with intrinsic calcifications
- Not just eroded bone fragments
- Imaging strategy
  - CT: Detects calcification, joint changes
    - Distinguishes lesion as bone or joint process
  - MR: May allow better lesion characterization

Helpful Clues for Common Diagnoses
- **Degenerative Disease, TMJ**
  - Key facts
    - Primary degenerative joint disease (DJD): Older patients
    - Secondary DJD: Younger patients with trauma or chronic bruxism
    - Cartilage fragments → loose bodies
    - Fragments may ossify; may embed in synovium
  - Imaging
    - Narrow joint, osteophytes, subchondral cysts, sclerosis
    - Flattened condyle
    - Calcifications in disc or in loose bodies
- **Chondromatosis, Synovial, TMJ**
  - Key facts
    - Synovial membrane proliferation and metaplasia → hyaline cartilage nodules
    - Nodules calcify or ossify
    - Adolescents, young adults
  - Imaging
    - Early CT: Joint widened, may erode into middle cranial fossa; noncalcified nodules
    - Early MR: Nodules T1 dark, T2 bright
    - Later CT: Irregular coarse calcifications; may appear "cloud-like," mimicking CPPD
    - Later MR: Nodules hypointense, joint enhancement, normal disc position
- **Osteochondritis Dissecans, TMJ**
  - Key facts
    - Osteochondral bone fragmentation
    - Repeated trauma or overuse
  - Imaging
    - CT: Loose fragment often conforms to condylar defect
    - MR: Better detects noncalcified fragment

Helpful Clues for Less Common Diagnoses
- **Calcium Pyrophosphate Dehydrate Deposition Disease, TMJ**
  - Key facts
    - Abbreviation: CPPD
    - Crystalline arthropathy
    - Calcium pyrophosphate dihydrate crystals
    - Acute form is pseudogout
    - Chronic tophaceous form more common in TMJ
    - Hereditary, sporadic, metabolic, & post-traumatic forms
  - Imaging
    - CT: Disc & joint space calcification("cloud-like," linear, or irregular); bone erosion common
    - MR: Enhancing soft tissue around condyle; joint effusion, periarticular edema
- **Ankylosis, TMJ**
  - Key facts
    - Follows displaced condylar fracture
    - May follow juvenile idiopathic arthritis
  - Imaging
    - Incomplete obliteration of joint space
    - Fibrous or bony bridging across joint

CALCIFIED TMJ LESIONS

Helpful Clues for Rare Diagnoses

- **Foreign Body Giant Cell Reaction (Proplast Implant)**
  - Key facts
    - Complication of Proplast implant
    - No longer used
  - Imaging
    - CT: Enhancing mass ± calcifications; marked bone erosion; implant is hyperdense "sheet" along fossa
    - MR: Implant appears hypointense
- **Chondroblastoma, TMJ**
  - Key facts
    - Older patients compared to chondroblastoma in other locations
  - Imaging
    - CT: Multilobulated expansile lesion with narrow transition zone; mixed lucency, sclerosis, & central calcification
    - MR: T2 heterogeneity ± fluid levels mimicking aneurysmal bone cyst, C+ of solid components & septations
- **Osteosarcoma, TMJ**
  - Key facts
    - 5-10% of all osteosarcomas
    - Associated with Paget disease, fibrous dysplasia, radiation therapy
  - Imaging
    - CT: Lytic, blastic, or mixed lesions; poorly marginated osteolysis, "sunburst" pattern of new bone formation
    - MR: T2 hyperintense enhancing mass; bone spicules T2 hypointense

- **Chondrosarcoma, TMJ**
  - Key facts
    - M > F; most in 4th-7th decades
  - Imaging
    - CT: Arc, whorl, stippled Ca++ in mass
    - MR: T2 bright well-defined mass with marked C+; calcifications T2 hypointense
- **Osteochondroma, TMJ**
  - Key facts
    - Cartilage-capped, fungiform, benign bony outgrowth
    - Arises in condyle or coronoid process
  - Imaging
    - CT: Marrow space contiguous between lesion & parent bone
    - MR: Cartilaginous cap bright on T2
- **Synovitis, Pigmented Villonodular, TMJ**
  - Key facts
    - Chondroid metaplasia variant has hyaline cartilage nodules ± enchondral ossification
    - Hemosiderin and calcification
    - Indistinguishable from chondroblastoma
  - Imaging
    - CT: Scalloped condyle & condylar fossa, calcifications within soft tissue mass
    - MR: T1 & T2 hypointense, marked signal loss with GRE
- **Gout, TMJ**
  - Key facts
    - Crystalline arthropathy due to monosodium urate crystals
  - Imaging
    - Identical to CPPD

Degenerative Disease, TMJ

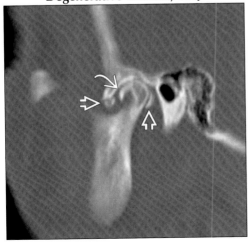

Sagittal oblique bone CT of advanced DJD shows severe joint space narrowing and deformity of condyle with beaking of anterior condylar margin ⤳. Note the multiple calcifications in joint spaces ⤳.

Degenerative Disease, TMJ

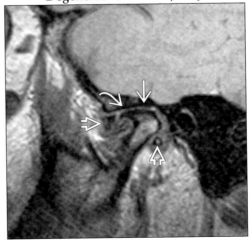

Sagittal PD FSE MR in same patient shows well-defined intraarticular calcifications ⤳ in association with severe DJD. Marked joint space narrowing ⤳ and beaking of mandibular condyle ⤳ are seen.

CALCIFIED TMJ LESIONS

(Left) Axial bone CT demonstrates multiple small calcified bodies ⮕ within the right temporomandibular joint, clustered posterior to the mandibular condyle ⮕. There is also subtle widening of the joint space ⮕. **(Right)** Axial T1 C+ FS MR in the same patient reveals intense synovial enhancement ⮕ around the right mandibular condyle. Intraarticular loose bodies ⮕ are seen as multiple ovoid hypointense foci within the TMJ.

Chondromatosis, Synovial, TMJ

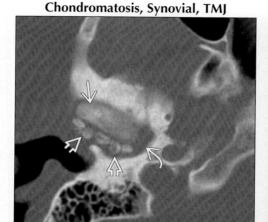

Chondromatosis, Synovial, TMJ

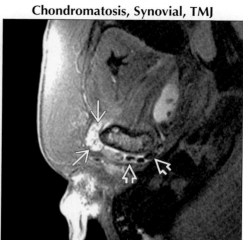

(Left) Axial bone CT demonstrates an amorphous mass-like appearance of the calcification with both "cloud-like" ⮕ and more well-defined dense nodular components ⮕. Marked deformity of the mandibular condyle ⮕ is also evident. **(Right)** Lateral 3D CT reformation in the same patient shows an irregular mass of calcified cartilaginous material ⮕ deforming the mandibular condyle ⮕ and widening the coronoid notch ⮕.

Chondromatosis, Synovial, TMJ

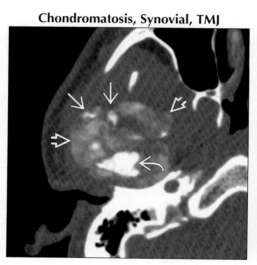

Chondromatosis, Synovial, TMJ

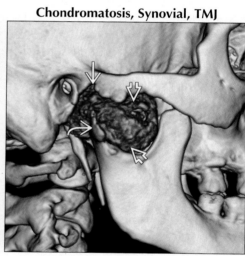

(Left) Axial NECT in a different patient demonstrates a more subtle soft tissue mass ⮕ anterior and medial to the subcondylar left mandible. The mass has multiple well-defined calcified nodules ⮕ within its substance. **(Right)** Axial bone CT shows a well-defined triangular-shaped osseous fragment ⮕ that "fits" into part of the larger triangular defect in the adjacent mandibular condyle ⮕.

Chondromatosis, Synovial, TMJ

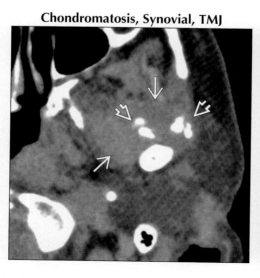

Osteochondritis Dissecans, TMJ

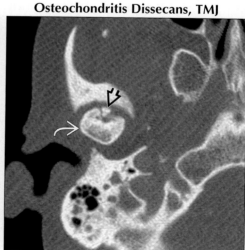

CALCIFIED TMJ LESIONS

Osteochondritis Dissecans, TMJ

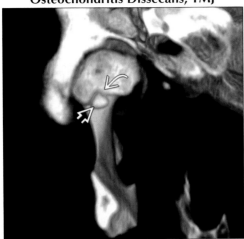

Osteochondritis Dissecans, TMJ

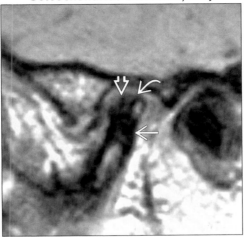

(Left) Anteroposterior subvolume 3D reformation from a CT shows an ossific fragment ⮊ that matches the defect in the adjacent mandibular condyle ⮊. *(Right)* Sagittal PD FSE MR in a different patient reveals a hypointense sclerotic osteocartilaginous fragment ⮊ within a larger triangular defect of the mandibular condyle ⮊. Note the other degenerative changes with sclerosis of the subcondylar neck ⮊.

Calcium Pyrophosphate Dehydrate Deposition Disease, TMJ

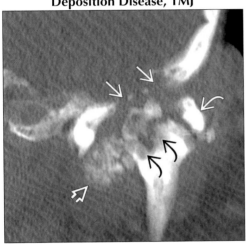

Calcium Pyrophosphate Dehydrate Deposition Disease, TMJ

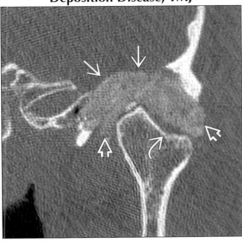

(Left) Coronal bone CT shows a grossly destructive chronic form of CPPD with extensive erosion of the condylar fossa roof ⮊ and the left mandibular condyle ⮊. There are prominent soft tissue calcifications ⮊ and separate bone fragments from the condyle ⮊. *(Right)* Coronal bone CT in a different patient shows homogeneous calcification ⮊ of a mass and extensive erosion of the TMJ condylar fossa ⮊ with remodeling of the condyle ⮊.

Calcium Pyrophosphate Dehydrate Deposition Disease, TMJ

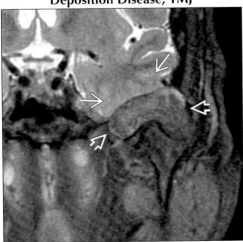

Calcium Pyrophosphate Dehydrate Deposition Disease, TMJ

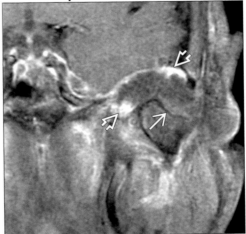

(Left) Coronal T2WI FS MR in the same patient reveals the homogeneous calcification to be diffusely low in signal. The left temporal lobe ⮊ is elevated by the mass ⮊, without parenchymal edema. *(Right)* Coronal T1 C+ FS MR in the same patient shows prominent enhancement of the peripheral inflamed synovium ⮊. Deformity of the condyle ⮊ is also clearly evident.

CALCIFIED TMJ LESIONS

(Left) Coronal bone CT shows overgrowth of the right TMJ, representing ankylosis occurring after an old medially displaced condylar fracture ➡. A bone osteophyte ➡ bridges the lateral aspect of the narrowed joint space ➡.
(Right) Coronal bone CT in a young adult reveals complete bilateral ankylosis ➡ of the temporomandibular joints. This patient had a history of severe juvenile idiopathic arthritis.

Ankylosis, TMJ

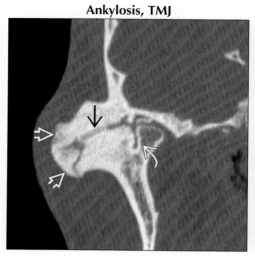

Ankylosis, TMJ

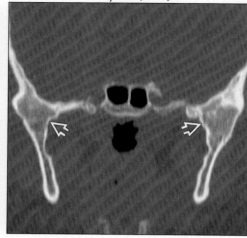

(Left) Axial bone CT in a patient with a prior Proplast implant demonstrates multiple calcifications ➡ within disorganized right TMJ. There is marked remodeling of both the condyle ➡ and glenoid fossa ➡. **(Right)** Sagittal PD FSE MR shows marked deformity of the TMJ with low intensity calcified debris ➡ anterior and posterior to the eroded condyle ➡. The condylar fossa ➡ appears flattened with erosion, nearly perforating the floor of the middle fossa.

**Foreign Body Giant Cell Reaction
(Proplast Implant)**

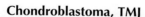
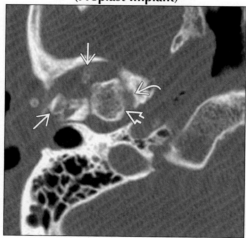

**Foreign Body Giant Cell Reaction
(Proplast Implant)**

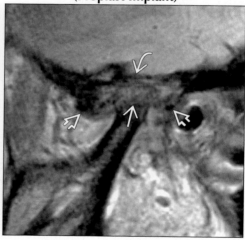

(Left) Coronal bone CT shows a mixed lucent & calcified lesion ➡ arising from and destroying the roof of the condylar fossa and extending into the TMJ. The condyle appears intact ➡. (Courtesy R. Kurokawa, MD.) **(Right)** Coronal T2WI FS MR demonstrates an expansile mass arising from the right temporal bone above condylar fossa. The mass has a markedly low peripheral signal ➡ & more central hyperintensity ➡. Temporal lobe ➡ is elevated without cerebral edema.

Chondroblastoma, TMJ

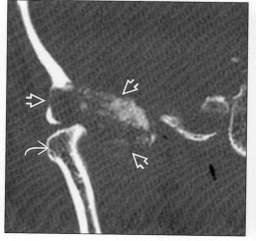

Chondroblastoma, TMJ

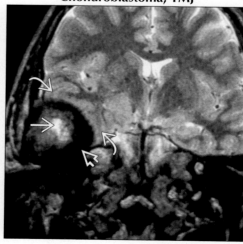

CALCIFIED TMJ LESIONS

Osteosarcoma, TMJ

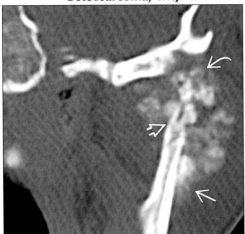

Osteosarcoma, TMJ

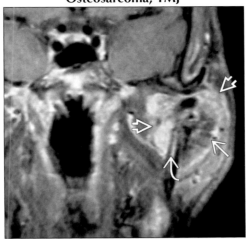

(Left) Coronal bone CT reveals an osteosarcoma of the mandibular ramus ➡, neck ➡, and condyle ➡. The "sunburst" periosteal reaction indicates an aggressive bone-forming process. (Right) Coronal T1 C+ FS MR reveals homogeneous enhancement of the soft tissue component ➡, with calcification appearing as regions of lower signal intensity ➡. Note the infiltration of the mandibular marrow ➡ with abnormal enhancement.

Chondrosarcoma, TMJ

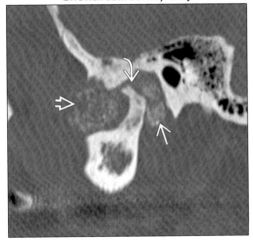

Chondrosarcoma, TMJ

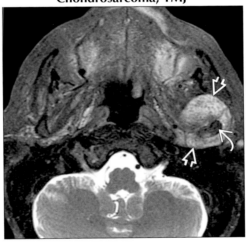

(Left) Sagittal bone CT reformation shows a soft tissue mass within & around the temporomandibular joint, containing stippled ➡ & more well-defined calcifications ➡. Condylar remodeling is also evident ➡. (Right) Axial T2WI FS MR in the same patient demonstrates a hyperintense mass ➡ surrounding the left mandibular condyle ➡. Innumerable tiny foci of hypointensity are evident, which correspond to fine calcifications evident on CT (not shown).

Osteochondroma, TMJ

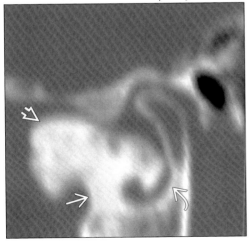

Synovitis, Pigmented Villonodular, TMJ

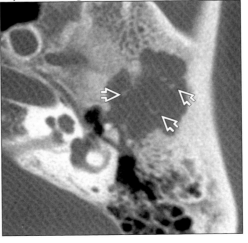

(Left) Sagittal oblique bone CT demonstrates a large osteochondroma ➡ immediately anterior to TMJ, arising from the coronoid process ➡. This bony outgrowth appears to thin and remodel the neck of the mandible ➡. (Right) Axial bone CT shows a lucent lesion eroding the roof of the condylar fossa. Multiple small calcifications ➡ are evident within the mass. This is an unusual appearance for PVNS, which is typically lucent. (Courtesy Y. Oda, MD.)

Suprahyoid & Infrahyoid

TMJ CYSTS

DIFFERENTIAL DIAGNOSIS

Common
- Joint Effusion
- Subchondral Cyst (Geode)
- Simple Bone Cyst (Traumatic)

Less Common
- Parotid Cyst
- Ganglion Cyst
- Synovial Chondromatosis
- Pigmented Villonodular Synovitis

Rare but Important
- Synovial Cyst
- Abscess

ESSENTIAL INFORMATION

Key Differential Diagnosis Issues
- Wide range of pathology responsible for cystic TMJ lesion
- Cyst may arise from
  - Temporomandibular joint itself
  - Mandibular condyle or neck
  - Skull base
  - Parotid gland
- Imaging strategy
  - CT: Cyst = low-density lesion
    - Bone CT for mandible/skull base lesion
    - CECT may differentiate parotid cyst
  - MR: T2 hyperintense, rim enhancement
    - Better definition of joint disc morphology
    - May better show small joint cysts
    - May better characterize parotid mass

Helpful Clues for Common Diagnoses
- **Joint Effusion**
  - Key facts
    - May be seen with many arthritides
    - Inflammatory or reactive most common
    - Also seen with degenerative, pyogenic, rheumatoid, psoriatic arthritis
    - Uncommonly post-traumatic
    - Effusion correlates with pain
  - Imaging
    - MR: Joint collection with variable signal depending on protein content
    - Closed mouth views: Often largest in anterior joint
    - Open mouth views: Shifts to posterior joint space

- **Subchondral Cyst (Geode)**
  - Key facts
    - Intrusion of synovium through cartilage-denuded articular bone surface
    - Rheumatoid (RA) or osteoarthritis (OA)
  - Imaging
    - Sharply marginated subcortical condylar lucency with thin sclerotic margins
    - Found beneath pressure segment of joint adjacent to area of maximal joint narrowing
    - RA: Begins at chondro-osseous junction
    - Other OA findings: Joint space narrowing, articular sclerosis, osteophytes
- **Simple Bone Cyst (Traumatic)**
  - Key facts
    - Synonym: Traumatic bone cavity
    - Fluid-filled intraosseous pseudocyst
    - No epithelial lining
  - Imaging
    - CT: Thin irregular well-corticated margin, minimal bone expansion
    - MR: T2 hyperintense focal lesion

Helpful Clues for Less Common Diagnoses
- **Parotid Cyst**
  - Key facts
    - May be single, multiple, uni- or bilateral
    - Key distinguishing feature: Arises within parotid tissue
    - Many causes of parotid cysts
    - Congenital (1st branchial cleft), inflammatory (sialocele, BLEL, HIV, Sjögren), neoplastic (Warthin, acinic cell)
  - Imaging
    - CT: Sharply defined low-density cyst ± blood-fluid levels
    - MR: T2 hyperintense, well-defined lesion with surrounding parotid tissue
- **Ganglion Cyst**
  - Key facts
    - Pseudocyst: Myxoid degeneration of collagenous joint capsule wall
    - Does not communicate with joint space
    - Lies within wall or superficial to joint capsule
    - Filled with viscid or gelatinous material
    - May be secondary to trauma
    - 70% of patients between 2nd & 4th decade
  - Imaging

- ≤ 2 cm cyst adjacent to joint
- No effusion within joint itself
- CT: May remodel bone; rarely may erode into condyle or roof of fossa
- MR: T2 hyperintense mass adjacent to joint

- **Synovial Chondromatosis**
  - Key facts
    - Synovial membrane proliferation and metaplasia → hyaline cartilage nodules
    - Nodules calcify
    - Adolescents, young adults
  - Imaging
    - Early CT: Joint widened, may erode into middle cranial fossa
    - Noncalcified nodules initially; lesion appears cystic at this stage
    - Early MR: Rim-enhancing cystic joint mass; nodules T1 dark, T2 bright
- **Pigmented Villonodular Synovitis**
  - Key facts
    - Benign synovial proliferation
    - Unknown etiology
    - Hemosiderin and calcium deposition
  - Imaging
    - CT: Scalloped condyle and condylar fossa, calcifications within soft tissue mass
    - MR: Cystic and solid; variable signal intensity
    - Peripheral low signal with T2 & GRE

Helpful Clues for Rare Diagnoses
- **Synovial Cyst**

  - Key facts
    - True cyst with synovial cell lining
    - Contains synovial fluid
    - May arise by herniation of synovial lining through joint capsule wall
    - Displacement of synovial tissue during embryogenesis may predispose to synovial cyst formation
    - Associated with inflammation: RA, osteoarthritis, prior trauma
  - Imaging
    - Usually communicates with joint space
    - CT: Low-density fluid collection appears contiguous with joint
    - MR: T2 hyperintense mass
    - May peripherally enhance if infected or associated with inflammatory arthropathy
- **Abscess**
  - Key facts
    - Most often secondary involvement from malignant otitis externa (MOE) or coalescent mastoiditis
    - Less commonly hematogenous septic arthritis
  - Imaging
    - MOE: Widened TMJ space, destruction of anterior wall EAC
    - Periauricular swelling & phlegmon
    - Mastoiditis: Air cell opacity with breakdown of septations
    - Mastoid and occipital inflammation
    - Must evaluate for intracranial spread of infection!

Joint Effusion

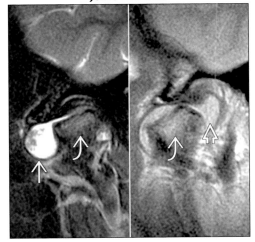

Sagittal T2WI MR closed mouth view (left) shows large effusion ➡ mimicking a cyst, anterior to degenerated condyle ⤳. Cyst partially reduces to posterior joint space ➡ on open mouth PD FSE MR view (right).

Joint Effusion

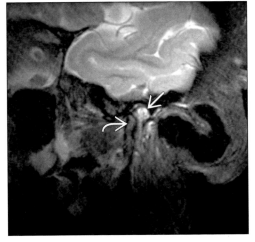

Sagittal T2WI FS MR in a patient with a history of rheumatoid arthritis demonstrates small effusion ➡ posterior to the condyle ⤳. Patient also has nonreducible bilateral anterior disc displacement.

TMJ CYSTS

(Left) Coronal T2WI MR reveals a focal cyst ➥ within the mandibular condyle. TMJ degeneration is so advanced in this patient that there is no residual joint space, and the deformed condylar head abuts the eroded middle fossa. (Right) Sagittal bone CT shows advanced degenerative change with a prominent subchondral geode ➥. Note the marked loss of joint space with remodeling and scalloping of the fossa. Also observe the small anterior condylar osteophyte ➥.

Subchondral Cyst (Geode)

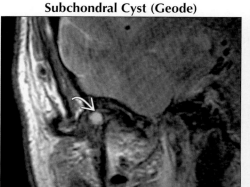

Subchondral Cyst (Geode)

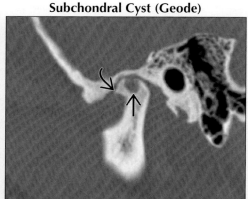

(Left) Axial bone CT demonstrates a sharply circumscribed expansile lucent lesion in the right mandibular condyle and subcondylar neck ➥. The overlying cortex is thinned but intact, and there is no abnormal matrix ossification or extraosseous soft tissue. (Right) Sagittal oblique ray-sum 3D CT rendering subvolume shows the same cystic lesion ➥ in the ramus of the mandible with mildly scalloped appearance of cyst wall. This reformation suggests partial septations.

Simple Bone Cyst (Traumatic)

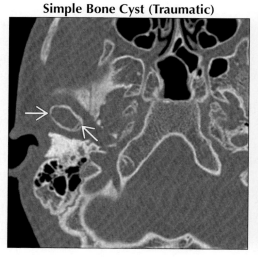

Simple Bone Cyst (Traumatic)

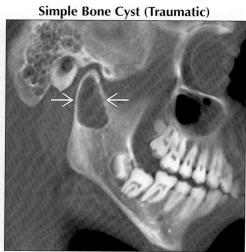

(Left) Axial CECT shows a well-defined rim-enhancing cystic mass ➥ immediately inferior and slightly anterior to the left TMJ. This sialocele is surrounded by parotid tissue, which is the clue to its true origin. (Right) Axial T2WI FS MR in a different patient shows a cystic intraparotid sialocele ➥ with hemorrhagic fluid level, abutting the right posterior ramus ➥ and inferior to the TMJ.

Parotid Cyst

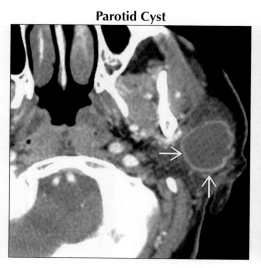

Parotid Cyst

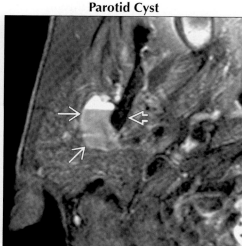

TMJ CYSTS

Ganglion Cyst

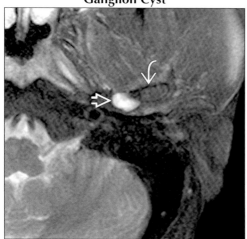

Ganglion Cyst

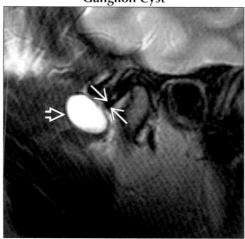

(Left) Axial T2WI FS MR demonstrates a small uniform intensity oval-shaped cyst ⊉ at the medial aspect of the left condyle ➡. The joint otherwise appears normal with minor degenerative changes and no joint effusion. *(Right)* Sagittal T2WI MR in a different patient demonstrates a much larger ganglion cyst ➡ anterior to the TMJ and specifically anterior to the disc ➡. There is no joint effusion and only minor degenerative joint changes.

Synovial Chondromatosis

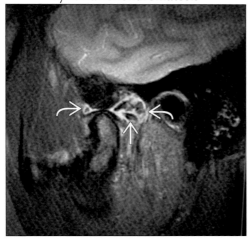

Pigmented Villonodular Synovitis

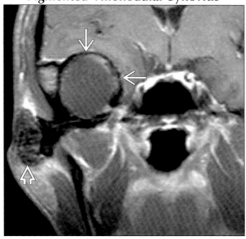

(Left) Sagittal oblique T2WI FS MR demonstrates multiple small low intensity bodies ➡ within hyperintense fluid of distended TMJ ➡. Condyle is sclerotic and slightly irregular due to degenerative change. *(Right)* Coronal T1 C+ FS MR demonstrates 2 masses centered around the right TMJ. The intracranial mass is cystic ➡, and the extracranial mass ⊉ is solid and low signal intensity. Both masses have a low signal intensity periphery and no significant enhancement.

Synovial Cyst

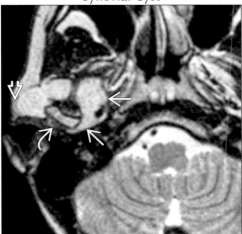

Abscess

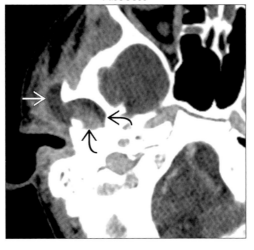

(Left) Axial T2WI MR shows a large lobulated hyperintense cyst ➡ surrounding and involving the right TMJ and extending laterally to result in a palpable cheek mass ⊉. Though the mass is intimately related to TMJ, no free fluid is evident in the joint space ➡. *(Right)* Axial CECT shows a distended TMJ space projecting laterally into the anterior parotid tissue ➡ as well as pus filling enlarged joint space of TMJ ➡. The joint was seeded from acute otomastoiditis.

DIFFUSE PAROTID DISEASE

DIFFERENTIAL DIAGNOSIS

Common
- Parotiditis, Acute
- Parotiditis, Chronic
- Sjögren Syndrome, Parotid
- Sarcoidosis, Parotid
- Benign Lymphoepithelial Lesions-HIV

Less Common
- Sialosis, Parotid
- Mucoepidermoid Carcinoma, Parotid
- Adenoid Cystic Carcinoma, Parotid

Rare but Important
- Non-Hodgkin Lymphoma, Parotid

ESSENTIAL INFORMATION

Key Differential Diagnosis Issues
- If unilateral: Think acute infection or malignancy (carcinoma vs. primary NHL)
  - If acute infection: Look for calculi along parotid duct; look for drainable abscess
- If bilateral: Look for ductal calculi, abnormality in other salivary glands or imaging evidence of HIV disease

Helpful Clues for Common Diagnoses
- **Parotiditis, Acute**
  - Either bacterial or viral, or acute-on-chronic with calculus disease (recurrent sialadenitis)
  - Acute viral parotiditis
    - Clinical diagnosis; rarely imaged

- Acute bacterial parotiditis often seen in neonates & elderly, debilitated patients
    - Unilateral enlargement of hyperdense parotid with subcutaneous fat stranding
    - Must look for abscess to be drained
- **Parotiditis, Chronic**
  - Bilateral, heterogeneous small glands
  - Dilated intraglandular ducts and may see ductal calculi
- **Sjögren Syndrome, Parotid**
  - Variable-sized cysts and small calcifications
    - Submandibular, sublingual, or lacrimal gland may be involved also
  - Look carefully for solid lesions since increased risk of primary parotid NHL
- **Sarcoidosis, Parotid**
  - Often indistinguishable from Sjögren syndrome at imaging
  - No increased risk for malignancy
- **Benign Lymphoepithelial Lesions-HIV**
  - Solid and cystic lesions that mimic Sjögren or sarcoid but other glands normal
    - Look for adenoidal hypertrophy and reactive neck nodes of HIV disease

Other Essential Information
- **Parotid Primary Malignancies**
  - When high grade, can diffusely infiltrate parotid
- **Non-Hodgkin Lymphoma, Parotid**
  - Usually part of systemic NHL with unilateral or bilateral solid nodules
  - Primary NHL much less common but can mimic unilateral primary neoplasm

Parotiditis, Acute

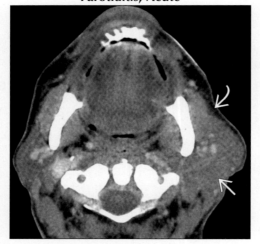

Axial CECT shows acute parotiditis with a diffusely enlarged and hyperdense left parotid gland ➡ with subcutaneous fat stranding ➡. No calculi or abscesses are evident.

Parotiditis, Acute

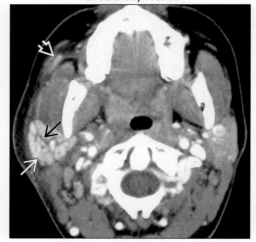

Axial CECT shows acute-on-chronic parotiditis (sialadenitis) with enhancement of the right parotid ➡ and intraglandular duct dilatation ➡. Calculi are noted in the Stensen duct ➡.

DIFFUSE PAROTID DISEASE

Parotiditis, Chronic

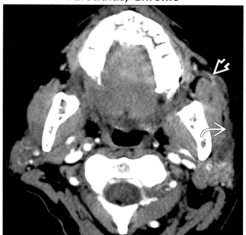

Sjögren Syndrome, Parotid

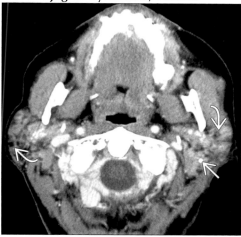

(Left) Axial CECT shows marked dilatation along the length of the left parotid duct ➡. Irregular enhancement of the distal duct ⬦ may be a stricture. No calculi or acute inflammatory change is seen. (Right) Axial CECT shows diffusely abnormal heterogeneous parotid glands with small round cystic regions ➡ and foci of calcification ➡. Abnormal submandibular glands were also present (not shown).

Sarcoidosis, Parotid

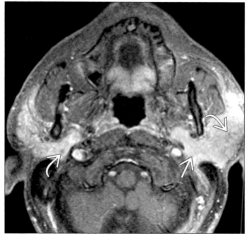

Benign Lymphoepithelial Lesions-HIV

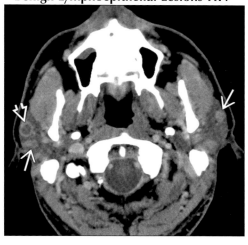

(Left) Axial T1 C+ FS MR shows bilateral parotid enlargement with diffuse infiltration of the glands ➡ and subtle small foci of cystic change ➡. (Right) Axial CECT shows diffuse bilateral parotid disease with small, solid, enhancing masses ➡ and mixed solid-cystic ⬦ lesions with mildly enlarged parotid glands.

Sialosis, Parotid

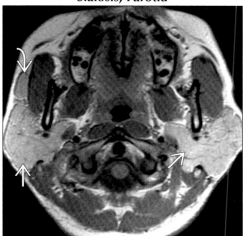

Mucoepidermoid Carcinoma, Parotid

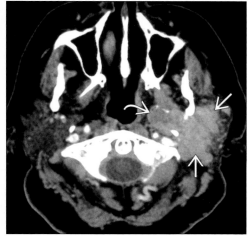

(Left) Axial T1WI MR reveals diffusely enlarged but homogeneously T1 hyperintense parotid glands ➡. There is also enlargement of the right accessory parotid ➡ on the masseter muscle surface. (Right) Axial CECT shows diffuse infiltration of the left parotid ➡, which appears markedly enlarged and hyperdense. This high-grade tumor also involves the deep lobe of the parotid ➡.

MULTIPLE PAROTID MASSES

DIFFERENTIAL DIAGNOSIS

Common
- Metastatic Disease, Nodal, Parotid
- Non-Hodgkin Lymphoma, Parotid
- Warthin Tumor

Less Common
- Benign Mixed Tumor, Parotid, Recurrent
- Sjögren Syndrome, Parotid
- Benign Lymphoepithelial Lesions-HIV

Rare but Important
- Sarcoidosis, Parotid
- Oncocytoma, Parotid

ESSENTIAL INFORMATION

Key Differential Diagnosis Issues
- Imaging strategies
  - CT most often 1st line imaging tool
  - When multiple lesions found
    - Determine if uni-/bilateral & if remainder of parotids are normal
    - Check rest of neck scan for adenoidal hypertrophy, abnormality of submandibular & sublingual glands, neck adenopathy, abnormal lung apices

Helpful Clues for Common Diagnoses
- **Metastatic Disease, Nodal, Parotid**
  - Ipsilateral skin/scalp SCCa or melanoma
  - May have "hairy" margins, necrosis, or form confluent masses
  - Level V nodes often also found
- **Non-Hodgkin Lymphoma, Parotid**
  - Nodules 2° to intraparotid nodes
  - Homogeneous, usually circumscribed
  - Associated with neck adenopathy
- **Warthin Tumor**
  - Most often tail of parotid; ≤ 20% bilateral
  - Cystic, solid, or mixed solid-cystic masses

Helpful Clues for Less Common Diagnoses
- **Benign Mixed Tumor, Parotid, Recurrent**
  - "Seeding" from operative cell spillage
  - Nodules best seen on T2 FS & T1 C+ FS MR
- **Sjögren Syndrome, Parotid**
  - Multiple cystic lesions, variably sized
  - Usually bilateral; other salivary glands also
    - Solid mass with Sjögren concerning for lymphoma
- **Benign Lymphoepithelial Lesions-HIV**
  - Bilateral solid and cystic lesions
  - May appear identical to Sjögren but does not involve other salivary glands
  - Look for other manifestations of HIV: Adenoidal hypertrophy, reactive nodes

Helpful Clues for Rare Diagnoses
- **Sarcoidosis, Parotid**
  - Painless bilateral swelling & dry mouth
  - Small parotid nodules (granulomas)
    - Later stage with small cysts may be identical to Sjögren & benign lymphoepithelial lesions-HIV
- **Oncocytoma, Parotid**
  - Uni- or bilateral, loss of normal architecture with multiple predominantly solid nodules
    - Dominant nodule may be oncocytoma

Metastatic Disease, Nodal, Parotid

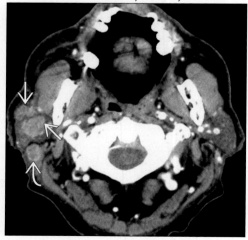

Axial CECT shows multiple nodules ➡ in the right parotid gland and an additional periparotid metastatic node ➡. All lesions have ill-defined, "hairy" margins and heterogeneous density.

Non-Hodgkin Lymphoma, Parotid

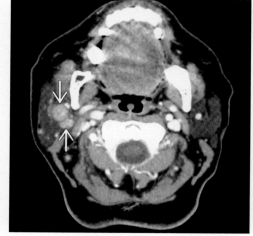

Axial CECT demonstrates multiple, uniformly enhancing, well-defined lymph nodes ➡ within the right parotid gland.

MULTIPLE PAROTID MASSES

Warthin Tumor
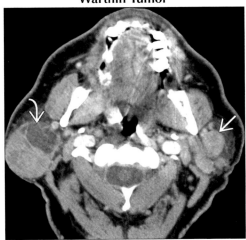

Benign Mixed Tumor, Parotid, Recurrent
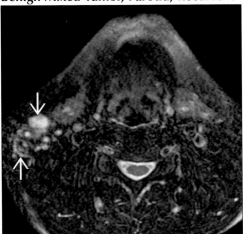

(Left) Axial CECT reveals multiple solid ➡ and partially cystic ➡ enhancing masses within the parotid glands bilaterally. The masses also vary in size but are all well circumscribed. *(Right)* Axial T2WI FS MR shows a recurrent benign mixed tumor from intraoperative cell spillage at the time of initial BMT resection. There are multiple small nodules ➡ within the tail of the right parotid gland that are markedly hyperintense.

Sjögren Syndrome, Parotid
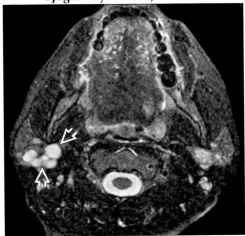

Benign Lymphoepithelial Lesions-HIV
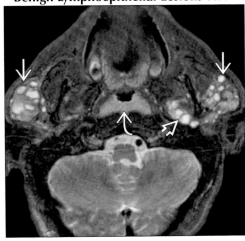

(Left) Axial T1WI FS MR shows multiple cystic nodules ➡ in the right parotid gland. Both glands appear more heterogeneous than normal. *(Right)* Axial T2WI FS MR of an adult patient shows enlarged parotid glands containing multiple small hyperintense cysts. These involve both the superficial ➡ and deep lobes ➡. Note the hyperplasia of the nasopharyngeal tonsillar tissue ➡, which is typical in patients with HIV.

Sarcoidosis, Parotid
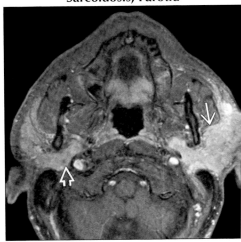

Oncocytoma, Parotid
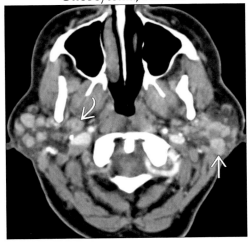

(Left) Axial T1 C+ FS MR demonstrates diffuse enlargement of the left parotid with avid enhancement ➡. On the right, the gland enhances mildly throughout, but the avidly enhancing region is confined to the deep lobe ➡. *(Right)* Axial CECT shows multiple solid nodules in the superficial ➡ and deep ➡ lobes of the parotid glands bilaterally. These lobulated nodules vary in size.

FOCAL RETROPHARYNGEAL SPACE MASS

DIFFERENTIAL DIAGNOSIS

Common
- Reactive Adenopathy, Retropharyngeal Space (RPS)
- Suppurative Adenopathy, RPS
- SCCa, Nodal, RPS
- Metastatic Node, Non-SCCa, RPS
- Non-Hodgkin Lymphoma, Nodal, RPS
- Carotid Artery, Tortuous, Neck

Less Common
- Multinodular Goiter
- Lipoma

Rare but Important
- Schwannoma, Sympathetic
- Adenoma, Parathyroid, Ectopic

ESSENTIAL INFORMATION

Key Differential Diagnosis Issues
- RPS mass located posterior to pharynx and anterior to prevertebral muscles
- Focal masses most often in high RPS, medial to internal carotid artery (ICA)
- In children, large homogeneous RPS nodes are normal finding
  - Typically larger than adjacent ICA
- In adult with oval RPS lesion, main differential is node vs. schwannoma
  - Abnormal node in adult if > 8 mm
  - History or imaging evidence of tonsillitis suggests reactive or suppurative node
  - If patient not acutely unwell, first consideration is metastatic node
    - Main differential: Nasopharyngeal carcinoma, SCCa, lymphoma, sinonasal tumor, thyroid carcinoma
  - Schwannoma usually arises in medial carotid sheath but appears to be in RPS
    - Diagnosis may require transfacial biopsy
- Imaging considerations
  - Metastatic retropharyngeal nodes not palpable so not clinically evident
  - CECT: RPS node isodense to prevertebral muscle and often missed
  - MR: T2 hyperintense to muscle; more readily identifiable

Helpful Clues for Common Diagnoses
- **Reactive Adenopathy, Retropharyngeal Space (RPS)**

- Key facts
  - Typically associated with pharyngitis &/or tonsillitis
  - Common finding in children even without obvious acute infection
- Imaging
  - Well defined, oval or round, solid
  - Often enlarged level II nodes
- **Suppurative Adenopathy, RPS**
  - Key facts
    - Most frequently seen with tonsillitis
    - Patient usually toxic, ill
  - Imaging
    - Cystic RPS node with surrounding inflammatory changes
    - Adjacent ICA may be narrowed; reversible
    - Primary infection often evident as enlarged, enhancing tonsils
- **SCCa, Nodal, RPS**
  - Key facts
    - Most commonly from nasopharyngeal carcinoma (NPC), which is actually undifferentiated tumor
    - Primary NPC arises in fossa of Rosenmüller; commonly drains to RPS, level II
    - SCCa arising in naso-, oro-, or hypopharynx may metastasize to RPS
    - Search for RPS node especially if posterior pharyngeal wall SCCa
  - Imaging
    - Variable density/intensity: May be large without necrosis if due to NPC
    - Metastatic node from true SCCa more likely to have necrosis
- **Metastatic Node, Non-SCCa, RPS**
  - Key facts
    - Both sinonasal and thyroid tumors may drain to RPS
    - Important to find RPS node for otherwise resectable sinonasal tumor
  - Imaging
    - Variable size and density/intensity
    - ± Calcification in thyroid metastasis
- **Non-Hodgkin Lymphoma, Nodal, RPS**
  - Key facts
    - Often in association with extensive adenopathy ± Waldeyer ring disease
  - Imaging
    - Variable size node medial to ICA

1

FOCAL RETROPHARYNGEAL SPACE MASS

- Frequently remains solid and homogeneous despite large size
- **Carotid Artery, Tortuous, Neck**
  - Key facts
    - Tortuous course of common or internal carotid artery
    - Uni- or bilateral
    - Arteries may be normal caliber or ectatic
    - May be incidental clinical or imaging finding
    - Warn clinicians so as to avoid biopsy
  - Imaging
    - In cross-section slice mimics RPS node
    - Readily apparent as artery on review of multiple slices or reformatted images
    - May have atherosclerotic calcium, arterial phase enhancement

Helpful Clues for Less Common Diagnoses
- **Multinodular Goiter**
  - Key facts
    - Common lower neck mass
    - Diffuse gland enlargement
    - Adenomatous change, fibrosis, calcification, hemorrhage, ± cystic change resulting in nodularity
    - Patients usually euthyroid
  - Imaging
    - Often wraps around pharynx to RPS as MNG enlarges in cranial direction
    - Review of multiple images reveals RPS mass to arise from enlarged thyroid
    - 90% of MNG have calcifications
- **Lipoma**

- Key facts
  - Benign, congenital mass that may enlarge with ↑ in body size
- Imaging
  - CT: Fat-density, well-defined mass
  - MR: Well-defined T1 hyperintense mass with signal loss on fat-saturation sequence

Helpful Clues for Rare Diagnoses
- **Schwannoma, Sympathetic**
  - Key facts
    - Often incidental imaging finding
    - Sympathetic chain tumor in medial carotid sheath; looks like RPS mass
    - Slow growing; stable over months
  - Imaging
    - Fusiform enhancing mass medial to ICA
- **Adenoma, Parathyroid, Ectopic**
  - Key facts
    - Adenoma most commonly found at posterior aspect thyroid or tracheoesophageal groove
    - May be anywhere from angle of mandible to mediastinum
  - Imaging
    - Difficult imaging diagnosis as mimics lymph node in any location
    - Arterial phase enhancement evident when dynamic imaging performed
    - Tc-99m-Sestamibi shows uptake which persists on delayed scans
    - SPECT best for accurate localization

Reactive Adenopathy, Retropharyngeal Space (RPS)
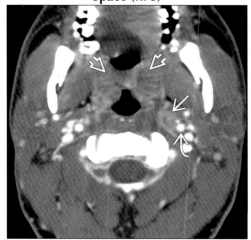

Axial CECT shows an enlarged, enhancing left retropharyngeal node ➡ medial to ICA ➡. There is also bilateral tonsillar inflammation and enlargement ➡, representing acute tonsillitis.

Suppurative Adenopathy, RPS
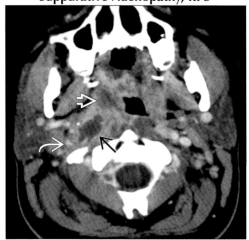

Axial CECT shows fluid density right RPS collection ➡ with surrounding inflammatory change and narrowing of the right ICA ➡. The ipsilateral inflamed tonsil ➡ is probable site of primary infection.

FOCAL RETROPHARYNGEAL SPACE MASS

(Left) Axial T1 C+ FS MR through nasopharynx reveals soft tissue distension of right fossa of Rosenmüller by primary nasopharyngeal carcinoma ➡. Immediately posterolateral is a left retropharyngeal metastatic node ➡. (Right) Axial CECT shows a low-density necrotic mass ➡ medial to right ICA. Primary SCCa is in left lateral and posterior oropharyngeal wall ➡ extending to left tongue base ➡. Additional level II low-density adenopathy is noted ➡.

SCCa, Nodal, RPS

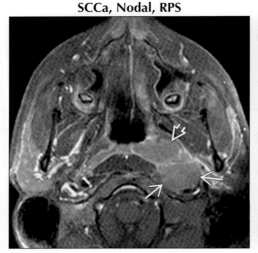

SCCa, Nodal, RPS

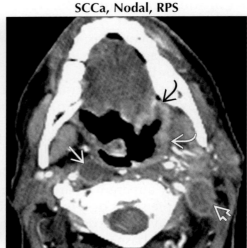

(Left) Axial CECT in a patient with primary SCCa of nasal vault shows bilateral subtle soft tissue masses ➡ medial to internal carotid arteries and displacing parapharyngeal fat anteriorly. The masses are reasonably symmetric and almost isodense to muscle, but clearly abnormal. (Right) Axial T2WI MR in the same patient better delineates same bilateral retropharyngeal nodes ➡, which are clearly of higher signal intensity than adjacent prevertebral muscles.

Metastatic Node, Non-SCCa, RPS

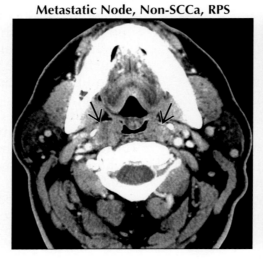

Metastatic Node, Non-SCCa, RPS

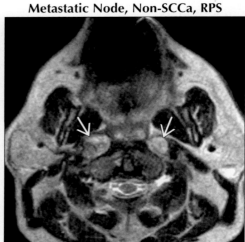

(Left) Axial CECT demonstrates a solid right retropharyngeal node ➡. Node is isodense to muscle and not well defined, but it is apparent on imaging because of deformity of adjacent airway. Note also bilateral posterior cervical nodes ➡. (Right) Axial CECT reveals markedly medial course of right internal carotid artery ➡, anterior to vertebral body and deforming posterior pharyngeal contour. The right internal jugular vein ➡ is normally located.

Non-Hodgkin Lymphoma, Nodal, RPS

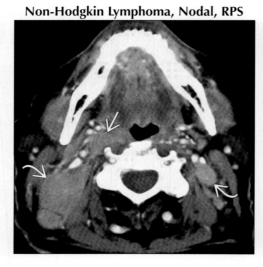

Carotid Artery, Tortuous, Neck

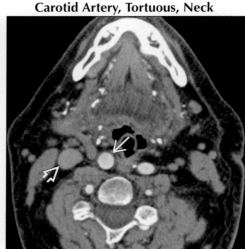

1

FOCAL RETROPHARYNGEAL SPACE MASS

Carotid Artery, Tortuous, Neck

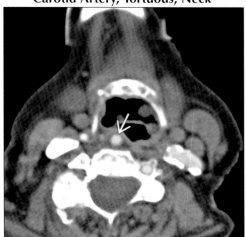

Multinodular Goiter

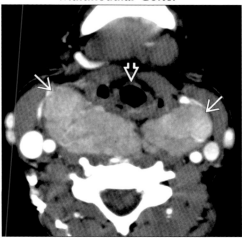

Lipoma

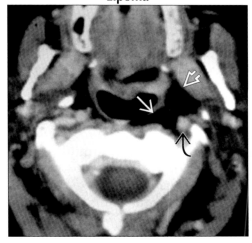

Schwannoma, Sympathetic

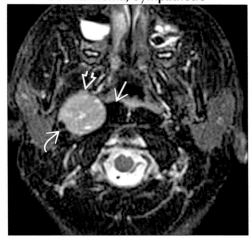

Schwannoma, Sympathetic

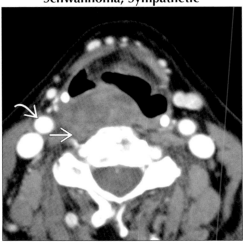

Adenoma, Parathyroid, Ectopic

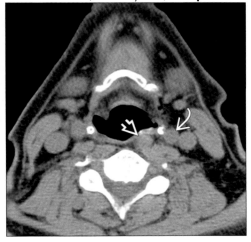

(Left) Axial CECT with arterial phase of contrast injection shows the right carotid artery ➡ nearly reaching the midline in the retropharyngeal space behind the hypopharynx. (Right) Axial CECT shows superior and retropharyngeal extension of a large goiter. Two lobes ➡ meet in the midline posteriorly and displace the hypopharynx and larynx ➡ anteriorly and the carotid sheaths laterally.

(Left) Axial CECT shows a fat-density, well-circumscribed mass ➡ within the left retropharyngeal space, medial to ICA ➡ with anterolateral extension to the parapharyngeal space ➡. (Right) Axial T2WI FS MR shows a well-defined mass ➡ medial to ICA ➡ and lateral to the right prevertebral muscle ➡. This sympathetic chain schwannoma mimics a RPS mass.

(Left) Axial CECT shows a heterogeneous, poorly enhancing mass in the retropharyngeal space, medial to carotid artery ➡, & anterior to prevertebral muscle ➡. Schwannoma displaces hypopharynx anteriorly. (Right) Axial NECT performed for anatomic localization after MIBI scan shows a well-defined mass ➡ in left retropharyngeal space, medial to CCA ➡. Patient had hypercalcemia after prior surgery with ultrasound unable to locate adenoma.

Suprahyoid & Infrahyoid

101

DIFFUSE RETROPHARYNGEAL SPACE DISEASE

DIFFERENTIAL DIAGNOSIS

Common
- Abscess, Retropharyngeal Space
- Effusion, Retropharyngeal Space

Less Common
- Longus Colli Tendonitis
- Neurofibromatosis Type 1
- Venous Malformation
- Lymphatic Malformation
- Multinodular Goiter

Rare but Important
- SCCa, Hypopharynx
- Lipoma

ESSENTIAL INFORMATION

Key Differential Diagnosis Issues
- Retropharyngeal space (RPS) is immediately posterior to pharynx & anterior to prevertebral muscles
- Distension of space results in biconvex, bow tie, or oval configurations
- Plain film cannot distinguish RPS from prevertebral space process
- Consider abscess 1st in differential of low density RPS mass
  - Delay in diagnosis and treatment can have grave consequences
    - Airway compromise
    - Abscess spreads to danger space and then mediastinum

Helpful Clues for Common Diagnoses
- **Abscess, Retropharyngeal Space**
  - Key facts
    - Most commonly results from pharyngitis or tonsillitis, which has seeded RPS nodes
    - Less commonly from anterior spread of prevertebral space infection
    - Typically pediatric age group
    - Increasingly in older patients with immunocompromised state, diabetes, alcoholism
  - Imaging
    - Low density, rim-enhancing RPS fluid
    - Often stranding of adjacent fat planes
  - Mass effect on adjacent tissues
    - Displaced or narrowed pharynx
    - Flattened prevertebral muscles

- **Effusion, Retropharyngeal Space**
  - Key facts
    - Benign fluid from excess lymph production or impaired lymph drainage
    - Most common causes: Internal jugular vein thrombosis (IJV) or new IJV resection, neck radiation therapy, pharyngitis
  - Imaging
    - Nonenhancing low density collection in retropharyngeal space
    - Only mild mass effect on adjacent tissues
    - Minimal displacement of pharynx
    - Uncommonly results in airway compromise
    - Uncommonly results in prevertebral muscle compression
  - Look for potential cause
    - Thrombosed IJV or evidence of IJV resection
    - Diffusely edematous tissues from radiation therapy
    - Pharyngitis/tonsillitis

Helpful Clues for Less Common Diagnoses
- **Longus Colli Tendonitis**
  - Key facts
    - Acute inflammatory process
    - Neck pain, stiffness, ± low grade fever
    - Pathologically: Calcium hydroxyapatite deposition in longus colli insertion, reactive RPS effusion
    - Resolves with anti-inflammatory therapy
  - Imaging
    - Nonenhancing fluid collection with smooth contours, minimal mass effect
    - KEY: Presence of focal prevertebral muscle calcifications at C1-C2 level
- **Neurofibromatosis Type 1**
  - Key facts
    - Neurocutaneous syndrome, chromosome 17 defect
    - RPS plexiform neurofibroma is one of many possible H&N manifestations
  - Imaging
    - Multilobulated trans-spatial mass
    - CT: Mild to moderately enhancing soft tissue masses
    - MR: T2 heterogeneously hyperintense with classic whorled appearance
    - Look for skin nodules or spine lesions as further evidence of NF1

DIFFUSE RETROPHARYNGEAL SPACE DISEASE

- **Venous Malformation**
  - Key facts
    - Congenital vascular malformation occurring in any space(s) in H&N
    - Characterized by multiple vascular pools
  - Imaging
    - Multilobulated trans-spatial masses
    - C+ distinguishes this from lymphatic malformation
    - CT: Intensely enhancing vascular spaces; calcified phleboliths
    - MR: T2 hyperintense with focal areas of signal loss from phleboliths; typically more hyperintense than neurofibromas
- **Lymphatic Malformation**
  - Key facts
    - Congenital malformation occurring in any space or multiple spaces in H&N
    - Cystic appearance with variable number and size of components
  - Imaging
    - MR: CSF signal intensity lesion insinuating in or through spaces with minimal mass effect
    - No significant enhancement unless venolymphatic component
- **Multinodular Goiter**
  - Key facts
    - Goiter is common thyroid pathology
    - When large, goiter spreads into RPS
  - Imaging
    - Multilobulated, heterogeneous enhancing masses that appear to meet in midline RPS

- Focal calcifications may be present
- Thyroid origin is key to diagnosis

Helpful Clues for Rare Diagnoses
- **SCCa, Hypopharynx**
  - Key facts
    - Posterior wall or pyriform sinus primary SCCa extends posteriorly into RPS
    - Caveat: Look for retropharyngeal nodes to level of skull base
  - Imaging
    - Solid enhancing tissue originating from posterior hypopharyngeal wall
    - Invades & distends RPS
    - Look for prevertebral involvement (nonoperative) & associated RPS nodes
- **Lipoma**
  - Key facts
    - Uncommon congenital or acquired lesion that may be incidental finding or present with pharyngeal mass effect
    - May enlarge with increased body weight
  - Imaging
    - Fat density or MR signal intensity mass displacing pharynx anteriorly
    - Confined to RPS or involves adjacent spaces, particularly carotid space

SELECTED REFERENCES

1. Davis WL et al: Retropharyngeal space: evaluation of normal anatomy and diseases with CT and MR imaging. Radiology. 174(1):59-64, 1990

Abscess, Retropharyngeal Space

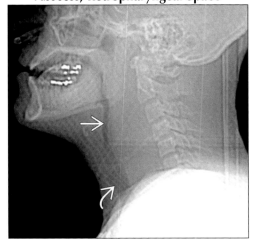

Lateral scout prior to CT scan in this immunocompromised patient reveals markedly expanded prevertebral soft tissues, displacing the pharynx ➡ and esophagus & trachea ➡ anteriorly.

Abscess, Retropharyngeal Space

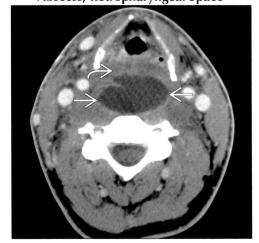

Axial CECT in the same patient shows a large fluid-attenuation mass ➡ displacing the hypopharynx ➡ anteriorly. Mass is anterior to prevertebral muscles and is thus located in the retropharyngeal space.

DIFFUSE RETROPHARYNGEAL SPACE DISEASE

(Left) Axial CECT shows a fluid-density mildly distended retropharyngeal space ➡ without enhancement. Reactive nodes ➡, secondary to the patient's tonsillitis, are also seen in the neck. (Right) Axial CECT shows fluid filling the retropharyngeal space ➡, which is subtly distended. Fluid extends bilaterally to the carotid sheaths. Notice the absence of normal venous enhancement, indicating a thrombosed right internal jugular vein ➡.

Effusion, Retropharyngeal Space

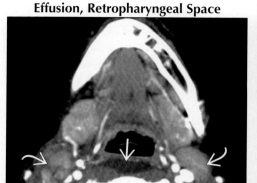

Effusion, Retropharyngeal Space

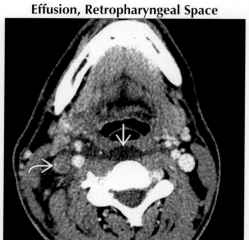

(Left) Sagittal T2WI MR reveals hyperintense retropharyngeal space edema ➡ extending from skull base to C4 level. There is subtle T2 hypointensity of the proximal aspect of the longus colli muscle ➡. (Right) Axial bone CT in the same patient reveals focal calcifications in proximal longus colli tendon ➡, anterior to C1-C2 level. CT is much more sensitive than MR for detection of the calcifications to make diagnosis of calcific tendonitis.

Longus Colli Tendonitis

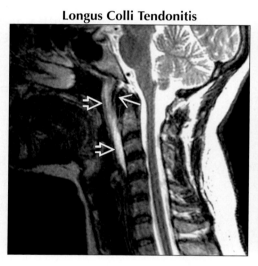

Longus Colli Tendonitis

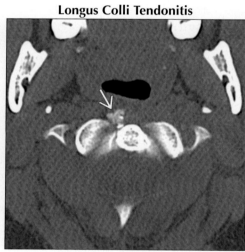

(Left) Axial STIR MR shows hyperintense trans-spatial masses surrounding both internal carotid arteries ➡ and infiltrating medially to involve the retropharyngeal space ➡ and prevertebral muscles. (Right) Axial T2WI FS MR reveals venous malformation diffusely involving the retropharyngeal space ➡ and extending between both carotid sheaths. Malformation infiltrates larynx also ➡ as a trans-spatial mass. Focal low signal intensity ➡ correlates with phleboliths.

Neurofibromatosis Type 1

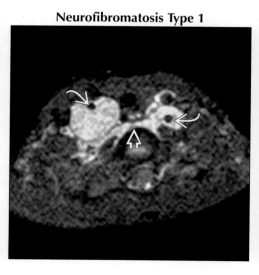

Venous Malformation

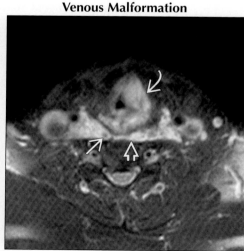

DIFFUSE RETROPHARYNGEAL SPACE DISEASE

Lymphatic Malformation

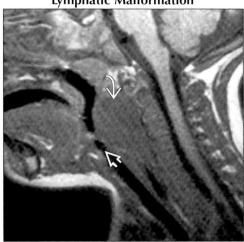

Lymphatic Malformation

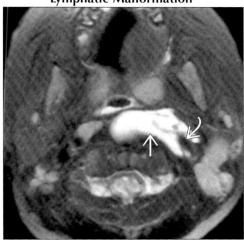

(Left) Sagittal T1WI MR in a child shows distension of retropharyngeal space by a low signal intensity mass ➡ anterior to vertebral bodies. The mass results in significant oropharyngeal narrowing ➡. (Right) Axial T2WI FS MR in the same child shows the retropharyngeal space mass ➡ to be hyperintense following fluid signal. On the axial plane, the lesion is clearly retropharyngeal and extends laterally around the left carotid artery ➡.

Multinodular Goiter

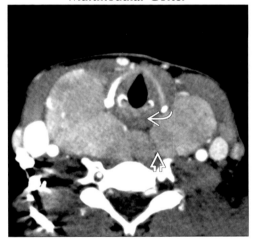

SCCa, Hypopharynx

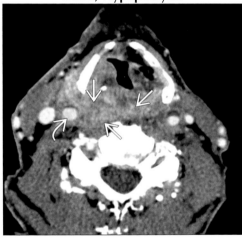

(Left) Axial CECT shows diffuse thyroid enlargement with both lobes meeting in midline in the retropharyngeal space ➡, displacing hypopharynx ➡ and larynx anteriorly. Thyroid lobes remain sharply defined with no evidence of invasion of adjacent soft tissues. (Right) Axial CECT through level of supraglottic larynx reveals enhancing tissue in hypopharynx ➡ that extends posteriorly to thickened retropharyngeal space and also laterally to the carotid artery ➡.

Lipoma

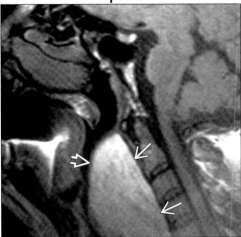

Lipoma

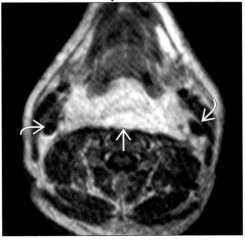

(Left) Sagittal T1WI MR shows a large, homogeneously hyperintense mass ➡ anterior to the cervical spine, protruding into the oropharynx ➡. The lesion is well defined & of fat intensity; there is no soft tissue nodularity or internal stranding. (Right) Axial T1WI MR in the same patient shows prevertebral muscle flattening by a lipoma ➡ & anterior oropharynx displacement, indicating lipoma is retropharyngeal. Carotid vessels are displaced laterally ➡.

DIFFUSE THYROID ENLARGEMENT

DIFFERENTIAL DIAGNOSIS

Common
• Multinodular Goiter

Less Common
• Thyroiditis, Chronic Lymphocytic (Hashimoto)
• Non-Hodgkin Lymphoma, Thyroid
• Anaplastic Carcinoma, Thyroid

Rare but Important
• 4th Branchial Anomaly
• Thyroiditis, Invasive Fibrous (Riedel)
• Thyroiditis, Granulomatous (de Quervain)
• Autoimmune Hyperthyroidism (Graves)

ESSENTIAL INFORMATION

Key Differential Diagnosis Issues
• Diffuse thyroid enlargement implies goiter (generalized enlargement of thyroid gland)
  ○ May be homogeneous or nodular goiter
  ○ Multinodular goiter (MNG) most common
• Homogeneous goiter
  ○ MNG, but nodules not evident on CT/MR
  ○ Thyroiditis, chronic lymphocytic
  ○ Non-Hodgkin lymphoma, thyroid
  ○ Anaplastic carcinoma, thyroid
  ○ Thyroiditis, invasive fibrous
  ○ Autoimmune hyperthyroidism
• Nodular goiter
  ○ Multinodular goiter
  ○ 4th branchial anomaly
  ○ Thyroiditis, granulomatous

Helpful Clues for Common Diagnoses
• **Multinodular Goiter**
  ○ Key facts
    ▪ Lower neck mass
    ▪ Diffuse gland enlargement with adenomatous change, fibrosis, calcification, hemorrhage ± cystic change resulting in nodularity
    ▪ Patients usually euthyroid
  ○ Imaging
    ▪ For surgical planning, important to evaluate entire extent, particularly inferior aspect of MNG
    ▪ CECT/MR: Heterogeneous multilobulated enlarged gland
    ▪ CT: 90% have calcifications (curvilinear, ring-like, or amorphous)

  ▪ MR: Variable T1 & T2 signal intensity, heterogeneous enhancement

Helpful Clues for Less Common Diagnoses
• **Thyroiditis, Chronic Lymphocytic (Hashimoto)**
  ○ Key facts
    ▪ Autoimmune-mediated lymphocytic inflammation of thyroid
    ▪ Thyroid enlarges, later shrinks
    ▪ Marked ↑ risk of primary thyroid non-Hodgkin lymphoma (NHL)
    ▪ Patients often euthyroid, 20% hypothyroid
  ○ Imaging
    ▪ Early stage: Symmetric thyroid enlargement
    ▪ Later stage: Small, fibrotic gland
    ▪ NECT: Iso-/hypodense to muscle
    ▪ CECT: Diffusely reduced density; may appear heterogeneous
    ▪ MR: Heterogeneous or diffusely high signal with lower signal bands
    ▪ FDG PET: Diffuse uptake typically found even in patients receiving thyroid hormone replacement
• **Non-Hodgkin Lymphoma, Thyroid**
  ○ Key facts
    ▪ Thyroid gland primary NHL site
    ▪ Usually diffuse large B-cell lymphoma
    ▪ Rapidly enlarging neck mass
    ▪ Older women, frequently with history of Hashimoto thyroiditis
    ▪ 30-40% of patients hypothyroid
  ○ Imaging
    ▪ 3 morphologic patterns found: Single large mass (80%), multiple thyroid masses, diffusely enlarged thyroid
    ▪ CECT: Tumor tends to be hypodense
    ▪ Necrosis or calcification uncommon
    ▪ Adenopathy tends to be low density
    ▪ MR: Tumor T2 hyperintense to normal gland but shows less enhancement
    ▪ Adenopathy shows little enhancement
• **Anaplastic Carcinoma, Thyroid**
  ○ Key facts
    ▪ Aggressive, rapidly growing, undifferentiated carcinoma
    ▪ Arises in multinodular goiter or differentiated thyroid carcinoma
    ▪ Associated with prior neck irradiation
  ○ Imaging

DIFFUSE THYROID ENLARGEMENT

- Large infiltrative mass with invasion of adjacent tissues
- Necrosis, hemorrhage, and calcification are common features
- CECT: Heterogeneous, infiltrating; nodes often centrally hypodense
- MR: Mixed signal, heterogeneous enhancement

Helpful Clues for Rare Diagnoses

- **4th Branchial Anomaly**
  - Key facts
    - Congenital developmental defect
    - Often presents as suppurative thyroiditis
    - Consider CT with oral barium after acute inflammation subsides
    - Tract from pyriform sinus to LEFT lobe
  - Imaging
    - CECT: Heterogeneous low-density thyroid; may be only left lobe
    - May see focal intrathyroidal collection with overlying inflammatory changes
- **Thyroiditis, Invasive Fibrous (Riedel)**
  - Key facts
    - Synonym: Riedel thyroiditis
    - Chronic inflammation with thyroid fibrosis extending beyond capsule to invade adjacent tissues
    - Rare, > 80% female
    - Rapidly enlarging, painless, hard mass
    - Postulated to be part of systemic multifocal fibrosclerosis
    - 1/3 develop other manifestations such as retroperitoneal fibrosis

- 30% hypothyroid; most euthyroid, rarely hyperthyroid
- FNA often nondiagnostic (difficult to obtain cells)
  - Imaging
    - Mimics diffuse neoplastic process but homogeneous; no adenopathy
    - Enlarged gland with compression and invasion of surrounding tissues
    - CECT: Reduced thyroid density; usually poor contrast enhancement
    - MR: Decreased signal intensity T1 & T2
- **Thyroiditis, Granulomatous (de Quervain)**
  - Key facts
    - Synonyms: de Quervain, subacute thyroiditis
    - Viral or postviral thyroid inflammation
    - Not an autoimmune process
    - Triphasic: Hyper-, hypo-, then euthyroid
  - Imaging
    - Not typically evaluated by CT or MR
    - I-123/I-131/Tc-99m nuclear scan: Low uptake
- **Autoimmune Hyperthyroidism (Graves)**
  - Key facts
    - Synonym: Graves disease
    - Most common cause of thyrotoxicosis
    - Autoimmune thyroiditis
    - Much more common in females
  - Imaging
    - Nonspecific thyroid enlargement without adenopathy or tissue invasion
    - I-123 nuclear scan: Elevated uptake

Multinodular Goiter

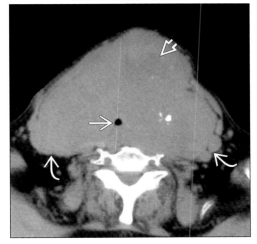

Axial NECT in a patient with dysphagia reveals a large mass encircling the trachea ➡ as it displaces vessels laterally ➡. The mass is heterogeneous with focal calcifications and low density anteriorly ➡.

Multinodular Goiter

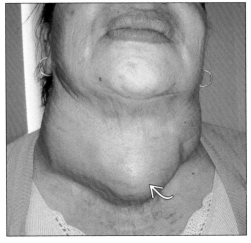

Clinical photograph of the same patient shows diffuse marked enlargement of neck from goiter with a more prominent central protuberance ➡. Patient reported that the mass had been present for many years.

DIFFUSE THYROID ENLARGEMENT

Multinodular Goiter

Multinodular Goiter

(Left) Axial T1WI MR shows a diffusely enlarged thyroid gland. Despite heterogeneity, the goiter remains sharply circumscribed, distorting the trachea ➡ and displacing the left common carotid ➡ and right vertebral arteries ➡. *(Right)* Coronal T2WI FS MR in the same patient shows diffuse heterogeneity of an enlarged thyroid gland. T2 sequence better illustrates goiter heterogeneity than the T1 image. It also better reveals the more focal right lobe nodularity ➡.

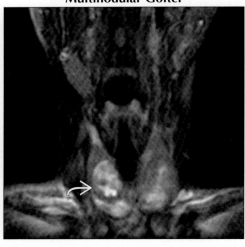

Thyroiditis, Chronic Lymphocytic (Hashimoto)

Thyroiditis, Chronic Lymphocytic (Hashimoto)

(Left) Axial NECT through the lower neck demonstrates smooth diffuse enlargement of thyroid lobes and isthmus ➡, surrounding the trachea and without invasion of adjacent structures. Note thyroid is lower in density than pectoralis muscle ➡. *(Right)* Axial T2WI MR in a different patient with a history of thyroidectomy shows homogeneous signal of "regrown" lobes ➡ except for a subtle linear hypointense band ➡ in the right lobe. This is believed to be fibrous tissue.

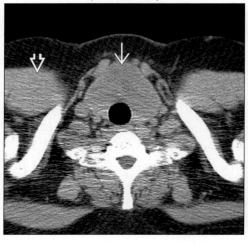

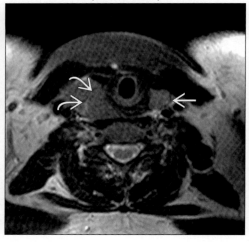

Thyroiditis, Chronic Lymphocytic (Hashimoto)

Thyroiditis, Chronic Lymphocytic (Hashimoto)

(Left) Axial NECT through lower neck shows a thyroid goiter, with both lobes ➡ appearing homogeneously enlarged but remaining well defined. The thyroid is isodense to skeletal muscle. *(Right)* Axial PET FDG scan in the same patient reveals diffusely increased uptake in enlarged thyroid lobes ➡. This was an incidental finding in a study performed to evaluate metastatic melanoma in a patient with a known history of thyroiditis and thyroxine therapy.

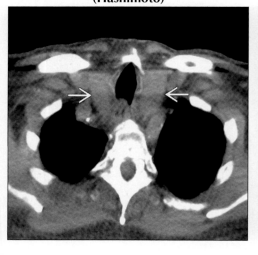

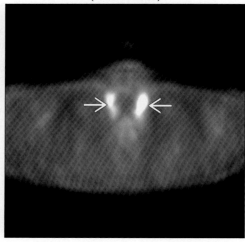

DIFFUSE THYROID ENLARGEMENT

Non-Hodgkin Lymphoma, Thyroid

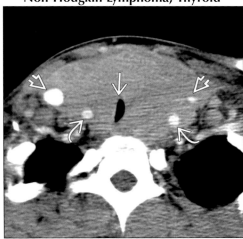

Non-Hodgkin Lymphoma, Thyroid

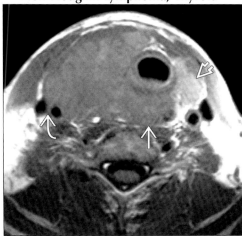

(Left) Axial CECT reveals a homogeneous infiltrative tumor engulfing thyroid and adjacent tissues. The tumor infiltrates carotid sheaths around and between the carotid ➡ and jugular vein ➡. Note that the trachea is compressed ➡. *(Right)* Axial T1WI MR shows a homogeneous hypointense mass infiltrating the right thyroid with preservation of the left ➡. The mass is relatively well circumscribed but infiltrates carotid sheath ➡ and is inseparable from esophagus ➡.

Anaplastic Carcinoma, Thyroid

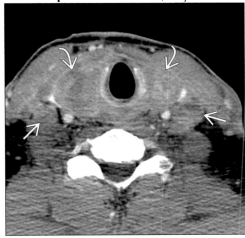

Anaplastic Carcinoma, Thyroid

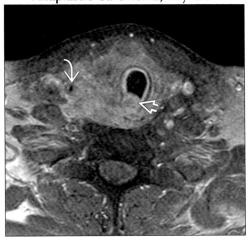

(Left) Axial CECT reveals a heterogeneous diffusely enlarged thyroid gland ➡, which is isodense & hypodense to the adjacent muscles. Also note the bilateral nodal metastases ➡. *(Right)* Axial T1 C+ FS MR demonstrates an anaplastic carcinoma invading the right neck soft tissue. The tumor infiltrates the right carotid space, narrows the carotid artery ➡, and invades the trachea ➡.

4th Branchial Anomaly

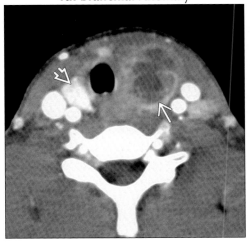

Thyroiditis, Invasive Fibrous (Riedel)

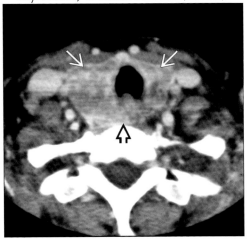

(Left) Axial CECT demonstrates marked heterogeneity of enlarged left thyroid lobe ➡ and relatively normal right lobe ➡. Heterogeneity indicates thyroid collection, although there is little evidence of overlying inflammation. Left unilaterality is another key finding. *(Right)* Axial CECT shows a diffusely heterogeneous but predominantly hypoenhancing thyroid gland ➡. There is no plane of separation between the tumor and esophagus ➡.

1

FOCAL THYROID MASS

DIFFERENTIAL DIAGNOSIS

Common
- Adenoma, Thyroid
- Colloid Cyst, Thyroid
- Multinodular Goiter
- Differentiated Carcinoma, Thyroid

Less Common
- Medullary Carcinoma, Thyroid
- Adenoma, Parathyroid, Visceral Space

Rare but Important
- Metastasis, Thyroid
- Paraganglioma, Thyroid

ESSENTIAL INFORMATION

Key Differential Diagnosis Issues
- CT and MR usually not definitive in evaluation of focal thyroid mass
  - No specificity of imaging appearance unless invasive features or adenopathy, which suggest malignancy
  - If multiple neck nodes, especially cystic, calcified, or heterogeneous, look carefully for focal thyroid primary malignancy
- Focal thyroid mass frequent incidental finding on neck CT or MR
  - Up to 16% of CT neck cases
  - Consider further evaluation by ultrasound for patient < 35 years or if punctate calcifications on CT

Helpful Clues for Common Diagnoses
- **Adenoma, Thyroid**
  - Key facts
    - Up to 75% of thyroid nodules
    - Usually multiple when present
  - Imaging
    - Variable imaging appearances
    - Solid lesions often appear poorly defined
    - Cystic degeneration or calcification results in heterogeneity of lesion
    - Imaging cannot distinguish from low grade primary thyroid malignancy
    - Diagnosis may be suggested by FNA
    - Diagnosis not proven without complete resection of mass
- **Colloid Cyst, Thyroid**
  - Key facts

- May be dominant mass in multinodular goiter presenting with sudden enlargement
    - Degeneration of adenomatous nodules; contains blood, colloid, or serous fluid
  - Imaging
    - Well-defined intrathyroid cystic mass; may be very large
    - Blood products result in variability of T1 MR signal intensity & CT density
- **Multinodular Goiter**
  - Key facts
    - Typically presents in euthyroid patient as large lower neck mass
    - May present as focal nodule, which at imaging is found to be largest of multinodular goiter
    - Diffuse heterogeneity of thyroid with adenomatous change, fibrosis, calcifications, & hemorrhage
    - May asymmetrically involve lobes or predominate in isthmus
  - Imaging
    - Thyroid enlarged & heterogeneous with multiple focal nodules and often focal calcifications
    - Thyroid gland remains well delineated from adjacent tissues
    - Cannot distinguish focal malignancy by imaging
    - Value of CT/MR is to evaluate airway compromise & full extent of lesion, including mediastinal involvement
- **Differentiated Carcinoma, Thyroid**
  - Key facts
    - Papillary carcinoma is most common form; follicular carcinoma 2nd
    - Term "differentiated thyroid carcinoma" encompasses both papillary and follicular carcinomas
    - Presentation may be focal thyroid mass or neck adenopathy
  - Imaging
    - Primary thyroid lesion may be small compared to adenopathy
    - Primary thyroid lesion may appear identical to adenoma unless invasion of adjacent tissues present
    - Larger focal intrathyroid lesions have ill-defined margin with normal thyroid
    - Nodal metastases: Cystic, solid, or mixed

FOCAL THYROID MASS

- Nodal variability in CT density/MR intensity from blood products, colloid, & calcification
- Calcifications found in primary lesion or nodes, especially with papillary type

Helpful Clues for Less Common Diagnoses

- **Medullary Carcinoma, Thyroid**
  - Key facts
    - Up to 10% of thyroid malignancies
    - Presents as painless thyroid nodule
    - Rare presentation with hypercalcitonin symptoms, paraneoplastic Cushing, or carcinoid syndromes
    - Familial form usually multifocal & bilateral; more indolent clinical course
    - May be part of MEN 2A & 2B syndromes
  - Imaging
    - Nonspecific imaging appearances
    - Usually well-circumscribed solid intrathyroidal mass
    - Calcification in primary lesion or nodes much less common than in differentiated carcinoma; typically fine, punctate
- **Adenoma, Parathyroid, Visceral Space**
  - Key facts
    - Most commonly found at posterior aspect of thyroid gland
    - Tracheoesophageal groove
    - Rarely intrathyroid location, mimicking thyroid adenoma
  - Imaging
    - Ultrasound primary imaging exam

- No distinguishing imaging features
- Diagnosis made by FNA of thyroid mass

Helpful Clues for Rare Diagnoses

- **Metastasis, Thyroid**
  - Key facts
    - Rare clinical thyroid mass; not uncommonly found at autopsy
    - Most frequently from breast, kidney, colon, or lung carcinoma or melanoma
  - Imaging
    - No distinguishing imaging features
    - May be found incidentally on FDG PET
    - In FDG PET, unexpected focal thyroid uptake in 2-3%; 45% of these lesions are metastases or malignant thyroid tumor
- **Paraganglioma, Thyroid**
  - Key facts
    - Typically presents as asymptomatic thyroid nodule; may be pulsatile
  - Imaging
    - As with paragangliomas elsewhere, hypervascular, intrathyroidal lesion
    - Mass enhances homogeneously and as intensely as normal thyroid
    - Prominent perithyroidal arteries, intralesional flow voids (MR), and avid enhancement; rarely seen in other thyroid masses
    - Caveat: Thyroid adenoma with paraganglioma-like features (PLAT) may mimic paraganglioma
    - PLAT lacks paraganglioma histochemical markers

Adenoma, Thyroid

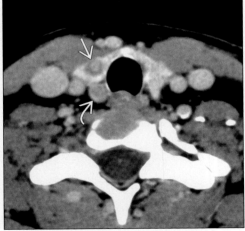

Axial CECT shows a well-defined heterogeneous but predominantly hypodense mass in the thyroid ➡. The 2nd low-density, well-defined lesion ➡ proved at surgery to be an exophytic right adenoma.

Adenoma, Thyroid

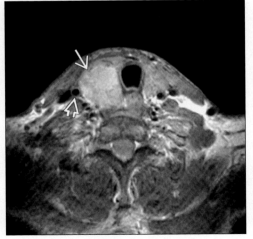

Axial T1 C+ MR reveals a large, well-circumscribed, uniform, mildly enhancing nodule ➡ replacing much of the right lobe of the thyroid gland. Note the clear delineation of the mass carotid artery laterally ➡.

FOCAL THYROID MASS

(Left) Axial CECT demonstrates a large heterogeneous cyst arising from the right thyroid lobe ➡. Higher density in the dependent portion ➡ suggests recent hemorrhage, which explains the rapid change in size. *(Right)* Axial CECT shows a large cystic mass ➡ arising from the left thyroid lobe, displacing the airway ➡ to the right. The cyst has an irregular thick rim and undulating contour, but there is no evidence of inflammatory change.

Colloid Cyst, Thyroid

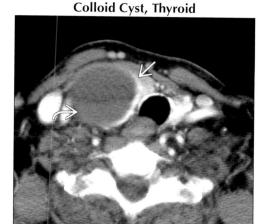

Colloid Cyst, Thyroid

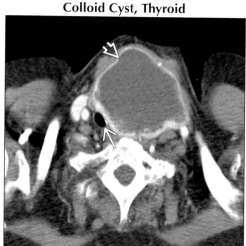

(Left) Axial CECT shows large masses distorting the trachea and asymmetrically deforming neck contour. Focal normal tissue ➡ clarifies that masses originate from thyroid gland. Lack of invasion of adjacent tissue favors benign disease. *(Right)* Axial T1 C+ FS MR reveals an asymmetrically enlarged right thyroid lobe ➡ with heterogeneous enhancement, representing 1 nodule in a multinodular goiter. The mildly enlarged left thyroid lobe ➡ is more homogeneous.

Multinodular Goiter

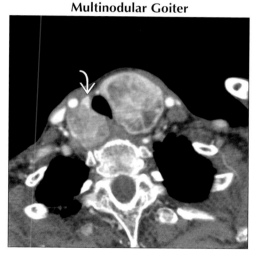

Multinodular Goiter

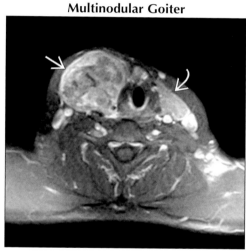

(Left) Axial CECT reveals a large low-density left neck nodal mass ➡ with peripheral nodular and linear enhancement. Low density in the left thyroid lobe ➡ is primary thyroid carcinoma, which is ill-defined but does not invade adjacent tissues. *(Right)* Axial T2WI MR demonstrates a heterogeneous thyroid gland that contains multiple nodules at the isthmus ➡. The large, fluid intensity, right neck node ➡ is a metastatic tumor from this papillary carcinoma.

Differentiated Carcinoma, Thyroid

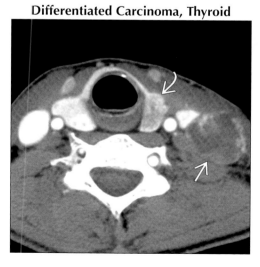

Differentiated Carcinoma, Thyroid

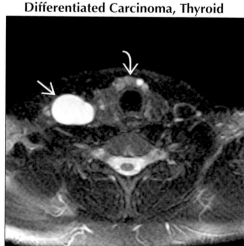

FOCAL THYROID MASS

Medullary Carcinoma, Thyroid

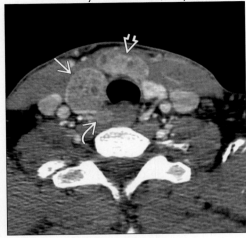

Medullary Carcinoma, Thyroid

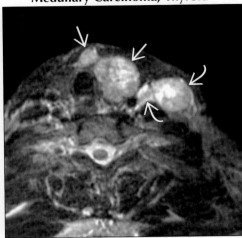

(Left) Axial CECT shows lobulated & heterogeneous appearance of right thyroid lobe ➡ & thyroid isthmus ➡. Round mass in right tracheoesophageal groove ➡ represents nodal metastasis or exophytic portion of gland. *(Right)* Axial T2WI FS MR reveals 2 heterogeneous but otherwise nonspecific focal thyroid masses ➡. Though the right thyroid node appears normal, more concerning are the enlarged left medullary carcinoma nodal metastases ➡.

Adenoma, Parathyroid, Visceral Space

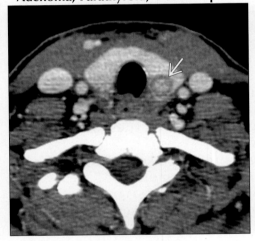

Metastasis, Thyroid

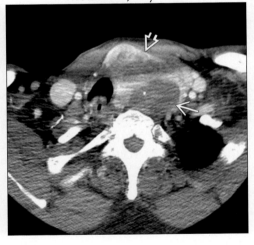

(Left) Axial CECT 2nd pass shows the target-like appearance of a focal intrathyroid lesion ➡ with peripheral washout but some residual central enhancement. Imaging appearances are otherwise nonspecific. *(Right)* Axial CECT demonstrates a markedly enlarged heterogeneous left thyroid gland with ill-defined lesion anteriorly ➡ and mixed solid-cystic lesion posteriorly ➡. This was colon carcinoma metastatic to thyroid.

Paraganglioma, Thyroid

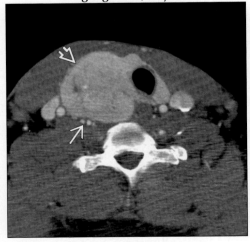

Paraganglioma, Thyroid

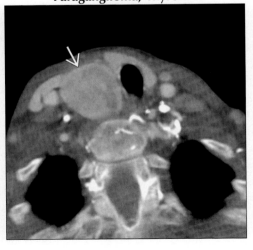

(Left) Axial CECT reveals a large enhancing mass ➡ with slightly irregular margins arising from the right thyroid gland. The mass is enhancing as intensely as normal gland, and many large feeding vessels ➡ are seen posterior to the right thyroid lobe. *(Right)* Axial CECT shows an avidly enhancing right thyroid mass ➡ with well-circumscribed borders. Thyroid paraganglioma shows homogeneous enhancement that is comparable or greater than the normal thyroid gland.

INVASIVE THYROID MASS

DIFFERENTIAL DIAGNOSIS

Common
- Anaplastic Carcinoma, Thyroid
- Non-Hodgkin Lymphoma, Thyroid
- Differentiated Carcinoma, Thyroid

Less Common
- Medullary Carcinoma, Thyroid
- Esophageal Carcinoma, Cervical
- SCCa, Hypopharynx
- SCCa, Larynx, Subglottic

Rare but Important
- 4th Branchial Anomaly + Suppurative Thyroiditis

ESSENTIAL INFORMATION

Key Differential Diagnosis Issues
- Large invasive thyroid mass not common
- May be difficult to differentiate by imaging
- Clinical history of rapidly growing mass favors anaplastic thyroid carcinoma (ATCa)
  - Main differential is thyroid lymphoma
- In these patients, diagnosis of non-Hodgkin lymphoma (NHL) favored by absence of
  - Calcification or necrosis
  - Invasion of surrounding structures
- Large cervical esophageal carcinomas may infiltrate visceral space, mimicking thyroid tumor

Helpful Clues for Common Diagnoses
- **Anaplastic Carcinoma, Thyroid**
  - Key facts: Rapidly growing mass, typically > 5 cm in diameter at presentation
    - Highly aggressive course
    - Mean survival 6 months
    - Arises in 50-60s, an older age group than differentiated thyroid cancer (DTCa)
    - Tendency to arise in multinodular goiter (MNG) or dedifferentiation of DTCa
    - Associated with prior neck irradiation
  - Imaging: CT often 1st line study; MR may give better delineation of tumor extent
    - CT/MR: Heterogeneous large mass associated with necrosis, invading surrounding tissues
    - CT: ± Calcifications from prior MNG
    - FDG PET: Useful for distant metastases
    - I-131: Not useful, as tumor does not concentrate iodine

- **Non-Hodgkin Lymphoma, Thyroid**
  - Key facts: Thyroid as primary site of NHL
    - Most commonly diffuse large B cell
    - Clinically mimics ATCa with rapidly enlarging mass in older patient
    - Markedly better prognosis!
    - Strong association with chronic lymphocytic thyroiditis (Hashimoto)
  - Imaging: Cross-sectional imaging to assess primary and nodal disease
  - CT/MR: 3 morphologic/imaging patterns may be found
    - 1) Single large mass (80%), 2) multiple thyroid masses, & 3) diffusely enlarged thyroid gland
    - Tumor tends to be homogeneous, usually without calcification or necrosis
    - Typically less invasive than ATCa
  - FDG PET: May be useful for distant metastases

- **Differentiated Carcinoma, Thyroid**
  - Key facts: 90% of thyroid malignancies, most commonly papillary or follicular
    - More common in women
    - Aged in 20s & 30s
    - Associated with prior radiation exposure
    - Generally excellent prognosis
  - Imaging: MR best; if CT must be used, avoid contrast
    - Iodine contrast uptake by tumor delays I-131 therapy 3-6 months
  - NECT/MR: Heterogeneous mass, calcifications may be present
    - Nodal metastases frequently heterogeneous, cystic, or solid
    - MR: Better delineates local invasion and nodal disease

Helpful Clues for Less Common Diagnoses
- **Medullary Carcinoma, Thyroid**
  - Key facts: Neuroendocrine malignancy
    - 5-10% thyroid malignancies
    - Most cases sporadic, multifocal
  - MEN 2A syndrome
    - Multifocal medullary thyroid carcinoma (MTC), pheochromocytoma, parathyroid hyperplasia with hyperparathyroidism
  - MEN 2B syndrome
    - Multifocal MTC, pheochromocytoma, mucosal neuromas of lips, tongue, GI tract, conjunctiva
    - Younger patients, aggressive course

- ○ Familial MTC syndrome
  - Autosomal dominant
  - Often multifocal MTC; later onset
  - No other somatic tumors
- ○ Imaging: Typically solid, circumscribed thyroid mass with adenopathy
  - Tendency for familial/inherited cases to be more infiltrative
  - CECT: No contraindication to iodine
  - May see punctate calcifications in primary ± nodes
- **Esophageal Carcinoma, Cervical**
  - ○ Key facts: Most often squamous cell carcinoma (SCCa), associated with
    - Tobacco & alcohol abuse
    - Achalasia, radiation, caustic stricture
    - 15% have synchronous or metachronous tumors (especially H&N SCCa, lung carcinoma)
  - ○ Imaging: Concentric or eccentric thickening of esophagus
    - Variable-sized, but once large typically invades adjacent structures
    - Can be difficult to determine whether primary is esophageal or thyroid
    - Tumor centered posterior to trachea
- **SCCa, Hypopharynx**
  - ○ Key facts: Mucosal primary, most often arising in pyriform sinus
    - Strong association with tobacco & alcohol abuse
    - Increased risk with radiation exposure
    - Presentation: Otalgia, dysphagia
    - Invasion of neck structures = T4 tumor

- ○ Imaging: CECT or MR for staging
  - Moderately enhancing infiltrating mass
  - Lateral spread of pyriform sinus tumor may invade thyroid, carotid sheath
  - Adenopathy common
- **SCCa, Larynx, Subglottic**
  - ○ Key facts: Least common of larynx sites
    - Mucosal tumor growing below true cords
    - 50% present with extralaryngeal spread
    - Strong association with tobacco use
  - ○ Imaging: CECT typically easier to obtain for patient comfort
    - Invasive mildly enhancing mass occupying subglottic airway and destroying cricoid cartilage
    - Infiltration of thyroid gland mimics primary thyroid tumor

Helpful Clues for Rare Diagnoses

- **4th Branchial Anomaly + Suppurative Thyroiditis**
  - ○ Key facts: Rare site for infection if no penetrating injury or FNA history
    - If isolated suppurative thyroiditis, 4th branchial anomaly present
    - Sinus tract from pyriform sinus apex to left thyroid lobe present
  - ○ Imaging: Heterogeneous, low-density left thyroid ± collection & overlying inflammatory changes (CECT)
    - When acute inflammation treated, CT with oral contrast may outline tract

Anaplastic Carcinoma, Thyroid

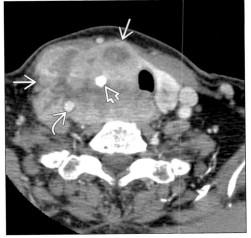

Axial CECT shows a large heterogeneous mass arising from the right thyroid ➔ but invading the adjacent tissues and surrounding the right common carotid artery ➔. Large calcification ➔ is also present.

Anaplastic Carcinoma, Thyroid

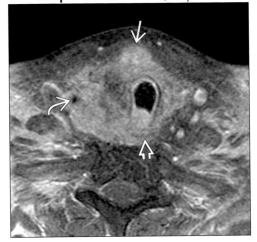

Axial T1 C+ FS MR reveals a tumor invading the right thyroid lobe and isthmus ➔ with extrathyroid infiltration engulfing the right carotid space ➔. The mass is inseparable from the cervical esophagus ➔.

INVASIVE THYROID MASS

(Left) Axial CECT shows multiple low-density masses ➡ expanding and encasing the thyroid gland with deep invasion of adjacent muscle ⬌. This is unusual for primary thyroid non-Hodgkin lymphoma, which tends to compress adjacent tissues without invasion. *(Right)* Axial T1WI MR reveals a large solid mass ➡ infiltrating the right thyroid lobe and adjacent carotid space ⬌. The tumor also displaces the trachea and cervical esophagus ⬌ to the left.

Non-Hodgkin Lymphoma, Thyroid

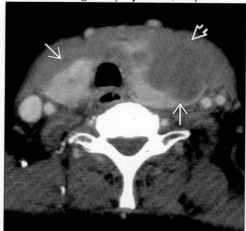

Non-Hodgkin Lymphoma, Thyroid

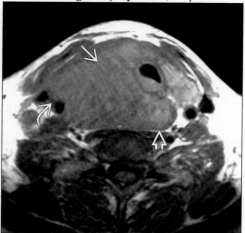

(Left) Axial NECT demonstrates a large infiltrative mass ➡ arising from the left thyroid lobe and involving many surrounding tissues, including cervical esophagus ⬌. Note small calcifications ➡ within the body of tumor. *(Right)* Axial CECT reveals a large heterogeneous noncalcified mass ➡ that arises in the right thyroid but extends across midline of gland and involves surrounding soft tissues. Tracheal invasion ⬌ was found at surgery.

Differentiated Carcinoma, Thyroid

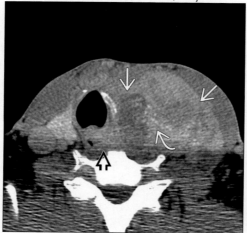

Differentiated Carcinoma, Thyroid

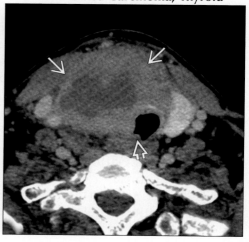

(Left) Axial CECT shows lobulated heterogeneous appearance of right thyroid lobe ➡ and more invasive appearance of heterogeneous isthmus ➡ involving strap muscles. Note an additional small enhancing heterogeneous node ➡. *(Right)* Axial T2WI MR through lower neck shows a heterogeneous left thyroid mass ➡. Though appearing well defined, mass could not be separated from trachea at surgery. Tracheal nodules ➡ were found to be tumor invasion.

Medullary Carcinoma, Thyroid

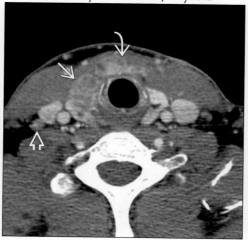

Medullary Carcinoma, Thyroid

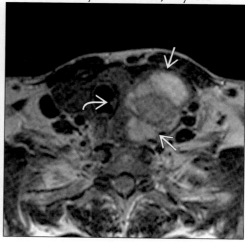

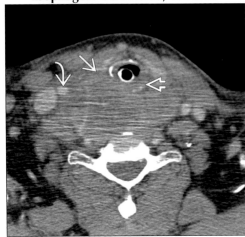

INVASIVE THYROID MASS

Esophageal Carcinoma, Cervical

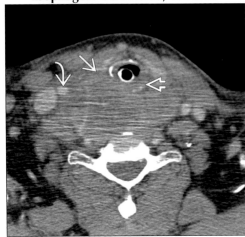

Esophageal Carcinoma, Cervical

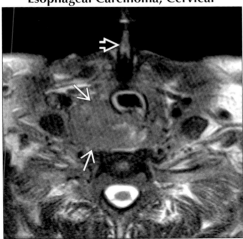

(Left) Axial CECT shows a bulky heterogeneous lower neck retrotracheal mass infiltrating inferior thyroid gland ➡, posterior cricoid ➡, and right carotid artery ➡. This invasive mass proved to arise from upper cervical esophagus. (Right) Axial T2WI MR reveals a large mass ➡ behind the trachea & lower thyroid. Thyroid gland is inseparable from esophagus, making primary site determination difficult. Note patient has tracheostomy ➡ from airway compromise.

SCCa, Hypopharynx

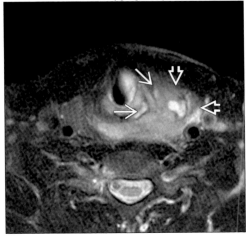

SCCa, Larynx, Subglottic

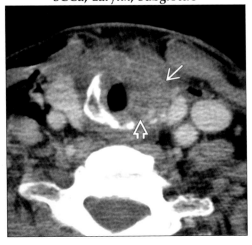

(Left) Axial T2WI FS MR shows a large infiltrative T2 hyperintense mass, which appears centered in the left thyroid, but actually arose as a left hypopharyngeal SCCa with invasion of thyroid ➡ and laryngeal cartilages ➡. (Right) Axial CECT shows an infiltrative mass in the lower neck involving the left thyroid gland ➡ and left part of cricoid cartilage ➡. Mass was determined to be subglottic SCCa, 50% of which present with extralaryngeal tumor spread (T4).

4th Branchial Anomaly + Suppurative Thyroiditis

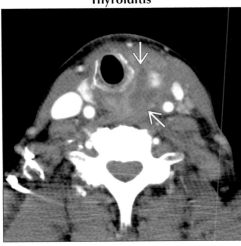

4th Branchial Anomaly + Suppurative Thyroiditis

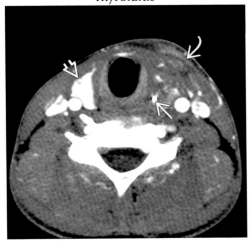

(Left) Axial CECT shows a heterogeneous fluid collection ➡ involving left thyroid lobe & distorting left neck with overlying acute inflammatory changes. When left-sided thyroiditis is present, pyriform sinus tract must be sought (4th branchial anomaly). (Right) Axial CECT shows a normal dense enhancing right thyroid ➡ but a heterogeneous left thyroid with overlying inflammatory change ➡. Dense focus ➡ is barium along pyriform sinus tract to thyroid.

CHEEK MASS

DIFFERENTIAL DIAGNOSIS

Common
- Abscess, Masticator Space
- Benign Mixed Tumor, Parotid
- Accessory Parotid Gland
- Venous Malformation
- Infantile Hemangioma
- SCCa, Buccal Mucosa
- SCCa, Nodes, Facial
- Warthin Tumor
- Benign Masticator Muscle Hypertrophy

Less Common
- Mucoepidermoid Carcinoma, Parotid
- Adenoid Cystic Carcinoma, Parotid
- Metastasis, Mandible-Maxilla
- Ameloblastoma
- Osteosarcoma, Mandible-Maxilla
- Juvenile Angiofibroma
- Chondrosarcoma, Masticator Space

Rare but Important
- Minor Salivary Gland Malignancy, Oral
- Schwannoma, Parotid
- Pigmented Villonodular Synovitis, TMJ
- Chondromatosis, Synovial, TMJ
- Sarcoma, Other, Masticator Space

ESSENTIAL INFORMATION

Key Differential Diagnosis Issues
- Imaging strategies for cheek mass
  ○ CT or MR appropriate 1st line modality
  ○ Beware artifact from dental amalgam obscuring buccal space on either CT/MR
  ○ Clinical history of "cheek mass" covers large anatomic area of anterolateral face
    ▪ Premolar region to preauricular area
    ▪ Zygomatic arch to angle of mandible
  ○ Lesion arise from masticator (MS), parotid (PS), & buccal (BS) spaces

Helpful Clues for Common Diagnoses
- **Abscess, Masticator Space**
  ○ Suggestive presentation: Acute swelling, pain, tenderness ± recent dental extraction
  ○ CECT: Enlargement of masticator muscles, stranding of overlying fat & thick platysma
    ▪ Focal low-density pus collection may be subtle; look carefully!
  ○ Bone CT: Look for dental infection
- **Benign Mixed Tumor, Parotid**

○ Preauricular mass; often longstanding
○ CECT: Mildly C+ superficial parotid mass
  ▪ Ca++ ± focal low density possible
  ▪ If large, replacing much of parotid, mass may look isodense to muscle
- **Accessory Parotid Gland**
  ○ Clenching teeth makes mass palpable
  ○ CT/MR: Lenticular soft tissue of similar density/intensity & C+ as normal parotid
  ○ Normal parotid tissue may be diseased
    ▪ Sjögren, salivary neoplasms, etc.
    ▪ Lesion arises from accessory gland if on masseter surface
- **Venous Malformation**
  ○ Mass often longstanding
    ▪ Bluish discoloration of skin possible
  ○ CECT: Ill-defined lobulated mass; often trans-spatial
    ▪ Presence of phleboliths diagnostic
  ○ MR: T2 hyperintense, C+, infiltrative mass
    ▪ Phleboliths hypointense on T2 MR
- **Infantile Hemangioma**
  ○ Rapidly enlarging cheek mass in infant
  ○ CT/MR: Avid C+ well-defined mass
    ▪ Large vessels in center of lesion
- **SCCa, Buccal Mucosa**
  ○ Clinically evident mucosal mass
    ▪ Invasive SCCa if palpable cheek mass
  ○ CT/MR: Mass invades laterally to buccal fat
    ▪ "Puff-cheek" CT shows lesion best as this separates buccal from gingival mucosa
- **SCCa, Nodes, Facial**
  ○ Facial nodes, skin, or oral mucosal SCCa
  ○ CT/MR: Nodal mass in buccal fat pad
- **Warthin Tumor**
  ○ Inferior cheek mass; smoker
  ○ CT/MR: Frequently cystic or mixed cystic-solid masses
    ▪ Multiple or bilateral (20%)
- **Benign Masticator Muscle Hypertrophy**
  ○ When unilateral, facial asymmetry
  ○ CT/MR: Enlargement of muscles of mastication
    ▪ Same density/intensity as other muscles; similar C+

Helpful Clues for Less Common Diagnoses
- **Mucoepidermoid Carcinoma, Parotid**
  ○ CT/MR: Invasive parotid tumor
- **Adenoid Cystic Carcinoma, Parotid**
  ○ CT/MR: Invasive parotid tumor
    ▪ Potential for CN7 perineural spread

- **Metastasis, Mandible-Maxilla**
  - Known malignancy history
  - CT/MR: Destructive bony lesion
- **Ameloblastoma**
  - CT/MR: "Bubbly," mixed cystic-solid mass in mandibular ramus associated with unerupted 3rd molar tooth
- **Osteosarcoma, Mandible-Maxilla**
  - CT/MR: Destructive lesion with periosteal elevation & osseous tumor matrix
- **Juvenile Angiofibroma**
  - Adolescent male
  - CT/MR: C+ nasal tumor extends through pterygopalatine fossa into MS & BS
- **Chondrosarcoma, Masticator Space**
  - CT/MR: Chondroid matrix in MS tumor

Helpful Clues for Rare Diagnoses
- **Minor Salivary Gland Malignancy, Oral**
  - CT/MR: Buccal mucosa invasive tumor
- **Schwannoma, Parotid**
  - CT/MR: Fusiform C+ well-circumscribed PS mass ± intramural cysts
- **Pigmented Villonodular Synovitis, TMJ**
  - MR: Enhancing nodular TMJ masses
  - T1 & T2 low signal from hemosiderin deposits
- **Chondromatosis, Synovial, TMJ**
  - Synovial membrane nodular proliferation
  - CT/MR: Fragments calcify/ossify
- **Sarcoma, Other, Masticator Space**
  - CT/MR: Invasive MS mass

Alternative Differential Approaches
- Anatomic spatial approach to cheek masses

  - Cheek mass may be from BS, MS, or PS
- **Buccal space lesions**
  - SCCa, buccal mucosa
  - SCCa, nodes, facial
  - Minor salivary gland malignancy, oral
- **Masticator space lesions**
  - Abscess, masticator space
  - Muscle mass
    - Benign masticator muscle hypertrophy
    - Sarcoma, other, masticator space
  - Bone mass (mandible or maxilla)
    - Metastasis, mandible-maxilla
    - Ameloblastoma
    - Osteosarcoma, mandible-maxilla
    - Chondrosarcoma, masticator space
  - TMJ-origin mass
    - Chondromatosis, synovial, TMJ
    - Synovitis, pigmented villonodular, TMJ
- **Parotid space lesions**
  - Benign mixed tumor, parotid
  - Accessory parotid gland
  - Warthin tumor
  - Mucoepidermoid carcinoma, parotid
  - Adenoid cystic carcinoma, parotid
  - Schwannoma, parotid
- **Trans-spatial lesions**
  - Involves multiple contiguous spaces
  - Any malignant tumor from BS, MS, PS
  - Advanced abscess; often inadequately treated with oral antibiotics
  - Congenital or developmental lesions
    - Venous malformation
    - Infantile hemangioma

Abscess, Masticator Space

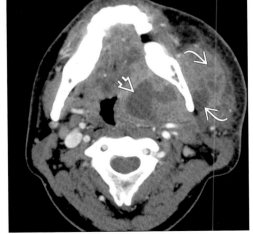

Axial CECT shows marked swelling of left cheek with multifocal abscesses in the masseter muscle ➋ and infiltration of subcutaneous fat. A large abscess in the medial pterygoid ➋ narrows the oropharynx.

Abscess, Masticator Space

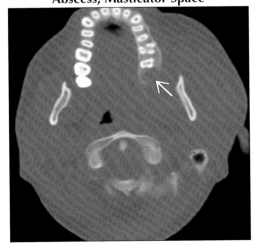

Axial bone CT demonstrates the origin of masticator space abscesses as the maxillary molar root socket. Note the alveolar bone loss ➋. Most masticator space infections are of dental origin.

CHEEK MASS

(Left) Axial T2WI FS MR shows a lobulated heterogeneous mass ➡️ sharply delineated from adjacent tissues, suggesting benign process. Lesion is predominantly hyperintense as expected with benign mixed tumor. (Right) Axial T1 C+ FS MR shows a heterogeneous peripherally enhancing mass ➡️ in parotid, distending left cheek. No overlying inflammatory features seen to suggest abscess. Areas lacking enhancement are often mistaken for necrosis.

Benign Mixed Tumor, Parotid

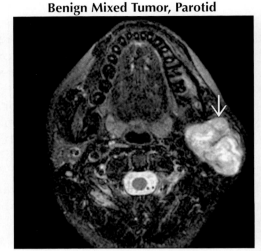

Benign Mixed Tumor, Parotid

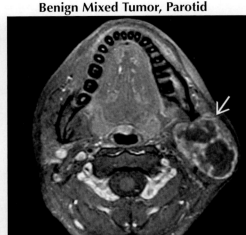

(Left) Axial CECT shows bilateral accessory parotid glands ➡️ overlying masseter muscles. Their location is characteristic, and the density, texture, and enhancement are similar to parotids. Accessory glands, when present, are not always bilateral. (Right) Axial CECT demonstrates a mildly enhancing heterogeneous mass ➡️ distending cheek. Focal calcification noted within lesion anteriorly ➡️. The mass arises from accessory parotid tissue on surface of masseter.

Accessory Parotid Gland

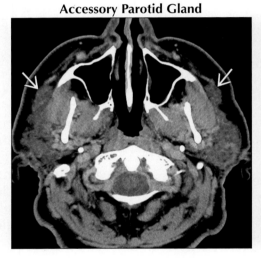

Accessory Parotid Gland

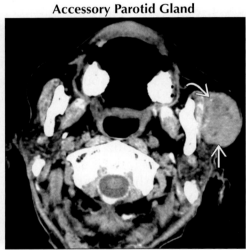

(Left) Axial STIR MR shows an infiltrative T2 hyperintense mass expanding cheek & predominantly involving buccal space ➡️, though deep component extends to parapharyngeal fat ➡️ & oral cavity ➡️. The well-defined oval low intensity foci are phleboliths. (Right) Axial T2WI FS MR shows a large markedly hyperintense mass distending cheek & replacing superficial ➡️ & deep ➡️ lobes of parotid. Note the prominent intralesional vessels ➡️.

Venous Malformation

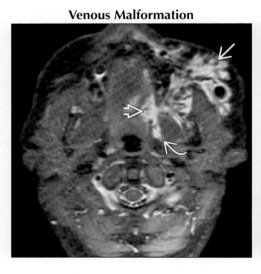

Infantile Hemangioma

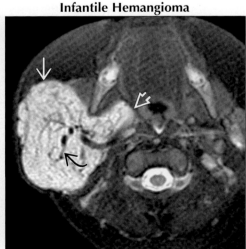

SCCa, Buccal Mucosa

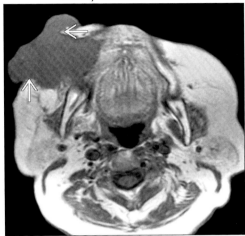

SCCa, Nodes, Facial

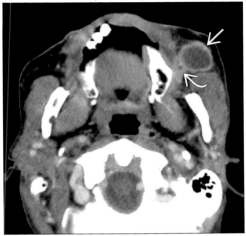

(Left) Axial T1WI MR shows an unusually large SCCa of the right buccal mucosa extending through the buccal fat and subcutaneous cheek tissues to the skin surface ➡, where it forms a fungating mass. *(Right)* Axial CECT shows a rim-enhancing cystic mass ➡ in the left buccal space anterior to the parotid and immediately abutting the facial vein and distal parotid duct ➡. This was a metastatic tumor from prior resected left cheek skin SCCa.

Warthin Tumor

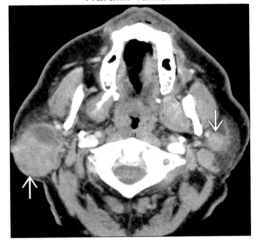

Warthin Tumor

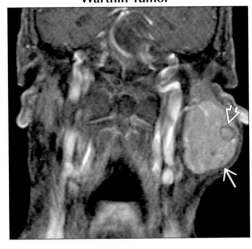

(Left) Axial CECT reveals bilateral, mixed solid & cystic, circumscribed, enhancing masses ➡ within the parotid glands. There is no cervical adenopathy in this smoker who presented with a right cheek mass. *(Right)* Coronal T1 C+ FS MR shows a large, enhancing, sharply marginated Warthin tumor projecting inferiorly off the parotid tail ➡. Note the low signal ring of calcification seen in the lateral margin of the tumor ➡.

Benign Masticator Muscle Hypertrophy

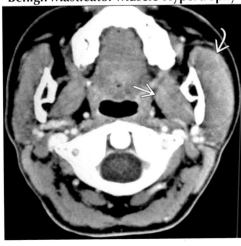

Benign Masticator Muscle Hypertrophy

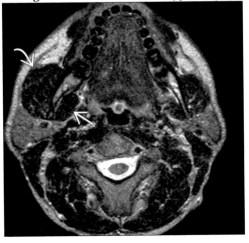

(Left) Axial CECT shows asymmetric enlargement of the masseter ➡. Enhancement is similar to other muscles. Note also the enlargement of ipsilateral medial pterygoid muscle ➡. *(Right)* Axial T2WI MR shows asymmetric enlargement of the right masseter muscle ➡ in a different patient. Masseter remains isointense to other muscles of mastication, and there is no underlying mass. Additionally, note the subtle enlargement of the right medial pterygoid ➡.

CHEEK MASS

(Left) Coronal T1 C+ FS MR shows a poorly defined enhancing mass ➡ replacing much of the right superficial parotid lobe. The margins and metastatic cervical adenopathy ➡ suggest a malignant neoplasm. *(Right)* Axial T2WI MR shows ill-defined increased signal throughout the superficial parotid lobe ➡ that is causing enlargement of left cheek. The mass extends to deep lobe also ➡. The lesion's ill-defined contour suggests malignant primary neoplasm.

Mucoepidermoid Carcinoma, Parotid

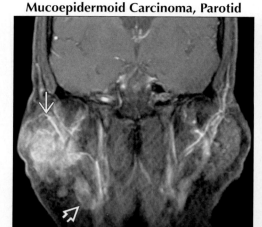

Adenoid Cystic Carcinoma, Parotid

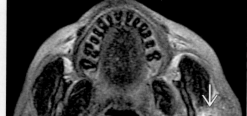

(Left) Axial T1 C+ FS MR reveals destruction of the mandibular angle ➡ by a metastatic lesion with a subtly enhancing soft tissue mass enlarging the medial pterygoid ➡ & masseter, distending the cheek. *(Right)* Axial CECT shows a expansile solid and cystic mass at left angle of mandible, with marked thinning of the mandible cortex and focal areas of cortical destruction ➡. There is no involvement of the adjacent parotid gland and no neck adenopathy.

Metastasis, Mandible-Maxilla

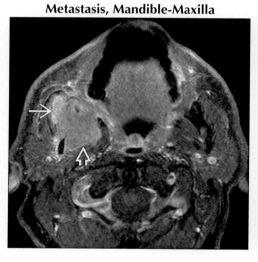

Ameloblastoma

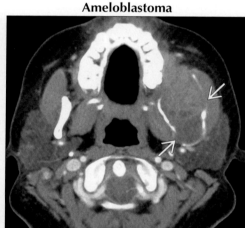

(Left) Axial CECT reveals a large, dense mass arising from angle of mandible and invading masseter ➡ and medial pterygoid ➡ muscles. *(Right)* Axial CECT reveals a large heterogeneous mass ➡ distinct from parotid, filling the left buccal space. This mass had "herniated" through the pterygopalatine fossa and pterygomaxillary fissure to the masticator and buccal spaces, arising originally in the lateral nose.

Osteosarcoma, Mandible-Maxilla

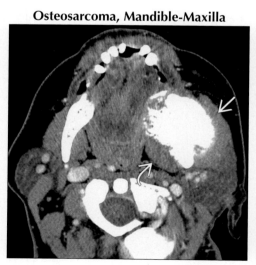

Juvenile Angiofibroma

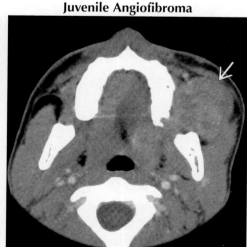

Chondrosarcoma, Masticator Space

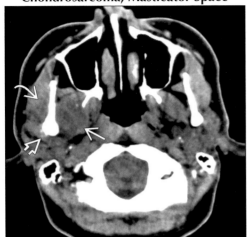

Minor Salivary Gland Malignancy, Oral

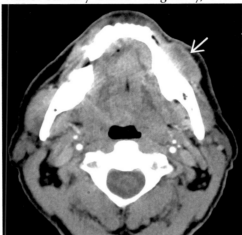

(Left) Axial NECT shows a low-density mass in the lateral pterygoid ➡ and masseter ➡ muscles, suggesting the process arises from mandibular body and ramus. Subtle calcifications ➡ make metastasis unlikely. (Right) Axial CECT shows a relatively well-circumscribed mass lateral to the mandible ➡, distorting lower cheek contour. The mass appears to be invasive, arising from the buccal mucosa. The lesion is better defined than might be expected for SCCa.

Schwannoma, Parotid

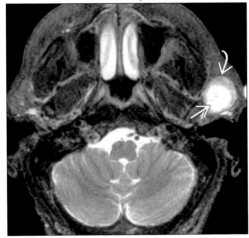

Pigmented Villonodular Synovitis, TMJ

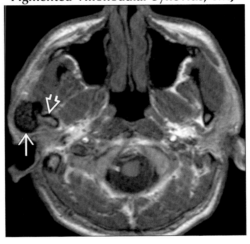

(Left) Axial T2WI FS MR shows a centrally hyperintense mass ➡ with peripheral intermediate signal rim in superficial parotid ➡. This target-like feature may also be seen on post-contrast images and suggests a schwannoma. (Right) Axial T1WI MR shows a low signal intensity mass ➡ just lateral to mandibular condyle ➡ with markedly lower peripheral signal intensity. Low signal intensity is secondary to blood products, especially hemosiderin.

Chondromatosis, Synovial, TMJ

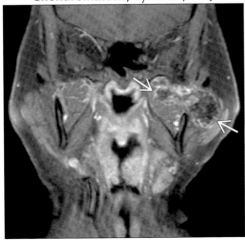

Sarcoma, Other, Masticator Space

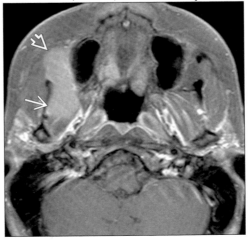

(Left) Coronal T1 C+ FS MR demonstrates a heterogeneously enhancing mass ➡ in the left temporomandibular joint with multiple foci of low signal within its lateral component. This low signal is secondary to calcifications within the lesion. (Right) Axial T1 C+ FS MR shows an enhancing masticator ➡ and buccal space ➡ mass in a patient without mucosal SCCa. Biopsy specimen revealed fibrosarcoma.

TRISMUS

DIFFERENTIAL DIAGNOSIS

Common
- Fracture, Mandible
- Trauma/Dislocation, TMJ
- Abscess, Palatine Tonsil
- Abscess, Masticator Space
- SCCa, Retromolar Trigone
- SCCa, Palatine Tonsil
- Radiation Changes, Acute
- Radiation Changes, Chronic

Less Common
- Sarcoma, Other, Masticator Space
- Osteosarcoma, Mandible-Maxilla
- Chondrosarcoma, Masticator Space
- Osteoradionecrosis, Mandible-Maxilla

Rare but Important
- Chondromatosis, Synovial, TMJ
- Synovitis, Pigmented Villonodular, TMJ
- Chondrocalcinosis, TMJ
- Perineural Tumor, CNV3, MS

ESSENTIAL INFORMATION

Key Differential Diagnosis Issues
- Trismus: Restricted opening of mouth from prolonged jaw muscle contraction
- Most frequent causes
  - Abnormalities of mandible ± TMJ
    - Trauma or TMJ arthropathies
  - Processes involving muscles of mastication ± deep face
    - Inflammation: Dental or peritonsillar abscess; radiation
    - Primary neoplasms: Sarcomas of muscles, mandible, or TMJ
    - Invasive neoplasms: SCCa invading deeply from oral cavity or oropharynx
  - Processes in which imaging usually not required/obtained
    - Tetanus, malignant hyperthermia
    - Side effect of methamphetamines and neuroleptics
- Imaging strategy
  - CT best 1st line study
    - Bone CT: Trauma, arthropathies
    - CECT: Infection, tumors
  - MR complementary
    - Tumor evaluation/characterization
    - Helps with skull base & perineural tumor spread

Helpful Clues for Common Diagnoses
- **Fracture, Mandible**
  - Key facts
    - Mandible analogous to pelvic ring; search for 2nd fracture or TMJ dislocation
    - 50% bilateral; 15% other facial fractures
  - Imaging
    - Bone CT: Linear lucency
- **Trauma/Dislocation, TMJ**
  - Key facts
    - Uni- or bilateral; unable to close mouth; masseteric spasm
    - Isolated or with mandibular fracture
  - Imaging
    - Displacement of condyle from fossa
- **Abscess, Palatine Tonsil**
  - Key facts
    - Tonsillitis first: Sore throat & fever
    - Onset of trismus suggests abscess
  - Imaging
    - CECT: Low-density collection or multiple small collections
- **Abscess, Masticator Space**
  - Key facts
    - Usually follows recent molar extraction
  - Imaging
    - CECT: Swollen masticator muscles
    - Focal abscesses may NOT have rim enhancement
    - May see small low density pockets
- **SCCa, Retromolar Trigone**
  - Key facts
    - Tends to invade mandible early (T4)
    - Anterolateral spread along buccinator
    - Posteromedially to oral cavity & medial pterygoid muscle
  - Imaging
    - CECT/MR: May only see loss of buccal fat & "full" buccinator or pterygoids
- **SCCa, Palatine Tonsil**
  - Key facts
    - Associated with alcohol abuse & tobacco
    - Up to 50% associated with HPV infection
  - Imaging
    - CECT/MR: Enlarged, enhancing tonsil
    - Look for deep extension to masticator muscles and carotid artery
- **Radiation Changes, Acute**
  - Key facts
    - Edema of soft tissues post-radiation

○ Imaging
  ▪ CECT: Swelling and loss of clarity of muscle fibers
  ▪ MR: T2 hyperintensity, muscle enhancement
- **Radiation Changes, Chronic**
  ○ Key facts
    ▪ Radiation-induced soft tissue fibrosis
    ▪ Severity dictated by radiation dose
  ○ Imaging
    ▪ Atrophy of muscles with loss of normal striations, paucity of fat

Helpful Clues for Less Common Diagnoses
- **Sarcoma, Other, Masticator Space**
  ○ Key facts
    ▪ Rhabdomyosarcoma most common
  ○ Imaging
    ▪ Aggressive, poorly defined mass
- **Osteosarcoma, Mandible-Maxilla**
  ○ Key facts
    ▪ Malignant tumor with osteoid matrix
  ○ Imaging
    ▪ Bone formation ± aggressive periosteal reaction
- **Chondrosarcoma, Masticator Space**
  ○ Key facts
    ▪ Arises in TMJ or masticator muscles
  ○ Imaging
    ▪ CECT: Invasive mass, ± calcifications
    ▪ MR: Typically T2 hyperintense, invasive
- **Osteoradionecrosis, Mandible-Maxilla**
  ○ Key facts
    ▪ Loss of bone vitality after radiation

▪ Often accompanied by infection
○ Imaging
  ▪ CT: Lytic permeative change, cortical loss
  ▪ MR: Marrow bright on T2, dark on T1

Helpful Clues for Rare Diagnoses
- **Chondromatosis, Synovial, TMJ**
  ○ Key facts
    ▪ Benign calcifying synovial metaplasia
  ○ Imaging
    ▪ CT: Calcified loose bodies in TMJ
    ▪ MR: Focal signal voids T1 & T2
- **Synovitis, Pigmented Villonodular, TMJ**
  ○ Key facts
    ▪ Monoarticular inflammatory arthropathy
  ○ Imaging
    ▪ Bone CT: Articular erosions, cysts
    ▪ MR: Heterogeneous mass, dark T2 signal
- **Chondrocalcinosis, TMJ**
  ○ Key facts
    ▪ Calcium pyrophosphate dihydrate deposition (CPPD) in joint
  ○ Imaging
    ▪ CT: Calcified mass involving joint space with degenerative changes
    ▪ MR: Low T2 periarticular signal with inhomogeneous enhancement
- **Perineural Tumor, CNV3, MS**
  ○ Key facts
    ▪ Facial pain/dysesthesias ⇒ trismus
  ○ Imaging
    ▪ CECT: Often subtle; enlarged inferior alveolar canal or foramen ovale
    ▪ MR: Thickening, enhancement of CNV3

Fracture, Mandible

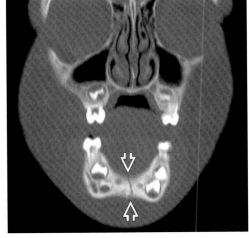

Coronal bone CT in a child with unwitnessed trauma reveals symphyseal fracture ⇨ without displacement. Mandible fractures often come in pairs; a 2nd fracture or TMJ dislocation should be sought.

Trauma/Dislocation, TMJ

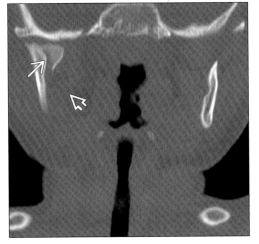

Coronal bone CT in the same patient shows condylar intraarticular fracture ⇨ with TMJ dislocation. Swelling of the right face and stranding of the medial pterygoid ⇨ is subtle on bone CT.

TRISMUS

Abscess, Palatine Tonsil

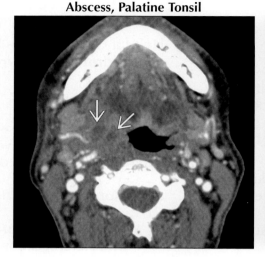

Abscess, Palatine Tonsil

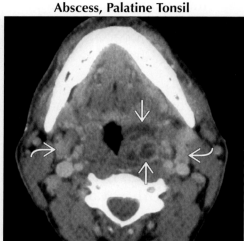

(Left) Axial CECT demonstrates asymmetric soft tissue fullness in the right oropharynx with deformity of the airway. Ill-defined regions of low density ➡ indicate pockets of pus within enlarged palatine tonsil. (Right) Axial CECT shows a more complex left tonsillar abscess with a multilocular collection involving the left palatine tonsil ➡. The airway is deformed and multiple bilateral reactive nodes are noted ➡.

Abscess, Masticator Space

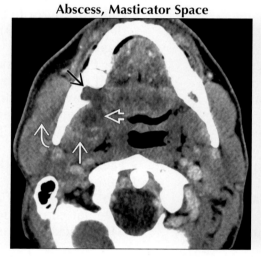

Abscess, Masticator Space

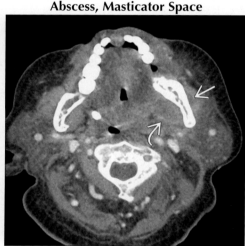

(Left) Axial CECT shows a low density collection ➡ in the right deep face contiguous with socket of extracted tooth ➡. Swelling & enlargement of the right medial pterygoid ➡, masseter ➡, & overlying subcutaneous fat stranding are consistent with infection. (Right) Axial CECT in a more subtle case shows swelling of the medial pterygoid ➡ but marked edema extending deep into parapharyngeal fat. Crescentic low density ➡ abutting mandibular ramus is typical of abscess.

SCCa, Retromolar Trigone

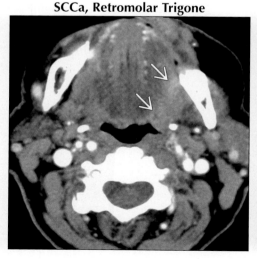

SCCa, Retromolar Trigone

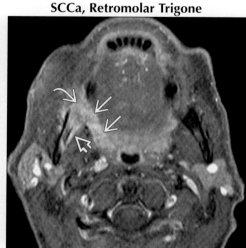

(Left) Axial CECT reveals asymmetric enhancement in the left oral cavity representing posteromedial extension of a retromolar trigone tumor ➡. (Right) Axial T1 C+ FS MR in a different patient shows an enhancing tumor arising in the right retromolar trigone ➡ and spreading posteromedially ➡. Invasion of the mandibular marrow and infiltration along the medial margin of the mandible ➡ is also present.

SCCa, Palatine Tonsil

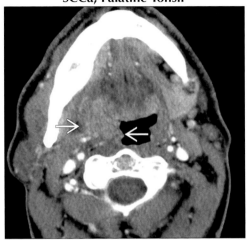

SCCa, Palatine Tonsil

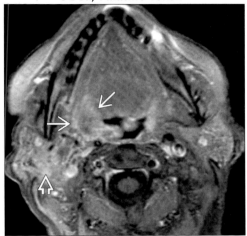

(Left) Axial CECT shows a large right enhancing tonsil ➡ with an ill-defined deep margin. This patient presented with trismus and a palpable ipsilateral level II node. *(Right)* Axial T1 C+ FS MR in a different patient reveals a heterogeneous, large, irregular mass in the right palatine tonsil ➡ extending toward the right tongue base. A heterogeneous enhancing mass in the right neck ➡ is the superior aspect of the nodal mass.

Radiation Changes, Acute

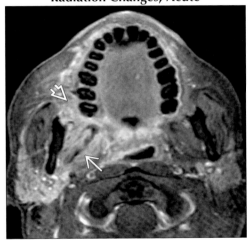

Radiation Changes, Acute

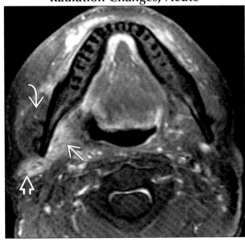

(Left) Axial T1 C+ FS MR 3 months after radiation therapy for palatine tonsillar SCCa shows intense enhancement of large right medial pterygoid muscle ➡, parotid gland, and oral cavity mucosa ➡. The oropharyngeal airway is deformed due to edema. *(Right)* Axial T1 C+ FS MR inferiorly shows marked enhancement of the medial pterygoid ➡ and parotid tail ➡. Relative preservation of the masseter muscle ➡ signal argues against denervation injury.

Radiation Changes, Chronic

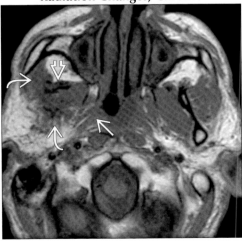

Radiation Changes, Chronic

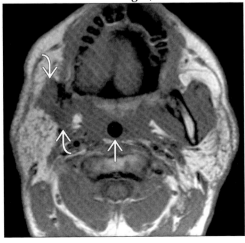

(Left) Axial T1WI MR in a patient radiated 9 years prior for nasopharyngeal carcinoma shows marked degeneration of the mandible from osteoradionecrosis with only a portion of the coronoid process visible ➡. Note the atrophic & scarred right muscles of mastication ➡ & the right nasopharynx ➡. *(Right)* Axial T1WI MR in the same patient shows similar atrophic, scarred appearance of the masticator muscles ➡ & deep facial tissues, with oropharyngeal stenosis ➡.

TRISMUS

Sarcoma, Other, Masticator Space

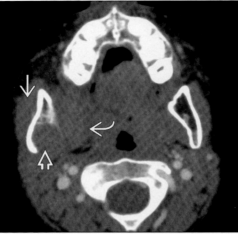

Sarcoma, Other, Masticator Space

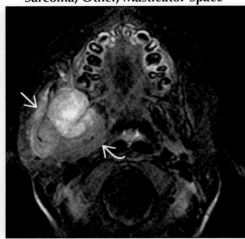

(Left) Axial CECT in a child shows a large, minimally enhancing rhabdomyosarcoma involving the right mandible ➡. Medial pterygoid ➡ & masseter ➡ involvement is subtle. *(Right)* Axial T2WI FS MR in the same patient allows better determination of the extent of soft tissue component. Masseteric ➡ & medial pterygoid ➡ involvement are more clearly evident with a tumor that is quite hyperintense relative to normal contralateral muscles.

Chondrosarcoma, Masticator Space

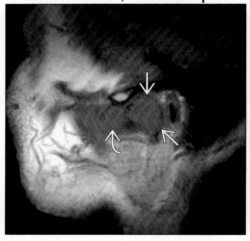

Chondrosarcoma, Masticator Space

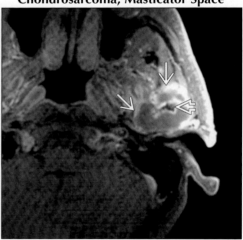

(Left) Sagittal T1WI MR through TMJ reveals a soft tissue mass encompassing & destroying the condylar head ➡ & filling glenoid fossa. Anterior extension into lateral pterygoid muscle ➡ evident with loss of normal muscle striations. *(Right)* Axial T1 C+ FS MR in the same patient shows rim enhancement of TMJ mass ➡ & focal low intensity residual condyle ➡. Soft tissue invasion suggests aggressive process. Lack of overlying inflammatory changes rules out infection.

Osteoradionecrosis, Mandible-Maxilla

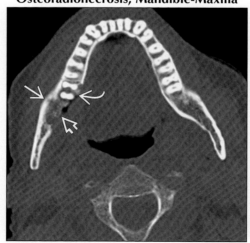

Osteoradionecrosis, Mandible-Maxilla

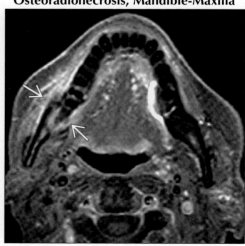

(Left) Axial bone CT in a patient with previous history of melanoma metastasis radiation demonstrates a destructive process affecting the posterior mandibular body ➡ with medial cortex loss ➡, punctate air and lucency around the posterior mandibular molar ➡. These findings are typical for mandibular osteoradionecrosis. *(Right)* Axial T1 C+ FS MR in the same patient shows enhancing tissue surrounding and within the radiated mandible ➡.

Chondromatosis, Synovial, TMJ

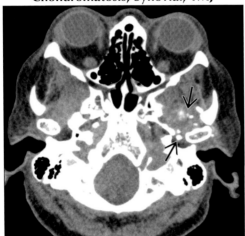

Chondromatosis, Synovial, TMJ

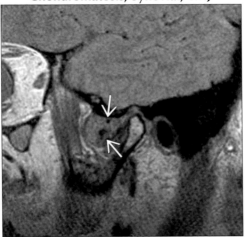

(Left) Axial NECT reveals a lesion in the left temporomandibular joint with multiple punctate calcifications ➡, typical of synovial chondromatosis. *(Right)* Sagittal T1WI MR shows a mass lesion in the anterior temporomandibular joint with multiple low signal foci ➡, secondary to calcified loose bodies, found in synovial chondromatosis.

Synovitis, Pigmented Villonodular, TMJ

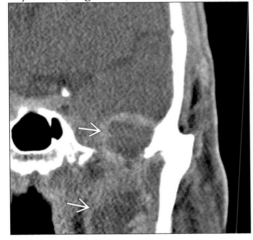

Synovitis, Pigmented Villonodular, TMJ

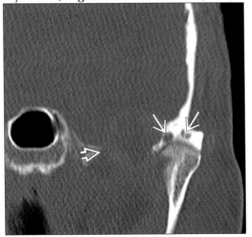

(Left) Coronal CECT shows a multicystic bilobed pigmented villonodular synovitis lesion affecting the medial aspect of the left TMJ ➡. *(Right)* Coronal bone CT in the same patient demonstrates a subarticular cystic change ➡ associated with a broad area of bony floor of middle cranial fossa dehiscence ➡.

Chondrocalcinosis, TMJ

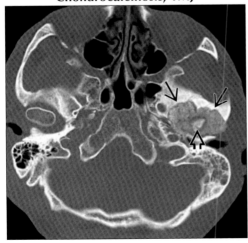

Perineural Tumor, CNV3, MS

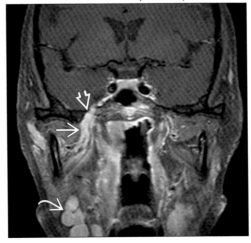

(Left) Axial bone CT demonstrates a calcified mass in the left TMJ that erodes and enlarges the condylar fossa ➡. The mandibular condyle has been remodeled ➡ by this focus of chondrocalcinosis. *(Right)* Coronal T1 C+ FS MR shows perineural NHL as an enlarged tubular enhancing mandibular division of the trigeminal nerve ➡ poking into the foramen ovale ➡. Note also the multiple large, uniformly enhancing jugulodigastric lymphoma nodes ➡.

SECTION 2
Oral Cavity, Mandible & Maxilla

Anatomically Based Differentials

Generic Imaging Patterns

Modality-Specific Imaging Findings

DIFFERENTIAL DIAGNOSIS

Common
- SCCa, Oral Tongue
- SCCa, Floor of Mouth
- SCCa, Retromolar Trigone
- SCCa, Mandibular or Maxillary Alveolar Ridge
- SCCa, Buccal Mucosa
- Denture Paste

Less Common
- Torus Palatinus
- Torus Mandibularis
- Torus Maxillaris
- Minor Salivary Gland Malignancy, Oral
- Benign Mixed Tumor, Oral

Rare but Important
- SCCa, Hard Palate
- Mucositis, Radiation

ESSENTIAL INFORMATION

Key Differential Diagnosis Issues
- Physical examination often reveals diagnosis
- Patient signs & symptoms
  - "Sore" in mouth
  - Boring pain (bone involvement)
  - Dysesthesias (perineural tumor)
- Oral cavity SCCa subsites (nearby locations with different treatment & prognosis)
  - SCCa of oral tongue, floor of mouth (FOM), buccal mucosa surgically treated with wide resection
  - SCCa of retromolar trigone, alveolar ridge, hard palate treated with composite resection (bone resected in addition to soft tissues & mucosal surface)
- Imaging must stage primary & nodes
  - Usually in levels IA, IB, & IIA/B
- Best work-up: MR for primary tumor; CECT for nodal disease
  - Imaging used for deep tongue & bone invasion + nodal metastases
  - CECT dental amalgam artifact obscures primary tumor; better than MR for detecting metastatic lymph nodes
  - MR better for interface between tumor & normal tissue

Helpful Clues for Common Diagnoses
- SCCa, Oral Tongue

- Key facts: Most common oral cavity SCCa
  - Lateral tongue subsite most common
  - When small, resection alone used
  - If > 2 mm below mucosal surface, neck dissection performed
- Imaging: Enhancing mass on oral tongue
  - Depth of invasion or extension to other subsites important
  - Small or superficial lesions difficult to detect with imaging
  - Larger lesions > 3 cm require more extensive surgery; staging MR best study
- **SCCa, Floor of Mouth**
  - Key facts: Mucosal covered space over mylohyoid & hyoglossus muscles
    - Undersurface of tongue, extending to anterior tonsillar pillar
    - Hyoglossus muscle in sublingual portion of FOM important landmark as it marks neurovascular bundle (CN12)
  - Imaging: Note size & extent of tumor
    - Check if lingual mandible cortex eroded
    - Does tumor cross lingual septum?
    - Involvement of neurovascular bundle affects surgical approach; check for tumor near hyoglossus muscle
- **SCCa, Retromolar Trigone**
  - Key facts: Small triangular area behind 3rd mandibular molar
    - Multiple potential sites of spread
    - Pterygomandibular raphe spread reaches hamulus of medial pterygoid plate
  - Imaging: Note size & extent of tumor
    - Check for spread anteriorly along mandibular alveolar ridge, lateral to buccal sulcus, medial to lingual sulcus, & FOM
    - Look for posterior extension to anterior tonsillar pillar, superior extension to pterygoid plates or buccal space
    - Bone windows may show buccal or lingual mandibular invasion, erosion of pterygoid plates, maxillary tuberosity, or posterior maxillary sinus wall
- **SCCa, Mandibular or Maxillary Alveolar Ridge**
  - Key facts: Superficial mucosal lesion may present with "loose tooth"
    - New pain from dentures also possible
    - Extent of lesion best assessed clinically

- Imaging: Best for mandible or maxilla bone invasion
  - Simultaneous nodal metastasis assessment done at time of imaging
- **SCCa, Buccal Mucosa**
  - Key facts: Tobacco/alcohol use risk factors for all oral cavity SCCa
    - Betel nut chewing (popular in South Africa & Asia) predisposes to buccal SCCa
  - Imaging: May be very hard to see on CECT because of dental amalgam artifact
    - Look for extension to buccinator muscle, subcutaneous fat, skin
    - Check for posterior spread into buccal space during image review
- **Denture Paste**
  - Key facts: Patient should remove dentures prior to CECT to avoid artifact
  - Imaging: Paste is high density, thin symmetric line along alveolar ridge mucosa

Helpful Clues for Less Common Diagnoses
- **Torus Palatinus**
  - Key facts: Incidental midline hard palate submucosal mass
  - Imaging: Midline lobulated cortical & subcortical bone thickening on oral surface of hard palate
- **Torus Mandibularis**
  - Key facts: Incidental submucosal mass on lingual or buccal surface of mandible
  - Imaging: Lobulated cortical bone thickening, uni- or bilateral, on lingual or buccal mandibular cortex
- **Torus Maxillaris**
  - Key facts: Incidental submucosal mass on oral or buccal surface of maxilla
  - Imaging: Lobulated cortical bone on oral or buccal cortex of maxilla
- **Minor Salivary Gland Malignancy, Oral**
  - Key facts: 2nd most common primary oral cavity malignancy
  - Imaging: Submucosal, so imaging needed to stage tumor
    - Determine local extension, presence of perineural spread
    - Palate most common location; look for CN5-V2 branch tumor spread
- **Benign Mixed Tumor, Oral**
  - Key facts: Most common location is submucosal hard/soft palate
  - Imaging: Smooth enhancing submucosal mass of hard palate
    - May also occur in sublingual space; rare in other oral cavity subsites

Helpful Clues for Rare Diagnoses
- **SCCa, Hard Palate**
  - Key facts: Rarest oral cavity SCCa subsite
  - Imaging: Invasive hard palate mass
- **Mucositis, Radiation**
  - Key facts: Acute-subacute radiation phase
  - Imaging: Diffuse mucosal enhancement

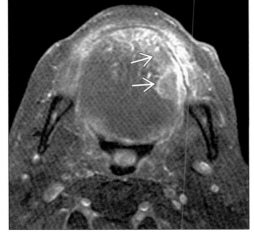

SCCa, Oral Tongue

Axial T1 C+ FS MR shows left lateral tongue SCCa ➡. The primary tumor is T1 (< 2 cm), but the depth of invasion is > 2 mm, so neck dissection for level I and II nodes will be performed.

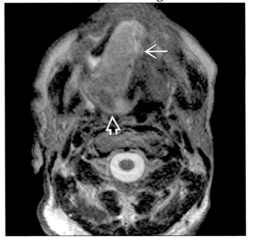

SCCa, Oral Tongue

Axial T2WI MR demonstrates a large right oral tongue SCCa, which crosses midline ➡ and extends posterior to the base of the tongue/lingual tonsil area ➡.

ORAL MUCOSAL SPACE/SURFACE LESION

(Left) Axial CECT demonstrates an enhancing midline anterior floor of mouth SCCa ➡. Invasion through the cortical bone ➡ makes this a T4 lesion. *(Right)* Axial T1WI MR reveals a bulky left retromolar trigone (RMT) SCCa spilling into buccal sulcus ➡ and lingual sulcus and invading lateral oral tongue ➡. Low signal in bone ➡ is secondary to invasion of RMT and proximal mandibular ramus.

SCCa, Floor of Mouth

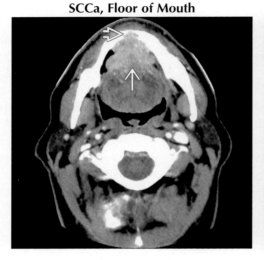

SCCa, Retromolar Trigone

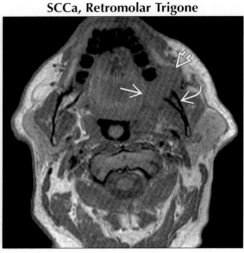

(Left) Axial CECT shows mandibular alveolar ridge SCCa with destruction of mandibular body. Note tumor has spilled into both buccal ➡ & lingual ➡ sulcus, with extension to lateral floor of mouth ➡. *(Right)* Axial T1WI MR shows a small left buccal mucosa SCCa ➡. Note the loss of fat beneath buccinator muscle ➡ and erosion of maxilla ➡. The lesion is so subtle that it probably would have been missed if clinical examination results were not available.

SCCa, Mandibular or Maxillary Alveolar Ridge

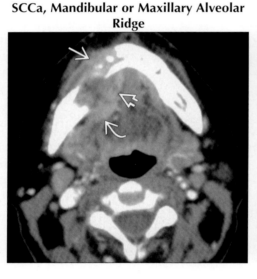

SCCa, Buccal Mucosa

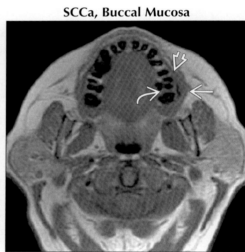

(Left) Axial CECT shows a thin straight line of high density ➡ on the buccal side of sulcus in a patient who removed dentures prior to CT. *(Right)* Coronal bone CT reveals lobulated bilateral paramedian bone excrescences ➡ from the oral cavity side of the hard palate. Note that the nasal cavity side of the palate is normal ➡.

Denture Paste

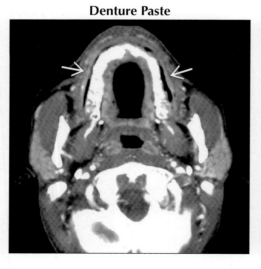

Torus Palatinus

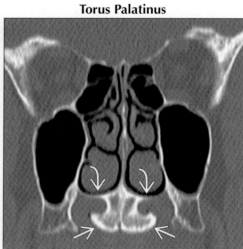

Torus Mandibularis
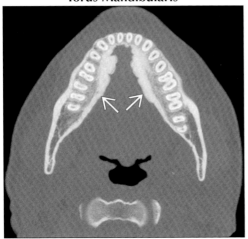

Torus Maxillaris
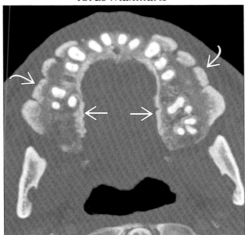

(Left) Axial bone CT demonstrates smoothly lobulated, densely calcified lesions arising from the lingual surfaces of the mandible ➡ bilaterally. Tori are submucosal and incidental, although they may affect the fit of dentures. *(Right)* Axial bone CT shows lobular but well-circumscribed bone excrescences on both the palatal ➡ and buccal ➡ sides of the otherwise normal maxilla. As with other tori, they are benign, submucosal, and incidental.

Minor Salivary Gland Malignancy, Oral
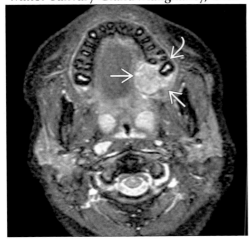

Benign Mixed Tumor, Oral
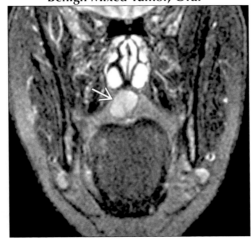

(Left) Axial T2WI FS MR reveals a high intensity mass ➡ in the lateral hard palate, involving the distal molars ➡, in a 15 year old girl. Despite smooth borders, the mass was mucoepidermoid carcinoma, the most common salivary gland malignancy in children. *(Right)* Coronal T2WI FS MR shows a well-circumscribed submucosal mass ➡ that is hyperintense compared to soft palate. Minor salivary glands are known to normally cluster in this anatomic area.

SCCa, Hard Palate
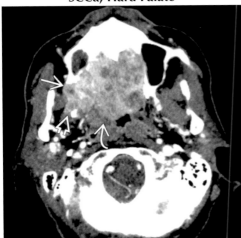

Radiation Mucositis
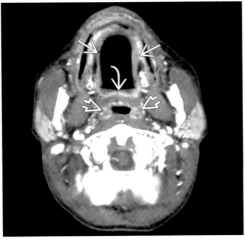

(Left) Axial CECT shows a large enhancing hard palate SCCa. Note extension into the deep right buccal space ➡, masticator space ➡, & anterior nasopharyngeal wall ➡. *(Right)* Axial CECT reveals continuous mucosal enhancement at hard ➡ & soft ➡ palate. Note similar mucosal enhancement of the nasopharyngeal surface ➡. Radiation & chemotherapy treatment had finished 8 weeks prior to this restaging scan with physical exam showing red edematous mucosa.

SUBLINGUAL SPACE LESION

DIFFERENTIAL DIAGNOSIS

Common
- Simple Ranula
- Abscess, Oral Cavity, SLS
- Dilated Submandibular Gland Duct
- SCCa, Floor of Mouth
- SCCa, Oral Tongue, Invasive
- Sialadenitis, Sublingual Gland
- Radiation Changes, Sublingual Gland, Acute

Less Common
- SLS Sialocele
- Atrophy, Hypoglossal Nerve
- Dermoid and Epidermoid, SLS
- Venous Malformation, SLS
- Lymphatic Malformation, SLS

Rare but Important
- Carcinoma, Sublingual Gland
- Benign Mixed Tumor, Sublingual Gland

ESSENTIAL INFORMATION

Key Differential Diagnosis Issues
- Boundaries of sublingual space (SLS)
  - Inferolateral: Mylohyoid muscle
  - Medial: Genioglossus-geniohyoid complex
  - No fascial encapsulation: Communicates with posterosuperior submandibular space & inferior parapharyngeal space
  - Anterior isthmus allows SLS communication with contralateral side
- Sublingual space contents
  - Anterosuperior hypoglossus muscle
  - Lingual nerve (distal CNV3 & chordae tympani branch CN7), distal CN9, CN12
  - Lingual artery & vein
  - Sublingual glands, minor salivary glands
  - Deep submandibular gland & duct
- Imaging recommendations
  - CECT with coronal reformations best
    - Dental amalgam artifact is problematic
  - MR less affected by amalgam artifact

Helpful Clues for Common Diagnoses
- **Simple Ranula**
  - Key facts: Postinflammatory, unilateral sublingual gland mucous retention cyst
    - Closely mimics lymphatic malformation, epidermoid, & sialocele
  - Imaging: Cystic lesion in SLS
- **Abscess, Oral Cavity, SLS**
  - Key facts: Caused by tooth abscess or submandibular duct (SMD) calculus
  - Imaging: Rim-enhancing fluid collection ± SMD calculus ± tooth abscess
- **Dilated Submandibular Gland Duct**
  - Key facts: SMD enlargement secondary to stone or stenosis
  - Imaging
    - CT/MR: High density/low intensity calculus causes proximal SMD enlargement with swollen, enhancing submandibular gland (sialadenitis)
- **SCCa, Floor of Mouth**
  - Key facts: Invasive SCCa under anterior tongue invades SLS
  - Imaging
    - CT/MR: Enhancing anterior sublingual SCCa directly invades SLS
- **SCCa, Oral Tongue, Invasive**
  - Key facts: SCCa on epithelial surface of oral tongue invades SLS
    - Assess mandibular cortex, hyoglossus & mylohyoid invasion, contralateral spread
    - 70% malignant nodes at presentation
  - Imaging
    - CT/MR: Enhancing tongue SCCa follows hyoglossus into SLS
- **Sialadenitis, Sublingual Gland**
  - Key facts: Focal inflammation of sublingual glands in SLS
  - Imaging: Enlarged, enhancing sublingual glands
- **Radiation Changes, Sublingual Gland, Acute**
  - Key facts: Suprahyoid radiation causes sialadenitis of all salivary glands (SLG)
    - Acute inflammation → xerostomia
  - Imaging
    - CT/MR: Enhancing, enlarged SLGs
    - Skin thickened; adjacent edema

Helpful Clues for Less Common Diagnoses
- **SLS Sialocele**
  - Key facts: SLS cystic lesion secondary to trauma, surgery, obstructing stone, or stenosis of SMGD
    - True sialocele: Distended SMGD
    - False sialocele: Ruptured duct, extravasated saliva develops pseudocyst
  - Imaging
    - CT/MR: Fluid density/intensity in dilated SMGD (true) or adjacent to duct (false)

- May peripherally enhance after 2 weeks
- **Atrophy, Hypoglossal Nerve**
  - Key facts: Unilateral atrophy of tongue, secondary CN12 dysfunction
    - Evaluate course of CN12 from medulla to sublingual space
    - Contralateral muscular hypertrophy may be hypermetabolic on PET
  - Imaging
    - CT/MR: Fatty replacement of genioglossus-geniohyoid
- **Dermoid and Epidermoid, SLS**
  - Key facts: Tissue rests in SLS
    - Epidermoid: Ectoderm only
    - Dermoid: Ectoderm & mesoderm
  - Imaging (CT/MR)
    - Epidermoid: Fluid density/intensity; DWI restriction, high signal
    - Dermoid: Mixed density/intensity; fatty or calcified elements possible
- **Venous Malformation, SLS**
  - Key facts: Poorly circumscribed dilated venous channels, trans-spatial
    - Slow flow; invisible on angiography
    - No enlarged feeding arteries
  - Imaging: Trans-spatial variably enhancing lesion & phleboliths
- **Lymphatic Malformation, SLS**
  - Key facts: Varied spectrum of dilated lymphatic spaces
    - Presentation: Pediatric, early adult
  - Imaging (CT/MR)
    - Cystic, nonenhancing lesion with imperceptible walls

- Multilocular; often trans-spatial
- Fluid-fluid levels possible
- Insinuates with no mass effect when small

Helpful Clues for Rare Diagnoses

- **Carcinoma, Sublingual Gland**
  - Key facts: SLG masses 90% malignant
    - Most commonly adenoid cystic, mucoepidermoid, or acinic cell carcinoma
  - Imaging (CT/MR)
    - Invasive SLS mass with heterogeneous density/intensity
    - Variable enhancement but present
    - 5-10 year follow-up; late recurrence
- **Benign Mixed Tumor, Sublingual Gland**
  - Key facts
    - Synonym: Pleomorphic adenoma
    - Arises from SLG or minor salivary gland within sublingual space
  - Imaging (CT/MR)
    - Well-circumscribed SLS lesion with homogeneous enhancement
    - MR: T2/STIR high signal

Alternative Differential Approaches

- Imaging appearance
  - Trans-spatial lesions: Lymphatic & venous malformations
  - Cystic lesions: Ranula, sialocele, lymphatic malformation, epidermoid
  - Solid lesions: Sialadenitis, squamous cell carcinoma, benign mixed tumor, tongue atrophy

Simple Ranula

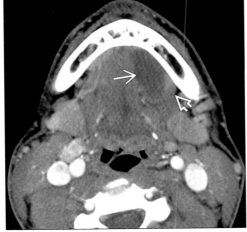

Axial CECT demonstrates a cystic mass ➡ with imperceptible walls in the anterior sublingual space. Notice that the left mylohyoid muscle is displaced posterolaterally ⧫.

Abscess, Oral Cavity, SLS

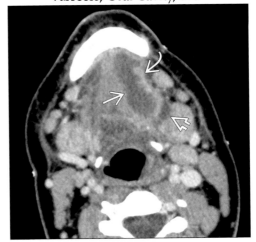

Axial CECT shows a sublingual space abscess ➡ with submandibular space extension ➡ Note the shaggy, subtly enhancing borders of the mylohyoid muscle ➡.

SUBLINGUAL SPACE LESION

(Left) Axial CECT reveals an enlarged submandibular duct ➡ secondary to a calculus (not shown) with associated submandibular gland postobstructive sialadenitis ⮊. *(Right)* Axial CECT reveals extensive invasion of the left sublingual space by squamous cell carcinoma ➡ in the left floor of the mouth. The submandibular duct ⮊ is obstructed by the tumor with enlargement and secondary submandibular sialadenitis visible.

Dilated Submandibular Gland Duct

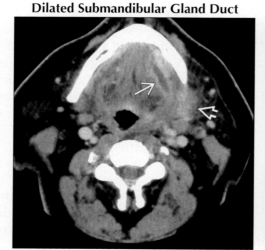

SCCa, Floor of Mouth

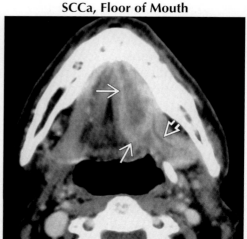

(Left) Coronal T1 C+ FS MR demonstrates an enhancing SCCa primary tumor extending inferiorly from the lateral oral tongue ➡ into the sublingual space ⮊. *(Right)* Axial CECT shows enlarged, enhancing left submandibular ⮊ and sublingual ➡ glands secondary to SMGD obstruction (not seen). Note loss of distinction of normal SLS fat separating genioglossus-geniohyoid from sublingual gland secondary to inflammatory stranding.

SCCa, Oral Tongue, Invasive

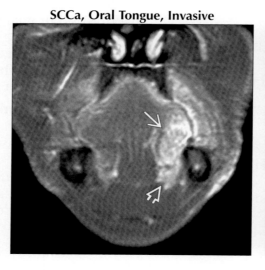

Sialadenitis, Sublingual Gland

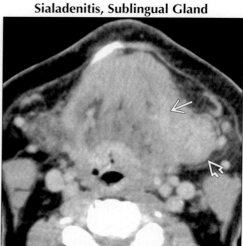

(Left) Axial CECT reveals enhancing sublingual glands ➡, submandibular glands ⮊, and lingual tonsils ➡. Note the diffuse stranding of the subcutaneous fat. *(Right)* Axial CECT reveals a dilated submandibular duct ➡ secondary to a distal ductal stenosis. Larger fluid density within the right sublingual space ⮊ represents the resulting "false sialocele" from submandibular ductal rupture & extravasated saliva contained within a fibrous pseudocapsule.

Radiation Changes, Sublingual Gland, Acute

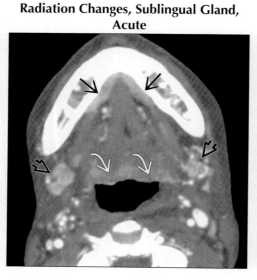

SLS Sialocele

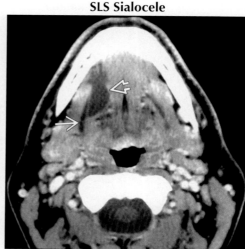

Atrophy, Hypoglossal Nerve

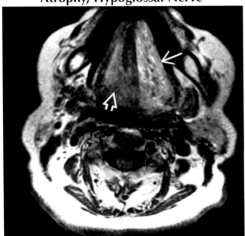

Dermoid and Epidermoid, SLS

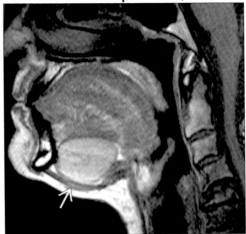

(Left) Axial T1WI MR shows atrophy & fatty replacement of left hyoglossus & genioglossus-geniohyoid musculature ➔. Note the mild hypertrophy of the contralateral root of tongue musculature ➔ & the relative collapse of the left oropharynx. Atrophy was secondary to a proximal CN12 schwannoma. *(Right)* Sagittal T1WI MR shows sublingual space epidermoid with ↑ T1 secondary to high protein content. Note attenuated mylohyoid muscle ➔.

Venous Malformation, SLS

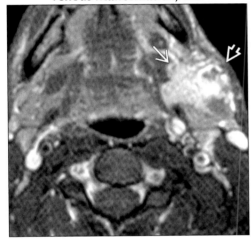

Lymphatic Malformation, SLS

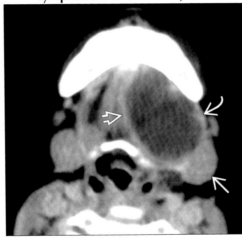

(Left) Axial T1 C+ FS MR shows an enhancing trans-spatial venous malformation that involves both the sublingual ➔ and submandibular ➔ spaces. *(Right)* Axial CECT shows a well-circumscribed fluid density lesion within the left sublingual space, extending posteriorly into the submandibular space and abutting the submandibular gland ➔. The genioglossus muscle is displaced medially ➔, and the thinned mylohyoid muscle inferolaterally ➔.

Carcinoma, Sublingual Gland

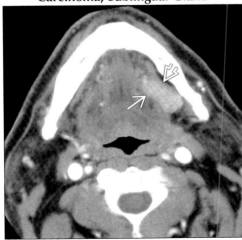

Benign Mixed Tumor, Sublingual Gland

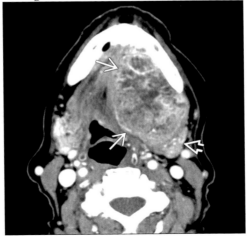

(Left) Axial CECT shows an invasive enhancing SLS carcinoma ➔ medial to the left mylohyoid muscle ➔. Final pathology revealed mucoepidermoid carcinoma of the sublingual gland. *(Right)* Axial CECT demonstrates a large heterogeneous mass in the left sublingual space ➔ that displaces the submandibular gland posterolaterally ➔. The mylohyoid muscle is hard to see laterally as it has been thinned over many years.

SUBMANDIBULAR SPACE LESION

DIFFERENTIAL DIAGNOSIS

Common
- Reactive Lymph Nodes, SMS
- SCCa, Nodal, SMS
- Accessory Salivary Tissue, SMS
- Sialadenitis, Submandibular Gland
- Benign Mixed Tumor, Parotid Tail
- Ranula, Diving
- Abscess, Oral Cavity, SMS
- Benign Mixed Tumor, Submandibular Gland
- Carcinoma, Submandibular Gland
- Suppurative Lymph Nodes, SMS

Less Common
- Non-Hodgkin Lymphoma, Nodal, SMS
- Aplasia-Hypoplasia, Submandibular Gland
- Non-TB Mycobacterium, Lymph Nodes, SMS
- Tuberculosis, Lymph Nodes, SMS
- SCCa, Oral Tongue, Invasive into SMS

Rare but Important
- 2nd Branchial Cleft Cyst
- Dermoid and Epidermoid, Oral Cavity, SMS
- Lymphatic Malformation, Oral Cavity, SMS
- Venous Malformation, SMS

ESSENTIAL INFORMATION

Key Differential Diagnosis Issues
- In addition to statistical DDx list above, consider alternative differential diagnosis approach to organize SMS lesions by structure of origin

Helpful Clues for Common Diagnoses
- **Reactive Lymph Nodes, SMS**
  - Key facts: Common in patient < 20; accompany upper respiratory infection
  - CT/MR: Multiple, ovoid nodes with enhancing, linear markings
- **SCCa, Nodal, SMS**
  - Key facts: Oral cavity SCCa drains to level I SMS nodes
  - CT/MR: Enhancing, round to ovoid node(s) > 15 mm ± central nodal necrosis
- **Accessory Salivary Tissue, SMS**
  - Key facts: Clinician may palpate mass, or radiologist may identify as abnormal
  - CT/MR: Similar density/intensity as adjacent submandibular gland
    - Lenticular mass projects into anterior SMS from mylohyoid cleft

- **Sialadenitis, Submandibular Gland**
  - Key facts: Acutely presents with swelling, pain in SMS
  - CT/MR: Swollen SMG with enlarged duct ± calcified intraductal calculus in SLS
    - Chronic: Atrophic SMG
- **Benign Mixed Tumor, Parotid Tail**
  - Key facts: Inferiorly projecting BMT may be mistaken for nonparotid neck mass with biopsy causing facial nerve branch injury
  - CT/MR: Ovoid mass "hangs" from parotid tail into posterior SMS
    - MR: Uniform T2 hyperintense mass with homogeneous enhancement
- **Ranula, Diving**
  - Key facts: Simple ranula of SLS ruptures into SMS creating pseudocyst
  - CT/MR: Comet-shaped, unilocular thin walled SLS mass, with tail collapsed in SLS
    - MR: Low T1 & high T2 signal with T1 C+ thin wall enhancement
- **Abscess, Oral Cavity, SMS**
  - Key facts: Painful SMS mass associated with tooth decay, ductal calculus or suppurative nodes
  - CECT: Rim-enhancing, low-density fluid collection in SMS; may be trans-spatial
- **Benign Mixed Tumor, Submandibular Gland**
  - Key facts: ~ 50% SMG tumors are BMT
  - CT/MR: Smooth margined mass projects from SMG margin; heterogeneous appearance when large
    - CT: Variable enhancement
    - MR: Low T1, high T2 signal
- **Carcinoma, Submandibular Gland**
  - Key facts: Firm, sometimes fixed SMS mass
  - CT/MR: Invasive mass emerging from SMG
- **Suppurative Lymph Nodes, SMS**
  - Key facts: Nodes seeded from tooth, SMG calculus, or pharyngeal infection
    - Suppurative node = intranodal abscess
  - CT/MR: Rim-enhancing nodal masses with fluid/pus center

Helpful Clues for Less Common Diagnoses
- **Non-Hodgkin Lymphoma, Nodal, SMS**
  - CT/MR: Multiple large nonnecrotic nodes
- **Aplasia-Hypoplasia, Submandibular Gland**
  - CT/MR: Unilateral small or absent SMG

SUBMANDIBULAR SPACE LESION

- **Non-TB Mycobacterium, Lymph Nodes, SMS**
  - CT/MR: Multiple large nonnecrotic nodes in a child
- **Tuberculosis, Lymph Nodes, SMS**
  - Key facts: PPD positive, often chronically ill patient
  - CT/MR: Round nodes with central cystic caseous necrosis
- **SCCa, Oral Tongue, Invasive into SMS**
  - Key facts: Primary tumor invades through mylohyoid muscle into SMS
  - CT/MR: Heterogeneous, invasive enhancing mass involves tongue, floor of mouth, & SMS

Helpful Clues for Rare Diagnoses
- **2nd Branchial Cleft Cyst**
  - CT/MR: Cystic mass in posterior SMS of child
- **Dermoid and Epidermoid, Oral Cavity, SMS**
  - CT/MR (dermoid): Mixed density/intensity ovoid SMS mass; T1 high signal from fat
  - CT/MR(epidermoid): Fluid density/intensity ovoid SMS mass
- **Lymphatic Malformation, Oral Cavity, SMS**
  - CT/MR: Multilocular cystic mass
- **Venous Malformation, SMS**
  - CT/MR: Trans-spatial mixed cystic, solid enhancing mass in SMS + phleboliths

Alternative Differential Approaches
- Another approach to submandibular space DDx is to consider structure of origin
  - Structure of origin analysis: Submandibular gland proper, submandibular nodes, & adjacent oral cavity structures
  - Add congenital lesions to these 3 structures of origin to complete this alternative differential diagnosis
- Submandibular gland lesions
  - Sialadenitis, submandibular gland
  - Benign mixed tumor, SMG
  - Carcinoma, submandibular gland
- Submandibular node lesions
  - Reactive lymph nodes, SMS
  - SCCa, nodal, SMS
  - Abscess, oral cavity, SMS
  - Suppurative lymph nodes, SMS
  - Non-Hodgkin lymphoma, nodal, SMS
  - Non-TB mycobacterium, lymph nodes
  - Tuberculosis, lymph nodes, SMS
- Lesions from adjacent oral cavity
  - Benign mixed tumor, parotid tail
  - Ranula, diving
  - SCCa, oral tongue
- Congenital lesions
  - Accessory salivary tissue, SMS
  - Aplasia-hypoplasia, submandibular gland
  - 2nd branchial cleft cyst
  - Dermoid and epidermoid, oral cavity
  - Lymphatic malformation, oral cavity
  - Venous malformation, SMS

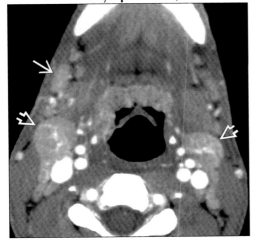

Reactive Lymph Nodes, SMS

Axial CECT through level of low oropharynx reveals a reactive right submandibular node → associated with bilateral reactive jugulodigastric nodes →.

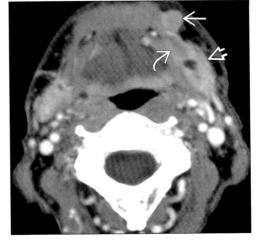

SCCa, Nodal, SMS

Axial CECT shows enlarged, enhancing metastatic level IA node → and an inflamed submandibular gland → with dilated duct →. This patient had known anterior floor of mouth squamous cell carcinoma.

SUBMANDIBULAR SPACE LESION

Accessory Salivary Tissue, SMS

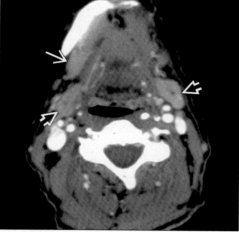

Accessory Salivary Tissue, SMS

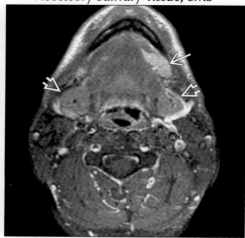

(Left) Axial CECT shows accessory salivary gland tissue ➡ anterior to normal submandibular glands ➡. The density of the accessory salivary tissue is identical to the normal submandibular glands. *(Right)* Axial T1 C+ FS MR reveals an enhancing pear-shaped accessory salivary gland ➡ emerging from the normal cleft in the mylohyoid muscle to fill the anterior submandibular space. Note the normal submandibular glands ➡.

Sialadenitis, Submandibular Gland

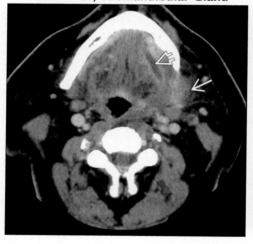

Sialadenitis, Submandibular Gland

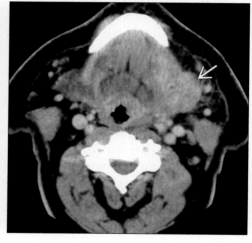

(Left) Axial CECT reveals inflamed, enhancing left submandibular gland ➡ with associated ductal dilation ➡. Notice the cellulitis in the tissues adjacent to the submandibular gland. *(Right)* Axial CECT reveals an enlarged, enhancing left submandibular gland ➡ secondary to ductal calculus (not shown). Clinically these patients may present with neck tenderness and fever, suspicious for oral cavity abscess.

Benign Mixed Tumor, Parotid Tail

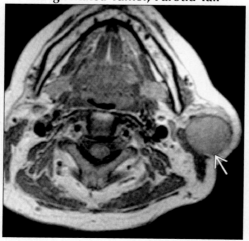

Benign Mixed Tumor, Parotid Tail

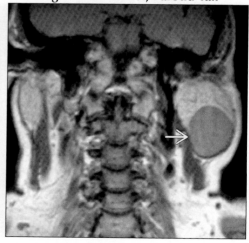

(Left) Axial T1WI MR demonstrates a large benign mixed tumor ➡ protruding from the inferolateral parotid (parotid tail) into the most posterolateral aspect of the submandibular space. *(Right)* Coronal T1WI MR shows a benign mixed tumor ➡ in the parotid tail hanging as an "earring" lesion into the posterior aspect of the submandibular space. These lesions may be mistaken for a cervical neck mass; biopsy or removal is complicated by facial nerve injury.

SUBMANDIBULAR SPACE LESION

Oral Cavity, Mandible & Maxilla

Ranula, Diving

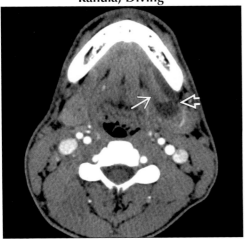

Abscess, Oral Cavity, SMS

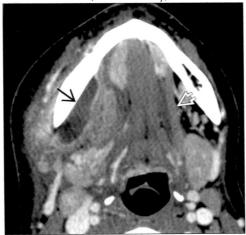

(Left) Axial CECT reveals a linear low density collapsed ranula tail in the posterior sublingual space ➡. This simple ranula has ruptured into the submandibular space to form a pseudocyst ➡. *(Right)* Axial CECT reveals a submandibular space abscess ➡ wedged between the mylohyoid muscle and the medial mandibular cortex. The opposite normal mylohyoid muscle ➡ can be seen medial to the SMS.

Benign Mixed Tumor, Submandibular Gland

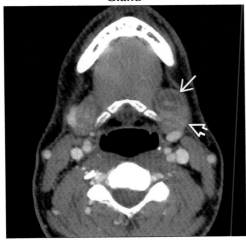

Carcinoma, Submandibular Gland

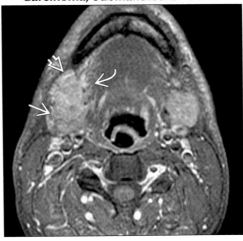

(Left) Axial CECT reveals a low-density, well-defined mass ➡ projecting from the anterior submandibular gland ➡. The absence of a fat plane between BMT & the gland excludes lymph node diagnosis. *(Right)* Axial T1 C+ FS MR shows an enhancing soft tissue mass arising from the right submandibular gland ➡ and invading anteriorly into the submandibular space ➡. This adenoid cystic carcinoma also invades the mylohyoid muscle ➡.

Suppurative Lymph Nodes, SMS

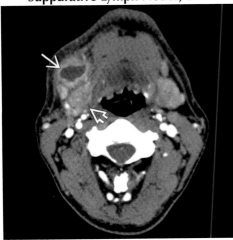

Suppurative Lymph Nodes, SMS

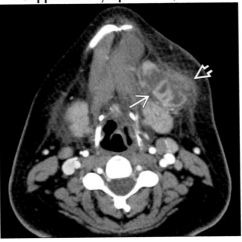

(Left) Axial CECT shows an irregular, rim-enhancing, thick-walled, suppurative lymph node ➡ anterior to the submandibular gland ➡. This node will shortly rupture to form a SMS abscess. *(Right)* Axial CECT through low submandibular space shows a suppurative nodal conglomerate ➡ with extensive cellulitis in the adjacent soft tissues ➡. Dental infection (not shown) seeded this submandibular nodal group with subsequent intranodal abscess development.

2

13

SUBMANDIBULAR SPACE LESION

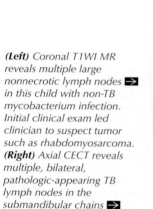

(Left) Axial CECT shows multiple, smoothly marginated, enlarged submandibular nodes ➡ in the submandibular space in a patient with systemic non-Hodgkin lymphoma. Note the homogeneous density of the adenopathy. *(Right)* Axial CECT demonstrates a normal, minimally enlarged right gland ➡ and the absence of the left submandibular gland ➡. The left submandibular space is filled with fat.

(Left) Coronal T1WI MR reveals multiple large nonnecrotic lymph nodes ➡ in this child with non-TB mycobacterium infection. Initial clinical exam led clinician to suspect tumor such as rhabdomyosarcoma. *(Right)* Axial CECT reveals multiple, bilateral, pathologic-appearing TB lymph nodes in the submandibular chains ➡ and internal jugular chains ➡.

(Left) Axial CECT shows a lateral oral tongue SCCa extending into the lateral sulcus ➡ and extending down the mylohyoid muscle to invade the superficial aspect of the submandibular space ➡. *(Right)* Axial CECT shows contiguous inferolateral spread from an oral tongue SCCa through the mylohyoid muscle to engulf the submandibular gland ➡ and anterior submandibular space ➡.

Non-Hodgkin Lymphoma, Nodal, SMS

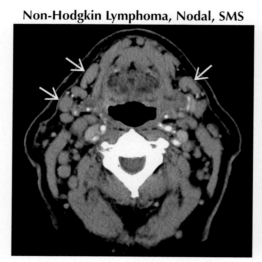

Aplasia-Hypoplasia, Submandibular Gland

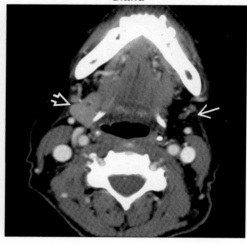

Non-TB Mycobacterium, Lymph Nodes, SMS

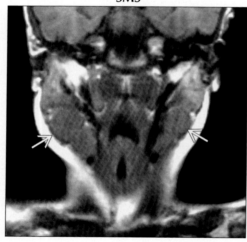

Tuberculosis, Lymph Nodes, SMS

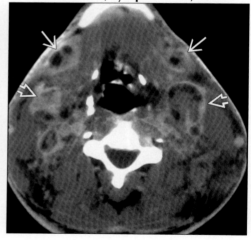

SCCa, Oral Tongue, Invasive into SMS

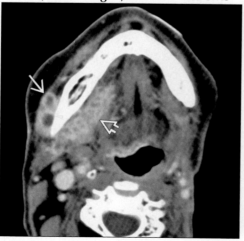

SCCa, Oral Tongue, Invasive into SMS

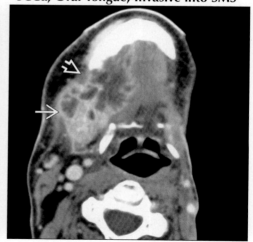

2nd Branchial Cleft Cyst

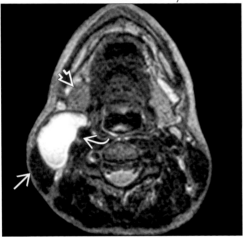

2nd Branchial Cleft Cyst

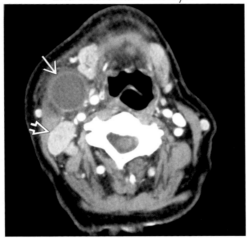

(Left) Axial T2WI MR demonstrates a well-defined hyperintense mass anterior to the sternomastoid muscle ➡, posterolateral to the submandibular gland ➡, & abutting the carotid space ➡. This is the typical 2nd BCC location. (Right) Axial CECT reveals a classic 2nd branchial cleft cyst ➡ in the posterior submandibular space. Note the large internal jugular chain node ➡ posterolateral to the cyst. Patient had both a branchial cleft cyst and non-Hodgkin lymphoma.

Dermoid and Epidermoid, Oral Cavity, SMS

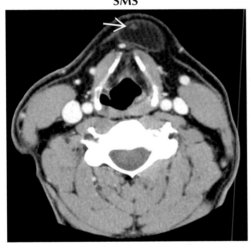

Dermoid and Epidermoid, Oral Cavity, SMS

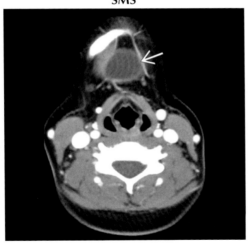

(Left) Axial CECT shows a submandibular space ovoid dermoid with both fluid density & a focus of higher density material ➡. It is possible to suggest the diagnosis of dermoid from the CT images because of the tissue density foci in the lesion. (Right) Axial CECT shows a cyst ➡ between the anterior bellies of digastric muscle in the SMS. This surgically proven dermoid is uniform higher than normal fluid density. Either dermoid or epidermoid could have this appearance.

Lymphatic Malformation, Oral Cavity, SMS

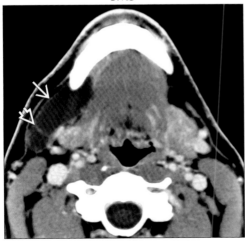

Venous Malformation, SMS

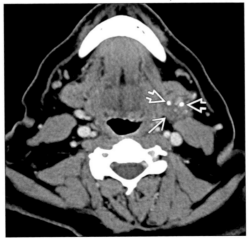

(Left) Axial CECT reveals a cystic submandibular space mass ➡ with internal septations ➡, characteristic of a lymphatic malformation. The lesion is lateral to the submandibular gland and deep to the platysma muscle. (Right) Axial CECT shows a poorly defined, mixed density mass in the left submandibular space ➡ involving the posterior margin of the submandibular gland. Notice the multiple phleboliths ➡ typical of a venous malformation.

SUBMANDIBULAR GLAND LESION

DIFFERENTIAL DIAGNOSIS

Common
- Accessory Salivary Tissue, SMS
- Sialadenitis, Submandibular Gland
- Benign Mixed Tumor, Submandibular Gland
- Carcinoma, Submandibular Gland

Less Common
- Radiation Changes, Acute, Submandibular Gland
- Atrophy, Submandibular Gland
- Benign Lymphoepithelial Lesions-HIV
- Aplasia-Hypoplasia, Submandibular Gland

Rare but Important
- Sjögren Syndrome, Submandibular Gland
- Sarcoidosis, Submandibular Gland
- Trauma, Submandibular Gland
- Mucocele, Submandibular Gland

ESSENTIAL INFORMATION

Key Differential Diagnosis Issues
- Submandibular gland (SMG) lesions DDx should be distinguished from submandibular space (SMS) lesions DDx
- SMG lesion DDx confined to those lesions arising from gland itself
- SMS lesion DDx includes lesions that arise from space itself
  - Nodal lesions are key part of SMS DDx but are not part of SMG DDx, as there are no lymph nodes within gland
  - SMG undergoes early encapsulation in embryogenesis resulting in absence of lymphoid aggregates/nodes
  - Parotid gland undergoes late encapsulation resulting in lymphoid aggregates/nodes within gland

Helpful Clues for Common Diagnoses
- **Accessory Salivary Tissue, SMS**
  - Key facts: Clinician may palpate mass or radiologist may identify as abnormal
    - Most commonly incidental finding
    - Any SMG pathology can occur within accessory SMG tissue
  - CT/MR: Benign-appearing SMS lesion with density & intensity similar to SMG
    - Located in anterior SMS
    - Lenticular mass projecting from mylohyoid cleft

- **Sialadenitis, Submandibular Gland**
  - Key facts: Acute presentation with painful SMG swelling
    - Secondary to SMG duct calculus or stenosis
  - CT/MR: May see dilatation of intraglandular ductal system
    - Acute SMG sialadenitis: Enlarged SMG + cellulitis with ductal dilatation ± calculus
    - Chronic SMG sialadenitis: Atrophic gland with ductal dilatation ± calculus
  - Plain film: Calcified calculus visible (90%)

- **Benign Mixed Tumor, Submandibular Gland**
  - Key facts: Benign heterogeneous tumor of SMG origin, composed of epithelial, myoepithelial, & stromal components
    - ~ 50% SMG tumors are BMT
  - CT/MR: Well-circumscribed SMG mass
    - Small BMT: Usually solitary, ovoid, & well circumscribed
    - Large BMT: Often heterogeneous & multiloculated with focal calcifications, hemorrhage, & necrosis
    - CECT: Variable enhancement
    - MR: Low T1, high T2 signal intensity
  - Ultrasound: SMG mass is well defined, solid, & hypoechoic compared to adjacent salivary tissue

- **Carcinoma, Submandibular Gland**
  - Key facts: 2 major carcinomas of SMG, adenoid cystic carcinoma (ACCa) & mucoepidermoid Ca (MECa)
    - Clinical presentation: Firm ± fixed submandibular gland mass
    - Metastatic disease accounts for 30% of deaths; whole body PET/CT has valuable role in follow-up
    - 5 year survival: 50%
    - Evaluate for perineural spread in ACCa
  - CT/MR: Invasive mass emerges from SMG
    - Submandibular and high internal jugular malignant nodes may be present

Helpful Clues for Less Common Diagnoses
- **Radiation Changes, Acute, Submandibular Gland**
  - Key facts: SMG, sublingual gland, & parotid all react to radiation if in field
  - CT/MR: Diffusely enhancing enlarged SMGs
- **Atrophy, Submandibular Gland**

- Key facts: Occurs with chronic ductal obstruction (calculus, postinfectious stenosis)
- CT/MR: SMG shrinks, + fatty infiltrates
  - SMG is visible, just partially or completely fatty infiltrated
  - Compare this to aplasia where no gland is seen in SMS
- **Benign Lymphoepithelial Lesions-HIV**
  - Key facts: More commonly present within parotid gland
  - CT/MR: Multiple cystic & solid masses enlarging both submandibular glands
    - Thin rim enhancement of cystic lesions with heterogeneous enhancement of solid lesions
    - Parotid lesions present if SMG affected
    - Associated with tonsillar hyperplasia & cervical reactive adenopathy
- **Aplasia-Hypoplasia, Submandibular Gland**
  - Key facts: Asymmetry may be confusing
    - Especially true with unilateral hypoplasia or complete absence of SMG
  - CT/MR: Hypoplasia of small gland
    - Aplasia: Absence of SMG at its expected location
    - Aplasia may be associated with contralateral hypertrophy of SMG or prominent salivary tissue in SLS

Helpful Clues for Rare Diagnoses
- **Sjögren Syndrome, Submandibular Gland**

- Key facts: Parotid, lacrimal, submandibular, & sublingual glands all affected by Sjögren inflammation
- CT/MR: Multiple phases from acute inflammatory to chronic involution
  - Acute: Enlarged SMGs with inflammatory foci
  - Chronic: Small, fibrosed submandibular glands with fatty infiltration
- **Sarcoidosis, Submandibular Gland**
  - Key facts: Parotid & submandibular glands may both be affected
  - CT/MR: Acute change shows enlarged, enhancing SMGs
- **Trauma, Submandibular Gland**
  - Key facts: Occurs with mandibular fracture
  - CT/MR: SMG contusion or rupture possible
- **Mucocele, Submandibular Gland**
  - Key facts: Benign cyst within SMG
    - Also called SMG retention cyst & sialocele
  - CT/MR: Benign-appearing, fluid density, or intensity cystic structure within SMG
    - No surrounding aggressive features

SELECTED REFERENCES

1. Alyas F et al: Diseases of the submandibular gland as demonstrated using high resolution ultrasound. Br J Radiol. 78(928):362-9, 2005
2. Cohen EG et al: Fine-needle aspiration biopsy of salivary gland lesions in a selected patient population. Arch Otolaryngol Head Neck Surg. 130(6):773-8, 2004
3. Bentz BG et al: Masses of the salivary gland region in children. Arch Otolaryngol Head Neck Surg. 126(12):1435-9, 2000

Accessory Salivary Tissue, SMS

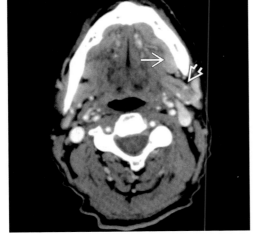

Axial CECT image demonstrates accessory salivary gland tissue ➡ seen anterior and medial to the normal submandibular gland ➡ and lateral to the neurovascular pedicle of the sublingual space.

Accessory Salivary Tissue, SMS

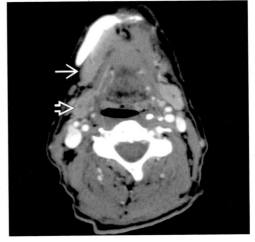

Axial CECT image through the submandibular glands demonstrates right-sided accessory salivary gland tissue ➡ seen anterior and medial to the normal right submandibular gland ➡.

SUBMANDIBULAR GLAND LESION

(Left) Axial CECT image shows acute sialadenitis as an enhancing, enlarged right submandibular gland ➡ secondary to stone in the distal duct by the ductal papilla ➡. Notice the density of the opposite normal submandibular gland is near muscle density.
(Right) Axial CECT reveals chronic sialadenitis as fatty infiltration of the submandibular gland ➡ due to a chronic submandibular duct calculus ➡.

Sialadenitis, Submandibular Gland
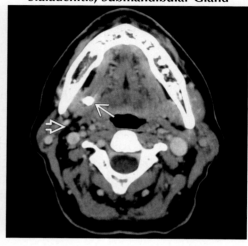

Sialadenitis, Submandibular Gland

(Left) Axial CECT image shows a mass within the right submandibular gland mass ➡. This benign mixed tumor is well defined and low density in comparison to the submandibular gland.
(Right) Axial CECT demonstrates abnormal enhancement and enlargement of the right SMG ➡, later found to be a SMG carcinoma. There were several pathologic nodes also identified ➡.

Benign Mixed Tumor, Submandibular Gland
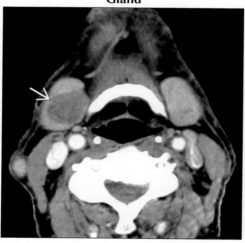

Carcinoma, Submandibular Gland
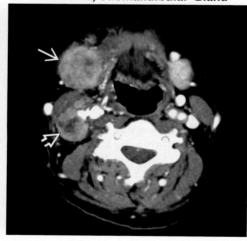

(Left) Axial CECT shows postoperative changes from extended right radical neck dissection, with absence of right internal jugular vein, sternocleidomastoid muscle, & submandibular gland ➡. Left SMG shows post-radiation changes as an enlarged enhancing gland ➡, anterior to the sternocleidomastoid muscle ➡. (Right) Axial CECT reveals fatty atrophy of the left submandibular gland ➡ secondary to chronic submandibular duct stone (not shown).

Radiation Changes, Acute, Submandibular Gland
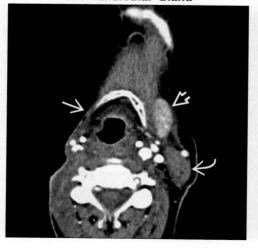

Atrophy, Submandibular Gland
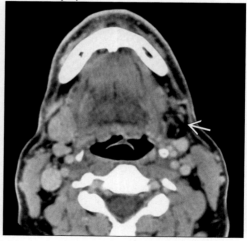

SUBMANDIBULAR GLAND LESION

Benign Lymphoepithelial Lesions-HIV

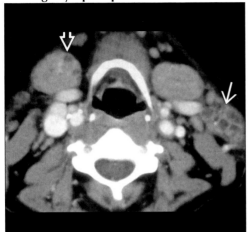

Aplasia-Hypoplasia, Submandibular Gland

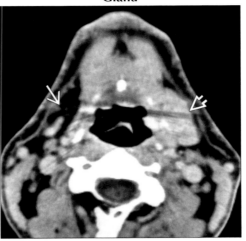

(Left) Axial CECT shows benign lymphoepithelial lesions in both the left parotid tail ➡ and the right submandibular gland ➡ in this patient with known HIV. Submandibular gland involvement with such lesions is rare. *(Right)* Axial CECT demonstrates absence of the right submandibular gland ➡ with slight hypertrophy of the left submandibular gland ➡.

Sjögren Syndrome, Submandibular Gland

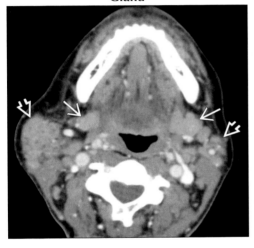

Sarcoidosis, Submandibular Gland

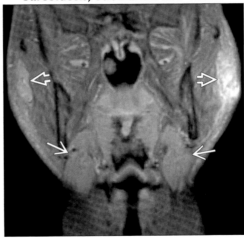

(Left) Axial CECT reveals bilateral submandibular gland enhancement ➡. The left gland is multilobular and enlarged. Note the enlarged right > left parotid tails with extensive enhancing lymphoid aggregates ➡ associated with Sjögren syndrome. *(Right)* Coronal T1 C+ FS MR shows bilateral diffuse enlargement of the parotid ➡ and the submandibular glands ➡. The accessory parotids enhance more than the submandibular glands.

Trauma, Submandibular Gland

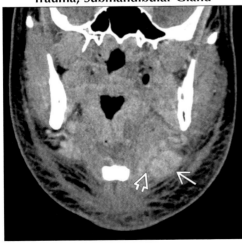

Mucocele, Submandibular Gland

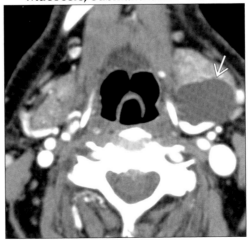

(Left) Coronal CECT demonstrates a swollen, ruptured left submandibular gland ➡ in association with mandibular fracture (not shown). The low density fluid/blood is visible between the pieces of the ruptured gland ➡. *(Right)* Axial CECT reveals a cystic lesion arising from the left submandibular gland ➡. Submandibular gland mucocele has also been referred to as submandibular gland retention cyst and sialocele.

ROOT OF TONGUE LESION

DIFFERENTIAL DIAGNOSIS

Common
- Abscess, Oral Cavity
- SCCa, Floor of Mouth
- SCCa, Oral Tongue

Less Common
- Dermoid and Epidermoid, Oral Cavity
- Thyroglossal Duct Cyst
- Ectopic Thyroid

Rare but Important
- Lymphatic Malformation, Oral Cavity
- Venous Malformation
- Foregut Duplication Cyst, Tongue

ESSENTIAL INFORMATION

Key Differential Diagnosis Issues
- Root of tongue (ROT) anatomic definition
  - Region encompassing genioglossus & geniohyoid muscles and lingual septum
  - ROT boundaries
    - Posterior: Base of tongue (lingual tonsil)
    - Anterior: Genu of mandible
    - Lateral: Sublingual space
    - Inferior: Mylohyoid muscle
    - Superior: Intrinsic muscles of tongue

Helpful Clues for Common Diagnoses
- **Abscess, Oral Cavity**
  - Key facts: No nodes in tongue root
    - Abscess results from hematogenous spread or local injury (i.e., tongue piercing)
  - CECT: Best imaging modality; review in soft tissue & bone algorithms
    - Rim-enhancing fluid density mass splays genioglossus muscles
    - Adjacent myositis with muscular enlargement & enhancement may be present
- **SCCa, Floor of Mouth**
  - Key facts: Infiltrating mass originating in area of oral cavity under anterior tongue
    - Local invasion most frequently to sublingual space, followed by ROT
    - Lymphatic spread most commonly to subdigastric, submaxillary, or midjugular nodes
  - MR: Best to assess for local invasion & nodal spread

- Low T1 & high T2 signal; avid enhancement on T1 C+
- T1 C+ shows anterior floor of mouth primary SCCa extending into ROT
- **SCCa, Oral Tongue**
  - Key facts: Invasive enhancing mass arising from surface of oral tongue with exclusion of lingual tonsil
    - Incidence of metastases at presentation > other intraoral carcinomas (70%)
    - Spread into floor of mouth through invasion of hyoglossus, genioglossus, or mylohyoid muscles
    - Spread across midline to opposite side of tongue
  - MR: Preferred imaging modality
    - T1 C+ shows primary oral tongue tumor invading ROT

Helpful Clues for Less Common Diagnoses
- **Dermoid and Epidermoid, Oral Cavity**
  - Key facts: Cystic ROT lesion derived from congenital epithelial rests
    - Epidermoid: Only epithelial elements
    - Dermoid: Both epithelial & dermal elements
  - CT: Hypodense unilocular mass usually with thin imperceptible wall
    - Homogeneous fluid density: Epidermoid
    - If fatty or mixed density or Ca++: Dermoid
  - MR: Low T1, high T2, DWI restricted diffusion (epidermoid)
    - Areas of high T1 (fat), very low signal Ca++ (dermoid)
- **Thyroglossal Duct Cyst**
  - Key facts: Unilocular ROT cystic mass without complex elements such as fat or calcifications
    - Results from failure of involution of thyroglossal duct with continued secretion by epithelial lining
  - Imaging: Appearance mimics epidermoid cyst
    - CT: Hypodense mass with thin rim of peripheral enhancement
    - MR: Hypointense on T1; may become hyperintense if proteinaceous contents
    - MR: Nonenhancing cyst on T1 C+
- **Ectopic Thyroid**

- Key facts: Well-circumscribed ROT mass with density/intensity similar to normal thyroid tissue
  - May grow rapidly at puberty
  - Potential for goitrous or carcinomatous transformation (3%)
  - May be only normal thyroid tissue
- CT: High-density lesion on NECT
  - Marked homogeneous enhancement
  - Lower neck images may reveal no normal thyroid
- MR: T1 & T2 hyperintense to tongue musculature
- Nuclear medicine: Avoid iodinated contrast if I-123 scan scheduled
  - I-123 required to evaluate for functional cervical thyroid

Helpful Clues for Rare Diagnoses
- **Lymphatic Malformation, Oral Cavity**
  - Key facts: Congenital, frequently trans-spatial lesion consisting of dilated lymphatic channels
  - Imaging: Uni- or multiloculated, nonenhancing cystic mass that splays genioglossus muscles
    - CT: Trans-spatial multilocular mass involves ROT ± sublingual or submandibular spaces
    - MR: Low intensity T1, high intensity T2; nonenhancing unless venous malformation elements
- **Venous Malformation**

- Key facts: Congenital slow-flow post-capillary lesion containing dilated endothelial-lined vascular channels
  - Mass enlarges with Valsalva, crying, bending over
- CT: Lobulated isodense to muscle mass
  - Rounded calcifications (phleboliths) common
  - Variable enhancement pattern related to flow rate through lesion
  - No enlarged feeding arteries evident on CTA
  - Frequent drainage by enlarged veins
- MR: Trans-spatial enhancing mass
  - T1 and T2 intermediate signal
  - Focal low signal foci on all sequences (phleboliths)
- **Foregut Duplication Cyst, Tongue**
  - Key facts: Congenital cystic lesion located between genioglossus muscles and lined with alimentary tract epithelium
    - May lead to feeding difficulty, especially in infants
  - CT: Circumscribed lesion with well-defined, thick, enhancing wall
    - Variable cyst contents, potentially fluid-debris levels & blood products
    - Frequently indistinguishable from dermoid cyst due to proteinaceous contents
  - MR: Isointense to muscle on T1; hyperintense if proteinaceous fluid or blood products present
  - Ultrasound: Bowel wall signature

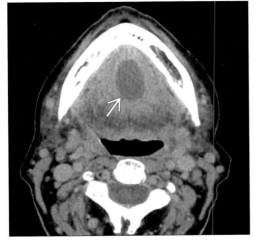

Abscess, Oral Cavity

Axial CECT in a patient after dental extraction shows a root of tongue abscess as a centrally located, peripherally enhancing lesion ➡. The normal adjacent anatomy is obscured by cellulitis.

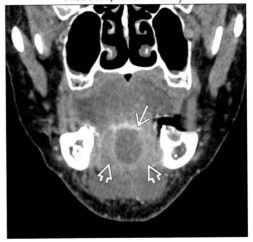

Abscess, Oral Cavity

Coronal CECT in the same patient demonstrates a hypodense rim-enhancing root of tongue abscess ➡ between the genioglossus muscles ➡.

ROOT OF TONGUE LESION

(Left) Axial CECT reveals a heterogeneously enhancing eccentric mass ➡ in the right floor of the mouth. The tumor has invaded through the right genioglossus into the lingual septum ➡ of the root of the tongue. *(Right)* Coronal CECT in the same patient shows a floor of mouth squamous cell carcinoma filling the right sublingual space ➡ and invading medially into the lingual septum ➡ portion of the root of the tongue.

SCCa, Floor of Mouth

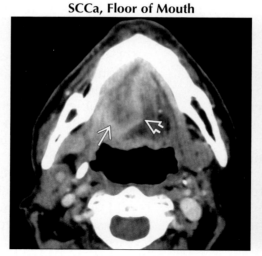

SCCa, Floor of Mouth

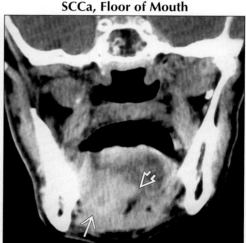

(Left) Axial T1 C+ FS MR shows a large lesion involving the entire right tongue ➡ with extension to the left of midline ➡. The midline fatty lingual septum is replaced by the tumor. *(Right)* Coronal T1 C+ MR depicts an enhancing SCCa of the left oral tongue that crosses the lingual septum into the contralateral tongue ➡ and invades the left sublingual space ➡. Notice that the left genioglossus ➡ is also invaded inferiorly.

SCCa, Oral Tongue

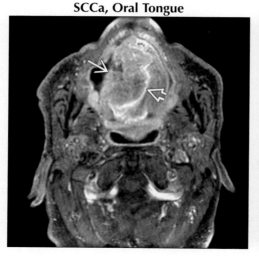

SCCa, Oral Tongue

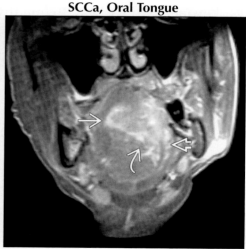

(Left) Axial T2WI MR shows a large homogeneously hyperintense dermoid ➡ imbedded in the intrinsic oral tongue muscles ➡. The absence of complex elements, such as fat or calcifications, makes the dermoid indistinguishable from an epidermoid cyst by imaging. *(Right)* Sagittal T1 C+ MR in the same patient reveals a nonenhancing dermoid cyst ➡ within the root of the tongue. The signal characteristics of the lesion follow fluid intensity.

Dermoid and Epidermoid, Oral Cavity

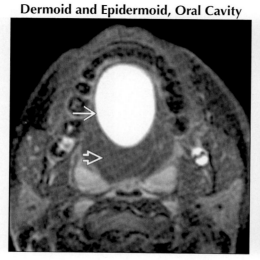

Dermoid and Epidermoid, Oral Cavity

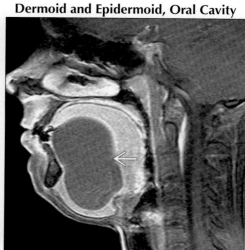

Oral Cavity, Mandible & Maxilla

Thyroglossal Duct Cyst
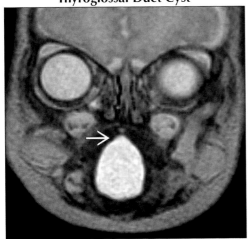

Thyroglossal Duct Cyst
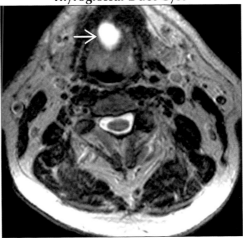

(Left) Coronal T2WI MR demonstrates a well-defined homogeneous root of tongue thyroglossal duct cyst ➔. Signal characteristics are typical of uncomplicated fluid contents. This lesion can be difficult to distinguish from an epidermoid cyst. *(Right)* Axial T2WI MR shows a thyroglossal duct cyst centered in the anterior aspect of the root of the tongue ➔.

Ectopic Thyroid
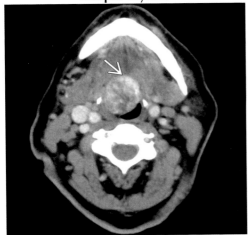

Lymphatic Malformation, Oral Cavity
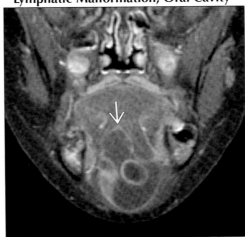

(Left) Axial CECT shows a lingual thyroid with a goiter. The lesion involves both the oropharyngeal mucosal space (lingual tonsil) and the posterior root of tongue ➔. No thyroid tissue was seen in the thyroid bed. *(Right)* Coronal T1 C+ FS MR reveals a complex root of tongue cystic mass ➔ with enhancing septations. No significant enhancement of the rest of the lesion was present after the administration of contrast.

Venous Malformation
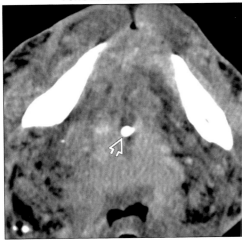

Foregut Duplication Cyst, Tongue
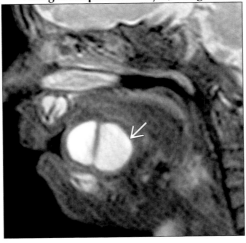

(Left) Axial NECT shows a trans-spatial venous malformation involving the sublingual & submandibular spaces bilaterally. A lingual septum phlebolith ➔ indicates involvement of the root of tongue. *(Right)* Sagittal T2WI FS MR shows a septated foregut duplication cyst ➔ located in the root of tongue. The homogeneously thick wall may suggest the differentiation from other ROT cystic lesions, such as an epidermoid cyst or a thyroglossal duct cyst.

DIFFERENTIAL DIAGNOSIS

Common
- Torus Palatinus
- SCCa, Hard Palate
- Fracture, Complex Midfacial
- Benign Mixed Tumor, Palate
- Minor Salivary Gland Malignancy, Oral

Less Common
- Cyst, Nasopalatine Duct
- Giant Cell Granuloma, Mandible-Maxilla
- Odontogenic Keratocyst
- Osteomyelitis, Mandible-Maxilla

Rare but Important
- Fibrous Dysplasia, Sinonasal
- Osteosarcoma, Mandible-Maxilla
- Metastasis, Mandible-Maxilla

ESSENTIAL INFORMATION

Key Differential Diagnosis Issues
- Bony hard palate often involved in maxilla and oral mucosal lesions

Helpful Clues for Common Diagnoses
- **Torus Palatinus**
  - Key facts: Midline bony exostosis of mature dense cancellous bone with rim of cortical bone of variable thickness
  - Imaging: Osseous projection into oral cavity from hard palate
    - Occasionally shows pedunculated protuberance
- **SCCa, Hard Palate**
  - Key facts: 1/2 of all hard palate cancers are squamous cell carcinomas (SCCa)
    - SCCa (53%), adenoid cystic carcinoma (15%), mucoepidermoid carcinoma (10%), adenocarcinoma (4%), anaplastic carcinoma (4%), other (14%)
    - Majority of patients ≥ 60 years
    - Posterior extension involves soft palate, with possible velopharyngeal insufficiency & hypernasal speech
    - Dental numbness may indicate perineural invasion
    - Dental sockets provide pathway of invasion to alveolar process of maxillary bone & into maxillary sinus
  - Imaging: CECT must include cervical node staging; MR for perineural disease
    - Invasive hard palate mucosal mass may reach maxillary sinus or nose
    - Greater palatine nerve perineural tumor spreads to pterygopalatine fossa
- **Fracture, Complex Midfacial**
  - Key facts: Hard palate fractures relatively rare with facial trauma
  - Imaging: Lucent line through hard palate
- **Benign Mixed Tumor, Palate**
  - Key facts: Composed of both epithelial & mesenchymal tissues
    - Most commonly arises in parotid or submandibular glands
    - Rarely arises from minor salivary glands localized in hard palate & other parts of oral mucosa
    - Slowly growing, painless mass, usually presents in 4-5th decade
    - Benign mixed tumor of oral cavity lacks well-defined fibrous capsule, feature associated with high recurrence rate
  - Imaging: Avid enhancement
    - Well-defined lobulated mass
    - Bone CT: Remodeling of bone
    - MR: Heterogeneous low to intermediate T1 signal intensity & intermediate to high T2 signal
- **Minor Salivary Gland Malignancy, Oral**
  - Key facts: Palatal tumors of minor salivary gland origin are often submucosal & may lack symptoms
    - Symptoms from perineural tumor spread from palate include facial pain/paresthesias
  - Imaging: Well-circumscribed or invasive margins
    - Enhancing mucosal mass superficial to hard palate
    - Greater palatine nerve perineural tumor possible

Helpful Clues for Less Common Diagnoses
- **Cyst, Nasopalatine Duct**
  - Key facts: Nasopalatine duct > 6 mm
    - Expands bone, or may extend into nasal cavity
    - Developmental nonneoplastic cyst; usually asymptomatic
    - Midline cyst develops from proliferation of trapped epithelial cells of incisive canal that secrete mucoid material within incisive canal

○ Imaging: Incisive foramen or canal will appear enlarged
  ▪ CT: Sharp sclerotic margin
- **Giant Cell Granuloma, Mandible-Maxilla**
  ○ Key facts: Benign disease process; can also be locally destructive
    ▪ < 7% of all benign lesions of mandible and maxilla in tooth-bearing areas
    ▪ Mandible, anterior to 1st molar teeth, is most commonly affected site
  ○ Imaging: Varied appearance from undefined destructive lesions to well-defined multilocular appearance
    ▪ Teeth or roots displacement
    ▪ CT: Bone wall thinning & lytic destruction
    ▪ MR: Hypointense on both T1 & T2 MR and avid homogeneous enhancement
- **Odontogenic Keratocyst**
  ○ Key facts: Multiple lesions seen in basal nevus syndrome
    ▪ High recurrence rate
    ▪ Not associated with tooth crown or unerupted tooth
  ○ Imaging: Expansile multilocular lucency
    ▪ 75% near 3rd molar
    ▪ 50% lucent, unilocular, well defined with sclerotic rim, scalloped border
    ▪ Internal high attenuation due to hemorrhage ± protein
- **Osteomyelitis, Mandible-Maxilla**
  ○ Key facts: May develop as sequelae of odontogenic infection or underlying systemic diseases

○ Imaging: Marked erosive process with mucoperiosteal thickening
  ▪ Look for dental source

Helpful Clues for Rare Diagnoses
- **Fibrous Dysplasia, Sinonasal**
  ○ Key facts: Normal bone replaced by fibrous-woven bone
    ▪ Active growth < 30 years of age
  ○ Imaging: Appearance depends on amount of fibrous tissue present
    ▪ Expansile lesion of medullary cavity
    ▪ "Ground-glass" appearance classic
    ▪ If more fibrous tissue, mixed lucent-sclerotic
- **Osteosarcoma, Mandible-Maxilla**
  ○ Key facts: Peak incidence, 3rd decade
    ▪ Mandible affected more than maxilla
  ○ Imaging: Lytic bone destruction with indefinite margins (osteolytic type), area of sclerosis (osteoblastic type), or mixed type
- **Metastasis, Mandible-Maxilla**
  ○ Key facts: Mandible metastasis 4x more frequent than in maxilla
    ▪ Most common primaries: Breast, lung, kidney, thyroid, prostate, stomach
  ○ Imaging: Destruction may be localized, bilateral, or diffuse

SELECTED REFERENCES
1. Ginsberg LE et al: Imaging of perineural tumor spread from palatal carcinoma. AJNR Am J Neuroradiol. 19(8):1417-22, 1998

Torus Palatinus

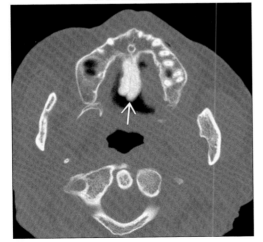

Axial bone CT shows a midline irregular sclerotic bone ➡ protruding inferiorly into the oral cavity. The marrow is contiguous with the maxilla, and there are no aggressive changes.

SCCa, Hard Palate

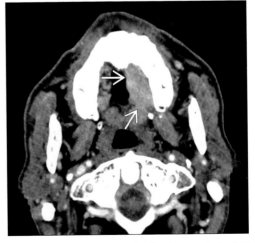

Axial CECT demonstrates a focal enhancing lesion ➡ involving the mucosa & overlying the hard palate. The left greater palatine nerve is at risk for perineural tumor spread based on the primary tumor location.

HARD PALATE LESION

(Left) *Axial bone CT reveals an irregular lucency through the hard palate, extending from anterior to posterior ➡, consistent with a hard palate fracture in this trauma patient.* **(Right)** *Axial CECT shows a focal heterogeneous mass ➡ remodeling the posterior hard palate ⇒, found to be a benign mixed tumor (pleomorphic adenoma).*

Fracture, Complex Midfacial

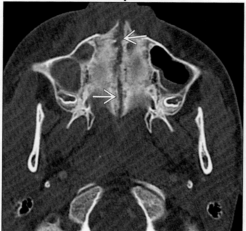

Benign Mixed Tumor, Palate

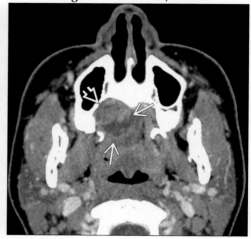

(Left) *Coronal NECT reveals a poorly defined invasive malignancy ➡ eroding the hard palate ⇒. Initial diagnosis of squamous cell carcinoma gave way to the surgical-pathology diagnosis of adenoid cystic carcinoma.* **(Right)** *Coronal STIR MR shows a focal high signal intensity adenoid cystic carcinoma within the mucosa overlying the right hard palate ➡, with minimal osseous changes. Imaging differentiation from benign mixed tumor is difficult.*

Minor Salivary Gland Malignancy, Oral

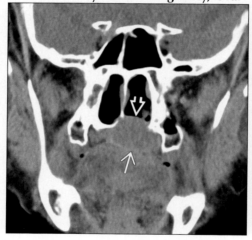

Minor Salivary Gland Malignancy, Oral

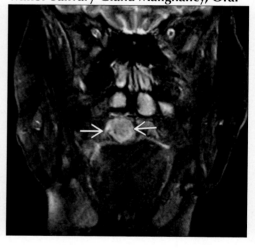

(Left) *Coronal T1 C+ MR demonstrates an invasive heterogeneously enhancing mucoepidermoid carcinoma of minor salivary gland origin in the left hard palate mucosa ➡. Subtle hard palate erosion is visible as enhancing tissue ⇒ in the nasal floor.* **(Right)** *Axial bone CT shows a radiolucent region of the anterior hard palate ➡. As expected, this nasopalatine cyst reveals no aggressive changes, and no internal matrix is seen.*

Minor Salivary Gland Malignancy, Oral

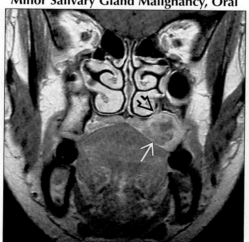

Cyst, Nasopalatine Duct

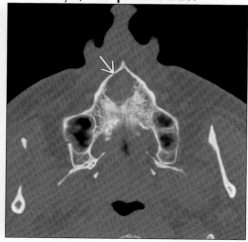

HARD PALATE LESION

Giant Cell Granuloma, Mandible-Maxilla

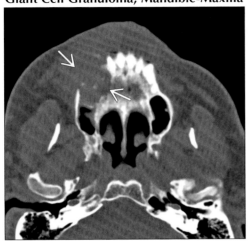

Odontogenic Keratocyst

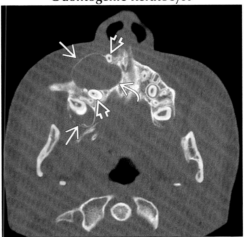

(Left) Axial bone CT shows an expansile-destructive giant cell granuloma in the hard palate involving the nasal floor and maxillary sinus ➡. Ossific flecks are seen in the lesion matrix, which are probably due to pieces of floating bone. *(Right)* Axial bone CT shows multiple maxillary ridge odontogenic keratocysts ➡ in a patient with basal cell nevus syndrome. The anterior lesion splays the maxillary teeth ➡ and enlarges into the hard palate ➡.

Osteomyelitis, Mandible-Maxilla

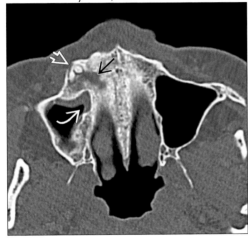

Fibrous Dysplasia, Sinonasal

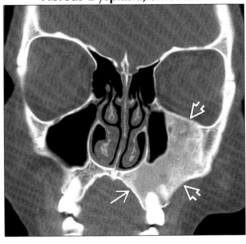

(Left) Axial bone CT shows a diseased maxillary tooth with lucency around its root, causing hard palate osteomyelitis ➡, superficial cortical loss ➡, & sympathetic maxillary sinus inflammation ➡. *(Right)* Coronal bone CT demonstrates marked bone thickening, with a uniform density of the thickened bone ➡, which has the typical "ground-glass" appearance of fibrous dysplasia. The hard palate is involved ➡ with expansion flattening its arch.

Osteosarcoma, Mandible-Maxilla

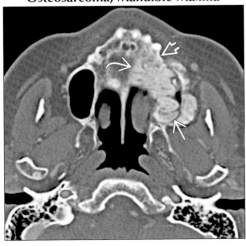

Metastasis, Mandible-Maxilla

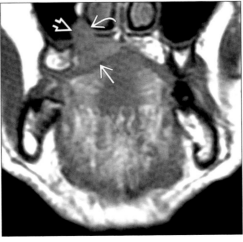

(Left) Axial bone scan demonstrates an osteoblastic osteosarcoma involving the maxillary sinus ➡, ridge ➡, and hard palate ➡. *(Right)* Coronal T1WI MR reveals a hard palate metastasis ➡ from primary breast carcinoma destroying the bone and communicating superiorly with the nose ➡ and maxillary sinus ➡.

MAXILLARY BONE LESION

DIFFERENTIAL DIAGNOSIS

Common
- Cyst, Periapical (Radicular)
- Cyst, Nasopalatine Duct
- Fracture, Zygomaticomaxillary Complex
- Cyst, Dentigerous (Follicular)
- Torus Maxillaris

Less Common
- Odontogenic Keratocyst
- SCCa, Hard Palate
- Fibrous Dysplasia, Mandible-Maxilla
- Osteomyelitis, Mandible-Maxilla
- Osteonecrosis, Mandible-Maxilla
- Ameloblastoma
- Burkitt Lymphoma, Mandible-Maxilla

Rare but Important
- Hemangioma, Facial Bones
- Osteosarcoma, Mandible-Maxilla
- Giant Cell Granuloma, Mandible-Maxilla
- Basal Cell Nevus Syndrome
- Cherubism, Mandible-Maxilla

ESSENTIAL INFORMATION

Key Differential Diagnosis Issues
- Similar pathologies affect maxilla and mandible
- Determination of odontogenic vs. nonodontogenic origin narrows differential
- Use CT for cortical bone involvement/matrix evaluation, MR for marrow and adjacent soft tissue extension

Helpful Clues for Common Diagnoses
- **Cyst, Periapical (Radicular)**
  - Key facts: Arises at apex of infected tooth as sequelae to periapical granuloma
  - Imaging: Sharply circumscribed radiolucency at tooth apex with thin sclerotic rim
    - Look for dehiscence of maxillary sinus floor & odontogenic sinusitis
- **Cyst, Nasopalatine Duct**
  - Key facts: Developmental, nonneoplastic cyst; most common nonodontogenic cyst
    - Location in anterior midline maxilla pathognomonic (incisive foramen)
  - Imaging: Expansile cyst in midline anterior maxilla with sharp sclerotic margins
    - Increased T2 signal

- **Fracture, Zygomaticomaxillary Complex**
  - Key facts: < 25% of all facial fractures (fxs)
    - Maxillary fxs most common in zygomaticomaxillary complex fxs
    - Also seen in alveolar ridge, complex midfacial & transfacial (Le Fort) fxs
  - Imaging: Determine if fracture is isolated or part of complex
    - Degree of comminution & involvement of vascular & neural structures important to note
- **Cyst, Dentigerous (Follicular)**
  - Key facts: Benign odontogenic cyst associated with crown of unerupted/partially erupted tooth
  - Imaging: Well-circumscribed, expansile lucent cyst containing tooth crown
    - Fluid signal on MR with hypointense tooth crown
- **Torus Maxillaris**
  - Key facts: Localized outgrowth of bone from alveolar portion of maxilla
  - Imaging
    - Internus: Arises along lingual surface of dental arch opposite roots of molars; may coalesce into lobular masses
    - Externus: Broader expansions along buccal aspect of superior alveolar ridge

Helpful Clues for Less Common Diagnoses
- **Odontogenic Keratocyst**
  - Key facts: Posterior mandible affected 2-4x greater than maxilla
    - Multiple in basal cell nevus syndrome
  - Imaging: Unilocular cystic lesion with thin sclerotic rim
    - May be associated with crown of tooth
- **SCCa, Hard Palate**
  - Key facts: SCCa accounts for 50% of palate cancers
  - CT: Soft tissue mass with destructive bony changes
    - Cortical involvement best shown on CT
  - MR: Soft tissue replaces marrow fat
    - Look for perineural spread on palatine nerves
- **Fibrous Dysplasia, Mandible-Maxilla**
  - Key facts: Normal medullary bone replaced by weak fibroosseous tissue
  - CT: Expansion of marrow with "ground-glass" ± fibrous density
  - MR: Tendency for ↓ T1 & T2 signal

- Enhancement varies with amount of fibrous tissue
- **Osteomyelitis, Mandible-Maxilla**
  - Key facts: Sequelae of odontogenic infection
  - CT: Erosion of maxillary alveolus near carious teeth
  - MR: ↓ T1, ↑ T2 & STIR
    - Avid enhancement of marrow & adjacent soft tissues
- **Osteonecrosis, Mandible-Maxilla**
  - Key facts: Often related to IV bisphosphonate use
    - Maxilla < mandible
  - Imaging: Mixed lytic & sclerotic
    - Mimics osteomyelitis
    - Look for pathologic fx, sequestra, oroantral fistulae
- **Ameloblastoma**
  - Key facts: Benign odontogenic neoplasm
    - Predilection for molar region
    - Mandible 4x more common than maxilla
  - Imaging: Expansile multilocular lesion with cortical thinning
    - ↑ T2 with enhancing wall + nodules
- **Burkitt Lymphoma, Mandible-Maxilla**
  - Key facts: High-grade B-cell lymphoma
  - Imaging: Mottled permeative pattern of bone destruction
    - Homogeneous with diffuse enhancement

Helpful Clues for Rare Diagnoses
- **Hemangioma, Facial Bones**

- Key facts: May involve maxilla, mandible, nasal bones
- Imaging: Sharply marginated; expansile with "sunburst," "honeycomb," or "soap bubble" pattern
- **Osteosarcoma, Mandible-Maxilla**
  - Key facts: High-grade bone malignancy
  - CT: Aggressive periosteal reaction and bone formation
  - MR: Heterogeneous T1/T2 signal & enhancement
    - Invasion of adjacent tissues
- **Giant Cell Granuloma, Mandible-Maxilla**
  - Key facts: Nonodontogenic intraosseous lesion
  - Imaging: Expansile mass within marrow space
    - ↓ T1/T2 signal with avid enhancement
- **Basal Cell Nevus Syndrome**
  - Key facts: Autosomal dominant syndrome involving multiple organ systems (skin, dental, CNS, GU)
  - Imaging: Multiple odontogenic keratocysts in mandible & maxilla
- **Cherubism, Mandible-Maxilla**
  - Key facts: Genetic condition distinct from fibrous dysplasia
    - May involute at puberty
  - Imaging: Marked polyostotic bone expansion with mixed density & coarse trabecular pattern

Cyst, Periapical (Radicular)

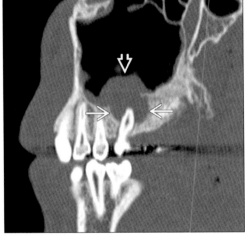

Sagittal oblique bone CT shows a halo of lucency ➡ at the apex of the root of the 2nd maxillary premolar. The bone demineralization secondary to dental caries produced sinus mucosal disease ➡.

Cyst, Nasopalatine Duct

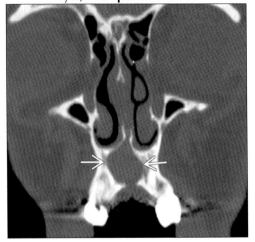

Coronal bone CT shows a typical appearance of an incisive canal cyst. There is an expansile cyst ➡ in the anterior midline, maxilla pathognomonic of this lesion.

(Left) Axial bone CT shows focal linear fractures of the anterior and posterior walls ➡ of the left maxillary sinus in a patient with a zygomaticomaxillary complex fracture. Note the foreign bodies in the soft tissues of the cheek ⬧➡. (Right) Axial bone CT shows an expansile unilocular cystic lesion ➡ associated with the crown of an unerupted tooth ➡ in the superior alveolus of the right maxilla.

Fracture, Zygomaticomaxillary Complex

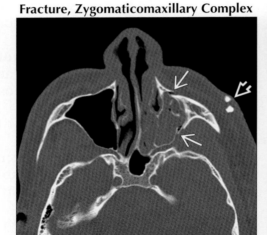

Cyst, Dentigerous (Follicular)

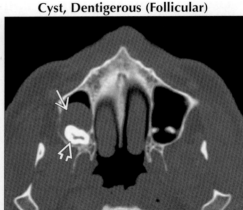

(Left) Axial bone CT shows a medially directed torus maxillaris ➡ on the right. There is contiguity of the marrow into this benign osseous lesion. There are also bilateral maxillary buccal exostoses ➡. (Right) Axial bone CT shows an expansile cyst arising from the left maxillary alveolus with smooth scalloping and thinning of its walls ➡. The cyst is displacing an unerupted left maxillary canine tooth superiorly, medially, and anteriorly ➡.

Torus Maxillaris

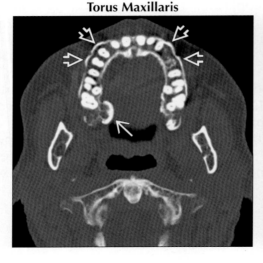

Odontogenic Keratocyst

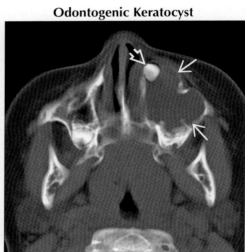

(Left) Coronal T1WI MR shows a focal, destructive, marrow-replacing lesion in the anterior right maxilla ➡, found to be a small maxilla squamous cell carcinoma. Note the normal fatty marrow signal in the left maxilla ➡. (Right) Axial bone CT shows markedly expanded maxillary bone of variable attenuation. There are areas of characteristic "ground-glass" density ➡ interspersed with more soft tissue density (fibrous) areas ➡.

SCCa, Hard Palate

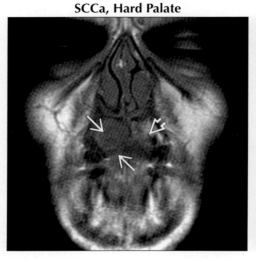

Fibrous Dysplasia, Mandible-Maxilla

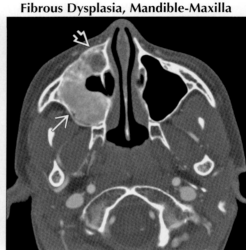

Osteomyelitis, Mandible-Maxilla

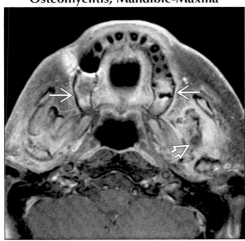

Osteonecrosis, Mandible-Maxilla

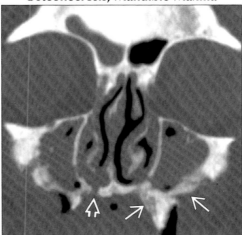

(Left) Axial T1 C+ FS MR shows diffuse maxillary alveolar and parosteal soft tissue enhancement ➡. There are fluid collections ➡ present near the left mandibular ramus in this patient with osteomyelitis. *(Right)* Coronal bone CT shows a mottled predominantly lytic pattern of osteonecrosis of the maxilla ➡ in this patient treated with bisphosphonates for breast carcinoma skeletal metastases. Note the oroantral fistula ➡.

Ameloblastoma

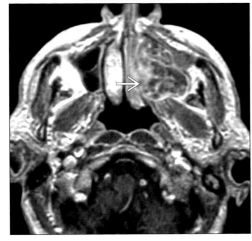

Burkitt Lymphoma, Mandible-Maxilla

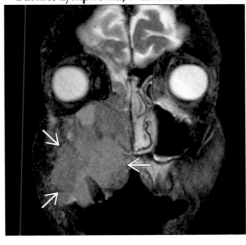

(Left) Axial T1 C+ MR shows a heterogeneous expansile mass in the maxillary alveolus with both solid and cystic components and enhancing septations ➡, found to be an ameloblastoma. *(Right)* Coronal T2WI FS MR shows a large, intermediate signal intensity mass ➡ arising from the right maxillary alveolus and extending cephalad into the right maxillary antrum. The homogeneous low signal of the lesion is characteristic of lymphoma.

Hemangioma, Facial Bones

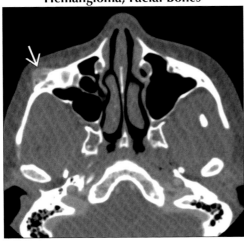

Osteosarcoma, Mandible-Maxilla

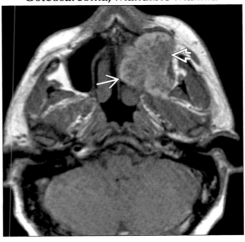

(Left) Axial CECT shows a lesion ➡ arising from the right maxillary bone at the malar eminence. This intraosseous hemangioma shows the classic "soap bubble" appearance frequently reported with these tumors. *(Right)* Axial T1WI MR shows a tumor arising from the left maxillary ridge, involving the nasal cavity ➡ and maxillary sinus ➡. The "sunburst" architecture of this mass is suggestive of osteosarcoma but would be better demonstrated on CT.

TOOTH-RELATED MASS, SCLEROTIC

DIFFERENTIAL DIAGNOSIS

Common
- Condensing Osteitis, Mandible-Maxilla
- Odontoma
- Cemento-Osseous Dysplasia, Periapical

Less Common
- Cemento-Osseous Dysplasia, Florid
- Dental Implantation
- Osteosclerosis, Mandible-Maxilla, Idiopathic

Rare but Important
- Ameloblastic Fibro-Odontoma
- Cementoblastoma
- Calcifying Epithelial Odontogenic Tumor

ESSENTIAL INFORMATION

Key Differential Diagnosis Issues
- Predominantly sclerotic lesions arising in tooth-bearing portions of jaw
- Intimately associated with dental crowns or roots, therefore located above mandibular canal
- Best imaging tools
  ○ Unenhanced bone CT
  ○ Panoramic and bitewing radiographs remain mainstays of screening

Helpful Clues for Common Diagnoses
- **Condensing Osteitis, Mandible-Maxilla**
  ○ Key facts
    - Periapical inflammation due to dental pulp infection
  ○ Imaging
    - Poorly marginated periapical bone sclerosis associated with carious or restored tooth
- **Odontoma**
  ○ Key facts
    - Arise in childhood to early adulthood
    - 50% associated with impacted tooth
    - May cause dental resorption
  ○ Imaging
    - Sclerotic with lucent rim (initially lucent, later calcified)
    - Compound odontoma: Contain tooth components (abortive teeth, a.k.a. "denticles"), more common anteriorly (canine region)

- Complex odontoma: Amorphous mass of dental tissue with relatively homogeneous calcification, more common posteriorly (premolar or molar region)
- **Cemento-Osseous Dysplasia, Periapical**
  ○ Key facts
    - Most arise in women in 4th-5th decade; Blacks and Asians > > Caucasians
  ○ Imaging
    - Often multifocal, between adjacent teeth, usually < 1 cm
    - Initially lucent, progressing to sclerosis with lucent margin
    - May be accompanied by bone cysts

Helpful Clues for Less Common Diagnoses
- **Cemento-Osseous Dysplasia, Florid**
  ○ Key facts
    - Diffuse form of periapical cemento-osseous dysplasia
  ○ Imaging
    - "Fluffy" sclerotic lesions in periapical alveolar bone or in edentulous areas
    - 2 or more quadrants affected; often symmetric and expansile; larger than periapical form
    - May be accompanied by bone cysts or complicated by osteomyelitis
- **Dental Implantation**
  ○ Key facts
    - Bone grafted into/above alveolus to provide base for dental implantation, typically mixed with hydroxyapatite or tricalcium phosphate
  ○ Imaging
    - Uniform speckled pattern of density immediately against alveolus; denser than native alveolar bone
    - Implant may not yet be present as clue to diagnosis
- **Osteosclerosis, Mandible-Maxilla, Idiopathic**
  ○ Key facts
    - Asymptomatic, incidental finding of unknown origin, not 2° to infection or systemic disease (e.g., pulp infection, Gardner syndrome)
  ○ Imaging

- Well-defined round or oval radiopacity associated with healthy tooth, most commonly associated with 1st molar or 2nd premolar
- No lucent rim; usually more radiopaque than condensing osteitis
- May enlarge in young patients; tends to stabilize with age; may disappear on follow-up
- No bone expansion, tooth erosion, or root displacement (suggests against central osteoma)

Helpful Clues for Rare Diagnoses

- **Ameloblastic Fibro-Odontoma**
  - Key facts
    - Usually in patients ≤ 20 years
    - Predilection for premolar or molar region of either jaw
    - Can be associated with crown of unerupted tooth
  - Imaging
    - Variable amounts of calcified vs. noncalcified tissue (influences radiographic appearance)
    - Sharply circumscribed with lucent rim regardless of calcification pattern
    - Randomly arranged central Ca++ of irregular size and shape or more solid Ca++ lesion with radiating, striated Ca++
- **Cementoblastoma**
  - Key facts
    - Patients ≤ 30 years
    - Arises from periodontal ligament

- Periapical lesion associated with mandibular premolar or 1st molar (never involves anterior dentition)
- Produces mass of cementum or cementum-like tissue fused to tooth root; usually removed en bloc with tooth
  - Imaging
    - Well-demarcated, rounded, or irregular lesion; mottled or sunburst Ca++ pattern; lucent rim
    - Obscures periodontal ligament space
- **Calcifying Epithelial Odontogenic Tumor**
  - Key facts
    - Rare benign lesion of unknown etiology, usually asymptomatic, but can be expansile
    - Arises in 3rd or 4th decade; 2/3 arise in mandible (premolar or molar regions)
    - Associated with impacted tooth in 50%
  - Imaging
    - Unilocular or multilocular radiolucency with scattered calcifications ("driven-snow" appearance)
    - Focally expansile with thinning of bone

SELECTED REFERENCES

1. Theodorou SJ et al: Imaging characteristics of neoplasms and other lesions of the jawbones: part 1. Odontogenic tumors and tumorlike lesions. Clin Imaging. 31(2):114-9, 2007
2. Theodorou SJ et al: Imaging characteristics of neoplasms and other lesions of the jawbones: part 2. Odontogenic tumor-mimickers and tumor-like lesions. Clin Imaging. 31(2):120-6, 2007
3. Yonetsu K et al: CT of calcifying jaw bone diseases. AJR Am J Roentgenol. 177(4):937-43, 2001

Condensing Osteitis, Mandible-Maxilla

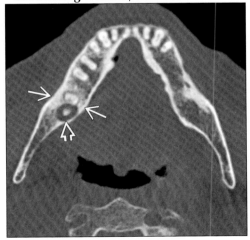

Axial bone CT demonstrates poorly marginated bone sclerosis ➡ surrounding periapical lucency associated with a carious tooth ➡.

Odontoma

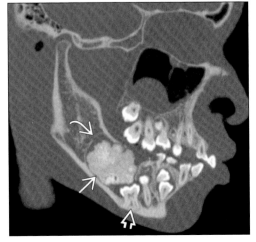

Sagittal oblique bone CT shows a lobulated, densely calcified complex odontoma ➡ associated with an impacted tooth ➡. Note lucent halo surrounding the calcified component ➡.

TOOTH-RELATED MASS, SCLEROTIC

Odontoma

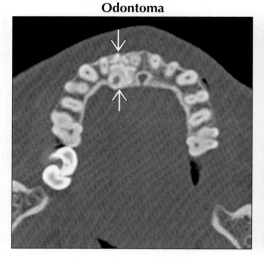

Odontoma

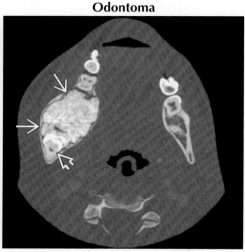

(Left) Axial bone CT reveals a cluster of small tooth-like calcifications (denticles) ➡ splaying the roots of the right maxillary incisors in this compound odontoma. *(Right)* Axial bone CT shows a complex odontoma with significant bone expansion. Note amorphous calcified material in the odontoma ➡ and associated impacted tooth ➡. There is a thin but intact lucent rim surrounding the lesion.

Cemento-Osseous Dysplasia, Periapical

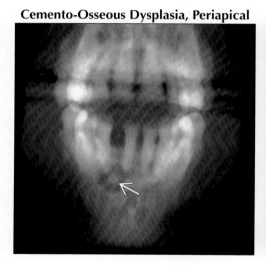

Cemento-Osseous Dysplasia, Periapical

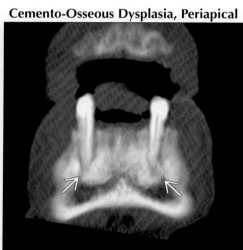

(Left) Anteroposterior 3D CT image shows an early phase of cemento-osseous dysplasia with a small nidus of calcification ➡ in an otherwise lucent periapical lesion. *(Right)* Coronal slab MPR CT shows bilateral foci of well-marginated bone sclerosis ➡ surrounding the roots of the mandibular canine teeth. Note the lucent zone separating the lesions from the tooth roots (contrast with cementoblastoma).

Cemento-Osseous Dysplasia, Florid

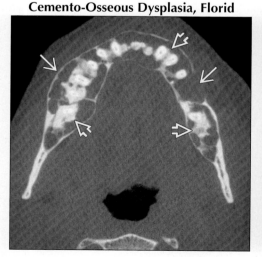

Cemento-Osseous Dysplasia, Florid

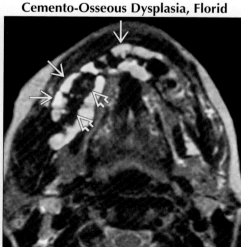

(Left) Axial bone CT demonstrates diffuse expansion of the mandible by simple bone cysts ➡ accompanying sclerotic lesions that surround the tooth apices ➡. *(Right)* Axial T2WI MR reveals fluid signal within the cysts ➡ and markedly hypointense signal surrounding the dental apices ➡.

Dental Implantation

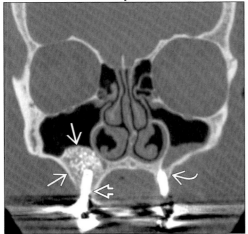

Osteosclerosis, Mandible-Maxilla, Idiopathic

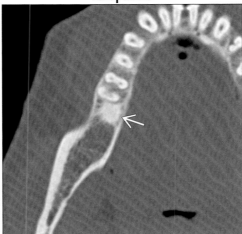

(Left) Coronal bone CT shows bone and hydroxyapatite ➡ that was surgically implanted in the right maxillary alveolus to provide sufficient bone to anchor a dental implant ➡. Note the markedly atrophic left maxillary alveolar ridge ➡. The diagnosis may be less obvious when this finding is encountered before implant insertion. *(Right)* Axial bone CT shows a densely sclerotic lesion associated with a vital right mandibular 1st molar ➡. There is no lucent rim.

Ameloblastic Fibro-Odontoma

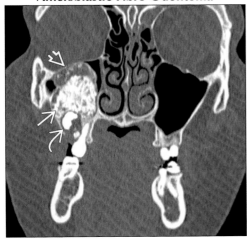

Ameloblastic Fibro-Odontoma

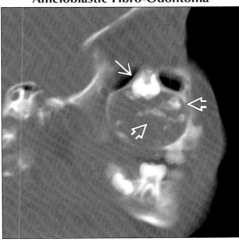

(Left) Coronal bone CT shows both densely calcified central ➡ and more peripheral lucent ➡ components of this lesion. Note the associated impacted tooth ➡. *(Right)* Sagittal bone CT thick ray-sum image demonstrates a more lucent example of this entity. Note the impacted tooth ➡ and multiple irregular calcifications ➡ in the lesion. The lesion appears cystic on CT, but a well-circumscribed soft tissue mass was found at surgery.

Cementoblastoma

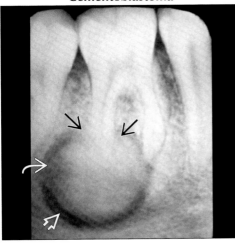

Calcifying Epithelial Odontogenic Tumor

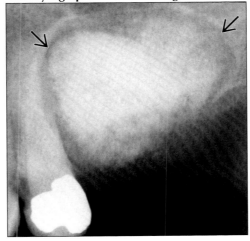

(Left) Bitewing film shows a sclerotic lesion surrounding a 1st molar root and obliterating the periodontal ligament space ➡. Note the peripheral lucent zone ➡. Sunburst calcification is visible in some portions ➡ of the lesion. (Courtesy C. Dunlap, MD.) *(Right)* Bitewing radiograph shows a sclerotic lesion with "fluffy" calcification and a lucent margin ➡. No impacted tooth was present in this patient. (Courtesy C. Dunlap, MD.)

TOOTH-RELATED MASS, CYSTIC

DIFFERENTIAL DIAGNOSIS

Common
- Cyst, Periapical (Radicular)
- Cyst, Dentigerous (Follicular)
- Odontogenic Keratocyst

Less Common
- Ameloblastoma, Cystic
- Cyst, Residual
- Cyst, Lateral Periodontal

Rare but Important
- Ameloblastic Fibro-Odontoma
- Calcifying Cystic Odontogenic Tumor

ESSENTIAL INFORMATION

Key Differential Diagnosis Issues
- Tooth-related: Abuts dental crown or roots

Helpful Clues for Common Diagnoses
- **Cyst, Periapical (Radicular)**
  - Associated with apex of carious or restored tooth, abuts lamina dura
  - May extend into maxillary sinus (odontogenic sinusitis)
- **Cyst, Dentigerous (Follicular)**
  - Surrounds crown of unerupted tooth (3rd mandibular molar or maxillary canine)
  - Attached to cemento-enamel junction
  - May displace tooth, erode roots, thin cortex, but does not usually expand bone
- **Odontogenic Keratocyst**
  - Posterior mandibular body/ramus near 3rd molar or in maxillary canine region

  - Multiloculated with daughter cysts
  - Longitudinal > transverse expansion, thin & expand bone > dentigerous cysts do
  - Mildly heterogeneous density (CT) or signal (MR) without enhancement
  - Multiple in basal cell nevus syndrome

Helpful Clues for Less Common Diagnoses
- **Ameloblastoma, Cystic**
  - Osseous expansion, erosion of tooth roots, thinning/dehiscence of cortex
  - "Soap bubble" or "honeycomb" appearance
  - Soft tissue component(s) with C+
- **Cyst, Residual**
  - Abuts alveolar crest at site of dental extraction; no associated tooth
- **Cyst, Lateral Periodontal**
  - Arises between & splay roots; not centered on tooth apex; vital teeth

Helpful Clues for Rare Diagnoses
- **Ameloblastic Fibro-Odontoma**
  - Multiloculated lucency without Ca++ (fibroma) or diffusely scattered coarse Ca++ (fibro-odontoma)
- **Calcifying Cystic Odontogenic Tumor**
  - Peripheral calcifications of irregular size/shape

SELECTED REFERENCES

1. Theodorou SJ et al: Imaging characteristics of neoplasms and other lesions of the jawbones: part 1. Odontogenic tumors and tumorlike lesions. Clin Imaging. 31(2):114-9, 2007

Cyst, Periapical (Radicular)

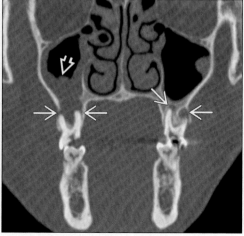

Coronal bone CT shows periapical cysts surrounding the apices of bilateral carious maxillary teeth ➡. Note associated sinusitis on the right ➡, possibly representing "odontogenic sinusitis."

Cyst, Dentigerous (Follicular)

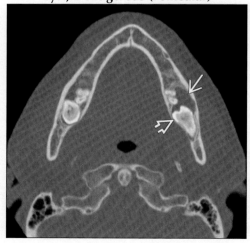

Axial bone CT reveals a well-circumscribed lucent lesion ➡ surrounding the crown of unerupted left mandibular 3rd molar ➡. The overlying cortex is intact. The adjacent tooth roots are preserved.

Odontogenic Keratocyst

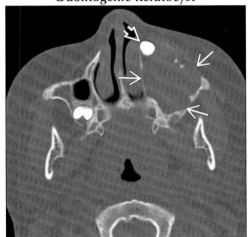

Ameloblastoma, Cystic

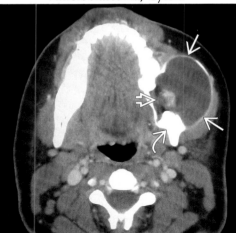

(Left) Axial bone CT shows a cystic lesion in the maxilla ➡. Note associated unerupted tooth ➡. The complex contour would be unusual for a dentigerous cyst. *(Right)* Axial CECT reveals a cystic-appearing posterior mandibular body lesion. Overlying bone is expanded & nearly dehiscent ➡. The soft tissue nodule ➡ is a clue to diagnosis of ameloblastoma. Absence of odontogenic keratocyst would be hard to exclude. Note associated unerupted 3rd molar ➡.

Cyst, Residual

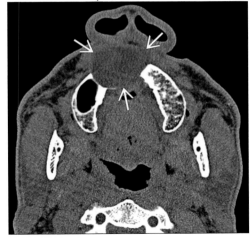

Cyst, Lateral Periodontal

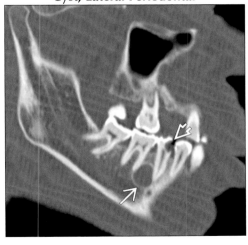

(Left) Axial bone CT demonstrates a large residual cyst ➡. It may be difficult to differentiate large premaxillary residual cysts from eccentric nasopalatine duct cysts. These 2 also share similar histological features. *(Right)* Sagittal oblique bone CT shows sharply marginated cyst ➡ splaying the apices of the mandibular 2nd bicuspid and 1st molar. The cyst is not centered on the tooth apex. The 2nd bicuspid ➡ is carious (not "classic").

Ameloblastic Fibro-Odontoma

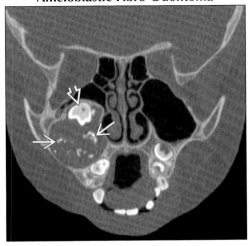

Calcifying Cystic Odontogenic Tumor

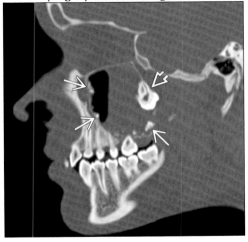

(Left) Coronal bone CT reveals a lucent lesion with central flocculent calcifications ➡ and a displaced unerupted tooth ➡. Note that this lesion only appears cystic on CT. A circumscribed soft tissue mass containing calcifications was encountered at surgery. *(Right)* Sagittal bone CT demonstrates a previously biopsied maxillary calcifying odontogenic cyst associated with peripheral calcifications ➡ and an unerupted tooth ➡.

LOW-DENSITY JAW LESION, SHARPLY MARGINATED (CT)

DIFFERENTIAL DIAGNOSIS

Common
- Cyst, Simple Bone (Traumatic)
- Cyst, Nasopalatine Duct

Less Common
- Ameloblastoma
- Giant Cell Granuloma, Mandible-Maxilla
- Cyst, Residual
- Aneurysmal Bone Cyst

Rare but Important
- Odontogenic Myxoma (Myxofibroma)
- Langerhans Histiocytosis, Mandible-Maxilla
- Cherubism, Mandible-Maxilla

ESSENTIAL INFORMATION

Key Differential Diagnosis Issues
- DDx refers to occasionally extensive lucent jaw lesions not strictly related to a tooth

Helpful Clues for Common Diagnoses
- **Cyst, Simple Bone (Traumatic)**
  - Key facts
    - Fluid-filled lesion with no epithelial lining, not associated with infection
    - May accompany other lesions (e.g., cemento-osseous dysplasia, osteomas)
  - Imaging
    - Mandibular or maxillary cyst with thin irregular corticated margin
    - Minimal buccolingual expansion or cortical thinning
- **Cyst, Nasopalatine Duct**
  - Key facts
    - Arises in incisive canal of maxilla
    - May span midline or lie unilaterally (due to splitting of incisive canal superiorly)
  - Imaging
    - Thin-walled sharply marginated cyst
    - Occasional displacement of incisor roots

Helpful Clues for Less Common Diagnoses
- **Ameloblastoma**
  - Key facts
    - Most common odontogenic tumor
    - Mandible (especially molar region & ramus) > maxilla
    - Multilocular > unilocular
  - Imaging
    - Osseous expansion with thinning and dehiscence of cortex

- Dental apical erosion
- "Soap bubble" or "honeycomb" appearance
- Variably sized cysts
- Mixed cystic & enhancing soft tissue components

- **Giant Cell Granuloma, Mandible-Maxilla**
  - Key facts
    - M < F, most patients < 20 years
    - Not true tumor; benign reactive proliferation of bone
    - May coexist with aneurysmal bone cyst
    - Histologically identical to brown tumor of hyperparathyroidism
  - Imaging
    - Expansile multilocular-appearing radiolucent lesion with thinning of surrounding cortical bone
    - Scattered calcification, soft tissue density on NECT
    - Prominent homogeneous enhancement
- **Cyst, Residual**
  - Key facts
    - Radicular cyst that remains following tooth extraction
  - Imaging
    - Sharply marginated lucent lesion
    - Apex reaches alveolar crest at site of missing tooth
- **Aneurysmal Bone Cyst**
  - Key facts
    - Primarily in patients < 20 years
    - Mandibular ramus > maxilla
    - Occur in isolation ± history of trauma (primary) or associated with other lesions such as giant cell tumors (secondary)
    - Not true cyst; no epithelial lining
    - Lined by fibrous connective tissue stroma surrounded with enlarged vascular spaces, hemosiderin deposition
    - No endothelium or basement membrane lining vascular spaces
  - Imaging
    - Appear unilocular > multilocular/"soap bubble"
    - Expansion, thinning, even dehiscence of bony cortex; fractures
    - Even when cortex disrupted, lesion appears sharply marginated and noninfiltrative

- Shell of reactive new bone may be observed
- Blood-fluid levels suggestive but not specific

Helpful Clues for Rare Diagnoses
- **Odontogenic Myxoma (Myxofibroma)**
  - Key facts
    - Locally invasive neoplasm
    - Typically arises in 2nd or 3rd decade
    - Mandibular molar area > maxilla
  - Imaging
    - "Tennis racket" appearance (created by multiple straight or mildly curvilinear interconnected thin septa)
    - Cortical thinning and dehiscence
    - Tooth displacement, occasional root resorption
- **Langerhans Histiocytosis, Mandible-Maxilla**
  - Key facts
    - Most patients present at < 15 years
    - May occur in isolation or in disseminated fashion
    - Most cases in children are solitary
    - Mandible > maxilla
  - Imaging
    - Uni- or multilocular lucent lesion with beveled edges, no marginal sclerosis or periosteal reaction
    - May see floating teeth, extraosseous soft tissue extension
- **Cherubism, Mandible-Maxilla**
  - Key facts

- Presents at 2-3 years with painless cheek swelling; proptosis
- NOT form of fibrous dysplasia
- Progression arrested at puberty, with subsequent partial or complete involution
- Both familial and sporadic cases reported
- Affects mandible, maxilla, or both, usually bilateral, with tooth displacement and loss
  - Imaging
    - Multiple bubbly circumscribed radiolucent areas
    - Marked bone expansion and cortical thinning
    - Appearance may vary depending on stage
    - Increased sclerosis during involution

SELECTED REFERENCES
1. Dunfee BL et al: Radiologic and pathologic characteristics of benign and malignant lesions of the mandible. Radiographics. 26(6):1751-68, 2006
2. Kaneda T et al: Benign odontogenic tumors of the mandible and maxilla. Neuroimaging Clin N Am. 13(3):495-507, 2003
3. Yoshiura K et al: Cystic lesions of the mandible and maxilla. Neuroimaging Clin N Am. 13(3):485-94, 2003
4. Scholl RJ et al: Cysts and cystic lesions of the mandible: clinical and radiologic-histopathologic review. Radiographics. 19(5):1107-24, 1999

Cyst, Simple Bone (Traumatic)

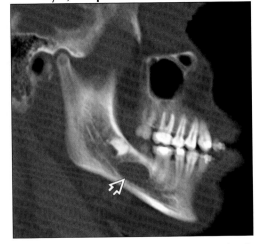

Lateral 3D CT subvolume shows a sharply circumscribed lucency in the right hemimandible ➡.

Cyst, Simple Bone (Traumatic)

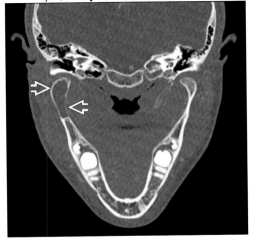

Coronal oblique bone CT demonstrates a sharply marginated lucency in the right mandibular condyle and subcondylar neck ➡. There is mild bone expansion in this patient with a simple bone cyst.

LOW-DENSITY JAW LESION, SHARPLY MARGINATED (CT)

(Left) Axial CECT reveals a bilateral expansile lesion centered in the premaxilla with thin ⇨ to dehiscent ➡ bony margins. This degree of anterior displacement of the buccal cortex and the bilaterality would be unusual for a radicular cyst. **(Right)** Coronal NECT shows a unilateral, sharply marginated lucent nasopalatine duct cyst ⇨ centered on the hard palate and abutting the midline at the upper end of the incisive canal ➡.

Cyst, Nasopalatine Duct

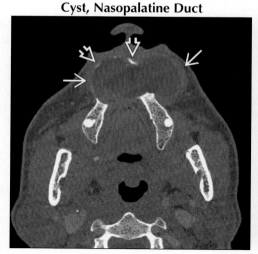

Cyst, Nasopalatine Duct

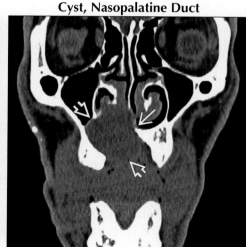

(Left) Axial CECT reveals a heterogeneously lucent mandibular ameloblastoma with narrow transition zones ⇨. There are both enhancing solid ➡ and cystic ➡ components. **(Right)** Axial T1 C+ FS MR shows a complex multiloculated lesion involving bilateral anterior mandible. Soft tissue components and cyst walls enhance prominently ⇨. The contents of unilocular cyst on the left ➡ were hyperintense on precontrast images (not shown).

Ameloblastoma

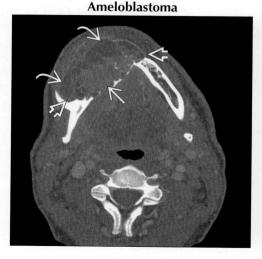

Ameloblastoma

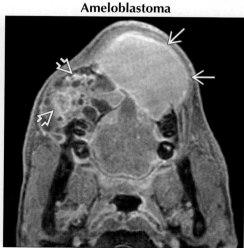

(Left) Coronal NECT shows an expansile giant cell granuloma of the right maxilla ⇨ protruding into the right nasal cavity ➡ and orbit ➡. Note similarities to aneurysmal bone cyst and soft tissue density of lesion. **(Right)** Axial NECT shows an expansile lesion of the left mandible with thin ⇨ or dehiscent ➡ margins. This lesion has septa ➡ reminiscent of an odontogenic myxoma. Differentiation of the 2 by imaging would be difficult.

Giant Cell Granuloma, Mandible-Maxilla

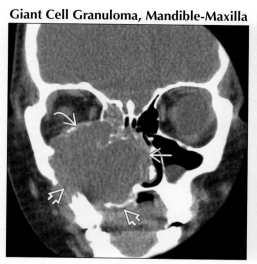

Giant Cell Granuloma, Mandible-Maxilla

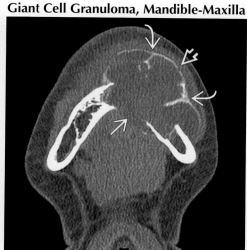

Cyst, Residual

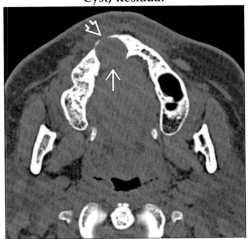

Aneurysmal Bone Cyst

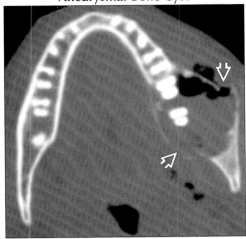

(Left) Axial NECT shows sharply marginated right paramedian lucent residual cyst expanding through the buccal ⇨ and lingual ⇨ cortex of the maxilla. *(Right)* Axial NECT demonstrates a pathologic fracture through a left mandibular aneurysmal bone cyst ⇨. Intralesional air implies that mucosal tearing has occurred.

Odontogenic Myxoma (Myxofibroma)

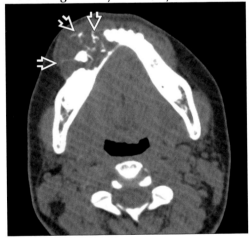

Langerhans Histiocytosis, Mandible-Maxilla

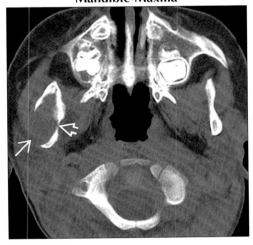

(Left) Axial bone CT reveals a typical appearance of mandibular odontogenic myxoma with characteristic multiple osseous septa ⇨. *(Right)* Axial bone CT in a child shows a single focus of Langerhans cell histiocytosis as a sharply marginated expansile lesion in the right mandibular ramus ⇨. The buccal cortex is dehiscent with a small extraosseous component ⇨. Note the absence of periosteal reaction or marginal sclerosis.

Cherubism, Mandible-Maxilla

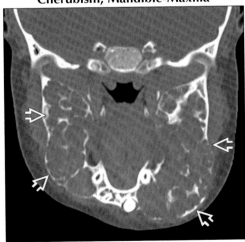

Cherubism, Mandible-Maxilla

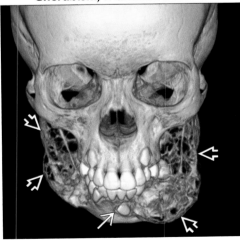

(Left) Coronal bone CT in a child shows bilateral, diffuse, "bubbly," cystic expansile mandibular process ⇨ highly suggestive of the diagnosis of cherubism. *(Right)* Anteroposterior 3D CT subvolume shows the diffuse, bilateral, multilocular, "bubbly" nature of bony abnormality ⇨. There was no maxillary involvement in this patient. This child's twin sister was similarly affected. Note the displaced permanent tooth ➡.

LOW-DENSITY JAW LESION, POORLY MARGINATED (CT)

DIFFERENTIAL DIAGNOSIS

Common
- SCCa, Alveolar Ridge
- Osteoradionecrosis, Mandible-Maxilla
- Osteomyelitis, Mandible-Maxilla
- Metastasis, Mandible-Maxilla
- Osteonecrosis, Mandible-Maxilla

Less Common
- Non-Hodgkin Lymphoma
- Multiple Myeloma
- Minor Salivary Gland Malignancy, Oral

Rare but Important
- Giant Cell Granuloma, Mandible-Maxilla
- Osteosarcoma, Mandible-Maxilla
- Sarcoma, Ewing, Mandible-Maxilla
- Leukemia

ESSENTIAL INFORMATION

Key Differential Diagnosis Issues
- Lucent lesions of mandible or maxilla
  - Wide transition zone
  - May be expansile
- Plain film (Panorex) used at initial imaging
- CT best evaluates bone destruction
- MR best shows soft tissue extent, often better delineates marrow abnormality
- Clinical history is key
  - Clinical primary mucosal tumor: SCCa, minor salivary gland tumor
  - Underlying systemic disease: Metastasis, NHL, myeloma, leukemia
  - Prior radiation: Osteoradionecrosis (ORN), radiation-induced sarcoma
  - Use of bisphosphonates: Osteonecrosis

Helpful Clues for Common Diagnoses
- **SCCa, Alveolar Ridge**
  - Key facts
    - > 90% oral cancers are SCCa
    - Associated with tobacco &/or alcohol abuse
    - Bone involvement upstages tumor, alters surgical management
    - Distinguish cortical erosion from marrow infiltration
  - Imaging
    - Maxillary or maxillary alveolar bone destruction with extraosseous mass
    - Usually no periosteal reaction or sclerosis

- **Osteoradionecrosis, Mandible-Maxilla**
  - Key facts
    - Up to 22% of patients with radiation therapy; peaking in 1st 6-12 months
    - Interstitial brachytherapy implants increase risk
    - 95% mandible
    - Swelling, pain, trismus, hypesthesia, ulceration, bone exposure
    - May develop fractures, fistulae
  - Imaging
    - Within radiotherapy portal
    - Cortical and medullary bone loss, sclerotic sequestra
    - Intraosseous or paraosseous gas
    - Soft tissue edema and inflammation
- **Osteomyelitis, Mandible-Maxilla**
  - Key facts
    - Mandible > > maxilla
    - Most often: Dental caries → pulpal and periapical infection, often polymicrobial
    - Pain, swelling, trismus, hypesthesia
  - Imaging
    - Appearance depends on chronicity
    - Plain films often normal in 1st 3-4 weeks
    - Early: Osseous lacunae and sinuses, paraosseous phlegmon or abscess
    - Late: Sclerosis, periosteal new bone formation, sequestra
- **Metastasis, Mandible-Maxilla**
  - Key facts
    - Mandible > > maxilla; molar region of mandible most common
    - Most often: Breast carcinoma in females; lung carcinoma in males
    - 30% occult primary tumor
  - Imaging
    - No distinguishing imaging features
    - Lytic lesions > sclerotic
    - ± Lesions in other bones
- **Osteonecrosis, Mandible-Maxilla**
  - Key facts
    - Biphosphonate therapy complication
    - Mandible > maxilla
    - Nonhealing lesion after dental visit
    - Inflammation, ulceration with exposed bone, cutaneous fistulas
    - ± Superinfection, often actinomycosis
  - Imaging
    - Sclerosis mixed with loss of cortical and cancellous bone

- May see periosteal reaction, fractures
- Uptake on bone scan, PET/CT

Helpful Clues for Less Common Diagnoses
- **Non-Hodgkin Lymphoma**
  - Key facts
    - May be primary site or with systemic disease
  - Imaging
    - Lytic lesion, loss of lamina dura
    - Marrow infiltration
    - ± Homogeneous bulky nodes
- **Multiple Myeloma**
  - Key facts
    - Older patients, 40-70 years
    - Jaw lesion heralds myeloma in 6%
  - Imaging
    - Lytic, "punched out" lesion
    - No sclerosis or bone expansion
    - Most lesions posterior mandible
- **Minor Salivary Gland Malignancy, Oral**
  - Key facts
    - Most frequent hard palate mucoepidermoid carcinoma
  - Imaging
    - CT: Lytic, indistinguishable from SCCa
    - MR: High signal intensity makes SCCa less likely

Helpful Clues for Rare Diagnoses
- **Giant Cell Granuloma, Mandible-Maxilla**
  - Key facts
    - Females in 2nd & 3rd decade
    - Radiographically & pathologically identical to brown tumor

- Imaging
  - Anterior mandible
  - Expansile, bone septa, root resorption
- **Osteosarcoma, Mandible-Maxilla**
  - Key facts
    - Mandible > maxilla
    - 30-40 years; older patients than with other osteosarcomas
    - Associated with Paget disease, fibrous dysplasia, radiotherapy
  - Imaging
    - Classic: Sunburst pattern of bone formation (radial spicules) or Codman triangle
    - Early: Widened periodontal ligament space, enlarged mandibular canal
    - Advanced: Lytic, blastic, or mixed
- **Sarcoma, Ewing, Mandible-Maxilla**
  - Key facts
    - While rare, mandible most common H&N site
    - Male > female; 5-25 years
  - Imaging
    - Permeative destruction
    - Sclerotic areas possible
    - May see sunburst periosteal pattern
    - Bulky extraosseous soft tissue component
- **Leukemia**
  - Key facts
    - Jaw lesions in up to 63% of patients with acute leukemia
  - Imaging
    - Loss of definition of lamina dura, lytic bone destruction, diffuse osteopenia

SCCa, Alveolar Ridge

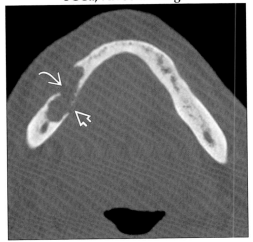

Axial bone CT shows a poorly marginated destructive lesion of the right mandibular alveolar ridge with destruction of both lingual ⊇ and buccal ⊅ cortex. Gingival squamous cell carcinoma was proven.

SCCa, Alveolar Ridge

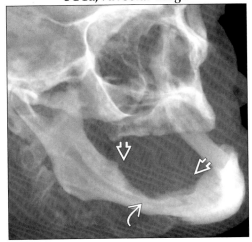

Right anterior oblique 3D CT reformation demonstrates saucer-shaped irregular destruction of the right mandibular alveolar ridge ⊇, nearly extending to the inferior alveolar canal ⊅.

LOW-DENSITY JAW LESION, POORLY MARGINATED (CT)

SCCa, Alveolar Ridge

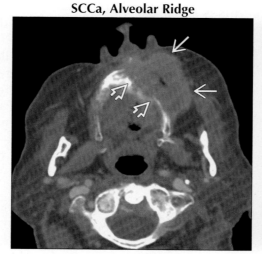

SCCa, Alveolar Ridge

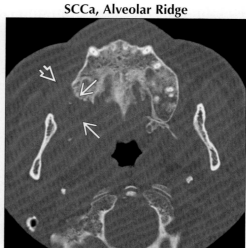

(Left) Axial CECT shows a large soft tissue mass arising from the left gingivobuccal sulcus ➡ and distorting the left cheek. The mass is producing irregular destruction of the left maxillary alveolar bone ➡. *(Right)* Axial bone CT in a different patient shows a lytic destructive process involving the posterior aspect of the right maxilla ➡ with destruction of pterygoid plates as well. The soft tissue component is subtly evident on bone CT ➡.

Osteoradionecrosis, Mandible-Maxilla

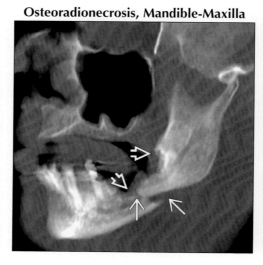

Osteoradionecrosis, Mandible-Maxilla

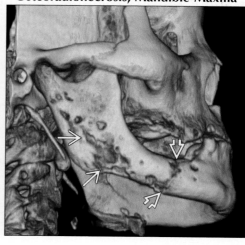

(Left) Lateral oblique thick multiplanar reconstruction from bone CT shows irregular bone density and multifocal cortical destruction ➡. Note also the clear evidence of pathologic fracture ➡ complicating the underlying osteoradionecrosis. *(Right)* Lateral oblique 3D CT reformation in a different patient demonstrates linear pathologic fracture ➡ and irregular lytic bone destruction ➡ in the right hemimandible.

Osteoradionecrosis, Mandible-Maxilla

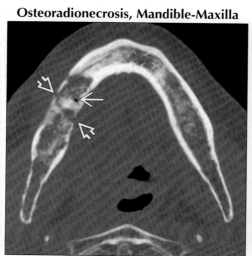

Osteomyelitis, Mandible-Maxilla

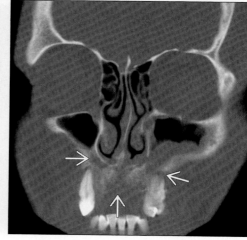

(Left) Axial bone CT shows osteolysis with mixed lucency and sclerosis involving much of the right hemimandible with a complicating pathologic fracture ➡. Note the intramedullary gas ➡ along the anterior margin of the lesion. *(Right)* Axial bone CT reveals an ill-defined lucency destroying the palate ➡. This immunocompromised patient did not have a mucosal lesion, and this was proven to be an unusual case of mucor osteomyelitis.

Osteomyelitis, Mandible-Maxilla

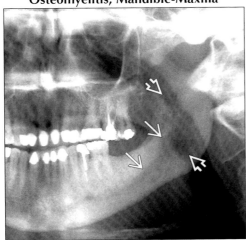

Osteomyelitis, Mandible-Maxilla

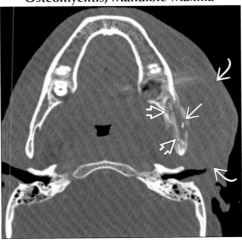

(Left) Panorex shows irregular sclerosis in the left mandible with loss of corticomedullary differentiation & mottled lucencies ➡. Note also the mandibular canal enlargement with demineralization of its margin ➡. *(Right)* Axial bone CT reveals poorly marginated, low attenuation process in left mandibular ramus ➡. Note osseous sequestrum ➡ within expanded mandible & marked left cheek swelling ➡ in this osteomyelitis case.

Metastasis, Mandible-Maxilla

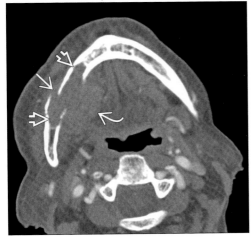

Metastasis, Mandible-Maxilla

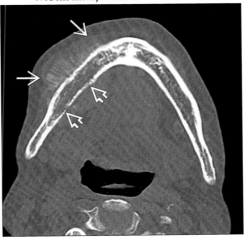

(Left) Axial CECT shows a poorly marginated intramedullary mandibular lesion ➡ in a patient with colon cancer. Note the associated pathologic fracture ➡ & extraosseous soft tissue component ➡ extending into floor of the mouth. *(Right)* Axial bone CT depicts a poorly marginated mandibular focus of metastatic adenocarcinoma ➡. Sunburst periosteal new bone formation pattern ➡ led to initial suspicion of osteosarcoma.

Osteonecrosis, Mandible-Maxilla

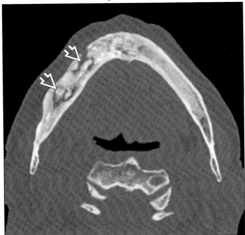

Osteonecrosis, Mandible-Maxilla

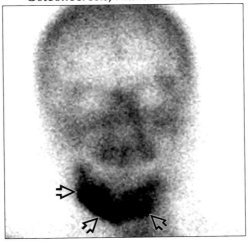

(Left) Axial bone CT reveals evolving osseous sequestrum ➡ within an otherwise diffusely sclerotic mandible in this case of mandibular osteonecrosis in a patient receiving bisphosphonate therapy. *(Right)* Anteroposterior bone scan in the same patient reveals diffuse tracer uptake ➡ in mandibular symphysis and markedly more in the right body of the mandible.

LOW-DENSITY JAW LESION, POORLY MARGINATED (CT)

Non-Hodgkin Lymphoma

Non-Hodgkin Lymphoma

(Left) Axial CECT with bone window demonstrates a poorly marginated lytic right hemimandibular lesion ⮞ with destruction of buccal cortex and sclerosis at the posterior margin ⮞. On careful examination of the bone windows, an associated soft tissue mass ⮞ is evident. *(Right)* Axial T1WI MR in the same patient better illustrates the soft tissue component ⮞ but also reveals more extensive marrow involvement ⮞. Markedly enlarged right level II node ⮞ is also evident.

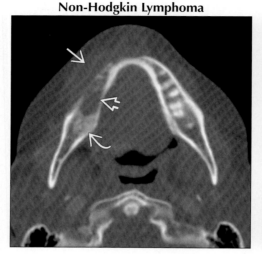

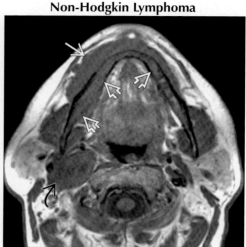

Multiple Myeloma

Minor Salivary Gland Malignancy, Oral

(Left) Axial bone CT shows a poorly marginated lytic lesion ⮞ in the left mandible with destruction of both lingual & buccal cortex. Note the associated extraosseous masses ⮞. *(Right)* AP Raysum CT slab shows a diffuse lytic mass involving the right mandibular body & symphysis ⮞. This was due to an extensive perineural tumor spread from a prior right parotid adenoid cystic carcinoma, coursing into the mandible along the inferior alveolar (V3) nerve.

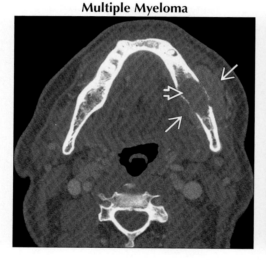

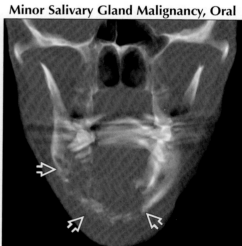

Minor Salivary Gland Malignancy, Oral

Minor Salivary Gland Malignancy, Oral

(Left) Coronal bone CT shows a multilobulated destructive maxillary lesion with poorly defined margins ⮞. The lesion involves the maxillary alveolar ridge and hard palate, projecting into both the right nasal cavity and right maxillary sinus ⮞. *(Right)* Coronal T2WI FS MR in the same patient reveals heterogeneous but predominantly high signal intensity of the maxillary mass ⮞. This high signal is less commonly encountered with squamous cell carcinoma.

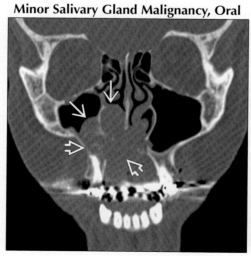

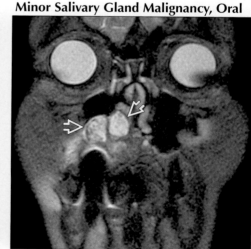

Giant Cell Granuloma, Mandible-Maxilla

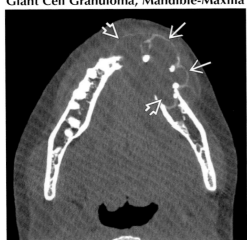

Osteosarcoma, Mandible-Maxilla

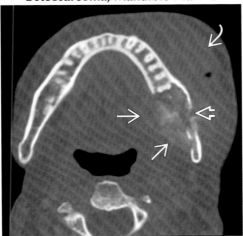

(Left) Axial bone CT shows a large left parasymphysial mandibular lesion ➡ with variably defined margins. The mass is expansile in some portions with thin "eggshell" cortical margins ➡. (Right) Axial CECT reveals a lucent-destructive lesion in the posterior body & ramus of the left hemimandible ➡ with ill-defined sunburst calcifications ➡. A large extraosseous component ➡ is also evident on the bone windows, with contained air from fine-needle aspiration.

Osteosarcoma, Mandible-Maxilla

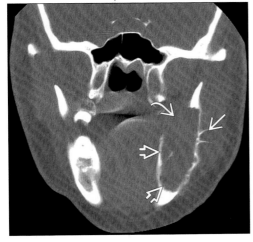

Sarcoma, Ewing, Mandible-Maxilla

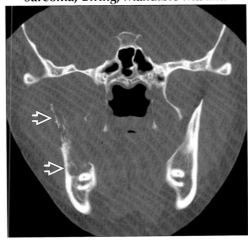

(Left) Coronal bone CT shows an expansile mass involving the mandibular body & ramus with irregular margins ➡ & cortical destruction ➡. Spiculated new bone formation ➡ along the buccal mandibular surface within extraosseous component is also seen in this rare low-grade osteosarcoma. (Right) Coronal bone CT reveals an ill-defined lytic lesion destroying mandibular ramus & coronoid process ➡. New bone formation is not evident.

Sarcoma, Ewing, Mandible-Maxilla

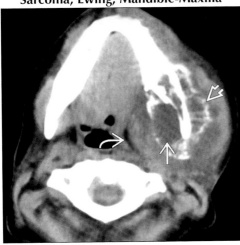

Leukemia

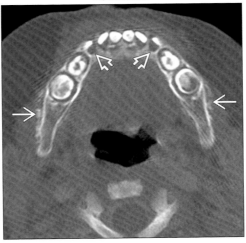

(Left) Axial NECT shows a distended left cheek with underlying lytic mandibular mass ➡. Sunburst periosteal new bone formation is evident within lateral extraosseous component ➡. Medial component displaces parapharyngeal fat ➡. (Right) Axial bone CT shows a loss of definition of the dental lamina dura & widening of periodontal ligament space around teeth ➡. Diffuse osseous lucency also evident with "hair on end" pattern of new bone formation ➡.

GROUND-GLASS LESIONS OF THE MANDIBLE & MAXILLA (CT)

DIFFERENTIAL DIAGNOSIS

Common
- Fibrous Dysplasia, Mandible-Maxilla
- Ossifying Fibroma, Mandible-Maxilla

Less Common
- Cemento-Osseous Dysplasia, Periapical
- Cemento-Osseous Dysplasia, Florid

Rare but Important
- Renal Osteodystrophy
- Paget Disease, Mandible-Maxilla

ESSENTIAL INFORMATION

Key Differential Diagnosis Issues
- "Ground-glass" lesions: Mass-like calcified matrix-producing bone lesions
  - May be homogeneous or heterogeneous intermediate CT attenuation
  - Fibroosseous lesions account for majority
  - Aggressive bone destruction, periosteal reactive new bone formation, & extraosseous soft tissue components absent

Helpful Clues for Common Diagnoses
- **Fibrous Dysplasia, Mandible-Maxilla**
  - Key facts
    - Histologically characterized by woven bone and absence of osteoblastic rimming of bone spicules
    - Most cases become quiescent at bone maturity (early adulthood)
    - Infrequently presents or reactivates in adulthood
    - Monostotic (80-85%), polyostotic (15-20%)
    - McCune-Albright syndrome in 3% of polyostotic FD
    - "Monostotic" term difficult to apply in craniofacial fibrous dysplasia (FD) where otherwise isolated FD may cross sutures to involve adjacent bones
    - Craniofacial region is most common site for sarcomatous degeneration of FD
  - Imaging: Radiographs & CT
    - Often less well defined, more radiopaque in craniofacial region than long bones
    - "Ground-glass" matrix expands involved bone (especially mandible) in fusiform fashion
    - Maintains native shape of affected bone unless complicated by cystic degeneration (aneurysmal bone cyst)
    - Maxillary expansion may encroach on maxillary sinus, orbit, nasal cavity
    - May encroach on neural & vascular foramina & canals
    - Intact bone cortex of variable thickness
    - FD and teeth: Periodontal ligament space narrowed; lamina dura involved
    - Teeth surrounded but often not displaced or eroded, though entire alveolar ridge may be displaced by massive disease
    - FD and sarcomatous degeneration: Permeative lytic pattern, destroyed cortex, widening of periodontal space, spiculated periosteal new bone formation
  - Imaging: MR
    - FD shows intermediate T1 signal, heterogeneous hypointensity on T2
    - Heterogeneous or marked enhancement
- **Ossifying Fibroma, Mandible-Maxilla**
  - Key facts
    - Clinical: Occurs predominantly in women; more common in African-Americans
    - Presents in 3rd-4th decade; later than FD
    - Histologically characterized by lamellar bone and osteoblastic rimming, cementum-like tissue
    - Most recent WHO classification views ossifying fibroma (OF) as subgroup of cemento-ossifying fibromas
    - Most grow slowly & do not recur
    - Juvenile subtype (arising in children under 15 years) may grow rapidly and tends to recur
    - Rarely OF lesions are multiple; may be confused with polyostotic FD
  - Imaging: Radiographs & CT
    - Circumscribed, spherical & focally more expansile than FD (due to centrifugal expansion) with thin intact cortex
    - Teeth often displaced and resorbed
    - Typical CT appearance: Radiolucent > lucent with central or peripheral radiopacities > entirely radiopaque
  - Imaging findings: MR
    - OF shows intermediate T1 & hypointense T2 signal

- Often enhances moderately

Helpful Clues for Less Common Diagnoses
- **Cemento-Osseous Dysplasia, Periapical**
  - Key facts
    - Most arise in women in 4th-5th decade
    - African-Americans, Asians > > Caucasians
    - Primarily found in alveolar process
  - Imaging: Radiographs & CT
    - Most common site = mandibular incisors
    - Often multifocal, between adjacent teeth, usually < 1 cm
    - Initially lucent, progressing to sclerosis with lucent margin
    - May be accompanied by bone cysts
- **Cemento-Osseous Dysplasia, Florid**
  - Key facts
    - Diffuse (2 or more quadrant) form of periapical cemento-osseous dysplasia
  - Imaging: Radiographs & CT
    - "Fluffy" sclerotic lesions in periapical alveolar bone or in edentulous areas
    - Often symmetric, expansile, lobulated, larger than periapical form
    - May be accompanied by bone cysts or complicated by osteomyelitis

Helpful Clues for Rare Diagnoses
- **Renal Osteodystrophy**
  - Key facts
    - Secondary hyperparathyroidism (chronic renal failure)
    - ↑ Osteoclast activity & population
    - Changes of osteitis fibrosa cystica reflect mixture of osteolysis & sclerosis

- Noncystic form mimics diffuse FD; with poor corticomedullary distinction
  - Imaging: Radiographs & CT
    - Diffuse demineralization, subperiosteal resorption, with ground-glass enlargement of mandible
    - Multifocal cortical thinning, loss of definition of lamina dura
    - Focal enlargement with brown tumor in osteitis fibrosa cystica
- **Paget Disease, Mandible-Maxilla**
  - Key facts
    - 17% of patients involve mandible or maxilla; older patients
    - Usually seen with skull involvement
  - Imaging: Radiographs & CT
    - Often bilateral and symmetric, maxilla involved 2x as commonly as mandible
    - Cortical and spongiosa trabecular thickening, "ground-glass" density interspersed with sclerotic islands of dense bone
    - May see hypercementosis around tooth roots mimicking cemento-osseous dysplasia, may obliterate periodontal ligament space

SELECTED REFERENCES

1. MacDonald-Jankowski DS: Fibro-osseous lesions of the face and jaws. Clin Radiol. 59(1):11-25, 2004
2. Mafee MF et al: Fibro-osseous and giant cell lesions, including brown tumor of the mandible, maxilla, and other craniofacial bones. Neuroimaging Clin N Am. 13(3):525-40, 2003

Fibrous Dysplasia, Mandible-Maxilla

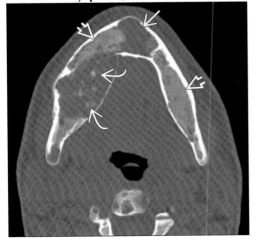

Axial bone CT shows diffuse mandibular expansion with "ground-glass" matrix ➡. Notice the lesion is inhomogeneous with focal areas that are purely cystic ➡ or cystic with multifocal ossification ➡.

Fibrous Dysplasia, Mandible-Maxilla

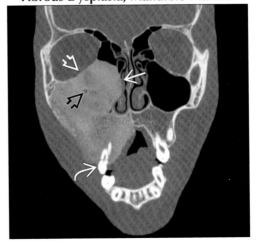

Coronal bone CT shows expansile maxillary bone lesion. Note orbital ➡ & nasal cavity ➡ encroachment, antral obliteration, depression of maxillary teeth ➡, & engulfed infraorbital nerve canal ➡.

GROUND-GLASS LESIONS OF THE MANDIBLE & MAXILLA (CT)

(Left) Coronal STIR MR demonstrates diffuse, predominantly low T2 signal in the maxillary fibrous dysplasia lesion ➡. *(Right)* Axial bone CT shows a mildly expansile, lucent yet not truly cystic-appearing, left mandibular lesion ➡. Ossifying fibromas can demonstrate variable attenuation depending on their stage of evolution. The mandibular cortex is thinned but intact.

Fibrous Dysplasia, Mandible-Maxilla

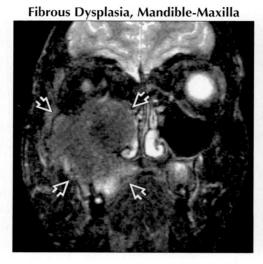

Ossifying Fibroma, Mandible-Maxilla

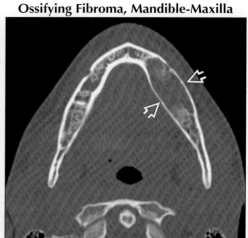

(Left) Left anterior oblique 3D CT shows a radiolucent lesion in the left hemimandible. Note the splaying of tooth roots ➡ and tapering/resorption of the root of the 2nd premolar ➡. *(Right)* Coronal bone CT reveals a bilobed ossifying fibroma with innumerable foci of psammomatoid calcifications ➡, most prominent along the lesion's periphery.

Ossifying Fibroma, Mandible-Maxilla

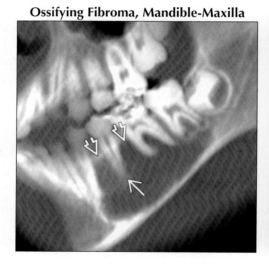

Ossifying Fibroma, Mandible-Maxilla

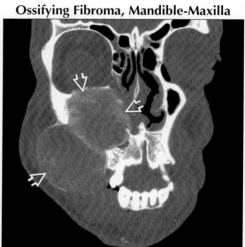

(Left) Axial CECT shows bilateral expansile ground-glass ossifying fibroma lesions ➡ in this patient with hyperparathyroidism due to a parathyroid carcinoma. While brown tumors are possible, there is also an association between ossifying fibromas and hyperparathyroidism. *(Right)* Axial bone CT reveals a focally expansile ground-glass density lesion ➡ with a central focus of coarse calcification ➡.

Ossifying Fibroma, Mandible-Maxilla

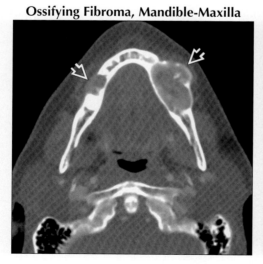

Ossifying Fibroma, Mandible-Maxilla

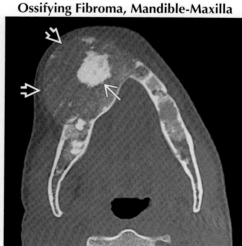

GROUND-GLASS LESIONS OF THE MANDIBLE & MAXILLA (CT)

Ossifying Fibroma, Mandible-Maxilla
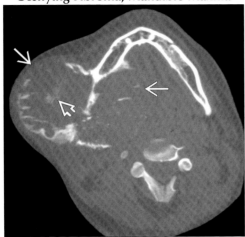

Cemento-Osseous Dysplasia, Periapical
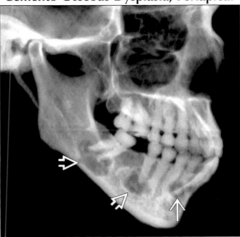

(Left) Axial bone CT reveals an aggressive-appearing mandibular mass with central increased density ➡ but multiple areas of apparent cortical breakthrough ➡. An osteosarcoma was suspected but juvenile aggressive ossifying fibroma was the final pathological diagnosis. *(Right)* Right anterior oblique 3D CT shows early pattern of periapical lucencies associated with vital teeth ➡. Subtle periapical calcification of 1 lesion ➡ is visible.

Cemento-Osseous Dysplasia, Florid
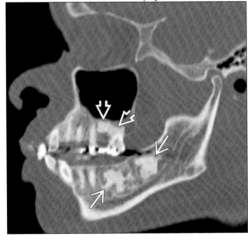

Cemento-Osseous Dysplasia, Florid
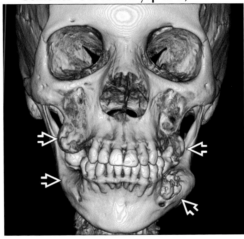

(Left) Sagittal oblique bone CT demonstrates patchy areas of increased density in the left hemimandible ➡ and left maxilla ➡. This example demonstrates the late-stage appearance of these lesions. *(Right)* Anteroposterior 3D CT shows expansile lobulated multi-quadrant lesions ➡, typical of florid cemento-osseous dysplasia.

Renal Osteodystrophy
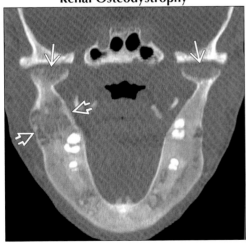

Paget Disease, Mandible-Maxilla
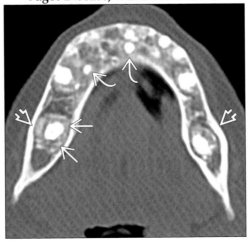

(Left) Coronal oblique bone CT shows diffuse expansion and uniform increased density of the mandible. Note more focal expansion on the right due to a coexisting brown tumor ➡. Note subperiosteal bone resorption in both mandibular condyles ➡. *(Right)* Axial bone CT shows diffuse expansion & heterogeneous increased density/cotton wool appearance of the mandible. Note thickened cortex ➡, periapical hypercementosis ➡, & sclerotic foci ➡.

SECTION 3
Hypopharynx & Larynx

Anatomically Based Differentials

Generic Imaging Patterns

Clinically Based Differentials

HYPOPHARYNGEAL LESION

DIFFERENTIAL DIAGNOSIS

Common
- Collapsed Pyriform Sinus, Normal Variant
- SCCa, Hypopharynx
- SCCa, Larynx, Supraglottic, HP Invasion
- Radiation Changes, Acute
- Radiation Changes, Chronic
- Vocal Cord Paralysis, Dilated Pyriform Sinus

Less Common
- Gastroesophageal Reflux
- Epiglottitis, Adult
- Diverticulum, Esophago-Pharyngeal
- Esophageal Carcinoma, Cervical

Rare but Important
- 4th Branchial Anomaly
- Lateral Hypopharyngeal Pouch
- Non-Hodgkin Lymphoma, Larynx-Hypopharynx
- Atonic Hypopharynx (CN10 Injury or Polio)

ESSENTIAL INFORMATION

Key Differential Diagnosis Issues
- Hypopharynx defined as caudal continuation of pharyngeal mucosal space/surface
  - Set between oropharynx above & cervical esophagus below
- Hypopharynx (HP) consists of 3 regions
  - Pyriform sinus
    - Anterolateral recess of HP
    - Pyriform sinus apex or inferior tip at level of true vocal cords
    - Anteromedial wall of pyriform sinus is posterolateral wall of aryepiglottic fold (marginal supraglottis)
  - Posterior wall
    - Inferior continuation of posterior wall of oropharynx
    - Inferior continuation into posterior wall esophagus
  - Post-cricoid region
    - Anterior wall of inferior HP
    - Common wall between HP & larynx
    - Extends from cricoarytenoid joints to lower edge of cricoid cartilage (cricopharyngeal muscle)
- History is critical in working through this differential diagnosis, especially if prior radiation therapy for H&N malignancy

- Diagnosis always confirmed with endoscopic findings

Helpful Clues for Common Diagnoses
- **Collapsed Pyriform Sinus, Normal Variant**
  - Key facts: Common incidental finding
  - Imaging: Asymmetry between pyriform sinuses, 1 aerated but other airless
    - Absence of associated mass important
- **SCCa, Hypopharynx**
  - Key facts: Mass originates in pyriform sinus, posterior HP wall, or post-cricoid HP
    - Clinically silent until late; often large at presentation
  - Imaging: C+ HP mass often involves larynx
    - Extends through aryepiglottic fold (AEF) into supraglottic larynx or by direct spread anteriorly into larynx
    - Unresectable if superior extension to posterior wall of oropharynx, inferior extension to cervical esophagus, or posterior extension into retropharyngeal space & prevertebral muscles
- **SCCa, Larynx, Supraglottic, HP Invasion**
  - Key facts: Laryngeal SCCa invading HP more common than primary HP Ca
  - Imaging: AEF SCCa invades pyriform sinus
    - Large supraglottic SCCa involves post-cricoid HP
- **Radiation Changes, Acute**
  - Key facts: Neck radiation history
  - Imaging: Mucosal surfaces, including AEF, appear symmetrically thickened, low density without enhancement
    - Pyriform sinus will be airless because AEFs are edematous
- **Radiation Changes, Chronic**
  - Key facts: Less severe form of acute radiation change
  - Imaging: Thickened AEF with airless pyriform sinus may be permanent
- **Vocal Cord Paralysis, Dilated Pyriform Sinus**
  - Key facts: Part of vagal neuropathy picture
  - Imaging: Asymmetric pyriform sinus dilatation
    - Other CN10 paralysis findings: Thickened AEF, enlarged ipsilateral laryngeal ventricle, vocal cord edema or atrophy, arytenoid cartilage displacement

HYPOPHARYNGEAL LESION

Helpful Clues for Less Common Diagnoses

- **Gastroesophageal Reflux**
  - Key facts: Best diagnosed with endoscopy, pH probes, upper GI
    - Symptoms: Dysphagia, reflux
  - Imaging: CT shows nonenhancing edematous mucosal surfaces
    - Posterior wall & post-cricoid portions of hypopharynx
- **Epiglottitis, Adult**
  - Key facts: Acutely ill, febrile, sore throat
  - Imaging: Diffuse edematous epiglottis, AEF with heterogeneous enhancement
    - Hypopharynx involved secondarily
- **Diverticulum, Esophago-Pharyngeal**
  - Key facts: a.k.a., Zenker diverticulum
    - Mucosa-lined outpouch of posterior HP
  - Imaging: Air-, debris-, or fluid-filled outpouching off posterior low HP
    - Located at C5-6 level, left of esophagus
- **Esophageal Carcinoma, Cervical**
  - Key facts: Upper cervical esophageal carcinoma spread superiorly into HP
  - Imaging: Invasive mass centered on esophagus behind trachea involves HP

Helpful Clues for Rare Diagnoses

- **4th Branchial Anomaly**
  - Key facts: Congenital sinus tract extends inferiorly from apex of pyriform sinus
    - Presentation: Recurrent thyroiditis, anterior left neck cervical neck mass
  - Imaging
    - Esophagram: Sinus tract extends inferiorly from pyriform sinus apex
    - CT: Cyst or abscess in left anterior cervical neck with left thyroid lobe inflammation/infection
- **Lateral Hypopharyngeal Pouch**
  - Key facts: Results from weak area of thyrohyoid membrane
    - Presentation: Globus (lump in throat), dysphagia, foreign body sensation
    - Post-deglutitive aspiration possible
  - Esophagram: Lateral HP pouches, often bilateral
- **Non-Hodgkin Lymphoma, Larynx-Hypopharynx**
  - Key facts: Extranodal, extralymphatic rare location for non-Hodgkin Lymphoma to occur
  - Imaging: Mimics SCCa
- **Atonic Hypopharynx (CN10 Injury or Polio)**
  - Key facts: CN10 pharyngeal plexus branch or polio affects constrictor muscle tone
  - Imaging: Unilateral patulous hypopharynx

SELECTED REFERENCES

1. Schmalfuss IM et al: Postcricoid region and cervical esophagus: normal appearance at CT and MR imaging. Radiology. 214(1):237-46, 2000
2. Silverman PM et al: Carcinoma of the larynx and hypopharynx: computed tomographic-histopathologic correlations. Radiology. 151(3):697-702, 1984

Collapsed Pyriform Sinus, Normal Variant

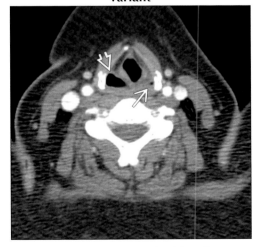

Axial CECT shows asymmetric airless left pyriform sinus ➡ with aryepiglottic fold located laterally in an asymptomatic patient with a normal endoscopy. Note the normal air-filled right pyriform sinus ➡.

SCCa, Hypopharynx

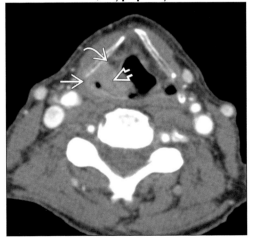

Axial CECT shows a bulky enhancing mass of the lateral pyriform sinus wall ➡ and marginal supraglottis ➡. Note anterior extension to the posterior paraglottic space ➡.

HYPOPHARYNGEAL LESION

(Left) Axial CECT shows posterior wall hypopharyngeal SCCa ➡. Note the extension of the tumor into the left paraglottic space ➡. *(Right)* Axial CECT shows bulky post-cricoid SCCa ➡. Cricoid cartilage is anteriorly displaced ➡, and the sclerotic arytenoid ➡ & thyroid cartilages are highly suspicious for laryngeal invasion.

SCCa, Hypopharynx

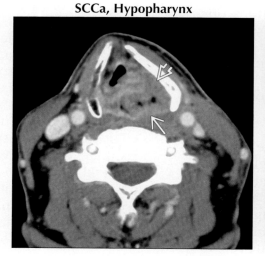

SCCa, Hypopharynx

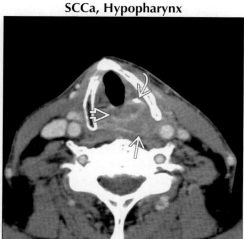

(Left) Axial CECT demonstrates a transglottic laryngeal SCCa, destroying part of the cricoid cartilage ➡ & extending from the posterior left true vocal cord posteriorly to involve the post-cricoid HP ➡. *(Right)* Axial CECT shows acute radiation change with mucosal enhancement in right pyriform sinus ➡ & edematous aryepiglottic fold ➡. Notice the avidly enhancing submandibular gland ➡, another manifestation of acute radiation change.

SCCa, Larynx, Supraglottic, HP Invasion

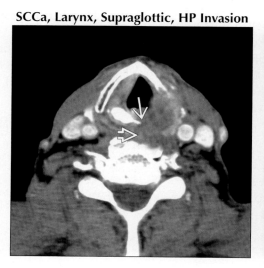

Radiation Changes, Acute

(Left) Axial CECT reveals a chronic radiation change seen 8 months after radiotherapy. Mucosal enhancement is not present, but the aryepiglottic fold remains thickened ➡. *(Right)* Axial CECT shows prominent air-filled left pyriform sinus ➡ and thickened paramedian aryepiglottic fold ➡. Both imaging findings are secondary to left vocal cord paralysis (not shown).

Radiation Changes, Chronic

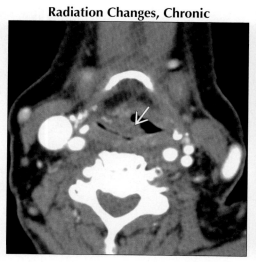

Vocal Cord Paralysis, Dilated Pyriform Sinus

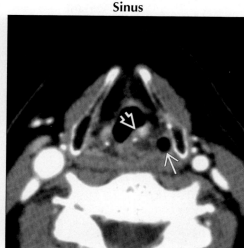

Gastroesophageal Reflux

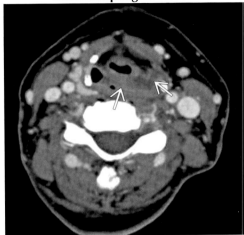

Epiglottitis, Adult

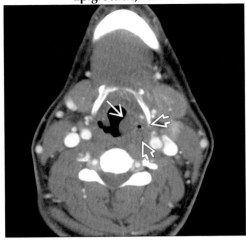

(Left) Axial CECT depicts a broad area of edematous tissue in the hypopharynx ➡. This patient presented with dysphagia and heartburn. Endoscopy showed obvious and severe gastroesophageal reflux. *(Right)* Axial CECT reveals an inflamed boggy left aryepiglottic fold ➡ with extension of the inflammation to involve walls of the left pyriform sinus ⮕.

Diverticulum, Esophago-Pharyngeal

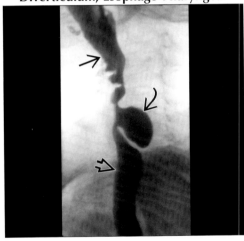

Esophageal Carcinoma, Cervical

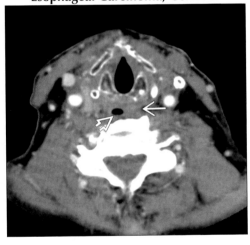

(Left) Lateral esophagram shows dense barium filling the pharynx ➡ & esophagus ⮕. The large posterior "bulge" represents Zenker diverticulum ⮕. Notice the bulge's emergence from the posterior low hypopharynx at ~ C5-6 as expected. *(Right)* Axial CECT depicts the superior margin of an esophageal carcinoma at the level of the post-cricoid hypopharynx. At this level, the only hint of invasion is the thick wall on the left ➡, along with the persistent luminal air ⮕.

4th Branchial Anomaly

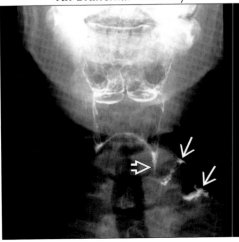

Lateral Hypopharyngeal Pouch

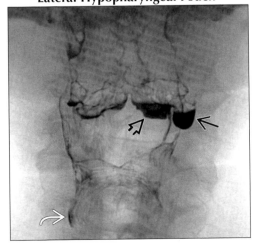

(Left) Anteroposterior radiograph demonstrates the classic pyriform sinus apex sinus tract in a patient with 4th branchial anomaly. The serpiginous sinus tract ➡ is seen leading inferiorly from the apex of the pyriform sinus ⮕. *(Right)* Anteroposterior esophagram demonstrates a typical left lateral hypopharyngeal diverticulum ➡, partially filled with barium. Note that it is lateral to the vallecula ⮕. The apex of normal pyriform sinus ➡ is also seen.

DIFFERENTIAL DIAGNOSIS

Common
- SCCa, Larynx, Supraglottic
- SCCa, Larynx, Glottic
- Vocal Cord Paralysis
- Radiated Larynx
- Laryngocele

Less Common
- Trauma, Larynx
- SCCa, Larynx, Subglottic
- Laryngohypopharyngeal Reflux
- Chondrosarcoma, Larynx

Rare but Important
- Rheumatoid Larynx
- Amyloidosis, Larynx
- Wegener Granulomatosis, Larynx
- Paraganglioma, Larynx
- Papilloma, Larynx
- Melanoma, Mucosal, Larynx
- Pseudotumor, Larynx
- Tracheopathia Osteochondroplastica
- Nodular Chondrometaplasia, Larynx

ESSENTIAL INFORMATION

Key Differential Diagnosis Issues
- Clinical history & endoscopy findings often provide clues to precise diagnosis
- Endoscopy performed for most laryngeal lesions, unless obviously incidental

Helpful Clues for Common Diagnoses
- **SCCa, Larynx, Supraglottic**
  - Endoscopy: Ulcerating mass on epiglottis, aryepiglottic fold (AEF), false cord
  - Imaging: Obtained to stage tumor & nodes
    - Check for mass on epiglottis, AEF, false cord; all subsites in supraglottic larynx
    - Determine involvement of laryngeal fat spaces: Preepiglottic & paraglottic
    - Important to note extension to glottic larynx or hypopharynx
    - Assume cartilage invasion if tumor on both sides of cartilage, cartilage destruction, or erosion
    - Metastatic adenopathy common as nodal drainage of supraglottic larynx is rich
- **SCCa, Larynx, Glottic**
  - Endoscopy: Mass or ulceration on true vocal cord in patient with hoarseness

- Imaging: Normal CECT/MR if lesion is small
  - Check for paraglottic space or subglottic extension & cartilage destruction
- **Vocal Cord Paralysis**
  - Endoscopy: Sluggish or fixed vocal cord
  - Imaging: Goal to determine reason for paralysis; laryngeal or neural origin
    - Paramedian or atrophied cord
    - Large air-filled pyriform sinus & laryngeal ventricle; paramedian AEF
    - Anteromedial arytenoid cartilage
    - Laryngeal carcinoma can invade cord → mechanical paralysis
    - Scan from medulla to carina on left, to clavicle on right
    - If normal larynx, work-up neural causes
- **Radiated Larynx**
  - Endoscopy: Edematous endolaryngeal soft tissues; radiation therapy history
  - Imaging
    - Thickened edematous free margin of epiglottis, AEF, false & true cords
    - Preepiglottic, paraglottic fat is "dirty"
    - Edematous mucosa may persist
- **Laryngocele**
  - Key facts
    - Congenital or acquired dilatation of laryngeal ventricle
    - If laryngeal tumor obstructs ventricle → acquired laryngocele
  - Imaging
    - Thin-walled air- or fluid-filled cyst communicating with laryngeal ventricle
    - Internal = entirely within larynx
    - Mixed = extends through thyrohyoid membrane

Helpful Clues for Less Common Diagnoses
- **Trauma, Larynx**
  - Key facts: Blunt or penetrating injury
  - Imaging: Cartilaginous disruption or soft tissue endolaryngeal injury
    - CT best imaging tool; use bone window to evaluate cartilage injury
    - Edema or hematoma of vocal cords with supraglottic swelling narrowing airway
- **SCCa, Larynx, Subglottic**
  - Key facts: Rare primary laryngeal lesion, poorly visualized at endoscopy
  - Imaging: Thin-slice CT with reformations is best imaging tool

- Extension to trachea must be noted so that tracheostomy does not go through tumor
- **Laryngohypopharyngeal Reflux**
  - Key facts: Acquired lesion on posterior laryngeal/hypopharyngeal wall, due to acidic stomach contents bathing mucosa
  - Imaging: Edema and diffuse mucosal enhancement; AEF, posterior or subglottic larynx, & hypopharynx
- **Chondrosarcoma, Larynx**
  - Key facts: Cartilage-producing neoplasm arising from cricoid or thyroid laryngeal cartilage with intact mucosa
  - Imaging: Expansile low density (CT)/hyperintense (T2 MR) nonenhancing mass with arc- or ring-like Ca++

Helpful Clues for Rare Diagnoses
- **Rheumatoid Larynx**
  - Key facts: Affects cricoarytenoid & cricothyroid joints (both synovial joints)
  - Imaging: Arytenoid sclerosis with vocal cord atrophy, fixation of joints
- **Amyloidosis, Larynx**
  - Key facts: Deposition of amyloid material in larynx with no mucosal lesion
  - Imaging: Submucosal enhancing mass without cartilage destruction or invasion
- **Wegener Granulomatosis, Larynx**
  - Key facts: Idiopathic systemic vasculitis that commonly involves respiratory tract
  - Imaging: Diffuse submucosal mass most common in subglottic larynx

- **Paraganglioma, Larynx**
  - Key facts: Vascular submucosal mass most common in supraglottic subsite of larynx
  - Imaging: Robustly enhancing well-circumscribed submucosal mass
- **Papilloma, Larynx**
  - Key facts: Benign but recurrent lesion, likely viral in etiology, most common in pediatric population
  - Imaging: CT/MR rarely necessary, but lesions are exophytic and frequently show airway compromise
- **Melanoma, Mucosal, Larynx**
  - Key facts: May be primary or metastatic
  - Imaging: Nonspecific asymmetric mucosal thickening & enhancement
- **Pseudotumor, Larynx**
  - Key facts: Benign lesion, also known as plasma cell granuloma, presenting with voice change or stridor
  - Imaging: Nonspecific enhancing laryngeal mass, usually subglottic in location
- **Tracheopathia Osteochondroplastica**
  - Key facts: Osteocartilaginous submucosal calcified nodules of unclear etiology found almost exclusively in adults
  - Imaging: Calcified nodules of anterior or lateral tracheal walls → airway compromise
- **Nodular Chondrometaplasia, Larynx**
  - Key facts: Benign cartilaginous submucosal mass following trauma or intubation
  - Imaging: Discrete mass arising from cartilage surface, no malignant features

SCCa, Larynx, Supraglottic

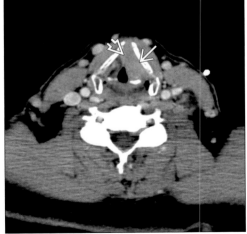

Axial CECT shows a mass ➡ *filling left paraglottic fat and crossing midline to involve right supraglottic larynx* ➡. *Left thyroid cartilage sclerosis, without destruction, is a nonspecific finding.*

SCCa, Larynx, Supraglottic

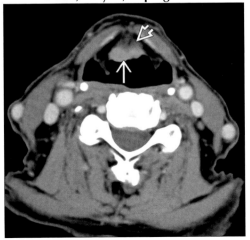

Axial CECT reveals a small mass ➡ *at the body of epiglottis with involvement of preepiglottic fat* ➡. *Even though the lesion is small, it is staged as T3 because of preepiglottic fat invasion.*

3

LARYNGEAL LESION

SCCa, Larynx, Glottic

(Left) Axial CECT shows a small left vocal cord lesion ➡, with extension to anterior commissure ⇉. Note that posterior commissure is normal ↘, with no thyroid cartilage destruction present. **(Right)** Axial CECT demonstrates an anterior commissure squamous cell carcinoma ➡ that affects the anteroinferior margins of both vocal cords with destruction of the thyroid cartilage ⇉.

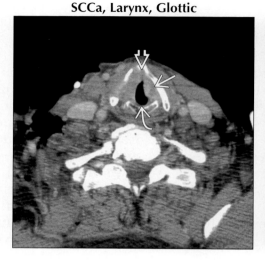
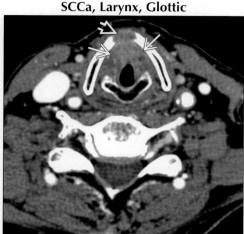

Vocal Cord Paralysis

(Left) Axial CECT shows vocal cord paralysis changes at the supraglottic level, with dilated ipsilateral pyriform sinus ➡, thickened aryepiglottic fold ⇉, and medially displaced arytenoid cartilage ⇉. **(Right)** Axial CECT demonstrates changes at the glottic level, including dilated laryngeal ventricle ➡ and atrophic true vocal cord ⇉. Note normal vocal cord on left. There is no laryngeal tumor that would explain the vocal cord paralysis.

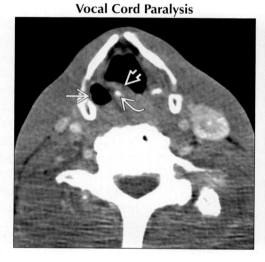
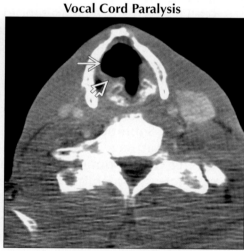

Radiated Larynx

(Left) Axial CECT reveals acute radiation mucositis as diffuse prominent mucosal enhancement of larynx ➡ and hypopharynx. **(Right)** Axial CECT reveals "dirty," indurated preepiglottic fat, thickened aryepiglottic fold ⇉, and airless pyriform sinus ⇉. These are all expected CECT post-radiation therapy subacute findings.

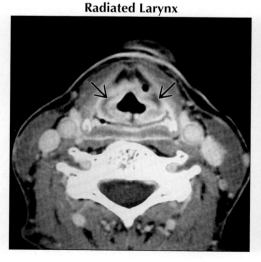
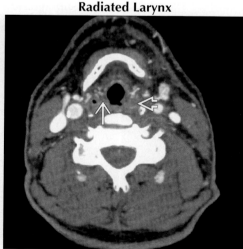

LARYNGEAL LESION

Laryngocele

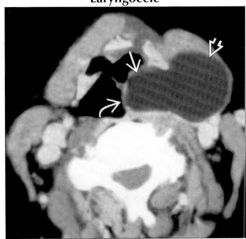

Laryngocele

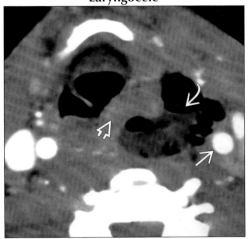

(Left) Axial CECT shows a mixed laryngocele, with both intra- ➡ and extralaryngeal ➡ components. The laryngocele contents are mucoid density. Notice the mild mass effect ➡ on the supraglottic airway. *(Right)* Axial CECT shows a mixed laryngocele ➡, filled with gas and pus, with typical lateral displacement of the carotid space ➡. Note inflamed, thickened left aryepiglottic fold ➡.

Trauma, Larynx

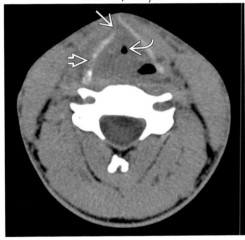

Trauma, Larynx

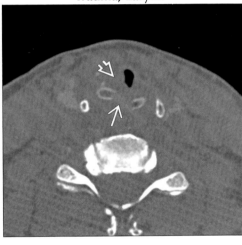

(Left) Axial NECT demonstrates a fracture at the superior thyroid notch ➡ and mid-lamina ➡, with diffuse swelling of the supraglottic laryngeal structures. Note airway narrowing ➡ from this supraglottic swelling and hematoma. *(Right)* Axial bone CT shows distracted cricoid cartilage ➡ fracture with endolaryngeal mucosal swelling/edema ➡. A direct blow to the neck can fracture the cricoid cartilage against the vertebral body.

SCCa, Larynx, Subglottic

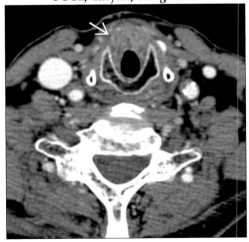

SCCa, Larynx, Subglottic

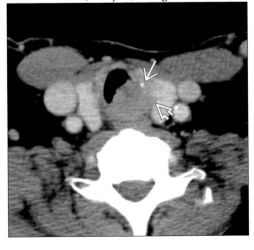

(Left) Axial CECT reveals an anterior subglottic mass destroying thyroid cartilage ➡ and invading infrahyoid strap muscles. No soft tissue should be present between the inner cartilage and the airway. *(Right)* Axial CECT shows bulky squamous cell carcinoma filling the subglottis and proximal cervical tracheal airway, with invasion of cartilage ➡. Note the lateral displacement of the left thyroid lobe from tumor invasion ➡.

LARYNGEAL LESION

(Left) Axial CECT reveals posterior laryngeal & hypopharyngeal edema. Note nonenhancing submucosal thickening of aryepiglottic fold (AEF), posterior paraglottic space, & posterior pharyngeal wall ➡. Swollen AEFs result in collapse of pyriform sinuses ⮞. (Right) Axial CECT shows a partially calcified cricoid cartilage mass displacing the larynx anteriorly. Note coarse bulky calcification ➡ & little enhancement in noncalcified portion of mass ⮞.

Laryngohypopharyngeal Reflux

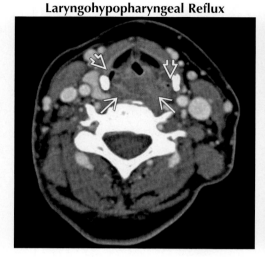

Chondrosarcoma, Larynx

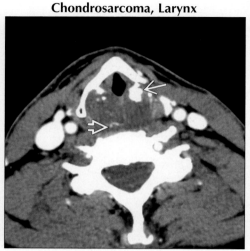

(Left) Axial CECT shows nonenhancing inflammatory changes ➡ in posterior right true vocal cord with frank erosion and sclerosis of residual cricoid cartilage ⮞. Severe rheumatoid arthritis can simulate malignancy, but history of arthritis and relative lack of enhancement are more suggestive of rheumatoid larynx. (Right) Axial CECT shows a rheumatoid lesion involving the right true vocal cord ➡, originally mistaken for squamous cell carcinoma.

Rheumatoid Larynx

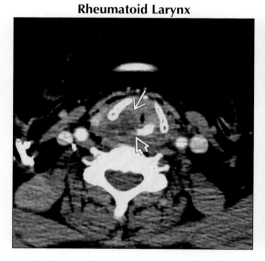

Rheumatoid Larynx

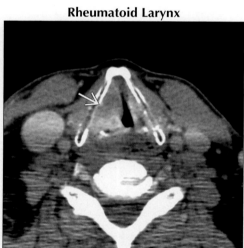

(Left) Axial T1WI MR depicts a discrete mass ➡ in the left paraglottic fat with minimal airway narrowing. The imaging appearance is nonspecific with biopsy the mainstay of diagnosis. (Right) Axial NECT shows circumferential laryngeal soft tissue with posterior web ➡. Note lack of laryngeal cartilage ossification, typical in pediatric larynx, which makes it nearly impossible to determine whether lesion is glottic or subglottic in location.

Amyloidosis, Larynx

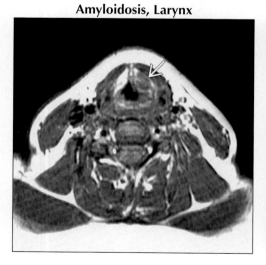

Wegener Granulomatosis, Larynx

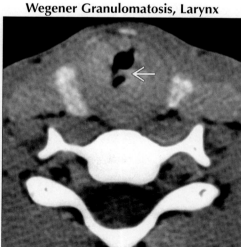

LARYNGEAL LESION

Paraganglioma, Larynx

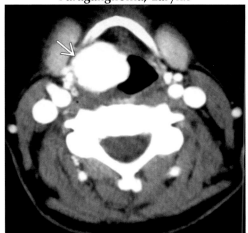

Papilloma, Larynx

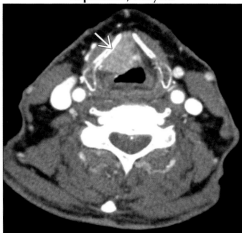

(Left) Axial CECT reveals a markedly enhancing well-circumscribed mass ➡ filling the right paraglottic space, with narrowing of the supraglottic airway. This amount of enhancement should suggest venous malformation, hemangioma, or paraganglioma. (Right) Axial CECT reveals an enhancing mass ➡ filling right paraglottic space in an adult with papillomatosis since childhood. The endoscopy results are necessary to differentiate from supraglottic SCCa.

Melanoma, Mucosal, Larynx

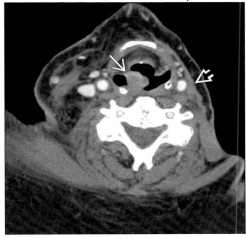

Pseudotumor, Larynx

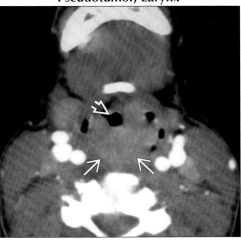

(Left) Axial CECT shows a bulky right aryepiglottic fold mass ➡ in this patient with melanoma. Note prior left neck dissection for treatment of nodal metastasis ➡. (Right) Axial CECT demonstrates a bulky mass involving left aryepiglottic fold, paraglottic fat, posterior laryngeal, and hypopharyngeal ➡ walls. Note the airway narrowing ➡.

Tracheopathia Osteochondroplastica

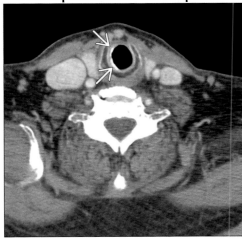

Nodular Chondrometaplasia, Larynx

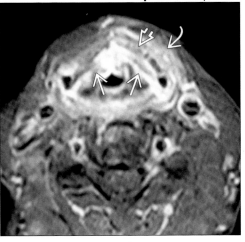

(Left) Axial CECT shows diffuse calcified subglottic mucosa ➡. Tracheopathia osteochondroplastica can be thin and non-nodular or more focal with discrete nodular ossification. (Right) Axial T1 C+ FS MR reveals diffuse inflammation of the larynx as abnormal enhancement in the paraglottic spaces ➡, left thyroid cartilage ➡, and strap muscles ➡. (Courtesy A. Chaturvedi, MD.)

EPIGLOTTIC ENLARGEMENT

DIFFERENTIAL DIAGNOSIS

Common
- SCCa, Larynx, Supraglottic
- Radiated Larynx

Less Common
- Epiglottitis, Adult
- Epiglottitis, Child
- Trauma, Larynx

Rare but Important
- Caustic or Thermal Injury
- Melanoma, Mucosal, Larynx
- Kaposi Sarcoma, Larynx

ESSENTIAL INFORMATION

Key Differential Diagnosis Issues
- Clinical setting & endoscopic results determine etiology of epiglottic enlargement
  - SCCa of epiglottis presents with mucosal lesion seen on endoscopy
  - Prior radiation therapy for H&N tumor essential information prior to image interpretation
  - Epiglottitis in adults or children presents with toxic febrile illness & sore throat, with inability to control secretions

Helpful Clues for Common Diagnoses
- **SCCa, Larynx, Supraglottic**
  - Key facts: Try to determine if lesion arises from lingual or laryngeal surface of epiglottis

  - CT/MR: Asymmetric > symmetric enhancing epiglottic mass
    - Preepiglottic space involvement (T3)
- **Radiated Larynx**
  - Key facts: History of radiation to H&N for primary tumor or lymphoma
  - CT/MR: Epiglottic/supraglottic thickening is diffuse, symmetric
    - CT: Low density, no enhancement
    - May persist for years

Helpful Clues for Less Common Diagnoses
- **Epiglottitis, Adult**
  - Key facts: Inflammation usually involves entire area, not just epiglottis
  - CT/MR: Entire supraglottic larynx, tongue base, & tonsils often thickened, edematous
    - Enhancing mucosa present
- **Epiglottitis, Child**
  - Key facts: Complete airway obstruction may occur abruptly
  - Lateral plain film: Edematous epiglottis, "thumb print" sign
- **Trauma, Larynx**
  - CT shows nonspecific findings of thickened, edematous epiglottis

Helpful Clues for Rare Diagnoses
- **Caustic or Thermal Injury**
  - History of injury essential to interpret imaging findings
- **Rare Mucosal Malignancy: Kaposi Sarcoma or Melanoma**
  - Enhancing asymmetric epiglottic mass has similar appearance regardless of histology

SCCa, Larynx, Supraglottic

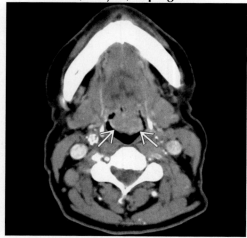

Axial CECT demonstrates a thickened enlarged enhancing mass ➡ completely replacing the normal epiglottis. Although usually asymmetric, mass may be difficult to see when smaller and symmetric.

SCCa, Larynx, Supraglottic

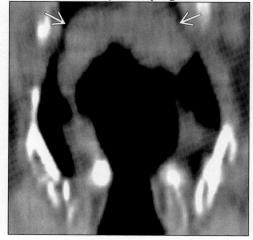

Coronal CECT reveals a globular epiglottis ➡ as a result of symmetric involvement with squamous cell carcinoma.

EPIGLOTTIC ENLARGEMENT

Radiated Larynx

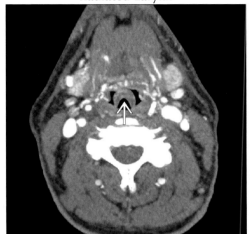

Radiated Larynx

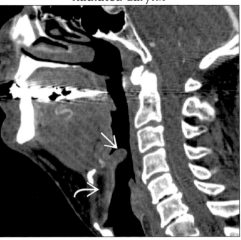

(Left) Axial CECT shows uniformly thickened, edematous nonenhancing suprahyoid epiglottis ➡ in a patient who finished radiation for tonsillar squamous cell carcinoma 8 weeks prior to CT examination. *(Right)* Sagittal CECT demonstrates nonenhancing edematous epiglottis ➡ on reformation. Note normal fat in the preepiglottic space ➡. This is the expected CECT appearance of the epiglottis after radiation treatment and may persist indefinitely.

Epiglottitis, Adult

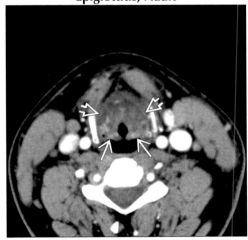

Epiglottitis, Adult

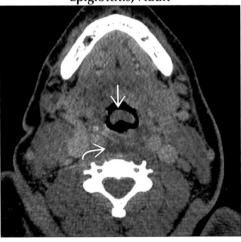

(Left) Axial CECT reveals a typical case of adult epiglottitis with edematous epiglottis and preepiglottic fat ➡. The aryepiglottic folds ➡ are also swollen and edematous. *(Right)* Axial CECT demonstrates nonenhancing swollen epiglottis ➡ in an immunocompromised patient with invasive fungal infection. Notice the fluid in the retropharyngeal space space ➡, likely sympathetic given lack of enhancement.

Epiglottitis, Child

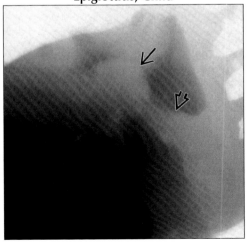

Caustic or Thermal Injury

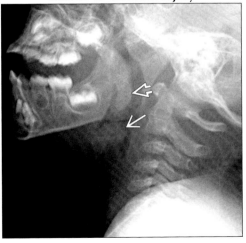

(Left) Lateral radiograph reveals marked thickening of the epiglottis ➡ and aryepiglottic folds ➡ in this child with fever, sore throat, and swollen epiglottis on clinical examination. *(Right)* Lateral radiograph shows thickening of epiglottis ➡ in a 17 month old who drank scalding hot soup. Notice otherwise normal airway with the associated swollen uvula ➡. Beefy red epiglottis was visualized on endoscopy.

DIFFERENTIAL DIAGNOSIS

Common
- Croup
- SCCa, Larynx, Supraglottic
- Radiated Larynx

Less Common
- Trauma, Larynx
- Epiglottitis, Adult
- Rheumatoid Larynx

Rare but Important
- Amyloidosis, Larynx
- Sarcoidosis, Larynx
- Wegener Granulomatosis, Larynx
- Non-Hodgkin Lymphoma, Larynx
- Pseudotumor, Larynx

ESSENTIAL INFORMATION

Key Differential Diagnosis Issues
- Malignant, inflammatory, or infectious etiologies in this group
- Chronic inflammatory lesions (rheumatoid arthritis, amyloidosis, sarcoidosis, Wegener granulomatosis), when involving larynx, may be difficult to tell apart

Helpful Clues for Common Diagnoses
- **Croup**
  - Key facts: Acute laryngotracheobronchitis
    - Clinical: "Barky" cough; 6 months of age to 3 years old, with peak at 1 year of age
    - Self-limited viral inflammation of upper airways
  - Imaging
    - AP plain film: Symmetric subglottic-tracheal narrowing → lack of normal "shouldering" of subglottic trachea → "steeple sign"
    - Lateral plain film: Hypopharyngeal distension with ill-defined narrow subglottic airway
- **SCCa, Larynx, Supraglottic**
  - Key facts: Normal supraglottis includes larynx superior to true vocal cords
    - Aryepiglottic folds (AEF), epiglottis, preepiglotticum, & paraglottic spaces
    - Lymphatic & vascular rich, resulting in frequent metastatic nodal disease
  - Imaging: Moderately enhancing infiltrating mass of supraglottis

- When large may extend in transglottic fashion to involve both glottic and subglottic larynx
- Often with associated pathologic adenopathy
- **Radiated Larynx**
  - Key facts: Acute & chronic phases
    - Acute phase: Mucositis with endolaryngeal swelling
    - Chronic phase: Diffuse endolaryngeal edema without discrete mass
    - Radionecrosis of laryngeal cartilage rare
    - Timing: Acute phase may be seen within months of radiation therapy
    - Chronic changes seen within 1 year of treatment; may persist for many years
  - Imaging
    - Acute changes: CECT shows mucosal enhancement with low-density swollen endolarynx
    - Chronic changes: CECT shows thickened, edematous free margin of epiglottis, AEF, false & true cords
    - Other chronic changes: Preepiglottic & paraglottic fat stranding; subcutaneous soft tissue stranding

Helpful Clues for Less Common Diagnoses
- **Trauma, Larynx**
  - Key facts: Trauma may be blunt or penetrating
    - Clinical assessment may be difficult
    - Imaging diagnosis also difficult if laryngeal cartilages are not ossified
  - Imaging: Offset of laryngeal cartilage contours
    - Associated soft tissue swelling of endolaryngeal or extralaryngeal soft tissues
    - Supraglottic edema/hematoma may compromise airway
    - Cricoarytenoid joint may be dislocated
- **Epiglottis, Adult**
  - Key facts: Seriously ill patient with difficulty speaking or swallowing
  - Imaging: CECT shows swollen, edematous supraglottis
    - If incompletely treated, may evolve into supraglottic or hypopharyngeal abscess
- **Rheumatoid Larynx**

DIFFUSE LARYNGEAL SWELLING

- ○ Key facts: 25% of rheumatoid arthritis patients have arthritis in cricoarytenoid ± cricothyroid joints
  - Both are synovial joints
- ○ Acute CECT findings
  - Cricoarytenoid or cricothyroid joint area swelling with associated cartilage erosion
  - Due to cartilage erosion, may mimic laryngeal squamous cell carcinoma
  - When severe, may cause supraglottic airway compromise
- ○ Chronic CECT findings
  - Vocal cord atrophy with cricoarytenoid joint fixation
  - Arytenoid cartilage sclerosis

Helpful Clues for Rare Diagnoses

- **Amyloidosis, Larynx**
  - ○ Key facts: Deposition of amyloid material in larynx with no mucosal lesion
    - Diffuse endolaryngeal soft tissue swelling
    - Primary form occurs here
    - May be found as secondary manifestation in patients with systemic multiple myeloma
  - ○ Imaging: Diffuse submucosal mass
    - No associated cartilage destruction or invasion
    - T2 hypointensity has been reported
- **Sarcoidosis, Larynx**
  - ○ Key facts: Head & neck manifestations seen in only 15% of patients with sarcoidosis
    - Laryngeal sarcoid in < 5%

- Often found in patients without pulmonary sarcoid
- ○ Imaging: Diffusively infiltrating submucosal mass
  - May present with glottic and supraglottic submucosal lesion
- **Wegener Granulomatosis, Larynx**
  - ○ Key facts: Systemic vasculitis, idiopathic
    - Commonly involves respiratory tract
  - ○ Imaging: Diffuse submucosal mass
    - Most commonly seen in subglottis
    - Trachea and bronchi may also be affected
- **Non-Hodgkin Lymphoma, Larynx**
  - ○ Key facts: Rare extranodal, extralymphatic site of non-Hodgkin lymphoma in H&N
  - ○ Imaging: Mimics squamous cell carcinoma
    - May be focal or transglottic
    - If nodes associated, large & non-necrotic
- **Pseudotumor, Larynx**
  - ○ Key facts: Benign lesion
    - a.k.a., plasma cell granuloma
    - Presents with voice change or stridor
  - ○ Imaging: Nonspecific diffuse endolaryngeal soft tissue
    - Enhancing lesion with subglottic predilection

SELECTED REFERENCES

1. Becker M et al: Imaging of the larynx and hypopharynx. Eur J Radiol. 66(3):460-79, 2008
2. Mukherji SK et al: Radiologic appearance of the irradiated larynx. Part II. Primary site response. Radiology. 193(1):149-54, 1994

Croup

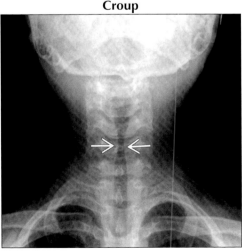

Sagittal oblique radiograph shows the symmetric narrowing of the subglottic larynx and trachea ➡, which causes the classic steeple appearance of croup.

Croup

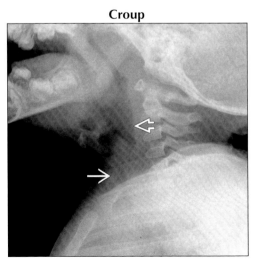

Lateral radiograph demonstrates subglottic narrowing ➡ with hyperdistention of the hypopharynx ➡, typical for croup.

DIFFUSE LARYNGEAL SWELLING

(Left) Axial CECT shows diffuse, bulky supraglottic squamous cell carcinoma involving the aryepiglottic folds (AEF) ➡ and the paraglottic spaces bilaterally ➡. Associated right level 3 metastatic lymph node ➡ is also visible. **(Right)** Axial CECT reveals a large supraglottic SCCa enlarging the left AEF ➡. Both paraglottic spaces ➡ are also invaded. Notice the extralaryngeal tumor spread into the infrahyoid strap muscles ➡.

SCCa, Larynx, Supraglottic

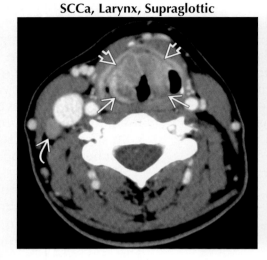

SCCa, Larynx, Supraglottic

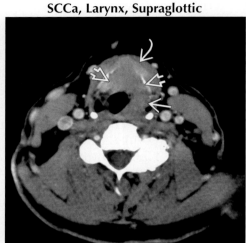

(Left) Axial CECT at the level of the true vocal cords reveals acute radiation-induced mucositis as diffuse mucosal enhancement of the hypopharynx ➡ and larynx. The surface of the right true vocal cord ➡ also enhances. The thickened enhancement of the left true vocal cord ➡ is due to tumor involvement of this area. **(Right)** Axial CECT shows diffuse soft tissue swelling ➡ of the supraglottic larynx secondary to radiation therapy.

Radiated Larynx

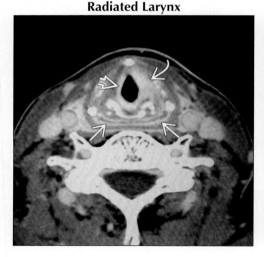

Radiated Larynx

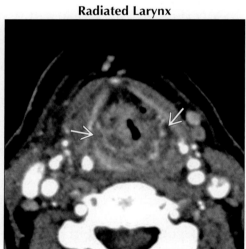

(Left) Axial NECT reveals a step-off at the superior thyroid notch ➡, secondary to thyroid lamina fracture. Diffuse supraglottic edema/hematoma ➡ narrows the airway. **(Right)** Axial CECT reveals reactive adenopathy ➡ associated with a swollen epiglottis ➡ and bilateral inflamed aryepiglottic folds ➡ in this patient with adult epiglottis. No focal abscess is seen.

Trauma, Larynx

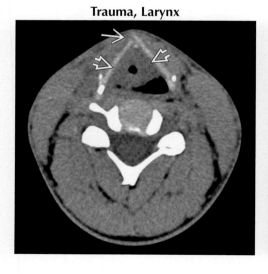

Epiglottitis, Adult

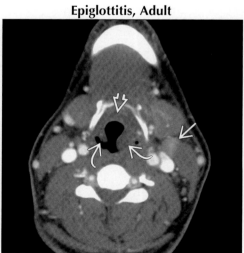

DIFFUSE LARYNGEAL SWELLING

Rheumatoid Larynx

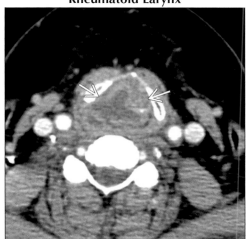

Amyloidosis, Larynx

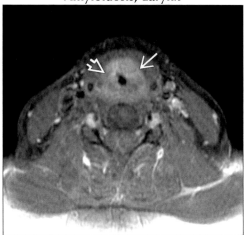

(Left) Axial CECT reveals minimally enhancing bilateral supraglottic soft tissue ➡. This represents inflammatory tissue emanating up from a severely inflamed right cricoarytenoid joint (not seen) in this patient with rheumatoid larynx. *(Right)* Axial T1 C+ FS MR shows left ➡ and, to a lesser extent, right ➡ false vocal cord enhancement due to primary laryngeal amyloidosis. T2 images (not shown) revealed the lesion to be hypointense.

Sarcoidosis, Larynx

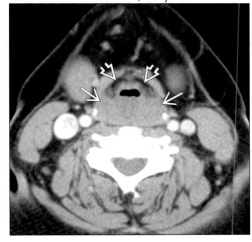

Wegener Granulomatosis, Larynx

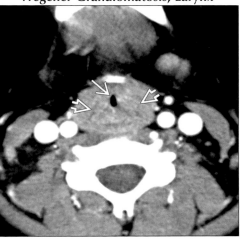

(Left) Axial CECT reveals posterior supraglottic involvement with sarcoidosis. Notice the thickened aryepiglottic folds ➡ with relative sparing of the preepiglottic space ➡. *(Right)* Axial CECT demonstrates diffuse laryngeal involvement in a child with severe systemic Wegener granulomatosis. Note the narrowed airway ➡ and bilateral increased supraglottic tissue ➡.

Non-Hodgkin Lymphoma, Larynx

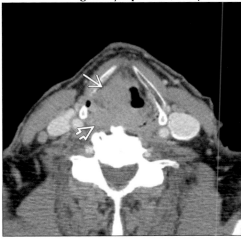

Pseudotumor, Larynx

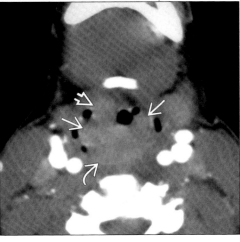

(Left) Axial CECT reveals extranodal, extralymphatic endolaryngeal non-Hodgkin lymphoma involving the right paraglottic space ➡ and hypopharynx ➡. *(Right)* Axial CECT shows a diffusely infiltrating mass involving the aryepiglottic folds ➡, right paraglottic space ➡, and hypopharynx ➡.

3

SUBGLOTTIC STENOSIS

DIFFERENTIAL DIAGNOSIS

Common
- Subglottic-Tracheal Stenosis, Iatrogenic
- Multinodular Goiter
- Non-Hodgkin Lymphoma, Thyroid
- Anaplastic Carcinoma, Thyroid
- Infantile Hemangioma

Less Common
- Trauma, Larynx
- Wegener Granulomatosis
- Sarcoidosis
- Subglottic-Tracheal Stenosis, Idiopathic
- SCCa, Larynx, Subglottic

Rare but Important
- Relapsing Polychondritis
- Amyloidosis, Larynx
- Schwannoma
- Mucopolysaccharidosis
- Subglottic-Tracheal Stenosis, Congenital

ESSENTIAL INFORMATION

Key Differential Diagnosis Issues
- Narrowing of short segment of airway
  - Below vocal cords to inferior cricoid ring
- Can be defined as extrinsic or intrinsic
  - Intrinsic: Primary subglottic process
    - Prior intubation or tracheostomy most common cause in all ages (~ 90%)
  - Extrinsic: Subglottic compression or invasion
    - Thyroid disease most common
- Imaging important to define etiology and extent of narrowing
  - May be critical when direct inspection difficult or unsafe

Helpful Clues for Common Diagnoses
- **Subglottic-Tracheal Stenosis, Iatrogenic**
  - Key facts
    - ~ 90% of all cases
    - Prolonged endotracheal intubation or tracheostomy
    - Pressure ischemia/necrosis with scarring
  - Imaging
    - Nonspecific soft tissue narrowing of lumen subglottis ± cervical trachea
    - May be circumferential or eccentric, smooth or irregular

- May see deformity of cricoid ring or of pretracheal tissues from tracheostomy
- **Multinodular Goiter**
  - Key facts
    - Diffuse gland enlargement may result in extrinsic compression of subglottis
    - Gland has adenomatous change, fibrosis, calcification, hemorrhage ± cysts
  - Imaging
    - Heterogeneous enlarged gland
    - 90% have calcifications
    - Important to assess complete extent of goiter
- **Non-Hodgkin Lymphoma, Thyroid**
  - Key facts
    - B-cell primary thyroid lymphoma
    - Rapidly enlarging neck mass may compress subglottis
  - Imaging
    - Homogeneous, without necrosis or calcifications
    - Tends to compress rather than invade
- **Anaplastic Carcinoma, Thyroid**
  - Key facts
    - Aggressive, invasive, rapidly growing primary thyroid neoplasm
  - Imaging
    - Heterogeneous mass invades adjacent structures
    - Destruction of cricoid cartilage to subglottis or tracheal rings to trachea
- **Infantile Hemangioma**
  - Key facts
    - Submucosal congenital lesion
    - Symptomatic in infancy during proliferative phase of growth
    - Typically biphasic stridor
    - May be clinically misdiagnosed as croup
    - Associated with superficial hemangiomas of H&N and cardiovascular anomalies
  - Imaging
    - Intensely enhancing mass internal to cricoid ring
    - May be circumferential or eccentric

Helpful Clues for Less Common Diagnoses
- **Trauma, Larynx**
  - Key facts
    - Cricoid ring usually fractures in 2 sites
  - Imaging
    - Fractures difficult to see in young patients with noncalcified cartilage

- Acute: Look for distorted cartilage, hematoma ± edema
- Chronic: Irregular thickened cricoid
- **Wegener Granulomatosis**
  - Key facts
    - Vasculitis with multiple necrotizing granulomas
    - Typically late manifestation of Wegener
  - Imaging
    - Nonspecific soft tissue narrowing lumen
    - Cartilage destruction
- **Sarcoidosis**
  - Key facts
    - Up to 3% of sarcoidosis patients
    - Submucosal granulomatous lesions
  - Imaging
    - Multifocal subglottic-tracheal wall thickening
- **Subglottic-Tracheal Stenosis, Idiopathic**
  - Key facts
    - Nonspecific chronic inflammatory tissue
    - Associated with gastroesophageal reflux
  - Imaging
    - Inflammatory thickening in subglottic-tracheal wall
- **SCCa, Larynx, Subglottic**
  - Key facts
    - Least common primary laryngeal site
    - Often presents with T4 stage disease
  - Imaging
    - Soft tissue mass infiltrating adjacent tissues

Helpful Clues for Rare Diagnoses
- **Relapsing Polychondritis**
  - Key facts: Idiopathic cartilage inflammation with fibrosis & calcifications
  - Imaging
    - Subglottic collapse with dynamic CT
- **Amyloidosis, Larynx**
  - Key facts
    - Diffuse or multifocal submucosal infiltrates or focal mass
  - Imaging
    - Luminal narrowing with focal or diffuse thickening of wall ± calcification
- **Schwannoma**
  - Key facts
    - Rare submucosal benign primary tumor
  - Imaging
    - Submucosal mass distorts lumen
    - Heterogeneous texture with larger lesion
- **Mucopolysaccharidosis**
  - Key facts: Mucopolysaccharide deposits in connective tissue
  - Imaging
    - Multilobulated luminal narrowing
- **Subglottic-Tracheal Stenosis, Congenital**
  - Key facts: Birth defect from incomplete formation of subglottis
    - Two forms: Membranous or cartilaginous
  - Imaging
    - Lumen < 4 mm in term infant
    - Membranous: Submucosal excess fibrous tissue narrows lumen
    - Cartilaginous: Malformed cricoid

Subglottic-Tracheal Stenosis, Iatrogenic

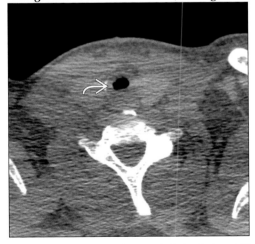

Axial NECT shows smooth, noncalcified soft tissue ➽ narrowing the subglottis circumferentially. No cartilage destruction is evident. This patient had a history of prior prolonged intubation.

Subglottic-Tracheal Stenosis, Iatrogenic

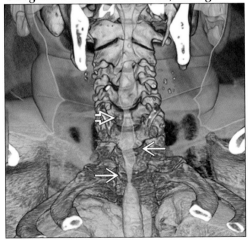

3D reformatted image from the same CT study demonstrates long segment irregularity to involve subglottis ➽ and cervical trachea ➽.

SUBGLOTTIC STENOSIS

(Left) Axial NECT at level of subglottis shows circumferential but predominantly posterior soft tissue internal to an irregular, poorly calcified cricoid ➡. Soft tissue is also evident between cricoid & thyroid ➡ cartilages, suggesting significant scarring in this patient. *(Right)* Sagittal NECT in the same patient shows marked narrowing of the subglottis ➡ with a smooth posterior soft tissue mass ➡. Cervical tracheal lumen ➡ is normal caliber & contour.

Subglottic-Tracheal Stenosis, Iatrogenic

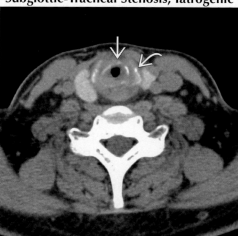

Subglottic-Tracheal Stenosis, Iatrogenic

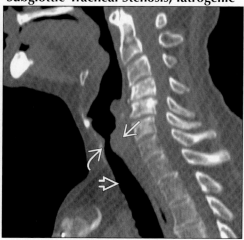

(Left) Axial CECT reveals markedly enlarged but only mildly heterogeneous thyroid lobes. Carotid ➡ and jugular vessels are displaced posterolaterally, sternocleidomastoid muscles laterally, and cricoid cartilage ➡ is compressed medially. *(Right)* Coronal CECT reformation in the same patient demonstrates subglottic luminal narrowing ➡ from enlarged thyroid lobes. Patient has already had cervical tracheal stent ➡ placed for severe stenosis.

Multinodular Goiter

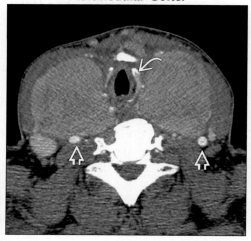

Multinodular Goiter

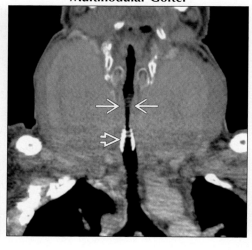

(Left) Sagittal radiograph performed in a patient with a rapidly enlarging neck mass reveals marked narrowing of subglottic lumen ➡ and cervical trachea ➡, with widening of prevertebral soft tissues. *(Right)* Axial CECT in the same patient reveals a low-density but heterogeneous mass infiltrating the right thyroid lobe ➡ & adjacent soft tissues and surrounding the upper airway ➡ with luminal narrowing & leftward displacement.

Non-Hodgkin Lymphoma, Thyroid

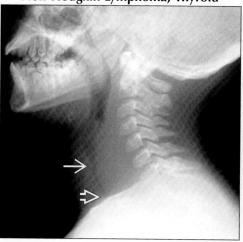

Non-Hodgkin Lymphoma, Thyroid

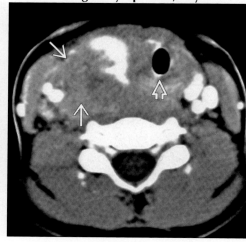

SUBGLOTTIC STENOSIS

Anaplastic Carcinoma, Thyroid

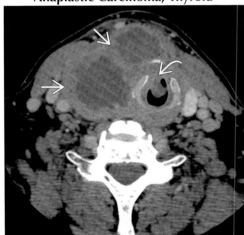

Anaplastic Carcinoma, Thyroid

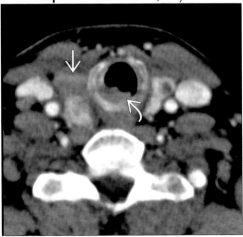

(Left) Axial CECT shows a heterogeneous, partially necrotic large mass ➡️ replacing the right thyroid & infiltrating adjacent tissues. Tumor invades cricoid with lobulated component in subglottic lumen ➡️. (Right) Axial CECT in a different patient reveals more subtle abnormal soft tissue ➡️ internal to cricoid ring in subglottic portion of larynx. Soft tissue is contiguous with homogeneous low-density infiltrating mass ➡️ arising in the right thyroid lobe.

Infantile Hemangioma

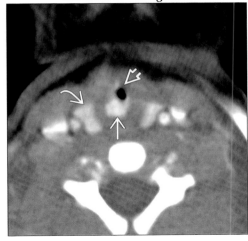

Infantile Hemangioma

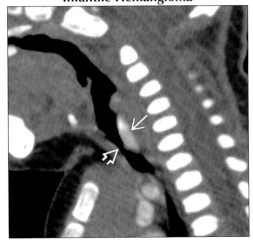

(Left) Axial CECT through an infant's neck at level of hyperdense thyroid gland ➡️ reveals markedly enhancing eccentric soft tissue mass ➡️, which results in significant narrowing of the subglottic airway ➡️. Note that hemangioma enhancement is similar to arterial contrast density. (Right) Sagittal CECT in the same patient demonstrates hemangioma as a predominantly posterior, markedly enhancing subglottic mass ➡️, resulting in airway narrowing ➡️.

Trauma, Larynx

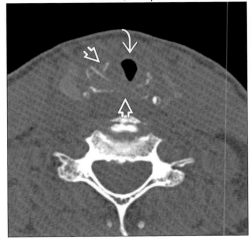

Trauma, Larynx

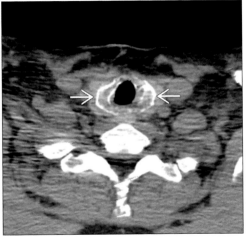

(Left) Axial bone CT following acute injury shows fragmentation of cricoid cartilage ➡️ with subglottic mucosal swelling and edema. This produces marked airway distortion and narrowing ➡️. Extensive swelling is noted in perilaryngeal tissues also. (Right) Axial NECT in a different patient with history of prior laryngeal fracture demonstrates marked thickening and deformity of cricoid ring ➡️, although only mild distortion of subglottic lumen is seen.

SUBGLOTTIC STENOSIS

(Left) Axial NECT at level of cricoid cartilage ➡ reveals extensive circumferential soft tissue, resulting in significant narrowing of subglottic lumen ➡. There is no evidence of cartilage destruction or distortion. (Right) Sagittal CECT shows thoracic tracheal wall thickening ➡ in combination with subglottic anterior wall soft tissue ➡, secondary to submucosal granulomatous lesions from systemic sarcoidosis.

Wegener Granulomatosis

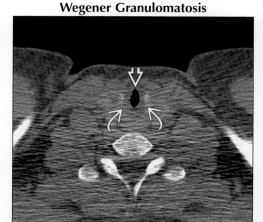

Sarcoidosis

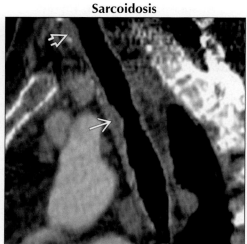

(Left) Axial NECT through level of cricoid ring reveals irregular circumferential soft tissue, thickest at the 7:00 o'clock position ➡, narrowing the subglottic lumen. This patient had no history of intubation or tracheostomy. (Right) Coronal NECT reformatted reveals extent of irregular subglottic tissue ➡ that narrows airway. Segment was resected, revealing nonspecific inflammatory tissue, negative for granulomatous diseases such as sarcoid & Wegener.

Subglottic-Tracheal Stenosis, Idiopathic

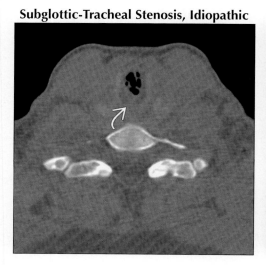

Subglottic-Tracheal Stenosis, Idiopathic

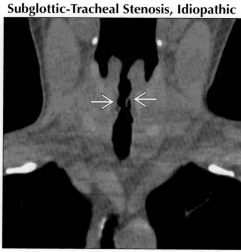

(Left) Axial CECT below the true cords reveals a large heterogeneous soft tissue mass markedly narrowing the subglottic lumen with destruction of cricoid ➡ & thyroid ➡ cartilages. (Right) Axial CECT shows smooth thick soft tissue ➡ at anterior margin of subglottis. Cricoid is intact, but lesion extended cephalad into true cords, indicating aggressive process. No adenopathy is evident. Glottic & supraglottic tumors may also spread inferiorly to subglottis.

SCCa, Larynx, Subglottic

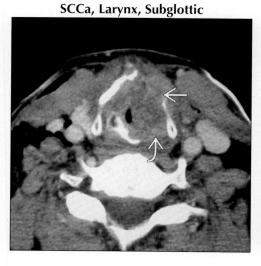

SCCa, Larynx, Subglottic

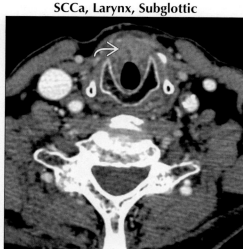

3

SUBGLOTTIC STENOSIS

Relapsing Polychondritis

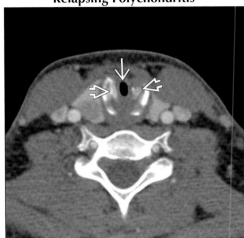

Amyloidosis, Larynx

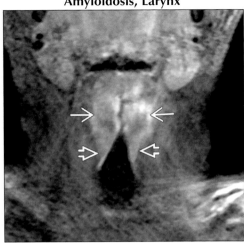

(Left) Axial CECT demonstrates subglottic stenosis ➡ from inflammatory tissue and calcifications ➡ in a patient with relapsing polychondritis. *(Right)* Coronal T1 C+ FS MR shows a bilateral paraglottic space mixed enhancing amyloid ➡ that causes supraglottic airway compromise. Note extension into the subglottic area ➡ with loss of glottic "shoulders," similar to croup.

Schwannoma

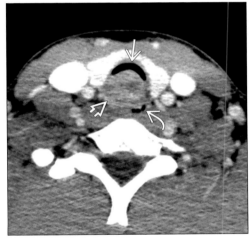

Schwannoma

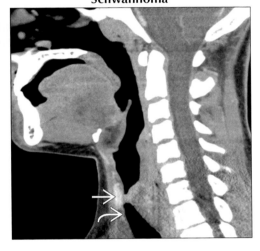

(Left) Axial CECT demonstrates a rounded heterogeneous mass ➡ producing crescentic narrowing of subglottic lumen ➡, which suggests submucosal origin. There is no evidence that mass invades adjacent soft tissues. Esophagus is compressed and displaced to the left ➡. *(Right)* Sagittal CECT reformatted image in the same patient demonstrates a focal posteriorly located mass narrowing the subglottis ➡ and proximal cervical trachea ➡.

Mucopolysaccharidosis

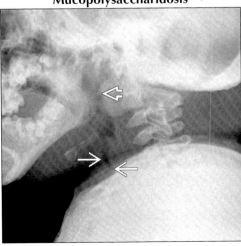

Mucopolysaccharidosis

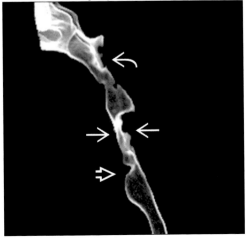

(Left) Lateral radiograph in a child with Hurler (type 2 mucopolysaccharidosis) reveals markedly irregular narrowing of subglottic airway ➡ and fullness of posterior oropharyngeal wall ➡. *(Right)* 3D reformation of CT demonstrates long segment irregularity of contour of subglottis ➡ and cervical trachea ➡ from submucosal deposits. Posterior oropharyngeal wall ➡ deposition is also evident.

VOCAL CORD PARALYSIS (LEFT)

DIFFERENTIAL DIAGNOSIS

Common
- SCCa, Nodes
- Paraganglioma, Glomus Jugulare
- Nasopharyngeal Carcinoma
- Acute Cerebral Ischemia-Infarction, PICA

Less Common
- Cavernous Malformation, Hemorrhagic
- Paraganglioma, Carotid Body
- Schwannoma, Jugular Foramen
- Dissection, Carotid Artery, Neck
- Paraganglioma, Glomus Vagale
- Schwannoma, Carotid Space
- Metastasis, Skull Base
- Differentiated Carcinoma, Thyroid
- Meningioma, Jugular Foramen
- Pancoast Tumor
- Lung Cancer, Non-Small Cell
- Esophageal Carcinoma, Cervical

Rare but Important
- Multiple Sclerosis, Brainstem
- Aneurysm, Aortic
- Chondrosarcoma, Skull Base
- Neurofibroma, Carotid Space
- Anaplastic Carcinoma, Thyroid

ESSENTIAL INFORMATION

Key Differential Diagnosis Issues
- Left vagus nerve extends into mediastinum; recurs via aortopulmonic window
  - Thoracic diagnoses therefore included in differential diagnosis list
- Left vocal cord paralysis (VCP) caused by diseases from medulla to AP window
  - If CN10 is affected below level of palate, VCP seen as simple, isolated finding
  - If CN10 is affected above level of palate, VCP occurs with other findings
    - Other cranial nerve dysfunction: CN9, CN11 ± CN12
    - Ipsilateral soft palate and pharyngeal constrictor malfunction (pharyngeal plexus injury)
- Best imaging modality
  - If unsure of location of lesion based on physical examination: CECT
  - If lesion confidently localized above level of palate: MR with contrast for posterior fossa, skull base, suprahyoid neck

Helpful Clues for Common Diagnoses
- **SCCa, Nodes**
  - Internal jugular chain extranodal extension into carotid space
- **Paraganglioma, Glomus Jugulare**
  - MR: Enhancing tumor with flow voids
    - Spreads superolaterally through middle ear floor to enter middle ear cavity
- **Nasopharyngeal Carcinoma**
  - Nasopharyngeal mucosal space tumor invades into carotid space (CS)
- **Acute Cerebral Ischemia-Infarction, PICA**
  - MR: DWI shows restricted diffusion in lateral medulla and inferior cerebellar hemisphere

Helpful Clues for Less Common Diagnoses
- **Cavernous Malformation, Hemorrhagic**
  - MR: GRE shows blooming lesion in medulla; multiple other lesions possible
- **Paraganglioma, Carotid Body**
  - MR: Enhancing tumor with flow voids splays ICA from ECA at bifurcation
- **Schwannoma, Jugular Foramen**
  - CT: Sharply marginated tumor enlarges jugular foramen
    - Spreads superomedially toward medulla
- **Dissection, Carotid Artery, Neck**
  - T1 MR with fat saturation: Intramural hematoma (hyperintense crescent adjacent to ICA lumen)
- **Paraganglioma, Glomus Vagale**
  - MR: Enhancing tumor in CS 1-2 cm below skull base with flow voids
- **Schwannoma, Carotid Space**
  - MR: Enhancing fusiform mass with intramural cysts possible
- **Metastasis, Skull Base**
  - CT/MR: Destructive, enhancing skull base lesion in vicinity of jugular foramen
- **Differentiated Carcinoma, Thyroid**
  - MR: Enhancing thyroid mass invades tracheoesophageal groove
- **Meningioma, Jugular Foramen**
  - CT: JF lesion causes permeative-sclerotic or hyperostotic bone changes
  - MR: Enhancing JF mass with dural tails, no flow voids; centrifugal spread pattern
- **Pancoast Tumor**
  - CT: Apical lung tumor invades mediastinum or cervical-thoracic inlet
- **Lung Cancer, Non-Small Cell**

○ CT: Mediastinal tumor invades aortopulmonic window
- **Esophageal Carcinoma, Cervical**
  - ○ CT: Cervical esophageal mass or paratracheal nodes invade tracheoesophageal groove

Helpful Clues for Rare Diagnoses
- **Multiple Sclerosis, Brainstem**
  - ○ MR: High signal lesions in white matter of suprasellar brain; medullary lesions may or may not be visible
- **Aneurysm, Aortic**
  - ○ CT: Aortic arch enlarges, stretches CN10 in aortopulmonic window
- **Chondrosarcoma, Skull Base**
  - ○ CT: Invasive SB mass centered in petrooccipital fissure; 50% chondroid matrix
  - ○ MR: Low T1, high T2 signal; enhances
- **Neurofibroma, Carotid Space**
  - ○ CT: Low-density ovoid or fusiform poorly enhancing mass in carotid space
- **Anaplastic Carcinoma, Thyroid**
  - ○ CT/MR: Large invasive enhancing thyroid mass in elderly patient; may have history of multinodular goiter

Alternative Differential Approaches
- Another approach to organizing causes of left vocal cord paralysis is to group lesions by ANATOMIC SEGMENT of LEFT CN10
  - ○ Intramedullary, skull base, carotid space, superior mediastinum, & tracheoesophageal groove causes

○ Intramedullary causes
  - Cerebral ischemia-infarction, acute
  - Cavernous malformation, hemorrhagic
  - Multiple sclerosis, brainstem
○ Skull base/jugular foramen causes
  - Paraganglioma, glomus jugulare
  - Schwannoma, jugular foramen
  - Metastasis, skull base
  - Meningioma, jugular foramen
  - Chondrosarcoma, skull base
○ Carotid space causes
  - Nasopharyngeal carcinoma
  - SCCa, nodes
  - Paraganglioma, carotid body
  - Paraganglioma, glomus vagale
  - Schwannoma, carotid space
  - Neurofibroma, carotid space
  - Dissection, carotid artery, neck
○ Superior mediastinal causes
  - Pancoast tumor
  - Aneurysm, aortic
  - Lung cancer, non-small cell
○ Visceral space/tracheoesophageal groove causes
  - Differentiated carcinoma, thyroid
  - Anaplastic carcinoma, thyroid
  - Esophageal carcinoma, cervical

SCCa, Nodes

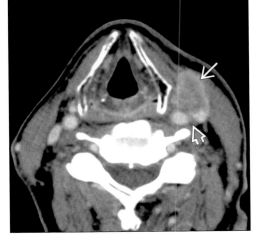

Axial CECT shows an amorphous squamous cell carcinoma lymph node ➡ invading the carotid space. Note the extranodal tumor surrounding the internal jugular vein and common carotid artery ➡.

Paraganglioma, Glomus Jugulare

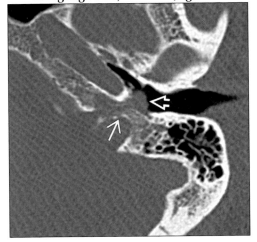

Axial bone CT reveals a middle ear mass ➡ connected through bone to the jugular foramen. Note the permeative-destructive bone changes ➡ along the lateral margin of the jugular foramen.

VOCAL CORD PARALYSIS (LEFT)

(Left) Axial T1 C+ FS MR reveals a left nasopharyngeal mucosal space tumor ⇨ that is deeply invasive. The enhancing tumor has reached the high nasopharyngeal carotid space ⇨ where CN10-12 reside. *(Right)* Axial DWI-B0 reveals restricted diffusion (high signal) in the lateral medulla ⇨ and inferior cerebellar hemisphere ⇨. ADC map (not shown) demonstrated corresponding low signal, signaling acute stroke.

Nasopharyngeal Carcinoma

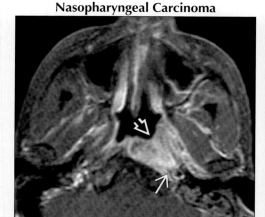

Acute Cerebral Ischemia-Infarction, PICA

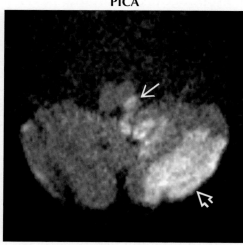

(Left) Sagittal T2WI MR demonstrates a giant posterior fossa cavernous malformation with multiple blood-filled "bubbles" within the 4th ventricle and vermis compressing the pons and medulla ⇨. *(Right)* Axial CECT reveals an enhancing left carotid space carotid body paraganglioma that splays the external ⇨ and internal ⇨ carotid arteries. Note a small contralateral second carotid body paraganglioma on right ⇨.

Cavernous Malformation, Hemorrhagic

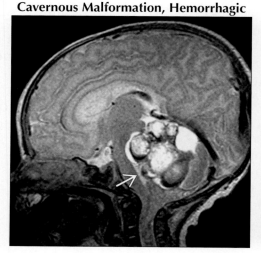

Paraganglioma, Carotid Body

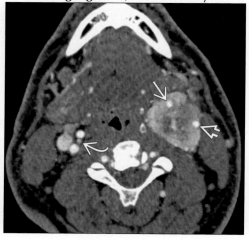

(Left) Axial bone CT demonstrates an enlarged jugular foramen with crisp, almost "surgical" margins ⇨. A jugular foramen schwannoma is the only lesion in this area that will create such a well-defined, remodeled-appearing jugular foramen. *(Right)* Axial T1 C+ FS MR reveals a well-circumscribed enhancing schwannoma extending superomedially from the enlarged jugular foramen toward the lateral medulla ⇨.

Schwannoma, Jugular Foramen

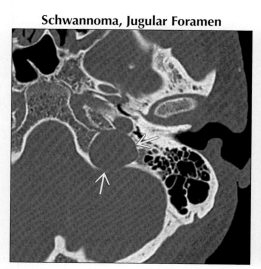

Schwannoma, Jugular Foramen

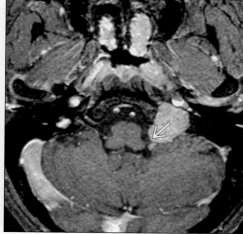

VOCAL CORD PARALYSIS (LEFT)

Dissection, Carotid Artery, Neck

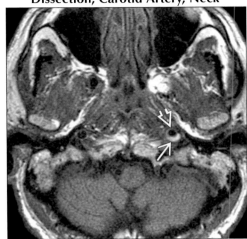

Dissection, Carotid Artery, Neck

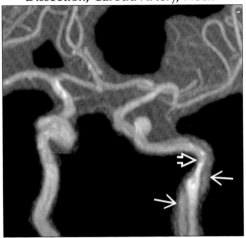

(Left) Axial T1WI MR shows a high signal subacute hemorrhage in the wall of the left internal carotid artery ➡ with secondary narrowing of the ICA lumen ⇒. This patient presented with acute onset of hoarseness and Horner syndrome. (Right) MRA reformation in the oblique-coronal plane demonstrates left internal carotid artery luminal narrowing ⇒ and an intramural high signal clot ➡ in the nasopharyngeal carotid space.

Paraganglioma, Glomus Vagale

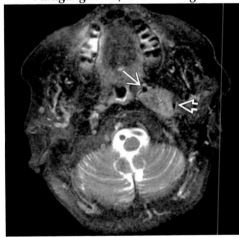

Schwannoma, Carotid Space

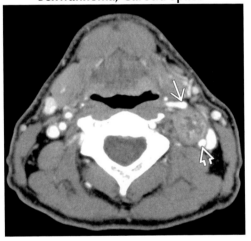

(Left) Axial T2WI FS MR shows a nasopharyngeal carotid space mass with anteromedial ICA ➡ and posterolateral internal jugular vein ⇒ displacement. Small signal voids are seen as focal black dots within the tumor. (Right) Axial CECT shows an unusual vagal schwannoma of the carotid space that splays the external ➡ and internal ⇒ carotid arteries and mimics a paraganglioma location. Even in this location, the lack of intense enhancement makes a paraganglioma unlikely.

Metastasis, Skull Base

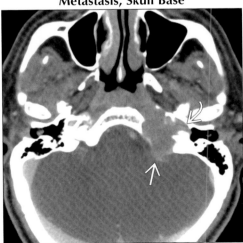

Differentiated Carcinoma, Thyroid

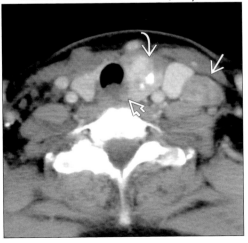

(Left) Axial CECT shows metastatic medullary thyroid carcinoma to the jugular foramen with extension cephalad into the low cerebellopontine angle cistern ⇒, anterior middle ear ➡, & nasopharyngeal carotid space (not shown). (Right) Axial CECT reveals a left partially calcified thyroid carcinoma ➡ invading the tracheoesophageal groove ⇒. A large inhomogeneously enhancing low internal jugular node is also present ➡.

VOCAL CORD PARALYSIS (LEFT)

(Left) Axial bone CT reveals an elliptical, faintly calcified meningioma ➡ emerging from the jugular foramen. Notice the mixed permeative-sclerotic pattern of bone change in the inferomedial temporal bone ➡ where the tumor has invaded bone. *(Right)* Axial T1 C+ MR shows a large en plaque meningioma centered in the jugular foramen with prominent dural tails ➡. This enhancing lesion exits inferiorly into the nasopharyngeal carotid space ➡.

Meningioma, Jugular Foramen

Meningioma, Jugular Foramen

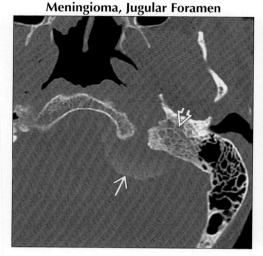

(Left) Coronal CECT shows an aggressive-appearing lung carcinoma of the left upper lobe apex ➡. The tumor invades cephalad into the visceral space of the neck ➡. The vagus nerve trunk and the recurrent laryngeal nerve both pass through this area. *(Right)* Axial CECT shows an enlarged 4R lymph node from bronchogenic carcinoma. The nodal conglomerate extends into the left aortopulmonic window ➡. This patient presented with hoarseness and hemoptysis.

Pancoast Tumor

Lung Cancer, Non-Small Cell

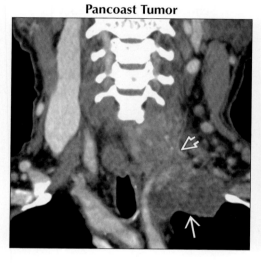

(Left) Axial CECT demonstrates left vocal cord paralysis in this patient with cervical esophageal carcinoma. Note the dilated ventricle ➡ and the paramedian left cord ➡. *(Right)* Axial CECT demonstrates a cervical esophageal primary adenocarcinoma that is invading the left tracheoesophageal groove ➡ where the recurrent laryngeal nerve is found. Left vocal cord paralysis caused hoarseness as a presenting symptom in this patient.

Esophageal Carcinoma, Cervical

Esophageal Carcinoma, Cervical

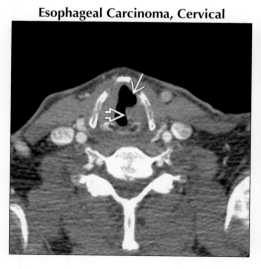
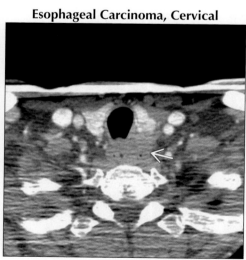

VOCAL CORD PARALYSIS (LEFT)

Multiple Sclerosis, Brainstem

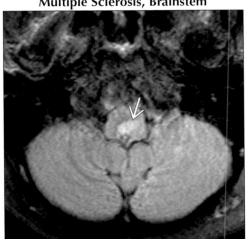

Aneurysm, Aortic

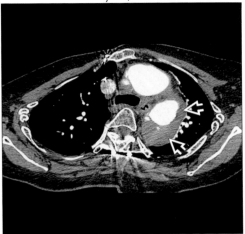

(Left) Axial FLAIR MR shows a dorsal medullary plaque ➡ extending asymmetrically into the left medullary parenchyma. Long tract signs as well as hoarseness were part of the clinical picture. (Right) Axial CTA reveals an aortic aneurysm in a patient with Marfan syndrome. Massive luminal dilatation with descending thoracic aorta wall thickening from thrombosed dissection ➡ is seen. Stretching of CN10 as it recurs in aortopulmonic window causes vocal cord paralysis.

Chondrosarcoma, Skull Base

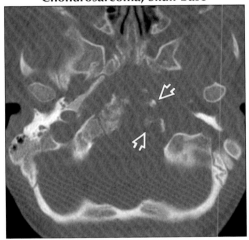

Chondrosarcoma, Skull Base

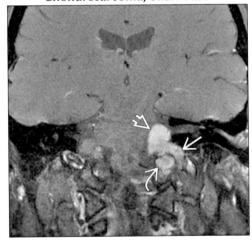

(Left) Axial bone CT shows a large skull base chondrosarcoma in a child with chondroid matrix ➡ within the tumor. This bulky lesion is centered in the petrooccipital fissure area. (Right) Coronal T1 C+ FS MR reveals an enhancing mass with components in cerebellopontine angle cistern ➡, jugular foramen ➡, and hypoglossal canal ➡. The lesion began in the petrooccipital fissure (not shown), invading inferolaterally to these more lateral structures.

Neurofibroma, Carotid Space

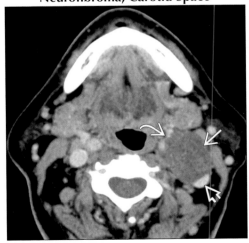

Anaplastic Carcinoma, Thyroid

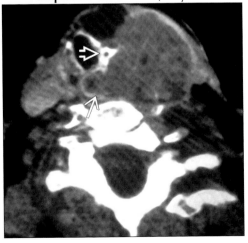

(Left) Axial CECT shows a well-circumscribed, low-density, soft tissue mass ➡ in the right carotid space. The right internal jugular vein is displaced posterolaterally ➡ and the carotid vessels anteromedially ➡. (Right) Axial CECT reveals a large, left thyroid lobe mass that invades the tracheoesophageal groove and cervical esophagus ➡. This anaplastic thyroid carcinoma causes cricoid cartilage sclerosis ➡ as it begins to invade the larynx.

VOCAL CORD PARALYSIS (RIGHT)

DIFFERENTIAL DIAGNOSIS

Common
- SCCa, Nodes
- Paraganglioma, Glomus Jugulare
- Nasopharyngeal Carcinoma
- Cerebral Ischemia-Infarction, Acute

Less Common
- Cavernous Malformation, Hemorrhagic
- Paraganglioma, Carotid Body
- Schwannoma, Jugular Foramen
- Dissection, Carotid Artery, Neck
- Paraganglioma, Glomus Vagale
- Schwannoma, Carotid Space
- Metastasis, Skull Base
- Differentiated Carcinoma, Thyroid
- Meningioma, Skull Base
- Esophageal Carcinoma, Cervical

Rare but Important
- Multiple Sclerosis, Brainstem
- Chondrosarcoma, Skull Base
- Neurofibroma, Carotid Space
- Anaplastic Carcinoma, Thyroid

ESSENTIAL INFORMATION

Key Differential Diagnosis Issues
- Right vagus nerve (CN10) extends from brainstem nuclei to level of clavicle
  - CN10 recurs around right subclavian artery
  - Thoracic diagnoses NOT part of differential diagnosis
- Right vocal cord paralysis (VCP) caused by diseases from medulla to clavicle
  - If CN10 is affected below level of palate, VCP alone is found without other clinical symptoms
  - If CN10 is affected above level of palate, VCP occurs with other symptoms
    - Other cranial nerve dysfunction: CN9, CN11 ± CN12
    - Ipsilateral soft palate and pharyngeal constrictor malfunction (pharyngeal plexus injury)
- Best imaging modality to evaluate CN10
  - CECT if unsure of location of lesion based on physical examination
  - Posterior fossa, skull base, suprahyoid neck contrast-enhanced MR best if lesion confidently localized above level of palate

Helpful Clues for Common Diagnoses
- **SCCa, Nodes**
  - CT/MR: Internal jugular chain extranodal tumor extends into carotid space
- **Paraganglioma, Glomus Jugulare**
  - Tumor spreads superolaterally through middle ear floor to enter middle ear cavity
  - CT: Permeative and destructive bony changes
  - MR: Enhancing tumor with flow voids
- **Nasopharyngeal Carcinoma**
  - Nasopharyngeal mucosal space tumor invades into posterolateral carotid space
- **Cerebral Ischemia-Infarction, Acute**
  - MR: DWI shows restricted diffusion in lateral medulla and inferior cerebellar hemisphere

Helpful Clues for Less Common Diagnoses
- **Cavernous Malformation, Hemorrhagic**
  - CT: Calcified lesion with high-density focal hemorrhage
  - MR: GRE shows blooming lesion in medulla
    - Multiple other lesions possible
- **Paraganglioma, Carotid Body**
  - CT: Avidly enhancing tumor in carotid bifurcation
  - MR: Enhancing tumor with flow voids splays ICA from ECA at bifurcation
- **Schwannoma, Jugular Foramen**
  - CT: Sharply marginated tumor enlarges jugular foramen
  - MR: Enhancing fusiform or ovoid lesion spreads superomedially toward medulla
    - Intramural cysts present if large
- **Dissection, Carotid Artery, Neck**
  - MR: T1 with fat saturation shows intramural hematoma (hyperintense crescent adjacent to ICA lumen)
  - MRA: Luminal narrowing; string sign
- **Paraganglioma, Glomus Vagale**
  - MR: Enhancing tumor in carotid space 1-2 cm below skull base with flow voids
- **Schwannoma, Carotid Space**
  - MR: Enhancing fusiform mass with intramural cysts possible
- **Metastasis, Skull Base**
  - CT: Destructive bone changes common
  - MR: Enhancing skull base lesion in vicinity of jugular foramen
- **Differentiated Carcinoma, Thyroid**

VOCAL CORD PARALYSIS (RIGHT)

- ○ CT: Enhancing thyroid mass with bizarre cystic nodular enhancing nodes
- ○ MR: Enhancing thyroid mass invades tracheoesophageal groove
- **Meningioma, Skull Base**
  - ○ CT: Jugular foramen (JF) lesion causes permeative-sclerotic or hyperostotic bone changes
  - ○ MR: Enhancing JF mass with dural tails, no flow voids; centrifugal spread pattern
- **Esophageal Carcinoma, Cervical**
  - ○ CT: Cervical esophageal mass or paratracheal nodes invade tracheoesophageal groove

Helpful Clues for Rare Diagnoses

- **Multiple Sclerosis, Brainstem**
  - ○ MR: High signal lesions in white matter of suprasellar brain
    - ▪ Medullary lesions not always visible
- **Chondrosarcoma, Skull Base**
  - ○ CT: Invasive skull base mass centered in petrooccipital fissure
    - ▪ 50% calcified matrix
  - ○ MR: Low T1, high T2 signal; enhances
- **Neurofibroma, Carotid Space**
  - ○ CT: Low-density ovoid or fusiform poorly enhancing mass in carotid space
- **Anaplastic Carcinoma, Thyroid**
  - ○ CT/MR: Large, invasive, enhancing thyroid mass in elderly patient
    - ▪ May have history of multinodular goiter

Alternative Differential Approaches

- Another approach to organizing causes of right vocal cord paralysis is to group lesions by ANATOMIC SEGMENT of RIGHT CN10
- Intramedullary, skull base, carotid space, & tracheoesophageal groove causes
- Intramedullary causes
  - ○ Cerebral ischemia-infarction, acute
  - ○ Cavernous malformation, hemorrhagic
  - ○ Multiple sclerosis, brainstem
- Skull base/jugular foramen causes
  - ○ Paraganglioma, glomus jugulare
  - ○ Schwannoma, jugular foramen
  - ○ Metastasis, skull base
  - ○ Meningioma, skull base
  - ○ Chondrosarcoma, skull base
- Carotid space causes
  - ○ SCCa, nodes
  - ○ Paraganglioma, glomus vagale
  - ○ Nasopharyngeal carcinoma
  - ○ Paraganglioma, carotid body
  - ○ Dissection, carotid artery, neck
  - ○ Schwannoma, carotid space
  - ○ Neurofibroma, carotid space
- Visceral space/tracheoesophageal groove
  - ○ Differentiated carcinoma, thyroid
  - ○ Esophageal carcinoma, cervical
  - ○ Anaplastic carcinoma, thyroid

SCCa, Nodes

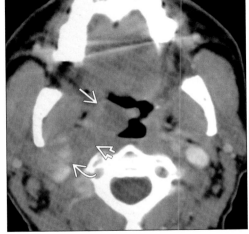

Axial CECT shows a right tonsillar SCCa ➡ with adjacent lateral retropharyngeal nodes ➡. The loss of soft tissue planes in the oropharyngeal carotid space indicates that an extranodal tumor is present ➡.

Paraganglioma, Glomus Jugulare

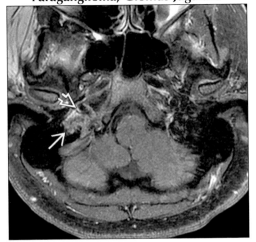

Coronal T1 C+ FS MR reveals an enhancing paraganglioma ➡ in the right jugular foramen, compressing the jugular bulb and abutting the horizontal petrous internal carotid artery ➡.

VOCAL CORD PARALYSIS (RIGHT)

(Left) Axial T1 C+ FS MR shows a large nasopharyngeal mucosal space mass that invades the right prevertebral muscles ➡ and carotid space ➡. CN9-11 were all affected at presentation. *(Right)* Axial FLAIR MR shows a lateral, medullary, subacute ischemic area secondary to vertebral artery dissection. The high signal area is confined to the lateral medulla ➡ without inferior cerebellar hemisphere involvement. Focal PICA embolus was suspected.

Nasopharyngeal Carcinoma

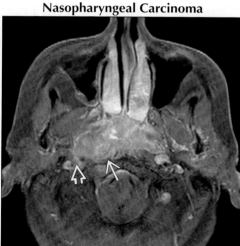

Cerebral Ischemia-Infarction, Acute

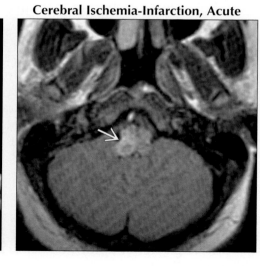

(Left) Sagittal T1 C+ MR shows a large posterior fossa hemorrhagic cavernous malformation with multiple blood-filled "bubbles" within the 4th ventricle and vermis. *(Right)* Axial CECT demonstrates clear definition of the avidly enhancing carotid body paraganglioma ➡ sitting in the notch between the external carotid artery ➡ and the internal carotid artery ➡. Vagal neuropathy is less common with this tumor than with glomus vagale paraganglioma.

Cavernous Malformation, Hemorrhagic

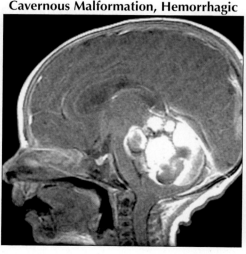

Paraganglioma, Carotid Body

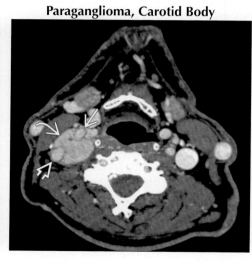

(Left) Axial T1 C+ MR shows a large enhancing mass in the right basal cistern ➡. This schwannoma can be followed inferolaterally into the jugular foramen ➡. *(Right)* Axial T1WI FS MR shows a tiny flow void ➡ in the right internal carotid artery with peripheral crescentic high signal from the intramural hemorrhage associated with this dissection. The opposite left internal carotid artery reveals normal size of flow void ➡.

Schwannoma, Jugular Foramen

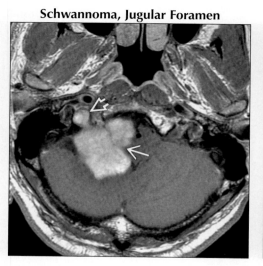

Dissection, Carotid Artery, Neck

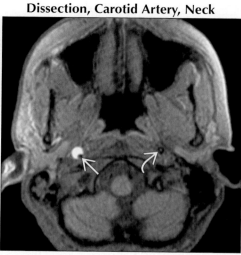

3

VOCAL CORD PARALYSIS (RIGHT)

Paraganglioma, Glomus Vagale
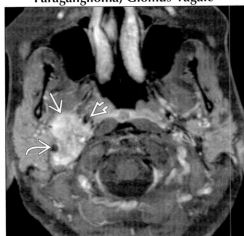

Schwannoma, Carotid Space
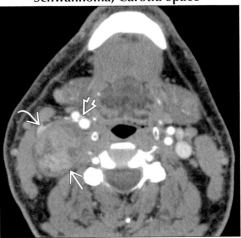

(Left) Axial T1 C+ FS MR reveals an enhancing nasopharyngeal carotid space mass ➡ on the right that elevates the internal carotid artery ➡ and displaces the styloid process laterally ➡. (Right) Axial CECT demonstrates an ovoid inhomogeneously enhancing right carotid space vagal schwannoma ➡. Notice the carotid arteries are displaced anteromedially ➡, although the internal jugular vein is flattened anterolaterally ➡.

Metastasis, Skull Base
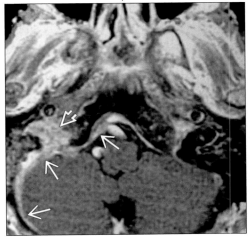

Differentiated Carcinoma, Thyroid
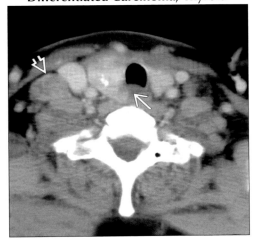

(Left) Axial T1 C+ MR reveals dural metastases in the posterior fossa ➡ with significant invasion of the right jugular foramen ➡. Rapid onset of 9-11 cranial neuropathy was the indication for this examination. (Right) Axial CECT demonstrates invasion of the right tracheoesophageal groove ➡ by this differentiated thyroid carcinoma. Also notice the low internal jugular malignant lymph node ➡ just lateral to the internal jugular vein.

Meningioma, Skull Base
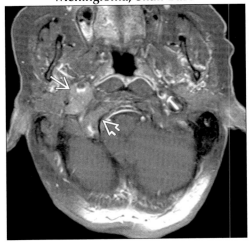

Esophageal Carcinoma, Cervical
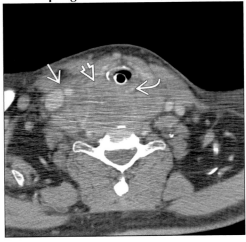

(Left) Axial T1 C+ FS MR shows extensive skull base meningioma that involves the right occipital bone ➡ and extends through the jugular foramen into the nasopharyngeal carotid space ➡. (Right) Axial CECT shows a bulky heterogeneous soft tissue mass that invades the right carotid space ➡ and tracheoesophageal groove ➡. Note the back of the trachea is destroyed ➡ by this aggressive esophageal malignancy.

DIFFERENTIAL DIAGNOSIS

Common
- Croup
- Foreign Body, Esophagus
- Exudative Tracheitis
- Subglottic Hemangioma

Less Common
- Innominate Artery Compression Syndrome
- Tracheal Stenosis, Congenital
- Tracheal Stenosis, Iatrogenic

Rare but Important
- Epiglottitis, Child
- Right Arch with Aberrant Left SCA
- Foreign Body, Trachea

ESSENTIAL INFORMATION

Key Differential Diagnosis Issues
- Stridor: Variably pitched respiratory sound caused by tissue vibration through area of respiratory tract of decreased caliber

Helpful Clues for Common Diagnoses
- **Croup**
  - Key facts
    - Viral etiology; barky cough
    - Most common age: 6 months-3 years; peak at 1 year
  - Imaging
    - AP plain film: Symmetric subglottic tracheal narrowing produces loss of normal "shouldering" of subglottic trachea; results in "steeple" sign
    - Lateral plain film: Hypopharyngeal distension & ill-defined narrow subglottic airway
    - Radiographs obtained to exclude other causes of stridor: Exudative tracheitis, epiglottitis, aspirated foreign body (FB), or subglottic hemangioma
- **Foreign Body, Esophagus**
  - Key facts
    - Coins are most common radiopaque FB in esophagus
    - If not passed, causes edema anterior to esophagus & around trachea; results in inspiratory stridor
    - Most common site upper thoracic esophagus followed by level of arch/carina & distal esophagus

- Button batteries have 2-layered margin on imaging; require emergent removal to prevent caustic esophageal injury
  - Imaging
    - If radiodense, see FB posterior to trachea
    - ± Thickening of soft tissue between esophagus & trachea
    - ± Anterior displacement of trachea
    - ± Tracheal narrowing at level of FB
- **Exudative Tracheitis**
  - Key facts
    - Purulent infection → intratracheal exudates may slough & occlude airway
    - Usually older than patients with croup
  - Imaging
    - Symmetric (or asymmetric) subglottic narrowing
    - ± Linear, soft tissue densities (membranes) within trachea ± tracheal wall irregularities (plaques)
- **Subglottic Hemangioma**
  - Key facts
    - Inspiratory stridor, airway obstruction, hoarseness or abnormal cry; usually younger than 6 months
    - Associated with cutaneous hemangiomas in up to 50% of patients
    - 7% of patients with PHACES syndrome have subglottic hemangioma
  - Imaging
    - Asymmetric subglottic tracheal narrowing on radiographs
    - Enhancing soft tissue mass on CT or MR

Helpful Clues for Less Common Diagnoses
- **Innominate Artery Compression Syndrome**
  - Key facts
    - Infantile trachea lacks rigidity
    - Symptoms: Stridor, apnea, dyspnea; usually resolve as child grows
    - Increased incidence with esophageal atresia; dilated esophageal pouch deviates trachea forward, innominate artery compresses anterior trachea
  - Imaging
    - Anterior tracheal narrowing at crossing innominate artery; below thoracic inlet
- **Tracheal Stenosis, Congenital**
  - Key facts

- Secondary to complete cartilaginous rings ± associated anomalies such as vascular ring
  - Imaging
    - Small caliber round (rather than horseshoe-shaped) trachea on cross sectional imaging
    - Inverted T-shaped carina on conventional radiograph or coronal reformatted CT images
    - Focal or diffuse stenosis possible
- **Tracheal Stenosis, Iatrogenic**
  - Key facts: History of prior endotracheal tube (ET) intubation, tracheostomy, or other injury
  - Imaging: Subglottic tracheal narrowing at level of prior ET tube or tracheostomy tube
    - Smooth focal narrowing (ET tube) or irregular longer narrowing (tracheostomy secondary to granulation tissue ± structural damage to tracheal rings)

Helpful Clues for Rare Diagnoses
- **Epiglottitis, Child**
  - Key facts
    - Life-threatening infections & edema of epiglottis & supraglottic structures
    - Abrupt onset of stridor, dysphagia, high fever, sore throat, dysphonia, hoarseness, and drooling
    - Symptoms of airway obstruction markedly increase when recumbent; do lateral radiograph in upright position

- Incidence markedly decreased since *H. influenzae* vaccination became universal
  - Imaging
    - Enlargement of epiglottis & thickening of aryepiglottic folds on lateral X-ray
- **Right Arch with Aberrant Left SCA**
  - Key facts: 0.1% of general population but usually asymptomatic
    - Rarely associated with tightly constricting left ligamentum arteriosum; presents with congenital stridor
    - Posterior esophageal indentation by aberrant subclavian artery (SCA) may cause dysphagia or feeding difficulties in infants
  - Imaging
    - Esophagram: Posterior esophageal indentation by aberrant SCA
    - CT/MR: Aberrant SCA coursing posterior to esophagus
- **Foreign Body, Trachea**
  - Key facts
    - Bronchial FB much more common than tracheal FB
    - Most airway FB not radiopaque; majority peanuts & carrots
    - Incident usually not witnessed
  - Imaging
    - If radiodense, identify FB in airway
    - When non-radiopaque FB aspiration, look for secondary signs: Hyperinflation, air-trapping, regional oligemia, atelectasis, pneumomediastinum, pneumothorax

Croup

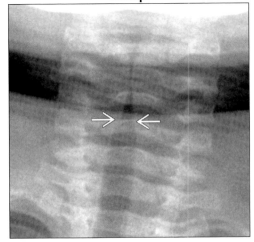

Anteroposterior radiograph shows loss of normal shouldering of the subglottic airway, producing a "steeple" sign .

Croup

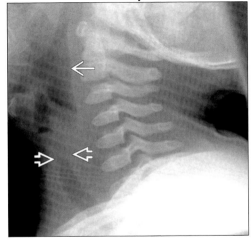

Lateral radiograph shows mild hypopharyngeal distention  *and a narrow subglottic airway* ➡.

INSPIRATORY STRIDOR IN CHILD

(Left) *Lateral radiograph shows a radiopaque coin in the esophagus ➡, dilated proximal esophagus ➡, and circumferential tracheal narrowing ➡ at the level of the coin.* **(Right)** *Lateral radiograph shows mild irregularity of the subglottic trachea ➡ with an intraluminal linear density related to a plaque ➡ in an older child with exudative tracheitis.*

Foreign Body, Esophagus

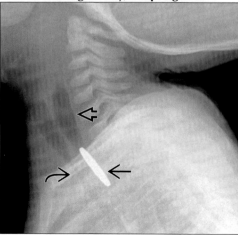

Exudative Tracheitis

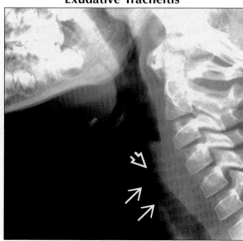

(Left) *Axial CECT demonstrates a small intensely enhancing subglottic mass ➡. On endoscopy a submucosal airway hemangioma was visible.* **(Right)** *Sagittal CECT shows the posterior enhancing mass ➡ resulting in focal tracheal narrowing ➡. Not surprisingly, the infant presented with stridor.*

Subglottic Hemangioma

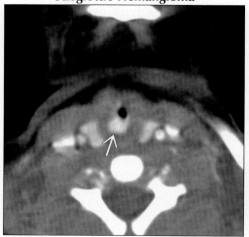

Subglottic Hemangioma

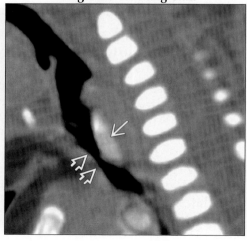

(Left) *Axial CECT reveals narrowing of the trachea ➡ at the level of the crossing innominate artery ➡. A pH probe is also seen in the upper thoracic esophagus ➡.* **(Right)** *Lateral esophagram shows anterior tracheal compression ➡ at the level of crossing innominate artery and an incidental small esophageal stricture ➡ in a patient with prior esophageal atresia repair.*

Innominate Artery Compression Syndrome

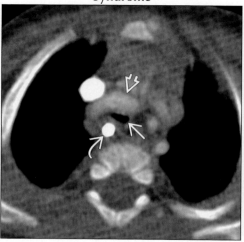

Innominate Artery Compression Syndrome

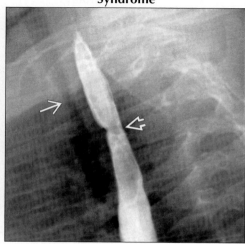

Tracheal Stenosis, Congenital

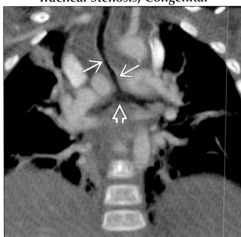

Tracheal Stenosis, Congenital

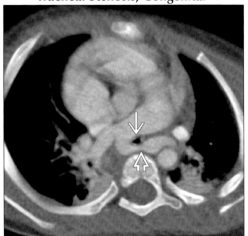

(Left) Coronal CECT shows distal intrathoracic tracheal narrowing ➡ with a nearly 180° angle between mainstem bronchi, resulting in an inverted-T appearance of the carina ⮞. *(Right)* Axial CECT reveals congenitally stenotic trachea ➡ in association with aberrant left pulmonary artery ⮞ arising from the right pulmonary artery and coursing posterior to the trachea.

Tracheal Stenosis, Iatrogenic

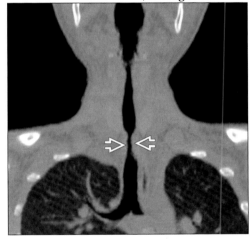

Epiglottitis, Child

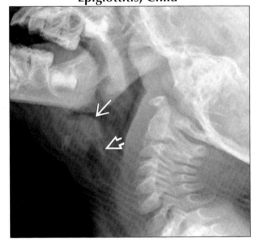

(Left) Coronal bone CT demonstrates an abrupt shelf that causes tracheal narrowing at the level of the thoracic inlet ⮞. This child had a prior history of prolonged endotracheal intubation. *(Right)* Anteroposterior radiograph shows a markedly swollen epiglottis ➡ and thickened aryepiglottic folds ⮞, diagnostic of epiglottitis.

Right Arch with Aberrant Left SCA

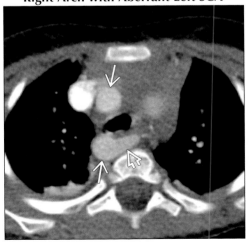

Foreign Body, Trachea

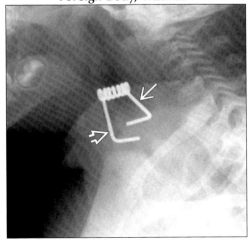

(Left) Axial CECT shows the congenital right arch ➡ associated with aberrant left subclavian artery ⮞ coursing posterior to the trachea. *(Right)* Lateral radiograph reveals a radiopaque spring from a wooden clothes pin in the hypopharynx ➡ and larynx ⮞.

SECTION 4
Lymph Nodes

Generic Imaging Patterns

ENLARGED LYMPH NODES IN NECK

DIFFERENTIAL DIAGNOSIS

Common
- Reactive Lymph Nodes
- SCCa Nodes
- Non-Hodgkin Lymphoma, Lymph Nodes
- Thyroid Carcinoma, Nodal
- Reactive Lymph Nodes, HIV Disease
- Suppurative Lymph Nodes
- Mononucleosis (EBV), Reactive Nodes
- Leukemia, Nodal Disease

Less Common
- Nasopharyngeal Carcinoma, Nodal Metastases
- Tuberculosis, Lymph Nodes
- Hodgkin Lymphoma, Lymph Nodes
- Sarcoidosis, Lymph Nodes
- Reactive Nodes, Cat Scratch Disease

Rare but Important
- Giant Lymph Node Hyperplasia (Castleman)
- Sinus Histiocytosis (Rosai-Dorfman)
- Kimura Disease
- Histiocytic Necrotizing Lymphadenitis (Kikuchi)

ESSENTIAL INFORMATION

Key Differential Diagnosis Issues
- Remember: Everyone has scattered small cervical nodes; 1st determine if too many nodes or if any node(s) are too big
- Key is to identify neck mass as node
  - Then describe characteristics: Homogeneous, cystic/necrotic, well circumscribed, extranodal spread
- Then interpret given clinical setting: Adult or child, febrile, HIV, known primary tumor
- Imaging appearance often nonspecific
  - Fine-needle aspiration if uncertainty persists

Helpful Clues for Common Diagnoses
- **Reactive Lymph Nodes**
  - Key facts: Normal nodes in upper neck
    - May enhance without neck infection
  - CECT/MR: Unilateral or bilateral, small to intermediate size, nonnecrotic C+ nodes
- **SCCa Nodes**
  - Key facts: Location of primary tumor determines nodal location

- Nodes in level I and II presumed metastatic if > 1.5 cm, all other levels presumed metastatic if > 1.0 cm
- Even though size is poor predictor of metastatic disease, it is routinely used to stage tumors
- Necrotic nodes always metastatic
- Perinodal stranding implies extracapsular extension
  - CECT/MR: Enlarged node at expected location for primary tumor; ± central necrosis
- **Non-Hodgkin Lymphoma, Lymph Nodes**
  - Key facts: 2 nodal patterns
    - 1 or 2 large nonnecrotic nodes
    - Multiple small homogeneous nodes involving different nodal neck groups
  - CECT/MR: Homogeneous nodes following 1 of patterns described
    - Occasionally node(s) may be centrally lucent
- **Thyroid Carcinoma, Nodal**
  - Key facts: Nodal metastases from papillary or follicular carcinomas
  - CECT: Solid enhancing nodules, cystic changes ± calcification in nodes
  - MR: If high T1 or T2 nodal signal, think of thyroid carcinoma
- **Reactive Lymph Nodes, HIV Disease**
  - Key facts: HIV patient + neck nodes creates concern for non-Hodgkin lymphoma (NHL)
  - CECT: Tonsillar diffuse hyperplasia with multiple intermediate-sized reactive-appearing nodes
    - Benign parotid lymphoepithelial lesions
- **Suppurative Lymph Nodes**
  - Key facts: Ill patient; tender neck masses
    - Suppurative node = intranodal abscess
  - CECT: Multiple intermediate-sized nodes with intranodal cystic/necrotic changes
- **Mononucleosis (EBV), Reactive Nodes**
  - Key facts: Ill teenagers
    - Epstein-Barr virus (EBV) is pathogen
  - CECT: Swollen edematous tonsils; reactive-appearing nodes
- **Leukemia, Nodal Disease**
  - Key facts: Myelocytic or lymphocytic precursor cells manifested within circulating blood compartment
  - CECT/MR: Similar to lymphoma nodes

ENLARGED LYMPH NODES IN NECK

- Intermediate to large nonnecrotic nodes

Helpful Clues for Less Common Diagnoses

- **Nasopharyngeal Carcinoma, Nodal Metastases**
  - Key facts: Nasopharynx + neck masses
  - CECT/MR: Single or multiple enlarged nodes, ± nodal necrosis
    - Spinal accessory nodes common
- **Tuberculosis, Lymph Nodes**
  - Key facts: Ill patient, often immunocompromised
    - Positive PPD; abnormal chest x-ray
  - CECT: Multiple neck nodes, both solid & cystic-necrotic in same patient
    - ± Soft tissue abscesses possible
- **Hodgkin Lymphoma, Lymph Nodes**
  - Key facts: Neoplasm of B-cell lymphocytes
    - Histopath marker: Reed-Sternberg cells
  - CT/MR: Similar to NHL
    - More likely to show intense nodal capsular enhancement, necrosis
    - Multiple large neck nodes
- **Sarcoidosis, Lymph Nodes**
  - Key facts: Self-limiting granulomatous disease of nodes, GI tract mucosa, parotid gland, lungs, liver, spleen, & skin
    - Unknown etiology
    - In USA, black:white ratio is 10:1
  - CECT: Reactive-appearing lymph nodes in lower cervical neck
    - Parotid inflammation possible
- **Reactive Nodes, Cat Scratch Disease**
  - Key facts: Organism = *Rochalimaea henselae*
    - Child; thorn scratch or cat bite
    - Fever, rash, headache, painful nodes
  - CECT: Large enhancing nodes in neck

Helpful Clues for Rare Diagnoses

- **Giant Lymph Node Hyperplasia (Castleman)**
  - Key facts: 2 types, hyaline-vascular type (90%) & plasma cell type
    - Unicentric or multicentric (rare)
  - CECT: Single large homogeneously C+ nodal mass most common
- **Sinus Histiocytosis (Rosai-Dorfman)**
  - Key facts: Lymphoproliferative disorder; unknown etiology
    - Unifocal: Solitary enhancing cervical or systemic node; benign clinical course
    - Multifocal: Multiple nodal masses; less common; aggressive clinical course
  - CECT: Large enhancing cervical node(s)
    - Dural-based enhancing masses
- **Kimura Disease**
  - Key facts: Presents with painless unilateral cervical lymphadenopathy
    - M:F = 6:1
  - CECT: Large inhomogeneously C+ nodes
    - Parotid infiltration; skin nodules
- **Histiocytic Necrotizing Lymphadenitis (Kikuchi)**
  - Key facts: Nodal inflammation; < 30 year old Japanese females
    - Resolves spontaneously in weeks
    - Presents with large, painful neck nodes
  - CECT: Multiple nonnecrotic nodal clusters

Reactive Lymph Nodes

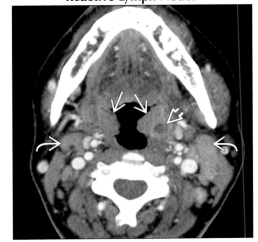

Axial CECT shows bilateral tonsillar inflammation ➡ with a small focus of intratonsillar abscess ➡ in a patient with pharyngitis. Bilateral reactive jugulodigastric nodes ➡ are present.

Reactive Lymph Nodes

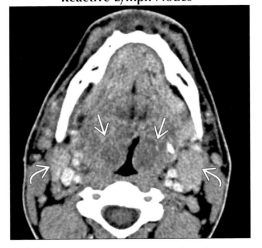

Axial CECT depicts bilateral high internal jugular reactive adenopathy ➡ in a patient with severe pharyngitis and bilateral inflamed edematous palatine tonsils ➡.

ENLARGED LYMPH NODES IN NECK

(Left) Axial CECT shows a large base of tongue tumor ➡ invading the floor of the mouth and sublingual space ➡. Note the bilateral metastatic enlarged necrotic level II nodes ➡. *(Right)* Axial CECT reveals a large SCCa filling the right vallecula ➡. A submandibular node (level IB) ➡ is poorly defined, suggesting extracapsular extension. Note the 2 jugulodigastric (level IIA) nodes ➡; 1 has central lucency, which implies necrosis.

SCCa Nodes

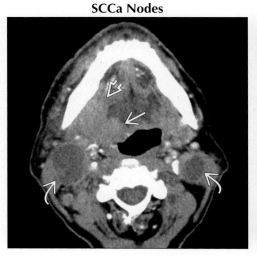

SCCa Nodes

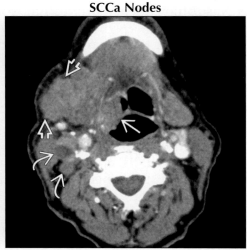

(Left) Axial CECT demonstrates large well-circumscribed homogeneous and nonnecrotic submandibular nodes ➡ in a patient with non-Hodgkin lymphoma. Both nodes are anterior to the submandibular glands ➡. *(Right)* Axial CECT depicts multiple bilateral small homogeneous nodes in virtually every nodal chain, including the submandibular ➡, internal jugular ➡, and spinal accessory chain ➡.

Non-Hodgkin Lymphoma, Lymph Nodes

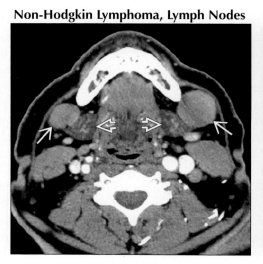

Non-Hodgkin Lymphoma, Lymph Nodes

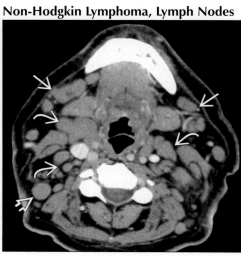

(Left) Axial CECT shows a pathologic right jugulodigastric node ➡ with unusual mixed cystic and solid enhancing ➡ components. Differentiated thyroid carcinoma CECT appearance may be solid enhancing, cystic, &/or calcified. *(Right)* Axial T1WI MR at the level of the thyroid bed shows a bizarre high signal internal jugular nodal mass ➡ adjacent to an irregular right thyroid lobe ➡, found to contain differentiated thyroid carcinoma.

Thyroid Carcinoma, Nodal

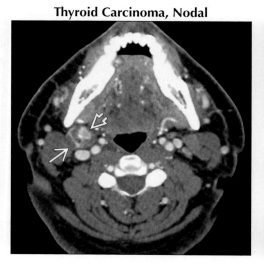

Thyroid Carcinoma, Nodal

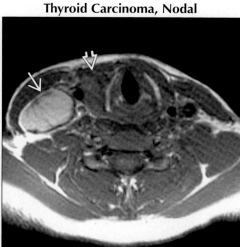

ENLARGED LYMPH NODES IN NECK

Reactive Lymph Nodes, HIV Disease
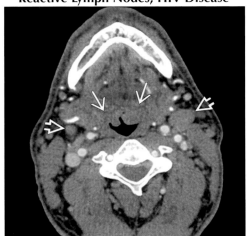

Reactive Lymph Nodes, HIV Disease
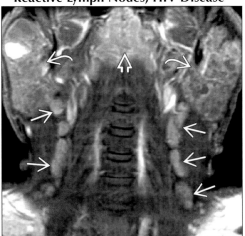

(Left) Axial CECT in a patient with known HIV demonstrates lingual tonsillar hypertrophy ➡ and reactive-appearing lymphadenopathy ➡. Both are common imaging manifestations of HIV. *(Right)* Coronal T1 C+ FS MR in a patient with HIV shows extensive reactive-appearing internal jugular chain nodes ➡ in association with adenoidal hypertrophy ➡ and benign lymphoepithelial lesions ➡ in the large parotid glands.

Suppurative Lymph Nodes
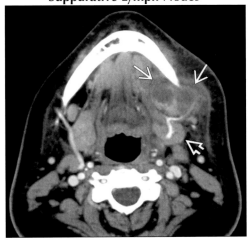

Suppurative Lymph Nodes
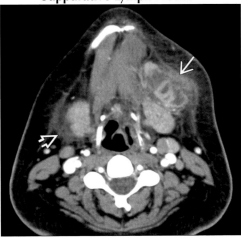

(Left) Axial CECT in a patient with an infected tongue stud shows a suppurative submandibular nodal conglomerate ➡ anterior to the submandibular gland ➡. Extensive cellulitic changes are present in surrounding soft tissues, signaling the nodal mass is inflammatory. *(Right)* Axial CECT in the same patient reveals the inferior portion of the suppurative nodes ➡. Cellulitic changes are seen diffusely. Note edema surrounding the right submandibular gland ➡.

Mononucleosis (EBV), Reactive Nodes
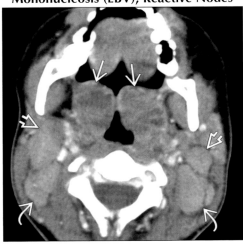

Mononucleosis (EBV), Reactive Nodes
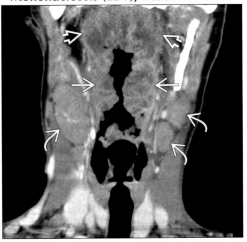

(Left) Axial NECT in a sick teenager shows swollen edematous palatine tonsils ➡ with large nonnecrotic reactive lymph nodes in the internal jugular ➡ and spinal accessory ➡ nodal groups. *(Right)* Coronal NECT in the same patient reveals badly swollen, edematous adenoids ➡ and palatine tonsils ➡. The internal jugular reactive nodes ➡ are very large in the coronal plane.

4

(Left) Axial CECT in a 15 month old infant with acute myelogenous leukemia shows nonnecrotic nodes ➡ and right parotid enlargement ⮆ from leukemic infiltration. *(Right)* Axial CECT in the same patient reveals multiple large nonnecrotic lymph nodes in the internal jugular ➡ and spinal accessory ⮆ chains. Differentiating leukemic and lymphomatous nodes is not possible with imaging.

Leukemia, Nodal Disease

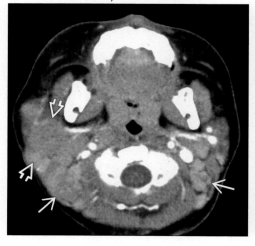

Leukemia, Nodal Disease

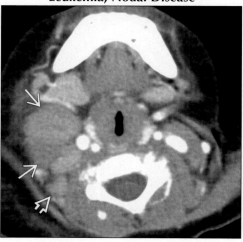

(Left) Axial CECT in a patient with a nasopharyngeal carcinoma and palpable neck masses shows bilateral inhomogeneously enhancing lymph node metastases ➡ from 1-4 centimeters in size. *(Right)* Axial CECT shows 2 metastatic lymph nodes from a primary nasopharyngeal carcinoma. The large, more anterior node ➡ is level IIB, while the more posterior node ⮆ is level VA. Although these nodes are nonnecrotic, this is not usually the case.

Nasopharyngeal Carcinoma, Nodal Metastases

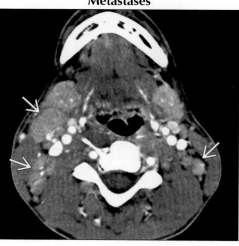

Nasopharyngeal Carcinoma, Nodal Metastases

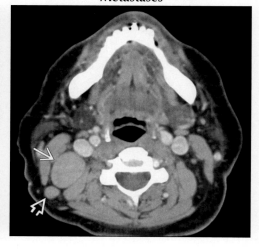

(Left) Axial CECT reveals a large inhomogeneously enhancing right jugulodigastric lymph node ➡ with adjacent inflammatory changes in the sternocleidomastoid muscle ⮆ & posterior submandibular space ➡. *(Right)* Axial CECT shows unilateral bulky Hodgkin lymphoma nodes ➡ in the lower cervical neck. The nodes are solid and homogeneously enhancing with the exception of 1 superficial necrotic node ➡. Appearance mimics NHL.

Tuberculosis, Lymph Nodes

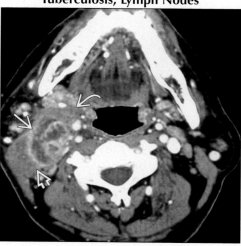

Hodgkin Lymphoma, Lymph Nodes

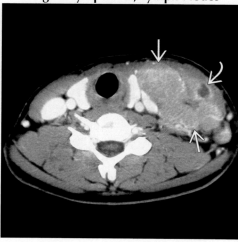

ENLARGED LYMPH NODES IN NECK

Sarcoidosis, Lymph Nodes

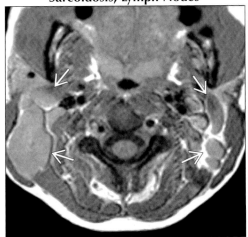

Reactive Nodes, Cat Scratch Disease

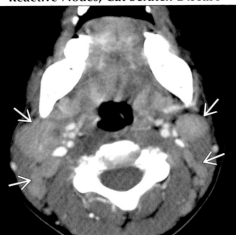

(Left) Axial T1WI MR reveals diffuse bilateral nodal sarcoidosis ➡. Mediastinal nodes & increased angiotensin converting enzyme in CSF suggest that nodes are from sarcoidosis. *(Right)* Axial CECT in a 3 year old with painful neck nodes, 2 weeks after a cat bite on tongue, shows large homogeneously enhancing lymph nodes ➡ in internal jugular & spinal accessory chains. These reactive nodes cannot be differentiated from reactive nodes from other infectious causes.

Giant Lymph Node Hyperplasia (Castleman)

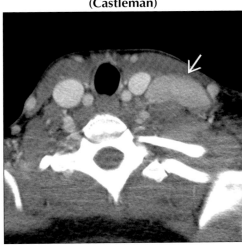

Sinus Histiocytosis (Rosai-Dorfman)

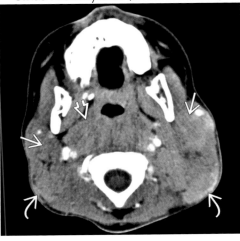

(Left) Axial CECT shows a large homogeneously and avidly enhancing left low internal jugular lymph node ➡ found to be giant lymph node hyperplasia at surgery. *(Right)* Axial CECT reveals massive bilateral lymphadenopathy involving the internal jugular ➡, spinal accessory ➡, and retropharyngeal ➡ nodal groups in this adolescent with painless neck masses.

Kimura Disease

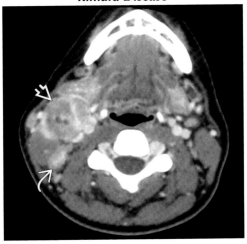

Histiocytic Necrotizing Lymphadenitis (Kikuchi)

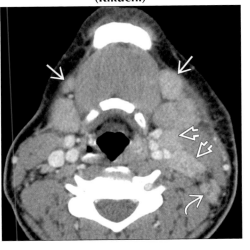

(Left) Axial CECT in a young non-Asian woman shows multiple enhancing ipsilateral nodes in the posterior cervical space ➡ & along the right internal jugular chain ➡. Parotid infiltration & skin nodules were present, though not seen on this image. *(Right)* Axial CECT in a 15 year old shows multiple nonnecrotic moderately enhancing nodes in the submandibular ➡, internal jugular ➡, & spinal accessory ➡ groups. Reactive nodes or NHL could look identical.

ENHANCING LYMPH NODES IN NECK

DIFFERENTIAL DIAGNOSIS

Common
- Reactive Lymph Nodes
- Suppurative Lymph Nodes
- SCCa, Nodes
- Differentiated Thyroid Carcinoma, Nodal
- Non-Hodgkin Lymphoma, Lymph Nodes
- Hodgkin Lymphoma, Lymph Nodes

Less Common
- Enhancing Lymph Node Mimics
- Metastases, Systemic, Nodal
- Tuberculosis, Lymph Nodes

Rare but Important
- Angiolymphoid Hyperplasia with Eosinophilia (Kimura)
- Giant Lymph Node Hyperplasia (Castleman)

ESSENTIAL INFORMATION

Key Differential Diagnosis Issues
- 1st step: Be sure mass is node & not nodal mimic
  - Paraganglioma, schwannoma, carotid artery pseudoaneurysm, & venous asymmetry could be misinterpreted as lymphadenopathy
    - Mimics usually solitary in carotid space (CS) behind or between artery & vein
    - Trace course of carotid artery & jugular vein to exclude vascular mimic (i.e., aneurysm, large asymmetric jugular vein, or diverticulum)
- Knowledge of clinical setting essential for differential of enhancing nodes
  - Even normal nodes may enhance
  - Size of node, presence of necrosis, & setting of infection or neoplasm help direct differential

Helpful Clues for Common Diagnoses
- **Reactive Lymph Nodes**
  - Key facts: Normal nodes, especially in levels I and II, may enhance even when there is no infection
    - When infection or abscess are present, small reactive nodes can enhance without being directly involved
  - Imaging: May be unilateral or bilateral; small or > 2 cm
- **Suppurative Lymph Nodes**
  - Key facts: Infected nodes often associated with neck abscess, especially in children
  - Imaging: Enhance homogeneously prior to suppuration, then become centrally low density
- **SCCa, Nodes**
  - Key facts: Size & presence of central necrosis more important criterion than enhancement when staging nodal metastases in H&N cancer
  - Imaging: > 1.5 cm in levels I and II; > 1.0 cm in all other levels in typical location for primary tumor
    - Enhancement in metastatic node after chemo- or radiation therapy does not mean persistent disease
    - Increase in size is better determinant of persistent disease
- **Differentiated Thyroid Carcinoma, Nodal**
  - Key facts: Nodal metastases from papillary or follicular carcinomas can enhance robustly
  - Imaging: Common nodal chains involved include visceral space, supraclavicular, levels IV and V
    - No standardized size criteria to determine nodal mets
    - Look for round T2-hyperintense enhancing nodes, often in small clusters
    - Primary lesion in thyroid gland may be small on CT or MR, or even microscopic
- **Non-Hodgkin Lymphoma, Lymph Nodes**
  - Key facts: More commonly low density without significant enhancement, but NHL should still be in differential of homogeneously enhancing cervical node
  - Imaging: Single or multiple cervical nodes, may be bilateral
    - When multiple, nodes often variable in appearance
    - Some enhance & others may be low density, almost cystic in appearance
- **Hodgkin Lymphoma, Lymph Nodes**
  - Key facts: Similar to NHL, enhancement generally exception, not most common appearance
  - Imaging: Usually dominant, enlarged well-circumscribed cervical node

Helpful Clues for Less Common Diagnoses
- **Enhancing Lymph Node Mimics**

- o Key facts: Multiple non-nodal lesions may mimic nodes in neck
  - List includes paraganglioma, schwannoma, venous asymmetry & variants, carotid artery pseudoaneurysms
  - o Imaging
    - Carotid body tumor: Splay ECA & ICA at bifurcation; + flow voids (MR)
    - Glomus vagale paraganglioma: Nasopharyngeal CS above area of internal jugular nodes; + flow voids (MR)
    - CS schwannoma: Displaces ICA anteriorly or medially; intramural cysts
    - Carotid artery pseudoaneurysm: Enhancing lumen ± subintimal clot, contiguous with carotid artery
    - Venous asymmetry: Tubular, contiguous with known veins
- **Metastases, Systemic, Nodal**
  - o Key facts: Metastases from melanoma, breast, lung, esophagus most common
    - Renal & gastrointestinal cancer nodal disease can also enhance
  - o Imaging: Low cervical nodes, including level V, usually involved
- **Tuberculosis, Lymph Nodes**
  - o Key facts: Clinically ill patient, possibly immunocompromised, with positive PPD & abnormal chest x-ray
    - Nontuberculous mycobacterial infection may occur in clinically well patient presenting with neck mass
  - o Imaging: Multiple nodes varying in size & enhancement pattern

- Both solid and centrally lucent nodes possible in same patient

Helpful Clues for Rare Diagnoses
- **Angiolymphoid Hyperplasia with Eosinophilia (Kimura)**
  - o Key facts: Chronic inflammatory disorder of H&N; primarily in young Asian males
    - Clinical triad of unilateral cervical adenopathy, systemic eosinophilia, elevated serum IgE
    - Subcutaneous nodules and parotid or submandibular gland masses usually present in addition to cervical adenopathy
  - o Imaging: Subcutaneous nodules, submandibular or parotid gland mass, & cervical adenopathy all enhance avidly
- **Giant Lymph Node Hyperplasia (Castleman)**
  - o Key facts: Lymphoproliferative disorder of unknown etiology characterized by nodal enlargement
  - o Unifocal: Presents as solitary enhancing cervical or systemic node; benign clinical course
  - o Multicentric: Multiple or diffuse nodal masses; aggressive clinical course, often fatal
    - Associated with AIDS
  - o Imaging: Well-circumscribed, enlarged, enhancing cervical node

Reactive Lymph Nodes

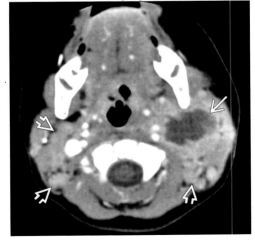

Axial CECT shows enhancing reactive nodes ⊟ associated with a large heterogeneous mass in the left neck ⊟, representing a matted group of suppurative left jugular chain lymph nodes.

Suppurative Lymph Nodes

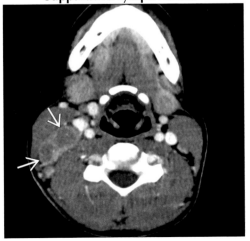

Axial CECT reveals multiple enlarged right internal jugular chain lymph nodes ⊟. Notice that the node centers are slightly lower density. This is the classic CECT appearance of early suppurative changes.

(Left) Axial CECT demonstrates an enhancing, centrally necrotic left level III node ➡ in a patient with recurrent SCCa. Note the nonenhancing edematous changes ➡ in the larynx from prior radiation. (Right) Axial CECT shows enhancing bilateral level III nodes ➡ from differentiated thyroid carcinoma. The posterior right level III node ➡ appears cystic. Heterogeneous solid and cystic nodes are common in this tumor.

SCCa, Nodes

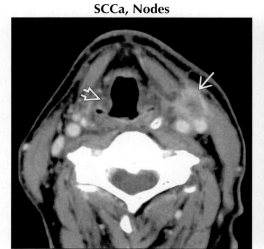

Differentiated Thyroid Carcinoma, Nodal

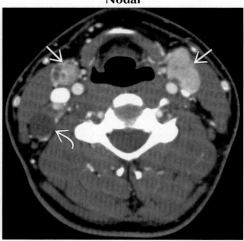

(Left) Axial T1 C+ MR shows multiple bilateral variable-sized enhancing nodes ➡ in levels IV and V, as well as paratracheal (VI) chain ➡. (Right) Axial CECT reveals multiple level IV ➡ and V ➡ heterogeneously enhancing lymph nodes. Hodgkin lymphoma frequently presents as unilateral nodes in contiguous nodal groups.

Non-Hodgkin Lymphoma, Lymph Nodes

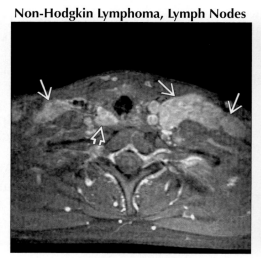

Hodgkin Lymphoma, Lymph Nodes

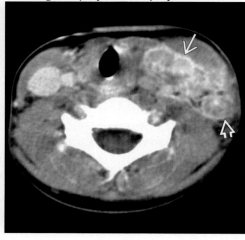

(Left) Axial CECT demonstrates a large right carotid body tumor splaying the internal ➡ and external ➡ carotid arteries. The lymph nodes do not insinuate themselves between the carotid artery branches. (Right) Axial CECT shows a large enhancing left carotid space mass. Medial displacement of internal ➡ and external ➡ carotid arteries and anterior deviation of internal jugular vein ➡ are typical for vagal schwannoma.

Enhancing Lymph Node Mimics

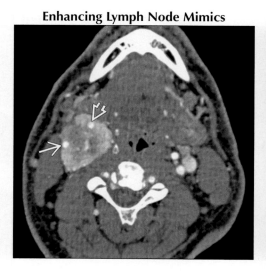

Enhancing Lymph Node Mimics

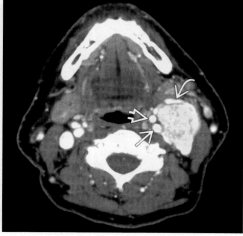

Enhancing Lymph Node Mimics

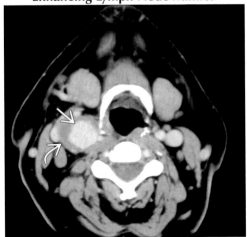

Enhancing Lymph Node Mimics

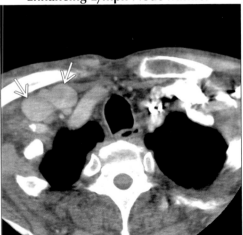

(Left) Axial CECT reveals a carotid artery pseudoaneurysm ➡ with enhancing central lumen and peripheral nonenhancing thrombus ➡. The location and central arterial enhancement help confirm a non-nodal diagnosis. *(Right)* Axial CECT demonstrates a tortuous, ectatic right subclavian vein ➡ that at 1st glance has the appearance of enhancing lymph nodes. However, contiguous images and multiplanar reconstructions confirmed its venous origin.

Metastases, Systemic, Nodal

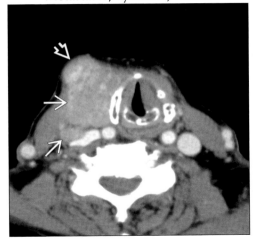

Tuberculosis, Lymph Nodes

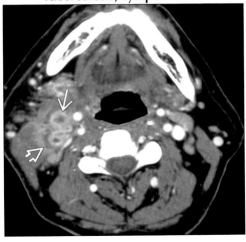

(Left) Axial CECT shows enhancing cervical adenopathy involving both the subcutaneous ➡ and level III ➡ nodes. *(Right)* Axial CECT reveals a complex nodal mass with intense circumferential enhancement ➡ around the central nodal abscesses. Note the extranodal enhancement and edema ➡, findings that suggest an inflammatory rather than neoplastic process.

Angiolymphoid Hyperplasia with Eosinophilia (Kimura)

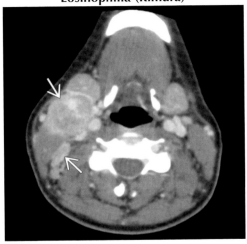

Giant Lymph Node Hyperplasia (Castleman)

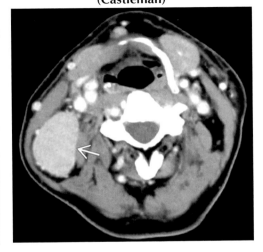

(Left) Axial CECT shows multiple enhancing nodes ➡ in a patient with Kimura disease. Findings are nonspecific, but if patient is a young Asian male with subcutaneous nodules & variable parotid gland density, Kimura disease should be considered. *(Right)* Axial CECT shows a single enlarged homogeneous enhancing node ➡ in unifocal disease. The mass is smooth with no perinodal induration. Biopsy is necessary to confirm diagnosis.

ENLARGED LYMPH NODES IN NECK OF CHILD

DIFFERENTIAL DIAGNOSIS

Common
- Reactive Lymph Nodes
- Suppurative Lymph Nodes
- Hodgkin Lymphoma, Lymph Nodes
- Cat Scratch Disease
- Non-Hodgkin Lymphoma, Lymph Nodes
- Non-TB Mycobacterium, Lymph Nodes

Less Common
- Neuroblastoma, Metastatic
- Lymphoproliferative Disorder, Post-Transplant
- Differentiated Thyroid Carcinoma, Nodal

Rare but Important
- Metastases, Systemic, Nodal
- Langerhans Histiocytosis, Nodal

ESSENTIAL INFORMATION

Helpful Clues for Common Diagnoses
- **Reactive Lymph Nodes**
  - Key facts
    - "Reactive" implies benign
    - Response to infection/inflammation, acute or chronic; any H&N nodal group
  - Imaging
    - Enlarged well-defined oval-shaped nodes with variable contrast enhancement
    - ± Cellulitis: Common with bacterial infection, usually absent in non-TB *Mycobacterium* (NTM)
    - ± Edema in adjacent muscles (myositis)
    - ± Necrosis: Bacterial, NTM, & cat scratch
- **Suppurative Lymph Nodes**
  - Key facts
    - Pus within node = intranodal abscess
    - If untreated, rupture ⇒ soft tissue abscess
  - Imaging
    - If thick enhancing walls + central hypodensity, suspect drainable abscess (phlegmon may have similar appearance)
    - Associated cellulitis: Common in bacterial infection, absent in NTM
    - Associated non-suppurative adenopathy
    - ± Thickening of muscles (myositis)
- **Hodgkin Lymphoma, Lymph Nodes**
  - Key facts
    - B-cell origin; histology shows Reed-Sternberg cells

- Most commonly involves cervical & mediastinal lymph nodes
    - Extranodal disease uncommon
    - Tumors are EBV positive in up to 50%
  - Imaging
    - Cannot distinguish Hodgkin lymphoma (HL) from non-Hodgkin lymphoma (NHL)
    - Round nodal masses with variable contrast enhancement, ± necrotic center
    - Single or multiple nodal chains
    - Calcification uncommon (unless treated)
    - FDG PET (or Ga-67) scans for staging & evaluating response to treatment
- **Cat Scratch Disease**
  - Key facts
    - Scratch or bite may precede development of adenopathy by 1-4 weeks
    - *Bartonella henselae* most common pathogen
  - Imaging
    - Homogeneous or necrotic lymphadenopathy
- **Non-Hodgkin Lymphoma, Lymph Nodes**
  - Key facts
    - Extranodal disease more common in NHL than HL
  - Imaging
    - Cannot distinguish NHL from HL
    - Single dominant node or multiple enlarged nonnecrotic nodes
    - Non-nodal lymphatic disease: Palatine, lingual, or adenoid tonsils
    - Non-nodal extralymphatic: Paranasal sinus, skull base, & thyroid gland
- **Non-TB Mycobacterium, Lymph Nodes**
  - Key facts
    - *M. avium-intracellulare* (MAI), *M. scrofulaceum, M. kansasii*
    - Usually nontender lymphadenopathy
  - Imaging
    - Necrotic lymphadenopathy common
    - Lack of surrounding cellulitis

Helpful Clues for Less Common Diagnoses
- **Neuroblastoma, Metastatic**
  - Key facts
    - Most cervical involvement with neuroblastoma is metastatic
  - Imaging
    - Large lymph nodes, rarely necrotic
    - ± Bilateral skull base metastasis common

- ± Enhancing masses with aggressive bone erosion
- **Lymphoproliferative Disorder, Post-Transplant**
  - Key facts
    - Spectrum: Benign hyperplasia to lymphoma
    - Most common in patients who are EBV seronegative prior to transplant
    - More common after heart or lung than after kidney transplant
    - Children > > > > adults
    - Abdomen, chest, allograft, H&N, CNS
  - Imaging
    - Cervical lymphadenopathy
    - Adenotonsillar hypertrophy; may lead to upper airway obstruction
    - ± Sinusitis, otitis media
- **Differentiated Thyroid Carcinoma, Nodal**
  - Key facts
    - Nodal spread common in papillary, distant spread common in follicular
    - 3x more common in women
    - Presents in 3rd & 4th decade; occasionally in adolescents, rare in young children
  - Imaging
    - Variable: Small to large nodes; homogeneous or heterogeneous; hemorrhagic or cystic necrosis
    - Focal calcifications & solid foci of enhancement may be present

Helpful Clues for Rare Diagnoses
- **Metastases, Systemic, Nodal**
  - Key facts
    - In children, primary malignancy is usually known
    - Neuroblastoma most common; other primary malignancies such as testicular carcinoma, hepatoblastoma, chordoma
    - Supraclavicular metastasis suggests chest or abdominal primary
  - Imaging
    - Single or multiple enlarged nodes
    - ± Necrosis
- **Langerhans Histiocytosis, Nodal**
  - Key facts
    - Focal, localized, or systemic disease
    - Unifocal > > multifocal
    - Skeletal involvement most common, adenopathy with systemic disease
  - Imaging
    - In acute disseminated disease (Letterer-Siwe), diffuse lymphadenopathy
    - + Hepatosplenomegaly, skin rash, marrow failure, & pulmonary disease

SELECTED REFERENCES

1. Malloy KM et al: Lack of association of CT findings and surgical drainage in pediatric neck abscesses. Int J Pediatr Otorhinolaryngol. 72(2):235-9, 2008
2. Herrmann BW et al: Otolaryngological manifestations of posttransplant lymphoproliferative disorder in pediatric thoracic transplant patients. Int J Pediatr Otorhinolaryngol. 70(2):303-10, 2006

Reactive Lymph Nodes

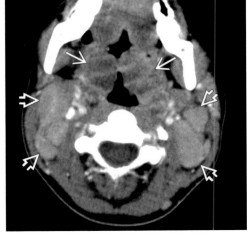

Axial CECT shows enlarged palatine tonsils ➡ and reactive cervical lymph nodes ➡ in a teenager with mononucleosis.

Reactive Lymph Nodes

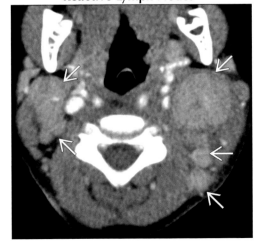

Axial CECT demonstrates left greater than right cervical adenopathy ➡ in a child with a throat swab positive for beta-hemolytic Streptococcus group A.

ENLARGED LYMPH NODES IN NECK OF CHILD

(Left) Axial CECT shows a well-defined low attenuation retropharyngeal abscess ➡ (secondary to a suppurative left lateral retropharyngeal lymph node) and nonsuppurative bilateral cervical adenopathy ➡. (Right) Axial CECT reveals a well-defined, rim-enhancing low attenuation intranodal abscess ➡ and significant soft tissue edema in the adjacent subcutaneous fat ➡.

Suppurative Lymph Nodes

Suppurative Lymph Nodes

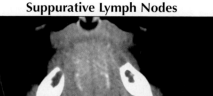
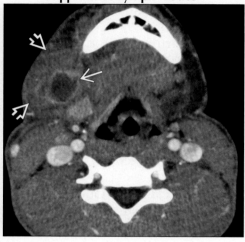

(Left) Axial CECT clearly defines a large moderately enhancing level IV cervical node ➡ along with a level V node ➡ in a teenager with Hodgkin lymphoma. (Right) Axial CECT demonstrates marked enlargement of the relatively low attenuation right cervical lymph nodes ➡ in another teenager with Hodgkin lymphoma.

Hodgkin Lymphoma, Lymph Nodes

Hodgkin Lymphoma, Lymph Nodes

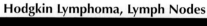
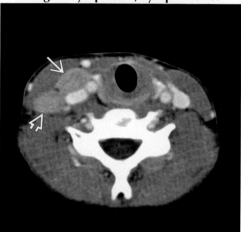
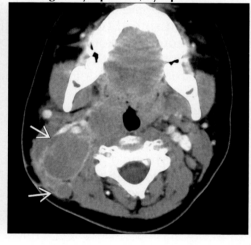

(Left) Axial CECT shows an ill-defined nodal mass ➡ with a small central area of necrosis ➡, adjacent to the left submandibular gland ➡. There is no significant surrounding soft tissue edema. (Right) Axial CECT clearly defines bilateral, symmetric enlargement of nonnecrotic cervical lymph nodes ➡ in a patient with T-cell lymphoma.

Cat Scratch Disease

Non-Hodgkin Lymphoma, Lymph Nodes

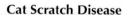
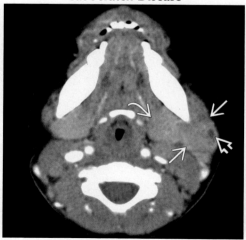
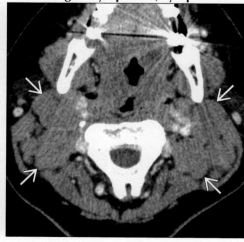

ENLARGED LYMPH NODES IN NECK OF CHILD

Non-TB Mycobacterium, Lymph Nodes

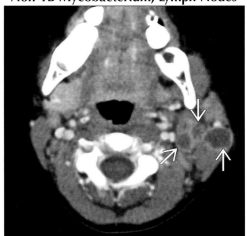

Neuroblastoma, Metastatic

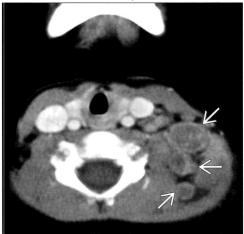

(Left) Axial CECT shows left-sided necrotic cervical lymph nodes ➔ without edema of the adjacent fat. This toddler presented with a left neck mass, without fever or elevated white blood cell count. The Mycobacterium avium intracellulare was isolated from the excision specimen. *(Right)* Axial CECT demonstrates several low attenuation left supraclavicular metastatic lymph nodes ➔ in a child with known neuroblastoma.

Lymphoproliferative Disorder, Post-Transplant

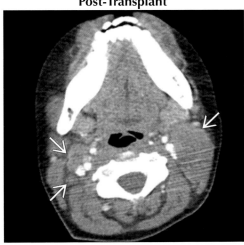

Differentiated Thyroid Carcinoma, Nodal

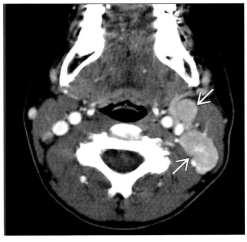

(Left) Axial CECT shows left greater than right cervical adenopathy ➔ in a 10 year old patient with a prior renal transplant. *(Right)* Axial CECT shows diffusely enhancing left cervical nodes ➔ in a teenager who presented with a left-sided neck mass that proved to be metastatic thyroid carcinoma.

Metastases, Systemic, Nodal

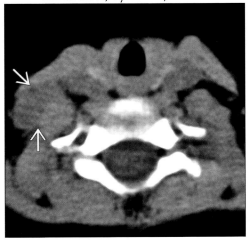

Langerhans Histiocytosis, Nodal

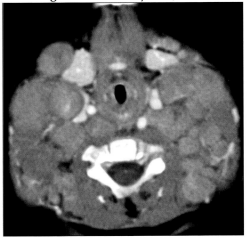

(Left) Axial CECT demonstrates a left supraclavicular metastatic nodal mass ➔ in a child with metastatic chordoma. *(Right)* Axial CECT reveals too numerous to count, massively enlarged anterior and posterior cervical lymph nodes in a child with extensive Langerhans cell histiocytosis.

SECTION 5
Trans-spatial, Multi-spatial in Head and Neck

Generic Imaging Patterns

Modality-Specific Imaging Findings

Clinically Based Differentials

AIR-CONTAINING LESIONS IN NECK

DIFFERENTIAL DIAGNOSIS

Common
- Trauma, General
- Abscess, Retropharyngeal Space (RPS)

Less Common
- Laryngocele
- Diverticulum, Esophago-Pharyngeal

Rare but Important
- 4th Branchial Anomaly
- Diverticulum, Lateral Cervical Esophageal
- Cervical Emphysema, Spontaneous

ESSENTIAL INFORMATION

Helpful Clues for Common Diagnoses
- **Trauma, General**
  - Key facts: Esophageal, pharyngeal, laryngeal, or superficial trauma
  - Imaging: Extraluminal air in neck ± laryngeal, hyoid, or facial fractures
- **Abscess, Retropharyngeal Space (RPS)**
  - Key facts: Posterior to pharyngeal mucosal space, anterior to prevertebral space
  - Imaging: Extranodal purulent fluid in RPS ± air in or adjacent to fluid collection ± extension to mediastinum

Helpful Clues for Less Common Diagnoses
- **Laryngocele**
  - Key facts: Lateral saccular cyst, laryngeal mucocele
  - Imaging: Air ± air-filled level
    - Internal laryngocele in paraglottic space
    - Mixed laryngocele in paraglottic & submandibular spaces
- **Diverticulum, Esophago-Pharyngeal**
  - Key facts: Zenker diverticulum = mucosal-lined outpouching of posterior hypopharynx
  - Imaging: Air-filled pouch posterior to esophagus; usually extends left of esophagus

Helpful Clues for Rare Diagnoses
- **4th Branchial Anomaly**
  - Key facts: 4th pharyngeal pouch remnant
    - Extends from apex of pyriform sinus to lower neck, anterior to left thyroid lobe
    - Present with recurrent thyroiditis or anterior neck abscess
  - Imaging
    - Abscess anterior to left thyroid lobe ± intrinsic inflammatory change in ipsilateral thyroid lobe
    - Inflamed pyriform sinus apex
    - Lack of aeration of pyriform sinus apex
- **Diverticulum, Lateral Cervical Esophageal**
  - Key facts: Mucosal-lined outpouching lateral to cervical esophagus
  - Imaging: Air-filled pouch lateral to cervical esophagus
- **Cervical Emphysema, Spontaneous**
  - Key facts: No history of vomiting, trauma, asthma, or other inciting event
  - Imaging: Pneumomediastinum & cervical emphysema

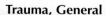

Trauma, General

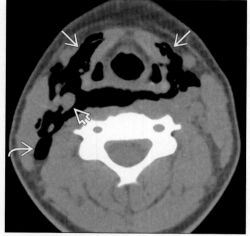

Axial CECT shows extensive air nearly surrounding the larynx ➡, the right carotid vessels ➡, and in the posterior triangle of the neck ➡ in a child who was thrown from a horse.

Trauma, General

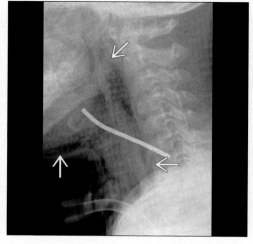

Lateral radiograph shows extensive subcutaneous and deep soft tissue air ➡ in a child who suffered direct penetrating injury from a piece of clothes hanger thrown from under a lawnmower.

AIR-CONTAINING LESIONS IN NECK

Abscess, Retropharyngeal Space (RPS)

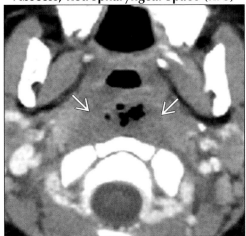

Laryngocele

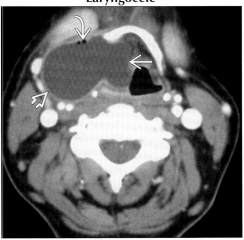

(Left) Axial CECT shows locules of gas within edematous retropharyngeal soft tissues ➡ secondary to abscess. *(Right)* Axial CECT shows mixed laryngocele involving both the paraglottic space ➡ and the anterior neck ➡. The mass is primarily fluid-filled but contains small bubbles of gas anteriorly ➡.

Diverticulum, Esophago-Pharyngeal

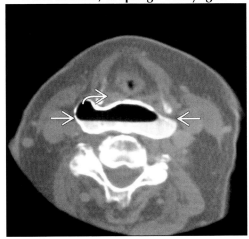

4th Branchial Anomaly

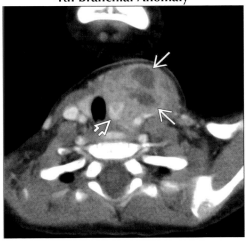

(Left) Axial NECT shows barium layering within the air-filled space ➡, displacing the pharynx anteriorly ➡, a variant of Zenker diverticulum. *(Right)* Axial CECT shows a large, irregularly shaped, heterogeneously enhancing abscess ➡ in the left neck, anterior to the left thyroid lobe ➡. This teenager had recurrent infections secondary to pyriform sinus tract, a 4th pharyngeal pouch remnant.

Diverticulum, Lateral Cervical Esophageal

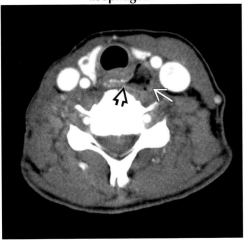

Cervical Emphysema, Spontaneous

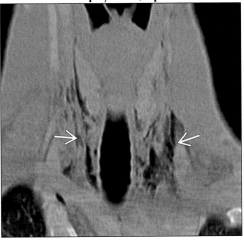

(Left) Axial CECT demonstrates a connection ➡ between the lateral esophageal wall and a lateral cervical diverticulum ➡. The diverticulum is filled with air and debris. *(Right)* Coronal CECT in lung window shows extensive cervical emphysema ➡ in a teenager with a history of neck fullness and chest pain. There was no history of trauma, asthma, vomiting, or other event that may have caused rupture of the trachea or esophagus.

SOLID NECK MASS IN INFANT

DIFFERENTIAL DIAGNOSIS

Common
- Fibromatosis Colli
- Reactive Lymph Nodes
- Infantile Hemangioma

Less Common
- Neurofibromatosis Type 1
- Teratoma

Rare but Important
- Langerhans Cell Histiocytosis, General
- Neuroblastoma, Metastatic
- Fibromatosis
- Neuroblastoma, Primary Cervical
- Thymus, Cervical

ESSENTIAL INFORMATION

Helpful Clues for Common Diagnoses
- **Fibromatosis Colli**
  - Key facts
    - Synonyms: Sternocleidomastoid (SCM) tumor of infancy, congenital muscular torticollis
    - Increased incidence in breech presentation and difficult deliveries
    - Present with neck mass ± torticollis, usually within first 2 weeks of life
    - Ultrasound preferred imaging modality
  - Imaging
    - Large SCM muscle, focal or diffuse
    - Almost always unilateral
    - Variable echogenicity, attenuation, signal intensity; heterogeneous contrast enhancement on MR
    - No associated adenopathy
    - No extramuscular extension of mass
- **Reactive Lymph Nodes**
  - Key facts
    - "Reactive" implies benign etiology
    - Acute or chronic
    - Any H&N nodal group
    - Response to infection/inflammation
  - Imaging
    - Enlarged oval-shaped lymph nodes
    - Variable enhancement, usually mild
    - ± Enlargement of lingual, faucial, or adenoid hypertrophy
    - ± Stranding of adjacent fat (cellulitis)
    - ± Edema in adjacent muscles (myositis)
    - ± Suppurative nodes or abscess

- **Infantile Hemangioma**
  - Key facts
    - Vacular neoplasm, NOT malformation
    - Usually not well seen at birth, more apparent within 1st few weeks of life
    - Proliferative phase 1st year of life
    - Involuting phase, 1-5 years
    - Involuted usually by 5-7 years
    - GLUT-1: Specific immunohistochemical marker expressed in all 3 phases of infantile hemangioma; also expressed in placenta, fetal, and embryonic tissue
    - Congenital hemangioma: Rare variant, present at birth or on prenatal imaging (fetal hemangioma); 2 subtypes, rapidly involuting (RICH) shows involution by 8-14 months, noninvoluting (NICH)
  - Imaging
    - Proliferative: Solid, intensely enhancing mass with intralesional high flow vessels
    - Involutional: Fatty infiltration, ↓ size
    - PHACES syndrome: Posterior fossa abnormalities, hemangiomas, arterial anomalies, cardiovascular defects, eye abnormalities, sternal clefts

Helpful Clues for Less Common Diagnoses
- **Neurofibromatosis Type 1**
  - Key facts
    - Carotid space, perivertebral space (brachial plexus) common
    - Localized, diffuse, or plexiform
    - Single or multiple
  - Imaging
    - Localized: Well-circumscribed, smooth, solid masses with variable enhancement
    - Diffuse: Plaque-like thickening of skin with poorly defined linear branching lesion in subcutaneous fat
    - Plexiform: Lobulated, tortuous, rope-like expansion in major nerve distribution; "tangle of worms" appearance
- **Teratoma**
  - Key facts
    - Contains all 3 germ layers
    - Mature or immature, rarely malignant in neonate
  - Imaging
    - Large, heterogeneous mass
    - Frequently with fat and calcium
    - Solid and cystic components

SOLID NECK MASS IN INFANT

Helpful Clues for Rare Diagnoses

- **Langerhans Cell Histiocytosis, General**
  - Key facts
    - Acute disseminated form (Letterer-Siwe) occurs in children < 1 year
    - Acute onset of hepatosplenomegaly, rash, lymphadenopathy, marrow failure
    - Skeletal involvement may be absent
  - Imaging
    - Large nonspecific cervical lymph nodes
    - Hepatosplenomegaly
- **Neuroblastoma, Metastatic**
  - Key facts
    - Most cervical disease is metastatic from retroperitoneal primary lesion
    - Metastatic cervical disease more common in older children
  - Imaging
    - Large metastatic lymph nodes
    - Bilateral skull base metastasis common
    - Skull base metastasis: Enhancing masses with osseous erosion ± intracranial or intraorbital extension
- **Fibromatosis**
  - Key facts
    - Synonyms: Desmoid or aggressive fibromatosis, infantile fibromatosis, extraabdominal desmoid tumor
    - Benign soft tissue tumor arising from musculoaponeurotic structures
    - Tendency to infiltrate adjacent tissues
    - Recurrence common
    - Does not metastasize

- Identified at all ages
- In infants, more common in retroperitoneum and extremity
  - Imaging
    - Well-defined or poorly marginated, infiltrative mass
    - Often trans-spatial enhancing mass
    - ± Erosion of adjacent bone
- **Neuroblastoma, Primary Cervical**
  - Key facts
    - < 5% are primary cervical lesions
    - In general, < 1 year = better prognosis
    - Young children may present with opsoclonus-myoclonus
  - Imaging findings
    - Solid mass closely associated with carotid sheath-space
    - Calcifications common
    - Foraminal or intraspinal extension
- **Thymus, Cervical**
  - Key facts
    - Remnants along thymopharyngeal duct
  - Imaging findings
    - Mildly enhancing soft tissue mass
    - Small dot-dash echoes on ultrasound, similar to mediastinal thymus

SELECTED REFERENCES

1. Greene AK et al: Intraosseous "hemangiomas" are malformations and not tumors. Plast Reconstr Surg. 119(6):1949-50; author reply 1950, 2007
2. Mulliken JB et al: Hemangiomas and vascular malformations in infants and children: a classification based on endothelial characteristics. Plast Reconstr Surg. 69(3):412-22, 1982

Fibromatosis Colli

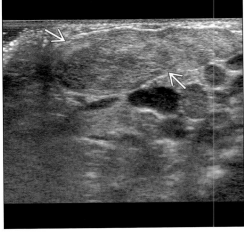

Longitudinal ultrasound shows fusiform enlargement of the left sternocleidomastoid muscle ➤ in a 2 month old with fibromatosis colli.

Fibromatosis Colli

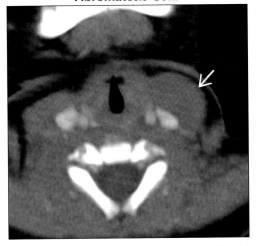

Axial CECT demonstrates diffuse enlargement of the left sternocleidomastoid muscle ➤ in a neonate after a difficult birth with palpable neck mass and torticollis.

SOLID NECK MASS IN INFANT

Reactive Lymph Nodes

(Left) Axial CECT shows bilateral nonsuppurative cervical lymph nodes ➡ and a large phlegmonous inflammatory mass in the left lateral retropharyngeal space ➡, in a 4 month old boy. *(Right)* Axial CECT reveals bilateral cervical adenopathy ➡ with surrounding stranding of the fat (cellulitis) and thickening of the right platysma muscle (myositis) ➡. There is also nonenhancing fluid ➡ surrounding the right sternocleidomastoid muscle.

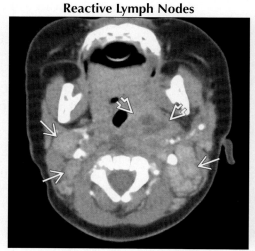

Reactive Lymph Nodes

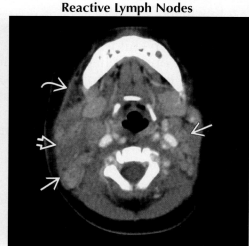

Infantile Hemangioma

(Left) Axial T2WI FS MR shows multiple enhancing hemangiomas ➡ in infant with PHACES syndrome. PHACES acronym: posterior fossa malformations, hemangiomas, arterial anomalies, coarctation of the aorta & cardiac defects, eye abnormalities, & sternal clefting. *(Right)* Axial T1 C+ FS MR reveals diffuse enlargement & intense enhancement of parotid hemangioma. Note the lesion is holoparotid, involving both the superficial ➡ & deep ➡ lobes.

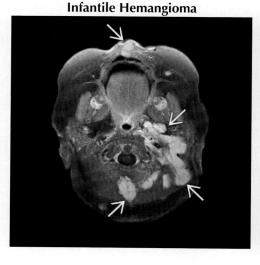

Infantile Hemangioma

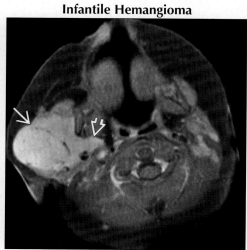

Neurofibromatosis Type 1

(Left) Axial T2WI MR depicts bilateral, hyperintense, carotid sheath neurofibromas ➡ that extend medially from the carotid sheath into the retropharyngeal space. *(Right)* Axial CECT shows a large heterogeneous trans-spatial neck mass in a 6 day old infant. Some areas are cystic ➡, others are more solid ➡, and there are small foci of calcifications ➡, consistent with congenital teratoma.

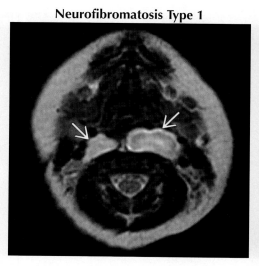

Teratoma

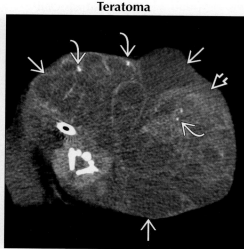

SOLID NECK MASS IN INFANT

Langerhans Cell Histiocytosis, General

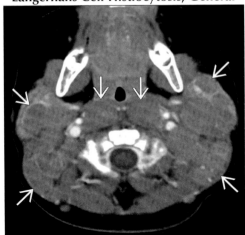

Neuroblastoma, Metastatic

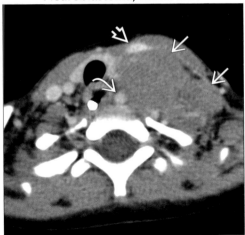

(Left) Axial CECT shows massive bilateral cervical adenopathy in all nodal groups ➡ in an 8 month old boy with an acute disseminated form of Langerhans cell histiocytosis. *(Right)* Axial CECT demonstrates a large conglomerate of metastatic left cervical lymph nodes in a girl with primary adrenal neuroblastoma ➡. The left jugular vein ➡ is displaced anteriorly, and the left carotid artery ➡ is deviated posteromedially.

Fibromatosis

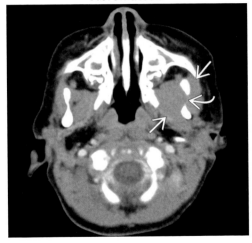

Neuroblastoma, Primary Cervical

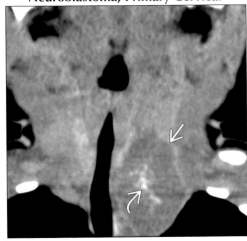

(Left) Axial CECT shows a soft tissue attenuation mass in the left masticator space ➡ with smooth thinning of the left mandible ramus ➡. The imaging diagnosis of possible sarcoma was replaced by surgical pathologic diagnosis of fibromatosis. *(Right)* Coronal CECT demonstrates a well-defined low attenuation left paratracheal neuroblastoma ➡ with central irregular calcifications ➡ in a 1 year old girl who presented with ataxia, opsoclonus-myoclonus.

Neuroblastoma, Primary Cervical

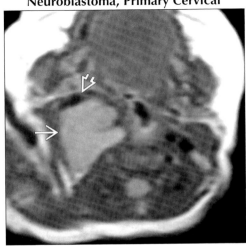

Thymus, Cervical

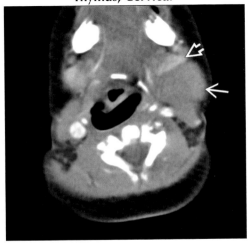

(Left) Axial PD FSE MR reveals a well-defined left carotid sheath primary cervical neuroblastoma ➡ without intraspinal extension. Notice the anterior displacement of the carotid artery and internal jugular vein ➡. *(Right)* Axial CECT shows a well-defined intermediate attenuation left anterior neck mass ➡ in a 3 month old with pathologically proven cervical thymus. The left submandibular gland ➡ is flattened anteriorly.

SOLID NECK MASS IN CHILD

DIFFERENTIAL DIAGNOSIS

Common
- Reactive Lymph Nodes
- Hodgkin Lymphoma, Lymph Nodes
- Infantile Hemangioma
- Neurofibromatosis Type 1
- Non-Hodgkin Lymphoma, Lymph Nodes

Less Common
- Lipoma
- Neuroblastoma, Metastatic
- Differentiated Thyroid Carcinoma, Nodal

Rare but Important
- Pilomatrixoma
- Neuroblastoma, Primary Cervical
- SCCa, Nodes
- Rhabdomyosarcoma
- Thymus, Cervical

ESSENTIAL INFORMATION

Helpful Clues for Common Diagnoses
- **Reactive Lymph Nodes**
  - Key facts
    - "Reactive" implies benign etiology
    - Acute or chronic; any H&N nodal group
    - Response to infection/inflammation
  - Imaging
    - Enlarged oval-shaped lymph nodes
    - ± Enlargement of lingual, faucial, or adenoidal hypertrophy
    - ± Stranding of adjacent fat (cellulitis)
    - ± Edema in adjacent muscles (myositis)
    - ± Suppurative nodes or abscess
    - Variable enhancement, usually mild
- **Hodgkin Lymphoma, Lymph Nodes**
  - Key facts
    - B-cell origin; histology shows Reed-Sternberg cells
    - Cervical & mediastinal nodes common
    - Waldeyer ring or extranodal < 1%
    - Tumors EBV positive in up to 50%
  - Imaging
    - Imaging cannot distinguish Hodgkin from non-Hodgkin lymphoma
    - Homogeneous lobulated nodal masses
    - Single or multiple nodal chain
    - Variable contrast enhancement
    - Necrotic center may be present
- **Infantile Hemangioma**
  - Key facts

- True vascular neoplasm
- Usually not present at birth; typically presents in 1st few months of life
- Rapid growth and spontaneous involution typical
  - Imaging
    - Solid, avidly enhancing mass
    - Intralesional high flow vessels
    - Fatty infiltration during involution
    - PHACES syndrome: Posterior fossa abnormalities, hemangiomas, arterial abnormalities, cardiovascular defects, eye abnormalities, sternal clefts
- **Neurofibromatosis Type 1**
  - Key facts
    - Carotid space, perivertebral space (brachial plexus) common
    - Localized, diffuse, or plexiform
    - Single or multiple
  - Imaging
    - Localized: Well-circumscribed, smooth, solid masses with variable enhancement
    - Diffuse: Plaque-like thickening of skin with poorly defined linear branching lesion in subcutaneous fat
    - Plexiform: Lobulated, tortuous, rope-like expansion in major nerve distribution; "tangle of worms" appearance
- **Non-Hodgkin Lymphoma, Lymph Nodes**
  - Key facts
    - All nodal chains involved
    - Extranodal 30%: Lymphatic (palatine or lingual tonsil & adenoids) or extralymphatic (paranasal sinuses, skull base, & thyroid)
  - Imaging
    - Cannot distinguish non-Hodgkin from Hodgkin lymphoma
    - Single dominant node or multiple nonnecrotic enlarged nodes

Helpful Clues for Less Common Diagnoses
- **Lipoma**
  - Key facts: Any space, may be trans-spatial
  - Imaging
    - Homogeneous fat density (CT) or signal (MR) without significant enhancement
    - If enhancement, suspect liposarcoma
- **Neuroblastoma, Metastatic**
  - Key facts
    - Most cervical disease is metastatic
  - Imaging

- Large lymph nodes, rarely necrotic
- Bilateral skull base metastasis common
- Enhancing masses with aggressive osseous erosion & intracranial/intraorbital extension
- **Differentiated Thyroid Carcinoma, Nodal**
  - Key facts
    - Nodal spread common in papillary, distant spread common in follicular
    - 3x more common in women
    - Usually 3rd & 4th decade, occasionally in adolescents, rare in young children
  - Imaging
    - Variable: Small to large, "reactive" in appearance or heterogeneous, hemorrhagic, or cystic necrosis
    - Focal calcifications & solid foci of enhancement may be present

Helpful Clues for Rare Diagnoses
- **Pilomatrixoma**
  - Key facts
    - Calcifying epithelioma of Malherbe
    - Usually benign in children
  - Imaging
    - Enhancing mass in subcutaneous fat
    - Variable calcification, adherent to skin
- **Neuroblastoma, Primary Cervical**
  - Key facts
    - < 5% of neuroblastomas are primary cervical lesions
    - Range from immature neuroblastoma to mature, benign ganglioneuroma
  - Imaging

- Well-defined solid mass closely associated with carotid sheath
- Intraspinal extension rare
- Calcifications may be present
- **SCCa, Nodes**
  - Key facts
    - Unknown primary SCCa rare in children
    - Nasopharyngeal carcinoma with adenopathy may occur in teenagers
  - Imaging
    - Enlarged, round nodes
    - May be heterogeneous ± multiple confluent nodes
- **Rhabdomyosarcoma**
  - Key facts
    - Most common location in H&N is parameningeal (middle ear, paranasal sinus, nasopharynx)
    - Intracranial extension in up to 55% of parameningeal lesions
  - Imaging
    - Soft tissue mass, variable enhancement
    - Bone erosion or nonaggressive bone remodeling
    - Cervical adenopathy may be associated
- **Thymus, Cervical**
  - Key facts: Thymic remnants along path of thymopharyngeal duct
  - Imaging: Mildly enhancing soft tissue mass along path of thymopharyngeal duct

Reactive Lymph Nodes

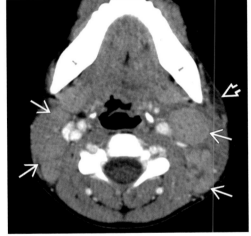

Axial CECT shows left greater than right, nonnecrotic, reactive cervical adenopathy ➡ and mild overlying soft tissue edema ➡ in a toddler with an elevated white blood cell count.

Hodgkin Lymphoma, Lymph Nodes

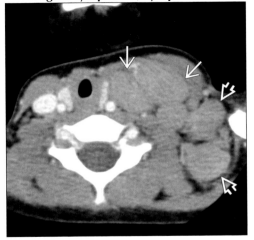

Axial CECT demonstrates multiple large supraclavicular cervical lymph nodes in a 4 year old with Hodgkin lymphoma. Both the internal jugular ➡ and spinal accessory ➡ chain nodes are involved.

SOLID NECK MASS IN CHILD

Infantile Hemangioma

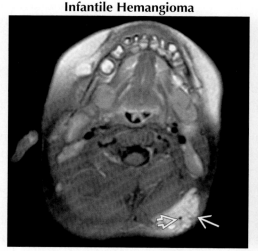

Infantile Hemangioma

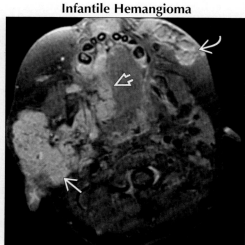

(Left) Axial T1 C+ FS MR reveals a homogeneously enhancing, lobulated infantile hemangioma ➡ in the posterior left subcutaneous fat with a single flow void ➡, consistent with a high flow intralesional vessel, typical of hemangioma. *(Right)* Axial T1 C+ FS MR shows multiple enhancing infantile hemangiomas in the right parotid gland ➡, right sublingual space ➡, and left cheek ➡ in a patient with PHACES syndrome.

Neurofibromatosis Type 1

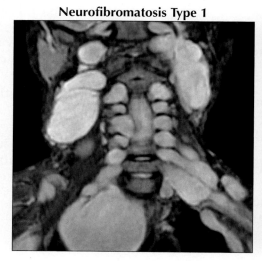

Non-Hodgkin Lymphoma, Lymph Nodes

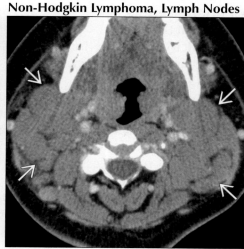

(Left) Coronal STIR MR demonstrates multiple bilateral neurofibromas involving the neck, neural foramina, cervical canal, brachial plexus, and thoracic inlet in a young child with neurofibromatosis type 1. *(Right)* Axial CECT reveals multiple bilateral internal jugular chain lymph nodes ➡ in a teenager with T-cell lymphoblastic lymphoma.

Lipoma

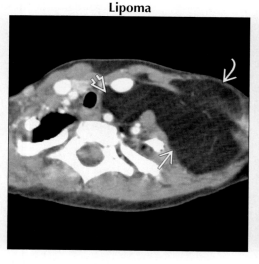

Neuroblastoma, Metastatic

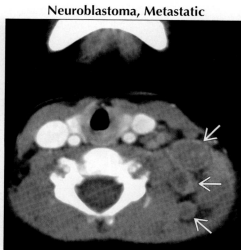

(Left) Axial CECT shows a trans-spatial left infrahyoid neck mass. The lipoma involves the carotid ➡, posterior cervical ➡, and superficial ➡ spaces of the infrahyoid neck. *(Right)* Coronal CECT reveals multiple partially necrotic left spinal accessory metastatic lymph nodes ➡ secondary to primary adrenal neuroblastoma.

SOLID NECK MASS IN CHILD

Differentiated Thyroid Carcinoma, Nodal

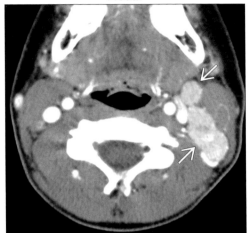

Pilomatrixoma

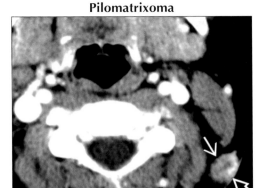

(Left) Axial CECT demonstrates high attenuation calcified metastatic papillary thyroid carcinoma nodal metastases ➡. Solid enhancing, cystic, or calcified components in neck nodes suggest differentiated thyroid carcinoma primary. *(Right)* Axial CECT reveals a well-defined, partially calcified pilomatrixoma ➡ in the subcutaneous fat of the left posterior neck, adherent to the skin ➡.

Neuroblastoma, Primary Cervical

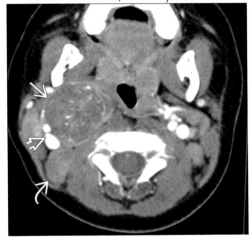

SCCa, Nodes

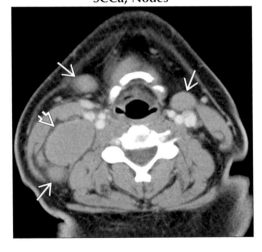

(Left) Axial NECT reveals a well-defined round mass ➡ with speckled intrinsic calcifications that deviates the carotid space laterally ➡. It proved to be a ganglioneuroblastoma, a mixture of neuroblastoma & ganglioneuroma. Nodal metastasis ➡. *(Right)* Axial CECT shows multiple enlarged, nonnecrotic cervical lymph nodes ➡; largest ➡ is deep to sternocleidomastoid muscle at level of hyoid bone in a teenager with metastatic nasopharyngeal carcinoma.

Rhabdomyosarcoma

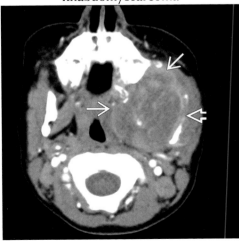

Thymus, Cervical

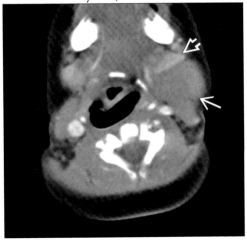

(Left) Axial CECT reveals a large heterogeneous left masticator space mass ➡ destroying the left mandible ➡ in a 3 year old with rhabdomyosarcoma. *(Right)* Axial CECT demonstrates an intermediate attenuation, solid-appearing mass ➡ posterior to the left submandibular gland ➡. Surgical pathology found the mass to be ectopic thymus.

CYSTIC NECK MASS IN CHILD

DIFFERENTIAL DIAGNOSIS

Common
- Suppurative Lymph Nodes
- Abscess
- Thyroglossal Duct Cyst
- Lymphatic Malformation
- Ranula
- 2nd Branchial Cleft Cyst

Less Common
- 1st Branchial Cleft Cyst
- Thymic Cyst

Rare but Important
- Dermoid and Epidermoid
- Teratoma

ESSENTIAL INFORMATION

Helpful Clues for Common Diagnoses
- **Suppurative Lymph Nodes**
  - Key facts
    - Pus in lymph node = intranodal abscess
  - Imaging
    - Thick enhancing nodal walls with central hypodensity
    - Edema in surrounding fat (cellulitis)
    - ± Thickening of muscles (myositis)
    - Associated nonsuppurative adenopathy
    - Nontuberculous mycobacterial adenitis lacks surrounding inflammatory changes
- **Abscess**
  - Key facts
    - Conglomeration of suppurative nodes or rupture of node ⇒ extranodal abscess
    - Superficial abscesses: Anterior or posterior cervical or submandibular space
    - Deep neck abscesses: Retropharyngeal, parapharyngeal, or tonsillar; may grow rapidly ⇒ airway compromise, ± mediastinal extension
    - If anterior to left thyroid lobe, think 4th branchial apparatus anomaly
    - Exclude dental infection & salivary gland calculus as cause of H&N infection
  - Imaging
    - Wide prevertebral soft tissue = cellulitis & edema ± frank abscess; false-positive in children, if neck not in extended position

- Rim-enhancing mass with low attenuation center; majority drainable pus, up to 25% may be phlegmon, without drainable pus
- Edema in surrounding fat (cellulitis); ± thickening of muscles (myositis); occasionally air in abscess cavity
- **Thyroglossal Duct Cyst**
  - Key facts
    - Remnant of thyroglossal duct, anywhere from foramen cecum at base of tongue to thyroid bed in infrahyoid neck
    - Treatment = resect cyst, tract, & midline hyoid bone (Sistrunk procedure)
  - Imaging
    - Cyst with minimal rim enhancement
    - At hyoid > suprahyoid = infrahyoid
    - Most in suprahyoid neck are midline; may be paramidline in infrahyoid neck
    - Infrahyoid embedded in strap muscles
    - May contain hyperechoic debris without hemorrhage or infection
    - Increased enhancement & surrounding inflammatory change when infected
    - ± Nodularity or calcifications if associated thyroid carcinoma (adults)
- **Lymphatic Malformation**
  - Key facts
    - Congenital vascular malformation
    - Variably sized lymphatic channels
    - Present at birth, grows with child
    - Hemorrhage ⇒ sudden increase in size
  - Imaging
    - Unilocular or multilocular; macrocystic or microcystic; 1 space or trans-spatial
    - Only septations enhance, unless associated with venous malformation
    - Lack high flow vessels on flow sensitive MR sequences & angiography
    - Fluid-fluid levels = hemorrhage
- **Ranula**
  - Key facts
    - Simple = postinflammatory retention cyst with epithelial lining; arising in sublingual gland or minor salivary gland, in sublingual space (SLS)
    - Diving = extravasation pseudocyst when ruptures out of SLS into submandibular space (SMS)
  - Imaging
    - Simple = well-defined cyst in SLS

- Diving = cyst in SLS & SMS; if SLS component collapsed ⇒ "tail"
- **2nd Branchial Cleft Cyst**
  - ○ Key facts
    - Characteristic location = at or inferior to angle of mandible, posterolateral to submandibular gland, lateral to carotid space, & anteromedial to sternocleidomastoid muscle (SCM)
    - Uncommon locations = parapharyngeal space, beaking in between internal & external carotid artery, anterior surface of infrahyoid carotid space
  - ○ Imaging
    - Well-defined unilocular cyst in typical location, with no significant contrast enhancement unless infected

Helpful Clues for Less Common Diagnoses
- **1st Branchial Cleft Cyst**
  - ○ Key facts
    - Remnant of 1st branchial apparatus
    - In or superficial to parotid gland, around pinna or external auditory canal; may extend to angle of mandible
    - Proximity to facial nerve important for surgical planning
  - ○ Imaging
    - Well-defined nonenhancing cyst; contrast-enhancing wall with surrounding inflammation if infected
- **Thymic Cyst**
  - ○ Key facts

- Remnant of thymopharyngeal duct, 3rd branchial pouch remnant
- Wall contains Hassall corpuscles
  - ○ Imaging
    - Cystic neck mass along course of thymopharyngeal duct ± solid enhancing thymic tissue
    - Closely associated with carotid sheath
    - May be connected to mediastinal thymus
    - Rarely ruptures into parapharyngeal space

Helpful Clues for Rare Diagnoses
- **Dermoid and Epidermoid**
  - ○ Key facts
    - Dermoid epithelial & dermal elements; epidermoid epithelial elements only
  - ○ Imaging
    - Well-defined cyst filled with fluid = dermoid OR epidermoid
    - Well-defined cyst with fatty material, mixed fluid ± calcification = dermoid
- **Teratoma**
  - ○ Key facts: All 3 germ cell lines; mature, immature, & malignant
  - ○ Imaging: Fat, calcium, cystic, & solid components

SELECTED REFERENCES

1. Koch BL: Cystic malformations of the neck in children. Pediatr Radiol. 35(5):463-77, 2005
2. Mulliken JB et al: Hemangiomas and vascular malformations in infants and children: a classification based on endothelial characteristics. Plast Reconstr Surg. 69(3):412-22, 1982

Suppurative Lymph Nodes

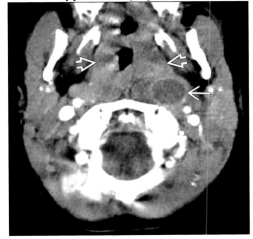

Axial CECT demonstrates a well-defined, rim-enhancing, suppurative left lateral retropharyngeal lymph node ➡ in a patient with pharyngitis. Note the swollen palatine tonsils ➡.

Suppurative Lymph Nodes

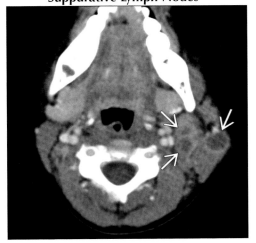

Axial CECT shows multiple necrotic left-sided cervical lymph nodes ➡, without inflammatory changes in the adjacent fat, in a 2 year old with mycobacterium avium intracellulare.

CYSTIC NECK MASS IN CHILD

Abscess

Abscess

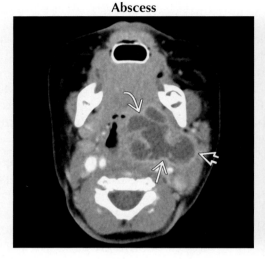
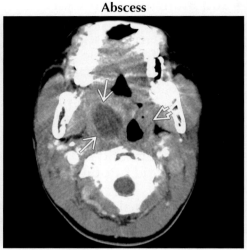

(Left) Axial CECT reveals a large, multiloculated abscess with a fairly well-defined rim of contrast enhancement in the left parapharyngeal ➡, deep parotid ⇨, and the oropharyngeal mucosal ➡ spaces in a 10 month old girl with persistent neck mass, despite oral antibiotics. *(Right)* Axial CECT demonstrates a well-defined, rim-enhancing, low attenuation abscess ➡ in the right palatine tonsil. Note the normal size of the left palatine tonsil ⇨.

Thyroglossal Duct Cyst

Thyroglossal Duct Cyst

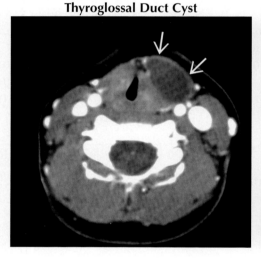
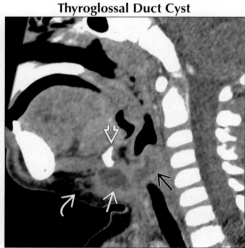

(Left) Axial CECT shows a sharply marginated, nonenhancing infrahyoid thyroglossal duct cyst ➡ embedded in the left strap muscles. The paramedian location of infrahyoid TGDC is characteristic. *(Right)* Sagittal CECT reveals an infected thyroglossal duct cyst ➡ along the inferior margin of the hyoid bone ⇨ with significant surrounding inflammatory changes ➡ and posterior rupture of the purulent material to the region of the aryepiglottic folds ➡.

Lymphatic Malformation

Lymphatic Malformation

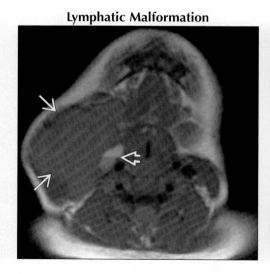
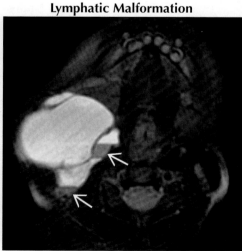

(Left) Axial T1WI MR shows a multiloculated macrocystic lymphatic malformation ➡. Fluid-fluid level ⇨ in medial locule is secondary to recent hemorrhage. *(Right)* Axial T2WI FS MR reveals the dependent blood products as the inferior component of fluid-fluid levels within 2 locules of the multiloculated, macrocystic lymphatic malformation ➡.

5

CYSTIC NECK MASS IN CHILD

Ranula

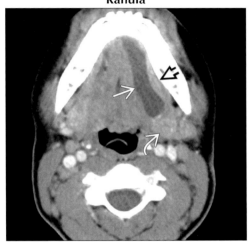

2nd Branchial Cleft Cyst

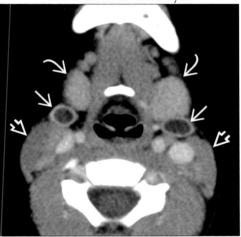

(Left) Axial CECT in a patient with a sublingual mass shows a low attenuation, nonenhancing ranula in the left sublingual space ➡. This is a simple ranula as it is confined to the sublingual space. Note also the submandibular gland ➡ and mylohyoid muscle ➡.
(Right) Axial CECT shows small bilateral 2nd branchial cleft cysts ➡ anterior to the sternocleidomastoid muscles ➡ and posterior to the submandibular glands ➡, in a child with branchiootorenal syndrome.

1st Branchial Cleft Cyst

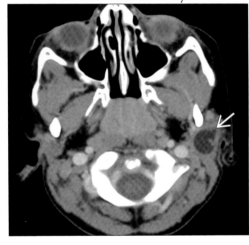

Thymic Cyst

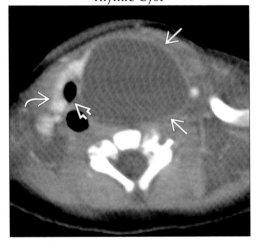

(Left) Axial NECT shows a low attenuation, nonenhancing cyst within the left parotid gland in a child with an intraparotid 1st branchial apparatus cyst ➡.
(Right) Axial CECT demonstrates a large simple thymic cyst in the left anterior neck ➡, significantly deviating the airway ➡ and thyroid gland ➡ to the right. In this patient, the cyst extended from the skull base to the upper mediastinum.

Dermoid and Epidermoid

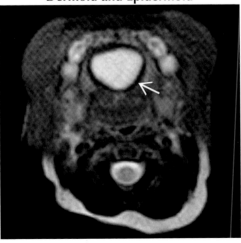

Teratoma

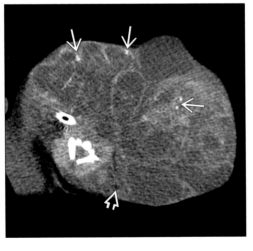

(Left) Axial T2WI MR shows a hyperintense midline dermoid cyst in the floor of the mouth ➡. Histology showed cyst lined by squamous epithelial and containing skin, adnexal structures, respiratory epithelium, and gastric epithelium. (Right) Axial CECT reveals a large, multiloculated cystic mass in the anterior neck of this infant with congenital teratoma. The lesion contains only tiny foci of fat ➡ and several foci of calcification ➡.

5

CYSTIC-APPEARING NECK MASSES IN ADULT

DIFFERENTIAL DIAGNOSIS

Common
- SCCa, Nodes
- Abscess
- Suppurative Lymph Nodes
- Differentiated Thyroid Carcinoma, Nodal
- Thrombosis, Jugular Vein, Neck
- Lymphatic Malformation
- Diving Ranula

Less Common
- Thyroglossal Duct Cyst
- 2nd Branchial Cleft Cyst
- Non-Hodgkin Lymphoma, Lymph Nodes
- Hodgkin Lymphoma, Lymph Nodes
- Metastases, Systemic, Nodal

Rare but Important
- Schwannoma, Cystic
- Diverticulum, Esophago-Pharyngeal (Zenker)

ESSENTIAL INFORMATION

Key Differential Diagnosis Issues
- Lesions in this differential diagnosis may be truly cystic, necrotic, or solid but cystic in imaging appearance
  - Intrathyroidal lesions excluded
- Patient's age determines differential
  - Congenital lesions more common in pediatric & young adult population
  - Cystic masses in adults commonly necrotic nodes (suppurative or SCCa) or lymphoma

Helpful Clues for Common Diagnoses
- **SCCa, Nodes**
  - Key facts: Nodes not truly cystic but H&N necrotic metastases from SCCa
    - Caveat: New "cystic" neck mass in adult with no history of neck mass is SCCa nodal metastasis until proven otherwise
    - 2nd branchial cleft cyst (BCC) is extremely unlikely in adult with no prior history of neck mass
  - Imaging: Thin-walled node, usually level II
    - Minimal wall enhancement
    - Small mural nodule common
- **Abscess**
  - Key facts: Patient will usually be toxic
    - Fever, elevated WBC count, hot tender neck are common symptoms

- Imaging: Peripherally enhancing mass with central low density surrounded by inflammatory stranding
- Evaluate for source
  - Look for rotted teeth, tonsillar infection, obstructing parotid or submandibular stones, sinus or mastoid infection
- **Suppurative Lymph Nodes**
  - Key facts: Multiple nodes with surrounding inflammatory changes in child or adult with hot, tender neck
  - Imaging: Submandibular, internal jugular chain nodes commonly affected in adults
    - Retropharyngeal nodes more commonly affected in children < 3 years; check for retropharyngeal fluid/abscess
- **Differentiated Thyroid Carcinoma, Nodal**
  - Key facts: Papillary thyroid carcinoma most common in middle-aged women
    - Nodal metastases may be present when thyroid gland is normal on physical exam & imaging
  - Imaging: Adenopathy often variable in appearance with cystic, solid, & enhancing nodes present in same patient
    - Nodal mets may be "upstream" from gland in levels II, III, as well as levels V, VI, and supraclavicular
- **Thrombosis, Jugular Vein, Neck**
  - Key facts: May be due to infected central line or idiopathic
  - Imaging: Surrounding induration usually present in acute thrombosis
    - Fat around vein appears normal in chronic state
  - Best confirmed with CECT or T2 MR
    - Reformations or coronal images confirm extent of thrombosis
- **Lymphatic Malformation**
  - Key facts: Doughy compressible chronic congenital neck mass in otherwise healthy patient
  - Imaging: May be unilocular, multilocular with septations, or trans-spatial
    - No significant enhancement in pure lymphatic malformation
    - Enhancement suggests lesion has venous component (lymphaticovenous malformation)
- **Diving Ranula**

○ Key facts: Soft compressible floor of mouth or submandibular space mass (diving ranula) in otherwise healthy patient
○ Imaging: Nonenhancing cystic mass arising in sublingual space
  ▪ Considered "diving" when lesion extends posterior & inferior to mylohyoid muscle into submandibular space

Helpful Clues for Less Common Diagnoses
• **Thyroglossal Duct Cyst**
  ○ Key facts: Lack of involution of thyroglossal duct
    ▪ Cyst located between foramen cecum and thyroid bed
  ○ Imaging: Midline or paramedian 2-3 cm nonenhancing cyst often wrapping around inferior hyoid bone
    ▪ If focal solid enhancing component, consider either associated thyroid remnant or differentiated thyroid carcinoma in thyroglossal duct cyst
• **2nd Branchial Cleft Cyst**
  ○ Key facts: Soft neck mass in child or young adult at angle of mandible
    ▪ 2nd BCC not a consideration in adult with no prior history of neck mass
  ○ Imaging: Nonenhancing cystic mass in embryologically defined location
    ▪ Between submandibular gland & sternocleidomastoid muscle
    ▪ Remember this is same location as jugulodigastric node
• **Non-Hodgkin Lymphoma, Lymph Nodes**

○ Key facts: 2nd most common neoplasm of head and neck in adults
○ Imaging: Multiple, often bilateral nonnecrotic nodes
  ▪ Variable density/signal intensity with some cystic in appearance; others solid
• **Hodgkin Lymphoma, Lymph Nodes**
  ○ Key facts: Neck common location for Hodgkin lymphoma nodes in young adult
  ○ Imaging: Multiple nonnecrotic nodes
    ▪ Variation in size, enhancement pattern, & density/intensity
• **Metastases, Systemic, Nodal**
  ○ Key facts: Nodal metastasis from breast, esophagus, lung can present in levels III, IV, V, and supraclavicular locations
  ○ Imaging: Single or multiple peripherally enhancing necrotic nodes, variable size
    ▪ Systemic metastases cluster in lower neck

Helpful Clues for Rare Diagnoses
• **Schwannoma, Cystic**
  ○ Key facts: Vagal origin most common; presents as carotid space mass
  ○ Imaging: Homogeneous low density nonenhancing tubular mass
    ▪ Well-circumscribed borders
• **Diverticulum, Esophago-Pharyngeal (Zenker)**
  ○ Key facts: Mucosa-lined outpouching of posterior hypopharynx at C5-C6
  ○ Imaging: Heterogeneous, sometimes air- and fluid-filled mass
    ▪ Posterior and left of esophagus

SCCa, Nodes

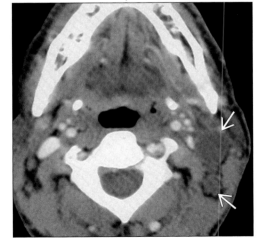

Axial CECT shows 2 cystic left neck masses ➡. Fine-needle aspiration demonstrated SCCa. The primary tumor was found in the left tonsil (not shown).

Abscess

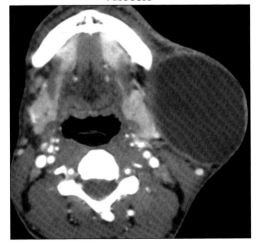

Axial CECT reveals an encapsulated nonenhancing large cystic left neck mass. Aspiration yielded pus from this cystic neck mass with overlying skin thickening.

CYSTIC-APPEARING NECK MASSES IN ADULT

(Left) *Axial CECT demonstrates a cystic left supraclavicular mass* ➡ *with peripheral enhancement in this patient with fever and induration over the lesion. Aspiration revealed Staph aureus within this intranodal abscess.* **(Right)** *Axial CECT shows multiple complex lymph nodes, with a cystic right level III node* ➡ *in this patient with papillary thyroid carcinoma. Notice the cystic-solid more anterior node* ⇒ *and contralateral solid enhancing node* ➡.

Suppurative Lymph Nodes

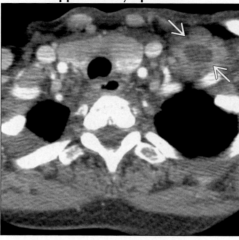

Differentiated Thyroid Carcinoma, Nodal

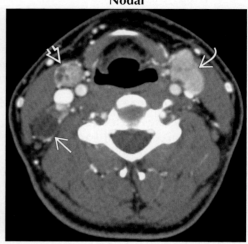

(Left) *Axial CECT reveals a peripherally enhancing right carotid space mass* ➡ *deep to the inflammatory phlegmon* ⇒ *and inflammatory skin thickening* ➡. *Acute jugular vein thrombosis may have a cystic appearance due to the nonenhancing luminal clot.* **(Right)** *Axial CECT shows a well-defined, nonenhancing low attenuation mass* ➡ *involving the left submandibular space, anterior to the left submandibular gland* ⇒.

Thrombosis, Jugular Vein, Neck

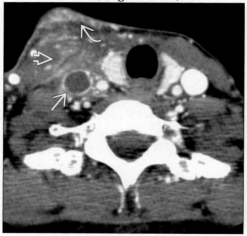

Lymphatic Malformation

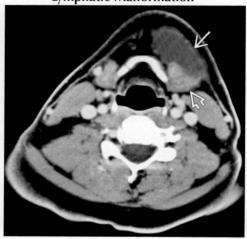

(Left) *Axial CECT demonstrates a large diving ranula with the typical sublingual space "tail"* ⇒ *accompanying the submandibular component* ➡ *within the posteroinferior submandibular space.* **(Right)** *Axial CECT reveals a simple paramedian thyroglossal duct cyst* ➡ *embedded in the left infrahyoid strap muscles.*

Diving Ranula

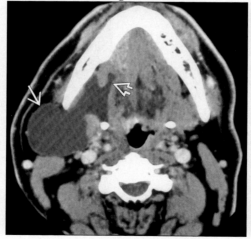

Thyroglossal Duct Cyst

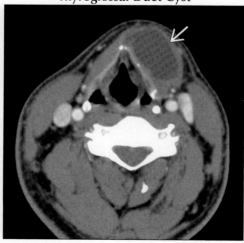

CYSTIC-APPEARING NECK MASSES IN ADULT

2nd Branchial Cleft Cyst
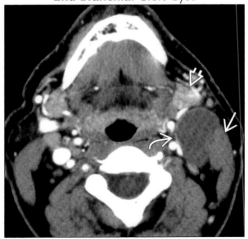

Non-Hodgkin Lymphoma, Lymph Nodes
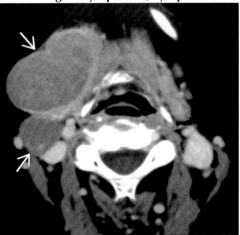

(Left) Axial CECT shows a nonenhancing low attenuation mass anterior to the sternocleidomastoid muscle ➡, posterior to the submandibular gland ➡, and lateral to the carotid space ➡. In an adult patient, a mass with this appearance could be nodal metastases from H&N SCCa, which is the diagnosis of exclusion. *(Right)* Axial CECT demonstrates 2 large low-density cystic-appearing NHL nodal masses ➡ in level IB and IIA nodal chains.

Hodgkin Lymphoma, Lymph Nodes
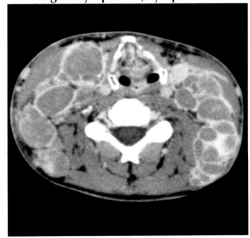

Metastases, Systemic, Nodal
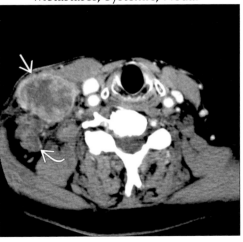

(Left) Axial CECT reveals massive cystic-appearing cervical nodes. All nodes are low density with peripheral enhancement. These nodes are really solid despite their cystic appearance. *(Right)* Axial CECT shows multiple nodal masses in levels III ➡ and V ➡ from a systemic malignancy. Necrosis in the larger node ➡ might suggest a cyst, but irregular capsule and heterogeneous central portion indicate malignancy.

Schwannoma, Cystic
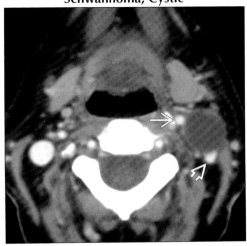

Diverticulum, Esophago-Pharyngeal (Zenker)
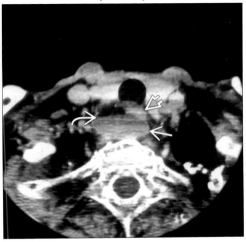

(Left) Axial CECT shows a nonenhancing "cystic" neck mass between the internal carotid artery ➡ and internal jugular vein ➡. The initial impression of neurofibroma was replaced by surgical confirmation of vagal schwannoma. *(Right)* Axial CECT shows a well-defined, oval-shaped midline mass ➡ posterior to the esophagus ➡. An air-fluid level ➡ suggests connection with either the trachea or esophagus.

TRANS-SPATIAL MASS IN CHILD

DIFFERENTIAL DIAGNOSIS

Common
- Abscess
- Lymphatic Malformation
- Venous Malformation
- Infantile Hemangioma
- Neurofibromatosis Type 1
- Rhabdomyosarcoma

Less Common
- Lipoma
- Thymic Cyst
- 4th Branchial Anomaly

Rare but Important
- Teratoma
- Fibromatosis

ESSENTIAL INFORMATION

Key Differential Diagnosis Issues
- Trans-spatial: Multiple contiguous spaces

Helpful Clues for Common Diagnoses
- **Abscess**
  - Key facts
    - Signs & symptoms of infection
    - May be in deep soft tissues of neck
    - May present with airway impingement
    - 75% drainable pus; 25% phlegmonous, nondrainable inflammatory tissue
  - Imaging
    - Low attenuation, rim-enhancing mass
    - Retropharyngeal edema common
    - May extend via danger space into mediastinum
- **Lymphatic Malformation**
  - Key facts
    - Most common cystic neck mass with spontaneous hemorrhage
    - Sudden increase in size secondary to hemorrhage or viral respiratory infection
  - Imaging
    - Unilocular or multilocular; macrocystic or microcystic; 1 space or trans-spatial
    - Insinuates morphology
    - Only septations enhance, unless associated with venous malformation
    - Lack high flow vessels on flow-sensitive MR sequences & angiography
    - Fluid-fluid levels secondary to intralesional hemorrhage common

- **Venous Malformation**
  - Key facts
    - Lobulated soft tissue mass; variably sized venous channels with phleboliths
    - Mass increases in size with Valsalva, crying, or bending over
  - Imaging
    - Intermediate attenuation/hyperintense T2 with variable contrast enhancement
    - No high flow vessels
- **Infantile Hemangioma**
  - Key facts
    - Neoplasm with spontaneous proliferation & involution
    - Present within 1st few weeks of life; usually not present at birth
    - May be multiple (PHACES syndrome)
  - Imaging
    - Lobulated mass, intense enhancement
    - High flow intralesional vessels
- **Neurofibromatosis Type 1**
  - Key facts
    - Localized neurofibroma (NF), diffuse NF, plexiform NF (PNF), or malignant peripheral nerve sheath tumor (PNST)
    - Multiple or plexiform, think NF1
  - Imaging
    - May be hypoattenuating on CT
    - Localized: Well-circumscribed, fusiform, solid masses & moderate enhancement ± dumbbell-shaped extension into neural foramina
    - Diffuse NF: Plaque-like subcutaneous lesion with poorly defined infiltrating margins, moderate enhancement
    - Plexiform NF: Lobulated, tortuous, rope-like enlargement in major nerve distribution; resembles tangle of worms
    - Malignant PNST: Benign vs. malignant difficult to differentiate on imaging; consider malignant if ≥ 5 cm, intensely enhancing with infiltrative margins
- **Rhabdomyosarcoma**
  - Key facts
    - Sites: Orbit, nasopharynx, temporal bone, sinonasal, cervical neck
  - Imaging
    - Soft tissue mass with variable contrast enhancement ± bone erosion
    - Coronal post-contrast fat-saturated T1 images best for intracranial extension

Helpful Clues for Less Common Diagnoses
- **Lipoma**
  - Key facts: Benign neoplasm, mature fat
  - Imaging
    - Well-circumscribed homogeneous mass of fat attenuation & signal intensity
    - Small minority of lesions will have a nonfatty soft tissue component
    - Any space of neck
    - Single space or trans-spatial
    - Imaging can not differentiate between lipoma & low grade liposarcoma
- **Thymic Cyst**
  - Key facts
    - Remnant of thymopharyngeal duct, 3rd branchial pouch remnant
    - Wall contains Hassall corpuscles
  - Imaging
    - Cystic neck mass along course of thymopharyngeal duct ± solid enhancing thymic tissue
    - Close association with carotid sheath
    - May be connected to mediastinal thymus directly or by fibrous cord
    - Rarely extends to skull base; may rupture into parapharyngeal space
- **4th Branchial Anomaly**
  - Key facts
    - Presents with recurrent thyroiditis or anterior neck abscess secondary to sinus tract extending from apex of pyriform sinus to lower anterior neck
  - Imaging
    - Cyst or abscess anterior to left thyroid lobe with associated thyroiditis
    - Barium swallow or post barium swallow CT may show sinus tract extending from apex of pyriform sinus to anterior lower neck

Helpful Clues for Rare Diagnoses
- **Teratoma**
  - Key facts
    - All 3 germ cell lines
    - Mature, immature, and malignant
  - Imaging: Fat, calcium, cystic, and solid components
- **Fibromatosis**
  - Key facts
    - Synonyms: Desmoid fibromatosis, extra-abdominal desmoid fibromatosis, infantile fibromatosis
    - Histologically benign fibroproliferative disorder with potentially aggressive clinical course & invasive growth
    - Associated with Gardner syndrome
  - Imaging
    - Poorly marginated trans-spatial mass
    - Moderate post-contrast enhancement
    - ± Bone erosion or invasion

SELECTED REFERENCES

1. Castellote A et al: Cervicothoracic lesions in infants and children. Radiographics. 19(3):583-600, 1999
2. Benson MT et al: Congenital anomalies of the branchial apparatus: embryology and pathologic anatomy. Radiographics. 12(5):943-60, 1992

Abscess

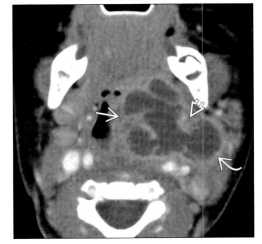

Axial CECT shows a large, multilobulated, rim-enhancing abscess arising from the left palatine tonsil ➡, spreading into the parapharyngeal space ➡ with extension to the deep parotid space ➡.

Lymphatic Malformation

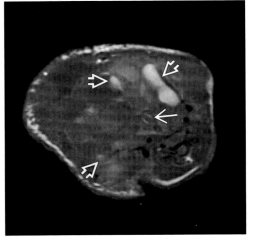

Axial T1WI MR shows an infiltrative, multiloculated, macrocystic neck lymphatic malformation, anterior to the suprastomal trachea ➡. Cysts contain hyperintense T1 signal fluid from hemorrhage ➡.

TRANS-SPATIAL MASS IN CHILD

(Left) Axial T1 C+ FS MR reveals a well-defined lobulated heterogeneously enhancing venous malformation involving the left masseter muscle ➡ and medial pterygoid muscle ➡. Note focal signal voids secondary to phleboliths in both the deep and superficial component ➡. *(Right)* Axial CECT shows a lobulated, heterogeneously enhancing venous malformation ➡ in the left cheek with a moderate amount of fat and multiple variably sized phleboliths ➡.

Venous Malformation

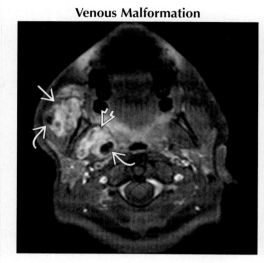

Venous Malformation

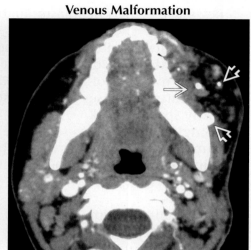

(Left) Axial T1 C+ FS MR demonstrates a homogeneously enhancing infantile hemangioma involving the left carotid space ➡, posterior cervical space of the neck ➡, and the left submandibular space ➡. *(Right)* Axial CECT shows an infiltrative low attenuation plexiform neurofibroma involving the retropharyngeal space ➡ and the left carotid space ➡ and extending between the compressed left pyriform sinus and hyoid bone ➡.

Infantile Hemangioma

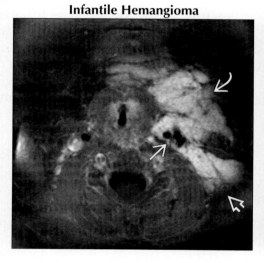

Neurofibromatosis Type 1

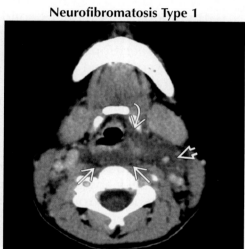

(Left) Axial STIR MR reveals an infiltrative hyperintense plexiform neurofibroma involving the retropharyngeal space ➡, the left carotid space ➡, & parapharyngeal space ➡. Plexiform neurofibroma signals neurofibromatosis 1. *(Right)* Axial T2WI FS MR shows a large heterogeneously enhancing rhabdomyosarcoma involving the left masticator space ➡ and deep parotid space ➡. Note the rhabdomyosarcoma erodes the mandible ➡.

Neurofibromatosis Type 1

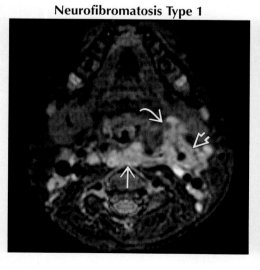

Rhabdomyosarcoma

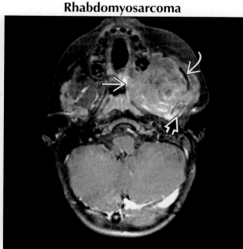

Lipoma

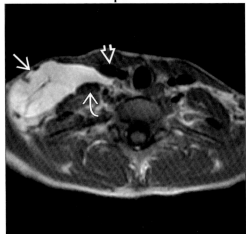

Thymic Cyst

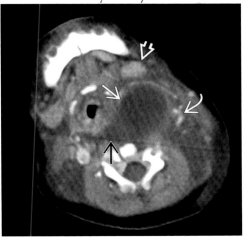

(Left) Axial T1WI MR demonstrates a well-defined right posterior cervical space lipoma ➔ insinuating between the internal jugular vein ➔ and the anterior scalene muscle ➔, resulting in mild leftward deviation of the trachea. (Right) Axial CECT reveals a large thymic cyst ➔ posterior to the left submandibular gland ➔, anteromedial to the carotid vessels ➔, and extending to the retropharyngeal space ➔.

Thymic Cyst

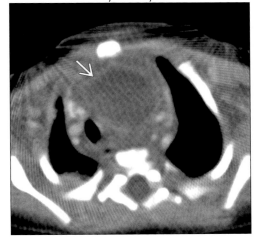

4th Branchial Anomaly

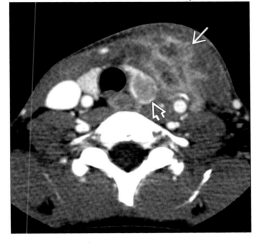

(Left) Axial CECT demonstrates a well-defined thymic cyst in the superior mediastinum ➔ that is contiguous with cyst in the left neck (not shown). (Right) Axial CECT reveals a heterogeneously enhancing inflammatory mass ➔ anterior to the left thyroid lobe, which contains a focal area of decreased enhancement consistent with focal thyroiditis ➔. Both are secondary to a 4th branchial pouch remnant (pyriform apex sinus tract).

Teratoma

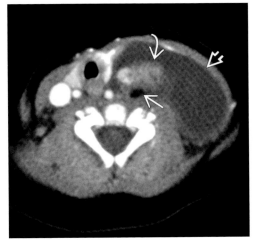

Fibromatosis

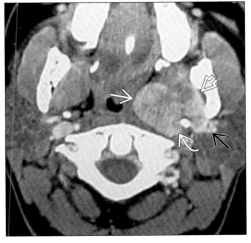

(Left) Axial CECT shows a low attenuation trans-spatial benign cystic teratoma that contains fat ➔, as well as cystic ➔ & solid ➔ components. The visceral, carotid, & posterior cervical spaces are all affected. (Right) Axial CECT reveals enhancing trans-spatial mass of the left parapharyngeal space ➔, masticator space ➔, carotid space ➔, & deep parotid space ➔. Pathologic diagnosis of fibromatosis was made in this patient with Gardner syndrome.

TRANS-SPATIAL NECK MASS

DIFFERENTIAL DIAGNOSIS

Common
- Abscess
- Venolymphatic Malformation
- Venous Malformation
- Lymphatic Malformation
- Squamous Cell Carcinoma
- Plexiform Neurofibroma

Less Common
- Infantile Hemangioma
- Lipoma
- Non-Hodgkin Lymphoma
- Anaplastic Carcinoma, Thyroid
- Non-Hodgkin Lymphoma, Thyroid

Rare but Important
- Fibromatosis
- Rhabdomyosarcoma

ESSENTIAL INFORMATION

Key Differential Diagnosis Issues
- Trans-spatial mass involves multiple contiguous spaces in neck
- Broadly divided into 2 groups of lesions
  - Congenital: Develop before deep cervical fascia fully formed
    - Venous &/or lymphatic malformation
    - Hemangioma
    - Plexiform neurofibroma
  - Acquired: Break through fascial layers
    - Aggressive infection
    - Malignant neoplasm
- Imaging strategies
  - CECT: 1st step for presumed infection
  - MR C+: May better characterize lesion
    - Best demonstrates full extent of congenital or neoplastic lesion

Helpful Clues for Common Diagnoses
- Abscess
  - Key facts
    - Most often of dental origin
    - Superficial infection may spread to deep face and narrow airway
    - Deep face infections may spread inferiorly to mediastinum
  - Imaging
    - CECT: Heterogeneously enhancing edematous tissues, ± focal fluid collection
    - Always assess airway & vascular patency

- Venolymphatic Malformation
  - Key facts
    - Congenital vascular malformation
    - Both venous & lymphatic components
  - Imaging
    - Lymphatic component: Saccular with fluid characteristics, ± blood-fluid levels
    - Venous component: Saccular or reticular with solid enhancement, ± phleboliths
    - MR: Both components T2 hyperintense, phleboliths hypointense
- Venous Malformation
  - Key facts
    - Congenital slow-flow vascular mass
    - Margins lobulated and infiltrative
  - Imaging
    - CT: Phleboliths are specific finding
    - MR: T2 hyperintense, infiltrative mass with moderate enhancement
- Lymphatic Malformation
  - Key facts
    - Congenital lymph tissue malformation
    - Uni- or multiloculated cystic mass
  - Imaging
    - CT: Fluid density well-defined thin-walled mass, ± blood-fluid levels
    - MR: Blood-fluid levels more readily apparent, no significant enhancement
- Squamous Cell Carcinoma
  - Key facts
    - Most common H&N neoplasm
    - Deep spread usually indicates T4 stage
    - Nodal conglomerates may also involve multiple spaces
  - Imaging
    - Mass arising from pharyngeal mucosa
    - Image with either CT or MR, but MR will better delineate deep extent
    - Adenopathy common; ± necrotic or cystic
- Plexiform Neurofibroma
  - Key facts
    - Benign Schwann cell tumor of small peripheral nerves
    - Diagnostic of neurofibromatosis type 1
  - Imaging
    - Infiltrating but lobulated mass
    - Mimics vascular malformation
    - CECT: "Cystic," minimally enhancing
    - T2 MR: Rounded lobules with central "target," moderate enhancement

Helpful Clues for Less Common Diagnoses

- **Infantile Hemangioma**
  - Key facts
    - Benign endothelial cell neoplasm
    - Presents in 1st 3 months, proliferates during 1st year, most involuted by age 9
  - Imaging
    - Changes with proliferative (PP) and involutional (IP) phase
    - PP: T2 hyperintense, marked enhancement, flow voids
    - IP: CT & MR heterogeneous texture with fatty replacement
- **Lipoma**
  - Key facts
    - Benign neoplasm of mature fat
    - Often found in posterior cervical & submandibular spaces
  - Imaging
    - CT: Nonenhancing homogeneous fat density mass
    - MR: Well-defined mass; always follows fat signal, no enhancement
- **Non-Hodgkin Lymphoma**
  - Key facts
    - Nodal disease may form large masses
    - Extranodal lymphatic disease (tonsils) may invade deep spaces
    - Extranodal extralymphatic disease may present as H&N mass
  - Imaging
    - Depends on form of non-Hodgkin lymphoma (NHL)
    - Homogeneous → heterogeneous with higher grade
- **Anaplastic Carcinoma, Thyroid**
  - Key facts
    - Aggressive undifferentiated tumor
  - Imaging
    - Heterogeneous infiltrative mass
    - Calcification and necrosis common
- **Non-Hodgkin Lymphoma, Thyroid**
  - Key facts
    - Thyroid is primary NHL site
  - Imaging
    - Single/multiple/diffuse thyroid forms
    - Tumor tends to be homogeneous without calcifications or necrosis

Helpful Clues for Rare Diagnoses

- **Fibromatosis**
  - Key facts
    - Benign neoplasm of fibroblast origin with infiltrative appearance
    - Often supraclavicular or masticator space
  - Imaging
    - CT: Homogeneous, mild enhancement
    - MR: T2 intermediate to low signal, moderate enhancement
- **Rhabdomyosarcoma**
  - Key facts
    - Skeletal cell soft tissue sarcoma
    - Children → young adults; 70% < 12 years
  - Imaging
    - CT: Muscle density infiltrative mass
    - MR: Heterogeneous signal & enhancement, ± hemorrhage

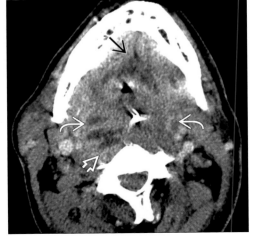

Abscess

Axial CECT through oral cavity demonstrates marked swelling & heterogeneity of floor of mouth ➔ and oropharyngeal ➔ & retropharyngeal spaces ➔ in a patient with a partially treated left dental infection.

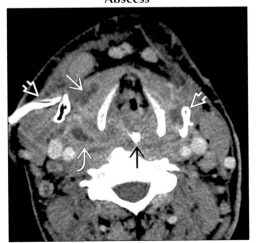

Abscess

Axial CECT in the same patient shows extensive swelling with involvement of visceral ➔ & carotid ➔ spaces. More inferior spread also resulted in mediastinitis. Note the presence of drains ➔ & nasogastric tube ➔.

TRANS-SPATIAL NECK MASS

(Left) Axial T2WI FS MR shows markedly hyperintense mass involving superficial neck tissues ⇨ but also infiltrating visceral ⇨ & left posterior cervical space ⇨. **(Right)** Axial T1 C+ FS MR in same patient reveals heterogeneous enhancement of lesion with solidly enhancing visceral space components ⇨, cystic components ⇨, and enhancement of thick septations. This is a recurrence of a partially resected venolymphatic malformation.

Venolymphatic Malformation

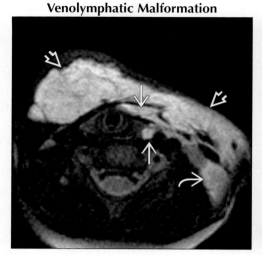

Venolymphatic Malformation

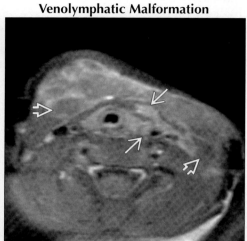

(Left) Axial NECT demonstrates a multilobulated mass with an almost infiltrative appearance, involving buccal ⇨ & masticator ⇨ spaces & superficial tissues of left face ⇨. Well-defined rounded phleboliths ⇨ are clearly evident within mass. **(Right)** Axial STIR MR better illustrates full extent of the trans-spatial mass. Deep extension to the oral cavity ⇨ & parapharyngeal space ⇨ are now seen. Phleboliths appear as hypointense rounded foci ⇨.

Venous Malformation

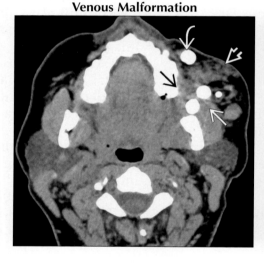

Venous Malformation

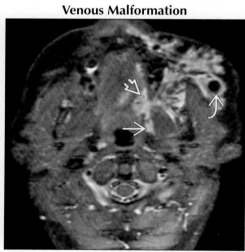

(Left) Axial CECT shows a nonenhancing fluid-density mass in the right neck crossing from submandibular ⇨ to parapharyngeal ⇨ to retropharyngeal space ⇨. The lack of enhancement or phleboliths indicates lesion is lymphatic only. **(Right)** Axial T2WI FS MR in a different patient reveals a multiseptated cystic mass centered in the left posterior cervical space with involvement of adjacent carotid ⇨, submandibular ⇨, and retropharyngeal ⇨ spaces.

Lymphatic Malformation

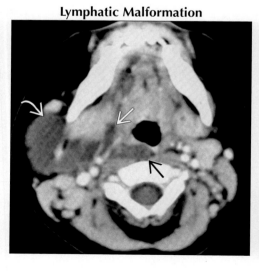

Lymphatic Malformation

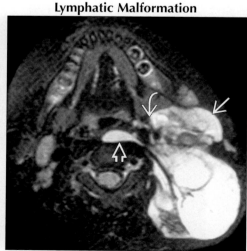

TRANS-SPATIAL NECK MASS

Squamous Cell Carcinoma

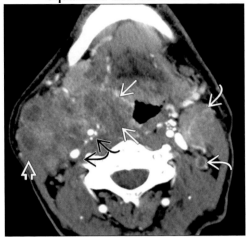

Squamous Cell Carcinoma

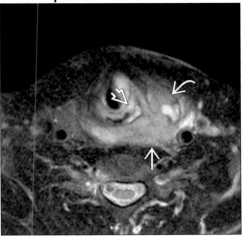

(Left) Axial CECT demonstrates a large heterogeneous mass in the right neck involving the sternocleidomastoid muscle ⮕ & carotid sheath ⮕. This nodal mass appears contiguous with tonsillar SCCa ⮕. Note contralateral nodal metastases also ⮕. *(Right)* Axial T2WI FS MR at level of cricoid cartilage ⮕ shows an infiltrative hypopharyngeal mass ⮕, invading the cartilage laterally into thyroid gland & posteriorly to retropharyngeal tissues ⮕.

Plexiform Neurofibroma

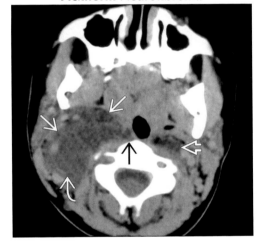

Plexiform Neurofibroma

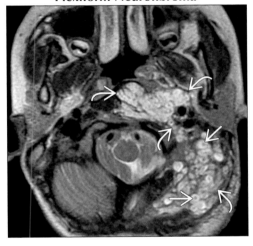

(Left) Axial NECT reveals a dominant right low-density neck mass ⮕ involving the right carotid space but also infiltrating posterior cervical ⮕, parapharyngeal, & retropharyngeal ⮕ spaces. A smaller well-circumscribed lesion of similar density is visible in left carotid space ⮕. *(Right)* Axial T2WI MR shows a trans-spatial hyperintense mass ⮕ composed of multiple contiguous small lobules with central low intensity ⮕, typical of plexiform neurofibroma.

Infantile Hemangioma

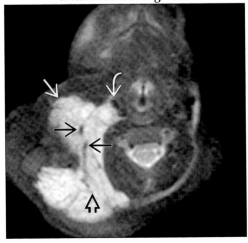

Infantile Hemangioma

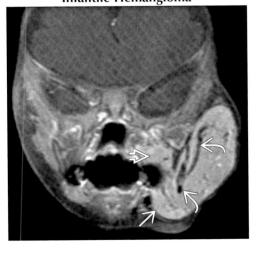

(Left) Axial T2WI FS MR reveals a markedly hyperintense & homogeneous neck mass involving anterior neck ⮕, posterior cervical ⮕ & carotid spaces ⮕. Note prominent central vessels ⮕ in this enlarging mass. *(Right)* Coronal T1 C+ FS MR in 4 month old demonstrates enhancing mass centered on parotid gland but also involving submandibular ⮕ & masticator ⮕ spaces. Note large vessels ⮕ during proliferative growth phase.

Trans-spatial, Multi-spatial in Head and Neck

5

Trans-spatial, Multi-spatial in Head and Neck

(Left) Axial CECT demonstrates a homogeneous low-density nonenhancing mass in the right parapharyngeal space ➡, extending laterally to submandibular space ➡, with posterior displacement of carotid vessels ➡. (Right) Coronal T1WI MR in the same patient reveals a homogeneously hyperintense lipoma as an extensive but well-defined mass involving superficial space ➡. Lipoma also extends around strap muscles ➡ to involve ipsilateral visceral space ➡.

Lipoma

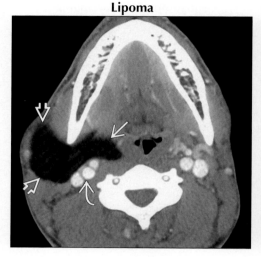

Lipoma

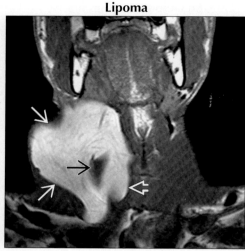

(Left) Axial CECT shows a large right nasopharyngeal mass ➡ extending inferiorly to oropharynx and infiltrating laterally to masticator space with full lateral pterygoid muscle ➡. (Right) Axial CECT shows a homogeneous right tonsillar mass ➡ and ipsilateral posterior cervical and carotid space mass that appears contiguous but which probably represents nodal metastases ➡. These nodal and lymphatic forms of NHL mimic SCCa but are more homogeneous.

Non-Hodgkin Lymphoma

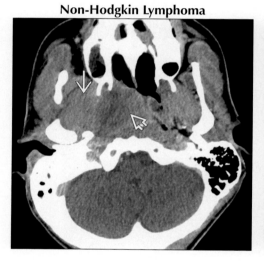

Non-Hodgkin Lymphoma

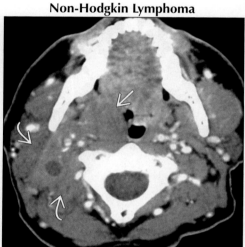

(Left) Axial CECT reveals heterogeneous partially necrotic mass ➡ arising from right thyroid lobe with infiltrating aggressive margins. Mass surrounds carotid ➡ & occludes internal jugular vein. Coarse calcifications ➡ suggest its origin in multinodular goiter. (Right) Axial CECT shows replacement of thyroid by tumor ➡. This heterogeneous mass appears to infiltrate adjacent anterior strap muscles & compresses jugular veins ➡ bilaterally.

Anaplastic Carcinoma, Thyroid

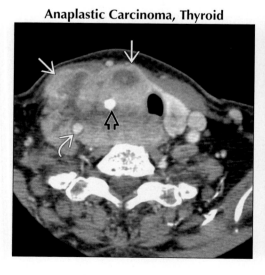

Anaplastic Carcinoma, Thyroid

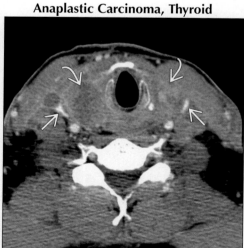

Non-Hodgkin Lymphoma, Thyroid

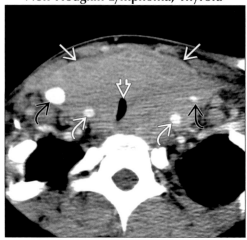

Fibromatosis

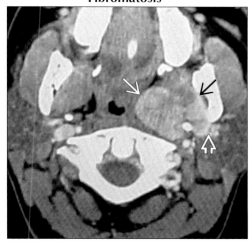

(Left) Axial CECT shows a homogeneous mass ➡ infiltrating adjacent spaces with encasement and displacement of common carotid ➡ and internal jugular veins ➡. The trachea is compressed ➡ also. (Right) Axial CECT demonstrates a moderately enhancing mass ➡ in left parapharyngeal space. While the medial margin is well defined, the lateral margin has infiltrative features with extension into masticator ➡ and carotid spaces and deep parotid lobe ➡.

Fibromatosis

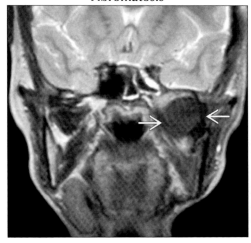

Fibromatosis

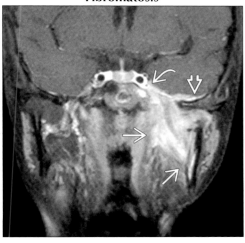

(Left) Coronal T2WI MR in a different patient reveals marked hypointensity and expansion of the left lateral pterygoid muscle ➡. Low signal intensity, when seen, is highly suggestive of fibromatosis. (Right) Coronal T1 C+ FS MR in the same patient shows diffuse enhancement ➡ in the masticator & parapharyngeal spaces, extending through the foramen ovale to the middle fossa ➡ & Meckel cave ➡, along the maxillary division of the trigeminal nerve.

Rhabdomyosarcoma

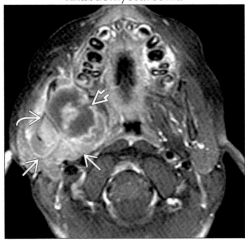

Rhabdomyosarcoma

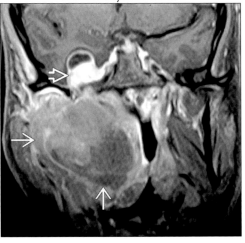

(Left) Axial T1 C+ FS MR shows a heterogeneous partially necrotic mass ➡ arising in the masticator space with mandible destruction ➡ and extensive infiltration of adjacent parotid tissue ➡. (Right) Coronal T1 C+ FS MR shows a markedly heterogeneous mass ➡ centered in the masticator space but infiltrating parapharyngeal space medially and parotid space laterally. The mass extends through foramen ovale and skull base to middle cranial fossa ➡.

HYPERDENSE NECK LESION (CT)

DIFFERENTIAL DIAGNOSIS

Common
- Atherosclerosis, Carotid Artery, Neck
- Multinodular Goiter
- Paraganglioma, Carotid Body
- Non-Hodgkin Lymphoma, Lymph Nodes
- Hodgkin Lymphoma, Lymph Nodes
- Paraganglioma, Glomus Vagale
- Schwannoma, Carotid Space

Less Common
- Infantile Hemangioma
- Chondrosarcoma, Larynx
- Thyroid, Ectopic
- Venous Malformation

Rare but Important
- Giant Lymph Node Hyperplasia (Castleman)
- Hemangiopericytoma
- Pseudoaneurysm, Carotid Artery, Neck
- Tuberculosis, Lymph Nodes
- Differentiated Thyroid Carcinoma, Nodal

ESSENTIAL INFORMATION

Key Differential Diagnosis Issues
- Hyperdense neck lesions on CT result from intrinsic hypercellularity, significant blood pool with avid enhancement, or intramural calcifications
  - High-density cellular lesions: Lymphoma & other nodal diseases
    - Uniform cellularity is a good clue for lymphoma
  - Lesions with significant blood pool effect: Paraganglioma, hemangioma, hemangiopericytoma, Castleman disease
    - Hypervascular lesions suggested by avid enhancement ± enlarged vascular structures
  - Lesions with intramural calcification: Chondroid or fibroosseous lesions, calcifications in granulomatous infections, or thyroid carcinoma adenopathy
- Associate mass with adjacent structures (nodes, thyroid, laryngeal cartilages, vascular structures) to narrow differential diagnosis
- Hypervascular masses may be identified by prominent arterial or venous structures in proximity to lesion
  - Identifying prominent arterial structures can significantly narrow differential diagnosis

Helpful Clues for Common Diagnoses
- **Atherosclerosis, Carotid Artery, Neck**
  - Key facts: Elderly population, association with peripheral & cardiovascular disease
  - Imaging: Circumferential or near-circumferential calcifications often with associated fibrofatty disease
    - Involves walls of carotid artery, predominant near bifurcation, narrows lumen of carotid artery
    - If diagnosis is in doubt, consider vascular imaging (CTA, MRA)
- **Multinodular Goiter**
  - Key facts: More common in elderly, but can be seen in all ages
  - Imaging: Typically involves entire thyroid gland
    - Heterogeneous high-density appearance of enlarged thyroid, with occasional calcifications & cysts
    - May result in significant tracheal & esophageal distortion
    - Despite significant size, remains well defined, does not invade adjacent structures
- **Paraganglioma, Carotid Body**
  - Key facts: 10% multiple if nonfamilial
  - Imaging: High-density lesion with avid enhancement, splays carotid bifurcation
    - May encase internal and external carotid arteries
- **Non-Hodgkin Lymphoma, Lymph Nodes**
  - Imaging: Typically large, uniform ovoid masses in nodal regions
    - Nodes may occasionally have low-density centers
    - Tends toward bilaterality more so than Hodgkin lymphoma
- **Hodgkin Lymphoma, Lymph Nodes**
  - Imaging: Typically large, uniform ovoid masses in nodal regions
    - More commonly unilateral than non-Hodgkin lymphoma
- **Paraganglioma, Glomus Vagale**
  - Key facts: Centered 1-2 cm below skull base in nasopharyngeal carotid space
    - Intimately associated with nodose ganglion of CN10

- Imaging: Carotid space mass with high density, avid enhancement
  - Contiguous enlarged vascular structures
- **Schwannoma, Carotid Space**
  - Key facts: Isolated or associated with NF2
  - Imaging: Enhancing carotid space mass
    - Intramural cysts, fusiform

Helpful Clues for Less Common Diagnoses

- **Infantile Hemangioma**
  - Key facts: Infant or child with skin discoloration
    - Mass usually involves with age
  - Imaging: Avidly enhancing, trans-spatial
- **Chondrosarcoma, Larynx**
  - Key facts: Hoarseness, voice change
  - Imaging: Arcs, rings, & whorls of Ca++
    - Most commonly involves cricoid
- **Thyroid, Ectopic**
  - Key facts: May be no other normal functioning thyroid tissue
  - Imaging: Found in midline in proximity to hyoid bone
    - May arise at tongue base or lateral neck below hyoid
- **Venous Malformation**
  - Key facts: Soft, pliable, longstanding lesion with occasional hyperpigmentation
    - No thrill or bruit; enlarged with Valsalva maneuver
  - Imaging: Phleboliths highly suggestive
    - Trans-spatial mass
    - No prominent arterial structures evident

Helpful Clues for Rare Diagnoses

- **Giant Lymph Node Hyperplasia (Castleman)**
  - Key facts: Nodal disease of neck & chest
  - Imaging: Avidly enhancing, multiple enlarged nodes
- **Hemangiopericytoma**
  - Key facts: Sinonasal, dural, perivertebral
  - Imaging: Hypervascular mass with prominent arterial & venous structures
- **Pseudoaneurysm, Carotid Artery, Neck**
  - Key facts: Organized, often lamellar layers of thrombus in wall of pseudoaneurysm
    - When found between bifurcation to skull base, dissection is suspected
  - Imaging: Follows arterial lumen into lesion
    - Avidly enhancing enlarged lumen with nonenhancing thick asymmetric "wall"
- **Tuberculosis, Lymph Nodes**
  - Key facts: Risk factors are HIV, weight loss, and travel to endemic regions
  - Imaging: Heterogeneous nodal masses with soft tissue abscesses
- **Differentiated Thyroid Carcinoma, Nodal**
  - Key facts: Primary tumor may be small
    - Nodes may be remote from visceral space
  - Imaging: Nodes with cystic, solid enhancement ± calcifications
    - Any nodal chain may be involved
    - Mistakes made in diagnosis when remote nodal involvement present with small primary tumor

---

Atherosclerosis, Carotid Artery, Neck

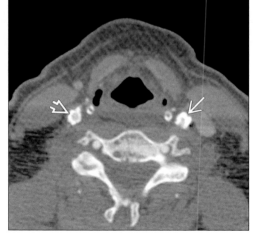

Axial CTA shows extensive calcifications of the left common carotid artery ➡️. *Patient has stent on contralateral side* ➡️. *Circumferential & eccentric calcifications are common in atherosclerotic vascular disease.*

Multinodular Goiter

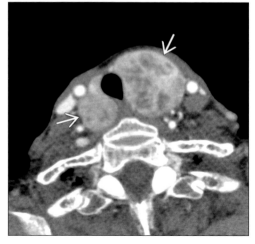

Axial CECT reveals heterogeneous multinodular goiter ➡️. *High density within goiter is due to enhancement, iodine, and calcifications. Bilateral enlargement of thyroid lobes occurs, but asymmetrically.*

HYPERDENSE NECK LESION (CT)

Paraganglioma, Carotid Body

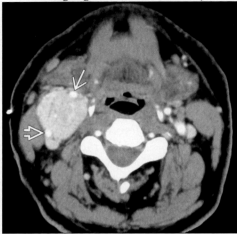

Non-Hodgkin Lymphoma, Lymph Nodes

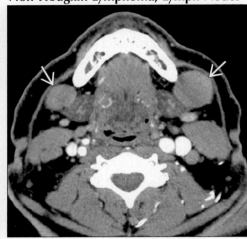

(Left) Axial CECT demonstrates a homogeneously enhancing carotid body paraganglioma splaying the external ➡ and internal ⇨ carotid arteries. This tumor type is often isodense to arteries and veins. *(Right)* Axial CECT shows multiple uniform submandibular lymph nodes ➡ that enhance slightly more than the neck muscles. Large nonnecrotic lymph nodes in unusual neck nodal chains are highly suggestive of lymphoma.

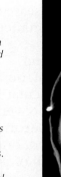

Hodgkin Lymphoma, Lymph Nodes

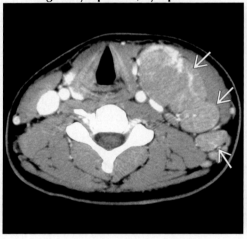

Paraganglioma, Glomus Vagale

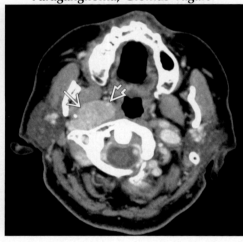

(Left) Axial CECT reveals unilateral bulky Hodgkin lymphoma nodes ➡ that enhance more avidly than the neck musculature does. This patient presented with night sweats, fevers, and neck masses. *(Right)* Axial CECT shows large glomus vagale paraganglioma ➡ as an enhancing mass in the nasopharyngeal carotid space. The tumor displaces the carotid artery ⇨ anteriorly and medially. Paraganglioma may appear similar to schwannoma in same location.

Schwannoma, Carotid Space

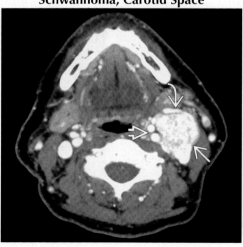

Infantile Hemangioma

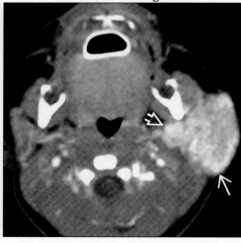

(Left) Axial CECT shows large carotid space vascular schwannoma mimicking paraganglioma. The avidly enhancing lobulated soft tissue mass ➡ does not splay carotids ⇨, which are displaced medially. Internal jugular vein ➡ is draped over the anterior surface of the schwannoma. *(Right)* Axial CECT demonstrates holoparotid infantile hemangioma as a diffusely enlarged left parotid gland that enhances both the superficial ➡ and deep ⇨ lobes.

5

Chondrosarcoma, Larynx
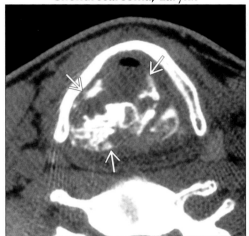

Thyroid, Ectopic
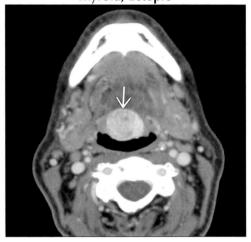

(Left) Axial NECT depicts cricoid chondrosarcoma as a lobulated mass with ring- & arc-like calcification, expansion, and sclerosis of cricoid cartilage ➡. Notice the near complete occlusion of the airway. *(Right)* Axial CECT reveals a large lingual thyroid ➡ as a round high-density mass at foramen cecum. The neck must be evaluated for normal thyroid tissue, as resection of ectopic tissue could result in acute profound hypothyroidism.

Venous Malformation
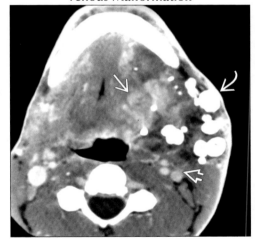

Giant Lymph Node Hyperplasia (Castleman)
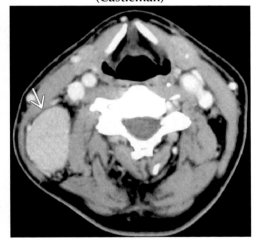

(Left) Axial CECT shows a trans-spatial venous malformation involving the left submandibular, sublingual ➡, & carotid ➡ spaces. The submandibular space contains the majority of the phleboliths ➡. *(Right)* Axial CECT reveals a large high-density enhancing node in the right spinal accessory chain ➡ in this patient with giant lymph node hyperplasia (Castleman disease).

Hemangiopericytoma
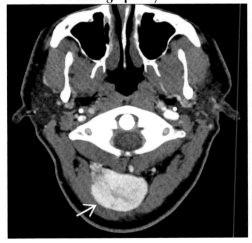

Pseudoaneurysm, Carotid Artery, Neck
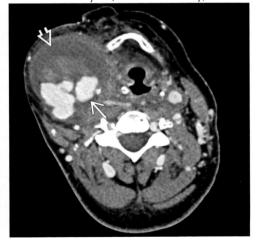

(Left) Axial CECT shows an avidly enhancing mass ➡ in the paraspinal aspect of the perivertebral space. Initially thought to be a vascular schwannoma, this lesion proved to be a hemangiopericytoma. *(Right)* Axial CECT shows a large complex pseudoaneurysm arising from the distal right common carotid artery with irregular filling of the enhancing hyperdense pseudoaneurysm lumen ➡. Lamellated thrombus is evident ➡, filling the pseudoaneurysm sac.

LOW-DENSITY NECK LESION (CT)

DIFFERENTIAL DIAGNOSIS

Common
- Tornwaldt Cyst
- SCCa, Nodes
- Abscess
- Suppurative Lymph Nodes

Less Common
- Thyroglossal Duct Cyst
- 2nd Branchial Cleft Cyst
- Lymphatic Malformation
- Lipoma
- Neurofibroma, Carotid Space
- Dermoid and Epidermoid
- Ranula

Rare but Important
- Thyroid Carcinoma, Nodal
- Tuberculosis, Lymph Nodes
- Thymic Cyst

ESSENTIAL INFORMATION

Key Differential Diagnosis Issues
- Low density on CT suggests either fluid or fatty density
  - Some solid lesions have characteristic low density (lipoma, neurofibroma)
- Presence of uniform low density or central low density may help suggest different diagnoses
- Peripheral enhancement should suggest necrosis & inflammatory/infectious lesions or tumor
- Developmental lesions may be midline or off-midline

Helpful Clues for Common Diagnoses
- **Tornwaldt Cyst**
  - Key facts: Seen incidentally on ~ 5% of all brain MRs; rarely symptomatic
  - Imaging: Midline nasopharyngeal cystic mass commonly of fluid density
    - Sits just anteromedial to prevertebral muscles in midline nasopharynx
- **SCCa, Nodes**
  - Key facts: Squamous cell carcinoma metastases from any H&N primary tumor in appropriate patient (history of smoking)
    - Caveat: 2nd branchial cleft cyst in adult should be considered cystic SCCa node until proven otherwise!

- Other malignancies may result in low-density nodes, i.e., thyroid carcinoma
  - Imaging: Round nodes with low density centers in drainage routes of known primary SCCa
- **Abscess**
  - Key facts: Abscess generally occurs in node-bearing spaces or adjacent to mandible
    - Node-bearing spaces: Retropharyngeal (RPS), parotid (PS), submandibular (SMS), posterior cervical (PCS)
    - Adjacent to mandible: Masticator (MS), sublingual space (SLS)
    - Sick patient with hot, tender neck mass
  - Imaging: Heterogeneous, irregular thick-walled collection with adjacent fat stranding
    - May be trans-spatial (multiple contiguous spaces)
- **Suppurative Lymph Nodes**
  - Key facts: Clinical history usually suggestive of infection
  - Imaging: Frequently found in clusters with adjacent fat stranding & fascial or skin thickening
    - Nodes may appear heterogeneous with low-density center

Helpful Clues for Less Common Diagnoses
- **Thyroglossal Duct Cyst**
  - Key facts: Child or young adult
    - Most common congenital lesion in neck
    - Found anywhere along thyroglossal duct from foramen cecum to infrahyoid neck
  - Imaging
    - Midline location (tongue base or perihyoid) or immediately paramedian in infrahyoid neck
    - Often intimately related to mid-body of hyoid bone
- **2nd Branchial Cleft Cyst**
  - Key facts: Should only considered as 1st diagnosis if young patient
  - Imaging: Embryologically defined location in posterior SMS
    - Well-defined, thin-rimmed cyst, typically located in posterior SMS
- **Lymphatic Malformation**
  - Key facts: May be found in any space in head and neck

- Often trans-spatial
  - Imaging findings: Heterogeneous, multilocular
    - May see fluid-debris levels in lesions
- **Lipoma**
  - Key facts: May be found in any space in head and neck
  - Imaging: Uniform fat density
    - Larger lesions may have some septations
- **Neurofibroma, Carotid Space**
  - Key facts: Isolated or in association with neurofibromatosis type 1 (NF1)
  - Imaging: Often has characteristic intermediate density (between soft tissue & fat)
    - If plexiform (complex, intertwined appearance), diagnostic of NF1
- **Dermoid and Epidermoid**
  - Key facts: Midline lesions that may occur in variety of locations
    - Locations include SLS, SMS, root of tongue, anterior neuropore, & roof of nasopharynx
  - Imaging: Dermoid & epidermoid may be indistinguishable
    - Epidermoid: DWI restricted diffusion; homogeneously cystic
    - Dermoid: Internal fatty elements or other mesenchymal components
- **Ranula**
  - Key facts
    - Simple ranula: SLS only; "bluish" mass under tongue

- Diving ranula: SLS & SMS; blottable mass in submandibular space
  - Imaging
    - Simple ranula: Ovoid cystic mass in SLS
    - Diving ranula: Cystic mass in SMS with SLS "tail"

Helpful Clues for Rare Diagnoses

- **Thyroid Carcinoma, Nodal**
  - Key facts: Nodal neck mass in 20-40 year old women
  - Imaging: Nodes with cystic and solid enhancing components
    - Primary thyroid tumor may be subtle
- **Tuberculosis, Lymph Nodes**
  - Key facts: Immunosuppressed patient, foreign national, traveler to endemic area
  - Imaging: Multiple cystic-necrotic nodes
    - May be accompanied by soft tissue abscesses with skin fistula
- **Thymic Cyst**
  - Key facts: More common in left neck, extend to mediastinum
  - Imaging: Left low cervical neck cyst between thyroid lobe and carotid space
    - May be large, bilobed with components in lower neck and mediastinum
    - Cervical-thoracic junction causes lesion to have "isthmus"

SELECTED REFERENCES

1. Turkington JR et al: Neck masses in children. Br J Radiol. 78(925):75-85, 2005

Tornwaldt Cyst

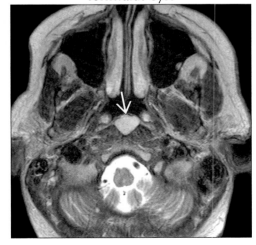

Axial T2WI MR reveals a medium-sized Tornwaldt cyst as a focal cyst in the midline of the nasopharyngeal mucosal space ➡. Note that the lesion sits between the prevertebral muscles.

SCCa, Nodes

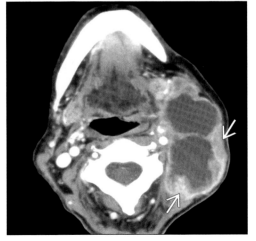

Axial CECT shows a typical case of multiple cystic SCCa nodal metastases. While nodes are largely cystic, the irregular peripheral enhancement ➡ suggests the diagnosis.

LOW-DENSITY NECK LESION (CT)

(Left) *Axial CECT demonstrates a rim-enhancing low-density abscess ➡ in the root of the tongue. Most neck abscesses will be accompanied by constitutional symptoms, i.e., leukocytosis, fever, and local inflammatory changes.* **(Right)** *Axial CECT shows a case of a large mass of matted suppurative nodes. Scans through the upper neck show a large mass in the left neck ➡ with central low density.*

Abscess

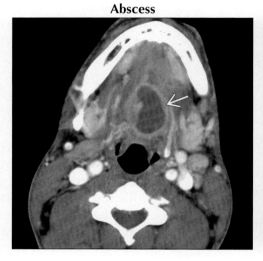

Suppurative Lymph Nodes

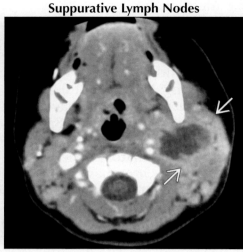

(Left) *Axial CECT shows the typical CT appearance of a suprahyoid thyroglossal duct cyst at tongue base in the area of the foramen cecum ➡.* **(Right)** *Axial CECT reveals a nonenhancing low-density cyst anterior to the sternocleidomastoid muscle ➡, lateral to the carotid space ➡, and posterior to the submandibular gland ➡. A cystic lesion in this location in a child is nearly always 2nd branchial apparatus cyst, or less likely, a lymphatic malformation.*

Thyroglossal Duct Cyst

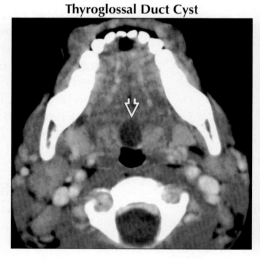

2nd Branchial Cleft Cyst

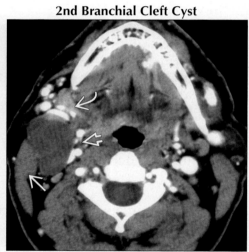

(Left) *Axial CECT demonstrates the appearance of lymphatic malformation of the submandibular and retropharyngeal spaces. This low attenuation, nonenhancing mass is trans-spatial, with extension into the right retropharyngeal space ➡.* **(Right)** *Axial CECT reveals a posterior cervical space lipoma. The mass is a well-defined fat density lesion ➡ with minimal internal septations. It tends to distort local anatomy.*

Lymphatic Malformation

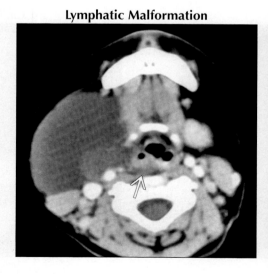

Lipoma

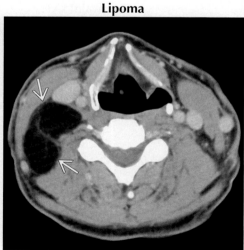

LOW-DENSITY NECK LESION (CT)

Neurofibroma, Carotid Space

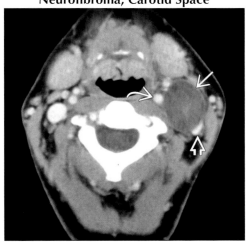

Dermoid and Epidermoid

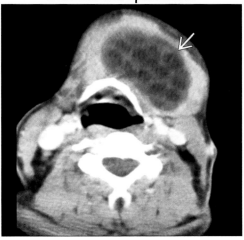

(Left) Axial CECT shows typical intermediate density appearance of a carotid space neurofibroma. Note the well-circumscribed low-density neurofibroma in the carotid space ➡ splaying the jugular vein ➡ and carotid artery ➡. (Right) Axial CECT reveals a large well-circumscribed, low-density dermoid with multiple rounded fatty density structures contained within the mass ➡.

Ranula

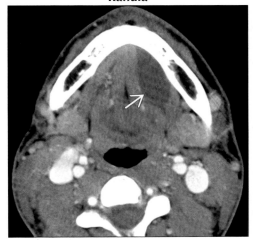

Thyroid Carcinoma, Nodal

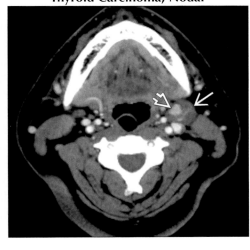

(Left) Axial CECT reveals a large simple ranula of the left sublingual space ➡. Note the lack of perceptible walls and the absence of spread into the submandibular space. (Right) Axial CECT shows a left jugulodigastric "cystic" node ➡ with nodular enhancement ➡ anteromedially. Careful review of the left thyroid lobe revealed a small primary differentiated thyroid carcinoma (not shown).

Tuberculosis, Lymph Nodes

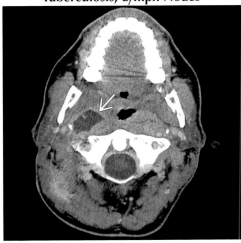

Thymic Cyst

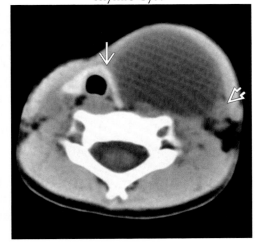

(Left) Axial CECT demonstrates a retropharyngeal node TB adenitis ➡ that is losing its ovoid configuration and will soon rupture into the rest of the retropharyngeal space. (Right) Axial NECT reveals a thymic cyst as a low-attenuation, well-defined mass in the left neck deviating the thyroid gland ➡ medially and the carotid space laterally ➡. CT appearance and location are classic for thymic cyst.

HYPERVASCULAR NECK LESION (CT/MR)

DIFFERENTIAL DIAGNOSIS

Common
• Paraganglioma, Carotid Body
• Paraganglioma, Glomus Vagale
• Schwannoma, Hypervascular Variant
• Venous Malformation
• Infantile Hemangioma

Less Common
• Metastasis
• Arteriovenous Malformation
• Thyroid Carcinoma, Nodal
• Hemangiopericytoma

Rare but Important
• Meningioma, Carotid Space
• Adenoma, Parathyroid, Visceral Space
• Adenoma, Parathyroid, Ectopic

ESSENTIAL INFORMATION

Key Differential Diagnosis Issues
• Hypervascularity suggested by presence of enhancing vessels on CT or MR or by numerous flow voids on MR
  ○ Flow voids on MR may appear as "pepper" (black dots or lines) on spin echo images
  ○ Prominent vascular structures may be seen adjacent to lesion, supporting hypervascular assessment
  ○ MR tends to be more sensitive & specific as to vascular nature of lesion
  ○ MRA can be useful on occasion
• Hypervascular lesion on CT may show particularly avid enhancement compared to noncontrast study
  ○ CTA also useful in defining vascular nature of suspect mass
  ○ Other useful tools include ultrasound & angiography

Helpful Clues for Common Diagnoses
• **Paraganglioma, Carotid Body**
  ○ Key facts: Characteristically splays ECA & ICA in carotid bifurcation
    ▪ Often multiple (> 10% in nonfamilial group)
  ○ Imaging: "Salt and pepper" MR appearance is highly suggestive of this diagnosis
    ▪ May see dilated arterial and venous structures in contiguity with lesion

  ▪ Careful evaluation of internal and external carotid important, as lesion may encase both proximal vessels
• **Paraganglioma, Glomus Vagale**
  ○ Key facts: Characteristic location is ~ 2 cm below skull base in nasopharyngeal carotid space
    ▪ Found in nodose ganglion of vagus nerve in this location
    ▪ Surgical removal will result in vagus nerve injury
  ○ Imaging: "Salt and pepper" MR appearance is highly suggestive of this diagnosis
    ▪ Angiography, often prelude to embolization, will demonstrate arteriovenous shunting
    ▪ Remember tendency for multiplicity; evaluate for additional lesions
• **Schwannoma, Hypervascular Variant**
  ○ Key facts: Locations along carotid sheath, perivertebral space, any region with typical neural structures
    ▪ Typically not hypervascular
    ▪ Occasional hypervascular variant schwannoma often misdiagnosed
  ○ Imaging: Hypervascular variant has prominent flow voids
    ▪ Characteristic "puddling" of contrast on angiography
    ▪ Note: Angiographic appearance may be best distinction between similar-appearing hypervascular vagal schwannoma & glomus vagale paraganglioma
    ▪ Schwannoma: "Puddling" of contrast
    ▪ Paraganglioma: Arteriovenous shunting
• **Venous Malformation**
  ○ Key facts: Lesion composed of enlarged, dysplastic venous structures without Arteriovenous shunting
    ▪ Clinical clues include soft, often "doughy" lesions with discoloration
  ○ Imaging: Often trans-spatial (multiple contiguous space involved)
    ▪ Phleboliths, absence of prominent arterial structures
• **Infantile Hemangioma**
  ○ Key facts: Present at or near birth
    ▪ Characteristic in clinical appearance
    ▪ Undergo proliferative phase, then progressively involute

○ Imaging: Often trans-spatial
  ▪ Diffuse avid enhancement is the rule
  ▪ No phleboliths

Helpful Clues for Less Common Diagnoses

• **Metastasis**
  ○ Key facts: Hypervascular tumors may give rise to hypervascular metastasis
    ▪ Nodal disease occasionally hypervascular with tumors
    ▪ Clinical clue: History of malignancy with tendency to hypervascularity, such as renal cell, choriocarcinoma, others
  ○ Imaging: Invasive soft tissue mass with prominent vascular flow voids (MR) or marked enhancement (CECT)

• **Arteriovenous Malformation**
  ○ Key facts: H&N hypervascular lesions with arteriovenous shunting uncommon
    ▪ Clinical clues: Palpable thrill or audible bruit over lesion = evidence of hyperdynamic flow
  ○ Imaging: Prominent arterial feeders, with dilated veins draining nidus are characteristic
    ▪ MRA or CTA may provide additional useful information
    ▪ Occasional calcifications in arterialized venous structures
    ▪ Careful angiographic study with embolization for either definitive therapy or pre-operative staging

• **Thyroid Carcinoma, Nodal**
  ○ Key facts: Mistaken for paraganglioma

○ Imaging: Flow voids (MR) or intense enhancement (CECT)
    ▪ Cystic component possible
• **Hemangiopericytoma**
  ○ Key facts: Perivertebral space mass common; any space possible
    ▪ Multiple other rare locations in H&N including orbit
  ○ Imaging: Prominent arterial feeders to avidly enhancing mass

Helpful Clues for Rare Diagnoses

• **Meningioma, Carotid Space**
  ○ Key facts: Dural-based mass extends contiguously into carotid space
  ○ Imaging: Hyperostosis of skull base in proximity to lesion = important clue
    ▪ Bilobed lesion from basal cistern to carotid space with jugular foramen waist
    ▪ Calcifications possible
• **Adenoma, Parathyroid, Visceral Space**
  ○ Key facts: Patient being imaged for hyperparathyroidism
  ○ Imaging: Intense enhancement of tracheoesophageal groove mass
• **Adenoma, Parathyroid, Ectopic**
  ○ Key facts: Adenoma outside visceral space
    ▪ Patient has hyperparathyroidism
  ○ Imaging: Intensely enhancing mass in cervicothoracic junction or superior mediastinum

Paraganglioma, Carotid Body

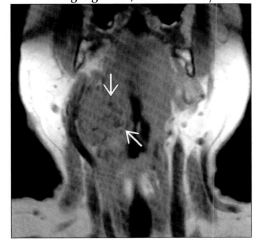

Coronal T1WI MR shows a large carotid body paraganglioma with multiple signal voids ➡. *Location at the carotid bifurcation is characteristic of this lesion with splaying of internal & external carotids.*

Paraganglioma, Carotid Body

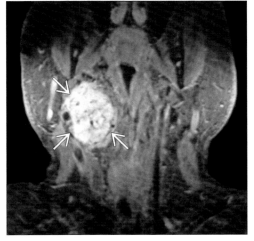

Coronal T1 C+ FS MR depicts an avidly enhancing carotid body paraganglioma ➡. *Despite contrast, multiple flow voids (black dots) remain apparent within paraganglioma parenchyma.*

HYPERVASCULAR NECK LESION (CT/MR)

(Left) *Axial T1 C+ FS MR shows a glomus vagale paraganglioma centered below the skull base in the nasopharyngeal carotid space. Prominent flow voids* ➡ *are evident within the avidly enhancing lesion and indicate its hypervascular nature.* *(Right)* *Coronal T1 C+ FS MR demonstrates an ovoid, avidly enhancing glomus vagale tumor centered below the skull base. Vessels in cross section are round or ovoid* ⊳, *while those in plane are linear in appearance* ➡.

Paraganglioma, Glomus Vagale

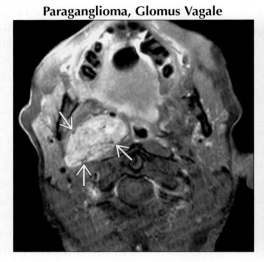

Paraganglioma, Glomus Vagale

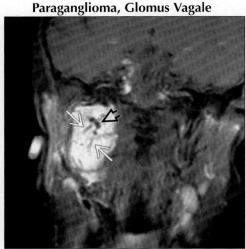

(Left) *Axial CECT reveals a carotid space schwannoma as an avidly enhancing soft tissue mass* ➡ *in the oropharyngeal carotid space, displacing the parapharyngeal space anteriorly.* *(Right)* *Sagittal oblique angiography demonstrates a right external carotid injection of a hypervascular schwannoma variant. Notice the "puddling" of contrast within the tumor parenchyma* ➡.

Schwannoma, Hypervascular Variant

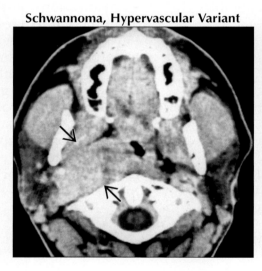

Schwannoma, Hypervascular Variant

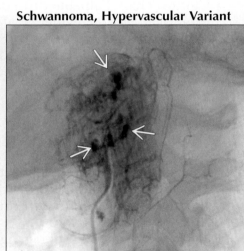

(Left) *Axial STIR MR shows a venous malformation involving oral mucosal, buccal, and masticator spaces. This trans-spatial lesion has multiple large flow voids* ➡ *on MR. On the CT (not shown), the lesion revealed phleboliths.* *(Right)* *Axial T2WI FS MR shows a typical appearance of parotid space infantile hemangioma with prominent branching flow voids* ➡ *within the lesion, defining the hypervascular nature of the lesion.*

Venous Malformation

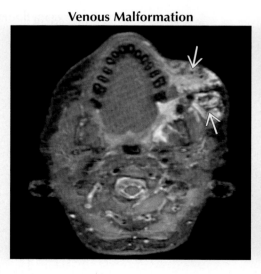

Infantile Hemangioma

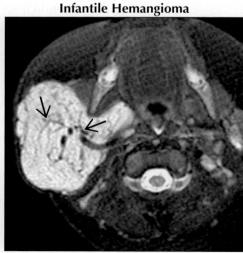

HYPERVASCULAR NECK LESION (CT/MR)

Metastasis

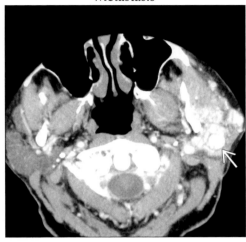

Arteriovenous Malformation

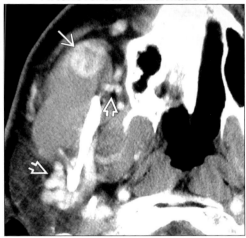

(Left) Axial CECT reveals renal cell carcinoma metastasis to parotid space as an intensely enhancing infiltrating mass. Note the prominent vascular enhancement within and at margins of the lesion. The retromandibular vein is enlarged ➡, secondary to high flow state. *(Right)* Axial CECT reveals prominent enhancement of the arteriovenous malformation nidus ➡ in anterior masseter muscle, with associated vascular structures ⇒ in the right masticator space.

Thyroid Carcinoma, Nodal

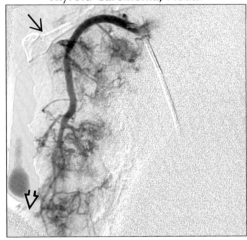

Hemangiopericytoma

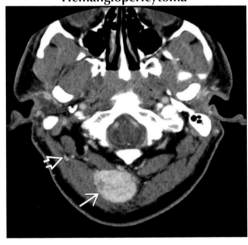

(Left) Lateral angiography of the external carotid artery branch shows hypervascular adenopathy from the level of the hyoid bone ➡ to the clavicle ⇒ in a patient with extensive differentiated thyroid carcinoma nodes. *(Right)* Axial CECT shows paraspinal hemangiopericytoma as a densely enhancing mass ➡ in the suboccipital musculature with prominent feeding arteries ⇒.

Meningioma, Carotid Space

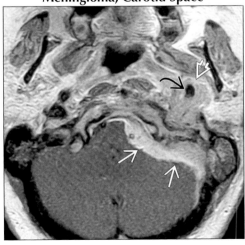

Adenoma, Parathyroid, Visceral Space

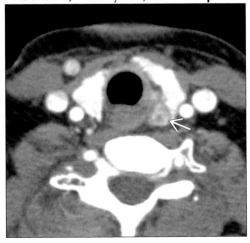

(Left) Axial T1 C+ MR shows carotid space meningioma with an extensive posterior fossa lesion ➡ extending through the jugular foramen into the nasopharyngeal carotid space ⇒. The lesion encases the internal carotid artery ➡. *(Right)* Axial CECT shows well-circumscribed enhancing parathyroid adenoma ➡ posterior and medial to the thyroid in the tracheoesophageal groove. The mass appears distinct from the thyroid.

DIFFERENTIAL DIAGNOSIS

Common
- Reactive Lymph Nodes, Jugulodigastric
- SCCa, Nodes, Jugulodigastric
- Benign Mixed Tumor, Parotid Tail
- Abscess, Masticator Space
- Mucoepidermoid Carcinoma, Parotid
- Adenoid Cystic Carcinoma, Parotid

Less Common
- Sialadenitis, Submandibular Gland
- Warthin Tumor, Parotid Tail
- Non-Hodgkin Lymphoma, Nodal
- Acute Parotiditis
- Ranula, Diving
- 2nd Branchial Cleft Cyst

Rare but Important
- Benign Mixed Tumor, Submandibular Gland
- Laryngocele, Mixed
- Carcinoma, Submandibular Gland
- Chondrosarcoma, Masticator Space

ESSENTIAL INFORMATION

Key Differential Diagnosis Issues
- Angle of mandible mass
  - Definition: Mass palpable just inferior to junction of body and ramus of mandible
  - Problem: Mass may arise from nodes, parotid tail, masticator space, submandibular space, or sublingual space
  - Imaging solution: Radiologist must 1st determine lesion space or structure of origin
- Major structures or spaces to consider when analyzing CT or MR images of lesion
  - Jugulodigastric nodal group
    - Reactive or suppurative node(s)
    - Malignant node: SCCa, NHL
  - Parotid tail lesion
    - Parotiditis
    - Benign mixed tumor, Warthin tumor
    - Parotid carcinoma: Mucoepidermoid or adenoid cystic
  - Masticator space lesion
    - Abscess
    - MS sarcoma
  - Submandibular space lesion
    - Submandibular gland sialadenitis
    - Submandibular gland benign mixed tumor

- Submandibular gland carcinoma
  - Sublingual space lesion
    - Diving ranula
  - Other miscellaneous lesions
    - 2nd branchial cleft cyst
    - Laryngocele, mixed type
- Caveat: Cystic angle of mandible mass in adult > 40 years old is cystic SCCa node until proven otherwise
  - Do not suggest 2nd branchial cleft cyst in this patient group!
  - Look for primary tumor instead

Helpful Clues for Common Diagnoses
- **Reactive Lymph Nodes, Jugulodigastric**
  - Key facts: Younger patients with URI
  - Imaging: Homogeneously enhancing jugulodigastric nodes
    - Inflammatory septa may be visibile with nodes when large
- **SCCa, Nodes, Jugulodigastric**
  - Key facts: SCCa node ↓ prognosis by 50%
    - Primary from tongue base or tonsil
  - Imaging: Cystic node just anterolateral to ICA with marginal enhancing soft tissue density
- **Benign Mixed Tumor, Parotid Tail**
  - Key facts: Most common parotid tumor
    - Tail of parotid lesions projects into posterior submandibular space (SMS)
    - Parotid tail masses may be clinically mistaken as submandibular in origin
    - Surgical approach to parotid tail masses via SMS may injure facial nerve
  - Imaging: Benign-appearing, well-encapsulated mass
    - MR: C+ mass with high T2 signal
- **Abscess, Masticator Space**
  - Key facts: From molar infection
  - Imaging: Enhancing abscess wall surrounds central pus
- **Mucoepidermoid Carcinoma, Parotid**
  - Key facts: Nodes often associated
  - Imaging: Well-circumscribed to invasive parotid tail mass
- **Adenoid Cystic Carcinoma, Parotid**
  - Key facts: Perineural tumor spread common
  - Imaging: Invasive, poorly enhancing parotid tail mass

Helpful Clues for Less Common Diagnoses
- **Sialadenitis, Submandibular Gland**

○ Key facts: Ductal calculus or stenosis
○ Imaging: Enlarged submandibular gland with enlarged duct ± calculus
• **Warthin Tumor, Parotid Tail**
  ○ Key facts: 20% have multiple tumors, synchronous or metachronous
    ▪ Common in smokers
  ○ Imaging: Well-circumscribed heterogeneous parotid tail mass
• **Non-Hodgkin Lymphoma, Nodal**
  ○ Key facts: Often involves multiple nodal chains including submandibular and internal jugular
  ○ Imaging: Nonnecrotic, large, C+ nodes
    ▪ Jugulodigastric or submandibular nodes
• **Acute Parotiditis**
  ○ Key facts: Unilateral (bacteria- or calculus-related) or bilateral (viral)
  ○ Imaging: Diffuse C+ enlarged parotid
• **Ranula, Diving**
  ○ Key facts: Postinflammatory retention cyst of sublingual space (SLS)
    ▪ Ruptures from posterior SLS into submandibular space (SMS)
  ○ Imaging: Cystic SMS mass with "tail" in SLS
• **2nd Branchial Cleft Cyst**
  ○ Key facts: Posterior to submandibular gland, lateral to carotid space (CS), anteromedial to sternocleidomastoid
    ▪ Most occur at mandible angle
  ○ Imaging: Well-defined cystic mass anterolateral to CS
    ▪ Same location of jugulodigastric node

Helpful Clues for Rare Diagnoses
• **Benign Mixed Tumor, Submandibular Gland**
  ○ Key facts: Intraglandular, slow-growing, painless mass
  ○ Imaging: Solitary ovoid or multilobular T2 hyperintense mass
    ▪ Mixed signal may be due to necrosis, hemorrhage, or calcification
• **Laryngocele, Mixed**
  ○ Key facts: Evaluate endolarynx for associated SCCa
  ○ Imaging: Cystic mass extends from paraglottic to submandibular space
• **Carcinoma, Submandibular Gland**
  ○ Key facts: Adenoid cystic or mucoepidermoid carcinoma
  ○ Imaging: Enhancing submandibular gland mass or exophytic growth with poorly defined margins
• **Chondrosarcoma, Masticator Space**
  ○ Key facts: Soft tissue mass with variable calcification patterns
  ○ Imaging: Presence & degree of calcification depend on tumor grade
    ▪ Rings & arcs: Low grade
    ▪ Amorphous calcification: High grade

SELECTED REFERENCES

1. Lowe LH et al: Swelling at the angle of the mandible: imaging of the pediatric parotid gland and periparotid region. Radiographics. 21(5):1211-27, 2001

Reactive Lymph Nodes, Jugulodigastric

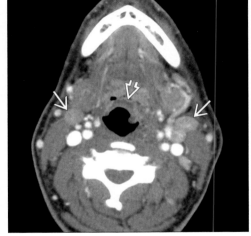

Axial CECT shows bilateral reactive adenopathy ➡ associated with a swollen epiglottis ➡. This patient presented with a palpable mass at the angle of the mandible.

SCCa, Nodes, Jugulodigastric

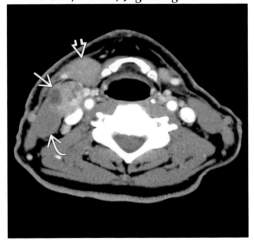

Axial CECT reveals a poorly circumscribed mass ➡, posterior to the submandibular gland ➡ and anterior to the sternocleidomastoid muscle ➡. Biopsy specimen showed jugulodigastric SCCa node.

ANGLE OF MANDIBLE MASS

(Left) Axial T1WI MR demonstrates an ovoid, uniform, intermediate signal benign mixed tumor of the parotid tail ➡, projecting inferiorly to the posterior submandibular space. (Right) Axial CECT shows abnormal soft tissue enhancement within the left masseter muscle ➡ from poor molar dentition ⧁, consistent with a phlegmon/abscess of the masticator space.

Benign Mixed Tumor, Parotid Tail

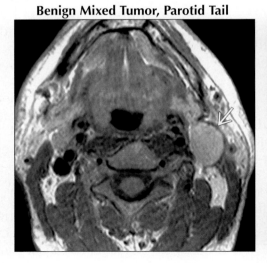

Abscess, Masticator Space

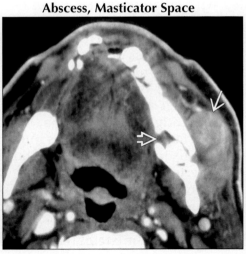

(Left) Coronal T1 C+ FS MR reveals high-grade infiltrative mucoepidermoid carcinoma extending inferiorly into the parotid tail ➡. (Right) Coronal T1 C+ MR demonstrates a large invasive left parotid mass that extends inferiorly into the parotid tail ➡ and involves the area of the angle of the mandible.

Mucoepidermoid Carcinoma, Parotid

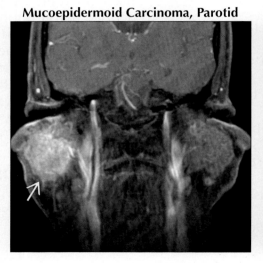

Adenoid Cystic Carcinoma, Parotid

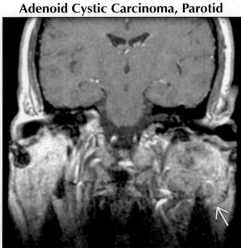

(Left) Axial CECT shows an enlarged right submandibular gland with a dense calculus ⧁ within the submandibular gland and intraglandular ductal dilatation ➡. (Right) Axial CECT demonstrates multiple, mixed solid and cystic, circumscribed, enhancing masses within the parotid glands bilaterally. The masses on the left appear solid ➡, while the right-sided parotid tail lesion has cystic regions ⧁.

Sialadenitis, Submandibular Gland

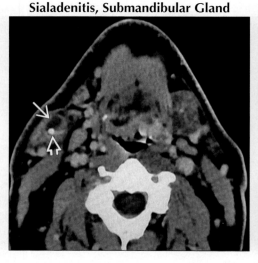

Warthin Tumor, Parotid Tail

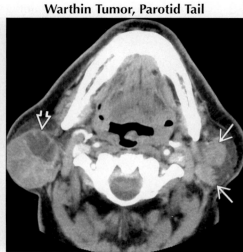

5

Non-Hodgkin Lymphoma, Nodal

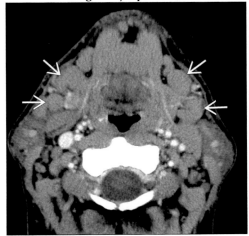

Acute Parotiditis

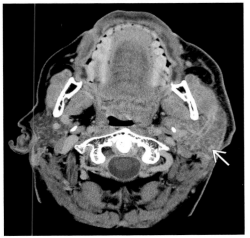

(Left) Axial CECT shows multiple bilateral solid nodes ➡ at the angle of the mandible, found to be non-Hodgkin lymphoma. There are no cystic regions within these nodes, which might be expected with squamous cell carcinoma. *(Right)* Axial CECT reveals diffuse enlargement of the left parotid gland ➡ with patchy enhancement of the gland, consistent with acute parotiditis.

Ranula, Diving

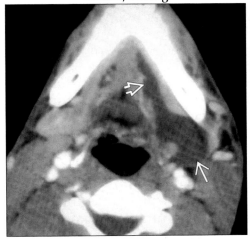

2nd Branchial Cleft Cyst

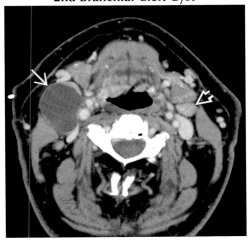

(Left) Axial CECT shows a classic ranula on the left, with a cystic mass extending with a "tail" into the submandibular space ➡ and a larger cystic region within the submandibular space ➡. *(Right)* Axial CECT reveals a 2nd BCC as a well-defined cystic mass ➡ anterior to the right sternomastoid muscle, posterolateral to the right submandibular gland & to the carotid space vessels. Note reactive left jugulodigastric node ➡ in the same location on the left.

Benign Mixed Tumor, Submandibular Gland

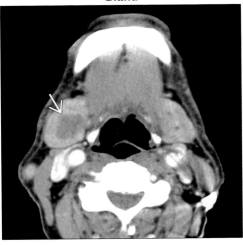

Laryngocele, Mixed

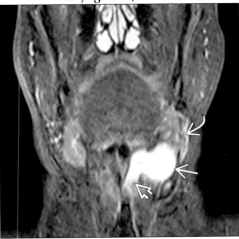

(Left) Axial CECT in patient with right angle of mandible mass shows a tumor within the submandibular gland ➡. This benign mixed tumor is well defined and low density in comparison to the remainder of the normal submandibular gland. *(Right)* Coronal T2WI FS MR reveals a mixed laryngocele ➡ extending laterally from the paraglottic space ➡ into the submandibular space, displacing the submandibular gland superiorly ➡.

SUPRACLAVICULAR MASS

DIFFERENTIAL DIAGNOSIS

Common
- Multinodular Goiter
- Differentiated Carcinoma, Thyroid
- SCCa, Nodes
- Differentiated Thyroid Carcinoma, Nodal
- Non-Hodgkin Lymphoma, Lymph Nodes
- Reactive Lymph Nodes

Less Common
- Lymphatic Malformation
- Metastases, Systemic, Nodal
- Lipoma
- Pancoast Tumor
- Neurofibromatosis Type 1
- Aneurysm, Subclavian Artery
- Fibromatosis Colli
- Hodgkin Lymphoma, Lymph Nodes
- Hypertrophy, Levator Scapulae Muscle
- Abscess

Rare but Important
- Anaplastic Carcinoma, Thyroid
- Non-Hodgkin Lymphoma, Thyroid
- Schwannoma, Brachial Plexus, PVS
- Esophageal Carcinoma, Cervical
- Liposarcoma

ESSENTIAL INFORMATION

Key Differential Diagnosis Issues
- Supraclavicular masses come from local structures or have congenital origins
  - Nodes, thyroid, esophagus, brachial plexus, subclavian artery

Helpful Clues for Common Diagnoses
- **Multinodular Goiter**
  - Key facts: Common neck mass in elderly
  - Imaging: Heterogeneous, multilobulated
    - 90% have calcifications
- **Differentiated Carcinoma, Thyroid**
  - Key facts: Female, < 40 years
    - 90% of all thyroid malignancies
  - Imaging: MR if possible
    - Avoid iodinated CT contrast as this study delays I-131 therapy
    - Tumor well defined or invasive ± nodes
- **SCCa, Nodes**
  - Key facts: Supraclavicular nodes drain from upper neck nodes
  - Imaging: Large, heterogeneous node(s)

- **Differentiated Thyroid Carcinoma, Nodal**
  - Key facts: Level IV, VB, & VI common nodal sites for differentiated thyroid nodes
  - CECT: Solid enhancing, cystic ± Ca++
  - MR: T1 high signal possible
- **Non-Hodgkin Lymphoma, Lymph Nodes**
  - Key facts: Low neck and mediastinal nodes often present simultaneously
  - Imaging: Multiple, bilateral, non-necrotic bulky nodes
    - Nodal density ≤ muscle density
    - Homogeneous with rim enhancement
- **Reactive Lymph Nodes**
  - Key facts: In setting of upper respiratory infection
  - Imaging: Oval-shaped, homogeneously enhancing, mildly enlarged nodes

Helpful Clues for Less Common Diagnoses
- **Lymphatic Malformation**
  - Key facts: Most present before age 5 years
    - 2nd smaller presentation peak between 20-30 years
  - Imaging: Fluid-filled mass with imperceptible wall ± septations
    - Uni- or multiloculated trans-spatial
    - Insinuates between normal structures
    - Fluid-fluid levels if hemorrhage has occurred
    - ± Enhancing component if mixed venous & lymphatic malformation
- **Metastases, Systemic, Nodal**
  - Key facts: Supraclavicular node from chest, abdomen, or pelvic primary tumor
    - Spreads to supraclavicular node(s) via thoracic duct, paratracheal chain, or hematogenous routes
  - Imaging: Necrotic, often extranodal mass
- **Lipoma**
  - Imaging: Fatty mass with minimal internal architecture
    - Thin smooth capsule
- **Pancoast Tumor**
  - Key facts: Lung SCCa or adenocarcinoma
    - Brachial plexopathy often associated
  - Imaging: Tumor invades lower neck from lung apex
- **Neurofibromatosis Type 1**
  - Key facts: Neurofibroma or plexiform neurofibroma
  - Imaging: Ovoid enhancing; "target" sign
    - Plexiform lesion irregular, enhancing

SUPRACLAVICULAR MASS

- **Aneurysm, Subclavian Artery**
  - Key facts: Pulsatile supraclavicular mass
  - Imaging: Focally enlarged subclavian artery
    - Variable lumen enhancement depending on size of intramural clot
- **Fibromatosis Colli**
  - Key facts: 70% present by 2 months after traumatic birth
  - Imaging: Fusiform sternocleidomastoid enlargement
    - Diffuse muscle enhancement without discrete mass
- **Hodgkin Lymphoma, Lymph Nodes**
  - Key facts: Unilateral supraclavicular node(s) common
  - Imaging: Bulky, homogeneous nodes
    - Cystic/necrotic nodes more common than in non-Hodgkin
- **Hypertrophy, Levator Scapulae Muscle**
  - Key facts: Occurs following neck node dissection
    - Levator scapulae muscle compensates for injured trapezius in lifting arm
  - Imaging: Enlarged asymmetric levator scapulae muscle
- **Abscess**
  - Key facts: Suppurative node rupture leads to abscess
  - Imaging: Single space or trans-spatial
    - Rim-enhancing fluid collection ± inflammation in adjacent soft tissues

Helpful Clues for Rare Diagnoses
- **Anaplastic Carcinoma, Thyroid**
  - Key facts: Arises from multinodular goiter or de novo
  - Imaging: Aggressive, invasive thyroid mass
- **Non-Hodgkin Lymphoma, Thyroid**
  - Key facts: Previous history of Hashimoto thyroiditis
  - Imaging: Aggressive, invasive thyroid mass
- **Schwannoma, Brachial Plexus, PVS**
  - Key facts: Painless, lateral supraclavicular mass
  - Imaging: Fusiform mass between anterior & middle scalene muscles
- **Esophageal Carcinoma, Cervical**
  - Key facts: Usually SCCa
  - Imaging: Invasive visceral space mass behind trachea
- **Liposarcoma**
  - Imaging: Well circumscribed, lobulated, or infiltrating
    - Soft tissue density in fatty mass
    - May have no visible fatty component

SELECTED REFERENCES
1. Ellison E et al: Supraclavicular masses: results of a series of 309 cases biopsied by fine needle aspiration. Head Neck. 21(3):239-46, 1999

Multinodular Goiter

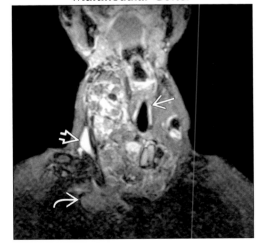

Coronal STIR MR shows a giant mixed signal multinodular goiter displacing the internal jugular vein laterally ➡, surrounding the trachea ➡, and extending inferiorly into the mediastinum ➡.

Multinodular Goiter

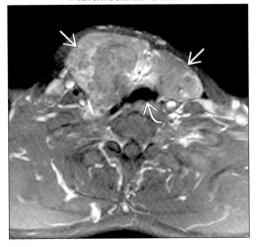

Axial T1 C+ FS MR in the same patient reveals that both lobes of the thyroid ➡ are greatly enlarged, causing compression of the trachea ➡.

SUPRACLAVICULAR MASS

Differentiated Carcinoma, Thyroid

(Left) Axial CECT demonstrates a large cystic-necrotic primary differentiated thyroid carcinoma ➡ in the left thyroid lobe. The tumor displaces the left carotid space ⬈ laterally. *(Right)* Coronal CECT in the same patient shows the large supraclavicular multi-cystic tumor ➡ arising from the left thyroid lobe. Note the incidental submandibular lipoma ⬈.

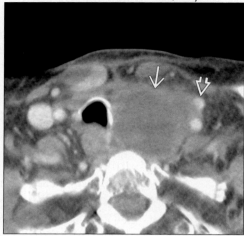

Differentiated Carcinoma, Thyroid

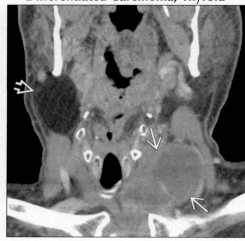

SCCa, Nodes

(Left) Axial CECT reveals an inhomogeneously enhancing left level IV internal jugular lymph node ➡ with invasive margins ⬈, signaling an extranodal component. Primary SCCa (not shown) is from pyriform sinus. *(Right)* Axial T1WI MR shows 2 focal nodes ➡, found to be SCCa nodes within the left supraclavicular fossa, in a patient with left preauricular skin squamous cell carcinoma.

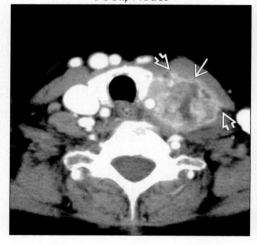

SCCa, Nodes

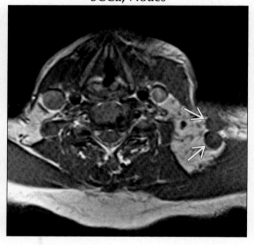

Differentiated Thyroid Carcinoma, Nodal

(Left) Axial CECT reveals primary differentiated thyroid carcinoma involving both thyroid lobes ⬈. Bilateral inhomogeneously enhancing low internal jugular metastatic nodes are also visible ➡. *(Right)* Axial T2WI MR shows enlarged right high signal supraclavicular metastatic nodes ➡. The thyroid gland demonstrates a heterogeneous appearance with multiple nodules ⬈, found to be differentiated thyroid carcinoma.

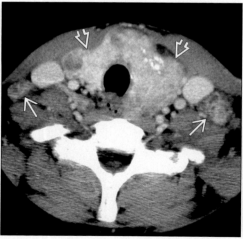

Differentiated Thyroid Carcinoma, Nodal

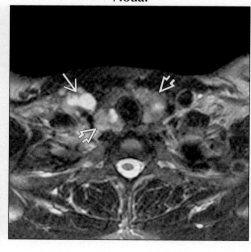

Non-Hodgkin Lymphoma, Lymph Nodes
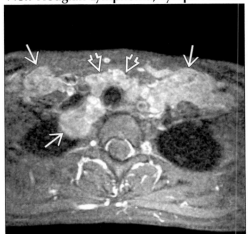

Non-Hodgkin Lymphoma, Lymph Nodes
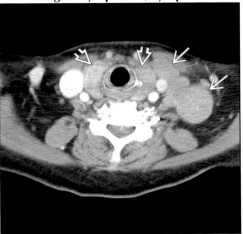

(Left) Axial T1 C+ FS MR reveals non-Hodgkin lymphoma supraclavicular nodal conglomerates ➡. Inhomogeneous enhancement of these nodal masses is typical. The thyroid lobes ➡ show mixed enhancing masses, suggesting that they are also involved by non-Hodgkin lymphoma. (Right) Axial NECT demonstrates multiple bulky level IV internal jugular non-Hodgkin lymphoma nodes ➡ associated with diffuse thyroid lymphoma ➡.

Reactive Lymph Nodes
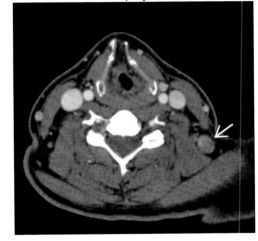

Lymphatic Malformation
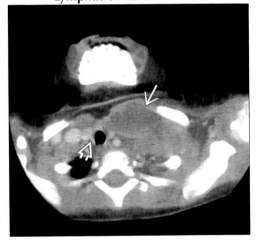

(Left) Axial CECT shows a focal round soft tissue density mass ➡ within the left supraclavicular fossa. Although there are no surrounding aggressive changes, this was found to be a reactive node. (Right) Axial CECT demonstrates a multilocular low-attenuation nonenhancing mass in the left supraclavicular fossa ➡. The mass deviates the thyroid gland and airway to the right ➡.

Metastases, Systemic, Nodal
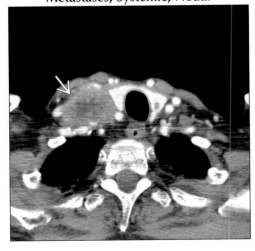

Lipoma
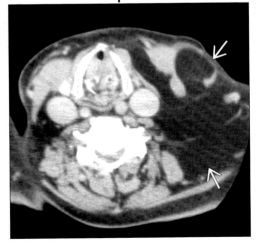

(Left) Axial CECT demonstrates metastatic nodal disease ➡ spreading to the right supraclavicular fossa from lung cancer in the right upper lobe of the lung. (Right) Axial CECT reveals a lipoma ➡ of the posterior cervical space of the left infrahyoid neck. The absence of significant soft tissue within the lipoma makes liposarcoma extremely unlikely.

SUPRACLAVICULAR MASS

(Left) Coronal CECT shows an invasive Pancoast tumor ➡ spreading superiorly into the perivertebral space ➡. *(Right)* Axial CECT shows multiple nonenhancing neurofibromas involving the brachial plexus ➡ bilaterally and surrounding both carotid arteries ➡.

Pancoast Tumor

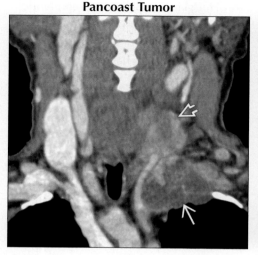

Neurofibromatosis Type 1

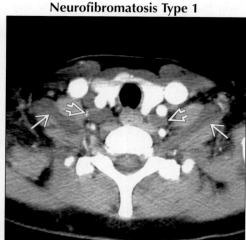

(Left) Coronal CECT demonstrates a large right subclavian artery aneurysm lumen ➡ projecting superiorly into the supraclavicular fossa. Note the very thick nonenhancing vessel wall ➡, which represents a subintimal clot. *(Right)* Coronal T1WI MR shows diffuse enlargement of the right sternocleidomastoid muscle ➡. The affected muscle is isointense to the contralateral noninvolved muscle ➡.

Aneurysm, Subclavian Artery

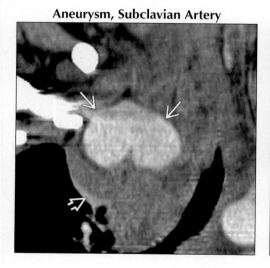

Fibromatosis Colli

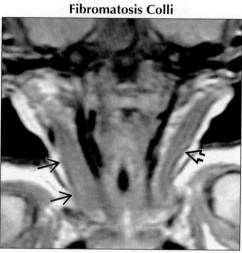

(Left) Axial CECT shows an ill-defined right supraclavicular heterogeneous soft tissue mass ➡. A matted nodal conglomerate of Hodgkin lymphoma was discovered at surgery. *(Right)* Axial CECT reveals a rounded & enlarged left levator scapulae muscle ➡. Surgical resection of the left internal jugular vein ➡ & sternocleidomastoid muscle, along with atrophy of the left trapezius muscle ➡, indicates previous left radical neck dissection with spinal accessory nerve injury.

Hodgkin Lymphoma, Lymph Nodes

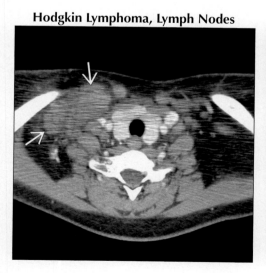

Hypertrophy, Levator Scapulae Muscle

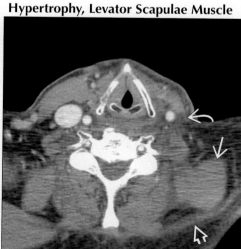

SUPRACLAVICULAR MASS

Abscess

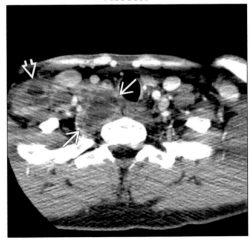

Anaplastic Carcinoma, Thyroid

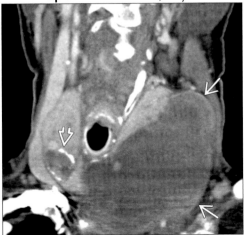

(Left) Axial CECT shows irregular rim-enhancing fluid in the perivertebral ➡ & supraclavicular ➡ areas. Aspiration revealed multiple soft tissue abscesses. *(Right)* Coronal CECT demonstrates an enlarged inhomogeneously enhancing thyroid gland with ring calcifications ➡, consistent with multinodular goiter. The left thyroid lobe shows a low-density cystic-necrotic anaplastic carcinoma ➡ arising from the multinodular goiter.

Non-Hodgkin Lymphoma, Thyroid

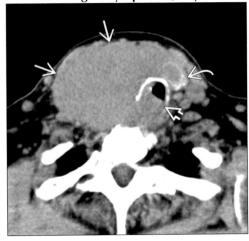

Schwannoma, Brachial Plexus, PVS

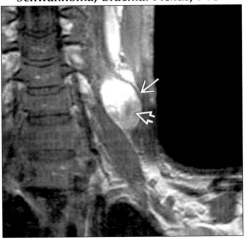

(Left) Axial NECT reveals a large thyroid non-Hodgkin lymphoma ➡ invading the trachea ➡. A small portion of the high-density left thyroid lobe is still visible ➡. *(Right)* Coronal T1 C+ MR demonstrates a fusiform schwannoma ➡ paralleling the extraforaminal brachial plexus. The lesion is avidly enhancing with evidence of intramural cystic change ➡. Needle biopsy caused the patient's arm to twitch.

Esophageal Carcinoma, Cervical

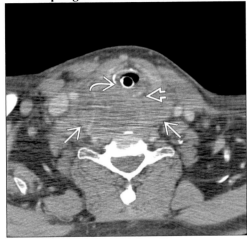

Liposarcoma

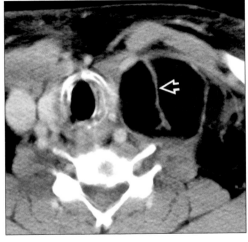

(Left) Axial CECT depicts an invasive cervical esophageal carcinoma as a bulky heterogeneous soft tissue mass ➡ that causes cricoid cartilage destruction ➡ and tracheal invasion ➡. *(Right)* Axial CECT shows a circumscribed, mixed fat and soft tissue density mass within the supraclavicular fossa. Nodular soft tissue & thick septae ➡ are imaging findings that suggest the diagnosis of liposarcoma rather than lipoma.

SECTION 6
Sinus & Nose

Anatomically Based Differentials

Generic Imaging Patterns

Modality-Specific Imaging Findings

Clinically Based Differentials

SINONASAL ANATOMIC VARIANTS

DIFFERENTIAL DIAGNOSIS

Common
- Nasal Septal Deviation
- Agger Nasi Cell
- Nasal Septal Spur
- Concha Bullosa
- Infraorbital Ethmoid (Haller) Cell
- Middle Turbinate, Paradoxical

Less Common
- Anterior Clinoid Process, Pneumatized
- Fovea Ethmoidalis, Asymmetric (Low)
- Uncinate Process, Pneumatized
- Frontal Cells
- Crista Galli, Pneumatized
- Supraorbital Ethmoid Cell
- Lamina Papyracea, Dehiscent

Rare but Important
- Sphenoethmoidal (Onodi) Cell
- Carotid Artery, Sphenoid Dehiscence

ESSENTIAL INFORMATION

Key Differential Diagnosis Issues
- Anatomic variants are rule rather than exception
- Multiple variants often present in same patient, so identify and report them!
- Variants may make patients prone to recurrent inflammatory disease and may increase risk of complications during functional endoscopic sinus surgery (FESS)

Helpful Clues for Common Diagnoses
- **Nasal Septal Deviation**
  - Most common variant; often associated with previous trauma; deviates from midline or "S-shaped;" impact on nasal airway patency depends on overall nasal cavity width
  - Measure maximum deviation from midline
- **Agger Nasi Cell**
  - Present in > 85% (really a variant?); most anterior extramural ethmoid air cell
  - Located anterior to frontal recess; at level of lacrimal sac or head of middle turbinate on coronal CT
- **Nasal Septal Spur**
  - Nearly always associated with septal deviation; often at ethmoid-vomer junction

- Document direction and length of spur; bony or cartilaginous; contact with lateral nasal wall structures or septum?
- **Concha Bullosa**
  - Pneumatization of conchal turn of middle turbinate; may narrow middle meatus
  - Can be diseased with mucosal thickening, fluid, retention cysts, osteoma
  - Inferior pneumatization is uncommon
- **Infraorbital Ethmoid (Haller) Cell**
  - Air cell located along inferior surface of orbital floor (antral roof); ↑ risk of orbital injury during FESS
  - Variable size; often bilateral; can narrow infundibulum and be diseased
- **Middle Turbinate, Paradoxical**
  - Concavity of turbinate concha directed toward septum; diffuse or focal; variable size; often "club-shaped"
  - Can narrow middle meatus and be diseased

Helpful Clues for Less Common Diagnoses
- **Anterior Clinoid Process, Pneumatized**
  - Position lateral to optic nerve ↑ risk of injury during sphenoid surgery
- **Fovea Ethmoidalis, Asymmetric (Low)**
  - Low position ↑ risk of skull base complication during ethmoidectomy resulting in CSF leak, encephalocele, or parenchymal brain injury
  - Report measurement of asymmetry in millimeters in dictation
- **Uncinate Process, Pneumatized**
  - May narrow either infundibulum or middle meatus
- **Frontal Cells**
  - Located anterior to frontal recess (above agger nasi cell) or within frontal sinus; 4 types (Bent classification); ↑ incidence of these cells with other variants (concha bullosa); types III & IV may be associated with ↑ disease in frontal sinus
    - Type I: Single cell above the agger nasi
    - Type II: Tier of two or more cells above agger nasi
    - Type III: Single large cell above agger nasi that extends superiorly into frontal recess
    - Type IV: Cell located completely within frontal sinus
- **Crista Galli, Pneumatized**

SINONASAL ANATOMIC VARIANTS

o Drains into one of frontal sinuses or frontal recess; mucocele formation and subsequent infection (mucopyocele) ↑ risk of anterior cranial fossa infection

- **Supraorbital Ethmoid Cell**
  o Cell within orbital plate of frontal bone; posterior to frontal sinus and frontal recess; best delineated on axial imaging
- **Lamina Papyracea, Dehiscent**
  o Post-traumatic or congenital; orbital fat or medial rectus muscle may herniate into ethmoid labyrinth; ↑ risk for orbital injury during FESS

Helpful Clues for Rare Diagnoses
- **Sphenoethmoidal (Onodi) Cell**
  o Pneumatization of posterior ethmoid cell superior to optic nerve; optic nerve at ↑ risk during posterior ethmoidectomy
  o Best seen on axial imaging
    - Look for horizontal septation on coronal images between this cell superiorly & sphenoid sinus inferiorly
- **Carotid Artery, Sphenoid Dehiscence**
  o Absence of bony covering over internal carotid artery; artery bulges into sphenoid sinus lumen; artery at ↑ risk for injury during sphenoid sinus surgery
  o Better delineated on axial imaging

Other Essential Information
- Anatomic variations can also be categorized based on location or anatomic structure involved
  o Frontal region variants

o Ethmoid region variants
o Middle turbinate variants
o Uncinate variants
o Sphenoethmoidal region variants
o Nasal septal variants
- Additional variants not mentioned above
  o Variable pneumatization (aplasia, hypoplasia, hyperpneumatization)
  o Intersinus septal cell (located within septum between frontal sinuses)
  o Fusion of uncinate to middle turbinate, lamina papyracea or skull base
  o Pneumatization of vertical lamella of middle turbinate
  o Septal recess (cell within posterior nasal septum)
  o Sphenoid sinus septations inserting on carotid canal
  o Pneumatization of dorsum sella

SELECTED REFERENCES

1. Aygun N et al: Imaging for functional endoscopic sinus surgery. Otolaryngol Clin North Am. 39(3):403-16, vii, 2006
2. DelGaudio JM et al: Multiplanar computed tomographic analysis of frontal recess cells: effect on frontal isthmus size and frontal sinusitis. Arch Otolaryngol Head Neck Surg. 131(3):230-5, 2005
3. Meyer TK et al: Coronal computed tomography analysis of frontal cells. Am J Rhinol. 17(3):163-8, 2003
4. Zeifer B: Update on sinonasal imaging: anatomy and inflammatory disease. Neuroimaging Clin N Am. 8(3):607-30, 1998
5. Melhem ER et al: Optimal CT evaluation for functional endoscopic sinus surgery. AJNR Am J Neuroradiol. 17(1):181-8, 1996
6. Earwaker J: Anatomic variants in sinonasal CT. Radiographics. 13(2):381-415, 1993

Nasal Septal Deviation

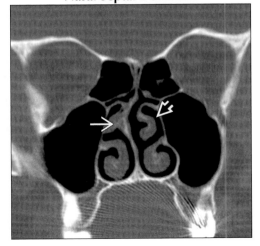

Coronal bone CT shows deviation of the nasal septum to the right with a small bony spur ➡. Also note paradoxical curvature of the middle turbinate ➡ on the left side.

Agger Nasi Cell

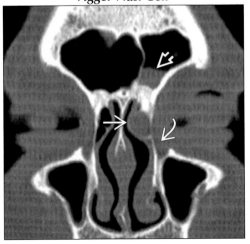

Coronal bone CT shows opacified agger nasi air cell ➡ on left with additional left frontal mucosal sinus disease ➡. This air cell is seen on the same coronal slice as the lacrimal sac ➡.

SINONASAL ANATOMIC VARIANTS

(Left) Coronal bone CT shows broad-based bony nasal septal spur ➡ directed towards the left with superolateral displacement of the middle turbinate ⟱. (Right) Coronal bone CT shows pneumatized left middle turbinate (concha bullosa) ➡. Also note septal deviation ⟱, pneumatized uncinate ⟱, and low left fovea ethmoidalis ⟱.

Nasal Septal Spur

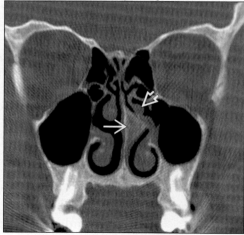

Concha Bullosa

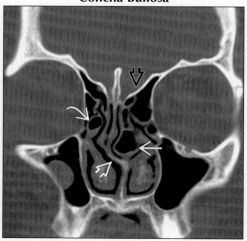

(Left) Coronal bone CT reveals a large infraorbital Haller cell ➡ on the right. The cell narrows the infundibulum ⟱. Note the infraorbital nerve ➡ location lateral to the air cell. (Right) Coronal bone CT shows bilateral paradoxical curvature of the middle turbinates ➡. The concavity of the conchae is directed toward the nasal septum. This patient had sinusitis at the time of imaging.

Infraorbital Ethmoid (Haller) Cell

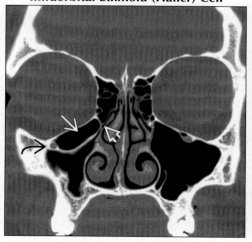

Middle Turbinate, Paradoxical

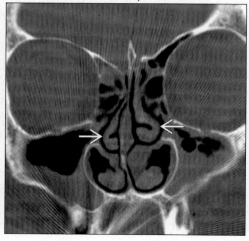

(Left) Axial bone CT demonstrates a well-aerated air cell within the left anterior clinoid process ➡. The optic nerve and internal carotid artery lie medial to this air cell. (Right) Coronal bone CT shows asymmetry in position of fovea ethmoidalis with left inferior in position compared to right sinus ➡. Infundibular pattern disease is seen on the left with a maxillary air-fluid level.

Anterior Clinoid Process, Pneumatized

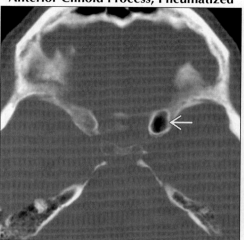

Fovea Ethmoidalis, Asymmetric (Low)

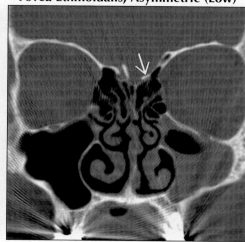

Uncinate Process, Pneumatized

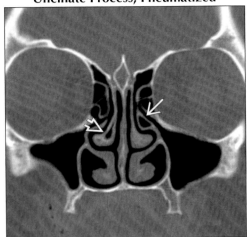

Frontal Cells

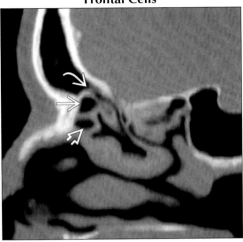

(Left) Coronal bone CT demonstrates an air cell within the left uncinate process ➡. A small concha bullosa is incidentally noted on the right ➡. *(Right)* Sagittal bone CT reveals a type I frontal cell ➡ superior to the agger nasi air cell ➡. The cell is located anterior to frontal recess and in this case is at level of the frontal ostium ➡.

Crista Galli, Pneumatized

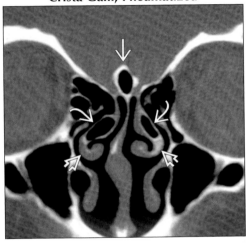

Supraorbital Ethmoid Cell

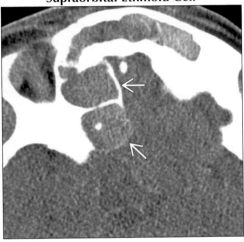

(Left) Coronal bone CT shows pneumatization of crista galli ➡. Note paradoxical curvature of the middle turbinates ➡ and pneumatization of the vertical lamellae ➡. *(Right)* Axial NECT shows two expanded opacified supraorbital ethmoid air cells ➡ in a patent with sinonasal polyposis. Note the position of these air cells posterior to the frontal sinus.

Lamina Papyracea, Dehiscent

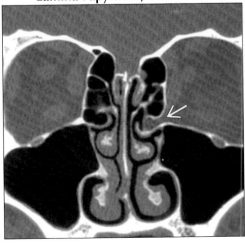

Sphenoethmoidal (Onodi) Cell

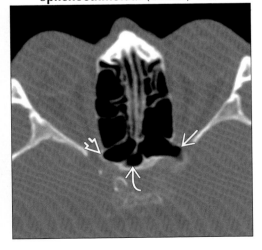

(Left) Coronal bone CT demonstrates dehiscence of the left lamina papyracea ➡ inferiorly with herniation of extraconal orbital fat through the defect into the ethmoid region. *(Right)* Axial bone CT shows a left sphenoethmoidal cell ➡ extending over the optic canal. A smaller cell is seen on the right ➡. Note the position of these cells superior to the sphenoid sinus ➡.

NASAL SEPTAL PERFORATION

DIFFERENTIAL DIAGNOSIS

Common
- Trauma
- Rhinitis Medicamentosa
- Cocaine Necrosis, Nose
- Wegener Granulomatosis, Sinonasal

Less Common
- Fungal Sinusitis, Invasive
- Sarcoidosis, Sinonasal
- SCCa, Sinonasal
- Non-Hodgkin Lymphoma, Sinonasal

Rare but Important
- Melanoma, Sinonasal
- Nasal Septal Abscess

ESSENTIAL INFORMATION

Key Differential Diagnosis Issues
- Insult to mucoperichondrium compromises blood supply to septal quadrangular cartilage, which leads to perforation
- Trauma & inhaled substances more common than infectious/neoplastic etiologies

Helpful Clues for Common Diagnoses
- **Trauma**
  - Septal fracture → hematoma → ischemic necrosis OR mucosal laceration with cartilage exposure
  - Iatrogenic: Post-septoplasty, intubation, packing, transsphenoidal & modified Lothrop surgical approaches
- **Rhinitis Medicamentosa**
  - Vasoconstrictive & steroid nasal sprays cause ischemic necrosis
- **Cocaine Necrosis, Nose**
  - Vasoconstriction leads to ischemic necrosis, chemical irritants damage mucosa
- **Wegener Granulomatosis, Sinonasal**
  - Vasculitis & necrotizing granulomatous disorder; nodular soft tissue erodes septum & turbinates

Helpful Clues for Less Common Diagnoses
- **Fungal Sinusitis, Invasive**
  - Angioinvasion compromises blood supply, or fungi directly invade septum
- **Sarcoidosis, Sinonasal**
  - Granulomatous disease with imaging features similar to Wegener
- **SCCa, Sinonasal**
  - 30-35% arise in nasal cavity and directly invade septum
- **Non-Hodgkin Lymphoma, Sinonasal**
  - Prefers nasal cavity over sinuses; dense on CT; ↓ T2 signal on MR

Helpful Clues for Rare Diagnoses
- **Melanoma, Sinonasal**
  - Nasal cavity preferred site of origin; may remodel or destroy septum
    - MR: ↑ T1, ↓ T2 signal
- **Nasal Septal Abscess**
  - Etiologies: Superinfected hematoma, sinusitis, or dental sources

Trauma

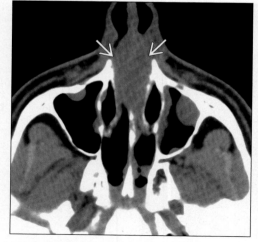

Axial NECT shows expansile lesion ➡ involving the cartilaginous and bony nasal septum, clinically consistent with a hematoma, although not hyperdense on CT. (Courtesy W. Smoker, MD.)

Cocaine Necrosis, Nose

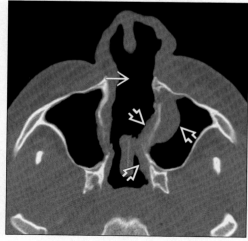

Axial bone CT shows a very large perforation of the cartilaginous and bony nasal septum ➡ related to cocaine abuse. Mucosal thickening ➡ is noted in the nasal cavity and maxillary antrum.

NASAL SEPTAL PERFORATION

Wegener Granulomatosis, Sinonasal

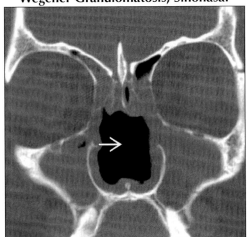

Fungal Sinusitis, Invasive

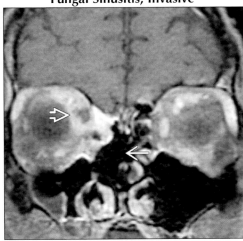

(Left) Coronal bone CT shows a large septal perforation ➡ in a patient with Wegener granulomatosis. There is middle and inferior turbinate erosion. Soft tissue is present in the adjacent sinuses. (Right) Coronal T1 C+ FS MR shows a septal perforation ➡ related to invasive fungal sinusitis. Disease persists in the right ethmoid sinuses, and there is extension into the orbit ➡.

Sarcoidosis, Sinonasal

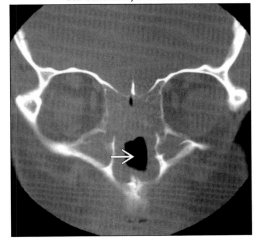

SCCa, Sinonasal

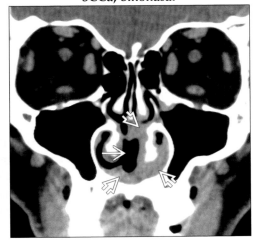

(Left) Coronal bone CT shows extensive sinus opacification and nasal cavity soft tissue thickening in a sarcoidosis patient. A large septal perforation is present anteriorly ➡. (Right) Coronal NECT shows inferior nasal septal perforation ➡ related to erosion caused by a squamous carcinoma ➡ of the floor of the nasal cavity and inferior turbinate.

Non-Hodgkin Lymphoma, Sinonasal

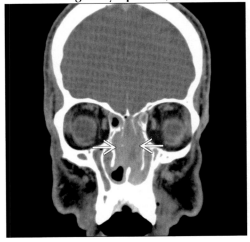

Melanoma, Sinonasal

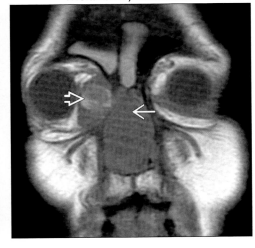

(Left) Coronal NECT shows a soft issue mass ➡ centered in the nasal cavity with destruction of the nasal septum. Nasal cavity location is characteristic for lymphoma in this region. (Right) Coronal T1WI MR shows a large sinonasal melanoma in the nasal cavity with destruction of the septum ➡. T1 shortening ➡ is noted in intraorbital tumor extension.

CONGENITAL MIDLINE NASAL LESION

DIFFERENTIAL DIAGNOSIS

Common
- Nasal Dermal Sinus
- Cephalocele, Frontoethmoidal
- Hemangioma, Sinonasal
- Choanal Atresia, Nasal

Less Common
- Nasal Glioma

Rare but Important
- Pyriform Aperture Stenosis

ESSENTIAL INFORMATION

Key Differential Diagnosis Issues
- Nasal dermal sinus & cephalocele: Intracranial extension and associated cysts/dermoids are important to identify at imaging
- MR is best imaging tool to evaluate extent of dermal sinuses and cephaloceles
- CT is modality of choice for evaluating bony narrowing in choanal atresia and pyriform aperture stenosis

Helpful Clues for Common Diagnoses
- **Nasal Dermal Sinus**
  - Clinical clue: Pit may be present along nasal dorsum
  - CT/MR: Fluid density or signal intensity tract from nasal tip to enlarged foramen cecum traversing nasal septum
    - Bifid crista galli may be present
  - Associated craniofacial anomalies possible
- **Cephalocele, Frontoethmoidal**
  - Clinical clue: Nasoglabellar or intranasal mass that may change in size with crying
  - MR: Extension of meninges, CSF & brain tissue through bony defect in cribriform plate or between frontal & nasal bones
- **Hemangioma, Sinonasal**
  - Clinical clue: Soft, reddish mass; capillary type most common; often arises from nasal septum
  - MR: Well-defined mass; T2 hyperintense; diffusely enhancing
- **Choanal Atresia, Nasal**
  - Clinical: Respiratory distress in newborn if bilateral; later presentation if unilateral
  - CT: Membranous or bony; unilateral or bilateral; thickened posterior vomer

Helpful Clues for Less Common Diagnoses
- **Nasal Glioma**
  - Clinical clues: Subcutaneous blue or red mass on nasal dorsum (extranasal type); polypoid submucosal mass (intranasal type)
  - MR: Intra- or extranasal soft tissue mass
    - MR signal typically NOT similar to brain parenchyma; no connection to intracranial contents

Helpful Clues for Rare Diagnoses
- **Pyriform Aperture Stenosis**
  - Anterior nasal bony stenosis
  - Look for central mega-incisor & midline intracranial anomalies

Nasal Dermal Sinus

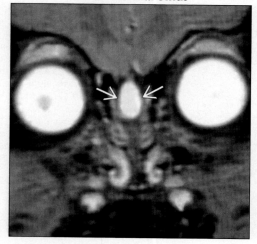

Coronal T2WI MR shows a portion of a nasal dermal sinus that extends from the skull base to the nasal tip. This image shows the hyperintense fluid-filled sinus ➡ within the nasal septum.

Cephalocele, Frontoethmoidal

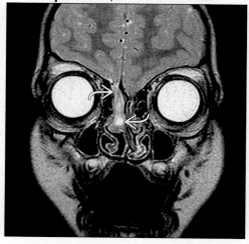

Coronal T2WI MR shows a cephalocele ➡ extending from the anterior cranial fossa through a skull base defect into the right nasal cavity. The meninges contain CSF and dysplastic brain tissue.

CONGENITAL MIDLINE NASAL LESION

Cephalocele, Frontoethmoidal

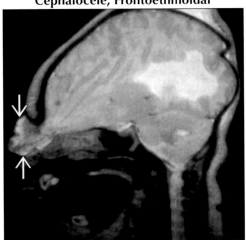

Hemangioma, Sinonasal

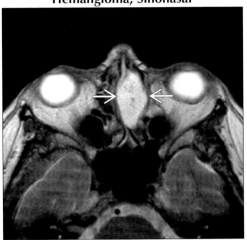

(Left) Sagittal T2WI MR shows a frontonasal type of cephalocele. Herniation of brain parenchyma ➡ through the fonticulus frontalis results from lack of fusion of the frontal and nasal bones. (Right) Axial T2WI MR shows a well-defined soft tissue mass in the left nasal cavity ➡. Hyperintense signal on this T2-weighted sequence is a characteristic feature of hemangiomas.

Choanal Atresia, Nasal

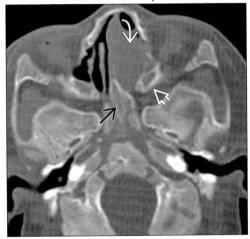

Nasal Glioma

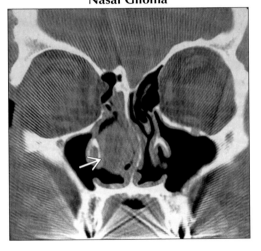

(Left) Axial bone CT shows unilateral choanal atresia with soft tissue in the left nasal cavity ➡ and narrowing of the left choana. The vomer is thickened ➡ and opposes the left maxilla ➡. (Right) Coronal bone CT shows an intranasal glioma ➡ not seen at the time of previous cephalocele repair. The anterior skull base is intact on this image.

Nasal Glioma

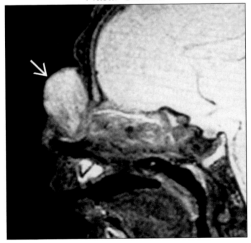

Pyriform Aperture Stenosis

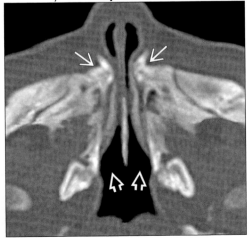

(Left) Sagittal T2WI MR shows an extranasal glioma over the nasal bridge, anterior to the expected location of the fused frontal and nasal bones ➡. (Right) Axial bone CT in a newborn shows pyriform aperture stenosis as a result of overgrowth of the nasal processes of the maxilla ➡ but no associated membranous atresia ➡.

FIBRO-OSSEOUS & CARTILAGINOUS LESIONS

DIFFERENTIAL DIAGNOSIS

Common
- Osteoma, Sinonasal
- Fibrous Dysplasia, Sinonasal
- Ossifying Fibroma, Sinus

Less Common
- Osteomyelitis, Mandible-Maxilla
- Chondrosarcoma, Sinonasal
- Osteosarcoma, Sinonasal

Rare but Important
- Chordoma, Clivus
- Giant Cell Granuloma, Mandible-Maxilla
- Cherubism, Mandible-Maxilla

ESSENTIAL INFORMATION

Key Differential Diagnosis Issues
- Fibro-osseous lesions may have similar imaging and histologic features

Helpful Clues for Common Diagnoses
- **Osteoma, Sinonasal**
  - Frontal > ethmoid > maxillary > sphenoid
  - CT: Density varies from dense (compact type) to less ossified (fibrous type)
- **Fibrous Dysplasia, Sinonasal**
  - Medullary bone replaced by woven bone
  - Facial bone involvement greater in polyostotic form
  - CT/MR: Appearance varies with amount of fibrous tissue (classic "ground-glass" appearance)
- **Ossifying Fibroma, Sinus**
  - Benign expansile tumor
  - Lesion ossifies from periphery
  - Better demarcated fibrous and osseous zones than fibrous dysplasia

Helpful Clues for Less Common Diagnoses
- **Osteomyelitis, Mandible-Maxilla**
  - Most often related to dental disease
  - Mandible > maxilla; lytic or sclerotic
  - ± Sequestra or periosteal reaction
- **Chondrosarcoma, Sinonasal**
  - Most in anterior maxillary alveolus
  - Expansile with bony remodeling
  - ± Ca++ tumor matrix; ↑ T2 signal
- **Osteosarcoma, Sinonasal**
  - ≤ 1% of sinonasal tumors
  - Imaging appearance varies with degree of osteo/chondroid/fibroblastic tumor
  - "Sunburst" periosteal reaction

Helpful Clues for Rare Diagnoses
- **Chordoma, Clivus**
  - Malignant notochordal tumor
  - Can extend into sphenoid sinus
  - Destructive midline mass with ↑ T2 signal
- **Giant Cell Granuloma, Mandible-Maxilla**
  - Arises from gingiva/alveolar mucosa
  - > 20 years, female, post-tooth extraction
  - Expansile and remodels bone
  - Low to intermediate T1/T2 MR signal
- **Cherubism, Mandible-Maxilla**
  - Autosomal dominant; M > F
  - Pathology = giant cell granuloma
  - Cystic expansion of mandible, then maxilla

Osteoma, Sinonasal

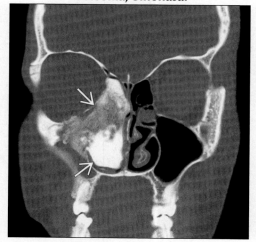

Coronal bone CT shows a large mixed osseous and soft tissue density mass within the nasal cavity and adjacent sinuses ➡. This osteoma could be confused with other fibro-osseous lesions.

Fibrous Dysplasia, Sinonasal

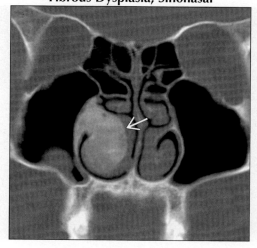

Coronal bone CT shows monostotic fibrous dysplasia involving the inferior turbinate ➡. The concha of the turbinate is expanded and has a "cotton wool" or "ground-glass" appearance.

FIBRO-OSSEOUS & CARTILAGINOUS LESIONS

Ossifying Fibroma, Sinus

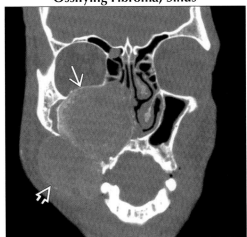

Osteomyelitis, Mandible-Maxilla

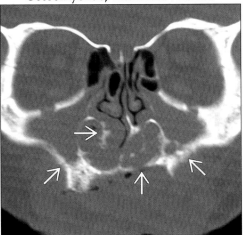

(Left) Coronal bone CT shows a bilobed lesion in the superficial soft tissues ➡ of the buccal space and maxillary sinus ➡. Note increased ossification along the superficial aspect of the maxillary sinus portion. *(Right)* Coronal bone CT shows a permeative bone erosion ➡ involving the palate, maxillary alveoli, sinus and lateral nasal walls, and inferior turbinates in this elderly patient with osteomyelitis.

Chondrosarcoma, Sinonasal

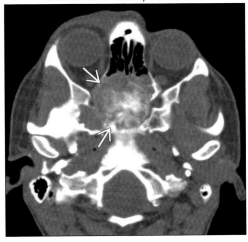

Osteosarcoma, Sinonasal

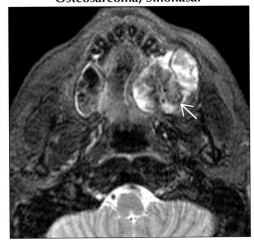

(Left) Axial bone CT shows a large vomer nasal septal chondrosarcoma ➡. The mass shows calcifications that are not characteristic of chondroid calcifications. *(Right)* Axial T2WI FS MR demonstrates an osteosarcoma arising within the left maxillary alveolus with extension into the antrum. The ossific matrix ➡ creates areas of hypointense signal on MR images.

Chordoma, Clivus

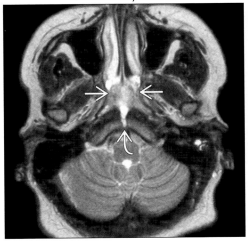

Giant Cell Granuloma, Mandible-Maxilla

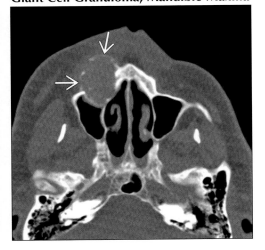

(Left) Axial T2WI MR shows an atypical chordoma ➡ presenting as a posterior nasal cavity/nasopharyngeal mass. The midline clival defect ➡ correlates with the path of the primitive notochord. *(Right)* Axial bone CT shows a maxillary giant cell granuloma ➡. An "eggshell" wall indicates its probable benign nature. A few ossific flecks can be seen in the lesion matrix.

INFLAMMATORY PATTERNS OF SINUSITIS

DIFFERENTIAL DIAGNOSIS

Common
- Sinusitis, Infundibular Pattern
- Sinusitis, Ostiomeatal Unit Pattern
- Sinusitis, Sporadic Pattern

Less Common
- Sinusitis, Sphenoethmoidal Recess Pattern
- Polyposis, Sinonasal
- Sinusitis, Frontal Recess Pattern

Rare but Important
- Sinusitis, Dental Source Pattern

ESSENTIAL INFORMATION

Key Differential Diagnosis Issues
- Patterns based upon routes of mucociliary drainage
- Surgery based on disease patterns & site of obstruction

Helpful Clues for Common Diagnoses
- **Sinusitis, Infundibular Pattern**
  - Disease limited to maxillary sinus; obstruction in ipsilateral ostium/infundibulum
  - Causes: Polyps, mucosal thickening, infraorbital ethmoid cells, atelectatic uncinate
- **Sinusitis, Ostiomeatal Unit Pattern**
  - Complete: Inflammation in ipsilateral maxillary, frontal & anterior ethmoid sinuses; occlusion at middle meatus

- Incomplete: Variable disease in frontal sinus and ostiomeatal unit
- Causes: Mucosal swelling, polyps, middle turbinate/septal variants
- **Sinusitis, Sporadic Pattern**
  - Not direct result of obstruction of mucociliary drainage
  - Random mucosal disease/fluid; includes retention cysts, mucoceles, surgical scarring

Helpful Clues for Less Common Diagnoses
- **Sinusitis, Sphenoethmoidal Recess Pattern**
  - Disease in ipsilateral sphenoid sinus ± posterior ethmoid cells
- **Polyposis, Sinonasal**
  - Not direct result of obstruction of mucociliary drainage
  - Polypoid sinonasal soft tissue lesions
- **Sinusitis, Frontal Recess Pattern**
  - Disease in frontal sinus; occlusion of ipsilateral frontal recess
  - Causes: Mucosal thickening, anatomic variants (frontal cells, agger nasi, supraorbital ethmoid), prior surgery

Helpful Clues for Rare Diagnoses
- **Sinusitis, Dental Source Pattern**
  - Maxillary disease with lucency/bone dehiscence around molar teeth below

SELECTED REFERENCES

1. Babbel RW et al: Recurring patterns of inflammatory sinonasal disease demonstrated on screening sinus CT. AJNR Am J Neuroradiol. 13(3):903-12, 1992

Sinusitis, Infundibular Pattern

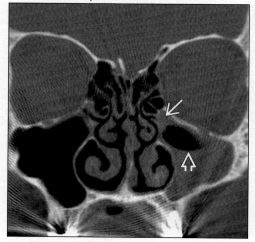

Coronal bone CT demonstrates mucosal thickening occluding the left infundibulum ➡. Mucosal thickening and an air-fluid level ➡ are present in the obstructed maxillary sinus.

Sinusitis, Ostiomeatal Unit Pattern

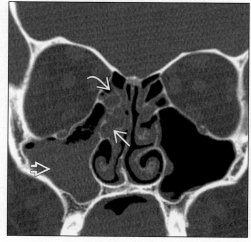

Coronal bone CT shows mucosal thickening occluding the middle meatus ➡ with obstructed secretions and mucosal thickening in the ipsilateral maxillary ➡ and anterior ethmoid sinuses ➡.

INFLAMMATORY PATTERNS OF SINUSITIS

Sinusitis, Sporadic Pattern

Sinusitis, Sphenoethmoidal Recess Pattern

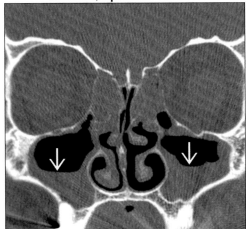

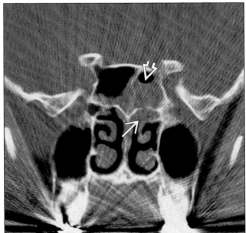

(Left) Coronal bone CT shows mucosal thickening in ethmoid and maxillary sinuses bilaterally with maxillary air-fluid levels ➡️. Frontal and sphenoid disease was noted on other images. *(Right)* Coronal bone CT shows typical case of sphenoethmoidal recess pattern disease. Mucosal thickening is seen in sphenoethmoidal recess ➡️ with an air-fluid level in the ipsilateral sphenoid sinus ➡️.

Polyposis, Sinonasal

Sinusitis, Frontal Recess Pattern

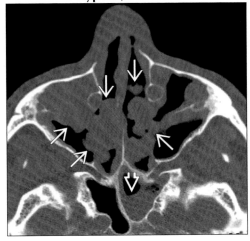

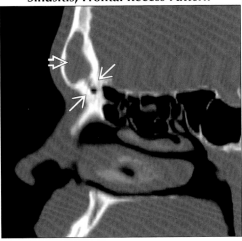

(Left) Axial bone CT shows multiple scattered soft tissue polyps ➡️ involving the nasal cavity and maxillary sinuses. Acute disease with an air-fluid level is seen in the left sphenoid sinus ➡️. *(Right)* Sagittal bone CT shows post-functional endoscopic sinus surgery neo-osteogenesis ➡️ narrowing the frontal recess and resulting in post-obstructive disease in the ipsilateral frontal sinus ➡️.

Sinusitis, Frontal Recess Pattern

Sinusitis, Dental Source Pattern

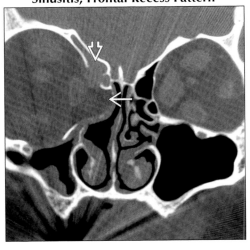

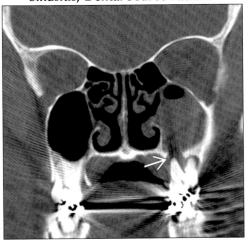

(Left) Coronal bone CT shows patient post-orbital decompression for Graves disease with herniated orbital fat ➡️ occluding the right frontal recess. Obstructed disease is seen in the ipsilateral frontal sinus ➡️. *(Right)* Coronal bone CT shows an air-fluid level in the left maxillary sinus. Lucency is noted surrounding a left molar tooth ➡️ that communicates with the alveolar recess. Multiple fillings are present.

MULTIPLE SINONASAL LESIONS

DIFFERENTIAL DIAGNOSIS

Common
- Rhinosinusitis, Acute
- Rhinosinusitis, Chronic
- Polyposis, Sinonasal
- Fungal Sinusitis, Allergic
- Retention Cyst, Sinonasal

Less Common
- Fungal Sinusitis, Invasive
- Wegener Granulomatosis, Sinonasal
- Sarcoidosis, Sinonasal

Rare but Important
- Fibrous Dysplasia, Sinonasal
- Osteoma, Sinonasal
- Metastasis
- Sinus Histiocytosis (Rosai-Dorfman)

ESSENTIAL INFORMATION

Key Differential Diagnosis Issues
- Infectious and inflammatory lesions are more likely to be multiple than neoplastic lesions

Helpful Clues for Common Diagnoses
- **Rhinosinusitis, Acute**
  - Key facts: Most common in ethmoid & maxillary sinuses
    - Most cases follow viral URI
    - Multiple sinus involvement less likely with odontogenic etiology
  - Imaging: Mucosal thickening ± air-fluid levels
    - Fluid levels may be difficult to detect in small sinuses (ethmoids)
- **Rhinosinusitis, Chronic**
  - Key facts: Multiple sinus involvement due to obstructing lesion at common drainage pathway (middle meatus, sphenoethmoidal recess) or underlying systemic condition
    - Cystic fibrosis, immunosuppression or compromised status, ciliary dysfunction
  - Imaging: Mucosal thickening; bone thickening & sclerosis (osteitis)
    - Decreased antral volume possible
- **Polyposis, Sinonasal**
  - Key facts: Non-neoplastic hyperplasia of sinus membranes

- ↑ Incidence in patients with asthma, aspirin intolerance, cystic fibrosis
  - Imaging: Polypoid soft tissue lesions in sinuses AND nasal cavity
    - Frequently arise near middle meatus & roof of nasal cavity
    - Usually multiple & bilateral
    - Often expansile; may be seen in allergic fungal sinusitis patients
- **Fungal Sinusitis, Allergic**
  - Key facts: Eosinophilic mucin & noninvasive fungal hyphae opacify & expand sinonasal cavities
    - Associated with allergies, polyps, chronic sinusitis; typically in young adults
  - Imaging: Opacified sinuses with expansion; often unilateral
    - ↑ Central and ↓ peripheral density on CT; ↓ T2 MR signal can mimic air
- **Retention Cyst, Sinonasal**
  - Key facts: Result from obstruction of submucosal mucinous glands
    - Occur in sinuses & uncommon in nasal cavity; rarely symptomatic
  - Imaging: Round or dome-shaped peripherally based sinus lesions
    - CT density/MR signal varies with water:protein ratio

Helpful Clues for Less Common Diagnoses
- **Fungal Sinusitis, Invasive**
  - Key facts: Aggressive infection seen in immunocompromised patients, diabetics
    - Angioinvasive fungi spread through bone & soft tissue along vessels
    - Maxillary > ethmoid > sphenoid
  - Imaging: Superficial or mass-like sinonasal soft tissue with bone erosion
    - Extension into adjacent compartments (orbit, skull base, masticator space)
- **Wegener Granulomatosis, Sinonasal**
  - Key facts: Necrotizing granulomatous disorder of sinonasal cavities
    - 90% show upper respiratory tract involvement
    - Prefers nasal septum and turbinates
  - Imaging: Nodular soft tissue lesions with mucosal ulcerations & bone erosion (septal perforation)
    - May extend beyond sinuses to orbits, meninges
- **Sarcoidosis, Sinonasal**

MULTIPLE SINONASAL LESIONS

○ Key facts: Granulomatous disorder with less frequent sinonasal involvement (3-20%) than Wegener
  ▪ Prefers nasal septum and turbinates
○ Imaging: Nodular soft tissue masses of nose and sinuses
  ▪ Less bone destruction than Wegener

Helpful Clues for Rare Diagnoses

- **Fibrous Dysplasia, Sinonasal**
  ○ Key facts: Mesenchymal developmental anomaly of bone
    ▪ Normal medullary bone replaced by weak osseous & fibrous tissue
    ▪ 75% of patients are < 30 years of age
    ▪ Polyostotic form: 20-30% of cases with 50% of those cases involving H&N
    ▪ Polyostotic form: ↑ in females
    ▪ Maxilla > mandible > frontal bone > ethmoid/sphenoid bone
  ○ Imaging: Ill-defined expansion of diploic space with "ground-glass" or mixed soft tissue and calcific density on CT
    ▪ Intermediate to low T1, ↓ T2 signal; variable enhancement
- **Osteoma, Sinonasal**
  ○ Key facts: Multiple osteomas seen in Gardner syndrome (autosomal dominant disease characterized by intestinal polyposis, osteomas & cutaneous and soft tissue tumors)
    ▪ Osteomas arise on average 17 years before appearance of polyps

○ Imaging: Densely ossified, well-defined lesion arising from bony wall
  ▪ Can show mixed density & mimic other fibro-osseous lesions
- **Metastasis**
  ○ Key facts: Widespread metastatic disease usually present
    ▪ 50% of metastases to H&N involve sinonasal cavities
    ▪ Renal & lung most common
  ○ Imaging: Lytic bone lesions in maxilla with soft tissue extension into sinuses & nose
- **Sinus Histiocytosis (Rosai-Dorfman)**
  ○ Key facts: Overproduction & accumulation of histiocytes in lymph nodes with extranodal sites; 3rd-4th decades
  ○ Imaging: Multiple enhancing soft tissue masses; look for cervical nodes

SELECTED REFERENCES

1. Alexander AA et al: Paranasal sinus osteomas and Gardner's syndrome. Ann Otol Rhinol Laryngol. 116(9):658-62, 2007
2. Aribandi M et al: Imaging features of invasive and noninvasive fungal sinusitis: a review. Radiographics. 27(5):1283-96, 2007
3. Hagemann M et al: Nasal and paranasal sinus manifestation of Rosai-Dorfman disease. Rhinology. 43(3):229-32, 2005
4. Braun JJ et al: Sinonasal sarcoidosis: review and report of fifteen cases. Laryngoscope. 114(11):1960-3, 2004
5. Mohammadi-Araghi H et al: Fibro-osseous lesions of craniofacial bones. The role of imaging. Radiol Clin North Am. 31(1):121-34, 1993
6. Som PM et al: Chronic inflammatory sinonasal diseases including fungal infections. The role of imaging. Radiol Clin North Am. 31(1):33-44, 1993

Rhinosinusitis, Acute

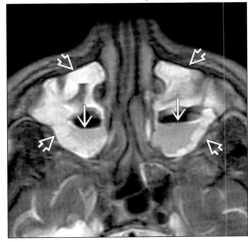

Axial T2WI MR shows bilateral maxillary air-fluid levels ➡ with peripheral edematous mucosa ⇥ in a patient with clinical symptoms of acute rhinosinusitis.

Rhinosinusitis, Chronic

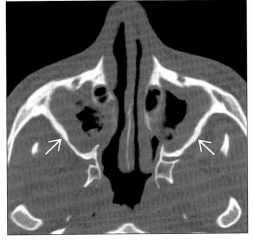

Axial bone CT shows bilateral maxillary sinus mucosal thickening with thickening & sclerosis of the bony sinus walls ➡ (chronic osteitis). This cystic fibrosis patient had recurrent sinus infections.

MULTIPLE SINONASAL LESIONS

(Left) Coronal bone CT shows multiple polypoid soft tissue lesions ➡ in the nasal cavities & paranasal sinuses, consistent with polyposis. The sphenoethmoidal recesses were occluded in this patient. *(Right)* Coronal T1 C+ FS MR shows markedly expansile polyps involving multiple sinuses and the nasal cavity. There is mass effect upon the right frontal lobe ➡ and the right orbit ⮕.

Polyposis, Sinonasal

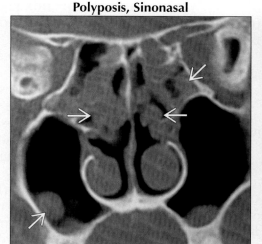

Polyposis, Sinonasal

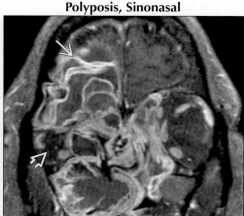

(Left) Axial NECT demonstrates a typical case of allergic fungal sinusitis involving the left nasal cavity, ethmoid, and sphenoid sinuses. Central high-density ➡ on CT is characteristic. *(Right)* Axial T1WI MR reveals marked expansion of ethmoid sinuses & left sphenoid sinus in a patient with allergic fungal sinusitis ➡. Trapped secretions are noted in the right sphenoid sinus ⮕.

Fungal Sinusitis, Allergic

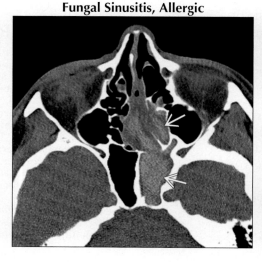

Fungal Sinusitis, Allergic

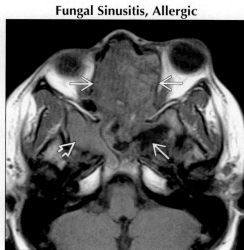

(Left) Axial T2WI MR shows mucous retention cysts ➡ in both maxillary sinuses. The signal characteristics vary depending on the protein and water content of the cysts. *(Right)* Axial T1 C+ FS MR reveals extensive Mucormycosis in a diabetic patient. The left maxillary and sphenoid sinuses are involved ➡, and there is extension into the masticator space ⮕.

Retention Cyst, Sinonasal

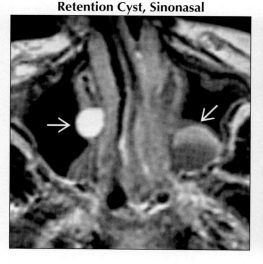

Fungal Sinusitis, Invasive

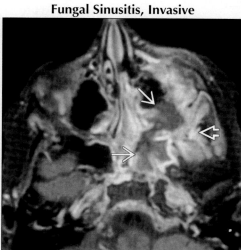

MULTIPLE SINONASAL LESIONS

Wegener Granulomatosis, Sinonasal
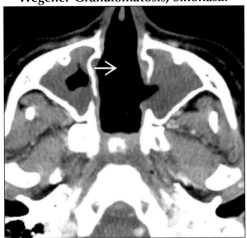

Sarcoidosis, Sinonasal
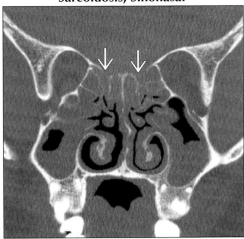

(Left) Axial CECT shows extensive maxillary sinuses mucosal thickening with chronic osteitis of the bony walls. A large septal perforation ➡ is seen in this patient with Wegener granulomatosis. *(Right)* Coronal bone CT shows pansinus mucosal disease in a sarcoidosis patient. Several foci of anterior skull base erosion ➡ are noted, and on MR imaging (not shown), intracranial disease was seen.

Fibrous Dysplasia, Sinonasal
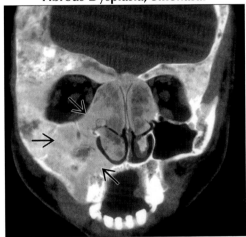

Osteoma, Sinonasal
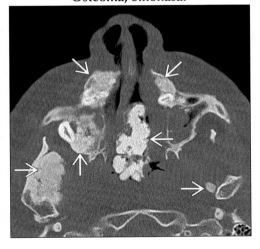

(Left) Coronal bone CT demonstrates polyostotic fibrous dysplasia of the cranium and midface. The typical ground-glass appearance of fibrous dysplasia is noted in multiple areas ➡. *(Right)* Axial bone CT reveals multiple dense osteomas ➡ arising from the maxilla, vomer, and mandible. Multiple osteomas are characteristic of Gardner syndrome. (Courtesy M. Castillo, MD.)

Metastasis
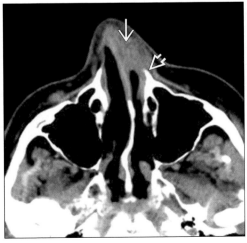

Sinus Histiocytosis (Rosai-Dorfman)
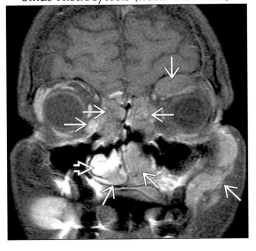

(Left) Axial NECT shows a left nasal vestibule ➡ metastasis from a GI carcinoma. Maxillary bone erosion ➡ is noted. A 2nd lesion was seen in the ethmoid sinuses on more superior images. *(Right)* Coronal T1 C+ FS MR shows multifocal histiocytosis ➡ of ethmoid sinuses, orbit, nasal cavity, and cheek soft tissues. Masses enhance less than nasal mucosa ➡. (Courtesy D. Shatzkes, MD.)

EXPANSILE SINONASAL LESION

DIFFERENTIAL DIAGNOSIS

Common
- Mucocele, Sinonasal
- Polyposis, Sinonasal
- Fungal Sinusitis, Allergic
- Ossifying Fibroma, Sinus
- Fibrous Dysplasia, Sinonasal

Less Common
- Polyps, Solitary, Sinonasal
- Cyst, Dentigerous (Follicular)
- Odontogenic Keratocyst
- Inverted Papilloma, Sinonasal
- Benign Mixed Tumor, Sinonasal

Rare but Important
- Nerve Sheath Tumor, Sinonasal
- Non-Hodgkin Lymphoma, Sinonasal
- Melanoma, Sinonasal
- Giant Cell Granuloma, Mandible-Maxilla
- Ameloblastoma

ESSENTIAL INFORMATION

Key Differential Diagnosis Issues
- Most of these lesions are benign and slow growing, causing bone remodeling or expansion

Helpful Clues for Common Diagnoses
- **Mucocele, Sinonasal**
  - Key facts: Most common expansile lesion
    - Results from obstruction of ostium or compartment of septated sinus
    - Frontal sinus (60-65%) > ethmoid (20-25%) > maxillary & sphenoid
  - Imaging
    - CT: Opacified, expanded sinus cavity with mucoid density
    - CT/MR: Enhancement of peripheral mucosa = mucopyocele
    - MR: Signal varies with protein:water ratio of secretions; generally ↓ T1, ↑ T2
- **Polyposis, Sinonasal**
  - Key facts: Inflamed mucous membranes with non-neoplastic hyperplasia
    - ↑ In allergy, aspirin sensitivity, CF
  - Imaging: Homogeneous masses with convex margins
    - Involve nasal cavity and sinuses
    - Bony remodeling & expansion when large

- Generally ↓ T1, ↑ T2 on MR, but varies with chronicity ± fungal presence
- **Fungal Sinusitis, Allergic**
  - Key facts: Form of sinusitis with viscous eosinophilic mucin & fungal hyphae
    - Immunocompetent patients; associated with allergy, asthma, polyposis
  - Imaging: Opacification & expansion of multiple sinuses; may be uni- or bilateral
    - CT: Central ↑ density, peripheral ↓ density
    - MR: ↓ T2 signal may mimic air
- **Ossifying Fibroma, Sinus**
  - Key facts: Benign, encapsulated fibro-osseous tumor
  - Imaging: Well-defined, expansile mass with central fibrous tissue & ossified rim (density ↑ with ↑ age of lesion)
- **Fibrous Dysplasia, Sinonasal**
  - Key facts: Developmental bone anomaly with formation of fibrous & osseous tissue
    - Monostotic and polyostotic forms
  - Imaging
    - Can be mixed osseous & fibrous
    - CT: Classic "ground-glass" appearance with expansion of medullary cavity

Helpful Clues for Less Common Diagnoses
- **Polyps, Solitary, Sinonasal**
  - Key facts: Inflammatory polyp without significant allergic history
    - Antrochoanal type most common
  - Imaging
    - CT: Well-defined, "dumbbell-shaped" mucoid density lesion extending from antrum ⇒ ostium ⇒ nasal cavity ⇒ nasopharynx
    - MR: Generally ↓ T1, ↑ T2 signal with only peripheral mucosal enhancement
- **Cyst, Dentigerous (Follicular)**
  - Key facts: Odontogenic cystic lesion
    - 2nd most common; mandible > maxilla
  - Imaging: Well-defined expansile unilocular cyst
    - Incorporating crown of unerupted tooth
- **Odontogenic Keratocyst**
  - Key facts: ~ 10% of odontogenic cysts
    - Mandible > maxilla; multiple (basal cell nevus syndrome)
  - Imaging: Uni- or multilocular cystic lesion
    - ± Crown of tooth (may mimic dentigerous cyst)

- **Inverted Papilloma, Sinonasal**
  - Key facts: 47% of nasal papillomas
    - Benign, but locally aggressive with malignant potential (SCCa)
    - 40-70 years, M:F = 2-4:1
  - Imaging
    - CT: Lobular mass on lateral nasal wall ± maxillary/ethmoid extension or intralesional Ca++
    - MR: "Convoluted," "cerebriform" architecture on T2 & post-gadolinium images; necrosis = coexistent carcinoma
- **Benign Mixed Tumor, Sinonasal**
  - Key facts: Arise from minor rests of salivary tissue most often in nasal septum
    - M < F; 30-60 years
  - Imaging: Septal mass
    - CT/MR: Variable enhancement
    - MR: ↑ T2 signal; larger lesions lobular with heterogeneous signal

Helpful Clues for Rare Diagnoses
- **Nerve Sheath Tumor, Sinonasal**
  - Key facts: 4% of H&N schwannomas
    - Schwannoma > > neurofibroma
    - Benign neoplasm; arise from CN5, V1 & V2 branches
  - Imaging: Well-circumscribed mass with bone remodeling (CT)
  - MR: Intermediate T1 signal
    - T2 varies with cellularity; large lesions ± cystic degeneration
- **Non-Hodgkin Lymphoma, Sinonasal**
  - Key facts: < 0.5% of extranodal NHL in Western populations (B-cell or NK/T-cell)
    - 2nd most common in areas of Asia (T-cell, EBV+); nasal cavity > sinuses
  - Imaging: Mass with bone remodeling ± destruction & extension into sinuses
    - MR: Homogeneous, ↓ T2 signal + diffuse enhancement
- **Melanoma, Sinonasal**
  - Key facts: Malignancy from mucosal melanocytes; nasal cavity > sinuses
    - Prognosis worse than cutaneous form
  - Imaging: Soft tissue mass with bone remodeling ± destruction
    - MR: ↑ T1 & ↓ T2 signal in melanotic form; enhance ± foci of hemorrhage
- **Giant Cell Granuloma, Mandible-Maxilla**
  - Key facts: Slow-growing, non-neoplastic lesion; may be related to trauma
    - ↑ Growth in pregnancy/post-partum
    - M:F = 1:2
    - Mandible & maxilla > skull base
  - Imaging: Heterogeneous soft tissue mass with avid enhancement
    - Bone remodeling ± destruction with intralesional mineralization
- **Ameloblastoma**
  - Key facts: Benign, locally aggressive odontogenic tumor
    - Mandible:maxilla = 4:1; arise near molars
    - Most present in 3rd-4th decades
  - Imaging: Expansile multilocular > unilocular cystic lesion; well-defined margins ("soap-bubble" or "honeycomb")

Mucocele, Sinonasal

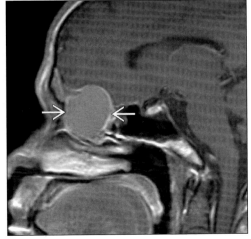

Sagittal T1 C+ MR shows a well-defined expansile lesion in the left ethmoid sinuses, consistent with a mucocele ➡. T1 shortening in the lesion suggests high protein content.

Polyposis, Sinonasal

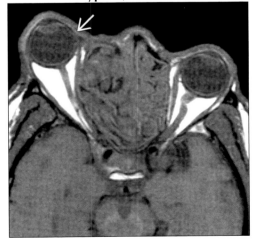

Axial T1WI MR shows severe sinonasal polyposis filling and expanding the ethmoid sinuses and resulting in right proptosis ➡. Heterogeneous signal may be due to decreased water or presence of fungi.

EXPANSILE SINONASAL LESION

(Left) Coronal bone CT shows the classic appearance of allergic fungal disease involving the left sinonasal cavities. The lamina papyracea is thin ➡, and the septum ⇉ is displaced to the right. (Right) Axial bone CT reveals a large ossifying fibroma of the left ethmoid sinuses and nasal cavity. The nasal septum ➡ and anterior sphenoid walls ⇉ are displaced by the mass but remain intact.

Fungal Sinusitis, Allergic

Ossifying Fibroma, Sinus

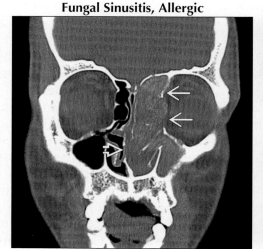

(Left) Coronal bone CT shows the classic appearance of fibrous dysplasia involving the left sphenoid bone. Obstructed secretions ➡ are seen in the left sphenoid sinus. Note small torus palatinus ⇉. (Right) Axial T2WI MR shows a T2 hyperintense antrochoanal polyp extending into the nasopharynx ➡. The polyp is hyperintense to turbinate mucosa ⇉. Note right maxillary retention cyst ➡.

Fibrous Dysplasia, Sinonasal

Polyps, Solitary, Sinonasal

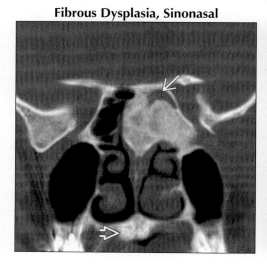

(Left) Axial CECT shows the typical CT appearance of a maxillary dentigerous cyst ➡ with displacement of an unerupted tooth ⇉. The lesion extends into the alveolar recess of the maxillary sinus. (Right) Coronal bone CT shows a maxillary odontogenic keratocyst (OKC) ➡ associated with supernumerary teeth ⇉ protruding into the floor of left maxillary antrum. This OKC mimics a dentigerous cyst.

Cyst, Dentigerous (Follicular)

Odontogenic Keratocyst

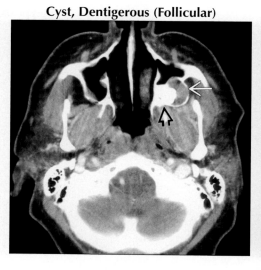
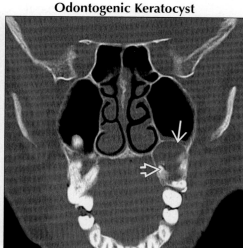

Inverted Papilloma, Sinonasal

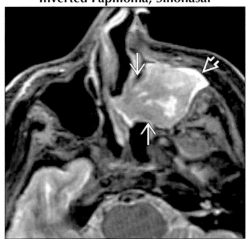

Benign Mixed Tumor, Sinonasal

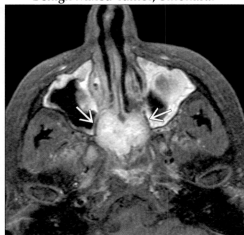

(Left) Axial T2WI MR shows a heterogeneous inverted papilloma expanding the left maxillary sinus, widening the ostium ➡, and involving the nasal cavity. Note peripheral trapped secretions ➡. *(Right)* Axial T1 C+ FS MR demonstrates a well-circumscribed uniformly enhancing pleomorphic adenoma in the posterior nasal cavity and nasopharynx splaying the medial maxillary walls ➡.

Nerve Sheath Tumor, Sinonasal

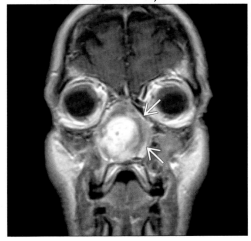

Non-Hodgkin Lymphoma, Sinonasal

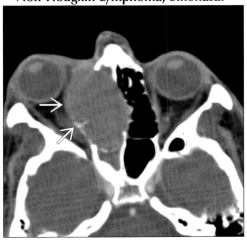

(Left) Coronal T1 C+ MR shows an expansile mass centered in the right nasal cavity displacing the nasal septum ➡ to the left. Central enhancement is prominent in this schwannoma. *(Right)* Axial CECT shows a sinonasal lymphoma filling the ethmoid sinuses and bulging into the right orbit ➡ (note proptosis). Lymphomas may cause more benign remodeling vs. destruction of bone.

Melanoma, Sinonasal

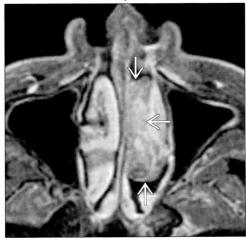

Giant Cell Granuloma, Mandible-Maxilla

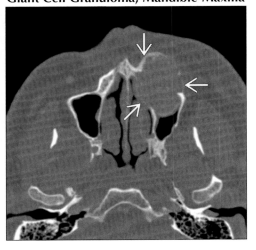

(Left) Axial T1 C+ FS MR shows a well-defined mucosal melanoma ➡ in the left nasal cavity displacing the turbinate laterally. The septum medial to the mass is intact. Melanomas may cause bone remodeling. *(Right)* Axial bone CT shows a typical case of a maxillary ridge giant cell granuloma. A thin rim of intact bone ➡ remains around the lesion, and matrix calcifications are visible.

NASAL LESION WITH BONE DESTRUCTION

DIFFERENTIAL DIAGNOSIS

Common
- SCCa, Sinonasal
- Non-Hodgkin Lymphoma, Sinonasal
- Inverted Papilloma, Sinonasal
- Fungal Sinusitis, Invasive
- Esthesioneuroblastoma

Less Common
- Wegener Granulomatosis, Sinonasal
- Adenocarcinoma, Sinonasal
- Undifferentiated Carcinoma, Sinonasal
- Sarcoidosis, Sinonasal
- Juvenile Angiofibroma
- Melanoma, Sinonasal

Rare but Important
- Chondrosarcoma, Sinonasal
- Osteosarcoma, Sinonasal
- Rhabdomyosarcoma
- Langerhans Histiocytosis, Skull Base
- Plasmacytoma, Skull Base
- Metastasis, Mandible-Maxilla

ESSENTIAL INFORMATION

Key Differential Diagnosis Issues
- Knowledge of patient demographics and clinical history is critical for narrowing differential diagnosis
- Presenting symptoms may be nonspecific and mimic chronic rhinosinusitis
- Best imaging tools
  - Sinonasal CT without contrast to identify Ca++ and early cortical bone destruction
  - Enhanced MR to determine vascularity, trans-spatial spread

Helpful Clues for Common Diagnoses
- **SCCa, Sinonasal**
  - Patient demographics: Adult patient (95% > 40 years); M > F
  - Maxillary antrum origin more common than nasal cavity, but most antral lesions involve the nasal cavity
  - Poorly defined with aggressive bone destruction; heterogeneous enhancement
- **Non-Hodgkin Lymphoma, Sinonasal**
  - Clinical clues: B-cell phenotype more common in North America and Europe; presents in 6th decade
  - Centered in nasal cavity with nasal septal destruction
  - CT: Homogeneous and may be hyperdense relative to other soft tissue
  - MR: Homogeneous signal and enhancement; decreased T2 signal due to high nuclear:cytoplasmic ratio of cells
- **Inverted Papilloma, Sinonasal**
  - Patient demographics: Adult male (40-70 years)
  - Rhinoscopy: Firm, vascular polypoid lesion on lateral nasal wall
  - CT: Polypoid mass near middle meatus with extension into maxillary antrum; intratumoral Ca++
  - MR: "Convoluted, cerebriform" architecture on T1 and T2 C+ sequences
- **Fungal Sinusitis, Invasive**
  - Clinical clue: Immunocompromised patient; rapidly progressive infection
  - Maxillary or ethmoid sinus origin with spread into nasal cavity
  - Infiltration of retroantral or premaxillary fat; decreased T2 signal due to fungal hyphae, metal chelates
- **Esthesioneuroblastoma**
  - Clinical clues: Adolescent or middle-aged patient with unilateral nasal obstruction and mild epistaxis; may bleed profusely on biopsy
  - Morphology: "Dumbbell-shaped" mass centered at cribriform plate
  - CT: Intralesional Ca++
  - MR: Avid enhancement; foci of hemorrhage; intracranial cyst formation

Helpful Clues for Less Common Diagnoses
- **Wegener Granulomatosis, Sinonasal**
  - Demographics: Wide age range (6th decade most common); M > F
  - CT: Lobular soft tissue lesions on nasal septum and turbinates; septal perforation is a common complication
- **Adenocarcinoma, Sinonasal**
  - Clinical clues: Adult (40-60 year old) male patient; indolent disease; may have occupational exposure history
  - Nonspecific imaging features, but may be more well defined than squamous cell carcinoma and esthesioneuroblastoma
- **Undifferentiated Carcinoma, Sinonasal**

NASAL LESION WITH BONE DESTRUCTION

- Clinical clue: Aggressive rapid growth pattern
- Nasal cavity and paranasal sinus involvement with spread into adjacent compartments
- **Sarcoidosis, Sinonasal**
  - Clinical clues: Usually a systemic disease with lung and kidney involvement; sinonasal involvement less often than Wegener
  - Nasal septum and turbinate involvement common; less "mass-like" with superficial, nodular soft tissue involvement
- **Juvenile Angiofibroma**
  - Clinical clues: Adolescent male patient with nasal obstruction and epistaxis
  - Location: Centered at sphenopalatine foramen with spread into pterygopalatine fossa, nasal cavity, and nasopharynx
  - Vascular mass with flow voids and avid enhancement
- **Melanoma, Sinonasal**
  - Clinical clues: Adult patient with epistaxis; pigmented lesion in nasal cavity at rhinoscopy
  - Attached to septum, lateral nasal wall, or inferior turbinate
  - CT: Bone may be remodeled or destroyed
  - MR: ↑ T1, ↓ T2 signal

Helpful Clues for Rare Diagnoses
- **Chondrosarcoma, Sinonasal**
  - Site of origin most often in skull base with secondary nasal cavity involvement

- Chondroid matrix of Ca++ on CT; T2 hyperintense
- **Osteosarcoma, Sinonasal**
  - Rare lesion; originates in maxilla or palate
  - CT: Osseous mass with periosteal reaction
- **Rhabdomyosarcoma**
  - Demographics: 70% < 12 years
  - Arise near skull base with extension into nasopharynx and nasal cavity
- **Langerhans Histiocytosis, Skull Base**
  - Demographics: Presents in 1st decade; gender: M > F
  - Originates in skull base or maxilla with extension into nasal cavity
- **Plasmacytoma, Skull Base**
  - Demographics: 5th to 9th decades; M > F; more common in African-Americans
  - Originates in skull base with extension into nasal cavity
- **Metastasis, Mandible-Maxilla**
  - Clinical clues: Breast and lung carcinoma most common primaries; widespread skeletal metastases present

Other Essential Information
- Although nodal spread from sinonasal malignancies is uncommon (< 20%), be sure to look at retropharyngeal and L2 and L3 nodes
- Imaging features of these lesions (particularly in adults) may be nonspecific and histologic confirmation is essential for diagnosis

SCCa, Sinonasal

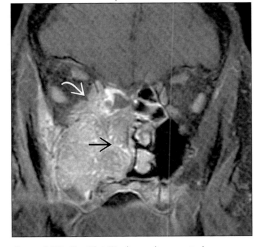

Coronal T1 C+ FS MR shows large antral squamous carcinoma with extension into the right nasal cavity → and orbit →. The middle and inferior turbinates are invaded by tumor.

Non-Hodgkin Lymphoma, Sinonasal

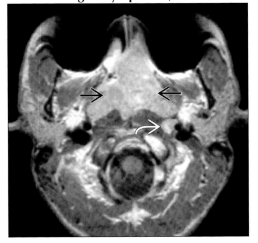

Axial T1 C+ MR shows the typical location and homogeneous enhancement pattern of sinonasal lymphoma with extension into the nasopharynx →. Note small retropharyngeal node on the left →.

NASAL LESION WITH BONE DESTRUCTION

(Left) Axial T1 C+ FS MR shows typical inverted papilloma centered near the middle meatus ⊡ extending into the antrum ➡ and nasal cavity ➡. A "convoluted" architecture is appreciated. *(Right)* Axial T2WI FS MR shows fungal sinusitis with spread from the antrum into the nasal cavity ⊡ and nasopharyngeal masticator space ➡. Decreased T2 signal and the mass-like appearance are typical.

Inverted Papilloma, Sinonasal

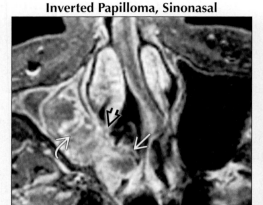

Fungal Sinusitis, Invasive

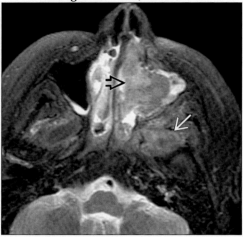

(Left) Coronal T1 C+ FS MR shows an invasive tumor with extension into the anterior cranial fossa. Diffuse enhancement is noted in this vascular neoplasm. Extension into the right orbit ➡ is present. *(Right)* Coronal bone CT shows lobular soft tissue centered on the septum and turbinates, characteristic of granulomatous diseases with septal perforation ➡. Lobular tissue ➡ is noted in the maxillary antrum.

Esthesioneuroblastoma

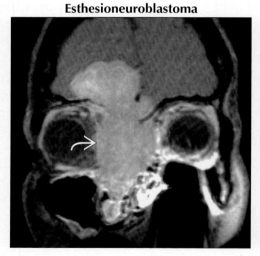

Wegener Granulomatosis, Sinonasal

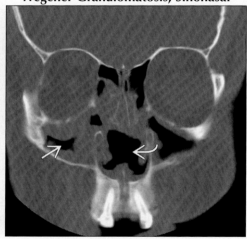

(Left) Coronal T1 C+ MR shows a large sinonasal adenocarcinoma with heterogeneous enhancement and marked intracranial extension ➡. The site of origin was likely the superior nasal cavity. *(Right)* Coronal bone CT shows a sinonasal undifferentiated carcinoma involving the nasal cavity and ethmoid sinuses with anterior skull base ➡ and orbital ➡ invasion.

Adenocarcinoma, Sinonasal

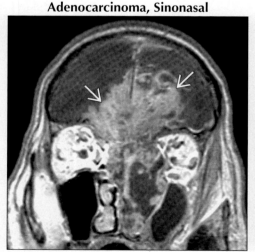

Undifferentiated Carcinoma, Sinonasal

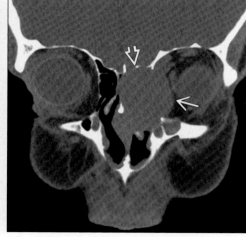

NASAL LESION WITH BONE DESTRUCTION

Sarcoidosis, Sinonasal

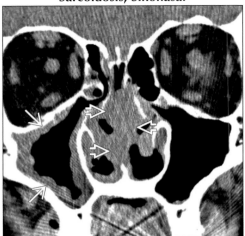

Juvenile Angiofibroma

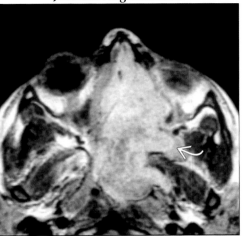

(Left) Coronal NECT shows typical appearance of sinonasal sarcoid involvement with lobular soft tissue along the nasal septum ➡ and involving the right maxillary sinus ➡. *(Right)* Axial T1 C+ MR shows large juvenile angiofibroma involving the nasal cavity, nasopharynx, and pterygopalatine fossa ➡. Diffuse enhancement is seen throughout this vascular lesion.

Melanoma, Sinonasal

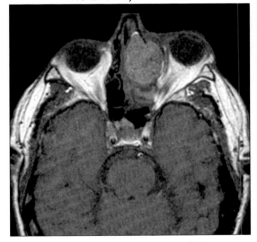

Chondrosarcoma, Sinonasal

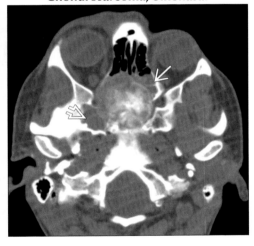

(Left) Axial T1WI MR shows fairly well-defined sinonasal melanoma involving the left ethmoids and upper nasal cavity. Note increased T1 signal in the mass relative to other soft tissue (muscle, brain). *(Right)* Axial bone CT shows a typical chondrosarcoma arising from the vomer area of the nasal septum with chondroid matrix. Note obstructed secretions in the sphenoid ➡ and ethmoid ➡ sinuses.

Osteosarcoma, Sinonasal

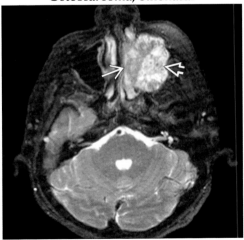

Rhabdomyosarcoma

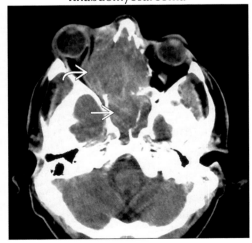

(Left) Axial T2WI FS MR reveals an osteosarcoma arising from the maxilla, involving the nasal cavity ➡ and maxillary antrum ➡. The ossific matrix creates low signal areas in the tumor matrix. *(Right)* Axial CECT shows aggressive midface alveolar rhabdomyosarcoma with bilateral nasal cavity involvement. There is extension into the sphenoid sinus ➡ and orbit ➡.

DIFFERENTIAL DIAGNOSIS

Common
- Polyposis, Sinonasal
- Fungal Sinusitis, Allergic
- Polyps, Solitary, Sinonasal
- Juvenile Angiofibroma
- Inverted Papilloma, Sinonasal

Less Common
- Osteoma, Sinonasal
- Nasolacrimal Duct Cyst
- Hemangioma, Sinonasal
- Benign Mixed Tumor, Sinonasal
- Rhinolith
- Non-Hodgkin Lymphoma, Sinonasal

Rare but Important
- Nerve Sheath Tumor, Sinonasal
- Melanoma, Sinonasal
- Giant Cell Granuloma, Mandible-Maxilla

ESSENTIAL INFORMATION

Key Differential Diagnosis Issues
- Patient demographics and findings at nasal endoscopy very helpful for narrowing differential diagnosis
- Imaging suggestions
  - CT is most useful modality for visualizing bone remodeling produced by these lesions
  - MR imaging is helpful for further characterizing lesions (signal characteristics, vascularity, architecture, presence of mucoid material or melanin)
    - For lesions in superior nasal cleft with possible cribriform plate erosion, MR is indicated to evaluate for intracranial extension & to exclude cephalocele
- In pediatric population, congenital lesions may also present as nasal mass without bone destruction
  - Nasal dermal sinus, nasal glioma, & nasoethmoidal cephaloceles included here

Helpful Clues for Common Diagnoses
- **Polyposis, Sinonasal**
  - Clinical clues: Patient > 20 years, often with history of allergies; when lesion is large & expansile can produce significant cosmetic deformity
  - Usually involves nasal cavity and paranasal sinuses; multiple and bilateral; anterior > posterior
- **Fungal Sinusitis, Allergic**
  - Clinical clues: Severe form of chronic rhinosinusitis most often seen in young adults
  - Unilateral or bilateral sinonasal opacification; multiple sinuses involved
  - CT: Central hyperdensity with low attenuation peripherally
  - MR: Signal variable on T1 related to protein/water content; hypointense on T2
- **Polyps, Solitary, Sinonasal**
  - Clinical clues: Teenager or young adult with unilateral nasal obstruction
  - Well-defined "dumbbell-shaped" lesion arising from antrum; widens middle meatus and extends into nasal cavity
  - CT: Mucoid density
  - MR: Low T1 and high T2 signal with peripheral enhancement
- **Juvenile Angiofibroma**
  - Clinical clues: Adolescent male patient presenting with unilateral nasal obstruction and epistaxis; vascular lesion in the nasal cavity on endoscopy
  - CT: Enhancing mass centered at sphenopalatine foramen with nasal cavity, nasopharyngeal, and pterygopalatine fossa extension; bone remodeling or erosion may be present
  - MR: Hyperintense on T2; "salt & pepper" appearance due to flow voids on T2 or post-contrast T1 sequences
- **Inverted Papilloma, Sinonasal**
  - Clinical clues: Male patient, 40-70 years of age; polypoid mass centered on lateral nasal wall near middle meatus
  - CT: Often involves both nasal cavity and maxillary antrum; may contain Ca++ and erode and remodel bone
  - MR: Convoluted "cerebriform" architecture

Helpful Clues for Less Common Diagnoses
- **Osteoma, Sinonasal**
  - Location: More common in paranasal sinuses than nasal cavity
  - CT: Attached to or arises within bones surrounding sinonasal cavities

- ▪ Dense "ivory" type is classic, but density variable due to mixture of fibrous and osseous components
  - ○ MR: T2 hypointense
- **Nasolacrimal Duct Cyst**
  - ○ Location: Anywhere along nasolacrimal apparatus from lacrimal sac to inferior meatus (valve of Hasner)
  - ○ CT/MR: Mucoid or fluid density/signal; expands nasolacrimal duct; cystic mass at sac or inferior meatus
- **Hemangioma, Sinonasal**
  - ○ Clinical clues: Soft red-blue mass usually in anterior nasal cavity arising from septum near Kiesselbach venous plexus; more common in pediatric population
  - ○ CT: Remodels adjacent bone; intraosseous form has a more permeative, lytic appearance
  - ○ MR: T2 hyperintense; diffuse enhancement
- **Benign Mixed Tumor, Sinonasal**
  - ○ Arises from minor rests of salivary tissue in nasal cavity or palate mucosa
  - ○ Well-defined mass; may contain Ca++ on CT; T2 hyperintensity characteristic on MR with variable enhancement
- **Rhinolith**
  - ○ Clinical issues: Usually found in children; chronic purulent rhinitis; imaging often not necessary
  - ○ CT is best imaging study, as calcium is deposited on the foreign body
- **Non-Hodgkin Lymphoma, Sinonasal**
  - ○ Clinical clues: Most common in older patients; prefers nasal cavity origin over paranasal sinuses
  - ○ CT: Although malignant, this tumor may show bone remodeling &/or bone destruction
  - ○ MR: Homogeneous; decreased T2 signal; homogeneous enhancement

Helpful Clues for Rare Diagnoses
- **Nerve Sheath Tumor, Sinonasal**
  - ○ Well-circumscribed mass with variable signal and enhancement on MR; schwannoma most common histology
- **Melanoma, Sinonasal**
  - ○ Nasal cavity site of origin more common than paranasal sinus
  - ○ CT: Although malignant, this tumor may show bone remodeling &/or bone destruction
  - ○ MR: T1 shortening in highly melanotic form (blood products, melanin); T2 hypointense (blood products, melanin, free radicals)
- **Giant Cell Granuloma, Mandible-Maxilla**
  - ○ Non-odontogenic tumor only occurring in maxilla and mandible; benign, but may be locally destructive
  - ○ CT: Well-defined soft tissue mass arising from maxilla with expansion into nasal cavity; thin "eggshell" periphery with central matrix calcifications

Polyposis, Sinonasal

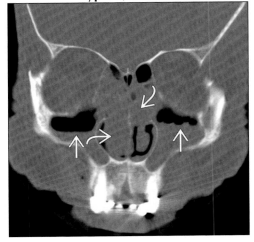

Coronal bone CT shows diffuse sinonasal polyposis with bilateral nasal polyps ⮞ and sinus mucosal thickening. There are maxillary fluid levels ⮞ consistent with acute inflammation.

Fungal Sinusitis, Allergic

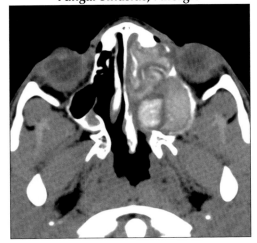

Axial NECT shows the typical appearance of allergic fungal sinusitis. Note unilateral expansion of the sinonasal cavities with central increased and peripheral low density material.

(Left) Axial T1 C+ MR shows an antrochoanal polyp extending from the maxillary antrum through the middle meatus ⇨ into the nasal cavity ⇨ and nasopharynx ⇨. *(Right)* Axial CECT shows a small juvenile angiofibroma of the left nasal cavity ⇨ projecting into the nasopharynx ⇨. Taken early in the injection, this image shows that the tumor enhances before the muscles enhance.

Polyps, Solitary, Sinonasal

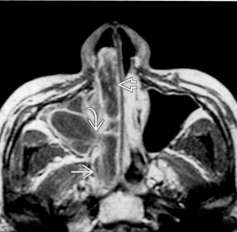

Juvenile Angiofibroma

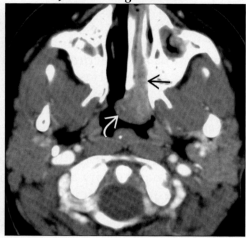

(Left) Coronal bone CT shows an inverted papilloma ⇨ arising near the middle meatus and extending into the maxillary antrum. The septum is slightly deviated toward the left. *(Right)* Coronal bone CT shows an osteoma of the left nasal cavity ⇨. This osteoma originated from the middle turbinate concha and is of mixed bone and soft tissue density.

Inverted Papilloma, Sinonasal

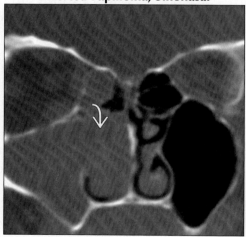

Osteoma, Sinonasal

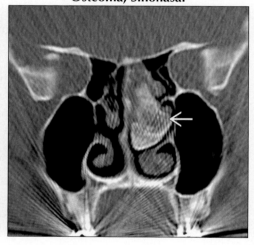

(Left) Coronal bone CT shows a nasolacrimal cyst ⇨ with expansion of the right nasolacrimal duct ⇨ and extension to the level of the inferior meatus ⇨ just beneath the inferior turbinate. *(Right)* Coronal CECT shows the features of a posterior nasal cavity hemangioma in an adult patient. Note a well-circumscribed lobular enhancing mass in the left nasal cavity ⇨ at the choana.

Nasolacrimal Duct Cyst

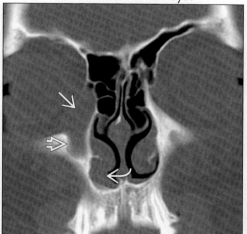

Hemangioma, Sinonasal

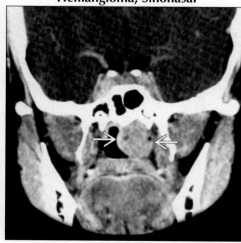

NASAL LESION WITHOUT BONE DESTRUCTION

Benign Mixed Tumor, Sinonasal
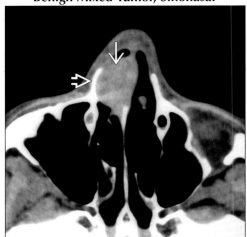

Rhinolith
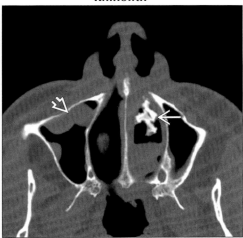

(Left) Axial NECT shows a benign mixed tumor (pleomorphic adenoma) in the right nasal vestibule ➡ arising from the septum. There is slight remodeling of the nasal process of the maxilla ➡. (Right) Axial bone CT shows an irregular dense rhinolith in the left nasal cavity ➡. Mucosal thickening is noted in the alveolar recess of the right maxillary sinus ➡.

Non-Hodgkin Lymphoma, Sinonasal
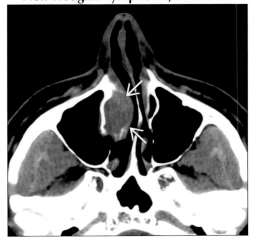

Nerve Sheath Tumor, Sinonasal
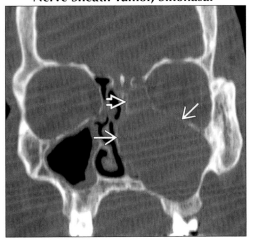

(Left) Axial NECT shows a homogeneous soft tissue mass ➡ in the right nasal cavity at the level of the inferior meatus. This lymphoma of the nasolacrimal duct expands the surrounding bone. (Right) Coronal bone CT shows a neurofibroma within the left maxillary sinus. There is remodeling of the sinus walls ➡. Obstructed secretions are noted in the left ethmoid sinuses ➡.

Melanoma, Sinonasal
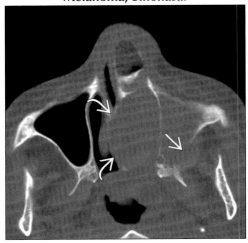

Giant Cell Granuloma, Mandible-Maxilla
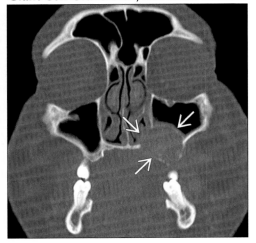

(Left) Axial bone CT shows a sinonasal melanoma with both bone remodeling ➡ and destruction ➡. Although highly malignant, melanoma may show benign changes within surrounding bone. (Right) Coronal bone CT shows a maxillary ridge giant cell granuloma bulging into the left nasal cavity. A thin rim of intact bone is seen at the periphery of the lesion ➡.

SINUS LESION WITHOUT BONE DESTRUCTION

DIFFERENTIAL DIAGNOSIS

Common
- Rhinosinusitis, Chronic
- Rhinosinusitis, Acute
- Mucocele, Sinonasal
- Polyposis, Sinonasal
- Fungal Sinusitis, Mycetoma
- Osteoma, Sinonasal

Less Common
- Fungal Sinusitis, Allergic
- Inverted Papilloma, Sinonasal
- Fibrous Dysplasia, Sinonasal
- Ossifying Fibroma, Sinus
- Polyps, Solitary, Sinonasal
- Juvenile Angiofibroma

Rare but Important
- Benign Mixed Tumor, Sinonasal
- Nerve Sheath Tumor, Sinonasal
- Silent Sinus Syndrome

ESSENTIAL INFORMATION

Key Differential Diagnosis Issues
- Infectious/inflammatory disorders & benign neoplasms comprise majority of lesions in this differential diagnosis
- Malignant neoplasms such as lymphoma & melanoma can cause bone remodeling rather than destruction

Helpful Clues for Common Diagnoses
- **Rhinosinusitis, Chronic**
  - Key facts: Involves multiple sinuses
    - Look for anatomic variants or obstructing lesions of drainage pathways
  - Imaging: Mucosal thickening, bone sclerosis, & thickening of sinus walls (osteitis)
- **Rhinosinusitis, Acute**
  - Key facts: Viral or bacterial infection
    - Look for odontogenic source if isolated to one maxillary sinus
  - Imaging: Normal-sized sinus lumen with mucosal thickening ± air-fluid levels
- **Mucocele, Sinonasal**
  - Key facts: Most common expansile sinus lesion arising from chronic obstruction
  - Imaging
    - CT: Opacified, expanded sinus with intact bony rim

- MR: ↓ T1, ↑ T2 with peripheral enhancement; if ↑ T1, high protein content secretions
- **Polyposis, Sinonasal**
  - Key facts: Commonly allergic patients
    - Involves nasal cavity and sinuses
  - Imaging: Lobular soft tissue lesions that can opacify and expand sinonasal cavities
- **Fungal Sinusitis, Mycetoma**
  - Key facts: Often asymptomatic
    - Colonization of obstructed secretions by noninvasive fungi in immunocompetent patient
  - Imaging: Opacified, nonexpanded sinus with increased density material ± calcifications
    - Maxillary > sphenoid
- **Osteoma, Sinonasal**
  - Key facts: Most common benign sinus tumor; frontal > ethmoid sinuses
  - Imaging: Well-defined, densely ossified mass attached to sinus wall
    - May be mixed fibrous & osseous

Helpful Clues for Less Common Diagnoses
- **Fungal Sinusitis, Allergic**
  - Key facts: Form of chronic sinusitis with eosinophilic mucin & noninvasive fungi
    - Often seen in allergic patients & those with polyposis
  - Imaging
    - CT: Opacified, expanded sinuses (unilateral or bilateral) with central ↑ density & peripheral ↓ density
    - MR signal variable; ↓ T2 signal mimics air
- **Inverted Papilloma, Sinonasal**
  - Key facts: Benign epithelial neoplasm with endophytic growth pattern
    - M:F = 4:1; nasal cavity > sinuses
    - May contain squamous cell carcinoma
  - Imaging: Lobular mass in nasal cavity near middle meatus with extension into antrum
    - "Convoluted" or "cerebriform" architecture on T2 or post-contrast MR
- **Fibrous Dysplasia, Sinonasal**
  - Key facts: Mesenchymal developmental anomaly forming weak woven bone
    - Mono- or polyostotic; focal or diffuse
  - Imaging
    - CT: Commonly expansile, ill-defined bony lesion with "ground-glass" matrix
    - MR: Variable signal; ↓ T2 common

SINUS LESION WITHOUT BONE DESTRUCTION

- **Ossifying Fibroma, Sinus**
  - Key facts: Benign fibro-osseous tumor of mature bone & fibrous tissue
    - Maxilla < mandible
  - Imaging
    - CT: Well-demarcated expansile mass with mixed soft tissue (central fibrous) & osseous (peripheral) density
    - MR: Fibrous component ↑ T2 & osseous ↓ T2 signal; heterogeneous enhancement
- **Polyps, Solitary, Sinonasal**
  - Key facts: Antrochoanal polyp common
  - Imaging
    - CT: Well-defined low-density lesion arising in antrum, widening ostium & protruding into nasal cavity/nasopharynx
    - MR: ↓ T1 & ↑ T2 signal with peripheral mucosal enhancement
- **Juvenile Angiofibroma**
  - Key facts: Benign, but locally invasive vascular neoplasm
    - Occurs in adolescent males with nasal obstruction and epistaxis
  - Imaging: Lesion centered in sphenopalatine foramen with extension into nasal cavity, nasopharynx, & pterygopalatine fossa
    - CT: Bone remodeling; pterygopalatine fossa expansion common
    - MR: Heterogeneous ↓ T1 & ↑ T2 MR signal with avid enhancement

Helpful Clues for Rare Diagnoses

- **Benign Mixed Tumor, Sinonasal**
  - Key facts: 8% of benign mixed tumors (pleomorphic adenoma) occur outside of major salivary glands
    - Most arise on nasal septum
    - 30-60 years at presentation
  - Imaging
    - CT: Well-defined mass with adjacent bone remodeling
    - MR: Intermediate T1 & ↑ T2 signal; variable enhancement
- **Nerve Sheath Tumor, Sinonasal**
  - Key facts: Benign tumors (schwannoma > neurofibroma)
    - ~ 10% of H&N schwannomas
    - Nasoethmoid > maxillary > nasal cavity > sphenoid
    - Neurofibroma more common in NF1
  - Imaging
    - CT: Well-defined mass with bone expansion/remodeling
    - MR: ↓ T1, ↑ T2 MR signal; variable enhancement; ± intramural cysts
- **Silent Sinus Syndrome**
  - Key facts: Chronic maxillary obstruction results in painless wall retraction from negative intrasinus pressure
  - Imaging: Opacified maxillary sinus with decreased volume & inward bowing of all walls + enophthalmos

Rhinosinusitis, Chronic

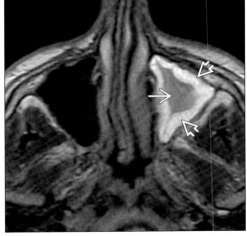

Axial T2WI MR shows an opacified left maxillary sinus. The sinus volume is decreased, the walls thickened, and central proteinaceous secretions ➡ *with peripheral edematous mucosa* ➡ *visible.*

Rhinosinusitis, Acute

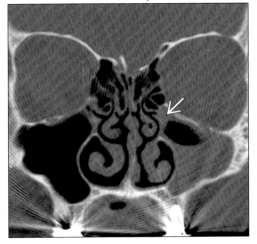

Coronal bone CT shows mucosal thickening and an air-fluid level in a patient with the clinical symptoms of acute sinusitis. There is occlusion of the ostiomeatal unit at the infundibulum ➡.

SINUS LESION WITHOUT BONE DESTRUCTION

(Left) Coronal bone CT shows an expanded opacified right maxillary sinus in a patient with Wegener granulomatosis. There is circumferential bony remodeling ➡ consistent with a mucocele. *(Right)* Coronal bone CT shows opacification and expansion of the right ethmoid cells ➡ and a polyp ⧓ in the nasal cavity. Bubbly secretions in the right maxillary sinus suggest acute inflammation.

Mucocele, Sinonasal

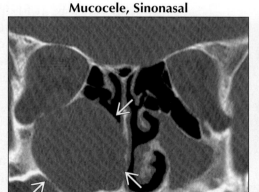

Polyposis, Sinonasal

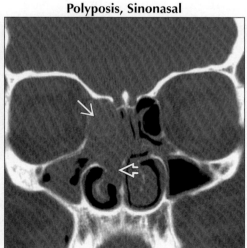

(Left) Axial NECT shows a high attenuation mycetoma (fungus ball) ➡ in the right maxillary sinus with multiple calcifications centrally. Mucosal thickening ⧓ is seen peripherally. *(Right)* Coronal bone CT shows a well-defined dense osseous lesion ➡ in the right frontal sinus, consistent with an osteoma. The lesion did not obstruct sinus drainage.

Fungal Sinusitis, Mycetoma

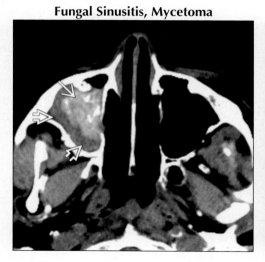

Osteoma, Sinonasal

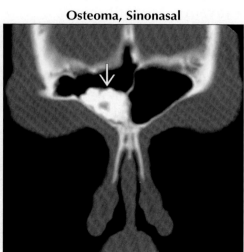

(Left) Axial bone CT shows opacified expanded right ethmoid sinuses ➡ with centrally dense material characteristic of allergic fungal sinusitis. The surrounding bone is remodeled, not destroyed. *(Right)* Axial NECT shows a nasal cavity inverted papilloma ➡ that has widened the maxillary ostium and extended into the left antrum. Secretions trapped anterior to the lesion ⧓ are less dense.

Fungal Sinusitis, Allergic

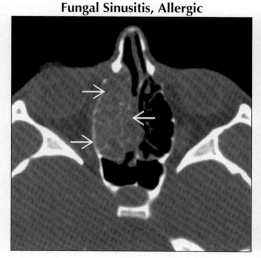

Inverted Papilloma, Sinonasal

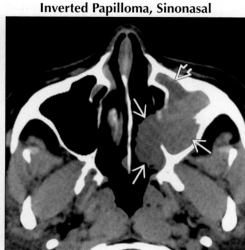

SINUS LESION WITHOUT BONE DESTRUCTION

Fibrous Dysplasia, Sinonasal

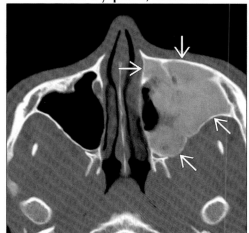

Ossifying Fibroma, Sinus

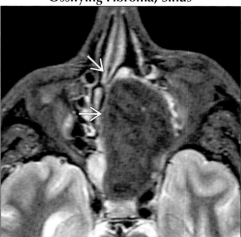

(Left) Axial bone CT shows a typical "ground-glass" appearance of fibrous dysplasia involving the left maxillary sinus. There is marked bone expansion, but the cortex ➡ remains intact. *(Right)* Axial T2WI MR shows a large hypointense left ethmoid ossifying fibroma. The nasal septum ➡ is deviated to the right. The low T2 signal is characteristic of an ossified lesion.

Polyps, Solitary, Sinonasal

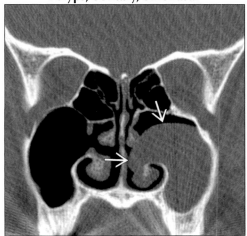

Juvenile Angiofibroma

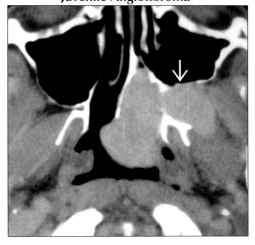

(Left) Coronal bone CT reveals a sharply marginated polyp ➡ arising from the left antrum and extending through a widened maxillary ostium into the left nasal cavity. *(Right)* Axial CECT reveals a "dumbbell-shaped" homogeneously enhancing juvenile angiofibroma in the left nasal cavity, nasopharynx, and pterygopalatine fossa and displacing the posterior maxillary wall ➡.

Benign Mixed Tumor, Sinonasal

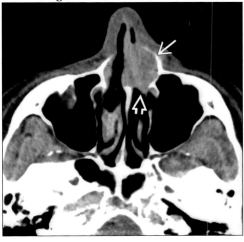

Nerve Sheath Tumor, Sinonasal

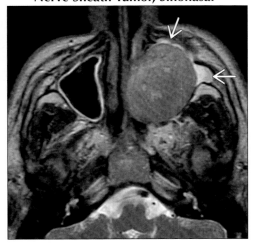

(Left) Axial CECT demonstrates a typical well-circumscribed anterior nasal benign mixed tumor ➡ with the left nasal bone remodeled and displaced laterally ➡. *(Right)* Axial T2WI MR shows a well-defined mass within the left maxillary antrum. This nerve sheath tumor was a neurofibroma histologically. Note trapped high signal secretions ➡ peripheral to the mass.

SINUS LESION WITH BONE DESTRUCTION

DIFFERENTIAL DIAGNOSIS

Common
- SCCa, Sinonasal
- Fungal Sinusitis, Invasive
- Esthesioneuroblastoma
- Non-Hodgkin Lymphoma, Sinonasal

Less Common
- Wegener Granulomatosis, Sinonasal
- Undifferentiated Carcinoma, Sinonasal
- Adenocarcinoma, Sinonasal
- Sarcoidosis, Sinonasal
- Rhabdomyosarcoma
- Adenoid Cystic Carcinoma, Sinonasal

Rare but Important
- Osteosarcoma, Sinonasal
- Chondrosarcoma, Sinonasal
- Langerhans Histiocytosis, Skull Base
- Metastasis

ESSENTIAL INFORMATION

Key Differential Diagnosis Issues
- This differential includes primarily neoplasms and aggressive infectious/granulomatous disorders

Helpful Clues for Common Diagnoses
- **SCCa, Sinonasal**
  - Key facts: Most common sinonasal (SN) malignancy
    - 80% involve antrum
    - May coexist in inverted papilloma
  - Imaging: Ill-defined mass
    - Aggressive bone destruction (rarely remodeling) & heterogeneous, mild enhancement
    - Large lesions with necrosis & hemorrhage
- **Fungal Sinusitis, Invasive**
  - Key facts: Aggressive infection in immunocompromised or debilitated patient
  - Aspergillus & mucormycosis most common
  - Imaging: Infiltrating mucosal or mass lesion ± bone destruction
    - ↓ T2 signal with spread into adjacent compartments
- **Esthesioneuroblastoma**

  - Key facts: Neural crest tumor of olfactory origin with good prognosis
    - 2 age peaks: 11-20 years & 50-60 years
    - Originates in superior nasal cavity
    - Presents with epistaxis or bleeding upon biopsy
  - Imaging: Avidly enhancing nasoethmoid mass
    - Intratumoral matrix calcification
    - Intracranial extension with cysts at tumor-brain interface
- **Non-Hodgkin Lymphoma, Sinonasal**
  - Key facts: < 50% of extranodal H&N non-Hodgkin Lymphoma arise in sinonasal cavities
  - Curable with radiotherapy; prefers nasal cavity site of origin
  - Imaging: High nucleus to cytoplasm ratio results in ↑ CT density & ↓ T2 MR signal
    - Homogeneously enhancing; causes bone remodeling or destruction

Helpful Clues for Less Common Diagnoses
- **Wegener Granulomatosis, Sinonasal**
  - Key facts: Necrotizing granulomatous disease with frequent nasal involvement
    - Prefers septum and turbinates
  - Imaging: Nodular soft tissue lesions in nasal cavity
    - Septal perforation and erosion of ethmoid septations
- **Undifferentiated Carcinoma, Sinonasal**
  - Key facts: Extremely malignant neoplasm with rapid growth, distant metastases, & poor prognosis
    - Presents at advanced stage
  - Imaging: Aggressive mass with ill-defined margins, bone destruction, & spread into adjacent compartments
- **Adenocarcinoma, Sinonasal**
  - Key facts: 10-20% of SN malignancies
    - Salivary & intestinal types; M > F
    - Higher incidence inhalational exposures
    - Predilection for nasoethmoid region
  - Imaging: Nonspecific; well- to poorly defined soft tissue mass with bone destruction
    - Variable MR signal with heterogeneous enhancement
- **Sarcoidosis, Sinonasal**

SINUS LESION WITH BONE DESTRUCTION

- ○ Key facts: Granulomatous disorder with less frequent SN involvement than Wegener, but similar features
- ○ Imaging: Nodular soft tissue lesions in nasal cavity > paranasal sinuses
- **Rhabdomyosarcoma**
  - ○ Key facts: Cancer of striated muscle
    - ▪ Most common childhood sarcoma
    - ▪ 40% in H&N (orbit, sinonasal, T-bone)
  - ○ Imaging: Soft tissue mass ± bone destruction with variable enhancement
    - ▪ MR best for evaluating perineural & intracranial spread
- **Adenoid Cystic Carcinoma, Sinonasal**
  - ○ Key facts: Accounts for < 10% of SN malignancies
    - ▪ Median age of incidence is 50 years
    - ▪ Palate primaries may extend into maxillary antrum & nasal cavity
    - ▪ Perineural spread, late recurrences, & distant metastases more common than other SN malignancies
    - ▪ Maxillary sinus & nasal cavity most common sites
  - ○ Imaging: Nonspecific; well- to poorly defined soft tissue mass ± bone destruction
    - ▪ Variable MR signal with heterogeneous enhancement
    - ▪ Look for perineural spread (may be extensive despite small primary site)

Helpful Clues for Rare Diagnoses
- **Osteosarcoma, Sinonasal**
  - ○ Key facts: ≤ 1% of SN tumors

- ▪ ↑ Risk if prior radiation therapy & ThO₂ (Thorotrast) exposure
    - ▪ Can arise in Paget, FD, or osteoblastoma
    - ▪ Males in 3rd & 4th decades
  - ○ Imaging
    - ▪ CT: Aggressive mass with bone destruction, irregular calcification ± osteoid matrix, "sunburst" periosteal reaction
    - ▪ MR: Low-to-intermediate T1 & T2 signal (ossified areas ↓ signal)
- **Chondrosarcoma, Sinonasal**
  - ○ Key facts: Most arise in maxilla anteriorly with antral extension; M:F = 3:2
  - ○ Imaging: Ca++ matrix (< 50%)
    - ▪ Expansile with variable bone destruction/remodeling
    - ▪ MR: ↑ T2 signal common
- **Langerhans Histiocytosis, Skull Base**
  - ○ Key facts: Skull & T-bone most common
    - ▪ Skull base, mandible-maxilla < common
    - ▪ Presents in 1st decade (more severe cases ⇒ earlier presentation)
  - ○ Imaging
    - ▪ CT: Focal or diffuse mass + bone destruction; punched out or irregular margins
    - ▪ MR: ↓ T1, ↑ T2 signal; heterogeneous enhancement ± blood products
- **Metastasis**
  - ○ Key facts: Very rare; renal > lung > breast; systemic metastases usually present
  - ○ Imaging: Aggressive bone-destroying soft tissue masses with variable enhancement

SCCa, Sinonasal

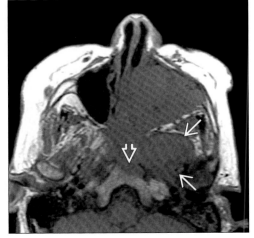

Axial T1WI MR shows a large maxillary squamous carcinoma. The lesion not only destroys the maxillary sinus walls but also invades the masticator space ➡ and clivus ➡.

Fungal Sinusitis, Invasive

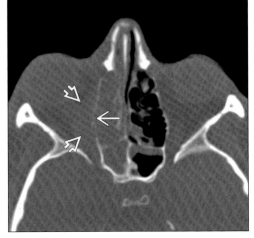

Axial bone CT shows extension of fungal sinusitis of the ethmoid sinuses into the orbit ➡. A small area of bone erosion by the fundus is noted in the lamina papyracea ➡.

SINUS LESION WITH BONE DESTRUCTION

(Left) *Axial CECT demonstrates a large esthesioneuroblastoma involving the ethmoid sinuses bilaterally and extending into the orbits* ➡️ *and anterior skull base* ➡️. **(Right)** *Coronal bone CT reveals a lymphoma originating in the nasal cavity and causing obstruction of multiple ethmoid air cells* ➡️. *Destruction of the bony nasal septum* ➡️ *is present.*

Esthesioneuroblastoma

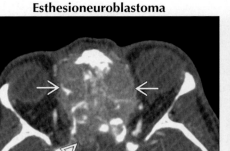

Non-Hodgkin Lymphoma, Sinonasal

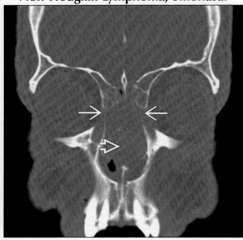

(Left) *Axial CECT shows extensive nodular soft tissue in the sinonasal cavities and bone destruction of the septum* ➡️ *and medial maxillary walls* ➡️ *related to Wegener granulomatosis.* **(Right)** *Coronal NECT demonstrates a very large sinonasal undifferentiated carcinoma that originated in the maxillary sinus and has spread into the nasal cavity* ➡️, *the orbit* ➡️, *and the soft tissues of the cheek.*

Wegener Granulomatosis, Sinonasal

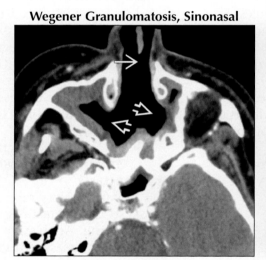

Undifferentiated Carcinoma, Sinonasal

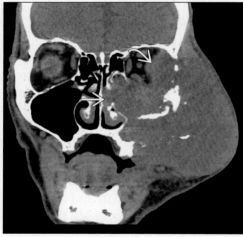

(Left) *Axial CECT shows a heterogeneous ethmoid sinus adenocarcinoma with cystic foci that invade the orbits* ➡️. *Invasion of the subcutaneous soft tissues is noted anteriorly* ➡️. **(Right)** *Coronal bone CT shows extensive sarcoidosis with nodular sinonasal soft tissue thickening. Large nasal septal perforation* ➡️ *is present with erosion of turbinates and ethmoid trabecula* ➡️.

Adenocarcinoma, Sinonasal

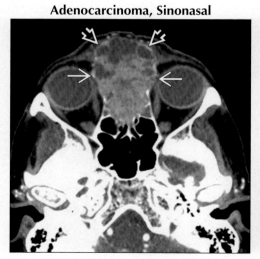

Sarcoidosis, Sinonasal

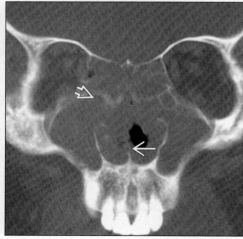

SINUS LESION WITH BONE DESTRUCTION

Rhabdomyosarcoma
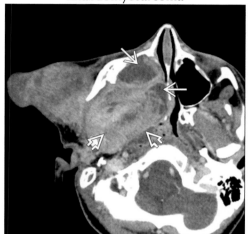

Adenoid Cystic Carcinoma, Sinonasal
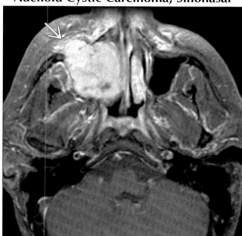

(Left) Axial CECT of a child reveals a large rhabdomyosarcoma involving the right maxillary antrum ➡, infratemporal fossa ➡, and soft tissues of the cheek. (Courtesy L. Ginsberg, MD.) *(Right)* Axial T1 C+ FS MR reveals a heterogeneously enhancing adenoid cystic carcinoma of the right maxillary antrum. There is extension through the anterior wall into soft tissues of the cheek ➡.

Osteosarcoma, Sinonasal
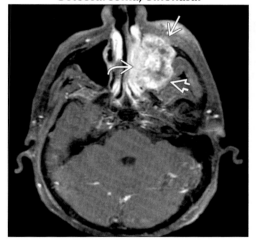

Chondrosarcoma, Sinonasal
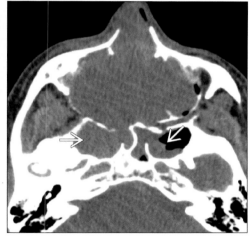

(Left) Axial T1 C+ FS MR shows a heterogeneously enhancing osteosarcoma involving the maxillary ridge, hard palate, and antrum. Note spread through anterior ➡, posterior ➡, and medial ➡ walls. *(Right)* Axial NECT shows large myxoid chondrosarcoma with bone destruction involving nasal cavity & maxillary sinuses. The nasal septum is eroded and trapped secretions are in sphenoid sinuses ➡.

Langerhans Histiocytosis, Skull Base
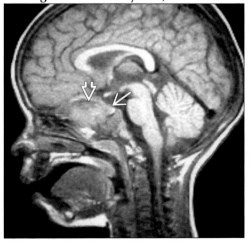

Metastasis
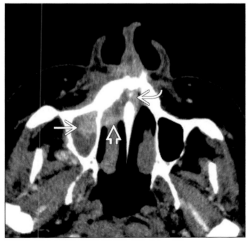

(Left) Sagittal T1WI MR in a child reveals Langerhans cell histiocytosis of the central skull base that invades the sella turcica ➡, anterior cranial fossa, and posterior ethmoid sinuses ➡. *(Right)* Axial CECT shows an enhancing lesion involving the right antrum ➡ and nasal cavity ➡. This prostate carcinoma metastasis erodes the septum ➡ and extends into the contralateral nasal cavity.

FACIAL BONE LESION

DIFFERENTIAL DIAGNOSIS

Common
- Fracture, General
- Fibrous Dysplasia, Sinonasal
- Osteoma, Sinonasal
- Ossifying Fibroma, Sinus
- Osteomyelitis, Mandible-Maxilla
- Cyst, Dentigerous (Follicular)

Less Common
- Odontogenic Keratocyst
- Osteonecrosis, Mandible-Maxilla
- Osteosarcoma, Mandible-Maxilla

Rare but Important
- Giant Cell Granuloma, Mandible-Maxilla
- Osteoradionecrosis, Mandible-Maxilla
- Hemangioma, Sinonasal
- Metastasis, Mandible-Maxilla

ESSENTIAL INFORMATION

Helpful Clues for Common Diagnoses
- **Fracture, General**
  - Key facts: Mechanisms include motor vehicle crashes, falls, assaults, occupational injuries, & gunshot wounds
    - Male (62%) > female (38%)
    - Mandible > nasal arch > zygomaticomaxillary > orbital > sphenotemporal > nasofrontoethmoidal > transfacial
  - Imaging: Best evaluated with CT to identify lucent fracture lines
    - Look for several of following: Fractures, skull base involvement, dural sinus & neurovascular canal involvement, fracture displacement, & foreign bodies
- **Fibrous Dysplasia, Sinonasal**
  - Key facts: Replacement of normal bone by fibrous-woven bone
    - Most common in first 3 decades
    - 3 forms ⇒ monostotic, polyostotic, Albright syndrome
    - Presents with painless facial swelling, cosmetic deformity, neurovascular compromise
  - Imaging: Variable depending upon amount of fibrous tissue present
    - Expansile lesion of medullary cavity
    - Classic "ground-glass" appearance

  - Can look similar to other fibro-osseous lesions (osteoma, ossifying fibroma) or Paget disease
- **Osteoma, Sinonasal**
  - Key facts: Benign neoplasm of compact or cancellous bone
    - M:F = 1:2
    - Sinuses (frontal & ethmoid) > jaws (mandible > maxilla)
    - Multiple in Gardner syndrome
  - Imaging: Well-defined sclerotic mass based on bone sessile or attached by pedicle
    - May have variable density with soft tissue components
- **Ossifying Fibroma, Sinus**
  - Key facts: Benign encapsulated fibrous tumor with various amounts of irregular trabeculae
    - Ossification ↑ as lesion matures
    - 3rd-4th decades; M < F
    - Situated at roots of teeth (periapical) in mandible
  - Imaging: Well-defined expansile lesion that progresses from predominantly lucent to ossified with maturation
- **Osteomyelitis, Mandible-Maxilla**
  - Key facts: Etiologies include odontogenic, post-traumatic, iatrogenic, & sinusitis-related
  - Imaging
    - CT: Mottled, irregular areas of bone lysis/sclerosis; sequestra may be painful & surrounded by areas of sclerosis
    - MR: Better for marrow & adjacent soft tissue involvement; ↓ T1, ↑ T2 signal + enhancement
- **Cyst, Dentigerous (Follicular)**
  - Key facts: 2nd most common odontogenic cyst (after radicular)
    - 75% in mandible; present in 3rd & 4th decades
  - Imaging: Circumscribed, unilocular expansile cystic lesion incorporating crown of unerupted tooth

Helpful Clues for Less Common Diagnoses
- **Odontogenic Keratocyst**
  - Key facts: Account for 3-11% of jaw cysts
    - Mandible:maxilla = 2:1; peak incidence in 2nd & 3rd decades
    - Multiple in basal cell nevus syndrome

○ Imaging: Multilocular or unilocular cystic lesion
  ▪ Often incorporates an impacted tooth
  ▪ Less expansile than dentigerous cyst
• **Osteonecrosis, Mandible-Maxilla**
  ○ Key facts: Caused by reduced local blood supply (ischemia) from multiple etiologies
    ▪ Bisphosphonate therapy, chronic infection, exogenous estrogen, heavy metals, & environmental pollutants
  ○ Imaging: Sclerotic > lytic bony changes in the mandible > maxilla
    ▪ Sequestra or pathologic fracture occurs
• **Osteosarcoma, Mandible-Maxilla**
  ○ Key facts: 6.5% arise in jaw (mandible > maxilla)
    ▪ Peak incidence in 3rd decade
  ○ Imaging: Osteolytic, osteoblastic, or mixed patterns
    ▪ "Sunburst" periosteal reaction
    ▪ Cortical breakthrough when large
    ▪ MR better defines soft tissue extent

Helpful Clues for Rare Diagnoses
• **Giant Cell Granuloma, Mandible-Maxilla**
  ○ Key facts: Probably reactive rather than neoplastic
    ▪ Mean age is 38-42 years at diagnosis
    ▪ 70% located in anterior jaws near incisor, canine, or premolar teeth
    ▪ Asymptomatic, but can grow rapidly
  ○ Imaging: Soft tissue mass located on alveolar mucosa/gingiva with remodeling of underlying alveolus

• **Osteoradionecrosis, Mandible-Maxilla**
  ○ Key facts: Reparative capacity of bone is insufficient to overcome radiation insult
    ▪ Incidence ~ 3%; rare when < 60 gray
    ▪ Incidence ↑ in those receiving combined chemo-/radiation therapy
  ○ Imaging
    ▪ CT: Cortical thinning, sclerosis, intraosseous air, pathologic fracture
    ▪ MR: ↓ T1, ↑ T2 signal + enhancement
• **Hemangioma, Sinonasal**
  ○ Key facts: Intraosseous hemangiomas < 1% of osseous tumors
    ▪ Calvaria & vertebra > facial bones (maxilla > mandible > nasal bones)
    ▪ Presents in 4th decade with painless swelling; M:F = 1:3
  ○ Imaging
    ▪ CT: Sharply marginated expansile lesion; intact inner & outer tables; "sunburst" pattern of radiating trabeculae; "soapbubble" & "honeycomb" appearance
    ▪ MR: Signal varies with blood flow & fat content
• **Metastasis, Mandible-Maxilla**
  ○ Key facts: Widespread disease usually present
    ▪ Breast & lung primaries most common
  ○ Imaging
    ▪ CT: Destructive lesion centered in medullary space with cortical erosion; lytic > blastic
    ▪ MR: ↓ T1, ↑ T2 signal with enhancement; MR better defines marrow involvement

Fracture, General

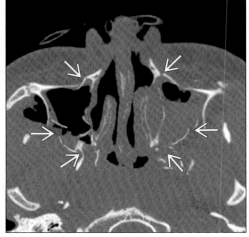

Axial bone CT shows extensive midface fractures (Le Fort II) ➡ *with hemorrhage layering in both maxillary sinuses. The maxillary walls, nasal septum, and pterygoid plates are fractured.*

Fibrous Dysplasia, Sinonasal

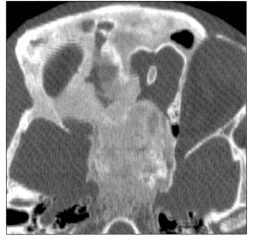

Axial bone CT shows extensive fibrous dysplasia involving the frontal, ethmoid, and sphenoid bones. The bones are expanded and show the classic ground-glass appearance.

FACIAL BONE LESION

(Left) Coronal bone CT shows typical appearance of an osteoma ➡ in a somewhat unusual location. The lesion arises from the maxillary alveolar ridge and protrudes into the maxillary sinus. **(Right)** Axial bone CT shows a bilobed ossifying fibroma with extension into the soft tissues of the buccal space from the maxilla. A peripheral rim of intact bone ➡ is present.

Osteoma, Sinonasal

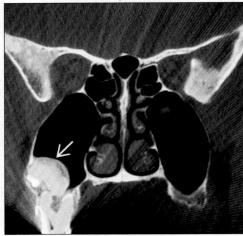

Ossifying Fibroma, Sinus

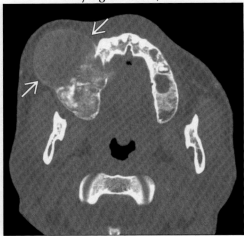

(Left) Axial bone CT shows abnormal sclerosis of the body of the mandible ➡ on the right, consistent with chronic osteomyelitis. A pathologic fracture ➡ is present in the weakened bone. **(Right)** Coronal bone CT shows a large maxillary dentigerous cyst presenting with a nasal and maxillary sinus extension. Note the crown of an unerupted upper molar tooth in the cyst ➡.

Osteomyelitis, Mandible-Maxilla

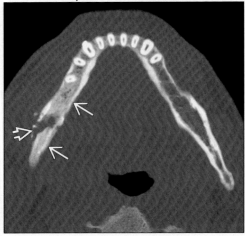

Cyst, Dentigerous (Follicular)

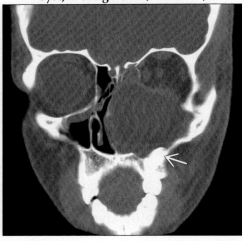

(Left) Coronal bone CT reveals an odontogenic keratocyst ➡ in a child with basal cell nevus syndrome. The lucent lesion smoothly expands and thins the surrounding bone. **(Right)** Axial bone CT shows sclerosis of mandible ➡ from left parasymphysial region through the right body. Pathologic fracture ➡ is seen in this case of bisphosphonate-related osteonecrosis.

Odontogenic Keratocyst

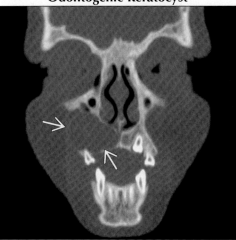

Osteonecrosis, Mandible-Maxilla

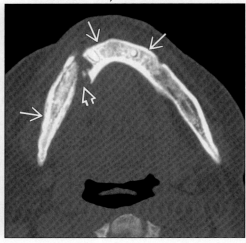

FACIAL BONE LESION

Osteosarcoma, Mandible-Maxilla

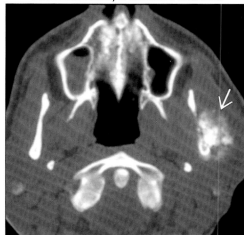

Giant Cell Granuloma, Mandible-Maxilla

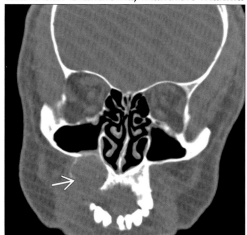

(Left) Axial bone CT demonstrates an aggressive mass with osseous matrix arising from the left mandibular ramus ➡. This type of periosteal reaction is typical of osteogenic sarcoma. (Right) Coronal bone CT reveals a well-defined bone lesion arising from the right maxillary alveolus ➡. An "eggshell" rim of bone remains intact around this giant cell granuloma.

Osteoradionecrosis, Mandible-Maxilla

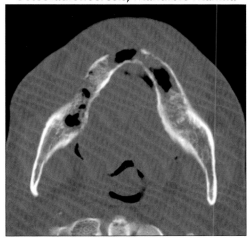

Hemangioma, Sinonasal

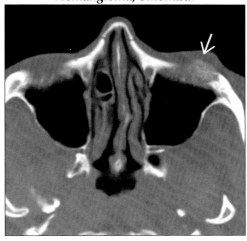

(Left) Axial bone CT shows diffuse mandibular osteopenia with multiple lytic foci and pockets of air within necrotic areas of bone. Radiation therapy was the cause of this osteonecrosis. (Right) Axial bone CT demonstrates a focal intraosseous hemangioma in the anterior wall of the left maxillary sinus ➡. A "lace-like" trabecular pattern is highly suggestive of this diagnosis.

Metastasis, Mandible-Maxilla

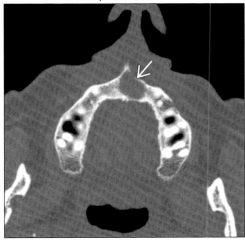

Metastasis, Mandible-Maxilla

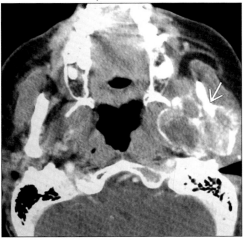

(Left) Axial bone CT shows a lytic lesion to the left of midline in the anterior aspect of the maxilla ➡. This was one of many lytic bony lesions present in this patient with multiple myeloma. (Right) Coronal CECT shows a neuroendocrine tumor metastasis to the ramus of the mandible on the left ➡. A large soft tissue component extends into the masticator muscles.

HYPERDENSE DISEASE IN SINUS LUMEN (CT)

DIFFERENTIAL DIAGNOSIS

Common
- Rhinosinusitis, Chronic
- Fungal Sinusitis, Mycetoma
- Osteoma, Sinonasal
- Fibrous Dysplasia, Sinonasal
- Fracture, General

Less Common
- Ossifying Fibroma, Sinus
- Fungal Sinusitis, Allergic
- Cyst, Dentigerous (Follicular)

Rare but Important
- Chondrosarcoma, Sinonasal
- Osteosarcoma, Sinonasal
- Meningioma, Skull Base

ESSENTIAL INFORMATION

Key Differential Diagnosis Issues
- Wide range of entities can produce increased density within paranasal sinuses including
  - Inflammatory diseases, neoplasms, bone disorders, trauma (including iatrogenic), & foreign bodies
- Increased density may be due to (presence of) calcifications, elevated protein ± decreased water content, fungal hyphae, chondroid or osseous matrix, or blood
- Clue to initial evaluation of a hyperdense sinus disease
  - Determine if hyperdense sinus lesion is arising primarily from bone surrounding sinus or from within sinus lumen
- Destruction of bony sinus walls surrounding dense lesion is suggestive of malignant neoplasm
- Bone expansion or remodeling most often indicates benign inflammatory (allergic fungal sinusitis) or neoplastic (ossifying fibroma) lesion

Helpful Clues for Common Diagnoses
- **Rhinosinusitis, Chronic**
  - Clinical clues: Numerous causes
    - History of underlying systemic disorder (cystic fibrosis, immotile cilia syndrome, immunodeficiency) or polyposis may be present
    - "Chronic" when disease persists for > 12 weeks and is recurrent

  - Increased density of sinus may be related to multiple factors
    - Elevated protein ± decreased water content of inspissated secretions
    - Presence of thickening and sclerosis of surrounding bony walls (chronic osteitis)
  - Sinus volume may decrease in size in longstanding disease ("silent sinus syndrome")
  - Look for lesions obstructing sinus drainage pathways (anatomic variants, polyps, neoplasms) that may be cause of recurrent inflammation
- **Fungal Sinusitis, Mycetoma**
  - Clinical clues: Patients are usually asymptomatic or experience mild pressure
    - Indolent course common
    - Occurs in all ages
    - Often found incidentally at imaging
    - Immunocompetent patients
  - Location: Maxillary > sphenoid (much less common in ethmoid and frontal sinuses)
  - Calcifications more common than chronic sinusitis
  - Increased density also related to fungal hyphae in the "fungus ball"
  - Nonexpansile lesion does not destroy bone but causes chronic osteitis similar to chronic sinusitis
- **Osteoma, Sinonasal**
  - Most common benign tumor of the paranasal sinuses
  - Usually asymptomatic unless obstructs sinus drainage
  - Solitary (multiple in Gardner syndrome)
  - Location: Frontal (80%), ethmoid (20%)
    - Uncommon in maxillary & sphenoid sinuses as well as nasal cavity
  - Dense "ivory" type is most common, but may contain fibrous tissue & mimic other fibro-osseous lesions
- **Fibrous Dysplasia, Sinonasal**
  - Clinical clues: Highest incidence between 3-15 years of age with 75% of cases presenting < 30 years
    - Symptoms may include painless facial swelling, sinusitis symptoms from obstruction, proptosis, headache, cranial nerve deficits depending on location
  - Monostotic or polyostotic

HYPERDENSE DISEASE IN SINUS LUMEN (CT)

- Affected bone is expanded with rim of intact cortex
    - Density of medullary cavity varies from classic "ground-glass" appearance to patchy areas of bone & soft tissue density
- **Fracture, General**
    - Many types of fractures may result in intrasinus hemorrhage
        - Frontal: Anterior or posterior frontal sinus walls; nasoethmoid complex
        - Ethmoid: Nasoethmoid complex; medial orbital blowout
        - Maxillary: Trimalar complex; orbital floor; Le Fort I & II; maxillary alveolar ridge
        - Sphenoid: Central skull base (often involves carotid canal)

Helpful Clues for Less Common Diagnoses

- **Ossifying Fibroma, Sinus**
    - Much more common in mandible than maxilla or other sinus walls
    - Well-circumscribed expansile lesion with varying amounts of fibrous & osseous tissue depending on lesion age
        - Classic appearance: Thick bony wall surrounding central fibrous tissue
    - Can be indistinguishable from mixed density osteoma or focal fibrous dysplasia
- **Fungal Sinusitis, Allergic**
    - Clinical clues: Occurs in immunocompetent, non-diabetic patients with longstanding chronic sinusitis
        - Frequent history of allergies ± polyposis

- Involves multiple sinuses & may be unilateral or bilateral
    - Expands affected sinuses
- Central increased density due to eosinophilic mucin, fungal hyphae, heavy metals, decreased water
    - Peripheral low-density rim of inflamed mucosa
- **Cyst, Dentigerous (Follicular)**
    - Maxillary alveolar lesions expand into antrum
    - Cyst with thin peripheral bony rim
        - Cyst often contains crown of immature tooth within its lumen

Helpful Clues for Rare Diagnoses

- **Chondrosarcoma, Sinonasal**
    - Most often arise from central skull base & grow into sphenoid & posterior ethmoid sinuses
        - Can primarily occur in nasal septum
    - Chondroid matrix is classic but may be only soft tissue density
- **Osteosarcoma, Sinonasal**
    - Osteosarcoma appears as highly aggressive soft tissue & osseous mass
    - "Sunburst" periosteal reaction is classic
- **Meningioma, Skull Base**
    - Usually extends from anterior or central skull base into sinuses below
    - Increased density due to hypercellularity of the tumor & hyperostosis in adjacent bone (approximately 30%)

Rhinosinusitis, Chronic

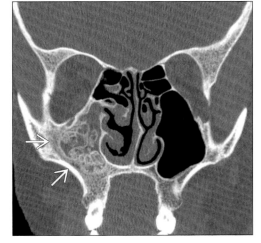

Coronal bone CT shows multiple foci of calcification in the maxillary antrum in this patient with chronic sinusitis and Wegener granulomatosis. Note osteitis of the maxillary walls ➜.

Fungal Sinusitis, Mycetoma

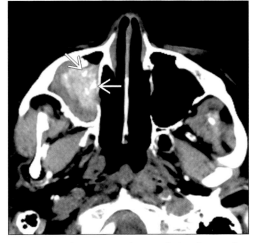

Axial NECT shows a nearly opacified right maxillary sinus with mixed density material. Multiple calcifications ➜ are seen within the more hyperdense portion of this mycetoma.

(Left) Axial bone CT shows a small, densely ossified lesion ➡️ in the right ethmoid labyrinth with the classic features of an "ivory" osteoma. *(Right)* Axial bone CT shows an osteoma in the maxillary sinus, a somewhat atypical location. Origin from the lateral maxillary wall is easily seen ➡️.

Osteoma, Sinonasal

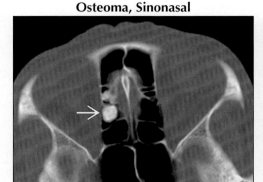

Osteoma, Sinonasal

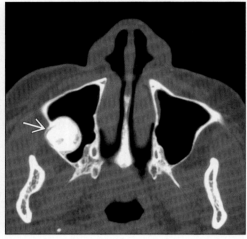

(Left) Axial bone CT shows the classic "ground-glass" expansile appearance of fibrous dysplasia involving the right ethmoid sinuses, sphenoid sinus, and nasal cavity. *(Right)* Coronal bone CT shows the typical appearance of fibrous dysplasia involving the left sphenoid sinus. Trapped secretions ➡️ are noted superior to the mass as it obstructs the sinus ostium.

Fibrous Dysplasia, Sinonasal

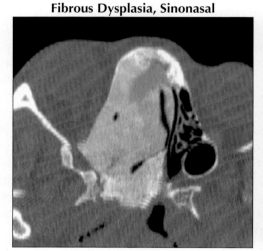

Fibrous Dysplasia, Sinonasal

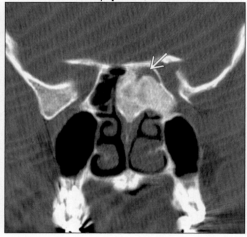

(Left) Axial NECT shows a dense air-fluid level in the left maxillary sinus, consistent with hemorrhage related to extensive midface fractures ➡️ involving the walls of the sinus. *(Right)* Coronal bone CT shows a large maxillary ossifying fibroma expanding the right half of the hard palate ➡️ and alveolar ridge. Mixed soft tissue and ossification are characteristic.

Fracture, General

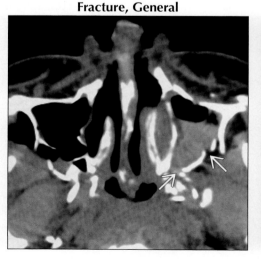

Ossifying Fibroma, Sinus

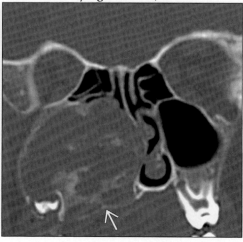

HYPERDENSE DISEASE IN SINUS LUMEN (CT)

Fungal Sinusitis, Allergic
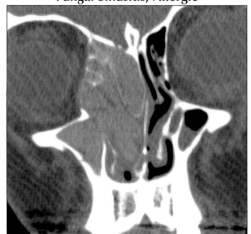

Fungal Sinusitis, Allergic
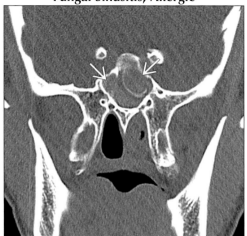

(Left) Coronal NECT shows marked expansion of the right sinonasal cavities by allergic fungal sinusitis. Centrally dense material with a low-density rim is classic. (Right) Coronal bone CT shows a classic case of allergic fungal sinusitis (AFS) with the mixed density material, characteristic of AFS opacifying the sphenoid sinuses ➡.

Cyst, Dentigerous (Follicular)
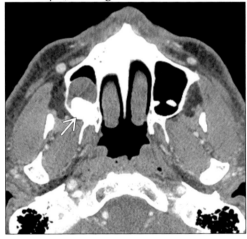

Chondrosarcoma, Sinonasal
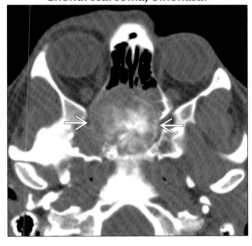

(Left) Axial CECT shows a cystic lesion in the alveolar recess of the right maxillary sinus containing the crown of an impacted tooth ➡. Findings are characteristic of a dentigerous cyst. (Right) Axial bone CT shows an expansile lesion ➡ involving the sphenoid sinus with central chondroid matrix typical of chondrosarcoma.

Osteosarcoma, Sinonasal
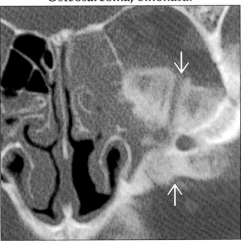

Meningioma, Skull Base
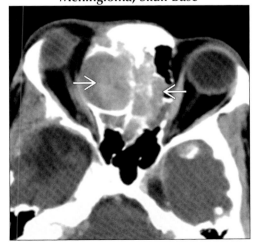

(Left) Coronal bone CT shows an aggressive maxillary osteogenic sarcoma ➡ of the left maxilla obliterating the antrum and showing "sunburst" periosteal reaction. (Right) Axial CECT shows a dense mass ➡ extending into the nasoethmoid region from the anterior cranial fossa. This patient with neurofibromatosis type 2 had multiple recurrent meningiomas.

CALCIFIED SINONASAL LESION (CT)

DIFFERENTIAL DIAGNOSIS

Common
- Osteoma, Sinonasal
- Ossifying Fibroma, Sinus
- Fungal Sinusitis, Mycetoma
- Fibrous Dysplasia, Sinonasal
- Rhinosinusitis, Chronic

Less Common
- Inverted Papilloma, Sinonasal
- Cyst, Dentigerous (Follicular)
- Esthesioneuroblastoma
- Rhinolith
- Chondrosarcoma, Sinonasal

Rare but Important
- Osteosarcoma, Sinonasal
- Adenocarcinoma, Sinonasal
- Meningioma, Skull Base

ESSENTIAL INFORMATION

Key Differential Diagnosis Issues
- 2 major calcified sinonasal lesions categories
  - Those arising primarily within sinonasal cavities containing calcification
  - Those arising primarily from sinonasal cavities bony walls
- Fibro-osseous lesions (osteoma, ossifying fibroma, fibrous dysplasia) can sometimes be indistinguishable at imaging

Helpful Clues for Common Diagnoses
- **Osteoma, Sinonasal**
  - Key facts: Most common benign sinus neoplasm
    - Arises from sinus walls; named by sinus that is invaded
    - Frontal (80%) > ethmoid (20%) > maxillary > sphenoid > nasal cavity
  - Imaging: Sessile or pedunculated, well-defined bone density mass
    - Occasionally mixed bone & soft tissue density
    - ↓ T2 MR signal; rarely obstructs sinus drainage pathways
- **Ossifying Fibroma, Sinus**
  - Key facts: In craniofacial skeleton mandible (75%), maxilla (10-20%)
    - Present at age 20-40 years; M < F; large lesions result in craniofacial deformity

- Imaging: Well-demarcated expansile mass with mixed soft tissue-fibrous center & osseous density
- **Fungal Sinusitis, Mycetoma**
  - Key facts: Colonization of obstructed secretions results in fungus ball
    - Indolent process with few symptoms (vague facial pressure)
    - Occurs in immunocompetent patients
    - Maxillary & sphenoid most common
  - Imaging: Single sinus containing hyperdense material
    - Chronic osteitis common; Ca++ more common than in chronic rhinosinusitis
- **Fibrous Dysplasia, Sinonasal**
  - Key facts: 75% of patients < 30 years
    - 70-80% monostotic; M < F polyostotic form
  - Imaging: Ill-defined expansion of diploic space with "ground-glass" density
    - May be heterogeneous with cystic areas
- **Rhinosinusitis, Chronic**
  - Key facts: Sinonasal infection/inflammation > 12 weeks in duration
    - Recurrent episodes; many predisposing conditions (CF, ciliary dysfunction, obstructing lesions)
  - Imaging: Mucosal thickening & dense inspissated secretions
    - Chronic osteitis of walls; Ca++ less common than with mycetoma

Helpful Clues for Less Common Diagnoses
- **Inverted Papilloma, Sinonasal**
  - Key facts: Adult male presents with symptoms similar to chronic rhinosinusitis
    - Tumor originates near middle meatus
    - Majority involve maxillary sinus; ~ 10% contain or degenerate into SCCa
  - Imaging: Lobular mass along lateral nasal wall
    - 10% show "tumorous Ca++"; 40% show "entrapped bone"
    - "Convoluted/cerebriform" architecture on T2 or T1 C+ MR
- **Cyst, Dentigerous (Follicular)**
  - Key facts: Also called "follicular cyst"
    - 25% in maxilla
    - Carcinoma, dermoid, ameloblastoma may arise from cyst wall

○ Imaging: Thin-walled, well-circumscribed unilocular cyst surrounding CROWN of unerupted tooth
  ▪ Bulges into maxillary sinus alveolar recess
  ▪ Displaces adjacent maxillary teeth
• **Esthesioneuroblastoma**
  ○ Key facts: Arises from olfactory epithelium near cribriform plate
    ▪ 2 incidence peaks (2nd and 6th decades)
    ▪ Vascular lesion presenting with nasal obstruction & intermittent epistaxis
    ▪ Excellent prognosis with multimodality therapy despite advanced stage
  ○ Imaging: Destructive soft tissue mass in upper nasal cavity/ethmoids
    ▪ Orbital invasion frequent
    ▪ Avid enhancement
    ▪ Intratumoral calcification unusual
    ▪ CYSTS at tumor-brain interface
• **Rhinolith**
  ○ Key facts: "Nasal cavity calculus" from salt deposition over time
    ▪ Core may be foreign body or chronic blood clot/ectopic tooth
  ○ Imaging: Calcific lesion in nasal cavity
    ▪ Not from bony septum or turbinate
• **Chondrosarcoma, Sinonasal**
  ○ Key facts: 10% of chondrosarcomas arise in H&N
    ▪ Typically present in 4th decade
    ▪ Site of origin usually skull base with secondary sinonasal cavity involvement

○ Imaging: Chondroid matrix with "ring-and-arc" pattern of Ca++
  ▪ May coalesce to form flocculent, fleck-like pattern
  ▪ ↑ T2 MR signal common

Helpful Clues for Rare Diagnoses
• **Osteosarcoma, Sinonasal**
  ○ Key facts: Rare sinonasal malignancy
    ▪ More common in mandible than maxilla
  ○ Imaging: Ill-defined mass arising from maxilla, extending into maxillary antrum & nasal cavity
    ▪ Mixed osteoid matrix & soft tissue components
    ▪ "Sunburst" periosteal reaction
• **Adenocarcinoma, Sinonasal**
  ○ Key facts: 10% of sinonasal tumors
    ▪ Arises from surface epithelium or seromucinous glands
    ▪ Mucinous (intestinal type) tumors more likely to contain Ca++
  ○ Imaging: Invasive mass into ethmoid sinuses & skull base; palate lesions extend into maxillary sinuses
• **Meningioma, Skull Base**
  ○ Key facts: Arise in anterior cranial fossa & extend intranasally through skull base
    ▪ Less often from meningothelial rests in sinus, nose, or orbits
  ○ Imaging: Avidly enhancing mass extending through skull base
    ▪ May contain calcifications ± cause hyperostosis of adjacent bone

Osteoma, Sinonasal

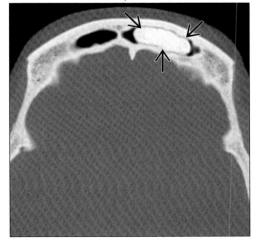

Axial bone CT shows the classic CT appearance of an "ivory" osteoma within the left frontal sinus ➡. The connection to the sinus wall is not seen on this image.

Ossifying Fibroma, Sinus

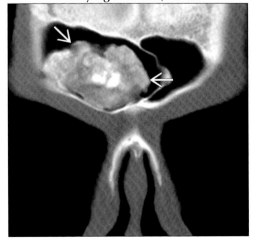

Coronal bone CT shows a lobular and diffusely but heterogeneously ossified mass ➡ nearly filling the right frontal sinus. This ossifying fibroma demonstrates nonspecific features.

(Left) Axial bone CT shows a fungal mycetoma with maxillary sinus expansion and dense calcifications ➡. There is extensive thickening and sclerosis of the walls of the sinus ➡. (Right) Axial NECT shows a dense right maxillary mycetoma with adjacent mucosal thickening ➡. Multiple coarse calcifications ➡ are seen. Chronic osteitis of the maxillary walls is present.

Fungal Sinusitis, Mycetoma

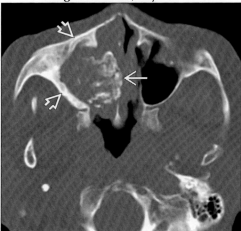

Fungal Sinusitis, Mycetoma

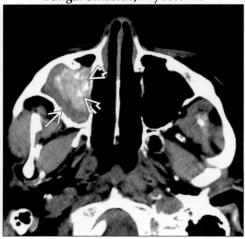

(Left) Coronal bone CT shows monostotic fibrous dysplasia that involves the maxilla ➡ and fills the maxillary sinus ➡. The bone thickening and "ground-glass" appearance are typical of fibrous dysplasia. (Right) Coronal bone CT shows a somewhat unusual case of chronic sinusitis of the maxillary sinuses with extensive bone thickening of the sinus walls ➡ and decreased antral volume.

Fibrous Dysplasia, Sinonasal

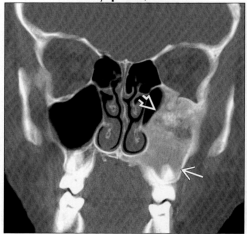

Rhinosinusitis, Chronic

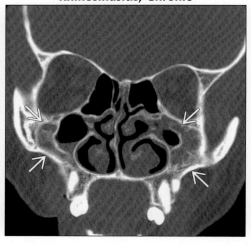

(Left) Axial NECT shows an inverted papilloma with classic middle meatus location with extension into the adjacent maxillary sinus. Several small calcifications ➡ are noted within the lesion. (Right) Axial bone CT demonstrates a unilocular dentigerous cyst ➡ of the left maxilla protruding into the antrum. Notice the impacted tooth ➡ within the anterior margin of the lesion.

Inverted Papilloma, Sinonasal

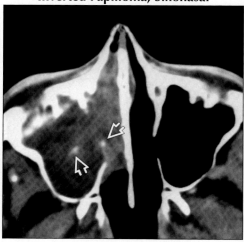

Cyst, Dentigerous (Follicular)

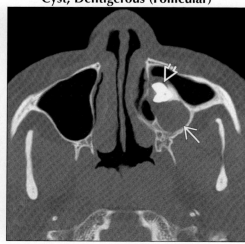

CALCIFIED SINONASAL LESION (CT)

Esthesioneuroblastoma

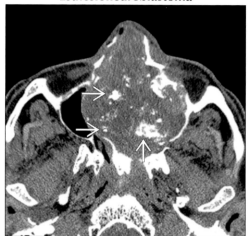

Rhinolith

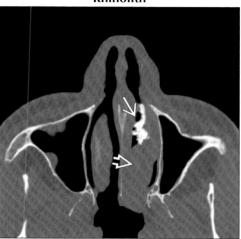

(Left) Axial NECT shows a large esthesioneuroblastoma centered in the nasal cavity with destruction of adjacent bone and containing multiple coarse calcifications ➡. (Courtesy W. Smoker, MD.) (Right) Axial bone CT shows a calcified foreign body (rhinolith) ➡ in the left nasal cavity medial to the inferior turbinate ➡. Several retention cysts are seen in the right maxillary sinus.

Chondrosarcoma, Sinonasal

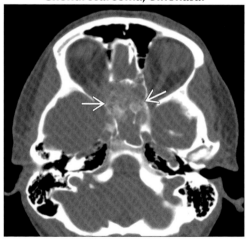

Osteosarcoma, Sinonasal

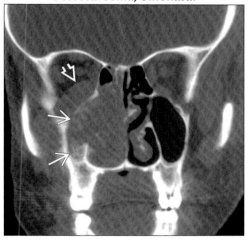

(Left) Axial bone CT shows a chondrosarcoma ➡ with posterior ethmoid and sphenoid sinus extension. The lesion shows the typical chondroid matrix of this cartilaginous neoplasm. (Right) Coronal bone CT shows a post-radiation sinonasal osteosarcoma in the maxillary sinus and nasal cavity with orbital invasion ➡. Note the calcified tumor matrix ➡.

Adenocarcinoma, Sinonasal

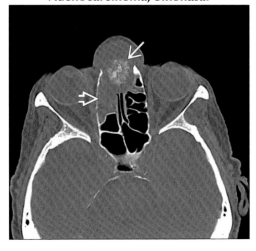

Meningioma, Skull Base

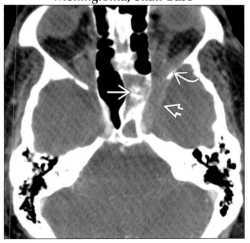

(Left) Axial bone CT shows an unusual adenocarcinoma of the upper nasal cavity and anterior ethmoid region with spiculated calcification ➡ centrally. Mucosal disease is noted posterior to mass ➡. (Right) Axial CECT shows a skull base meningioma extending into the left sphenoid sinus with central calcifications ➡. Left cavernous sinus ➡ and orbital ➡ involvement is present.

T2 HYPOINTENSE SINUS LESION (MR)

DIFFERENTIAL DIAGNOSIS

Common
- Rhinosinusitis, Chronic
- Fungal Sinusitis, Mycetoma
- Osteoma, Sinonasal
- Fungal Sinusitis, Allergic
- Polyposis, Sinonasal
- Hemorrhage, Sinonasal
- Ossifying Fibroma, Sinus

Less Common
- Fibrous Dysplasia, Sinonasal
- Fungal Sinusitis, Invasive
- Cyst, Dentigerous (Follicular)
- Non-Hodgkin Lymphoma, Sinonasal

Rare but Important
- Melanoma, Sinonasal
- Osteosarcoma, Sinonasal

ESSENTIAL INFORMATION

Key Differential Diagnosis Issues
- Lesions containing calcification, ossification, melanin, metal chelates, fungal elements, blood products can show decreased T2 signal
  - Lesions with high nuclear:cytoplasmic ratio can also show decreased T2 signal

Helpful Clues for Common Diagnoses
- **Rhinosinusitis, Chronic**
  - Key facts: Sinonasal (SN) inflammation lasting ≥ 12 weeks
    - Often recurrent; more common in ethmoid & maxillary sinuses
  - Imaging: ↓ T2 MR signal due to inspissated sections (↓ water, ↑ protein)
    - Thickened, sclerotic sinus walls (osteitis) also produce ↓ signal
    - Sinus volume normal or decreased
- **Fungal Sinusitis, Mycetoma**
  - Key facts: Also known as "fungus ball"
    - Secretion colonization by saprophytic fungi in immunocompetent patient
    - Asymptomatic or mild pressure sensation; can occur at any age
  - Imaging: Single, nonexpanded, sinus with complete or near complete opacification
    - Fungus ball is ↑ density on CT with Ca++
    - ↓ T2 MR signal due to fungal hyphae, metal chelates, & foci of Ca++
- **Osteoma, Sinonasal**
  - Key facts: Most common benign SN tumor
    - Frontal & ethmoid most common
    - Usually sporadic (if multiple consider Gardner syndrome)
  - Imaging: T2 signal varies with fibrous:osseous ratio
    - Uniform ↓ T2 signal in compact (ivory) type of osteoma
    - Patchy ↓ signal in cancellous/fibrous types of osteoma
    - CT helpful for characterization & relationship to sinus drainage pathways
- **Fungal Sinusitis, Allergic**
  - Key facts: Inflammation in immunocompetent patients with allergies
    - Eosinophilic mucin containing fungal hyphae opacifies & expands multiple sinuses; mostly unilateral
  - Imaging
    - MR: ↓ T2 signal from fungal concretions & heavy metal chelates; mimics air on T2
    - MR: Variable T1 signal (depends on protein:water ratio); peripheral mucosa is T2 hyperintense, enhances
    - CT: Centrally hyperdense with remodeling & expansion of sinus walls
- **Polyposis, Sinonasal**
  - Key facts: Hyperplasia of inflamed mucosa forms lobular soft tissue polyps
    - Pathogenesis: Chronic inflammation with allergy & fungal colonization
  - Imaging: Polypoid lesions of nasal cavity & sinuses
    - Can opacify & expand sinonasal cavities
    - Variable T1 & T2 MR signal depends on polyps age & presence of fungal elements
    - Chronic polyps with fungal colonization show ↓ T2 signal
- **Hemorrhage, Sinonasal**
  - Key facts: Etiologies include trauma (most common), bleeding disorders, vascular malformations, infections/granulomatous disorders, vascular neoplasms
  - Imaging: CT shows hyperdense fluid or focal collection in soft tissue mass
    - MR: Acute blood (deoxyhemoglobin) shows ↓ T2 & intermediate T1 signal
    - Subacute blood (intracellular methemoglobin): ↓ T2 & ↑ T1 signal; look for flow voids to determine vascularity
- **Ossifying Fibroma, Sinus**

○ Key facts: Benign expansile fibro-osseous sinus mass
○ Imaging: Expansile sinus lesion with central soft tissue density & peripheral ossification
  ▪ Areas of ossification show T2 hypointensity with hyperintense fibrous components

Helpful Clues for Less Common Diagnoses

• **Fibrous Dysplasia, Sinonasal**
  ○ Key facts: Developmental bone anomaly
    ▪ Bones of H&N involvement more common in polyostotic form
  ○ Imaging: ↓ T2 signal in areas of ossification
    ▪ CT: Expands medullary cavity; homogeneous (ground-glass) to matrix, ± heterogeneous
• **Fungal Sinusitis, Invasive**
  ○ Key facts: Aggressive fungal infection most commonly in immunocompromised or diabetic patients
  ○ Imaging: Infiltrating or mass-like soft tissue; fungal hyphae and heavy metals cause ↓ T2 MR signal
• **Cyst, Dentigerous (Follicular)**
  ○ Key facts: Unilocular; 75% in mandible
    ▪ Maxillary alveolar lesions expand into antrum
  ○ Imaging: Cystic lesion often containing crown of unerupted tooth
    ▪ Tooth crown looks like focal ↓ T2 signal within ↑ signal fluid cyst
• **Non-Hodgkin Lymphoma, Sinonasal**

○ Key facts: Slightly < 50% of H&N lymphomas occur in the SN cavities
  ▪ Prefers nasal cavity origin over sinuses
  ▪ B-cell, T-cell, and T/NK-cell types
○ Imaging: Small blue cell tumor with high nuclear:cytoplasmic ratio causes ↓ T2 MR signal
  ▪ Enhances homogeneously
  ▪ Remodels or destroys bone (turbinates/septum)

Helpful Clues for Rare Diagnoses

• **Melanoma, Sinonasal**
  ○ Key facts: Aggressive malignancy of melanocytes in nasal mucosa
    ▪ Worse prognosis than cutaneous forms
  ○ Imaging: Nasal cavity > paranasal sinus origin
    ▪ ↓ T2 signal due to presence of melanin, hemorrhage, & free radicals
    ▪ Melanin & blood cause ↑ T1 signal
    ▪ May remodel bone
• **Osteosarcoma, Sinonasal**
  ○ Key facts: Mandible > maxilla site of origin
    ▪ M > F, with mean age 35 years
  ○ Imaging
    ▪ Sunburst periosteal reaction better seen on CT
    ▪ MR: Ossified matrix causes ↓ T2 signal
    ▪ MR: Less ossified histologies have variable T2 signal

Rhinosinusitis, Chronic

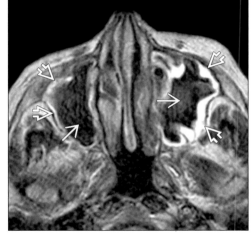

Axial T2WI MR shows low signal intensity inspissated secretions ⮕ in the maxillary sinuses mimicking the appearance of air. High signal inflamed mucosa ⮕ is noted at the periphery.

Fungal Sinusitis, Mycetoma

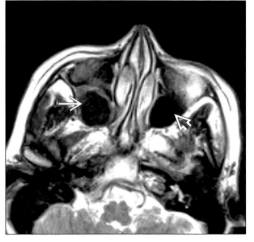

Axial T2WI MR shows a slightly expansile mycetoma within a septated right maxillary sinus ⮕. The hypointense signal mimics air but is slightly hyperintense to air on the normal contralateral side ⮕.

(Left) Coronal T2WI MR shows a heterogeneous naso-ethmoidal osteoma. Low signal osseous ➡ and higher signal fibrous ➡ areas are seen in this osteoma that was mixed density on CT (not shown). *(Right)* Axial T2WI MR shows expanded, opacified left ethmoid and sphenoid sinuses ➡ due to allergic fungal sinusitis. The signal mimics air. Hyperintense secretions and mucosa are noted on the right ➡.

Osteoma, Sinonasal

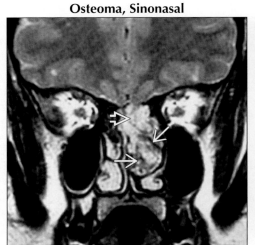

Fungal Sinusitis, Allergic

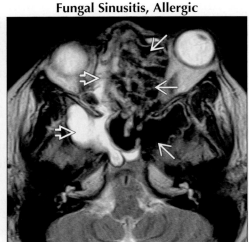

(Left) Coronal STIR MR shows marked expansion of the right frontal, ethmoid, and maxillary sinuses with hypointense polyps ➡. Trapped secretions ➡ of higher signal are seen bilaterally. *(Right)* Axial T2WI MR shows hypointense expansile polyps with peripheral high signal mucosa in the frontal sinuses and supraorbital ethmoid cells ➡.

Polyposis, Sinonasal

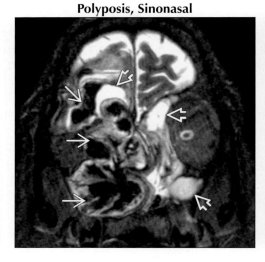

Polyposis, Sinonasal

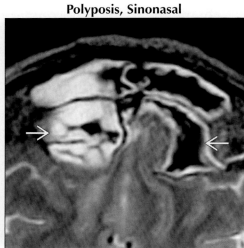

(Left) Coronal T2WI MR of a child shows a large cavernous hemangioma involving the nasal cavity, ethmoids, and maxillary sinus with hypointense foci of intralesional blood ➡. *(Right)* Axial T2WI MR shows heterogeneous, mixed signal ossifying fibroma in the left frontal sinus. The central fibrous portion ➡ is hyperintense compared to the peripheral osseous component ➡.

Hemorrhage, Sinonasal

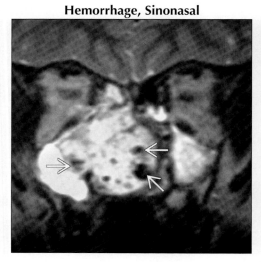

Ossifying Fibroma, Sinus

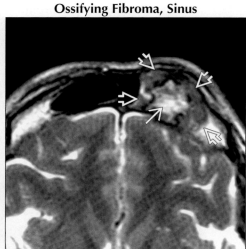

T2 HYPOINTENSE SINUS LESION (MR)

Fibrous Dysplasia, Sinonasal

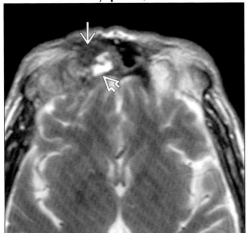

Fungal Sinusitis, Invasive

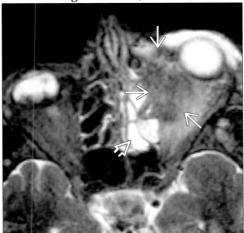

(Left) Axial T2WI FS MR shows focal fibrous dysplasia involving the right frontal sinus. Hypointense signal is seen in the lesion ➡ with trapped secretions ➡ posteriorly. (Right) Axial T2WI MR shows invasive Aspergillus fungal sinusitis extending from the left ethmoids into the orbit ➡. The fungal disease is hypointense compared to adjacent secretions and mucosa ➡.

Cyst, Dentigerous (Follicular)

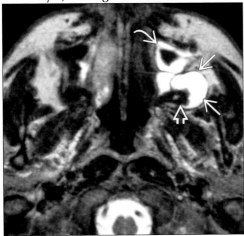

Non-Hodgkin Lymphoma, Sinonasal

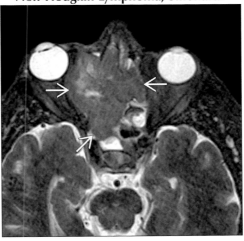

(Left) Axial T2WI MR shows a left maxillary dentigerous cyst ➡ with central hypointense impacted tooth ➡. Note antral mucosal thickening anteriorly ➡. (Courtesy W. Smoker, MD.) (Right) Axial STIR MR shows hypointense lymphoma ➡ in the upper nasal cavity and ethmoid sinuses with right orbital extension causing proptosis. Low T2 signal is characteristic of high nuclear:cytoplasmic ratio tumors.

Melanoma, Sinonasal

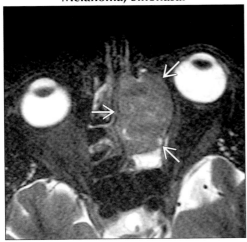

Osteosarcoma, Sinonasal

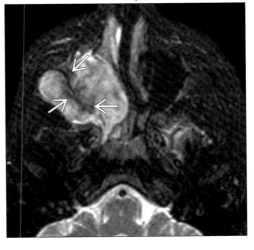

(Left) Axial STIR MR shows a typical melanoma ➡ centered in the left ethmoid sinuses with orbital extension. Hypointense signal is related to melanin, blood products, or free radicals. (Right) Axial T2WI FS MR shows a right maxillary osteosarcoma that was previously radiated. Hypointensity is seen in the central ossified portion of this aggressive mass ➡.

NASAL OBSTRUCTION IN NEWBORN

DIFFERENTIAL DIAGNOSIS

Common
- Nasolacrimal Duct Cyst
- Choanal Atresia, Nasal

Less Common
- Nasal Dermal Sinus
- Cephalocele, Frontoethmoidal
- Nasal Glioma
- Hemangioma, Sinonasal
- Tonsillar Tissue, Prominent/Asymmetric

Rare but Important
- Pyriform Aperture Stenosis
- Rhabdomyosarcoma

ESSENTIAL INFORMATION

Key Differential Diagnosis Issues
- Bilateral nasal cavity lesions in newborn produce respiratory distress as newborns are obligate nasal breathers
- Unilateral lesions that do not cause respiratory distress may present later in childhood

Helpful Clues for Common Diagnoses
- **Nasolacrimal Duct Cyst**
  - Inferior meatus location produces nasal obstruction
  - Well-defined cystic lesion below inferior turbinate; dilated nasolacrimal duct
- **Choanal Atresia, Nasal**
  - Stenosis > atresia; unilateral:bilateral = 2:1; bony (90%) & membranous (10%)
  - CT: Posterior nasal cavity narrowed by thickened vomer & medialized maxilla; soft tissue or bony plate occludes choanae

Helpful Clues for Less Common Diagnoses
- **Nasal Dermal Sinus**
  - Fluid-filled cyst or sinus tract from foramen cecum to nasal tip; within midline septum; bifid crista galli
- **Cephalocele, Frontoethmoidal**
  - Nasoethmoidal form presents as intranasal mass; may enlarge with crying; intracranial connection
- **Nasal Glioma**
  - Well-defined soft tissue mass with no connection intracranially
  - MR: Signal typically not similar to brain and may enhance
- **Hemangioma, Sinonasal**
  - Enhancing lesion along anterior nasal septum; T2 hyperintense
- **Tonsillar Tissue, Prominent/Asymmetric**
  - Midline nasopharyngeal soft tissue

Helpful Clues for Rare Diagnoses
- **Pyriform Aperture Stenosis**
  - Bony narrowing of anterior nasal passageway
  - Associated maxillary central mega-incisor and midline intracranial anomalies
- **Rhabdomyosarcoma**
  - Aggressive soft tissue malignancy; rare in newborn

Nasolacrimal Duct Cyst

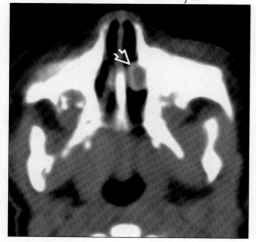

Axial NECT shows a mucoid-density nasolacrimal duct cyst ➡ at the level of the inferior meatus. Because this was a unilateral lesion, the infant did not present in respiratory distress.

Choanal Atresia, Nasal

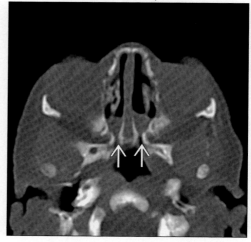

Axial bone CT shows bilateral membranous atresia with bony stenosis ➡. Note very small choanae and fluid layering in the nasal cavity. This newborn was in respiratory distress.

NASAL OBSTRUCTION IN NEWBORN

Nasal Dermal Sinus

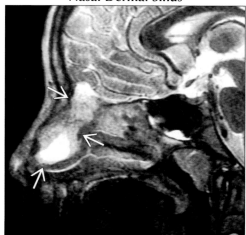

Cephalocele, Frontoethmoidal

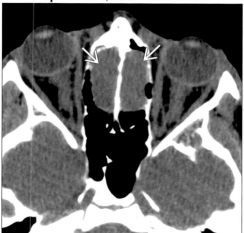

(Left) Sagittal T2WI MR shows a sinus tract ➡ extending from a widened foramen cecum in the anterior skull base towards the nasal tip. The lesion is hyperintense, consistent with fluid. *(Right)* Axial NECT shows bilateral frontoethmoidal encephaloceles of the nasoethmoidal type ➡. These cephaloceles protrude through the cribriform plates into the nasal cavity and ethmoid region.

Nasal Glioma

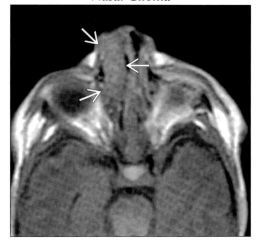

Hemangioma, Sinonasal

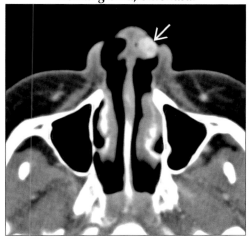

(Left) Axial T1WI MR reveals a nasal cavity mass ➡ obstructing the nasal airway in an infant. This intranasal glioma is isointense to brain on this sequence, but that is not always the case. *(Right)* Axial CECT shows a small enhancing capillary hemangioma in the left nasal vestibule ➡. The lesion was clinically visible within the nostril.

Pyriform Aperture Stenosis

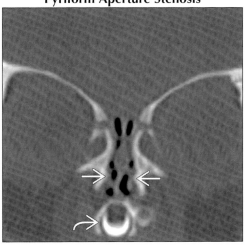

Rhabdomyosarcoma

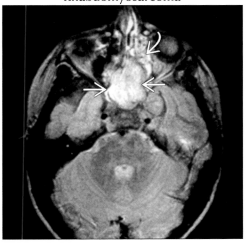

(Left) Coronal bone CT shows marked narrowing of the anterior nasal passage (pyriform aperture) ➡ and the associated finding of an unerupted central mega-incisor ➡. *(Right)* Axial FLAIR MR shows a hyperintense rhabdomyosarcoma ➡ in the nasopharynx extending into the posterior nasal cavity with obstructed left ethmoid sinus secretions ➡.

ANOSMIA-HYPOSMIA

DIFFERENTIAL DIAGNOSIS

Common
- Rhinosinusitis, Acute
- Rhinosinusitis, Chronic
- Cerebral Contusion
- Polyposis, Sinonasal
- Alzheimer Dementia
- Parkinson Disease

Less Common
- Fungal Sinusitis, Allergic
- Meningioma
- Wegener Granulomatosis, Sinonasal
- Non-Hodgkin Lymphoma, Sinonasal
- Esthesioneuroblastoma
- Adenocarcinoma, Sinonasal
- Sarcoidosis, Sinonasal

Rare but Important
- Melanoma, Sinonasal
- Cephalocele, Frontoethmoidal
- Kallmann Syndrome

ESSENTIAL INFORMATION

Key Differential Diagnosis Issues
- Disorders of olfactory dysfunction evaluated clinically with olfactory testing and nasal endoscopy
- Imaging helpful for further evaluating inflammatory or neoplastic etiologies seen on endoscopy
  - Also used to rule out intracranial causes if clinical examination is negative
- Toxic inhalants are common cause of olfactory disturbance but do not result in imaging abnormalities

Helpful Clues for Common Diagnoses
- **Rhinosinusitis, Acute**
  - Key facts: Olfactory dysfunction related to mucosal swelling in olfactory clefts, obstruction of nasal airflow
  - Imaging: Mucosal thickening & air-fluid levels
- **Rhinosinusitis, Chronic**
  - Key facts: Mucosal thickening & osteitis block airflow to olfactory clefts
    - Chronic inflammation damages CN1 fibers
  - Imaging: Mucosal thickening, thickening and sclerosis of bone

- **Cerebral Contusion**
  - Key facts: Shearing of olfactory fibers at cribriform plate causes olfactory dysfunction
  - Imaging: Bifrontal edema ± hemorrhage above orbital plates
- **Polyposis, Sinonasal**
  - Key facts: Occurs sporadically or in association with underlying conditions (CF, asthma, ciliary dysfunction)
    - Commonly arises in nasal cavity & block airflow to olfactory clefts
  - Imaging: Polypoid soft tissue in sinonasal cavities; may be expansile
- **Alzheimer Dementia**
  - Neurodegenerative disorder with dementia
  - Anosmia reported in up to 90%
- **Parkinson Disease**
  - Hyposmia is frequent complaint & may present years before motor symptoms
  - Related to nigrostriatal dopaminergic degeneration

Helpful Clues for Less Common Diagnoses
- **Fungal Sinusitis, Allergic**
  - Key facts: Form of chronic sinusitis with colonization of obstructed secretions or polyps by saprophytic fungi in immunocompetent patients
  - Imaging: Unilateral > bilateral sinonasal cavity opacification & expansion
    - Central ↑, peripheral ↓ density on CT
- **Meningioma**
  - Key facts: Olfactory groove location compresses olfactory tracts/bulbs & inferior frontal brain parenchyma
  - Imaging: Dural-based, extra-axial, enhancing mass above cribriform plate
    - "Dural tails" may be present
- **Wegener Granulomatosis, Sinonasal**
  - Key facts: Necrotizing sinonasal granulomatous disorder
  - Imaging: Nodular sinonasal soft tissue thickening
    - More often around septum & turbinates than olfactory clefts
- **Non-Hodgkin Lymphoma, Sinonasal**
  - Key facts: Prefers nasal cavity origin over sinuses; blocks olfactory cleft airflow or infiltrates olfactory mucosa

ANOSMIA-HYPOSMIA

○ Imaging: Homogeneous, ↑ CT density, ↓ T2 MR signal, diffuse enhancement without necrosis
• **Esthesioneuroblastoma**
  ○ Key facts: Olfactory epithelium malignancy arising near cribriform plate
    ▪ 2 incidence peaks: 2nd & 6th decades
  ○ Imaging: Enhancing mass in nasal cavity and ethmoids
    ▪ Extension into anterior fossa common
    ▪ Cysts at brain-tumor interface
• **Adenocarcinoma, Sinonasal**
  ○ Key facts: Inhalational risk factors include wood dust, chemicals used in textile and leather industries, nickel, and other metals
  ○ Imaging: Nonspecific invasive lesion
    ▪ Often involves ethmoids & superior nasal cavity
• **Sarcoidosis, Sinonasal**
  ○ Granulomatous disorder with sinonasal involvement less common than Wegener, but similar appearance
  ○ Nodular soft tissue in nasal cavity & sinuses blocks airflow to olfactory mucosa

Helpful Clues for Rare Diagnoses
• **Melanoma, Sinonasal**
  ○ Prefers nasal cavity site of origin
  ○ Bone remodeling or destruction; ↑ T1, ↓ T2 MR signal
• **Cephalocele, Frontoethmoidal**
  ○ Damage to herniated tissue in cephalocele or mass effect blocking airflow causes olfactory dysfunction

• **Kallmann Syndrome**
  ○ X-linked or autosomal dominant inherited disorder
  ○ Hypogonadotropic hypogonadism with anosmia
  ○ Absence of olfactory sulci, tracts, & bulbs
    ▪ Hypoplastic anterior pituitary gland

Alternative Differential Approaches
• Consider causes of anosmia-hyposmia by anatomic segments along olfactory nerve
• Intra-axial causes (injury, degeneration, or mal-development of intracranial olfactory apparatus)
  ○ Cerebral contusion
  ○ Alzheimer dementia
  ○ Parkinson disease
  ○ Kallmann syndrome
• Meningeal causes (compression of olfactory nerves/bulbs)
  ○ Meningioma
• Nasal causes (prevent olfactants from reaching the olfactory clefts)
  ○ Rhinosinusitis, acute
  ○ Rhinosinusitis, chronic
  ○ Polyposis, sinonasal
  ○ Fungal sinusitis, allergic
  ○ Wegener granulomatosis, sinonasal
  ○ Non-Hodgkin lymphoma, sinonasal
  ○ Esthesioneuroblastoma
  ○ Adenocarcinoma, sinonasal
  ○ Sarcoidosis, sinonasal
  ○ Melanoma, sinonasal
  ○ Cephalocele, frontoethmoidal

Rhinosinusitis, Acute

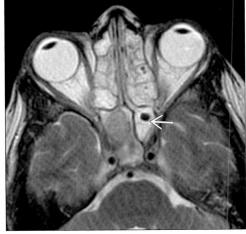

Axial T2WI MR shows extensive mucosal thickening in the ethmoid and sphenoid sinuses in a patient with acute or chronic sinusitis. A small fluid level is seen in the left sphenoid sinus ➡.

Rhinosinusitis, Chronic

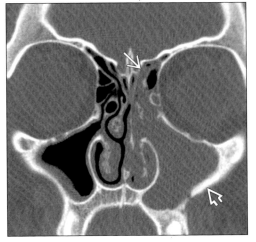

Coronal bone CT shows a left maxillary ethmoid frontal recess ➡ *and nasal cavity mucosal thickening in a patient with chronic inflammation. Note thickening of left maxillary wall* ➡.

(Left) Axial NECT shows frontal and temporal hemorrhagic contusions ➡ from acceleration/deceleration injury. Olfactory apparatus shearing occurs along the anterior skull base in this injury. *(Right)* Coronal bone CT reveals ethmoid, left maxillary sinus, and right infundibulum ➡ opacification with nasal polypoid tissue ➡. A right maxillary air-fluid level ➡ suggests acute disease.

Cerebral Contusion

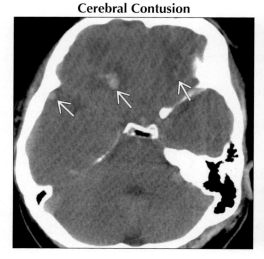

Polyposis, Sinonasal

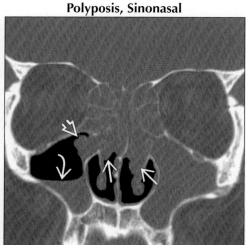

(Left) Axial NECT shows typical CT findings of Alzheimer dementia with bilateral hippocampal atrophy, indicated by enlarged temporal horns ➡ when compared to the lateral ventricular size. *(Right)* Axial T2WI MR shows classic midbrain findings in Parkinson disease with "blurring" and thinning of pars compacta ➡. There is hypointensity of the red nuclei and substantia nigra from iron deposition.

Alzheimer Dementia

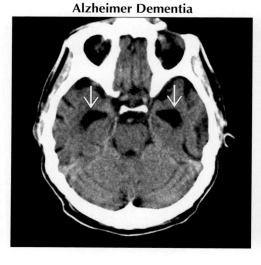

Parkinson Disease

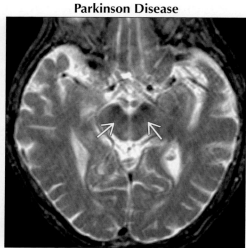

(Left) Coronal NECT demonstrates typical features of allergic fungal sinusitis (AFS) with bilateral sinus and nasal cavity ➡ involvement. Mixed density is characteristic of the secretions in AFS. *(Right)* Coronal T1 C+ FS MR reveals an olfactory meningioma filling the floor of the anterior fossa above the olfactory bulbs ➡. Note the diffuse enhancement within the mass.

Fungal Sinusitis, Allergic

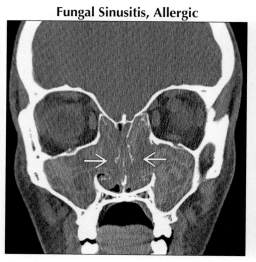

Meningioma

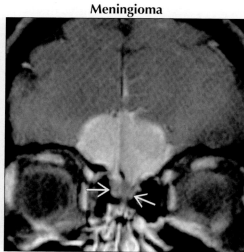

ANOSMIA-HYPOSMIA

Wegener Granulomatosis, Sinonasal

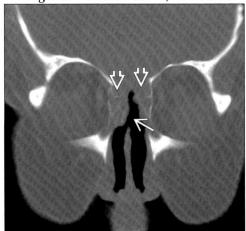

Non-Hodgkin Lymphoma, Sinonasal

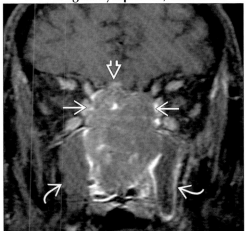

(Left) Coronal bone CT shows nodular soft tissue in the upper nasal cavity and ethmoids in a patient with Wegener granulomatosis. Erosion of the superior septum ➡ and anterior skull base ➡ is present. *(Right)* Coronal T1 C+ FS MR shows a large homogeneously enhancing lymphoma of the nasal cavity with orbital ➡ and skull base ➡ extension. Note the trapped secretions in the maxillary sinuses ➡.

Esthesioneuroblastoma

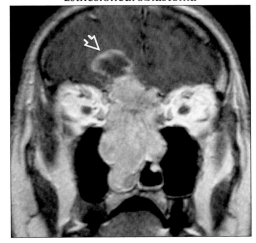

Adenocarcinoma, Sinonasal

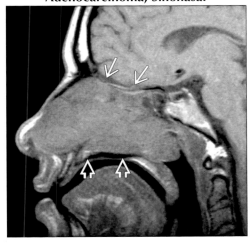

(Left) Coronal T1 C+ MR shows an esthesioneuroblastoma originating in the superior nasal cavities with a large intracranial component. A characteristic cyst is seen ➡ at the brain-tumor margin. *(Right)* Sagittal T1WI MR reveals an adenocarcinoma filling the nasal cavity and extending into the nasopharynx. Despite the lesion's aggressive nature, no skull base ➡ or palate ➡ invasion is present.

Sarcoidosis, Sinonasal

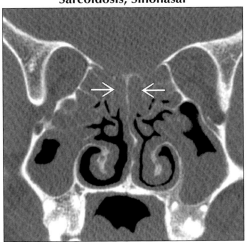

Melanoma, Sinonasal

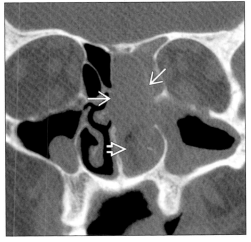

(Left) Coronal bone CT demonstrates extensive mucosal disease of the ethmoid and maxillary sinuses in a patient with sarcoidosis. Soft tissue fills the upper nasal cavity ➡ below the cribriform plates. *(Right)* Coronal bone CT shows a mass ➡ within the left nasal cavity, a trapped ethmoid, and maxillary secretions. Packing is present inferiorly ➡ due to bleeding of this vascular melanoma.

DIFFERENTIAL DIAGNOSIS

Common
- Fracture, General
- Juvenile Angiofibroma
- Hemangioma, Sinonasal
- Nasopharyngeal Carcinoma

Less Common
- Esthesioneuroblastoma
- Melanoma, Sinonasal
- SCCa, Sinonasal
- Fungal Sinusitis, Invasive
- Wegener Granulomatosis, Sinonasal
- Sarcoidosis, Sinonasal
- Rhinosinusitis, Acute
- Rhinosinusitis, Chronic

Rare but Important
- Hemangiopericytoma
- Hereditary Hemorrhagic Telangiectasia

ESSENTIAL INFORMATION

Key Differential Diagnosis Issues
- Trauma is most common etiology of nasal bleeding & may result from many types of fractures
- Vascular or aggressive neoplasms, aggressive infections, & granulomatous disorders comprise majority of remaining entities
- Caveat: Biopsy of vascular neoplasms under poorly controlled circumstances can result in life-threatening hemorrhage

Helpful Clues for Common Diagnoses
- **Fracture, General**
  - Key facts: Significant epistaxis results from fractures involving nasal septum, midface, & anterior skull base
    - Fractures of any bony sinus wall causing hemorrhage can result in nasal bleeding
  - Imaging: Fractures with intranasal or intrasinus hemorrhage
    - Look for focal soft tissue hematomas near fracture lines or extravascular contrast pooling on enhanced studies indicative of active bleeding
- **Juvenile Angiofibroma**
  - Key facts: Adolescent male patient presenting with nasal obstruction & intermittent unilateral nose bleeds

- Imaging: Mass centered at sphenopalatine foramen; extension into nasal cavity, nasopharynx, & infratemporal fossa
  - MR: Flow voids with "salt & pepper" on T2 & post-gad T1 sequences
- **Hemangioma, Sinonasal**
  - Key facts: Capillary more common than cavernous type; location: anterior nasal cavity origin, often from septum near Kiesselbach venous plexus
  - Imaging: MR: T2 hyperintense; diffuse contrast enhancement; large lesions may contain foci of hemorrhage
- **Nasopharyngeal Carcinoma**
  - Key facts: Most common cancer in Asian males, high incidence in Eskimos; < 50 years
    - Associated with EBV
    - Symptom triad is neck mass (adenopathy), serous otitis media, & bloody nasal discharge
  - Imaging: Mass centered in lateral pharyngeal recess; look for deep extension into skull base, retropharyngeal & cervical nodes, perineural spread

Helpful Clues for Less Common Diagnoses
- **Esthesioneuroblastoma**
  - Key facts: Malignancy arising from olfactory epithelium; excellent prognosis with combined therapy despite extent beyond sinonasal cavities
    - 2 age peaks of incidence in 2nd & 6th decades
  - Imaging: Avidly enhancing mass centered at cribriform plate; intratumoral Ca++
    - Cyst formation at tumor-brain interface for lesions with intercranial extent
- **Melanoma, Sinonasal**
  - Key facts: Aggressive malignancy typically arising in males 50-80 years of age; mean survival 24 months; pigmented mass at endoscopy
  - CT: Epicenter in nasal cavity along septum or inferior turbinate; may show bone destruction or remodeling
  - MR features: ↑ T1, ↓ T2 signal, avid enhancement
- **SCCa, Sinonasal**
  - Key facts: 30% arise in nasal cavity; friable tumor with bleeding mainly due to bone & vascular invasion

○ Imaging: Soft tissue mass with aggressive bone destruction; areas of necrosis in large lesions
- **Fungal Sinusitis, Invasive**
  ○ Key facts: Aggressive infection in immunocompromised patient or those with predisposing conditions (poorly controlled diabetics)
    ▪ Aspergillus & Mucormycosis most common organisms; angioinvasive
  ○ CT: Bone erosion typical, but need NOT be present for disease extension beyond sinus walls; can appear mass-like
  ○ MR: ↓ T2 signal due to fungal hyphae/metal chelates
- **Wegener Granulomatosis, Sinonasal**
  ○ Key facts: Necrotizing granulomatous disease preferentially affects septum & turbinates
    ▪ Septal ulceration & perforation can lead to "saddle nose" deformity
  ○ Imaging: Nodular soft tissue thickening in nasal cavity; osteitis; septal perforation
- **Sarcoidosis, Sinonasal**
  ○ Key facts: Granulomatous disorder; affects sinonasal cavities < Wegener, though similar appearance
  ○ Imaging: Nodular soft tissue thickening in nasal cavity; osteitis; may lead to septal perforation
- **Rhinosinusitis, Acute**
  ○ Key facts: Rarely results in significant nasal bleeding

▪ Influenza, measles, typhus, & catarrhalis in children & adolescents
  ○ Imaging: Mucosal thickening & air-fluid levels
- **Rhinosinusitis, Chronic**
  ○ Key facts: Significant epistaxis rare; crusting & nose-picking implicated
  ○ Imaging: Mucosal thickening, proteinaceous secretions, & osteitis

Helpful Clues for Rare Diagnoses
- **Hemangiopericytoma**
  ○ Key facts: Uncommon vascular neoplasm; sinus > nasal cavity
  ○ Imaging: Intensely enhancing mass; may contain bone or cartilage
- **Hereditary Hemorrhagic Telangiectasia**
  ○ Key facts: Autosomal dominant genetic disorder with formation of telangiectasias
    ▪ 95% have recurring nose bleeds (90% by age 21); multifocal bleeding common
  ○ Imaging: Lesions occult to cross-sectional imaging; angiography used for localization of telangiectasias and active bleeding & treatment

Other Essential Information
- Epistaxis is classified based on bleeding site (anterior or posterior)
  ○ Anterior bleeding often from septum (venous plexus) or inferior turbinate
  ○ Posterior bleeding from sphenopalatine artery branches in posterior nasal cavity or nasopharynx

Fracture, General

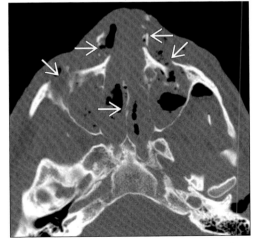

Axial bone CT shows multiple midface fractures ➡ in an assault patient. There is facial swelling, blood in the nasal cavity and sinuses, and soft tissue emphysema.

Juvenile Angiofibroma

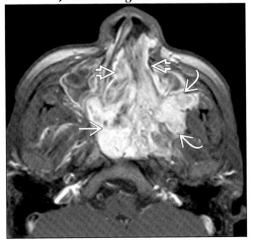

Axial T1 C+ FS MR shows an instance of a very large juvenile angiofibroma with extensive spread into the nasopharynx ➡, nasal cavity ➡, and infratemporal fossa ➡.

(Left) Sagittal T1 C+ MR shows a homogeneously enhancing hemangioma ➡ within the nasal cavity superiorly. Obstructed secretions are seen in the frontal sinus ➡. *(Right)* Axial CECT shows an enhancing mass in the nasopharynx ➡ centered to the right of midline, effacing the fossa of Rosenmüller, and eroding the medial pterygoid plate ➡.

Hemangioma, Sinonasal

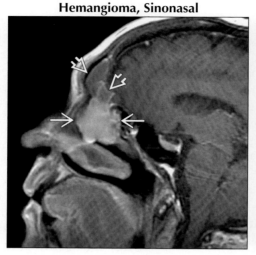

Nasopharyngeal Carcinoma

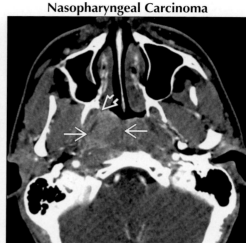

(Left) Coronal T1 C+ MR shows an avidly enhancing esthesioneuroblastoma involving the nasal cavity and extending into the anterior cranial fossa. A cyst is noted at the tumor-brain interface ➡. *(Right)* Coronal T1 C+ FS MR reveals a sinonasal melanoma with both intracranial and orbital extension. The mass enhances diffusely, and trapped secretions ➡ in the frontal sinus are noted superiorly.

Esthesioneuroblastoma

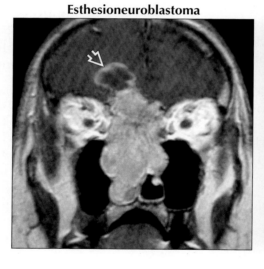

Melanoma, Sinonasal

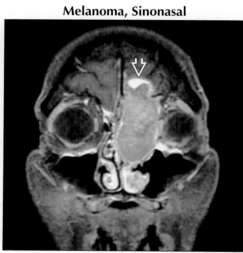

(Left) Axial T1WI MR shows an advanced maxillary squamous carcinoma ➡ that involves the orbit and skull base. The mass extends posteriorly into the skull base ➡ and left cavernous sinus ➡. *(Right)* Axial T1 C+ FS MR shows a case of invasive fungal sinusitis with orbital ➡ and cavernous sinus ➡ invasion. Ethmoidectomy changes from prior Mucormycosis debridement are present.

SCCa, Sinonasal

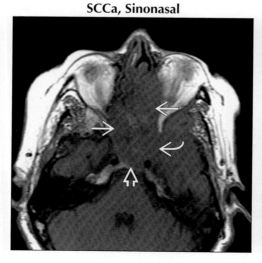

Fungal Sinusitis, Invasive

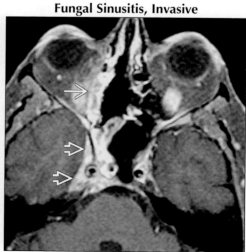

EPISTAXIS

Wegener Granulomatosis, Sinonasal

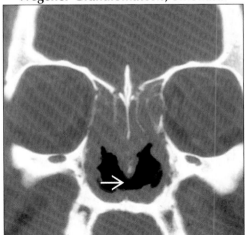

Sarcoidosis, Sinonasal

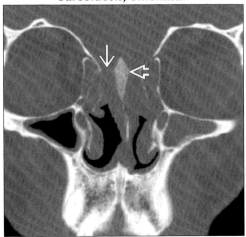

(Left) Coronal bone CT shows nodular soft tissue within the nasal cavity and ethmoid sinuses. A nasal septal perforation ➡, a common complication of sinonasal granulomatous disease, is present. *(Right)* Coronal bone CT shows nodular soft tissue sarcoid involvement of the nasal clefts. Skull base erosion ➡ is seen in this patient with intracranial disease as well as crista galli osteitis ➡.

Rhinosinusitis, Acute

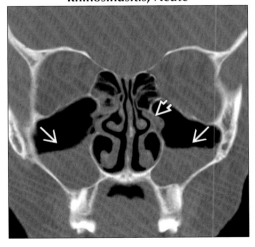

Rhinosinusitis, Chronic

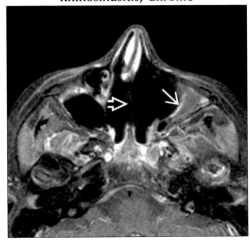

(Left) Coronal bone CT shows bilateral maxillary air-fluid levels ➡ in a patient with acute rhinosinusitis. The left ostiomeatal unit is occluded by mucosal thickening ➡. *(Right)* Axial T1 C+ FS MR shows bilateral antrostomy defects and markedly decreased left antral volume ➡ due to chronic rhinosinusitis. A large septal perforation ➡ is also present.

Hemangiopericytoma

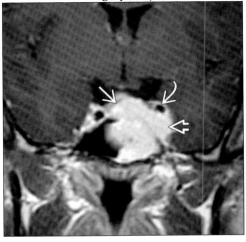

Hereditary Hemorrhagic Telangiectasia

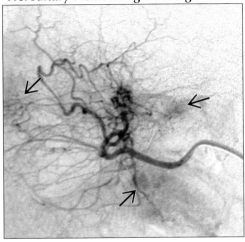

(Left) Coronal T1 C+ MR shows an intensely enhancing sphenoid hemangiopericytoma extending into the sella ➡ and cavernous sinus ➡. The left internal carotid artery ➡ is slightly compressed. *(Right)* Lateral angiography shows multiple foci of contrast accumulation ➡ in mucosal telangiectasias in the nasal cavity and nasopharynx in a patient with hereditary hemorrhagic telangiectasia.

TRAUMATIC LESIONS OF FACE

DIFFERENTIAL DIAGNOSIS

Common
- Fracture, Nasal Bone
- Fracture, Mandible
- Fracture, Zygomaticomaxillary Complex
- Fracture, Inferior Orbital
- Fracture, Medial Orbital Blowout

Less Common
- Fracture, Nasoethmoid Complex
- Fracture, Frontal Sinus
- Fracture, Transfacial (Le Fort)

Rare but Important
- Fracture, Complex Midfacial
- Trauma/Dislocation, TMJ

ESSENTIAL INFORMATION

Key Differential Diagnosis Issues
- 75% of facial fractures (fx) occur in mandible, zygoma, & nose
- Mechanisms: Auto accidents > assaults > falls > sports injuries
  - Penetrating trauma less common fx cause
- Force required to fx facial bones classified as high or low impact
  - High impact fxs: Supraorbital rim, mandibular symphysis, fronto-glabellar, mandibular angle
    - Incidence of other major injuries ≈ 50%
  - Low impact fxs: Zygoma, nasal bones
- Imaging recommendations
  - High-resolution MDCT is modality of choice for rapid evaluation of facial trauma
  - 3D images helpful for surgical planning
  - Plain films used in focal trauma (nasal fx)

Helpful Clues for Common Diagnoses
- **Fracture, Nasal Bone**
  - Most common facial fx
    - Less force required to fracture nasal bone compared to other bones
  - Most are diagnosed clinically
    - Imaging obtained to plan repair if deformity persists after edema resolves
  - Imaging: Evaluate for associated septal hematoma requiring evacuation
- **Fracture, Mandible**
  - Frequently multiple ± bilateral on opposite sides of symphysis
  - Essentially "ring of bone" with "fixation" at TMJs
  - Degree of fx displacement depends on fx orientation & muscle attachments
  - Locations: Condylar > coronoid process > ramus > angle > body > parasymphyseal > symphyseal > alveolar process
  - Associated imaging: TMJ dislocation (condylar/subcondylar fx)
    - Hypesthesia over chin with fx through alveolar foramen (parasymphyseal)
    - 15% have at least 1 other facial bone fx
- **Fracture, Zygomaticomaxillary Complex**
  - Zygoma is exposed facial bone
    - Fx results from forceful blow to cheek
    - Central depression with fx at both ends
    - Isolated zygoma fx is rare
  - Trismus results from impingement on temporalis muscle
    - Lateral orbital fx fragments may impinge lateral rectus
  - Imaging: "Tripod" or "tetrapod" fx involves separation of 3 major attachments of zygoma from face
    - Fx of maxillary sinus & lateral orbital wall (diastasis of zygomaticofrontal suture) in addition to zygoma
    - Look for involvement of orbital apex/optic canal
- **Fracture, Inferior Orbital**
  - "Blowout" term used with floor fx & intact infraorbital rim
  - Orbital muscle entrapment is clinical diagnosis
  - Typically results from blunt trauma
    - Infraorbital rim & orbital floor are thin; most common sites of orbital fracture
    - May be associated with zygomaticomaxillary complex fx
    - Look for associated lamina papyracea fx (medial orbital blowout)
  - Imaging: Suspect orbital floor fracture if hemorrhage or "trapdoor" or "fallen fragment" noted on axial head CT
    - Other findings: Pneumo-orbita, ocular injury (24%); chronic enophthalmos
- **Fracture, Medial Orbital Blowout**
  - Results from blunt trauma
  - Imaging: Medial displacement of lamina papyracea

6

TRAUMATIC LESIONS OF FACE

- Herniation of extraconal fat ± medial rectus muscle into defect
- Orbital floor fracture may be associated

Helpful Clues for Less Common Diagnoses
- **Fracture, Nasoethmoid Complex**
  - Results from trauma to nasal bridge
    - Fx extends into nose through ethmoids
  - Widening of nasal bridge on physical examination
  - More serious than isolated nasal bone fx
  - Imaging: Fx of nasal bone & ethmoid sinuses ± cribriform plate
    - Cribriform plate fx ⇒ CSF rhinorrhea
- **Fracture, Frontal Sinus**
  - Anterior wall fx with depression ⇒ cosmetic deformity & hypesthesia in distribution of supraorbital nerve
  - Posterior wall fx ⇒ CSF leak, meningitis, or parenchymal brain injury
- **Fracture, Transfacial (Le Fort)**
  - Complex, bilateral fx with large unstable fragment ("floating face")
    - Invariably involves pterygoid plates
  - Pure Le Fort fx rarely seen & may vary from side-to-side
  - Facial distortion (elongated face), mobile maxilla, malocclusion, or midface instability may be present clinically
  - Le Fort I: Transverse fx of maxilla above maxillary teeth
    - Involves medial & lateral maxillary sinus walls, septum, pterygoid plates
    - Most common Le Fort type
      - Mobile hard palate on physical exam
  - Le Fort II: Pyramid fx of maxilla
    - Apex above nasal bridge with inferolateral extension through infraorbital rims
    - Mobile maxilla & subconjunctival hemorrhages on physical exam
  - Le Fort III: Craniofacial disruption
    - Requires significant causative force
    - Fx involves maxilla, zygoma, lateral orbital walls
    - Mobility of all facial bones relative to cranium on physical exam

Helpful Clues for Rare Diagnoses
- **Fracture, Complex Midfacial**
  - Account for ≈ 5% of facial fx
    - Synonym = "smash" fx
    - Severe facial comminution
    - Includes several varieties of otherwise unclassifiable fxs
  - Patients often in unstable condition with axial & appendicular skeletal injuries
- **Trauma/Dislocation, TMJ**
  - May be associated with contralateral mandible fx (body or angle)
  - May be dislocated without fx (spontaneously during large yawn)
  - Imaging: Look for condylar/subcondylar fx (fracture fragment pulled medially by medial pterygoid muscle)
    - "Empty TMJ" sign on CT suggests dislocation of condyle from glenoid fossa

Fracture, Nasal Bone

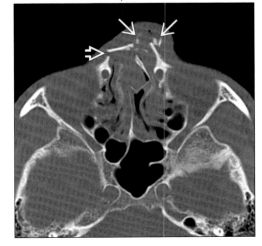

Axial bone CT shows comminuted nasal bone fractures ➡️ with displacement of fragments to the left, resulting in clinical deformity. A fracture of the nasal process of the maxilla is noted ➡️.

Fracture, Nasal Bone

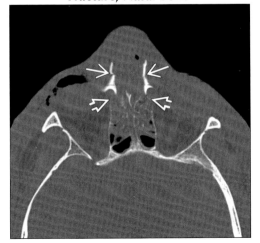

Axial bone CT shows bilateral nasal bone fractures ➡️ associated with bilateral anterior ethmoid fractures ➡️. Patient is at risk for CSF leak from associated cribriform plate fracture (not shown).

TRAUMATIC LESIONS OF FACE

(Left) Axial NECT reveals a fracture through the posterior left mandibular body ➡ associated with extensive facial air. Look for a contralateral condyle/subcondylar region second fracture in such a case. (Right) Sagittal NECT 3D reformatted image shows a mildly diastased, oblique fracture ➘ at the junction of the body and angle of the mandible. As this fracture traverses the inferior alveolar foramen, chin hypesthesia is likely in this patient.

Fracture, Mandible

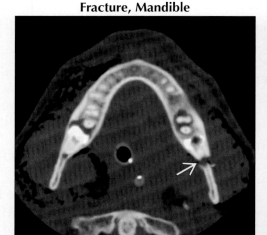

Fracture, Mandible

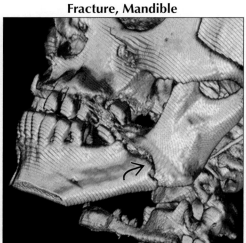

(Left) Axial bone CT shows the classic features of a zygomaticomaxillary fracture with fractures involving the anterior and posterior maxillary sinus walls ➡ and the left zygomatic arch ➘. (Right) Axial bone CT through orbits in the same patient shows a comminuted fracture of the left lateral orbital wall ➡ with slight diastasis and angulation. The fracture fragments do not impinge on the lateral rectus muscle.

Fracture, Zygomaticomaxillary Complex

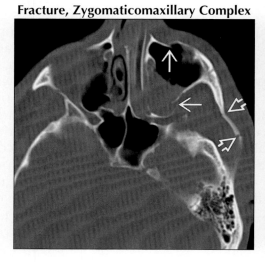

Fracture, Zygomaticomaxillary Complex

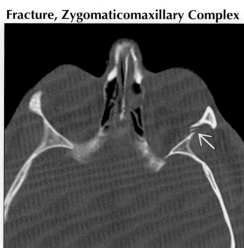

(Left) Axial NECT shows a fluid-hemorrhage level in the left maxillary sinus in a trauma patient. There is a bony fragment ➡ in the fluid. This "fallen fragment" should raise suspicion for an orbital floor fracture. (Right) Coronal bone CT in the same patient shows a large defect in the floor of the left orbit with a fracture fragment ➡ displaced into the maxillary antrum. The fracture does not involve the infraorbital foramen ➘.

Fracture, Inferior Orbital

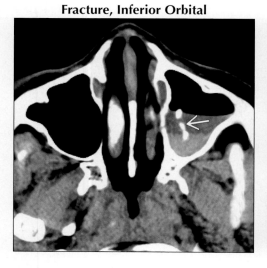

Fracture, Inferior Orbital

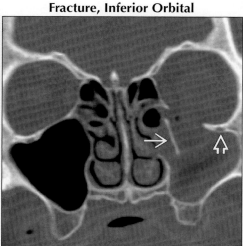

TRAUMATIC LESIONS OF FACE

Fracture, Medial Orbital Blowout

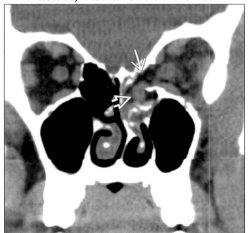

Fracture, Frontal Sinus

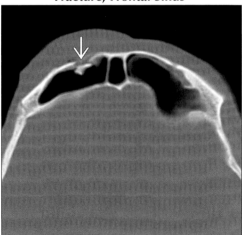

(Left) Coronal NECT demonstrates a large defect in the medial wall of the left orbit ➜ with herniation of extraconal fat and the left medial rectus muscle ➜ into the left ethmoid sinuses. *(Right)* Axial bone CT shows a slightly depressed fracture of the anterior wall of the right frontal sinus ➜. There is overlying soft tissue swelling, and the posterior wall is intact.

Fracture, Transfacial (Le Fort)

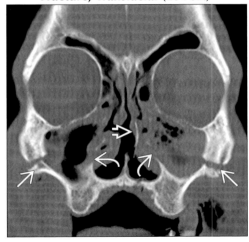

Fracture, Transfacial (Le Fort)

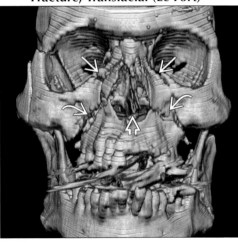

(Left) Coronal bone CT shows fractures through the lateral ➜ and medial ➜ walls of the maxillary sinuses with a displaced nasal septal fracture ➜. The palate is separated from the rest of the face (Le Fort I fracture). *(Right)* Anteroposterior 3D reformation reveals features of Le Fort type II transfacial fracture. A pyramidal fragment encompassing the maxilla is inferiorly displaced. Fractures involve the infraorbital rims ➜, maxilla ➜, and nasal septum ➜.

Fracture, Complex Midfacial

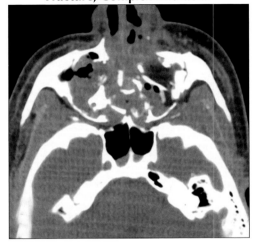

Trauma/Dislocation, TMJ

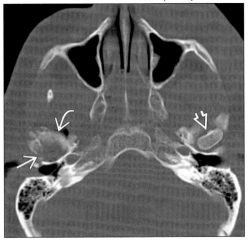

(Left) Axial NECT shows extensive comminuted fractures of the midface consistent with a facial "smash" injury. There is significant hemorrhage within the sinonasal cavities and facial swelling. *(Right)* Axial bone CT demonstrates "empty TMJ" sign ➜ with anterior dislocation of the fractured condyle ➜ with respect to the glenoid fossa. A small amount of air is seen in the joint space. Note the normal appearance of the left TMJ ➜.

SECTION 7
Orbit

Anatomically Based Differentials

Generic Imaging Patterns

Modality-Specific Imaging Findings

Clinically Based Differentials

DIFFERENTIAL DIAGNOSIS

Common
- Cellulitis, Orbit
- Abscess, Subperiosteal, Orbit
- Infection, Other Pathogen, Orbit
- Dacryocystitis

Less Common
- Dacryoadenitis
- Dacryocystocele
- Infantile Hemangioma, Orbit
- Eyelid Cyst (Meibomian)
- Benign Neoplasm Lacrimal Gland
  - Benign Mixed Tumor, Lacrimal

Rare but Important
- Malignant Neoplasm Lacrimal Gland
  - Adenoid Cystic Carcinoma, Lacrimal
  - Non-Hodgkin Lymphoma, Lacrimal
- Sebaceous Carcinoma

ESSENTIAL INFORMATION

Key Differential Diagnosis Issues
- Orbital septum: Membranous sheet that acts as anterior boundary of orbit
  - Functions as barrier to entry into postseptal orbit for infection and tumor
- Preseptal orbit: Soft tissues superficial to orbital septum

Helpful Clues for Common Diagnoses
- **Cellulitis, Orbit**
  - Key facts: Secondary to trauma or cutaneous, hematogenous, or iatrogenic infection
  - Imaging
    - Increased density and enhancing periorbital soft tissues, lids, orbital septum
    - Look for retroseptal extraconal or intraconal direct extension or fat infiltration
- **Abscess, Subperiosteal, Orbit**
  - Key facts: Collection of pus between orbital wall & orbital periosteum due to adjacent focus of infection/inflammation
  - Imaging
    - CECT hypodense or MR T2 hyperintense lenticular rim-enhancing fluid collection extending from medial orbital wall or orbital roof

- Frequently displacement, enlargement, & enhancement of medial, superior, ± inferior rectus muscles
- Look for associated ethmoid or frontal sinus disease, periorbital cellulitis, cavernous sinus involvement
- **Infection, Other Pathogen, Orbit**
  - Key facts: From intraocular/orbital surgery, penetrating orbital injury, diabetes, IV drug use, renal failure
  - Imaging
    - CT: Periorbital cellulitis or abscess, thickened, enhancing infiltrative sclera
    - MR: Enhancing orbital septum, scleral-uveal enhancement
- **Dacryocystitis**
  - Key facts: Inflammation or infection secondary to obstruction of lacrimal sac
    - Congenital or acquired
  - Imaging
    - Soft tissue thickening and enhancement of medial epicanthus and preseptal space
    - Soft tissue obstructing nasolacrimal duct
    - May be associated dacryoliths

Helpful Clues for Less Common Diagnoses
- **Dacryoadenitis**
  - Key facts: Lacrimal gland infection/inflammation
  - Imaging
    - Enlargement, enhancement of lacrimal gland, involvement of orbital septum
    - Preseptal ± periorbital soft tissue thickening & enhancement
    - Typically no bone erosion, but periosteal reaction of lateral orbital wall adjacent to lacrimal fossa
- **Dacryocystocele**
  - Key facts: Cystic enlargement of lacrimal sac due to primary canalization failure or secondary obstruction
    - Most commonly congenital
  - Imaging
    - Cystic enlargement of lacrimal sac ± nasolacrimal duct
    - Preservation of anterior & posterior lacrimal crests
    - May have associated dacryocystitis or preseptal cellulitis
- **Infantile Hemangioma, Orbit**
  - Key facts: Capillary hemangioma

- Adults: Orbital endothelial cell neoplasm distinct from cavernous hemangiomas
  - Imaging
    - Most commonly in medial epicanthus; preseptal tissues often with postseptal extension
    - Discrete moderately well-marginated mass on nasal dorsum, preseptal tissues, or lids
    - Moderately to intensely enhancing; flow voids on MR
- **Eyelid Cyst (Meibomian)**
  - Key facts: Obstruction of meibomian glands posterior to eyelash in tarsal plate of upper or lower eyelid
  - Imaging
    - Typically diagnosed on physical exam; imaging performed to exclude postseptal involvement
    - Cystic-appearing mass or nodule in upper or lower eyelid or tarsal plate, often with surrounding blepharitis
- **Benign Mixed Tumor, Lacrimal**
  - Key facts: Pleomorphic adenoma
    - Most common benign neoplasm of lacrimal gland
    - Consists of epithelial & myoepithelial cells
  - Imaging
    - Round to ovoid, discrete well-circumscribed mass in lacrimal gland
    - Majority arise in orbital lobe of lacrimal gland in superolateral extraconal orbit

- Majority have associated bony remodeling
- Punctate calcifications may be present

Helpful Clues for Rare Diagnoses
- **Adenoid Cystic Carcinoma, Lacrimal**
  - Key facts: Most common primary lacrimal malignancy
    - Accounts for ~ 30% of all lacrimal tumors
    - Presents with preseptal mass, pain
  - Imaging
    - Diffuse irregular lacrimal gland enlargement & enhancement
    - Invades or less often erodes bone
- **Non-Hodgkin Lymphoma, Lacrimal**
  - Key facts: Primary non-Hodgkin lymphoma of lacrimal gland is rare
    - Accounts for ~ 3% of all lacrimal masses
  - Imaging
    - Homogeneous enlargement & mild enhancement of lacrimal gland
    - Does not typically erode bone
- **Sebaceous Carcinoma**
  - Key facts: Rare malignancy arising from meibomian glands in eyelid
    - Accounts for ~ 0.4-4% of epithelial orbital malignancies
    - 5% of eyelid malignancies
  - Imaging
    - Diffuse irregular enhancing area or mass involving eyelid and preseptal space
    - > 50% are associated with or present as chalazion or blepharoconjunctivitis

Cellulitis, Orbit

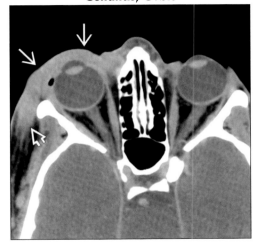

Axial CECT reveals swelling and infiltration of the skin and underlying soft tissues ➡ anterior to the right orbit and extending posteriorly toward the suprazygomatic masticator space ➡.

Abscess, Subperiosteal, Orbit

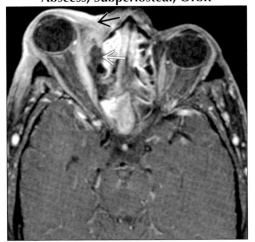

Axial T1 C+ MR shows proptosis of the right globe with diffuse enhancement involving the preseptal space ➡ with postseptal infiltration and abscess ➡ into the extraconal space.

(Left) Axial NECT demonstrates edema ⮞ and a large abscess ➡ involving the left preseptal space, lower eyelid, and skin. *(Right)* Axial CECT reveals soft tissue swelling and enhancement along the nasal dorsum ➡ and preseptal space ⮞ with soft tissue obstruction of an enlarged lacrimal sac ⮡.

Infection, Other Pathogen, Orbit

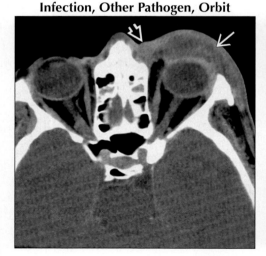

Dacryocystitis

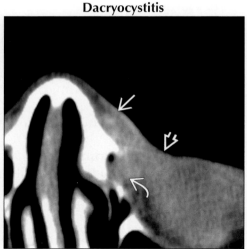

(Left) Axial CECT shows diffuse irregular enlargement and enhancement of the orbital and palpebral lobes of the lacrimal gland ➡ with extension to the orbital septum ⮥. Clinical symptoms would help to distinguish this from lacrimal malignancy. *(Right)* Axial CECT shows bilateral dacryocystoceles ➡ extending from the lacrimal sacs ⮞ in this patient with Wegner granulomatosis. Note that even the larger mass is confined by the intact orbital septum ➡.

Dacryoadenitis

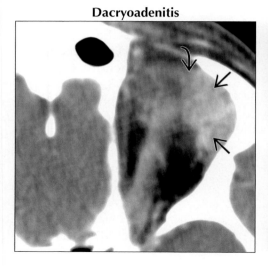

Dacryocystocele

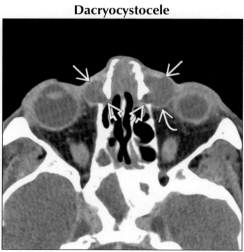

(Left) Axial CECT shows a well-defined enhancing ovoid infantile hemangioma ➡ adjacent to the lower eyelid at the medial canthus. Note the lack of significant surrounding blepharitis. *(Right)* Axial T1 C+ FS MR demonstrates a preseptal orbitonasal infantile hemangioma ➡ with marked contrast enhancement. Prominent punctate and linear flow voids are evident ⮥.

Infantile Hemangioma, Orbit

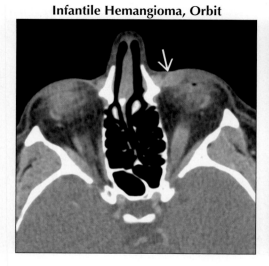

Infantile Hemangioma, Orbit

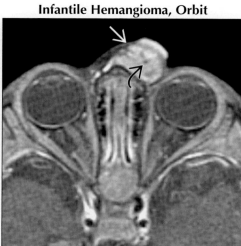

Eyelid Cyst (Meibomian)

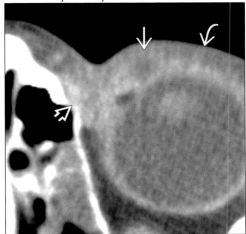

Eyelid Cyst (Meibomian)

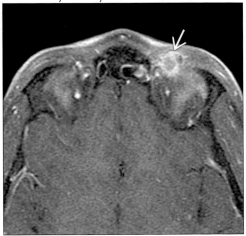

(Left) Axial CECT shows a small cystic mass ➡ in the eyelid of this patient with associated blepharitis ➡, preseptal cellulitis, and dacryocystitis ➡. (Right) Axial T1 C+ FS MR reveals an irregular rim-enhancing cystic mass ➡ in the superior aspect of the lid in the medial orbit. The irregularity of the posterior border is suggestive of rupture.

Benign Mixed Tumor, Lacrimal

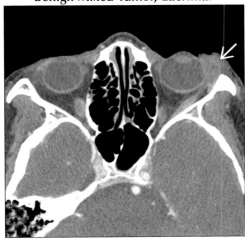

Adenoid Cystic Carcinoma, Lacrimal

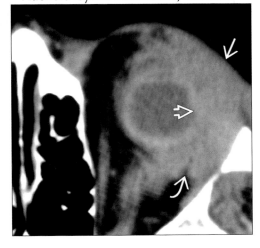

(Left) Axial CECT demonstrates unilateral fullness of the palpebral lobe of the left lacrimal gland ➡, which is also unusually hypodense. No calcifications are evident. (Right) Axial NECT shows an ill-defined mass centered in the left lacrimal gland. The mass shows significant local extension anteriorly into the preseptal space ➡ and dermis. Note the extension posteriorly into the retrobulbar orbit ➡, as well as into the sclera ➡.

Non-Hodgkin Lymphoma, Lacrimal

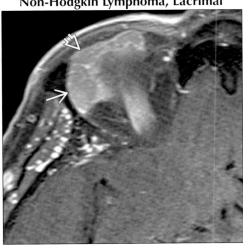

Sebaceous Carcinoma

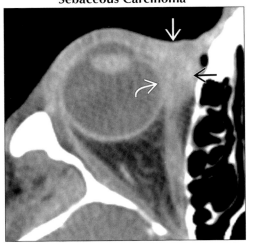

(Left) Axial T1WI FS MR reveals a mildly enhancing mass intrinsic to the right lacrimal gland ➡ with orbital septal and preseptal extension ➡. The homogeneous appearance and lack of significant enhancement would favor lymphoma. (Right) Axial CECT shows an enhancing mass extending from the eyelid ➡ through the orbital septum ➡ to encase the insertion of the medial rectus muscle. Note the extension to and infiltration of the sclera ➡.

DIFFERENTIAL DIAGNOSIS

Common
- Ocular Hemorrhage, Post-Traumatic
- Retinal or Choroidal Detachment
- Idiopathic Orbital Inflammatory Disease (Pseudotumor)
- Melanoma, Ocular

Less Common
- Infection, Other Pathogen, Orbit
- Staphyloma
- Choroidal Hemangioma (Hamartoma)
- Coloboma

Rare but Important
- Osteoma, Choroidal
- Metastases, Ocular

ESSENTIAL INFORMATION

Helpful Clues for Common Diagnoses
- **Ocular Hemorrhage, Post-Traumatic**
  - Key facts
    - Head/face trauma or orbit/ocular surgery → vitreal or suprachoroidal hemorrhage
    - In adults or children, accidental head trauma rarely → retinal hemorrhage
  - Imaging
    - CT: Patchy or lenticular hyperdensity in vitreous body or hyperdensity in suprachoroidal space
    - MR: Acute = hypointense T1/T2 mass in or appearing to compress vitreous body
    - ± Globe rupture, intraocular gas, shattered or dislocated lens
- **Retinal or Choroidal Detachment**
  - Key facts
    - Retinal: Detachment of sensory retina from retinal pigment epithelium
    - Choroidal: Accumulation of fluid or blood in suprachoroidal space
  - Imaging
    - Retinal: V-shaped abnormality with apex at optic disk; ends extend toward ciliary bodies
    - Choroidal: CT hyperdense, MR hypointense lines parallel to choroidal plane, do not converge at disk
    - Subretinal space has CT hyperdense or MR hyperintense fluid; ingress of vitreal fluid → decreased signal intensity

- **Idiopathic Orbital Inflammatory Disease (Pseudotumor)**
  - Key facts
    - Benign inflammatory process of unknown etiology
  - Imaging
    - Space-occupying infiltrative process involving any part of orbit
    - Ocular lesions: ↑ enhancement + irregular or nodular scleral thickening
    - Scleral involvement (part of anterior form) usually with optic nerve sheath involvement
- **Melanoma, Ocular**
  - Key facts
    - Majority are choroidal in location
    - Ciliary body & iris lesions less common
  - Imaging
    - Protuberant or dome-shaped solitary hyperdense and enhancing choroidal mass with broad choroidal base
    - MR: Hyperintense T1/hypointense T2 + enhancement; amelanotic lesions may be hypointense
    - May have associated T1 hyperintense, T2 hypointense choroidal detachment

Helpful Clues for Less Common Diagnoses
- **Infection, Other Pathogen, Orbit**
  - Key facts
    - Endophthalmitis: Inflammation of ocular space
    - Secondary to exogenous (surgery/trauma) or endogenous source
  - Imaging
    - Acute: Thickening and enhancement of uveal-scleral layers; ↑ density & enhancement of vitreous body; ± serous choroidal detachment
    - Chronic/late: Phthisis bulbi (small shrunken globe ± hyperdense vitreous, enhancing vitreous and scleral or vitreal calcification)
- **Staphyloma**
  - Key facts
    - Acquired buckling of scleral wall in posterior pole of globe
    - Associated with degenerative changes in severe myopia
  - Imaging

- Axially (anterior-posterior) enlarged globe + focal posterior globe bulge and associated uveal-scleral thinning
  - Peripapillary staphyloma: Rare congential defect of fundus from excavation of posterior wall of globe & vitreous outpouching; extends to normal optic nerve head, associated chorioretinal coloboma
- **Choroidal Hemangioma (Hamartoma)**
  - Key facts
    - Congenital vascular hamartoma
    - Typically presents in middle-aged/elderly
    - Isolated or part of Sturge-Weber syndrome
  - Imaging
    - Solitary or diffuse
    - CT: Lenticular hyperdense mass in juxtapapillary or macular region; avidly enhances
    - MR: T1 & T2 hyperintense; avid contrast enhancement, > in melanoma cases
- **Coloboma**
  - Key facts
    - Congenital gap or defect in layers of scleral wall caused by failure of fetal fissure to close
  - Imaging
    - Focal defect in posterior scleral wall at optic nerve head with outpouching of vitreous
    - Bilateral > > unilateral
    - Typically in pediatric patients, may be incidentally identified in adults

Helpful Clues for Rare Diagnoses
- **Osteoma, Choroidal**
  - Key facts
    - Benign ossifying tumor of choroid
    - Young women (20-30 years)
    - 75% unilateral
  - Imaging
    - CT: Well-defined lenticular calcification in choroidal-retinal layer of posterior pole of globe
    - MR: T1 hyperintense, T2 hypointense; marked enhancement
- **Metastases, Ocular**
  - Key facts: Breast & lung carcinoma most common
  - Imaging
    - Usually involves posterior globe, typically uvea, and extends along choroidal plane
    - 1/3 bilateral uveal lesions
    - MR: T2 hypointense and enhancing irregularities of choroid ± associated choroidal or retinal detachment
    - Moderate to marked enhancement suggests extraocular melanoma, thyroid, or renal cell carcinoma primary lesions

SELECTED REFERENCES

1. Smoker WR et al: Vascular lesions of the orbit: more than meets the eye. Radiographics. 28(1):185-204; quiz 325, 2008
2. Lane JI et al: Retinal detachment: imaging of surgical treatments and complications. Radiographics. 23(4):983-94, 2003

Ocular Hemorrhage, Post-Traumatic

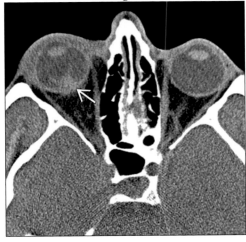

Axial NECT shows a vitreal hemorrhage ➡ at the posterior attachment of the vitreous body to the retina in a patient with perforating open globe injury.

Retinal or Choroidal Detachment

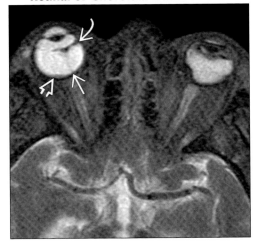

Axial T2WI FS MR reveals retinal detachment with retinal "leaves" attaching at the apex ➡ & the ora serrata ➡. Subhyaloid effusion ➡ & complete retinal detachment are apparent in the right globe.

(Left) Axial T2WI FS MR shows a choroidal detachment with a biconcave expansion of the suprachoroidal space ➡ extending anteriorly from the limbus ⇥ to the posterior attachment. *(Right)* Axial CECT shows thickening & enhancement of the sclera ➡, as well as the optic nerve sheath ⇗, in a patient with the anterior form of idiopathic orbital inflammatory disease. Note that the choroidal layer has normal dimensions ⇥.

Retinal or Choroidal Detachment

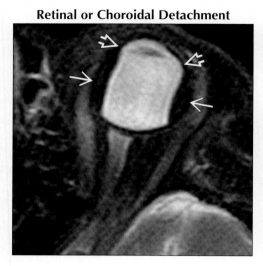

Idiopathic Orbital Inflammatory Disease (Pseudotumor)

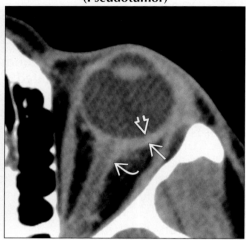

(Left) Axial T1 C+ FS MR reveals a significantly enhancing broad-based choroidal mass ➡ arising near the limbic junction. The hypointense scleral ⇗ and retinal layers ⇥ are preserved. *(Right)* Sagittal T1WI MR shows a well-defined hyperintense choroidal-based melanoma ➡. This classic appearance of intrinsic high signal on pre-contrast T1 is secondary to the paramagnetic properties of melanin.

Melanoma, Ocular

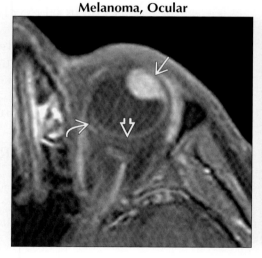

Melanoma, Ocular

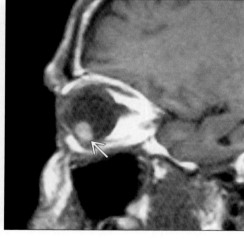

(Left) Axial CECT demonstrates mildly enhancing nodularity of the sclera ➡ and a serous choroidal effusions ⇥ in a patient with pseudomonas scleritis. *(Right)* Axial CECT reveals a mildly rim-enhancing mass involving the choroidal-retinal layer ➡. This finding resulted from endogenous spread of a hepatic abscess.

Infection, Other Pathogen, Orbit

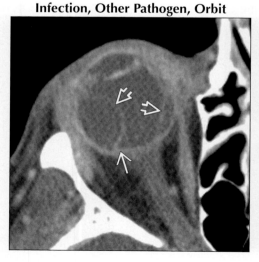

Infection, Other Pathogen, Orbit

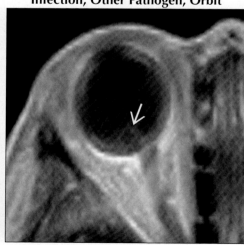

Staphyloma

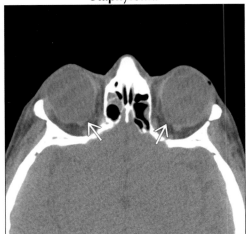

Choroidal Hemangioma (Hamartoma)

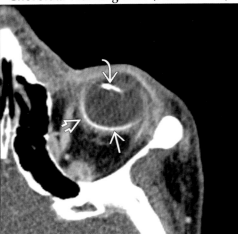

(Left) Axial NECT in a 65 year old patient with severe myopia demonstrates bilateral axial elongation of the globes with thinning & outpouching of the sclera ➡. *(Right)* Axial CECT reveals intense enhancement of the choroid ➡, representing diffuse choroidal hemangioma (hamartoma). Note calcification of lens ➡ & soft tissue thickening surrounding the sclera, reflecting angiomatosis of periscleral plexus ⇒ in a patient with Sturge-Weber syndrome.

Coloboma

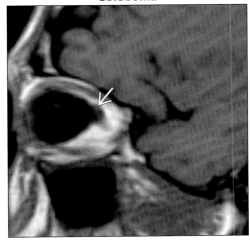

Osteoma, Choroidal

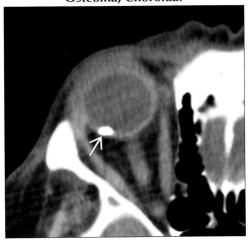

(Left) Sagittal T1WI MR shows an elongated globe with posterior vitreous protrusion through the scleral cleft ➡ in a middle-aged patient. *(Right)* Axial NECT shows a well-defined calcification centered within the choroidal layer ➡. Note that this lies lateral to the optic nerve head, distinguishing it from optic nerve drusen.

Metastases, Ocular

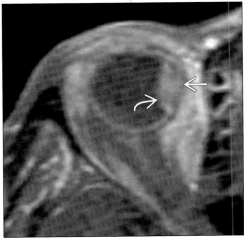

Metastases, Ocular

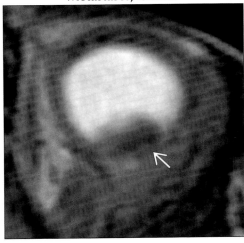

(Left) Axial T1WI FS MR reveals mildly moderately enhancing, heterogeneous choroidal-based breast carcinoma metastases ➡ with flattened dome-shaped retinal margin ➡, suggesting the integrity of Bruch membrane may be preserved. *(Right)* Axial T2WI MR in the same patient shows an additional choroidal-based hypointense mass ➡ at posterior pole of the opposite globe. Irregularity of this margin is concerning for violation of the retinal layer.

DIFFERENTIAL DIAGNOSIS

Common
- Retinoblastoma
- Persistent Hyperplastic Primary Vitreous
- Retinopathy of Prematurity
- Cataract, Congenital

Less Common
- Coats Disease
- Coloboma
- Toxocariasis, Orbit
- Microphthalmos, Congenital

Rare but Important
- Astrocytoma, Retinal
- Norrie Disease
- Walker-Warburg Syndrome

ESSENTIAL INFORMATION

Helpful Clues for Common Diagnoses
- **Retinoblastoma**
  - Key facts: Malignant tumor arising from neuroectodermal cells of retina
    - Classified as primitive neuroectodermal tumor (PNET)
    - Most common intraocular tumor of childhood
    - Most common cause of leukocoria
    - Rare trilateral or quadrilateral form involves bilateral globes + pineal, or pineal + suprasellar tumor
  - Imaging
    - Unilateral (70-75%)
    - CT: Punctate or speckled calcified intraocular mass
    - MR: T1 mildly hyperintense, T2 moderately hypointense (cf. vitreous); moderate to marked heterogeneous enhancement
- **Persistent Hyperplastic Primary Vitreous**
  - Key facts: Congenital lesion due to incomplete regression of embryonic vitreous and blood supply
    - 2nd most common cause of leukocoria
  - Imaging
    - Hyperdense or hyperintense small globe: No calcification
    - Retrolental enhancing soft tissue, classically with "martini glass" shape
    - Associated retinal detachments common
- **Retinopathy of Prematurity**
  - Key facts: Occurs due to prolonged exposure to supplemental oxygen in premature infants
    - Premature birth interrupts normal vasculogenesis ⇒ incomplete vascularization of retina ⇒ hypoxia ⇒ abnormal neovascularization
  - Imaging
    - Usually bilateral
    - Hyperdense globe ± abnormal retrolental soft tissue
    - Early: Microphthalmia
    - Advanced: Vitreal calcification
- **Cataract, Congenital**
  - Key facts: Lens opacification
    - Most are sporadic and unilateral
    - ~ 20% familial
    - ~ 17% associated with systemic disease or syndrome: Trisomy 21, craniofacial syndromes, diabetes, etc.
  - Imaging
    - Small, hypodense lens
    - Lens may assume spherical shape (spherophakia), differentiating from acquired cataract

Helpful Clues for Less Common Diagnoses
- **Coats Disease**
  - Key facts: Primary retinal vascular anomaly with retinal telangiectasis and exudative retinal detachment
    - Unilateral in 80-90% of patients
    - Most patients male
  - Imaging
    - Advanced stages may appear to obliterate vitreous
    - CT: Mild diffusely and homogeneously hyperdense vitreous without calcification
    - MR: Retinal detachment with nonenhancing T1 and T2 hyperintense subretinal exudate
- **Coloboma**
  - Key facts: Defect in ocular tissue involving structures of embryonic cleft
    - Bilateral > unilateral
  - Imaging
    - Focal defect of posterior globe with outpouching of vitreous
    - Defect at optic nerve head insertion with funnel-shaped excavation
- **Toxocariasis, Orbit**

- Key facts: Eosinophilic granuloma caused by infection of larval nematode *Toxocara cani* or *cati*
- Imaging
  - CT: Diffuse hyperdensity in vitreous ± discrete mass; no calcification
  - MR: Enhancing, variable T1 hypo/isointense, T2 iso/hyperintense retrolental or vitreous mass
- **Microphthalmos, Congenital**
  - Key facts: Corneal diameter of < 11 mm and anteroposterior diameter of globe < 20 mm at birth
    - Isolated or associated with craniofacial anomalies, coloboma, persistent hyperplastic primary vitreous, retinopathy of prematurity
  - Imaging
    - Overall volume and dimension of globe < unaffected side or comparison normal
    - Simple microphthalmia: Structurally normal small eye or complex with associated findings, as above

Helpful Clues for Rare Diagnoses
- **Astrocytoma, Retinal**
  - Key facts: Retinal astrocytic hamartoma is ocular manifestation of tuberous sclerosis complex
  - Imaging
    - Enhancing exophytic juxtapapillary or epipapillary retinal mass
    - Mass may be multifocal ± bilateral

- Rarely may occur in isolation without tuberous sclerosis complex
- **Norrie Disease**
  - Key facts: X-linked recessive syndrome of retinal malformation, deafness, and mental retardation
  - Imaging
    - Bilateral hyperdense vitreous, small anterior chamber
    - Small lens without calcification
    - May have associated retrolental mass, retinal detachment, microphthalmia, optic nerve atrophy
- **Walker-Warburg Syndrome**
  - Key facts: Also known as HARD+E
    - **H**ydrocephaly, **a**gyria, **r**etinal **d**etachment ± **e**ncephalocele
  - Imaging
    - Bilateral retinal detachment
    - Vitreous ± subretinal hemorrhage
    - Associated hydrocephalus, agyria/dysgenesis of cerebral and cerebellar gray and white matter

SELECTED REFERENCES

1. Chung EM et al: From the archives of the AFIP: Pediatric orbit tumors and tumorlike lesions: neuroepithelial lesions of the ocular globe and optic nerve. Radiographics. 27(4):1159-86, 2007

Retinoblastoma

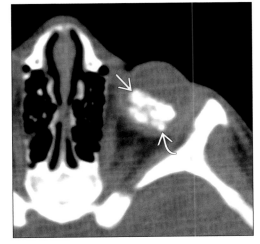

Axial NECT shows coarse calcifications typical of retinoblastoma in the posterior segment of the globe ➔ involving the vitreous body, as well as the choroidal-retinal layers ➔.

Retinoblastoma

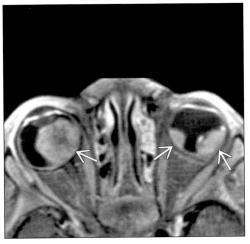

Axial T1WI FS MR shows bilateral enhancing retinal masses ➔ extending into the vitreous but not extending beyond the sclera into the optic nerve or intraconal orbit.

(Left) Axial T2WI FS MR reveals a hypointense retrolental "martini glass"-shaped mass ⮕ with associated fluid-fluid levels ⮕ in the vitreous body and a subretinal effusion ⮕. *(Right)* Axial CECT demonstrates an enhancing retrolental embryonic fibrovascular tissue ⮕ and right small globe (microphthalmia).

Persistent Hyperplastic Primary Vitreous

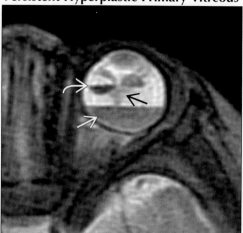

Persistent Hyperplastic Primary Vitreous

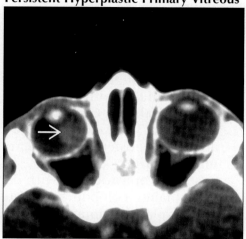

(Left) Axial CECT shows a small left globe with dense peripheral calcifications ⮕. Both lenses are also calcified. The right globe shows more punctate scattered calcifications ⮕ and fluid-fluid level ⮕, indicating retinal detachment. *(Right)* Axial T2WI MR in the same patient reveals fluid-fluid level ⮕ and peripheral low signal intensity from dense calcification ⮕. Note the deformed, low signal intensity calcified lens ⮕.

Retinopathy of Prematurity

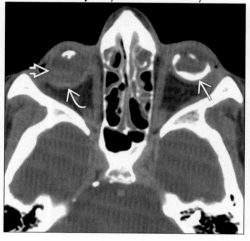

Retinopathy of Prematurity

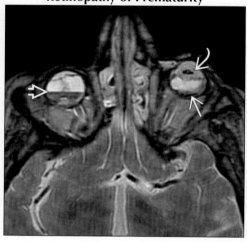

(Left) Axial CECT in a child with leukocoria shows significant thinning and loss of density from the right lens ⮕ with increased depth of the anterior chamber ⮕ compared to the opposite normal left globe. *(Right)* Axial NECT depicts diffuse homogeneous hyperdense vitreous of left globe ⮕ in a child with no history of trauma or surgery. Coats disease as a primary retinal vascular anomaly with retinal telangiectasis caused this exudative retinal detachment.

Cataract, Congenital

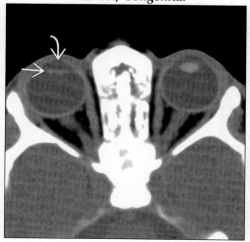

Coats Disease

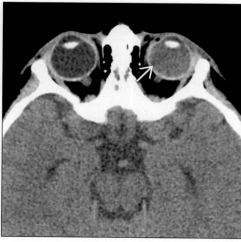

Coloboma

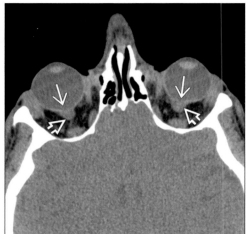

Toxocariasis, Orbit

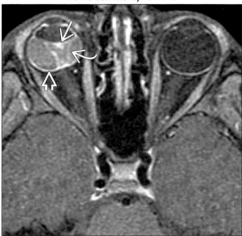

(Left) Axial NECT shows a defect in the posterior globes bilaterally ➡ with outpouching of the vitreous ⮕. (Right) Axial T1 C+ FS MR demonstrates hyperintensity of the right globe vitreous with an enhancing retrolental mass ⮕, retinal detachments ➡, and hypointense retinal and scleral nodules ⮕.

Microphthalmos, Congenital

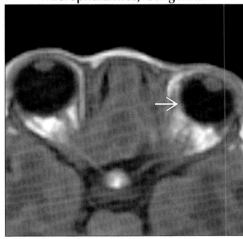

Astrocytoma, Retinal

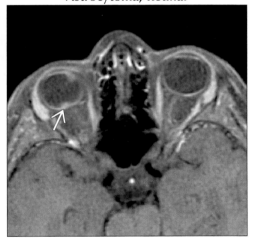

(Left) Axial T2WI MR shows an asymmetrically small left globe ➡ with otherwise normal lens, vitreous body, and choroidal-retinal layers. (Right) Axial T1 C+ FS MR reveals an enhancing nodular retinal astrocytoma ➡ at the optic nerve head in a child with tuberous sclerosis.

Norrie Disease

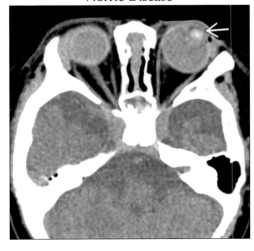

Walker-Warburg Syndrome

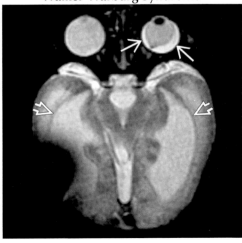

(Left) Axial NECT shows bilateral abnormal increase in globe density. Left globe & orbit are enlarged with decrease in size of anterior chamber ⮕. Norrie disease is diagnosed clinically when grayish-yellow fibrovascular masses are found in globes of an infant. (Right) Axial T2WI MR reveals a rim of (T2) hyperintensity along the posterior left globe ➡, suggestive of retinal dysplasia ± subretinal hemorrhage. Note the marked lateral ventricle dilatation ⮕.

OPTIC NERVE-SHEATH LESION

DIFFERENTIAL DIAGNOSIS

Common
- Optic Nerve Sheath Meningioma
- Optic Pathway Glioma

Less Common
- Lymphoproliferative Lesions, Orbit (NHL)
- Idiopathic Orbital Inflammatory Disease (IOID), Perineuritis
- Orbital Sarcoid
- Metastasis, Orbit
- Optic Neuritis

Rare but Important
- Optic Neuritis, Infectious

ESSENTIAL INFORMATION

Helpful Clues for Common Diagnoses
- **Optic Nerve Sheath Meningioma**
  - Key facts: Slow-growing benign tumor
    - Painless progressive vision loss
  - Imaging: Uniform nerve enhancement
    - Calcification in 30-50%
    - "Tram-track" appearance outlines sheath
    - Perioptic cyst behind optic nerve head
- **Optic Pathway Glioma**
  - Key facts: Benign tumor in children
    - 30-40% of patients have NF1
    - Malignant variant in adults rare
  - Imaging: Fusiform mass
    - Kinking or buckling common
    - May involve nerve, chiasm, tract, or central pathways

Helpful Clues for Less Common Diagnoses
- **Lymphoproliferative Lesions, Orbit (NHL)**
  - Key facts: MALT-type lymphoma
    - Responsive to treatment
  - Imaging: Solid tumor anywhere in orbit
    - Pliable tumor molds to normal structures
- **Idiopathic Orbital Inflammatory Disease (IOID), Perineuritis**
  - Key facts: Subtype of IOID (pseudotumor)
  - Imaging: Nerve involvement may be isolated or occur with other lesions
- **Orbital Sarcoid**
  - Key facts: Systemic disease common
  - Imaging: Nerve involvement may be isolated or occur with other lesions
- **Optic Neuritis**
  - Key facts: Acute vision loss
    - Inflammatory or autoimmune etiology
    - High prevalence of multiple sclerosis
  - Imaging: Unilateral in 70%
    - Diffuse enhancement without mass

Helpful Clues for Rare Diagnoses
- **Optic Neuritis, Infectious**
  - Key facts: Acute vision loss
    - CMV, HIV, herpes, other viruses
    - TB, Lyme, syphilis, toxoplasmosis
  - Imaging: Diffuse enhancement

Alternative Differential Approaches
- Concomitant lesions elsewhere in orbit
  - Idiopathic perineuritis (pseudotumor)
  - Sarcoidosis, orbit
  - Lymphoproliferative lesions, orbit (NHL)

Optic Nerve Sheath Meningioma

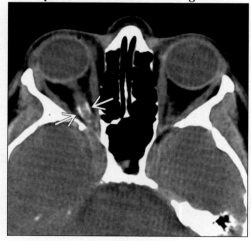

Axial NECT shows a small meningioma of the proximal right intraorbital optic nerve sheath with characteristic "tram-track" calcifications ➡.

Optic Pathway Glioma

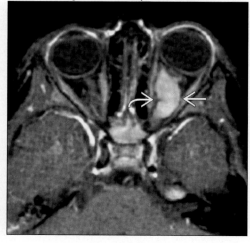

Axial T1 C+ FS MR shows a fusiform mass of the left intraorbital optic nerve ➡ with diffuse homogeneous enhancement. The kinked contour of this sausage-shaped tumor ➡ is typical.

OPTIC NERVE-SHEATH LESION

Lymphoproliferative Lesions, Orbit (NHL)

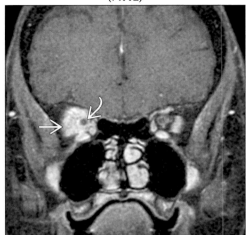

Idiopathic Orbital Inflammatory Disease (IOID), Perineuritis

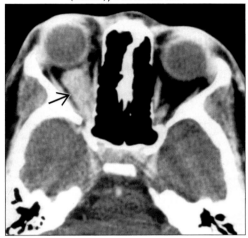

(Left) Coronal T1 C+ FS MR shows a homogeneously enhancing, somewhat lobulated intraconal mass ➡️ that surrounds the optic nerve ➡️. This appearance of "molding" around normal structures is typical of orbital lymphoma. (Right) Axial CECT shows a homogeneously enhancing intraconal mass ➡️ that is indistinguishable from the optic nerve-sheath complex. This example of idiopathic orbital inflammatory disease (pseudotumor) demonstrates isolated nerve involvement.

Orbital Sarcoid

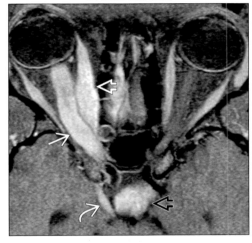

Metastasis, Orbit

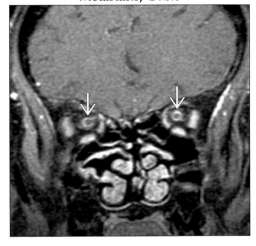

(Left) Axial T1 C+ FS MR shows marked diffuse thickening and enhancement of the right optic nerve ➡️. Oculomotor neuritis ➡️ is evident, as well as medial rectus ➡️ and suprasellar ➡️ involvement with sarcoid. (Right) Coronal T1 C+ FS MR in a patient with known gastric adenocarcinoma shows bilateral perioptic enhancement ➡️, indicating CSF disseminated carcinomatosis with metastatic deposits in the optic nerve sheaths.

Optic Neuritis

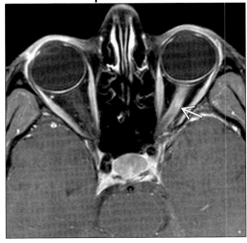

Optic Neuritis, Infectious

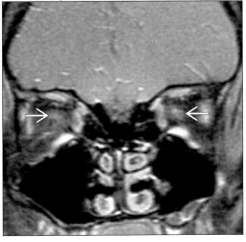

(Left) Axial T1 C+ FS MR shows enhancement and very mild diffuse thickening of the left optic nerve ➡️, without focal mass or nodularity. This patient was subsequently diagnosed with multiple sclerosis. (Right) Coronal T1 C+ FS MR shows bilateral somewhat ill-defined mild enhancement within the optic nerves ➡️ of a child with acute vision loss, due to viral optic neuritis.

DIFFERENTIAL DIAGNOSIS

Common
- Glioma, Optic Pathway
- Meningioma, Optic Nerve Sheath
- Idiopathic Orbital Inflammatory Disease (Pseudotumor)
- Cavernous Hemangioma, Orbit
- Retrobulbar Hematoma

Less Common
- Lymphoproliferative Lesions, Orbit
- Lymphatic Malformation, Orbit
- Thrombosis, Cavernous Sinus, Large Superior Ophthalmic Veins
- Venous Varix, Orbit
- Sarcoidosis, Orbit

Rare but Important
- Schwannoma, Orbit
- Coloboma
- Malignant Nerve Sheath Tumor
- Erdheim-Chester Disease, Orbit

ESSENTIAL INFORMATION

Helpful Clues for Common Diagnoses
- **Glioma, Optic Pathway**
  - Key facts: Primary neuroglial tumor most often associated with neurofibromatosis type 1 (NF1)
  - Imaging
    - Fusiform enlargement of optic nerve (CN2) with variable posterior optic pathway involvement
    - Characteristic kinking/buckling of CN2
    - Avid tumor enhancement common
- **Meningioma, Optic Nerve Sheath**
  - Key facts: Benign neoplasm of optic nerve sheath arising from arachnoid "cap" cells
  - Imaging
    - Enhancing mass surrounding optic nerve, often with calcification
    - "Tram-track" appearance due to enhancement/calcification of nerve sheath surrounding CN2
    - May have perioptic cyst: ↑ CSF within retrobulbar optic nerve sheath
- **Idiopathic Orbital Inflammatory Disease (Pseudotumor)**
  - Key facts: Nonspecific inflammatory process of unknown etiology
    - Presents with painful proptosis

- Imaging
  - Infiltrative or mass-like enhancing soft tissue involving any area of orbit
  - Intraconal space may show diffuse infiltration or more discrete irregular mass
  - Look for simultaneous extraocular muscle, lacrimal, or scleral involvement
- **Cavernous Hemangioma, Orbit**
  - Key facts: Encapsulated venous malformation typically seen in adults
    - Most common adult orbital mass
  - Imaging
    - Well-circumscribed ovoid enhancing mass
    - Heterogeneous early patchy central enhancement
    - Mass "fills in" on delayed images
- **Retrobulbar Hematoma**
  - Key facts: Due to rupture of infraorbital artery/branches following trauma or surgery
  - Imaging
    - Irregular soft tissue mass involving posterior globe surface & distal portion of intraorbital CN2

Helpful Clues for Less Common Diagnoses
- **Lymphoproliferative Lesions, Orbit**
  - Key facts: Most are non-Hodgkin lymphoma (NHL); primarily mucosa associated lymphoid tissue (MALT)
  - Imaging
    - Homogeneously enhancing solid mass
    - Intraconal location < < extraconal
    - Encases or molds to CN2 and other structures
- **Lymphatic Malformation, Orbit**
  - Key facts: Congenital, hamartomatous lymphatic malformation
  - Imaging
    - Lobulated, cystic, poorly marginated & rim-enhancing trans-spatial mass
    - Typically involves both intraconal & extraconal spaces
    - May have fluid-fluid levels (hemorrhage) but no flow voids
- **Thrombosis, Cavernous Sinus, Large Superior Ophthalmic Veins**
  - Key facts: Most commonly complication of rhinosinusitis or trauma
  - Imaging

- Uniform enlargement of superior ophthalmic veins spanning intraconal space
- Associated filling defects within enlarged cavernous sinus
• **Venous Varix, Orbit**
  ○ Key facts: Distensible low-flow venous malformation
  ○ Imaging
    - Significantly enhancing tubular or tortuous mass that distends with increased venous pressure
    - May have phleboliths or multiple varices
• **Sarcoidosis, Orbit**
  ○ Key facts: Systemic condition of noncaseating granulomas with orbital involvement in ~ 25% of cases
  ○ Imaging
    - Thickening and enhancement of CN2
    - Diffuse irregular soft tissue masses that may involve intraconal space
    - Mass-like lacrimal ± extraocular muscle infiltration

Helpful Clues for Rare Diagnoses
• **Schwannoma, Orbit**
  ○ Key facts: Arises from Schwann cells of sympathetic nerves adherent to optic nerve sheath
    - Also arises from cranial nerves 3, 4, 6, or V1
  ○ Imaging
    - Ovoid or fusiform intraconal mass with increased density on CT

- Moderate to marked typically homogeneous enhancement
• **Coloboma**
  ○ Key facts: Focal defect of posterior globe; bilateral > unilateral
  ○ Imaging
    - Defect in globe at optic nerve insertion with outpouching of vitreous
    - Retrobulbar colobomatous cyst is contiguous with globe
    - Contains nonenhancing fluid of vitreal density
• **Malignant Nerve Sheath Tumor**
  ○ Key facts: Rare in orbit
    - Most arise from V1
    - 70% associated with NF1
  ○ Imaging
    - Often with invasive margins
    - Intraconal solid mass with central hypodensity
    - Patchy, irregular peripheral enhancement
• **Erdheim-Chester Disease, Orbit**
  ○ Key facts: Non-Langerhans histiocytosis with orbital xanthogranulomatous deposits in ~ 30% of cases
  ○ Imaging
    - Infiltrative extra- ± intraconal masses; often bilateral
    - Iso- to hyperdense on CT
    - Hypointense on T1 & T2 MR
    - Heterogeneous enhancement

Glioma, Optic Pathway

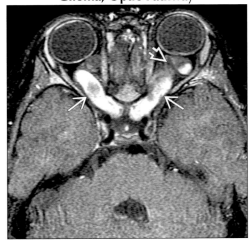

Axial T1 C+ FS MR shows that both optic nerves are tortuous, enlarged, and enhancing ➡ to the level of the optic chiasm. Characteristic kinking ➡ is seen anteriorly on the left.

Meningioma, Optic Nerve Sheath

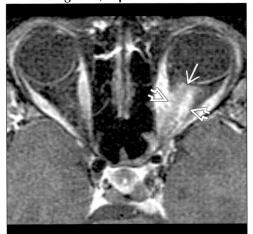

Axial T1 C+ FS MR demonstrates enlargement and enhancement of the intraorbital optic nerve sheath by meningioma ➡. The optic nerve remains normal in size and is nonenhancing ➡.

(Left) Axial T2WI FS MR reveals a diffuse hyperintense mass in the intraconal right orbit ➡ with mild enlargement of the optic nerve sheath ⇨. (Right) Axial CECT shows an irregular well-defined lobular intraconal mass ➡ that displaces the optic nerve ⇨ in a patient with Graves disease. Note the patchy central enhancement with subtle areas of rim enhancement within the cavernous hemangioma ➡.

Idiopathic Orbital Inflammatory Disease (Pseudotumor)

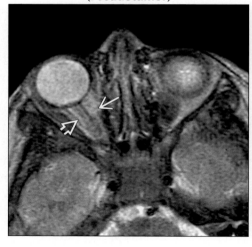

Cavernous Hemangioma, Orbit

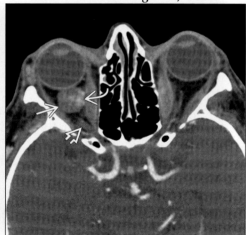

(Left) Axial NECT shows a hypodense to isodense soft tissue mass ➡ in the retrobulbar intraconal space in a patient following head trauma. There is stranding of the intraconal fat ⇨ and preseptal and periorbital edema and cellulitis ➡. (Right) Axial T1 C+ FS MR shows a homogeneously enhancing intraconal NHL wrapping around the optic nerve ➡. The adjacent ethmoid sinus is filled with NHL with the same signal intensity as intraconal disease ➡.

Retrobulbar Hematoma

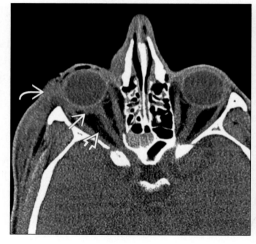

Lymphoproliferative Lesions, Orbit

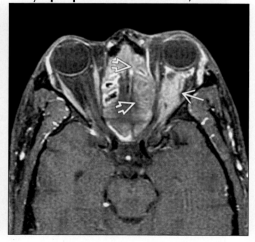

(Left) Axial T2WI MR shows an intraconal multilocular lymphatic malformation with multiple fluid-fluid levels ➡, indicating that hemorrhage into the lesion has occurred. (Right) Axial CECT shows a homogeneously enhancing tubular appearing "mass" ➡ that follows the course of the superior ophthalmic vein. Note that the mass is asymmetrically enlarged compared to the left side ➡ in this patient with cavernous sinus thrombosis.

Lymphatic Malformation, Orbit

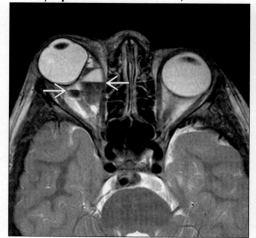

Thrombosis, Cavernous Sinus, Large Superior Ophthalmic Veins

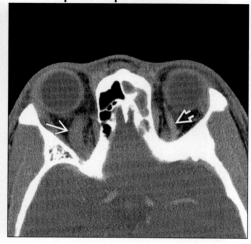

Venous Varix, Orbit

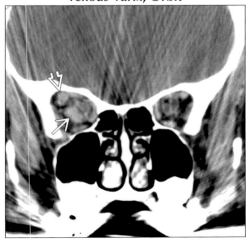

Sarcoidosis, Orbit

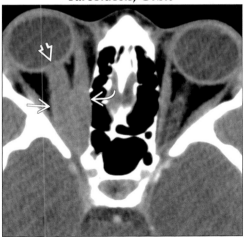

(Left) Coronal CECT shows an enhancing ovoid structure ➡ in the intraconal fat of the right orbit. The key associated feature is the asymmetric dilatation of the superior ophthalmic vein ➡. (Right) Axial CECT reveals proptosis of the right globe with an intraconal mass from optic nerve sheath sarcoid involvement ➡ that also indents the posterior globe ➡. The medial rectus muscle is also involved ➡.

Schwannoma, Orbit

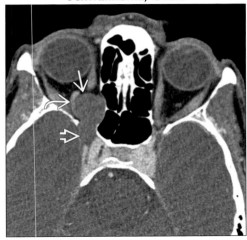

Coloboma

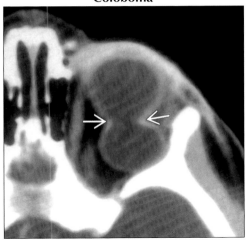

(Left) Axial NECT reveals a smoothly lobulated isodense schwannoma involving the intraconal space ➡. It displaces the adjacent vessel ➡ and is contiguous with the anterior cavernous sinus ➡. This lesion did not enhance on CT but homogeneously enhanced on MR (not shown). (Right) Axial CECT shows a large cystic intraconal mass that connects with the globe through a broad posterior wall defect ➡. Note that the coloboma is the same density as the vitreous.

Malignant Nerve Sheath Tumor

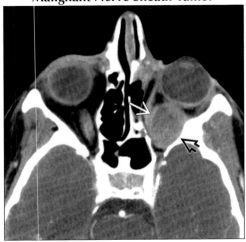

Erdheim-Chester Disease, Orbit

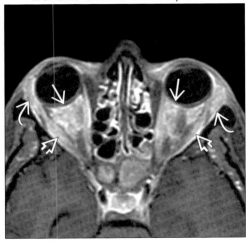

(Left) Axial CECT demonstrates a heterogeneously enhancing intraconal mass with a relatively hypodense center and somewhat patchy rim enhancement ➡. Note the remodeling of the lateral orbital wall ➡. (Right) Axial T1 C+ FS MR shows multiple foci of irregularly enhancing intraconal ➡, conal ➡, and extraconal ➡ masses.

DIFFERENTIAL DIAGNOSIS

Common
- Benign Mixed Tumor, Lacrimal
- Lymphoproliferative Lesions, Orbit
- Idiopathic Orbital Inflammatory Disease
- Hematoma, Orbit

Less Common
- Dermoid and Epidermoid, Orbit
- Mucocele, Sinonasal
- Dacryocystocele
- Subperiosteal Abscess, Orbit
- Sarcoidosis, Orbit
- Sjögren Syndrome, Orbit
- Lacrimal Cyst
- Adenoid Cystic Carcinoma, Lacrimal
- Malignant Mixed Tumor, Lacrimal
- Rhabdomyosarcoma, Orbit
- Sinonasal Malignancy
- Metastasis, Orbit
- Neurofibromatosis Type 1, Orbit
- Fibrous Dysplasia, Orbit
- Orbital Cavernous Hemangioma
- Infantile Hemangioendothelioma, Orbit
- Venous & Lymphatic Malformations
  - Lymphatic Malformation, Orbit
  - Venolymphatic Malformation, Orbit
  - Venous Varix, Orbit

Rare but Important
- Adenocarcinoma, Lacrimal
- Hemangiopericytoma, Orbit

ESSENTIAL INFORMATION

Helpful Clues for Common Diagnoses
- **Benign Mixed Tumor, Lacrimal**
  - Key facts: Most common orbital neoplasm
    - Slowly progressive painless proptosis
  - Imaging: Scalloped bony remodeling
    - Uniform mass with lobulations
- **Lymphoproliferative Lesions, Orbit**
  - Key facts: Lower grade MALT lymphoma
    - Very responsive to radiation therapy
  - Imaging: Anywhere in orbit, esp. lacrimal
    - Homogeneous pliable enhancing mass
- **Idiopathic Orbital Inflammatory Disease**
  - Key facts: Painful proptosis
    - Restricted eye movements
  - Imaging: Typically involves muscles
    - Multifocal mass-like or ill-defined enhancement anywhere in orbit

- **Hematoma, Orbit**
  - Key facts: Acute blood may threaten vision
    - May evolve into chronic hematic cyst
  - Imaging: ± fracture or foreign body
    - Dense irregular collection

Helpful Clues for Less Common Diagnoses
- **Dermoid and Epidermoid, Orbit**
  - Key facts: Congenital ectodermal inclusion
    - Acute inflammation with trauma/rupture
  - Imaging: Superotemporal most common
    - Dermoid shows fat density, Ca++, debris
    - Epidermoid shows homogeneous fluid
- **Mucocele, Sinonasal**
  - Key facts: Slowly progressive symptoms
    - Associated with polyposis or obstruction
  - Imaging: Frontal > ethmoid > sphenoid
    - Inspissated secretions, sinus expansion
- **Dacryocystocele**
  - Key facts: Nasolacrimal obstruction
    - Congenital in infants, acquired in adults
  - Imaging: Medial canthal cystic mass
    - Variable fluid signal
    - Duct enlarged if distal obstruction
- **Subperiosteal Abscess, Orbit**
  - Key facts: Related to ethmoid sinusitis
    - Requires immediate attention
  - Imaging: Medial rim-enhancing collection
    - Adjacent sinus opacification
- **Sarcoidosis, Orbit**
  - Key facts: 25% of patients with sarcoid
    - Noncaseating granulomas
  - Imaging: Multifocal inflammation
    - Mass-like lacrimal and muscle infiltration
    - May occur anywhere in orbit
- **Sjögren Syndrome, Orbit**
  - Key facts: Autoimmune exocrinopathy
    - Salivary and lacrimal involvement
  - Imaging: Hypertrophic or normal early
    - Atrophic and heterogeneous late
- **Lacrimal Cyst**
  - Key facts: Benign exocrine cyst (lacricele)
  - Imaging: Uncomplicated fluid lesion
- **Adenoid Cystic Carcinoma, Lacrimal**
  - Key facts: Painful mass
    - Insidious malignancy, poor prognosis
  - Imaging: Invasive solid lacrimal mass
    - Destructive bony changes very suggestive
    - May appear deceptively benign
- **Malignant Mixed Tumor, Lacrimal**
  - Key facts: Malignant transformation of benign mixed tumor

○ Imaging: Partially irregular margin
  ▪ Invasive features superimposed on previously benign mass
• **Rhabdomyosarcoma, Orbit**
  ○ Key facts: Most common childhood soft tissue malignancy
  ○ Imaging: Variably enhancing mass
    ▪ Superior and medial most common
    ▪ Bone destruction common
    ▪ May simulate benign lesion early
• **Sinonasal Malignancy**
  ○ Key facts: Squamous cell carcinoma, esthesioneuroblastoma, melanoma, etc.
  ○ Imaging: Destructive mass centered in sinuses with extension into orbit
• **Metastasis, Orbit**
  ○ Key facts: Breast most common
    ▪ Melanoma has propensity for orbit
  ○ Imaging: Anywhere in orbit
• **Neurofibromatosis Type 1, Orbit**
  ○ Key facts: Inherited tumor syndrome
  ○ Imaging: Plexiform neurofibromas
    ▪ Sphenoid dysplasia with herniation
• **Fibrous Dysplasia, Orbit**
  ○ Key facts: Abnormal bone formation in children and younger adults
  ○ Imaging: Expansile bone lesion
    ▪ Ground-glass matrix with mixed areas of sclerosis &/or lucency
    ▪ Active lesions show variably enhancing fibrovascular tissue
• **Orbital Cavernous Hemangioma**
  ○ Key facts: Common adult orbital mass
    ▪ Slowly progressive painless proptosis

○ Imaging: Vast majority are intraconal
  ▪ Extraconal apical lesions are uncommon
• **Infantile Hemangioendothelioma, Orbit**
  ○ Key facts: a.k.a. capillary hemangioma
    ▪ Proliferative vascular mass of infants
    ▪ Usually regresses spontaneously
  ○ Imaging: Intensely enhancing
    ▪ Irregular margins, often trans-spatial
    ▪ Anywhere; superomedial most common
• **Lymphatic Malformation, Orbit**
  ○ Key facts: Endothelial malformation
  ○ Imaging: Multilocular mass, prone to hemorrhage, fluid-blood levels
• **Venolymphatic Malformation, Orbit**
  ○ Key facts: Endothelial malformation
  ○ Imaging: Irregular mass with heterogeneous enhancement
• **Venous Varix, Orbit**
  ○ Key facts: Endothelial malformation
  ○ Imaging: Low-flow mixed malformation, distends dynamically with Valsalva

Helpful Clues for Rare Diagnoses
• **Adenocarcinoma, Lacrimal**
  ○ Key facts: Often aggressive and painful
    ▪ Includes undifferentiated, ductal, polymorphous, acinic, & basal types
  ○ Imaging: Locally invasive
    ▪ Solid or heterogeneous enhancing mass
• **Hemangiopericytoma, Orbit**
  ○ Key facts: Variably aggressive
    ▪ Local recurrence common
  ○ Imaging: Anywhere in orbit
    ▪ Solid, intensely enhancing mass

Benign Mixed Tumor, Lacrimal

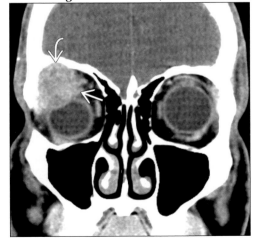

Coronal CECT shows a moderately enhancing, slightly lobulated, superotemporal right orbital mass ➔ that displaces the globe inferiorly. The overlying bone shows smooth scalloping ➔.

Lymphoproliferative Lesions, Orbit

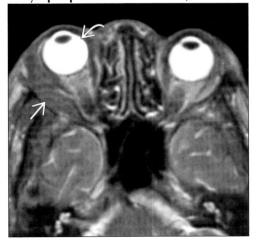

Axial T2WI FS MR shows a hypointense mass extending along the right lateral extraconal orbit ➔. The right eye is proptotic ➔. The low T2 signal is indicative of the high cellularity of lymphoma.

(Left) Axial T1 C+ MR shows a dominant mass centered in the lateral left extraconal orbit with intense, slightly heterogeneous enhancement ➡. The mass involves the lateral rectus itself. Note that the anterior tendinous insertion is also thickened ➡. (Right) Axial NECT in a trauma patient with orbitofacial fractures shows an extraconal hematoma in the lateral right orbit ➡. Small foci of ectopic areas ➡ are also evident.

Idiopathic Orbital Inflammatory Disease

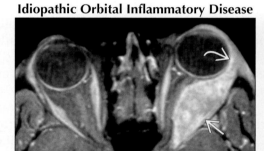

Hematoma, Orbit

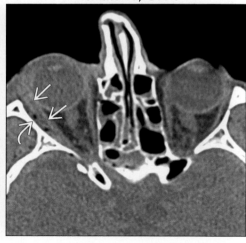

(Left) Coronal NECT shows a well-defined mass in the left superotemporal orbit ➡, showing internal fatty density with some heterogeneous debris. Benign remodeling of the bony orbit is evident ➡. (Right) Coronal NECT shows severe sinonasal polyposis with pansinus obstruction and dense inspissated secretions. Multiple mucoceles with dehiscence are present in the bilateral orbits ➡, as well as in the anterior cranial fossa ➡.

Dermoid and Epidermoid, Orbit

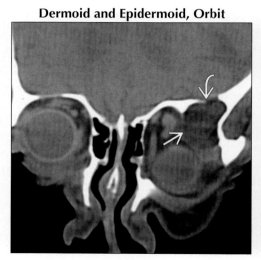

Mucocele, Sinonasal

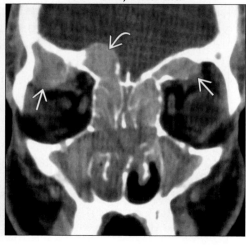

(Left) Axial CECT shows a rim-enhancing dacryocystocele centered in the lacrimal fossa ➡. The adjacent soft tissues are thickened ➡, indicating associated acute cellulitis. (Right) Coronal CECT shows a small fluid-density abscess in the right medial extraconal orbit ➡. The adjacent rectus muscle ➡ and orbital fat ➡ show inflammatory changes. Note the presence of ipsilateral ethmoid sinusitis ➡.

Dacryocystocele

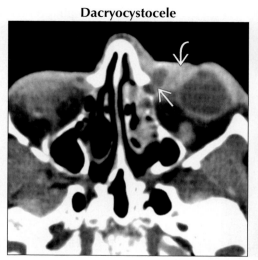

Subperiosteal Abscess, Orbit

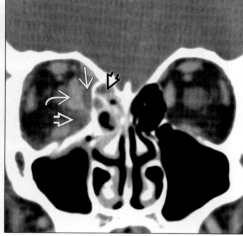

Sarcoidosis, Orbit

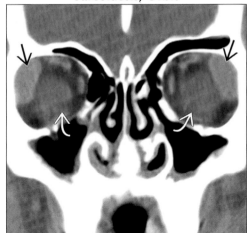

Sjögren Syndrome, Orbit

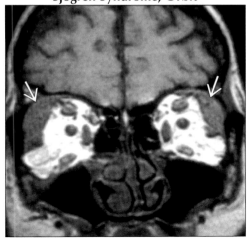

(Left) Coronal CECT reformation shows bilateral homogeneous enhancing superotemporal extraconal masses ➡, representing marked symmetric enlargement of the lacrimal glands. There is mild inferomedial displacement of the globes ➡. *(Right)* Coronal T1WI MR shows bilateral lacrimal gland enlargement ➡. Note the gland's fine heterogeneous texture. Enlargement with miliary appearance indicates intermediate disease stage.

Lacrimal Cyst

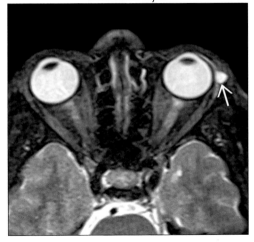

Adenoid Cystic Carcinoma, Lacrimal

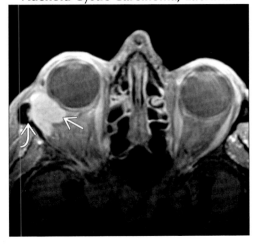

(Left) Axial T2WI FS MR shows a simple unilocular fluid signal lesion ➡ in the left lacrimal gland. The orbits are otherwise normal. *(Right)* Axial T1 C+ FS MR shows a homogeneously enhancing mass ➡ that fills and enlarges the right lacrimal gland. Early bone erosion is present in the lateral orbital wall ➡.

Malignant Mixed Tumor, Lacrimal

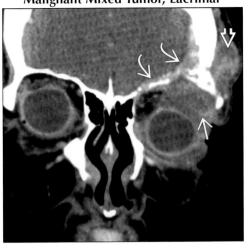

Rhabdomyosarcoma, Orbit

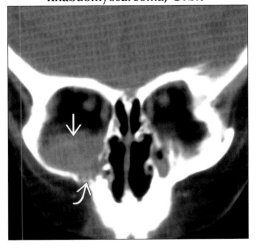

(Left) Coronal CECT shows an aggressive soft tissue mass ➡ centered in the left lacrimal gland. There is evidence of bone destruction with intracranial dural invasion ➡, as well as extension into the adjacent temporal fossa ➡. *(Right)* Coronal NECT reveals a large solid mass in the inferior right orbit ➡, which is inseparable from adjacent rectus muscle. Early bony destruction is seen in the orbital floor ➡.

EXTRACONAL MASS

(Left) Coronal T1 C+ FS MR in a patient with esthesioneuroblastoma shows an enhancing mass centered high in the nasal cavity. There is invasion into the extraconal orbits bilaterally ⇥ and into the anterior cranial fossa ⇗. Postobstructive secretions are evident in the right maxillary sinus ⇥. (Right) Axial T1 C+ FS MR in a patient with metastatic melanoma shows multiple masses in the bilateral extraconal, intraconal, and preseptal orbits ⇥.

Sinonasal Malignancy

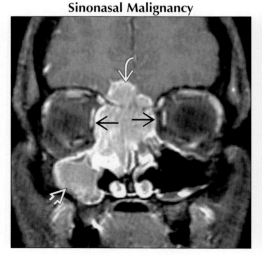

Metastasis, Orbit

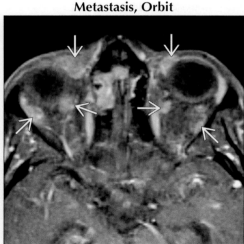

(Left) Axial CECT shows sphenoid dysplasia with herniation of the contents of the middle crania fossa into the orbit, including the brain ⇥ and an arachnoid cyst ⇥. Preseptal and extraconal enhancing masses represent plexiform neurofibromas ⇥. (Right) Coronal bone CT shows marked expansion of the left maxilla bowing up into the left orbit ⇥. The dysplastic bone shows areas of mixed ground-glass density ⇥ and fibrovascular lucency ⇥.

Neurofibromatosis Type 1, Orbit

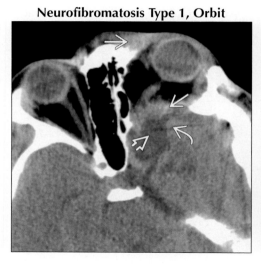

Fibrous Dysplasia, Orbit

Orbital Cavernous Hemangioma

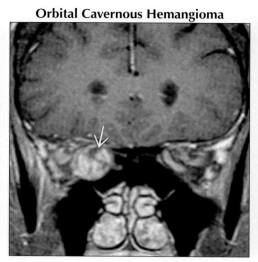

(Left) Coronal T1 C+ FS MR shows an atypical location for cavernous hemangioma in the extraconal right orbit near the apex ⇥. Remodeling of the medial orbital wall is seen bowing into the posterior ethmoid sinus. (Right) Axial T1 C+ FS MR shows multifocal irregular intensely enhancing vascular masses in the preseptal and postseptal extraconal space of the right orbit ⇥, as well as in the intraconal space ⇥ and high masticator space ⇥.

Infantile Hemangioendothelioma, Orbit

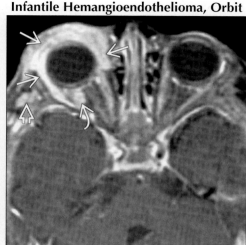

Lymphatic Malformation, Orbit

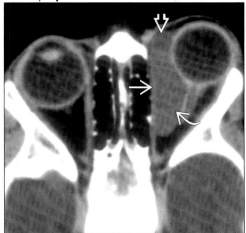

Venolymphatic Malformation, Orbit

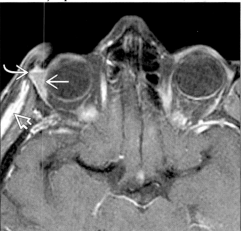

(Left) Axial CECT shows a cystic, mildly dense, nonenhancing mass with an imperceptible wall in the medial left orbit. The mass is trans-spatial with extraconal ➡, intraconal ➡, and preseptal ➡ components. (Right) Axial T1 C+ FS MR shows a small insinuating enhancing lesion ➡ in the right lateral extraconal orbit. Note the presence of a small fluid level ➡. Vascular malformation is also evident in the temporalis fossa ➡.

Venous Varix, Orbit

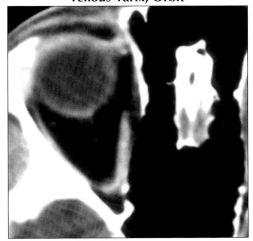

Venous Varix, Orbit

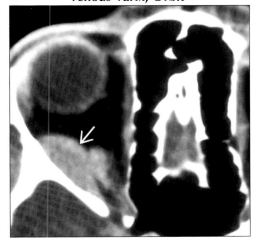

(Left) Axial CECT obtained during quiet respiration in a patient with intermittent proptosis shows a normal appearance to the right orbit without evidence of mass. (Right) Axial CECT obtained during Valsalva maneuver demonstrates an extraconal vascular mass ➡ that was not visible previously. The increased systemic venous pressure caused by Valsalva results in dynamic dilatation of the varix, with mild associated proptosis.

Adenocarcinoma, Lacrimal

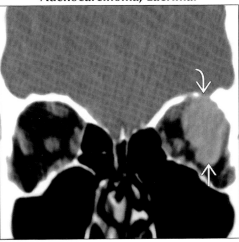

Hemangiopericytoma, Orbit

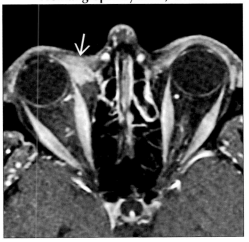

(Left) Coronal CECT shows a relatively well-defined, mildly enhancing, left extraconal mass within the lacrimal fossa ➡. There is associated erosion of the orbital roof ➡. (Right) Axial T1 C+ FS MR shows a brightly enhancing mass in the anterior medial extraconal right orbit ➡. Although the poorly defined margins suggest a more aggressive lesion than hemangiopericytoma, the diagnosis was confirmed by biopsy.

LACRIMAL GLAND LESION

DIFFERENTIAL DIAGNOSIS

Common
- Benign Mixed Tumor, Lacrimal
- Lymphoma, Lacrimal
- Idiopathic Orbital Inflammatory Disease

Less Common
- Adenoid Cystic Carcinoma, Lacrimal
- Sarcoidosis, Orbit
- Sjögren Syndrome, Orbit
- Dermoid and Epidermoid, Orbit

Rare but Important
- Carcinoma ex Pleomorphic Adenoma, Lacrimal

ESSENTIAL INFORMATION

Helpful Clues for Common Diagnoses
- **Benign Mixed Tumor, Lacrimal**
  - Key facts: Most common epithelial tumor
  - Imaging: Discrete mass, scalloped bone
- **Lymphoma, Lacrimal**
  - Key facts: MALT type common
  - Imaging: Pliable mass, extends posteriorly from gland, multiple masses
- **Idiopathic Orbital Inflammatory Disease**
  - Key facts: 25% have lacrimal pattern
  - Imaging: Diffuse gland enlargement

Helpful Clues for Less Common Diagnoses
- **Adenoid Cystic Carcinoma, Lacrimal**
  - Key facts: Painful mass; insidious tumor, poor prognosis
  - Imaging: Bony erosion is suggestive

- **Sarcoidosis, Orbit**
  - Key facts: 50% involve lacrimal gland, 25% bilateral
  - Imaging: Gland enlargement; associated ocular and orbital findings
- **Sjögren Syndrome, Orbit**
  - Key facts: Dry eyes and mouth
  - Imaging: Normal or enlarged early in disease; fat deposition later
- **Dermoid and Epidermoid, Orbit**
  - Key facts: Cystic inclusion arising at suture
  - Imaging: Bony remodeling, debris, and fat

Helpful Clues for Rare Diagnoses
- **Carcinoma ex Pleomorphic Adenoma, Lacrimal**
  - Key facts: Preexisting benign mixed tumor
  - Imaging: Benign &/or aggressive features

Other Essential Information
- Morphology
  - Tumors not distinct from gland, appear as diffuse enlargement even when benign

Alternative Differential Approaches
- Bilateral disease ⇒ systemic condition
  - Lymphoma, lacrimal
  - Sjögren syndrome, orbit
  - Sarcoidosis, orbit
- Concomitant lesions elsewhere in orbit
  - Idiopathic orbital inflammatory disease
  - Lymphoma, lacrimal
  - Sarcoidosis, orbit
- Pain typically present
  - Idiopathic orbital inflammatory disease
  - Adenoid cystic carcinoma, lacrimal

Benign Mixed Tumor, Lacrimal

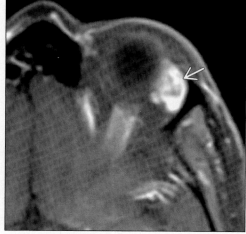

Axial T1 C+ FS MR shows a small discrete enhancing mass in the left lacrimal gland ➡. This tumor was found incidentally on MR of the brain.

Lymphoma, Lacrimal

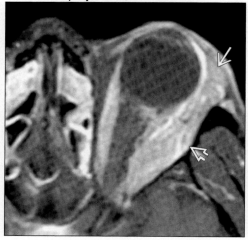

Axial T1 C+ FS MR shows a homogeneously enhancing mass involving the left lacrimal gland ➡ and extending posteriorly into the lateral extraconal space ➡.

LACRIMAL GLAND LESION

Idiopathic Orbital Inflammatory Disease
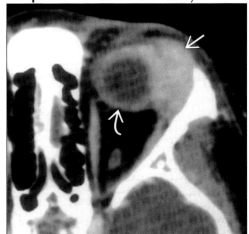

Adenoid Cystic Carcinoma, Lacrimal
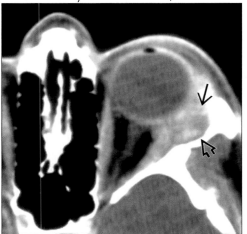

(Left) Axial CECT shows marked enlargement and increased homogeneous enhancement of the lacrimal gland ➡. Scleral thickening ➡ is also noted as a manifestation of orbital pseudotumor. *(Right)* Axial CECT shows an enhancing mass originating in the left lacrimal gland ➡. Erosion of the adjacent bony orbit ⊳ is a suspicious and ominous finding in this malignant tumor.

Sarcoidosis, Orbit
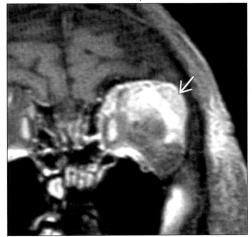

Sjögren Syndrome, Orbit
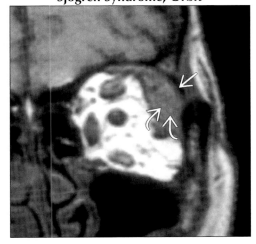

(Left) Coronal T1 C+ FS MR shows increased size and enhancement of the right lacrimal gland ➡, with ill-defined margins and infiltration into the adjacent orbital soft tissues. *(Right)* Coronal T1WI MR shows diffuse homogeneous enlargement of the left lacrimal gland ➡. Small hyperintense foci ➡ correlate with early fat deposition.

Dermoid and Epidermoid, Orbit
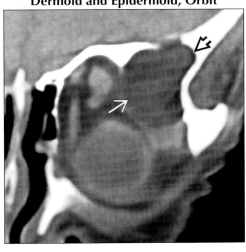

Carcinoma ex Pleomorphic Adenoma, Lacrimal
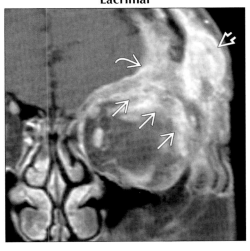

(Left) Coronal NECT shows a heterogeneous cyst with fat density contents ➡. The lesion arises not from the gland but from the frontozygomatic suture near the lacrimal fossa. Benign bony remodeling ⊳ reflects the developmental origin of this epithelial inclusion. *(Right)* Coronal T1 C+ FS MR shows an aggressive tumor originating in the left lacrimal gland ➡, with extensive regional invasion into the adjacent intracranial ➡ and extracranial ➡ spaces.

ORBITAL WALL LESION

DIFFERENTIAL DIAGNOSIS

Common
- Trauma, Orbit
- Mucocele, Sinonasal
- Abscess, Subperiosteal, Orbit
- Polyposis, Sinonasal
- SCCa, Sinonasal
- Esthesioneuroblastoma
- Undifferentiated Carcinoma, Sinonasal
- Metastasis, Orbit
- Dermoid and Epidermoid, Orbit

Less Common
- Rhabdomyosarcoma, Orbit
- Fibrous Dysplasia, Skull Base
- Paget Disease, Skull Base
- Langerhans Histiocytosis, Skull Base
- Silent Sinus Syndrome
- Meningioma, Skull Base
- Adenocarcinoma, Sinonasal

Rare but Important
- Wegener Granulomatosis, Orbit
- Neurofibromatosis Type 1, Orbit
- Osteosarcoma, Skull Base
- Cephalocele, Spheno-Orbital

ESSENTIAL INFORMATION

Key Differential Diagnosis Issues
- Most common pathology is trauma
  ○ Acute or chronic fracture
- Remainder is predominantly from sinuses, secondarily involving orbit
  ○ Acute sinus infection, chronic sinus inflammatory disease, sinus neoplasms
  ○ Medial orbital wall most vulnerable to ethmoid disease due to natural dehiscences
- Other consideration: Primary bone lesion
  ○ Metastases, dysplasia, or bone neoplasms
- Imaging strategy
  ○ Bone CT initial exam for orbital disease
  ○ MR best for differentiation of tumor from sinus secretions & to identify intracranial spread

Helpful Clues for Common Diagnoses
- **Trauma, Orbit**
  ○ Lateral orbital wall fracture frequently seen with other facial fractures
    ▪ Especially zygomatic arch & maxilla

  ○ Medial orbital & inferior orbital "blow-out" fractures most common
    ▪ Typically fluid level (blood) present in adjacent paranasal sinus
    ▪ May be isolated (medial blow-out & inferior blow-out) or complex with other facial fractures
    ▪ Look for herniation of orbital fat or extraocular muscle through defect orbital roof fractures
  ○ Orbital roof fractures less common but are anterior skull base fractures
    ▪ Carefully assess cribriform plate & frontal sinus for fractures & potential CSF leak
- **Mucocele, Sinonasal**
  ○ T1 & T2 MR: Markedly variable signal intensity reflecting mucus concentration
    ▪ T1 C+: Thin rim of enhancement
  ○ CECT: May see subtle rim enhancement
  ○ NECT: Low-density cystic expansion of paranasal sinus(es)
    ▪ Frontal/ethmoid > > sphenoid/maxillary
    ▪ Sinus (& therefore orbital) walls bowed
    ▪ Walls thinned & may be imperceptible, particularly medial orbital wall
- **Abscess, Subperiosteal, Orbit**
  ○ Rim-enhancing, lenticular fluid collection adjacent to opacified sinus
    ▪ Ethmoid sinus → medial orbital wall
    ▪ Superior (frontal sinusitis) less common
    ▪ Bone destruction not always evident
    ▪ Intracranial complications: Cavernous sinus thrombosis, subdural empyema, cerebritis, brain abscess
- **Polyposis, Sinonasal**
  ○ NECT: Pansinus opacification with bony remodeling as sinuses expand
    ▪ Typically bilateral, may be asymmetric
    ▪ Enlarged maxillary infundibula, loss of ethmoid trabeculae
    ▪ Bony dehiscence occurs with increasing sinus expansion
  ○ CECT: Polyps are low-density while surrounding mucosa enhances
  ○ T1 & T2 MR: Variable signal intensities from mucus between polyps
- **SCCa, Sinonasal**
  ○ Most common of sinonasal malignancies
  ○ Unilateral soft tissue mass with destruction of adjacent sinus ± orbit wall
  ○ Maxillary SCCa → orbital floor invasion

- Nasal/ethmoid SCCa → medial orbital wall
  - MR T1 C+: Heterogeneous enhancement
- **Esthesioneuroblastoma**
  - Arises from nasal vault, typically destroys cribriform plate & medial orbital walls
    - Often bilateral orbital invasion
  - NECT: Tumor expands nasal cavity; ± bony destruction
  - T1 C+: Homogeneous enhancement
- **Undifferentiated Carcinoma, Sinonasal**
  - Most often arise in ethmoids or nasal vault with medial orbital wall destruction
  - MR T1 C+: Heterogeneous enhancement
- **Metastasis, Orbit**
  - Destructive lesion centered on bone
  - Diagnosis suggested by multiple lesions
- **Dermoid & Epidermoid, Orbit**
  - Well-defined low density orbital mass, usually < 1 cm
  - Dermoid: Fat density, CT; fat intensity, MR
  - Benign bone remodeling
  - Most commonly superolateral orbit near zygomatico-frontal suture

Helpful Clues for Less Common Diagnoses
- **Rhabdomyosarcoma, Orbit**
  - Proptosis, decreased vision in < 15 year old
  - Rapidly growing, destructive orbital mass
- **Fibrous Dysplasia, Skull Base**
  - "Ground-glass" bony expansion
  - < 30 years of age
- **Paget Disease, Skull Base**
  - Heterogeneous bony expansion
  - > 50 years of age

- **Langerhans Histiocytosis, Skull Base**
  - Young male with proptosis
  - "Punched out" or destructive appearing bony lesion; 30% multiple
  - When multiple, mimics metastases
- **Silent Sinus Syndrome**
  - Enlarged orbital volume from ipsilateral "atelectatic" maxillary sinus
- **Meningioma, Skull Base**
  - Bony hyperostosis of orbital roof
  - CECT or MR show intracranial mass
- **Adenocarcinoma, Sinonasal**
  - Indistinguishable from sinonasal SCCa

Helpful Clues for Rare Diagnoses
- **Wegener Granulomatosis, Orbit**
  - Necrotizing granulomas of upper and lower respiratory tracts
  - Orbital invasion from maxillary & ethmoid sinus into extraconal orbit is late complication
  - Orbit involvement 1st extrasinonasal site
- **Neurofibromatosis Type 1, Orbit**
  - Characteristic findings: Sphenoid dysplasia, buphthalmos, plexiform neurofibroma ± optic nerve glioma
- **Osteosarcoma, Skull Base**
  - Destructive bony lesion with aggressive periosteal reaction and osteoid matrix
- **Cephalocele, Spheno-Orbital**
  - Greater wing of sphenoid-posterior orbital meningeal-brain protrusion
  - Very rare cephalocele type

Trauma, Orbit

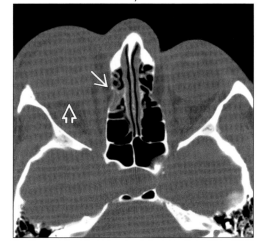

Axial bone CT shows a fracture of the middle 1/3 of the medial orbital wall ➡ with blood in the adjacent ethmoid air cells. Note also the misshapen ruptured globe ⊟.

Trauma, Orbit

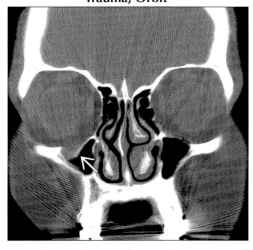

Coronal NECT shows a chronic inferior orbital wall fracture ➡. There is deformity of the right orbital floor depressed into the maxillary sinus. The lack of fluid in the adjacent sinuses suggests chronicity.

ORBITAL WALL LESION

(Left) Axial CECT shows an expansile fluid-density lesion ⇒ arising from the anterior left ethmoid air cells that markedly thins and distorts the left medial orbital wall. (Right) Axial CECT shows a right subperiosteal abscess ⇒, which developed from adjacent ethmoid sinusitis. This has also resulted in focal destruction of the medial orbital wall.

Mucocele, Sinonasal

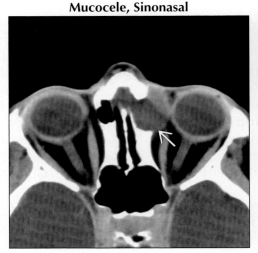

Abscess, Subperiosteal, Orbit

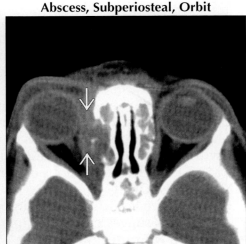

(Left) Axial T1WI MR shows an extreme example of deformity of the right medial orbital wall ⇒ from sinonasal polyposis. This chronic process has markedly expanded the ethmoid air cells. (Right) Coronal T1 C+ FS MR shows an aggressive heterogeneously enhancing mass arising from the sinuses and invading the right orbit through the inferior ⇒ and medial ⇒ orbital walls.

Polyposis, Sinonasal

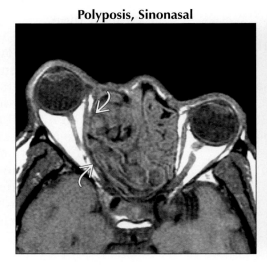

SCCa, Sinonasal

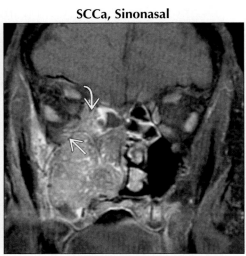

(Left) Coronal T1 C+ FS MR shows a homogeneous sinonasal mass expanding the nasal vault and destroying the right medial orbital wall ⇒. The tumor also invades the anterior cranial fossa. (Right) Coronal T1 C+ FS MR shows a heterogeneous mass destroying the medial orbital wall ⇒ to invade the orbit and surround the adjacent extraocular muscles. It also invades the anterior fossa.

Esthesioneuroblastoma

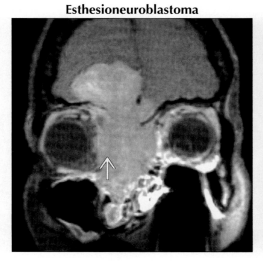

Undifferentiated Carcinoma, Sinonasal

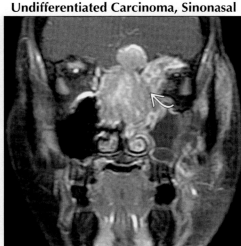

Metastasis, Orbit
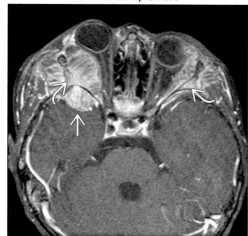

Dermoid and Epidermoid, Orbit
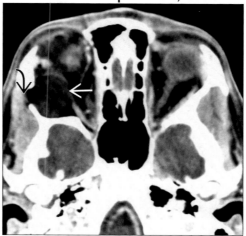

(Left) Axial T1 C+ FS MR shows bilateral neuroblastoma sphenoid wing metastases ➤ with soft tissue and orbital extension, marked right proptosis, and right-side intracranial disease ➤. *(Right)* Axial CECT shows an unusual dermoid ➤ expanding the superolateral orbital wall, which also has a focal defect ➤. The fatty mass is centered at the sphenozygomatic suture.

Rhabdomyosarcoma, Orbit
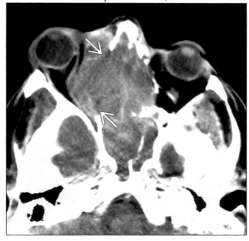

Fibrous Dysplasia, Skull Base
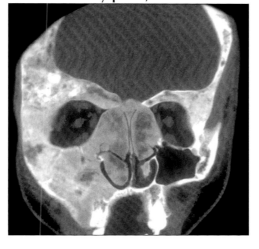

(Left) Axial CECT shows a homogeneous, mildly enhancing sinonasal mass destroying the right medial wall ➤ to invade the orbit and displace the globe laterally. *(Right)* Coronal bone CT shows extensive facial and skull base bony expansion with distortion of all walls of the right orbit. The left orbital floor is spared in this patient with McCune-Albright syndrome.

Langerhans Histiocytosis, Skull Base
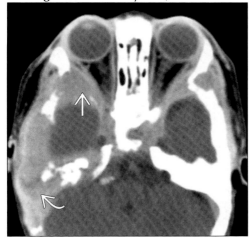

Silent Sinus Syndrome
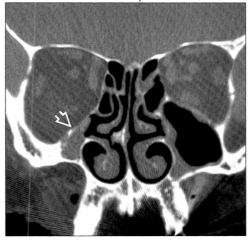

(Left) Axial CECT shows multifocal soft tissue lesions destroying the skull base, including the posterolateral orbital wall ➤ and the temporal bone ➤. *(Right)* Coronal bone CT shows a small opacified right maxillary sinus. The ipsilateral depressed orbital floor ➤ results in an enlarged orbital volume, which may manifest as enophthalmos.

DIFFERENTIAL DIAGNOSIS

Common
- Trauma, Orbit
- Retinopathy of Prematurity (ROP)
- Retinal Detachment
- Coloboma

Less Common
- Persistent Hyperplastic Primary Vitreous
- Microphthalmos, Congenital

Rare but Important
- Infection, Other Pathogen, Orbit
- Toxocariasis, Orbit

ESSENTIAL INFORMATION

Helpful Clues for Common Diagnoses
- **Trauma, Orbit**
  - Key facts
    - Any trauma may lead to globe rupture
  - Imaging
    - Small globe ± ocular hemorrhage or detachment ± gas within globe
    - If foreign body: BB common; wood may be air or intermediate attenuation
    - Posterior scleral rupture may lead to deep anterior chamber
- **Retinopathy of Prematurity (ROP)**
  - Key facts
    - Vasculoproliferative disorder in low birth weight premature infants
  - Imaging
    - Noncalcified, retrolental mass = retinal detachment (RD)
    - Bilateral microphthalmia, hyperdense globe ± calcification as late findings
- **Retinal Detachment**
  - Key facts: 3 potential spaces/ocular detachments
    - Posterior hyaloid (between posterior hyaloid membrane & inner sensory retina)
    - Subretinal (between inner sensory retina & outer retinal pigmented epithelium)
    - Posterior choroidal (between choroid & sclera)
    - Ocular detachments occur in trauma, persistent hyperplastic primary vitreous (PHPV), ROP, ocular masses, Coats disease, or infection
  - Imaging

- RD = V-shaped density
- Total RD may simulate PHPV
- **Coloboma**
  - Key facts
    - Gap or defect of ocular tissue; may involve any structures of embryonic cleft
    - Optic disc coloboma (ODC): Defect confined to optic disc
    - Choroidoretinal coloboma (CRC): Separate from or extends beyond disc, arises from globe wall
    - Morning glory disc anomaly (MGDA): Central tuft of glial tissue within defect
    - Peripapillary staphyloma (PPS): Congenital scleral defect at optic nerve head; nearly all unilateral
  - Imaging
    - Focal outpouching of vitreous
    - Bilateral or unilateral
    - Usually with microphthalmos, rarely with macrophthalmos
    - ± Optic tract and chiasm atrophy
    - Retrobulbar colobomatous cyst may communicate with globe
    - Sclera enhances, glial tuft in MGDA may enhance
    - Rarely dystrophic calcification at margins
    - ± Other abnormalities if associated with syndromes (Meckel, Walker Warburg, Aicardi, CHARGE), basal cephaloceles, midline facial clefting

Helpful Clues for Less Common Diagnoses
- **Persistent Hyperplastic Primary Vitreous**
  - Key facts
    - Remnants of primary vitreous and primitive hyaloid artery (failure of involution) occur along course of Cloquet canal: Anterior, posterior, or both (most common)
    - 2nd most common cause of leukocoria after retinoblastoma
    - Sporadic, unilateral; bilateral more common in association with syndromes (Walker-Warburg, Norrie)
  - Imaging
    - Noncalcified, tubular, cylindrical, or triangular-shaped enhancing tissue within vitreous compartment
    - Microphthalmos, retinal detachment ± ↑ attenuation of entire vitreous body common

MICROPHTHALMOS

- Small dysplastic lens and shallow anterior chamber with anterior involvement
- **Microphthalmos, Congenital**
  - Key facts
    - Microphthalmia = eye < 2/3 normal size, or < 16 mm axial dimension
    - Anophthalmia: Complete absence of globe or only vestigial remnant
  - Imaging
    - Small globe; unilateral or bilateral
    - ± Intracranial structural abnormalities (more common in bilateral)
    - ± Coloboma or cyst

Helpful Clues for Rare Diagnoses
- **Infection, Other Pathogen, Orbit**
  - Key facts
    - Viral (herpes simplex, herpes zoster, CMV, rubella, rubeola, mumps, EBV)
    - Bacterial (syphilis, Lyme, brucellosis, cat-scratch, *E. coli*)
    - Fungal (candidiasis) or parasitic (*Toxocara canis*)
    - Most patients are not imaged
    - Most treated without sequelae of microphthalmia
  - Imaging
    - Thickened, enhancing sclera (scleritis)
    - Thickened, enhancing uvea (uveitis)
    - ↑ Attenuation/signal of vitreous secondary to ↑ protein ± uveitis ± ocular detachment in endophthalmitis

- Endophthalmitis: Intraocular infectious or inflammatory process involving vitreous cavity or anterior chamber
- **Toxocariasis, Orbit**
  - Key facts
    - Inflammatory response to nematode *Toxocara canis* causes chorioretinitis
    - Granulomatous inflammation surrounds dead larvae
    - May appear as focal posterior or peripheral retinal granuloma
    - Most commonly unilateral
  - Imaging
    - Focal or diffuse thickening and enhancement of globe
    - Retinal detachment may be associated
    - ↑ Attenuation/intensity of vitreous possible

Other Essential Information
- End-stage damage to globe from any cause may ⇒ phthisis bulbi (calcified, small globe)

SELECTED REFERENCES

1. Apushkin MA et al: Retinoblastoma and simulating lesions: role of imaging. Neuroimaging Clin N Am. 15(1):49-67, 2005
2. Weissman JL et al: Enlarged anterior chamber: CT finding of a ruptured globe. AJNR Am J Neuroradiol. 16(4 Suppl):936-8, 1995

Trauma, Orbit

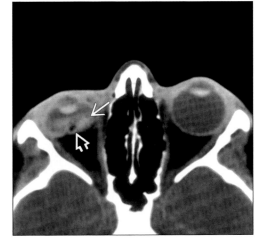

Axial NECT shows rupture of the right globe with decreased volume of vitreous cavity and high attenuation, consistent with hemorrhage ➡. Note also a small posterior bubble of gas ➡.

Trauma, Orbit

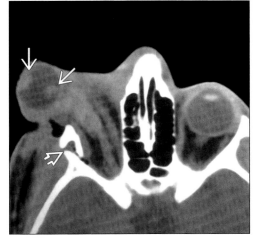

Axial NECT shows shattered pieces of lens ➡ within a small right globe. Also note the near complete post-traumatic enucleation from orbital wall fractures ➡ in a patient with severe head trauma.

MICROPHTHALMOS

(Left) *Axial CECT shows bilateral microphthalmia with increased attenuation secondary to chronic retinal detachment.* **(Right)** *Axial T2WI MR in an infant born prematurely demonstrates bilateral microphthalmia with hyperintense proteinaceous fluid nearly obliterating the vitreous cavity.*

Retinopathy of Prematurity (ROP)

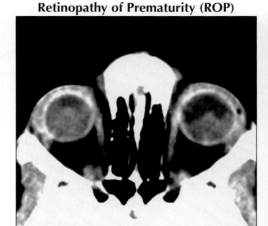

Retinopathy of Prematurity (ROP)

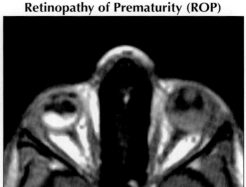

(Left) *Axial FLAIR MR reveals a small hyperintense right globe with near complete retinal detachment ➡, obliterating the vitreous cavity.* **(Right)** *Axial T1 C+ FS MR reveals a large right colobomatous cyst ➡ projecting off the posterior aspect of a microphthalmic globe ➡.*

Retinal Detachment

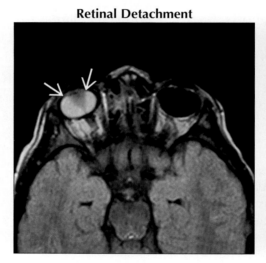

Coloboma

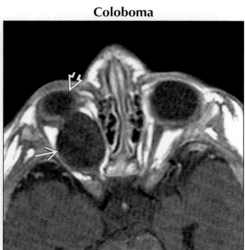

(Left) *Axial NECT shows bilateral microphthalmia with bilateral optic disc colobomas ➡. Note the large left-sided retrobulbar colobomatous cyst ➡.* **(Right)** *Axial T2WI MR reveals a small globe with a fluid level in the posterior vitreous ➡ & a linear hypointense structure ➡ extending from the posterior aspect of the lens to the optic nerve head. This linear structure represents the persistent Cloquet canal in a patient with Walker-Warburg syndrome.*

Coloboma

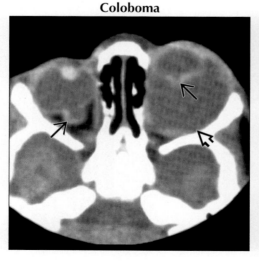

Persistent Hyperplastic Primary Vitreous

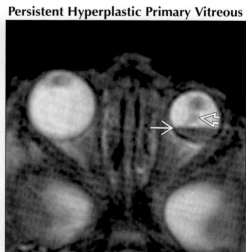

MICROPHTHALMOS

Microphthalmos, Congenital
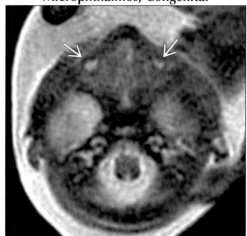

Microphthalmos, Congenital
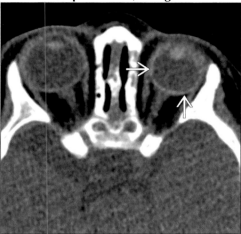

(Left) Axial T2WI MR in a 27 week fetus demonstrates severe bilateral microphthalmia ➡. *(Right)* Axial NECT in a 7 month old child demonstrates moderate left-sided microphthalmia ➡.

Microphthalmos, Congenital
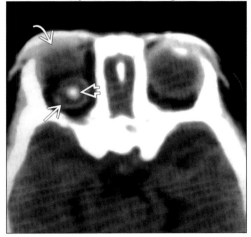

Microphthalmos, Congenital
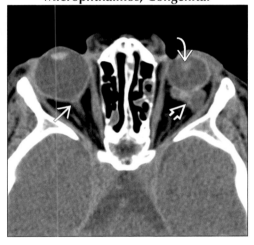

(Left) Axial NECT reveals a small microphthalmic right globe ➡ with a malpositioned lens ➡ and a large anterior cyst ➡. *(Right)* Axial NECT demonstrates a deformed right globe with a small optic disc coloboma ➡ and a small microphthalmic left globe with multiple small posterior colobomatous cysts ➡. Notice also the small left lens ➡.

Infection, Other Pathogen, Orbit
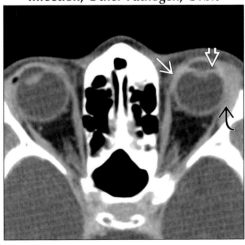

Toxocariasis, Orbit
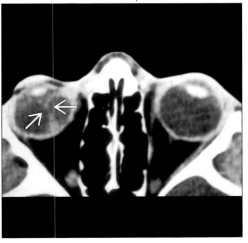

(Left) Axial CECT shows thick, enhancing sclera ➡ and ciliary body ➡ in association with a mild decrease in the size of the left globe and enlargement of the left lacrimal gland ➡ in a patient with nonspecific scleritis and uveitis. *(Right)* Axial NECT shows small right globe with complete retinal detachment ➡ secondary to toxocariasis.

DIFFERENTIAL DIAGNOSIS

Common
- Staphyloma
- Neurofibromatosis Type 1

Less Common
- Glaucoma, Acquired
- Glaucoma, Congenital

Rare but Important
- Myopia, Congenital
- Sturge-Weber Syndrome
- Congenital Cystic Eye
- Coloboma with Macrophthalmia

ESSENTIAL INFORMATION

Key Differential Diagnosis Issues
- Elongated globe in anteroposterior (AP) dimension may be secondary to myopia, staphyloma, or coloboma
- Diffuse enlargement of globe in AP and transverse dimension = buphthalmos ("ox eye" or "cow eye")
  - Buphthalmos may be present in congenital glaucoma, neurofibromatosis type 1 (NF1), Sturge-Weber, acquired glaucoma

Helpful Clues for Common Diagnoses
- **Staphyloma**
  - Key facts
    - Thinning and stretching of scleral-uveal layers of globe
    - Progressive myopia (nearsightedness) results in posterior staphyloma
    - Posterior staphyloma may also occur in glaucoma, connective tissue disorders, scleritis, necrotizing infection, or trauma
    - Anterior staphyloma may occur if infection or inflammation ⇒ corneal thinning
  - Imaging
    - Elongated globe, thinning of posterior wall, unilateral or bilateral
- **Neurofibromatosis Type 1**
  - Key facts
    - Congenital neurocutaneous syndrome
    - Mutation of gene on chromosome 17
    - Orbitofacial abnormalities in NF1 typically unilateral
    - Plexiform neurofibroma (PNF) diagnostic

- Up to 50% with facial and eyelid involvement have ipsilateral glaucoma
  - Imaging
    - Buphthalmos
    - Thickening of uveal & scleral layer; anterior rim enlargement
    - PNF orbit and skull base + sphenoid bony dysplasia ⇒ enlargement of orbital foramina and middle cranial fossa ⇒ herniation of intracranial contents into orbit ⇒ pulsatile exophthalmos
    - ± Enlargement, tortuosity, and enhancement of optic nerve glioma

Helpful Clues for Less Common Diagnoses
- **Glaucoma, Acquired**
  - Key facts
    - Leading cause of blindness in African-Americans and 2nd leading cause of blindness worldwide
    - > 4 million Americans have glaucoma; only 1/2 know they have it
    - Risk factors: African-American, > 60 years, family member with glaucoma, Hispanic, Asian, high myopia, diabetes mellitus, hypertension, trauma
    - Primary open angle > > angle closure
    - Diagnosis by tonometry (measures intraocular pressure), ophthalmoscopy (may show evidence of optic nerve atrophy), visual field tests (lose peripheral vision 1st), or gonioscopy (measure angle between iris and cornea)
  - Imaging
    - Less plasticity in globe of adults; therefore buphthalmos and deep anterior chamber uncommon
- **Glaucoma, Congenital**
  - Key facts
    - Incidence 1:5,000-1:10,000 live births; boys > > girls; bilateral in majority
    - Present at birth; usually diagnosed within 1st year of life
    - Clinical: Large eyes, excessive tearing, cloudy cornea, and light sensitivity
    - Obstruction to flow of aqueous humor from anterior chamber ⇒ elevated intraocular pressure, enlargement of globe and deep anterior chamber
    - Normal mean anterior chamber depth 3 mm; in congenital glaucoma mean anterior chamber depth 6.3 mm

- Complications: Subluxated lens, optic nerve atrophy
  - ○ Imaging
    - Enlarged AP dimension of globe
    - Deep anterior chamber

Helpful Clues for Rare Diagnoses
- **Myopia, Congenital**
  - ○ Key facts
    - Idiopathic globe enlargement (AP dimension) ⇒ convergence of light anterior to retina (nearsightedness)
  - ○ Imaging
    - Increased AP dimension of oval-shaped globe, unilateral or bilateral
- **Sturge-Weber Syndrome**
  - ○ Key facts
    - Sporadic congenital disorder of fetal cortical vein development ⇒ progressive venous occlusion and chronic venous ischemia
    - Up to 30% of patients have glaucoma
  - ○ Imaging
    - Contrast enhancement at site of choroidal angioma ⇒ ↑ intraocular pressure, glaucoma, & buphthalmos
    - ± Retinal telangiectatic vessels, scleral angioma, iris heterochromia
    - Serpentine leptomeningeal contrast enhancement of pial angiomatosis (80% unilateral)
    - Enlarged ipsilateral choroid plexus
    - Cortical calcification with parenchymal volume loss

- **Congenital Cystic Eye**
  - ○ Key facts
    - Synonym: Anophthalmos with cyst
    - Secondary to failure of involution of primary optic nerve vesicle early in embryologic development ⇒ cyst formation rather than a globe
    - Cyst filled with proliferating glial tissue, may ⇒ complex cyst
  - ○ Imaging
    - Large malformed cyst within orbit, without identifiable lens
    - ± Complex solid appearing components
- **Coloboma with Macrophthalmia**
  - ○ Key facts
    - Gap or defect of ocular tissue, usually with microphthalmia, rarely with macrophthalmia
    - Colobomatous macrophthalmia with microcornea syndrome: Autosomal dominant inheritance; gene linked to region of 2p23-p16
  - ○ Imaging
    - Axial enlargement of globe
    - Myopia and microcornea
    - Inferonasal iris coloboma
    - Chorioretinal coloboma

SELECTED REFERENCES
1. Elcioglu NH et al: Colobomatous macrophthalmia with microcornea syndrome maps to the 2p23-p16 region. Am J Med Genet A. 143A(12):1308-12, 2007

Staphyloma

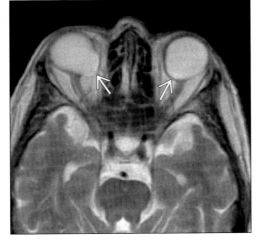

Axial T2WI MR shows bilateral longitudinal extension of the globes ➡ caused by degenerative weakness of the posterior sclera.

Staphyloma

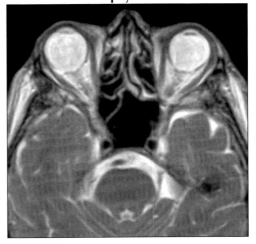

Axial T2WI MR demonstrates mild elongation of both globes in a patient with staphyloma.

MACROPHTHALMOS

(Left) Axial T2WI MR reveals mild enlargement of the right globe with bilateral lens dislocation in an adult with Marfan syndrome. (Right) Axial T1 C+ MR shows severe sphenoid dysplasia ➡, plexiform neurofibroma ➡, marked proptosis, and buphthalmos ➡.

Staphyloma

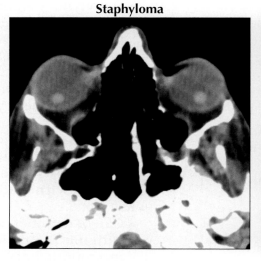

Neurofibromatosis Type 1

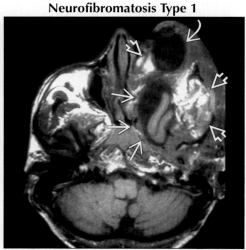

(Left) Axial T2WI MR demonstrates sphenoid wing dysplasia ➡ and infiltrative nodular hyperintense plexiform neurofibroma ➡ causing distortion of the orbit, proptosis, and buphthalmos ➡. (Right) Axial CECT shows right buphthalmos, dysplastic right sphenoid bone ➡, and plexiform neurofibroma that involves the right cavernous sinus ➡ and orbit ➡.

Neurofibromatosis Type 1

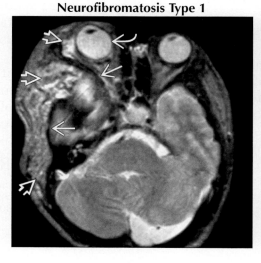

Neurofibromatosis Type 1

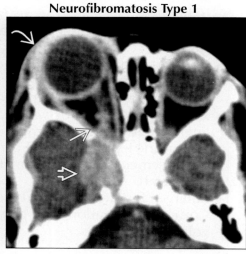

(Left) Axial T2WI FS MR reveals enlargement of the right globe ➡ with minimal asymmetry in the depth of the right anterior chamber. (Right) Axial T1WI MR demonstrates bilateral globe enlargement with increased depth of the anterior chambers ➡.

Glaucoma, Congenital

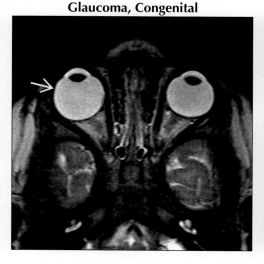

Glaucoma, Congenital

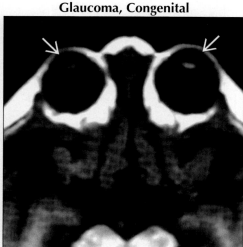

MACROPHTHALMOS

Glaucoma, Congenital
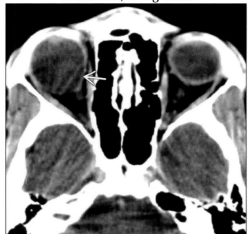

Myopia, Congenital
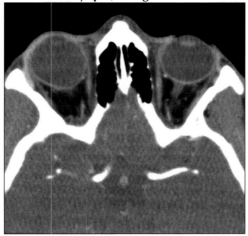

(Left) Axial CECT in this patient with congenital glaucoma reveals an elongated right globe ➡ (buphthalmos). *(Right)* Axial CECT shows an enlarged right globe in a patient with congenital myopia.

Sturge-Weber Syndrome
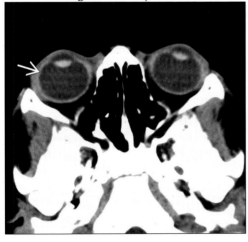

Sturge-Weber Syndrome
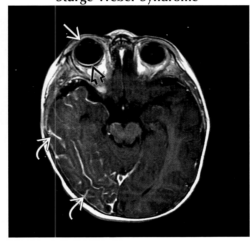

(Left) Axial NECT shows subtle enlargement of the right globe ➡, without visualized angioma, in a child with Sturge-Weber syndrome. *(Right)* Axial T1 C+ MR shows enlargement of right globe, deep anterior chamber ➡, mild thickening and contrast enhancement of choroidal angioma ➡, and diffuse abnormal leptomeningeal enhancement throughout the small right cerebral hemisphere ➡.

Congenital Cystic Eye
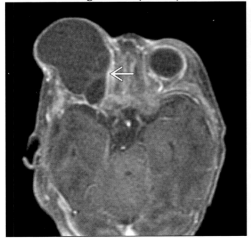

Coloboma with Macrophthalmia
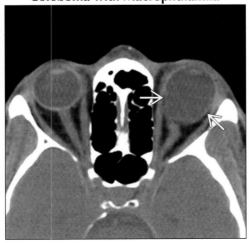

(Left) Axial T1 C+ FS MR shows a large cystic mass in the right orbit with complex elements posteromedially ➡, without an identifiable lens. *(Right)* Axial NECT reveals a broad-based coloboma defect ➡ involving the large left globe.

OPTIC NERVE SHEATH "TRAM TRACK" SIGN

DIFFERENTIAL DIAGNOSIS

Common
- Meningioma, Optic Nerve Sheath

Less Common
- Idiopathic Orbital Inflammatory Disease
- Optic Neuritis
- Sarcoidosis, Orbit
- Lymphoproliferative Lesions, Orbit

Rare but Important
- Metastasis, Orbit
- Erdheim-Chester Disease, Orbit

ESSENTIAL INFORMATION

Key Differential Diagnosis Issues
- "Tram track" appearance due to enhancement or Ca++ of optic nerve sheath

Helpful Clues for Common Diagnoses
- **Meningioma, Optic Nerve Sheath**
  - Key facts: Arises from arachnoid cap cells within optic nerve sheath
  - Imaging: Solid C+ tubular mass around intraorbital optic nerve ± Ca++

Helpful Clues for Less Common Diagnoses
- **Idiopathic Orbital Inflammatory Disease**
  - Key facts: Pseudotumor; benign inflammatory process involving any area of orbit
  - Imaging: Diffuse irregular enlargement & enhancement of optic nerve sheath with thickened sclera (anterior form)
- **Optic Neuritis**
  - Key facts: Acute neuritis associated with multiple sclerosis or idiopathic isolated form
  - Imaging: Enhancement of intraorbital optic nerve
    - Inflammatory C+ of nerve sheath
- **Sarcoidosis, Orbit**
  - Key facts: Systemic noncaseating granulomas affecting any part of orbit
  - Imaging: Perineuritic forms shows enhancement of nerve sheath
    - Look for involvement of optic nerve, extraocular muscles, fat
- **Lymphoproliferative Lesions, Orbit**
  - Key facts: Hyperplasia or lymphoma
  - Imaging: Uncommonly encases optic nerve ± exophytic mass

Helpful Clues for Rare Diagnoses
- **Metastasis, Orbit**
  - Key facts: Rare leptomeningeal carcinomatosis
    - Most common from breast, lung, GI
  - Imaging: Thickened enhancing optic nerve sheath
    - Look for other CNS lesions
- **Erdheim-Chester Disease, Orbit**
  - Key facts: Systemic disorder with xanthogranulomas
  - Imaging: Enhancement of optic nerve sheath
    - Look for multiple intraconal ± extraconal masses

Meningioma, Optic Nerve Sheath

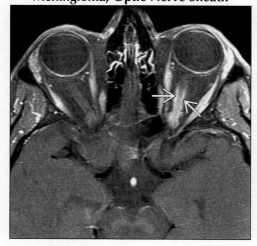

Axial T1 C+ FS MR shows enhancement of the nerve sheath ➡ outlining the nerve, resulting in the "tram track" appearance.

Meningioma, Optic Nerve Sheath

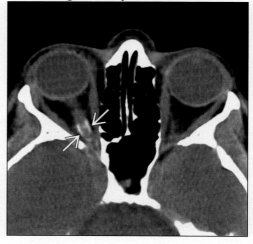

Axial NECT shows the typical "tram track" calcifications ➡ of a meningioma encasing the optic nerve. There is little soft tissue abnormality associated with the calcifications of the lesion.

OPTIC NERVE SHEATH "TRAM TRACK" SIGN

Idiopathic Orbital Inflammatory Disease

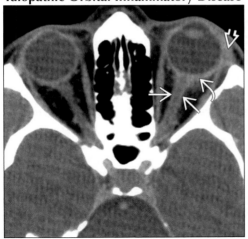

Optic Neuritis

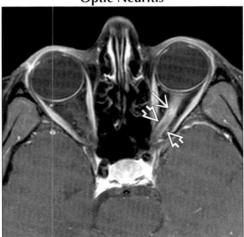

(Left) Axial CECT shows irregular thickening and enhancement of the optic nerve sheath ➡, giving it a "tram track" appearance. However, there is accompanying irregular thickening of the sclera ➡ and orbital septum ➡, which distinguishes this from meningioma. *(Right)* Axial T1 C+ FS MR shows enhancement of the optic nerve ➡ and modest enhancement of the nerve sheath ➡. Note the normal appearance of the orbital fat and extraocular muscles.

Sarcoidosis, Orbit

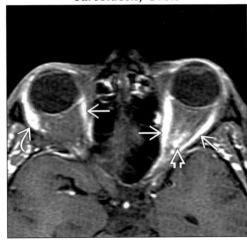

Lymphoproliferative Lesions, Orbit

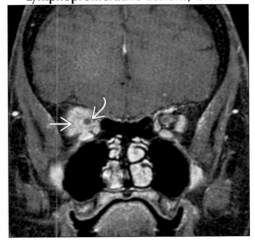

(Left) Axial T1 C+ FS MR shows abnormal enhancement along the left optic nerve sheath ➡, as well as abnormal enhancement of the extraocular muscles ➡ and lacrimal gland ➡. *(Right)* Coronal T1 C+ FS MR shows a uniformly enhancing mass ➡ that eccentrically surrounds the optic nerve ➡ and nearly fills the intraconal space.

Metastasis, Orbit

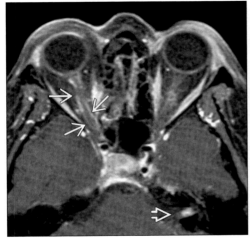

Erdheim-Chester Disease, Orbit

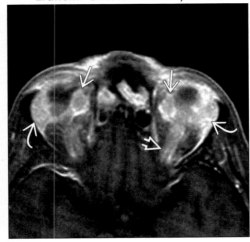

(Left) Axial T1 C+ FS MR shows enhancement on both sides of the intraorbital optic nerve ➡, and metastatic deposits in the IAC ➡. Diagnosis was central nervous system carcinomatosis from gastric adenocarcinoma. *(Right)* Axial T1 C+ FS MR shows patchy enhancement of the optic nerve sheath ➡. The multiple foci of enhancing intraconal ➡ & extraconal ➡ masses readily distinguish this from meningioma & would be unusual for IOID or lymphoma.

EXTRAOCULAR MUSCLE ENLARGEMENT

DIFFERENTIAL DIAGNOSIS

Common
- Thyroid-Associated Orbitopathy
- Idiopathic Orbital Inflammatory Disease (Pseudotumor)

Less Common
- Lymphoproliferative Lesions, Orbit
- Metastasis, Orbit
- Trauma, Orbit
- Cellulitis, Orbit
- Sarcoidosis, Orbit

Rare but Important
- Rhabdomyosarcoma, Orbit

ESSENTIAL INFORMATION

Helpful Clues for Common Diagnoses
- **Thyroid-Associated Orbitopathy**
  - ○ Key facts: Most common cause of exophthalmos in adults
  - ○ Imaging: Spares muscle tendons
    - ▪ "I'M SLOW" mnemonic for predilection
    - ▪ Inferior > medial > superior > lateral > obliques
- **Idiopathic Orbital Inflammatory Disease (Pseudotumor)**
  - ○ Key facts: Myositic pattern most common
    - ▪ Painful limited eye movement
  - ○ Imaging: Infiltrative muscle enlargement
    - ▪ May involve any part of orbit

Helpful Clues for Less Common Diagnoses
- **Lymphoproliferative Lesions, Orbit**
  - ○ Key facts: Lymphoid hyperplasia to NHL
  - ○ Imaging: Pliable mass anywhere in orbit
- **Metastasis, Orbit**
  - ○ Key facts: Breast, lung, melanoma
    - ▪ Sclerotic tissue suggests breast cancer
  - ○ Imaging: Solitary lesions common
    - ▪ May mimic other pathology
- **Trauma, Orbit**
  - ○ Key facts: Diplopia following trauma
  - ○ Imaging: Associated hematoma common
    - ▪ Muscle injury may occur without mechanical entrapment
- **Cellulitis, Orbit**
  - ○ Key facts: Secondary to sinusitis
    - ▪ Look for underlying cause or obstruction
  - ○ Imaging: Muscle and fat infiltration
    - ▪ Check for subperiosteal abscess
- **Sarcoidosis, Orbit**
  - ○ Key facts: Isolated muscle disease rare
    - ▪ Usually associated with lacrimal disease
  - ○ Imaging: Mass-like enlargement of muscle

Helpful Clues for Rare Diagnoses
- **Rhabdomyosarcoma, Orbit**
  - ○ Key facts: Childhood malignancy
    - ▪ Arises from orbital mesenchymal tissue, does not originate in muscle proper
  - ○ Imaging: Aggressive, destructive solid mass

Alternative Differential Approaches
- Multiple lesions elsewhere in orbit(s)
  - ○ Idiopathic orbital inflammatory disease
  - ○ Lymphoproliferative lesions, orbit
  - ○ Sarcoidosis, orbit
  - ○ Metastasis, orbit

Thyroid-Associated Orbitopathy

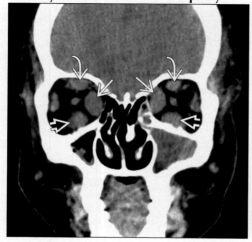

Coronal NECT shows symmetric enlargement of the medial rectus ➡, inferior rectus ➡, and, to a lesser extent, the superior rectus ➡ muscles. This is the expected pattern of EOM involvement.

Idiopathic Orbital Inflammatory Disease (Pseudotumor)

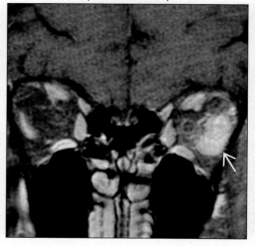

Coronal T1 C+ FS MR reveals asymmetric marked enlargement of the left lateral rectus muscle ➡. The margins of the muscle are ill defined, and the adjacent orbital fat shows inflammatory infiltration.

EXTRAOCULAR MUSCLE ENLARGEMENT

Lymphoproliferative Lesions, Orbit

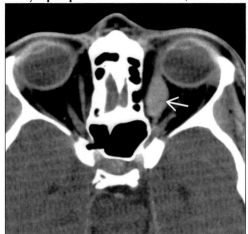

Metastasis, Orbit

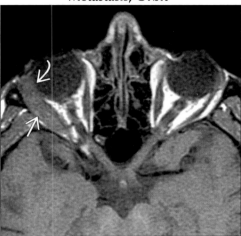

(Left) Axial CECT shows asymmetric mass-like enlargement of the left medial rectus muscle ➡. On pathology, the tumor cells were nonmonoclonal, indicating hyperplasia rather than overt lymphoma. *(Right)* Coronal T1WI MR in a patient with breast cancer demonstrates broad marked thickening of the right lateral rectus muscle ➡. Note that tumor involvement extends anteriorly to the muscle tendon ➡.

Trauma, Orbit

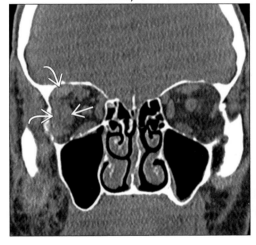

Cellulitis, Orbit

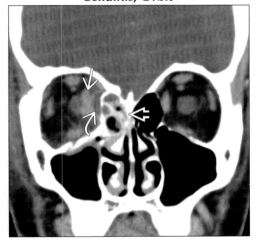

(Left) Coronal NECT reveals acute traumatic injury of the right orbit with enlargement of the right lateral rectus muscle ➡ and extraconal hematoma ➡. *(Right)* Coronal CECT depicts enlargement of the right medial rectus muscle ➡ with associated infiltration of the medial orbital fat. A small subperiosteal abscess is present ➡, and ipsilateral ethmoid sinusitis is evident ➡.

Sarcoidosis, Orbit

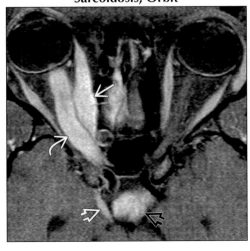

Rhabdomyosarcoma, Orbit

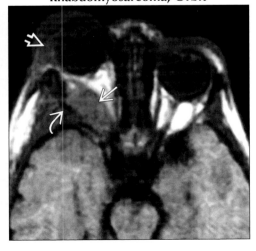

(Left) Axial T1WI FS MR shows asymmetric enlargement of the right medial rectus muscle ➡. Other features of orbital & intracranial sarcoid are evident, with involvement of the right optic nerve ➡, right oculomotor nerve ➡, & suprasellar region ➡. *(Right)* Axial T1WI MR reveals an intermediate signal mass extending laterally to the right lateral rectus ➡. Invasion into the lateral orbital wall is evident ➡, as is preseptal extension of the tumor ➡.

LARGE SUPERIOR OPHTHALMIC VEIN(S)

DIFFERENTIAL DIAGNOSIS

Common
- Carotid-Cavernous Fistula, Traumatic
- Thrombosis, Cavernous Sinus
- Carotid-Cavernous Fistula, Nontraumatic
- Large Superior Ophthalmic Vein, Normal Variant
- Venous Varix, Orbit

Less Common
- Dural A-V Fistula
- Schwannoma, Cavernous Sinus
- Meningioma, Cavernous Sinus
- Infantile Hemangioma, Orbit
- Arteriovenous Malformation

Rare but Important
- Raised Intracranial Pressure

ESSENTIAL INFORMATION

Key Differential Diagnosis Issues
- Superior ophthalmic veins (SOV) part of complex valveless orbital & periorbital venous system
  - Drain to cavernous sinus
- Enlarged veins most often due to cavernous sinus pathology
  - Arterialized sinus with retrograde flow along SOV, e.g., carotid-cavernous fistula
  - Increased venous pressure transmitted along SOV, e.g., cavernous sinus thrombosis (CST)
  - Increased SOV pressure from distended cavernous sinus, e.g., cavernous sinus mass
- Less often SOV enlarged as normal variant, venous varix, or AVM/dural AVF

Helpful Clues for Common Diagnoses
- **Carotid-Cavernous Fistula, Traumatic**
  - Key facts
    - M > F, 15-25 years
    - Usually clear clinical diagnosis: Recent trauma with orbital symptoms & signs
    - Direct fistula from leak of cavernous ICA
  - Imaging
    - CECT: Enlarged enhancing SOV & ipsilateral distended cavernous sinus
    - Ipsilateral proptosis, hazy orbital fat, enlarged ipsilateral pterygoid plexus
    - MR: Flow void in enlarged SOV & cavernous sinus

- Angio: Arterialized cavernous sinus from direct ICA flow → retrograde SOV flow
- **Thrombosis, Cavernous Sinus**
  - Key facts
    - Most often secondary to facial infection
    - Sinusitis, facial, orbital, or periorbital cellulitis with thrombophlebitis
  - Imaging
    - CECT/MR: Sinus filling defects
    - SOV may be distended & enhancing from venous hypertension OR
    - SOV may be thrombosed with filling defects
    - Must evaluate for ICA thrombosis and for intracranial complications: Cerebritis, subdural empyema
- **Carotid-Cavernous Fistula, Nontraumatic**
  - Key facts
    - F > M, classically middle-aged
    - Spontaneous, gradual onset
    - Indirect fistula from intracavernous branches of ICA
  - Imaging
    - CECT/MR: Usually unilateral enlarged SOV & cavernous sinus
    - Proptosis and orbital fat edema more subtle than with traumatic fistula
    - Angio: Cavernous sinus fills from small ICA branches → retrograde SOV flow
- **Large Superior Ophthalmic Vein, Normal Variant**
  - Key facts
    - Diagnosis of exclusion!
    - Ensure no clinical symptoms and no cavernous sinus imaging abnormality
  - Imaging
    - CECT/MR: Symmetric prominent SOV
    - No evidence of cavernous sinus mass or thrombosis
    - Normal appearance of retrobulbar fat
- **Venous Varix, Orbit**
  - Key facts
    - Low flow congenital venous malformation
  - Imaging
    - CECT/MR: Variable imaging appearance
    - From simple "beaded" SOV to extraconal enhancing mass
    - Distends with Valsalva maneuver or with patient prone

LARGE SUPERIOR OPHTHALMIC VEIN(S)

Helpful Clues for Less Common Diagnoses
- **Dural A-V Fistula**
  - Key facts
    - Abnormal communication between meningeal artery and vein or dural sinus
    - Usually acquired lesion
    - Arterialized venous flow may be direct to SOV or to cavernous sinus
  - Imaging
    - CECT/MR: Arterialized venous drainage results in prominent, asymmetric venous channels
    - Angio: Often required for definitive diagnosis and for endovascular treatment
- **Schwannoma, Cavernous Sinus**
  - Key facts
    - Benign tumor of Schwann cells
    - May arise from CN3, CN4, CNV1, CNV2, or CN6
  - Imaging
    - CECT/MR: Smooth unilateral cavernous sinus mass with convex lateral margin
    - May see anterior extension to orbit
    - May see posterior extension to Meckel cave (CN5), interpeduncular cistern (CN3/4), or prepontine cistern (CN6)
- **Meningioma, Cavernous Sinus**
  - Key facts
    - Benign, slow-growing tumor abutting dura
    - May present with cranial neuropathy or incidental imaging finding
  - Imaging
    - CECT/MR: Unilateral or bilateral cavernous sinus enlargement and enhancement
    - May see dural tail, narrowed ICA
    - SOV may be distended ipsilateral to meningioma
- **Infantile Hemangioma, Orbit**
  - Key facts
    - Endothelial neoplasm of infants
    - Proliferation during first 12 months
    - Involution over subsequent decade
    - Increased venous flow may distend SOV
  - Imaging
    - CECT/MR: Intensely enhancing mass with large vessels during proliferation
    - Heterogeneous mass with focal fat with involution
- **Arteriovenous Malformation**
  - Key facts
    - Congenital abnormal direct communication between arteries and veins with shunting of blood
  - Imaging
    - CECT/MR: Intracranial tangle of vessels
    - SOV may enlarge from direct drainage or from increased cavernous sinus flow

Helpful Clues for Rare Diagnoses
- **Raised Intracranial Pressure**
  - Key fact: Patient usually comatose
  - Imaging
    - Effacement of sulci, ventricles, and cisterns
    - Compression of dural venous sinuses

Carotid-Cavernous Fistula, Traumatic

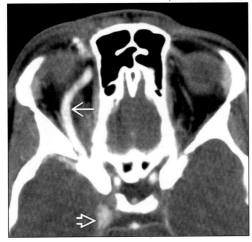

Axial CECT shows asymmetrically enlarged right superior ophthalmic vein ➡ with enlarged ipsilateral cavernous sinus ⧐ in a young patient with right proptosis and ophthalmoplegia.

Carotid-Cavernous Fistula, Traumatic

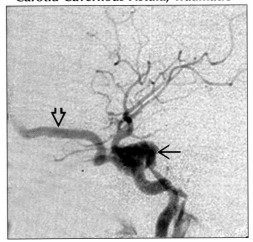

Lateral angiography during right ICA injection shows contrast filling the cavernous sinus ⧐ and retrograde flow markedly distending the superior ophthalmic vein ⧐ during the arterial phase of injection.

LARGE SUPERIOR OPHTHALMIC VEIN(S)

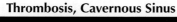

(Left) Axial CECT shows abnormally enlarged enhancing left SOV ➡ and minimal enhancement of enlarged thrombosed right SOV ➡ in a patient with fever, double vision, and right proptosis. *(Right)* Axial CECT shows filling defects bilaterally in a cavernous sinus ➡, indicating cavernous sinus thrombosis. The patient has bacterial sphenoethmoidal sinusitis ➡, a frequent cause of cavernous sinus thrombosis.

Thrombosis, Cavernous Sinus

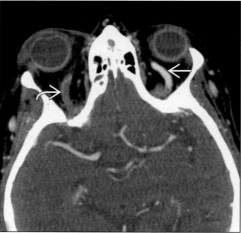

Thrombosis, Cavernous Sinus

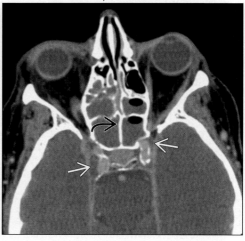

(Left) Lateral angiography during injection of left ICA shows pooling of contrast in the cavernous sinus ➡ and retrograde filling of the superior ophthalmic vein ➡. Note there is no large arterial feeder but rather small ICA branches responsible for fistula to sinus. *(Right)* Coronal CECT shows bilateral enlargement of superior ophthalmic veins ➡ as an incidental finding in a patient with a normal clinical examination and no evidence of intracranial abnormality.

Carotid-Cavernous Fistula, Nontraumatic

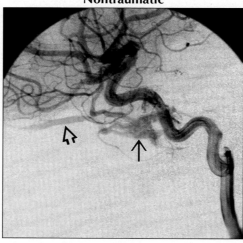

Large Superior Ophthalmic Vein, Normal Variant

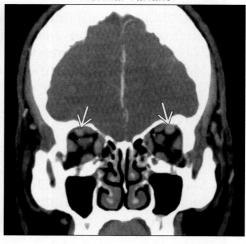

(Left) Axial CECT in a patient with mild proptosis reveals bilaterally enlarged superior orbital veins ➡ with "beaded" varicose appearance as an intermittent finding on different imaging studies. Valsalva maneuver may be needed to show varices. *(Right)* Coronal CECT shows asymmetric dilatation of the right superior ophthalmic vein ➡ as compared to the left ➡, in addition to other enhancing tubular structures in orbit, consistent with dilated veins ➡.

Venous Varix, Orbit

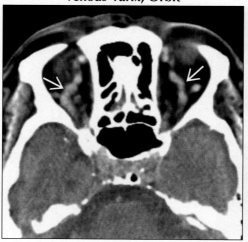

Venous Varix, Orbit

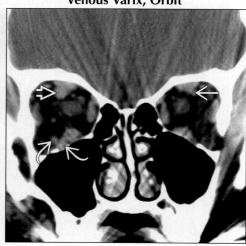

LARGE SUPERIOR OPHTHALMIC VEIN(S)

Dural A-V Fistula

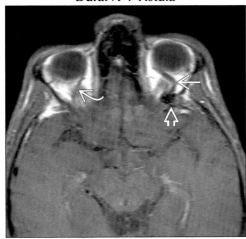

Dural A-V Fistula

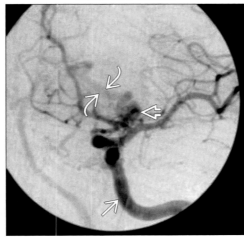

(Left) Axial T1 C+ MR shows flow void in enlarged left superior ophthalmic vein ➡ draining small dural A-V fistula ⏩ at posterior left orbit. Note the normal right superior orbital vein ➡. *(Right)* Angiography in the same patient with left ICA injection ➡ shows a tangle of vessels ⏩ and arterialized flow along the superior ophthalmic vein ➡. Dural AVF predominant supply was from middle meningeal artery, but this injection showed some ophthalmic artery supply.

Meningioma, Cavernous Sinus

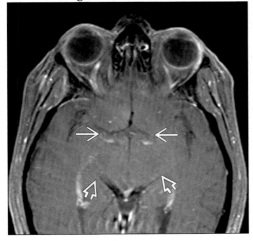

Meningioma, Cavernous Sinus

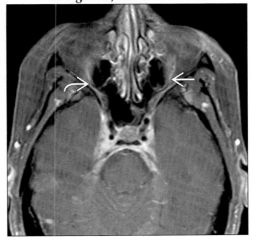

(Left) Axial T1 C+ FS MR shows bilaterally enlarged cavernous sinuses ➡ with dural enhancement extending along the posterior margin of the clivus and margin of the tentorium ⏩. Internal carotid arteries are of normal caliber. *(Right)* Axial T1 C+ FS MR in the same patient shows an asymmetrically enlarged right superior ophthalmic vein ➡, with normal appearance of the left side ➡. No abnormality of retrobulbar fat is evident.

Infantile Hemangioma, Orbit

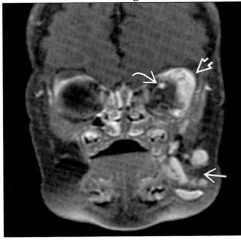

Raised Intracranial Pressure

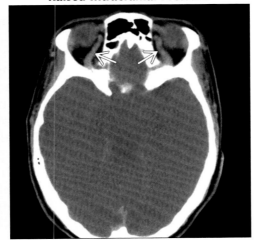

(Left) Coronal T1 C+ FS MR shows left facial ➡ and extraconal ⏩ infantile hemangiomas in a patient with PHACES syndrome. Note the large left superior ophthalmic vein ➡. *(Right)* Axial CECT demonstrates bilaterally distended superior ophthalmic veins ➡ in a patient with diffuse catastrophic hypoxia, which resulted in marked cerebral edema & raised intracranial pressure. Note effacement of cerebral sulci & cisterns with loss of gray-white differentiation.

DIFFERENTIAL DIAGNOSIS

Common
- Cellulitis, Orbit
- Idiopathic Orbital Inflammatory Disease (Pseudotumor)
- Infantile Hemangioma, Orbit
- Lymphatic Malformation, Orbit
- Plexiform Neurofibroma, Orbit

Less Common
- Lymphoproliferative Lesions, Orbit
- Rhabdomyosarcoma
- Sarcoidosis, Orbit
- Metastasis, Orbit

Rare but Important
- Wegener Granulomatosis, Orbit
- Hemangiopericytoma
- Erdheim-Chester Disease, Orbit

ESSENTIAL INFORMATION

Helpful Clues for Common Diagnoses
- **Cellulitis, Orbit**
  - Key facts: Secondary to trauma or cutaneous, hematogenous, or iatrogenic infection
  - Imaging
    - ↑ Density and enhancing periorbital soft tissue, lids, orbital septum
    - Retroseptal extraconal &/or intraconal fat infiltration
    - Intraconal involvement may compromise optic nerve
- **Idiopathic Orbital Inflammatory Disease (Pseudotumor)**
  - Key facts: Benign inflammatory process of unknown local or systemic etiology
    - Composed of lymphocytic infiltrates
  - Imaging: Space-occupying infiltrative process involving any part of orbit
    - Infiltrative or tumefactive enhancing mass that may involve retrobulbar, intraconal, and extraconal spaces
    - Does not distort or invade globe
    - Does not destroy bone
    - May involve lacrimal gland with diffuse irregular enlargement
- **Infantile Hemangioma, Orbit**
  - Key facts: Benign endothelial cell vascular neoplasm of infants, distinct from pediatric or adult cavernous hemangioma

  - Imaging: CT modality of choice to avoid sedation
    - Lobulated mass seen anywhere in orbit
    - Most common location superomedial extraconal, supranasal periorbita
    - 10% exclusively retrobulbar
    - CT: Mildly hyperdense, no calcification, intensely enhancing
    - MR: Heterogeneously hyperintense T1 and T2; diffuse avid enhancement; look for flow voids
- **Lymphatic Malformation, Orbit**
  - Key facts: Congenital hamartomatous lymphatic and venous malformation
  - Imaging
    - General: Irregular multilocular cystic mass typically trans-spatial with intraconal and extraconal components
    - MR: Variable T1, hyperintense T2; fluid-fluid levels; no flow voids
    - Enhanced MR: Variable enhancement, most commonly rim enhancement of cysts
- **Plexiform Neurofibroma, Orbit**
  - Key facts: Neurocutaneous disorder manifestation
    - Plexiform neurofibroma pathognomonic for neurofibromatosis type 1
  - Imaging
    - General: Serpentine, infiltrative, often trans-spatial masses involving muscles, nerve sheath, nerve branches, sclera
    - CT: Hypodense infiltrative mass
    - MR: Hypointense mass on T1, characteristic "target" appearance on T2 or T1 C+; variably enhancing

Helpful Clues for Less Common Diagnoses
- **Lymphoproliferative Lesions, Orbit**
  - Key facts: Spectrum of benign and malignant tumors (NHL)
  - Imaging
    - Homogeneously enhancing solid mass
    - Can be found anywhere in orbit, but typically extraconal
    - Predilection for lacrimal gland
    - May present as diffuse form with infiltration of intraconal space, muscles, or optic nerve sheath
- **Rhabdomyosarcoma**
  - Key facts: Most common primary malignant tumor of orbit in children

- Imaging
  - Proliferating phase: Infiltrative heterogeneously enhancing mass; involution phase: Fat infiltration & ↓ size
  - Destroys or remodels bone
- **Sarcoidosis, Orbit**
  - Key facts: Idiopathic systemic disease of noncaseating granulomas affecting orbit in ~ 20-25% of cases
  - Imaging
    - Thickening and enhancement of intraorbital &/or chiasmatic optic nerve
    - Can involve uveal-scleral coat or any other part of orbit (fat, EOM, lacrimal gland) with thickening and enlargement
    - May present with infiltrative mass identical to lymphoma
    - Look for systemic lesions or intracranial involvement: Parenchymal lesion, leptomeningeal, dural, or skull lesions
- **Metastasis, Orbit**
  - Key facts: Most commonly from breast, prostate, lung
  - Imaging
    - Usually diffuse, enhancing intraconal mass
    - Breast and lung may have 1 or more ocular masses

Helpful Clues for Rare Diagnoses
- **Wegener Granulomatosis, Orbit**
  - Key facts: Necrotizing granulomatous vasculitis affecting orbit ~ 20% of cases

- M:F = 3:2, ANCA antibody positive in more than 90% of cases
  - Imaging
    - Most common appearance: Irregular thickening and enhancement of sclera; often bilateral
    - Frequently presents as irregular ± enhancing soft tissue mass in orbit adjacent to sinus with soft tissue/mucosal disease and bone erosion
    - Adjacent paranasal sinus and nasal involvement present in majority of cases
- **Hemangiopericytoma**
  - Key facts: Vascular neoplasm arising from pericytes of Zimmerman
  - Imaging
    - Infiltrating strongly enhancing mass
    - Tendency for lateral extraconal orbital and bony invasion
- **Erdheim-Chester Disease, Orbit**
  - Key facts: Systemic disorder of osteosclerosis and xanthogranulomas
    - May involve pituitary, orbit, retroperitoneum, lung, heart
  - Imaging
    - Often bilateral involvement
    - Diffuse infiltrative mass most commonly involving intraconal space
    - May involve any other area in orbit
    - Moderately to significantly enhancing on CT and MR
    - Persistent enhancement for several days reported with gadolinium

Cellulitis, Orbit

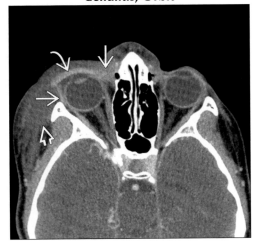

Axial CECT shows a thickened and enhancing orbital septum ➡ with postseptal extraconal edema, thickened enhancing lid and tarsal plate ➡, and periorbital soft tissue thickening ➡.

Idiopathic Orbital Inflammatory Disease (Pseudotumor)

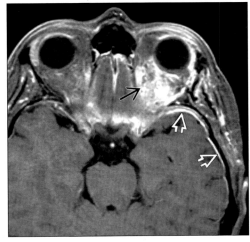

Axial T1 C+ FS MR reveals diffusely infiltrating, poorly marginated enhancement in the intraconal retrobulbar space ➡. Note the associated dura-arachnoid thickening ➡.

ILL-DEFINED ORBITAL MASS

Idiopathic Orbital Inflammatory Disease (Pseudotumor)

Infantile Hemangioma, Orbit

(Left) Axial CECT demonstrates an infiltrative moderately enhancing mass ➡ centered in the lateral left orbit. The mass is indistinguishable from the lateral rectus muscle and displaces and partially encases the optic nerve/sheath complex ➡. *(Right)* Axial T1WI MR shows a vascular retrobulbar intraconal mass ➡ with irregular lobulated margins. The key feature of this lesion is the numerous curvilinear and punctate high velocity flow voids ➡.

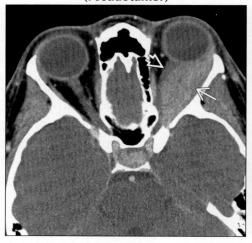

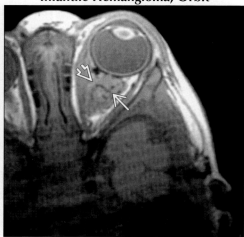

Lymphatic Malformation, Orbit

Plexiform Neurofibroma, Orbit

(Left) Axial T2WI MR shows a complex multiloculated mass in the right orbit with fluid-fluid levels ➡ resulting from previous hemorrhage. The mass has an infiltrative multicystic appearance involving most of the postseptal orbit. *(Right)* Axial T1WI FS MR shows multi-compartmental enhancing plexiform neurofibroma involving the extraconal ➡ and intraconal ➡ right orbit, along with the cavernous sinus ➡.

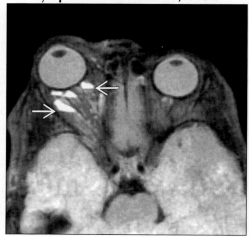

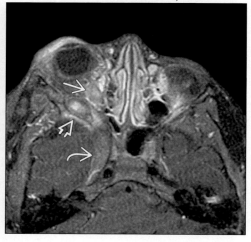

Lymphoproliferative Lesions, Orbit

Lymphoproliferative Lesions, Orbit

(Left) Axial NECT reveals a lobulated mass involving the sclera of the globe ➡ and lacrimal gland ➡. The scleral calcification is unrelated to the orbital non-Hodgkin lymphoma. *(Right)* Axial T1WI FS MR shows an irregular but homogeneously enhancing septal mass ➡ that extends postseptally into the extraconal space ➡. There is infiltrative enlargement and enhancement of the medial rectus muscle ➡ in this patient with non-Hodgkin lymphoma.

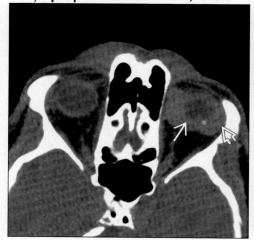

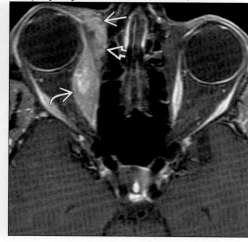

ILL-DEFINED ORBITAL MASS

Rhabdomyosarcoma

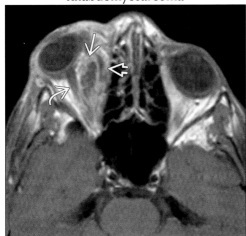

Sarcoidosis, Orbit

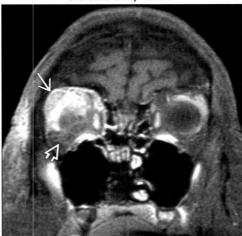

(Left) Axial T1 C+ MR in a child shows an infiltrative heterogeneously enhancing mass of the right orbit, involving the intraconal ➡ & extraconal spaces ➡ deforming the globe and displacing the optic nerve ➡. The heterogeneous enhancement makes lymphoma less likely. *(Right)* Coronal T1 C+ FS MR shows marked enhancement and irregular diffuse enlargement of the right lacrimal gland ➡ and a "stranded" appearance of the right retro-orbital fat ➡.

Metastasis, Orbit

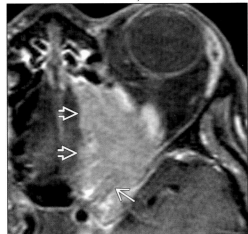

Wegener Granulomatosis, Orbit

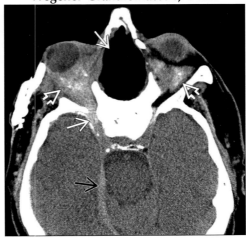

(Left) Axial T1WI FS MR demonstrates moderately enhancing intraconal & extraconal prostate carcinoma metastasis encasing the optic nerve ➡. Note extension through medial orbital wall ➡. *(Right)* Axial CECT reveals spread of Wegener granulomatosis into both orbits ➡ with associated complete destruction of the sinonasal bony structures ➡. Inflammatory process has spread through the right orbital apex & involves the tentorium cerebelli ➡.

Hemangiopericytoma

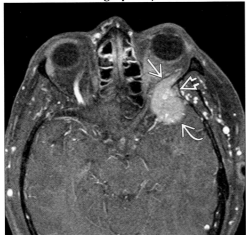

Erdheim-Chester Disease, Orbit

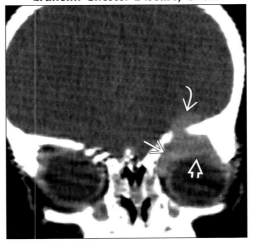

(Left) Axial T1WI FS MR reveals an enhancing hemangiopericytoma infiltrating the lateral orbital wall, lateral rectus, and extraconal space ➡. Note the infiltration of the sphenoid bone ➡ and the intracranial extension ➡. *(Right)* Coronal CECT shows an irregular enhancing mass in the superior orbit ➡ with infiltration of the sclera ➡, depression of the globe with adjacent destruction of the orbital roof, and intracranial extension ➡.

DIFFERENTIAL DIAGNOSIS

Common
- Dermoid and Epidermoid, Orbit
- Staphyloma
- Mucocele, Sinonasal
- Dacryocystocele
- Lacrimal Cyst
- Eyelid Cyst (Meibomian)

Less Common
- Abscess, Subperiosteal, Orbit
- Lymphatic Malformation, Orbit
- Trauma, Orbit
- Venous Varix, Orbit
- Coloboma

Rare but Important
- Cephalocele, Frontoethmoidal
- Congenital Cystic Eye
- Cephalocele, Spheno-Orbital

ESSENTIAL INFORMATION

Key Differential Diagnosis Issues
- Lesion location (intraocular, intraconal, extraconal, extraorbital) & patient demographics (age) narrow differential
- Dilatation of optic nerve sheath with CSF in papilledema, periopptic meningioma, dural ectasia (NF1) may appear as "cystic" mass

Helpful Clues for Common Diagnoses
- **Dermoid and Epidermoid, Orbit**
  - Key facts
    - Congenital inclusion of epithelial/dermal elements
  - Imaging
    - Well-defined extraconal mass
    - Superolateral at frontozygomatic suture or superonasal at frontolacrimal suture
    - Dermoid if fatty ± fluid-fluid levels
    - Punctate Ca++ (~ 15%); smooth osseous remodeling
- **Staphyloma**
  - Key facts: Abnormal protrusion of uveal tissue through weak point in globe
    - From inflammatory or degenerative condition
    - Posterior type results in myopia
  - Imaging: Focal outpouching of globe with scleral thinning
- **Mucocele, Sinonasal**
  - Key facts: Opacified expanded sinus due to chronic obstruction
    - Frontal & ethmoid sinuses
  - Imaging: Smooth, convex walls
    - Expanded sinus/air cell with homogeneous hypodense or soft tissue density material
    - Lamina papyracea, medial orbital wall, or orbital roof expanded & thinned or dehiscent
- **Dacryocystocele**
  - Key facts: Dilatation of lacrimal sac secondary to more distal obstruction in lacrimal apparatus
    - In newborns, frequently associated with dilatation of nasolacrimal duct (NLD mucocele)
  - Imaging: Fluid-filled mass centered at lacrimal sac with bony remodeling
    - ± Dilatation of nasal lacrimal canal & cystic intranasal mass (NLD mucocele)
- **Lacrimal Cyst**
  - Key facts: Arises from obstruction of excretory ducts of palpebral or orbital lobes of lacrimal gland
    - Arises spontaneously, or following trauma/surgery
  - Imaging
    - Well-defined cyst or cystic lesion in lacrimal parenchyma
    - Secondary obstruction due to benign or malignant lacrimal neoplasm indistinguishable
    - Look for enhancing or irregular parenchymal mass = neoplasm
- **Eyelid Cyst (Meibomian)**
  - Key facts: Obstruction of meibomian glands at base of eyelash in tarsal plate
    - Synonym: Chalazion
  - Imaging
    - Diagnosed on physical exam
    - Imaging performed to exclude orbital involvement
    - Cystic mass or nodule in upper/lower eyelid or tarsal plate
    - Surrounding inflammation (blepharitis)

Helpful Clues for Less Common Diagnoses
- **Abscess, Subperiosteal, Orbit**
  - Key facts: Collection of pus between orbital wall & periosteum due to adjacent focus of infection (sinusitis)

○ Imaging
  ▪ Medial orbital wall rim-enhancing focus
  ▪ Displacement of medial rectus & adjacent ethmoid sinusitis
• **Lymphatic Malformation, Orbit**
  ○ Key facts: Congenital vascular malformation
  ○ Imaging
    ▪ Irregular, lobulated extraconal ± intraconal cystic lesion
    ▪ Irregularly enhancing ± fluid-fluid levels
• **Trauma, Orbit**
  ○ Key facts: Chronic epithelial-lined hematoma (hematic cyst)
    ▪ Found following trauma adjacent to medial, lateral, or superior orbital walls
    ▪ Intralesional chronic blood products & cholesterol granules
  ○ Imaging
    ▪ Extraconal mass with hypo- to isodense internal contents
    ▪ Circumscribed ± enhancing rim
    ▪ May be ↑ signal on T1 MR
    ▪ Look for associated fracture, dehiscence, or erosion
• **Venous Varix, Orbit**
  ○ Key facts: Distensible venous low flow malformation
  ○ Imaging
    ▪ Enhancing extraconal retrobulbar mass
    ▪ Complex flow signal on MR that ↑ with Valsalva
    ▪ Tortuous or tubular distension may appear as cystic mass

• **Coloboma**
  ○ Key facts: Focal defect of globe with variable presentations
  ○ Imaging: Retrobulbar cyst isodense to vitreous
    ▪ Cyst communicates with globe

Helpful Clues for Rare Diagnoses
• **Cephalocele, Frontoethmoidal**
  ○ Key facts: Most common cephalocele
    ▪ If fronto-orbital type ⇒ orbital mass
  ○ Imaging
    ▪ Nonenhancing cystic or soft tissue mass extending from anterior fossa through skull base/lacrimal bone defect
    ▪ CT: Solid component isointense to brain parenchyma
    ▪ MR: Hyperintense CSF rim on T2
• **Congenital Cystic Eye**
  ○ Key facts: Arises from failure of primary optic vesicle to invaginate
  ○ Imaging: Absence of recognizable globe with cystic or mixed cystic/solid mass
• **Cephalocele, Spheno-Orbital**
  ○ Key facts: Herniation of meninges, CSF ± brain parenchyma through orbital apex, superior orbital fissure (SOF), or posterolateral wall
  ○ Imaging
    ▪ CT: Nonenhancing cystic or soft tissue density mass extending from apex, SOF, or posterolateral wall
    ▪ MR: Mass follows gray matter with CSF rim

Dermoid and Epidermoid, Orbit

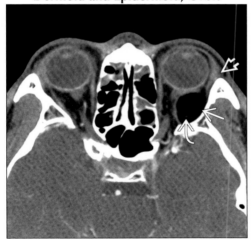

Axial CECT shows a well-defined fat density mass ➡ along the lateral orbital wall with scattered dense internal components ➡. Note that the mass is separate from the lacrimal gland ➡.

Dermoid and Epidermoid, Orbit

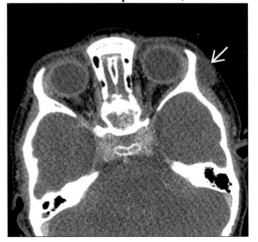

Axial NECT shows a cystic mass on the lateral orbital rim ➡. Note the apparent absence of bone erosion, suggestive of a benign process. This is a common site for dermoids involving the orbit.

CYSTIC ORBITAL LESIONS

(Left) Axial T2WI MR shows bilateral posterior senescent staphyloma ➡ incidentally found on a head MR. The lesions are medial to the optic nerves. Thinning of the sclera is most noticeable on the right. (Right) Axial NECT shows an expansile lesion extending from the ethmoid sinus through the medial orbital wall ➡ with displacement of the left globe. The lamina papyracea is dehiscent, and the medial rectus muscle is displaced ➡. Note the intact nasolacrimal duct ➡.

Staphyloma

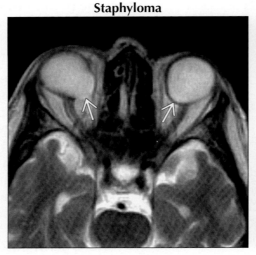

Mucocele, Sinonasal

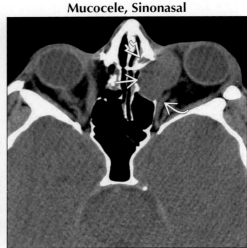

(Left) Axial NECT shows bilateral well-defined cysts ➡ in lacrimal sacs in an infant with clinically apparent medial orbit masses. Bony wall remodeling is evident. If associated with nasolacrimal duct mucoceles, patient presents with nasal obstruction secondary to intranasal component. (Right) Axial NECT shows cystic expansion of palpebral lobe of right lacrimal gland ➡ following orbital trauma. Note the adjacent periorbital hematoma ➡.

Dacryocystocele

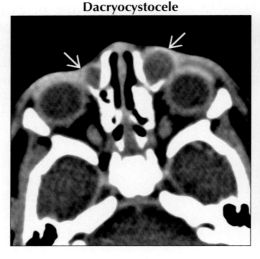

Lacrimal Cyst

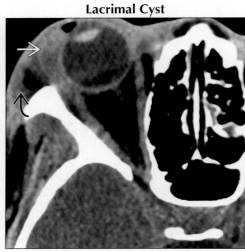

(Left) Axial T1 C+ FS MR shows a rim-enhancing cystic mass in the posterior-superior aspect of the upper eyelid tarsal plate ➡. The irregularity of the posterior margin suggests the possibility of rupture. (Right) Axial CECT shows a rim-enhancing fluid collection located in the extraconal space of the medial right orbit ➡. Note the associated significant mucosal disease in the ethmoid sinuses ➡ and displacement of the medial rectus muscle ➡.

Eyelid Cyst (Meibomian)

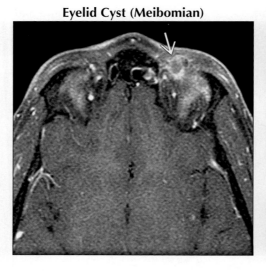

Abscess, Subperiosteal, Orbit

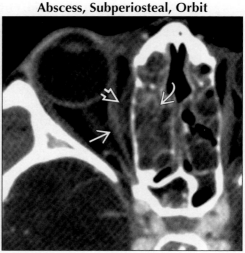

CYSTIC ORBITAL LESIONS

Lymphatic Malformation, Orbit

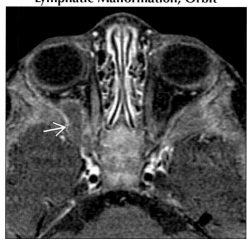

Trauma, Orbit

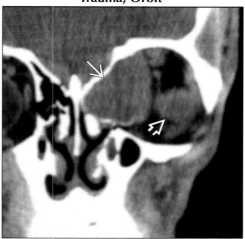

(Left) Axial T1WI FS MR reveals a nonenhancing cystic mass ➡ extending through the superior orbital fissure. The insinuation through the spaces of the orbit by a cystic-appearing mass is typical for lymphatic malformations. **(Right)** Coronal NECT shows a large hematic cyst ➡ with a hyperdense rim in a patient following orbital trauma. The medial orbital wall is absent, and the globe/optic nerve-sheath complex is displaced laterally ➡.

Venous Varix, Orbit

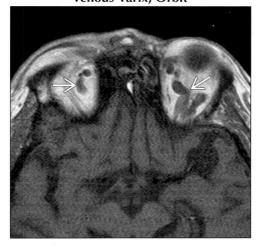

Coloboma

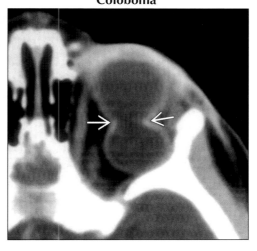

(Left) Axial T1WI MR demonstrates bilateral enlarged superior orbital vein varices ➡. Note that these "cystic masses" follow the course of ophthalmic vessels. These varices enhance avidly with contrast, differentiating them from other cystic lesions. **(Right)** Axial CECT shows a large posterior globe dehiscence through a broad defect ➡ centered on the upper margin of the optic disc. Notice that the retrobulbar cyst density is the same as the vitreous density.

Cephalocele, Frontoethmoidal

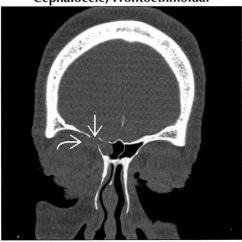

Congenital Cystic Eye

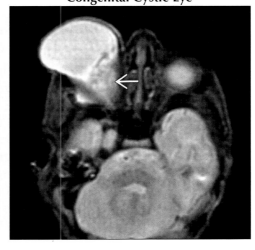

(Left) Coronal bone CT shows a cystic mass ➡ extending from a defect in the fovea ethmoidalis into the superomedial orbit ➡. This acquired cephalocele is superior in location compared to congenital naso-orbital cephaloceles. **(Right)** Axial T2WI FS MR reveals a large cystic mass in the right orbit in this newborn. There are some complex elements seen in the posteromedial aspect of the cyst ➡. No normal-appearing globe was visible in the orbit.

VASCULAR LESIONS OF ORBIT

DIFFERENTIAL DIAGNOSIS

Common
- Cavernous Hemangioma, Orbit

Less Common
- Infantile Hemangioma, Orbit
- Malformations with Spectrum of Mixed Venous &/or Lymphatic Components
  - Lymphatic Malformation, Orbit
  - Venolymphatic Malformation, Orbit
  - Venous Malformation, Orbit
  - Venous Varix, Orbit

Rare but Important
- Arteriovenous Connections
  - Arteriovenous Malformation, Orbit
  - Dural Arteriovenous Fistula, Orbit
  - Carotid-Cavernous Fistula
- Hemangiopericytoma, Orbit

ESSENTIAL INFORMATION

Helpful Clues for Common Diagnoses
- **Cavernous Hemangioma, Orbit**
  - Key facts
    - Most common adult orbital mass
    - Malformation, not true neoplasm
  - Imaging
    - Well-demarcated, ovoid
    - Usually intraconal, often lateral
    - Phleboliths atypical in orbit
    - Hemorrhage unusual
    - Characteristic patchy enhancement that fills in dynamically
  - Other useful information
    - Cavernous hemangioma of orbit unique compared to other locations
    - Physiologically like low flow AVM

Helpful Clues for Less Common Diagnoses
- **Infantile Hemangioma, Orbit**
  - Key facts
    - Synonyms: Capillary hemangioma, benign hemangioendothelioma
    - Most common benign orbital tumor of infancy
    - Proliferative mass, not malformation
    - Frequently regresses spontaneously
  - Imaging
    - Intensely enhancing vascular mass
    - Ultrasound for rapid bedside confirmation

- **Lymphatic Malformation, Orbit**
  - Key facts
    - Vascular malformation with lymphatic endothelial channels
    - Synonyms: Cystic hygroma, lymphangioma
  - Imaging
    - Multiloculated, irregular cystic mass
    - May be large and trans-spatial
    - Propensity to hemorrhage, with fluid-fluid levels
- **Venolymphatic Malformation, Orbit**
  - Key facts
    - Vascular malformation with mixed venous and lymphatic channels
  - Imaging
    - Lobulated, irregular trans-spatial mass
    - Blood and fluid levels
    - Heterogeneous enhancement
- **Venous Malformation, Orbit**
  - Key facts
    - Vascular malformation without lymphatic component
    - Less likely to hemorrhage
  - Imaging findings
    - More homogeneous enhancement
    - Trans-spatial with facial component
    - Similar to other head and neck lesions of same name
- **Venous Varix, Orbit**
  - Key facts
    - Distensible venous channel with systemic connection
    - May present with acute hemorrhage
    - Often associated with venolymphatic malformation
  - Imaging
    - Dynamic enlargement of lesion with provocative maneuver (e.g., Valsalva)
    - May not be visible when patient relaxed

Helpful Clues for Rare Diagnoses
- **Arteriovenous Malformation, Orbit**
  - Key facts
    - Direct arteriovenous connection
    - Typically fed by ophthalmic artery
    - External carotid supply may be minimal
  - Imaging
    - High flow characteristics
    - Demonstrable on CTA, MRA, or US
    - Enlarged superior ophthalmic vein
    - Often located anteriorly in orbit

VASCULAR LESIONS OF ORBIT

- **Dural Arteriovenous Fistula, Orbit**
  - Key facts
    - Extraorbital facial &/or intracranial shunt
    - Similar to indirect cavernous-carotid fistula
  - Imaging
    - Internal &/or external carotid supply
    - Early filling orbital veins
- **Carotid-Cavernous Fistula**
  - Key facts
    - May be due to trauma, venous thrombosis, or aneurysm
    - Arterialization of cavernous sinus and orbital veins
  - Imaging
    - Enlarged superior ophthalmic vein
- **Hemangiopericytoma, Orbit**
  - Key facts
    - Slowly growing hypervascular neoplasm
    - Ranges from benign to malignant; very rarely metastatic
  - Imaging
    - Usually circumscribed; often lobulated
    - May have infiltrative margins
    - Often medial adjacent to sinuses

Alternative Differential Approaches
- **Patient age vs. vascular orbital lesions**
  - Pediatric patients
    - Infantile hemangioma, orbit
    - Lymphatic malformation, orbit
    - Venolymphatic malformation, orbit
    - Venous malformation, orbit
  - Adult patients
    - Cavernous hemangioma, orbit
    - Venous varix, orbit
    - Arteriovenous malformation, orbit
    - Dural arteriovenous fistula, orbit
    - Carotid-cavernous fistula
    - Hemangiopericytoma, orbit
- **Classification of malformations**
  - Type 1: No flow
    - Lymphatic malformation, orbit
  - Type 2: Venous flow
  - 2A: Distensible
    - Venous varix, orbit
  - 2B: Nondistensible
    - Venous malformation, orbit
    - Venolymphatic malformation, orbit
  - 2C: Combined; features of both
  - Type 3: Arterial flow
  - 3A: High flow
    - Arteriovenous malformation
  - 3B: Low flow
    - Cavernous hemangioma
- **Ocular lesions** not discussed here include
  - Melanoma, ocular
  - Metastasis, ocular
  - Coats disease
  - Choroidal hemangioma

SELECTED REFERENCES
1. Smoker WR et al: Vascular lesions of the orbit: more than meets the eye. Radiographics. 28(1):185-204, 2008
2. Rootman J: Vascular malformations of the orbit: hemodynamic concepts. Orbit. 22(2):103-20, 2003

Cavernous Hemangioma, Orbit

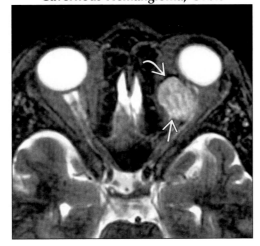

Axial T2WI FS MR shows the typical T2 hyperintensity of a cavernous hemangioma ➡. A chemical shift artifact can be seen at the well-defined margin between the mass and the orbital fat ➡.

Cavernous Hemangioma, Orbit

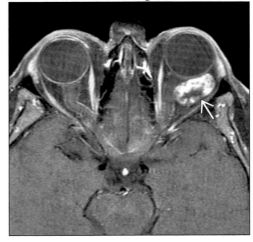

Axial T1 C+ FS MR shows a large intraconal cavernous hemangioma. Characteristic patchy enhancement of the lesion is seen after contrast administration ➡.

VASCULAR LESIONS OF ORBIT

(Left) Axial CECT demonstrates a large infiltrative orbitofacial infantile hemangioma. Preseptal ➡ and retrobulbar ➡ components are present, as well as involvement of the suprazygomatic masticator space ➡. **(Right)** Axial T1WI MR shows an infantile capillary hemangioma with an atypical, primarily retrobulbar location ➡. Numerous curvilinear and punctate high velocity flow voids ➡ are evident.

Infantile Hemangioma, Orbit

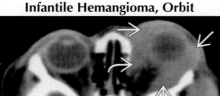

Infantile Hemangioma, Orbit

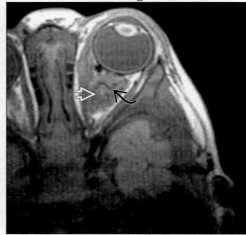

(Left) Axial CECT reveals a nonenhancing, low-density, mildly lobulated intraconal and extraconal lymphatic malformation ➡ without a significant venous component. **(Right)** Axial T2WI FS MR shows a multilocular mass typical of orbital lymphatic malformation. Characteristic fluid-fluid levels are present ➡, representing sequelae of prior hemorrhage.

Lymphatic Malformation, Orbit

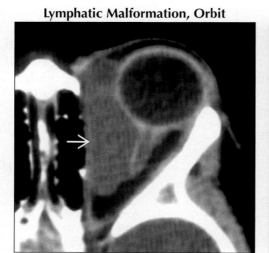

Lymphatic Malformation, Orbit

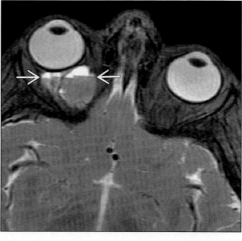

(Left) Axial T1 C+ FS MR shows a lobular intraconal mass ➡, isointense with mild irregular marginal enhancement ➡, indicating mixed lymphatic and venous vascular elements. **(Right)** Coronal T1 C+ FS MR demonstrates a somewhat lobular but homogeneously enhancing intraconal mass ➡, representing a venous malformation with a minimal lymphangiomatous component.

Venolymphatic Malformation, Orbit

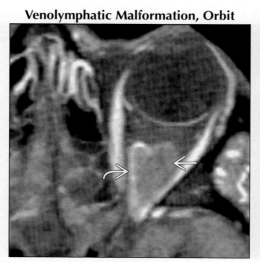

Venous Malformation, Orbit

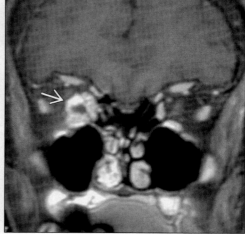

VASCULAR LESIONS OF ORBIT

Venous Varix, Orbit
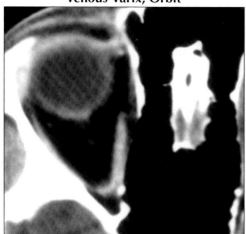

Venous Varix, Orbit
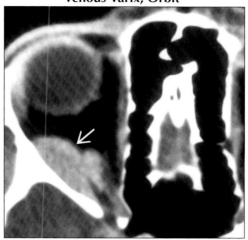

(Left) Axial CECT with patient breathing normally shows an essentially normal appearance of the orbit without a vascular mass evident. *(Right)* Axial CECT in the same patient during Valsalva maneuver shows a distensible venous varix ➡. The varix has contiguity with the systemic venous system and thus enlarges when venous outflow is impeded.

Arteriovenous Malformation, Orbit
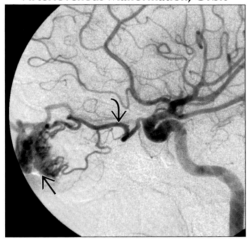

Dural Arteriovenous Fistula, Orbit
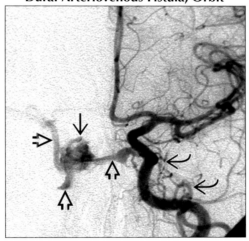

(Left) Lateral angiography reveals a large anterior orbital arteriovenous malformation ➡ with a dominant internal carotid supply via an enlarged ophthalmic artery ➡. *(Right)* Anteroposterior angiography shows an arteriovenous fistula of the orbit ➡ fed primarily via dural branches from the external carotid ➡, with characteristic early filling of orbital venous structures ➡.

Carotid-Cavernous Fistula
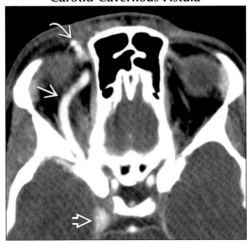

Hemangiopericytoma, Orbit
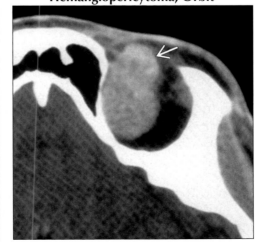

(Left) Axial CECT demonstrates an enlarged superior ophthalmic vein ➡, secondary to carotid-cavernous fistula. Distended cavernous sinus ➡ and orbital vessels ➡ typical of carotid-cavernous fistula are evident. *(Right)* Axial CECT shows a relatively well-defined hyperdense mass in the left orbit ➡, representing a hemangiopericytoma.

ACCIDENTAL FOREIGN BODIES IN ORBIT

DIFFERENTIAL DIAGNOSIS

Common
- Orbital Foreign Body, Metal

Less Common
- Orbital Foreign Body, Glass
- Orbital Foreign Body, Wood & Organic
- Orbital Foreign Body, Dirt & Debris
- Orbital Foreign Body, Miscellaneous

Rare but Important
- Orbital Foreign Body, Occult
- Orbital Foreign Body, Granuloma

ESSENTIAL INFORMATION

Key Differential Diagnosis Issues
- Imaging strategy
  - CT study of choice to detect & characterize orbital foreign body (FB)
    - Dedicated thin-section orbit; routine head CT inadequate resolution
    - Should not mistake physiologic or degenerative calcification for FB
    - Assess for occult FB in all trauma cases
    - Look for intracranial penetration whenever orbital FB present
    - CT also study of choice when screening patients for orbital metal prior to MR
  - Plain radiography insensitive for many FBs
  - Ultrasound (US) may be helpful but limited with posterior orbit FBs
  - MR contraindicated until FB known to be non-ferromagnetic
    - MR may be useful for assessing complications
- Location
  - Position of FB may influence whether removal is indicated
    - Removal of FB from posterior orbit has increased risk of visual or motor injury
  - FB within globe implies perforation
  - Intraocular FB typically passes through anterior segment to reside in posterior segment
- Composition
  - Metallic objects most dense and will have streak artifact on CT
  - Glass denser than bone and often visible on plain films
  - Wood, organic materials, and plastic often not visible with plain films

- Nature of FB may dictate whether removal is necessary
  - Some materials result in toxic effect on eye, such as infection, delayed granuloma

Helpful Clues for Common Diagnoses
- **Orbital Foreign Body, Metal**
  - Key facts
    - Often workplace related: Machined or hammered fragment
    - Firearm and air gun projectiles common
    - Most are biologically inert
    - Should remove elemental copper or iron
    - Copper incites inflammatory response and has toxic effect on retina
    - Iron dissolution causes siderosis and may damage retina
  - Imaging
    - CT: Extremely dense, beam-hardening artifact common
    - Not able to determine metal composition
    - US: Echodense and highly reflective
    - MR: NOT recommended because of risk of FB motion and further orbit damage

Helpful Clues for Less Common Diagnoses
- **Orbital Foreign Body, Glass**
  - Key facts
    - Automobile glass most common
    - Window panes & drinking glasses occasional sources
    - Frameless spectacles more likely to shatter; polycarbonate lenses lowest risk
    - Biologically inert but frequently symptomatic and may migrate
  - Imaging
    - CT: Readily detectable; usually does not induce beam-hardening artifact
    - Higher density than cortical bone, lower density than metal
    - MR: Often obscured by susceptibility artifact, depending on composition
    - US: Echodense and highly reflective
- **Orbital Foreign Body, Wood & Organic**
  - Key facts
    - Tree branches, pencils, chopsticks frequent
    - High risk of cellulitis and abscess
    - Requires exploration and removal
    - Wooden and organic FB similar or lower density than soft tissues; often MISSED on CT

- May have delayed presentation from complications: Cellulitis, abscess, granuloma, or chronic draining sinus
  - Imaging
    - CT: Treated wood has very low density, can be mistaken for air in orbit
    - 2 key differentiating features: Wood has defined linear contours, wood denser than air with wide windows: Window width = 1000, window length = -500
    - Living plant material may be similar to orbital soft tissues and less conspicuous
    - Pencil has characteristic target appearance with low-density periphery and dense graphite core
- **Orbital Foreign Body, Dirt & Debris**
  - Key facts
    - Typically in trauma setting
    - Usually fine or granular material: Dirt, sand, gravel
    - May be unsuspected if patient unconscious or has soft tissue swelling
  - Imaging
    - CT: Material often on surface of eye
    - Hyperdense: More dense than bone, less dense than metal
- **Orbital Foreign Body, Miscellaneous**
  - Key facts
    - Objects range from ordinary to bizarre
    - Blast injuries from explosions frequently cause significant eye injury
    - Animal bite may leave behind tooth
    - Identification of FB important to assess infection and toxin risk

- Imaging
  - CT/MR: Variable depending on object
  - Plastic has very low CT density, similar to air, & has signal void on MR
  - Animal teeth have bone density on CT, low signal on MR

Helpful Clues for Rare Diagnoses
- **Orbital Foreign Body, Occult**
  - Key facts
    - Most often children who may not recognize object penetration
    - Often preserved vision and motility
    - Entry wound may be small
    - All puncture wounds need exploration
  - Imaging
    - CT is study of choice
    - Occult FB may be found anywhere in eye or orbit
- **Orbital Foreign Body, Granuloma**
  - Key facts
    - Localized tissue reaction to foreign body with inflammatory response
    - Most common with organic material as it may penetrate eye unnoticed
    - May readily break with attempted removal; difficult to detect on CT
  - Imaging
    - Mass-like enhancement and surrounding edema associated with FB
    - May mimic orbital abscess or mass

Other Essential Information
- Penetrating trauma in eye, in orbit, in globe; foreign objects

Orbital Foreign Body, Metal

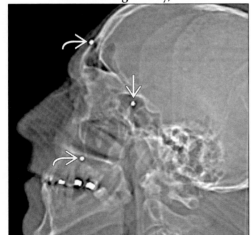

Lateral radiograph shows several small foreign bodies in the face of a shotgun victim ➡. One shot appears to project into the orbit ➡, but its location is indeterminate on this single plain radiograph.

Orbital Foreign Body, Metal

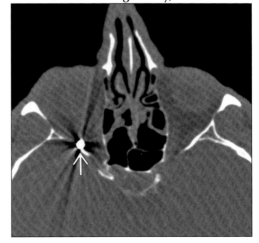

Axial bone CT confirms the location of 1 foreign body lateral to the right orbital apex ➡. The posterior position of object is a relative contraindication to surgical removal. Note the metallic streak artifact.

ACCIDENTAL FOREIGN BODIES IN ORBIT

(Left) Axial NECT shows a small intraocular metallic fragment ➡ with a subtle stellate streak artifact. Penetrating globe injuries commonly occur while hammering a metal object, as in this patient. MR is contraindicated. *(Right)* Bone CT MIPS projection in a different patient reveals a nail fragment ➡ traversing the medial aspect of the right orbit, coursing through the medial rectus muscle, & penetrating into the posterior ethmoid sinus.

Orbital Foreign Body, Metal

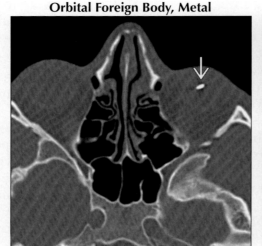

Orbital Foreign Body, Metal

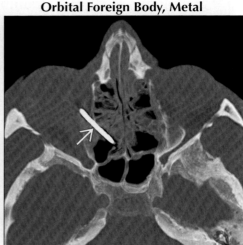

(Left) Axial bone CT demonstrates a hyperdense object in left preseptal tissues ➡. The object has multangular contour with attenuation higher than that of cortical bone but without streak artifact. This is typical for automobile glass. *(Right)* Axial bone CT in a different patient reveals multiple well-defined hyperdense shards of glass ➡ penetrating the left orbit & perforating globe. The patient had fallen face first onto a drinking glass while intoxicated.

Orbital Foreign Body, Glass

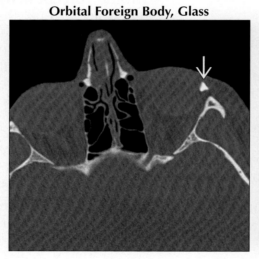

Orbital Foreign Body, Glass

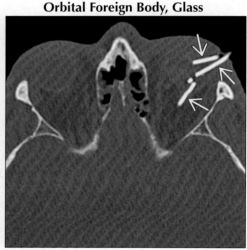

(Left) Coronal NECT demonstrates a pencil penetrating the inferior left extraconal orbit. In cross section, the pencil is a markedly low-density cylinder composed of treated wood ➡, with a hyperdense graphite core ➡. *(Right)* Axial bone CT shows a wooden stick penetrating right orbit and extending through lamina papyracea. Note that object is low in density. Outer layer of cellular material ➡ has soft tissue density, and inner pith has air density ➡.

Orbital Foreign Body, Wood & Organic

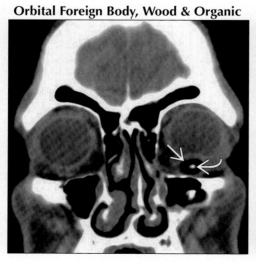

Orbital Foreign Body, Wood & Organic

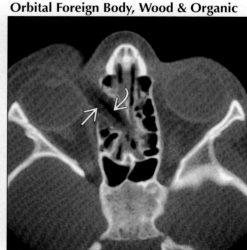

Orbital Foreign Body, Dirt & Debris

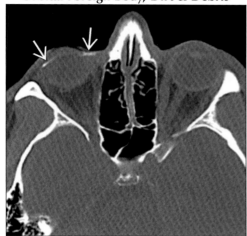

Orbital Foreign Body, Miscellaneous

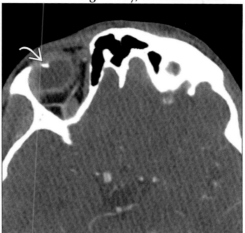

(Left) Axial NECT in a comatose motor vehicle crash victim shows fine hyperdense foreign material ➔ under eyelid. Sand was grossly visible on examination. The eye was irrigated, and the finding was absent on follow-up scan. (Right) Axial CECT through the right orbit in a patient who had been teasing his pet snake reveals a fang embedded in the sclera ➔. Object density is comparable to that of orbital bony walls.

Orbital Foreign Body, Miscellaneous

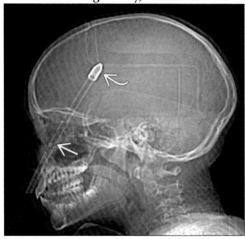

Orbital Foreign Body, Miscellaneous

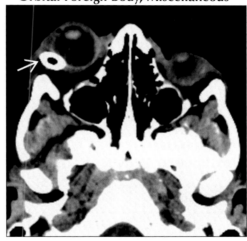

(Left) Lateral radiograph shows a long linear object, the shaft of an arrow, appearing to traverse the orbit ➔ & penetrate orbital roof. Bullet-point arrowhead typically used in target shooting ➔ is seen projecting inside cranium. (Right) Axial NECT in the same patient shows a hollow aluminum arrow shaft passing obliquely through lateral right orbit ➔. The shaft appears to graze sclera with some deformity of globe. Penetration of globe cannot be excluded.

Orbital Foreign Body, Occult

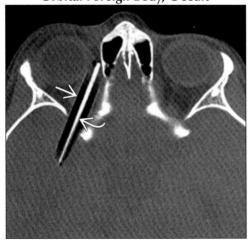

Orbital Foreign Body, Granuloma

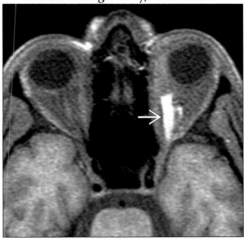

(Left) Axial bone CT in a young child with an unwitnessed fall at school & cut on right eyelid. CT reveals intraorbital pencil with central graphite core ➔ & peripheral wooden shaft ➔, which has a density similar to air. Remarkably there were no visual symptoms. (Right) Axial T1 C+ FS MR in a different patient shows an enhancing lesion in the intraconal orbit ➔. A small twig with granuloma, thought to be from an old hiking injury, was removed during surgery.

SURGICAL DEVICES & TREATMENT EFFECTS IN ORBIT

DIFFERENTIAL DIAGNOSIS

Common
- Surgical Device, Orbit, Intraocular Lens
- Surgical Device, Orbit, Scleral Buckle
- Surgical Device, Orbit, Microplate

Less Common
- Surgical Device, Orbit, Mesh Repair
- Surgical Device, Orbit, Prosthesis
- Surgical Device, Orbit, Vitreous Silicone
- Surgical Device, Orbit, Gas Tamponade

Rare but Important
- Surgical Device, Orbit, Granuloma

ESSENTIAL INFORMATION

Key Differential Diagnosis Issues
- Clinical history
  - Helps to differentiate foreign body from surgical implant
- Location
  - Position of implant usually determines nature of device
  - Malposition should be reported
- Calcification
  - Retinal or scleral physiological calcification may be mistaken for implant

Helpful Clues for Common Diagnoses
- **Surgical Device, Orbit, Intraocular Lens**
  - Key facts
    - Artificial lens placed following phakotomy for treatment of cataract
    - Extremely common in older patients
    - Consists of central optic component with peripheral haptic loops that fixate device within lens capsule
  - Imaging
    - Absence of native lens
    - Unilateral or bilateral
    - Plastic or silicone disc located in posterior chamber of anterior segment
    - Anterior chamber placement less common, just anterior to plane of iris
    - Artificial lens very thin compared to biological lens due to high refractive index of plastic
    - CT: Hyperdense thin short line; haptic loops may be visible as tiny dots in cross section

- MR: Signal void on most sequences; best demonstrated with T2 using contrast of humor fluid signal
- **Surgical Device, Orbit, Scleral Buckle**
  - Key facts
    - Most common conventional treatment for retinal detachment
    - Silicone or plastic device buckles sclera, relieving traction on torn retina, thus allowing it to heal
    - Alternative to less invasive laser photocoagulation for treatment of large or recurrent tears
  - Imaging
    - 2 types of silicone devices: Bands and sponges
    - Silicone band appears as thin dense line; may be circumferential or radial
    - Higher volume silicone sponge has low density; acts as volume filler, used for more severe detachments

- **Surgical Device, Orbit, Microplate**
  - Key facts
    - Very common in reconstructive surgery
    - Used in repair of trauma, correction of anomalies, and cosmetic reconstruction
    - Made of titanium, vitallium (alloy), and stainless steel
  - Imaging
    - Thin malleable metal plates with short fixation screws
    - Linear, L-shaped, X-shaped, T-shaped
    - Associated post-traumatic or congenital deformities

Helpful Clues for Less Common Diagnoses
- **Surgical Device, Orbit, Mesh Repair**
  - Key facts
    - Used to repair large bony orbital defect or severely comminuted fractures
    - Titanium mesh sheet with holes for fixation
  - Imaging
    - Appears as multiple lines in cross section across osseous defect
    - May be loaded with transplanted bone
- **Surgical Device, Orbit, Prosthesis**
  - Key facts
    - Restoration of orbital appearance from enucleation, phthisis, or malformation
    - Deep orbital implant component serves as volume filler

SURGICAL DEVICES & TREATMENT EFFECTS IN ORBIT

- Deep implant may be inert plastic (methylmethacrylate) or may be porous (hydroxyapatite) to allow for biological ingrowth and native movement
- Superficial ocular component provides cosmetic facade (painted plastic)
  ○ Imaging
    - Plastic intraorbital implant molds to contours of post-treatment socket
    - Plastic superficial ocular prosthesis is dome- or crescent-shaped
    - Plastic appears hyperdense on CT; hypointense on most MR sequences
    - Porous intraorbital implant shows enhancement on CT and MR due to vascular ingrowth
    - Fluid signal ellipsoid gel expanders also used for managing orbit volume
- **Surgical Device, Orbit, Vitreous Silicone**
  ○ Key facts
    - Treatment of retinal detachment particularly due to macular holes
    - Most common preparation is polydimethylsiloxane
    - Some risk of complication related to chemical effects of silicone and may be subsequently removed
  ○ Imaging
    - Hyperdense on CT compared to normal vitreous; due to silicone atoms
    - Hyperintense on T1 MR relative to normal vitreous
    - Significant variability of signal on T2 MR, dependent on oil viscosity

- Prominent chemical shift artifact characteristic
- Fat saturation may result in silicone suppression, depending on pulse width
- **Surgical Device, Orbit, Gas Tamponade**
  ○ Key facts
    - Treatment of retinal detachment particularly due to macular holes
    - Often in conjunction with vitrectomy
    - C3F8 perfluoropropane most common, slowly absorbed over several weeks
  ○ Imaging
    - Gas density within posterior segment
    - Concomitant scleral buckle, silicone oil, or other tamponade device often present

Helpful Clues for Rare Diagnoses
- **Surgical Device, Orbit, Granuloma**
  ○ Key facts
    - Localized tissue reaction to foreign body with inflammatory response
    - Fibrous tissue in chronic setting
  ○ Imaging
    - Surrounding edema and enhancement; may mimic abscess
    - Surgical device abuts granuloma

SELECTED REFERENCES
1. Lane JI et al: Retinal detachment: imaging of surgical treatments and complications. Radiographics. 23(4):983-94, 2003
2. Ainbinder DJ et al: Anophthalmic socket and orbital implants. Role of CT and MR imaging. Radiol Clin North Am. 36(6):1133-47, xi, 1998

Surgical Device, Orbit, Intraocular Lens

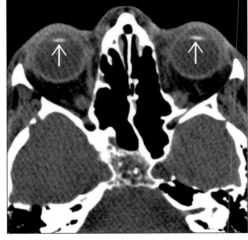

Axial NECT shows bilateral intraocular prosthetic lenses, seen as thin dense lines of acrylic plastic ➡ in the expected locations of the native lenses.

Surgical Device, Orbit, Intraocular Lens

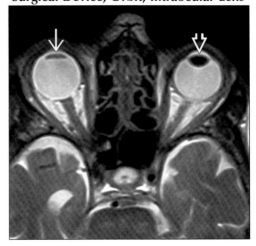

Axial T2WI MR demonstrates the typical appearance of a prosthetic lens as a thin disc of low signal in the right eye ➡. By comparison, the native lens in the left eye ➡ is much thicker.

SURGICAL DEVICES & TREATMENT EFFECTS IN ORBIT

(Left) Axial NECT shows 2 dense dots ➡ at the peripheral aspect of the anterior eye segment, representing cross sections of 1 of the haptic loops that fixates the artificial lens in the native lens capsule. (Right) Axial T2WI MR shows bilateral scleral bands ➡. Note the waist-like contour deformity of the globes caused by the circumferential constriction of the bands.

Surgical Device, Orbit, Intraocular Lens

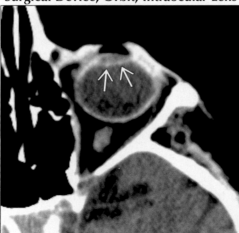

Surgical Device, Orbit, Scleral Buckle

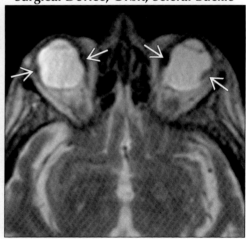

(Left) Axial NECT shows a typical scleral band on the right, seen as a thin high-density silicone circlet ➡. On the left, the band is augmented by a heterogeneous low-density silicone sponge ➡, which provides more bulk & creates a greater degree of scleral buckling. (Right) Axial NECT using MIPS projection shows internal fixation using microplates ➡ & short screws ➡ for repair of fractures involving inferior orbital rim & medial orbit near lacrimal fossa.

Surgical Device, Orbit, Scleral Buckle

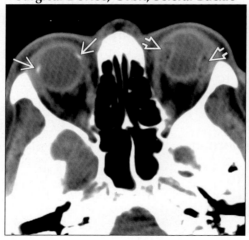

Surgical Device, Orbit, Microplate

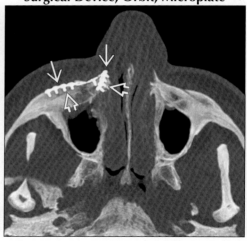

(Left) Bone CT with 3D rendering shows microplate fixation of extensive orbital and facial fractures. Surface rendering is useful for assessing the structural and cosmetic result of facial reconstruction. (Right) Coronal NECT shows segments of titanium mesh along the medial orbital wall ➡, used for repair of severe lamina papyracea fracture.

Surgical Device, Orbit, Microplate

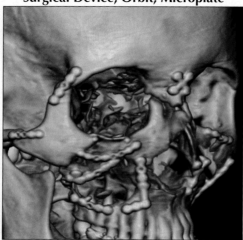

Surgical Device, Orbit, Mesh Repair

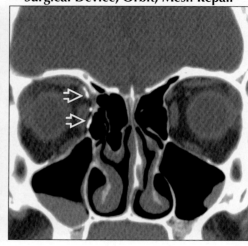

Surgical Device, Orbit, Prosthesis

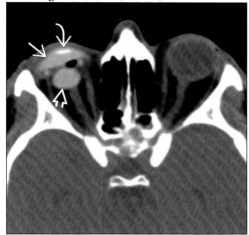

Surgical Device, Orbit, Prosthesis

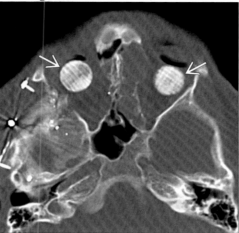

(Left) Axial NECT shows a right ocular prosthesis. The broad dome of plastic ➡ forms the cosmetic surface of the implant, with a custom painted iris ➡. The deeper component ➡ is a volume filler that molds to the contours of the post-treatment orbit. (Right) Axial bone CT shows bilateral ocular prostheses ➡. These spherical implants serve as volume fillers and can show native movement following extraocular muscle attachment & tissue ingrowth.

Surgical Device, Orbit, Vitreous Silicone

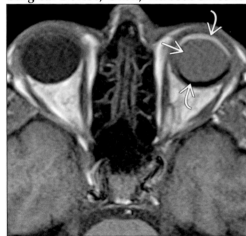

Surgical Device, Orbit, Vitreous Silicone

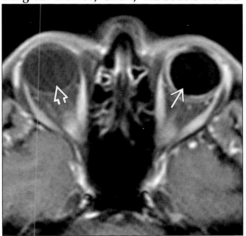

(Left) Axial T1WI MR shows abnormal intermediate signal in the left globe ➡ that is hyperintense compared to the contralateral vitreous, with associated striking chemical shift artifact ➡. (Right) Axial T1 C+ FS MR shows the markedly suppressed signal of the silicone oil due to fat-suppression pulse ➡. The right vitreous shows normal hypointensity ➡.

Surgical Device, Orbit, Gas Tamponade

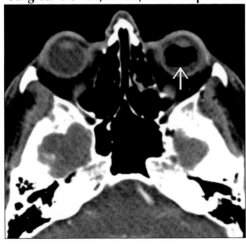

Surgical Device, Orbit, Granuloma

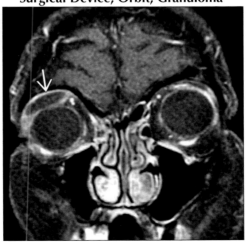

(Left) Axial CECT shows intravitreal gas density ➡ relating to tamponade for the treatment of retinal detachment. (Right) Coronal T2WI FS MR shows a lesion in the superolateral orbit with central low signal and rim enhancement ➡ that mimics an abscess. At surgery, granulomatous and fibrous reaction was found in association with a fragment of silicone scleral sponge (not shown).

INTRAOCULAR CALCIFICATIONS (CT)

DIFFERENTIAL DIAGNOSIS

Common
- Drusen

Less Common
- Retinoblastoma
- Phthisis Bulbi
- Ocular Calcification, Miscellaneous

Rare but Important
- Osteoma, Choroidal

ESSENTIAL INFORMATION

Helpful Clues for Common Diagnoses
- **Drusen**
  - Key facts: Hyaline calcific deposits
    - Common in elderly; 0.3% of patients
    - Usually incidental but may be associated with macular degeneration
  - Imaging: Punctate hyperdensity
    - Often at optic nerve head or macula but may occur anywhere along retina
    - No soft tissue mass but may be associated with retinal detachment

Helpful Clues for Less Common Diagnoses
- **Retinoblastoma**
  - Key facts: Primary retinal malignancy
    - Most common childhood ocular tumor
    - Presents with leukocoria
    - 60% sporadic; 40% inherited
  - Imaging: Calcification > 90%
    - Punctate, speckled, or flocculent Ca++
    - Avid enhancement

- Retinal detachment not unusual
- Unilateral in 75%
- Look for coincident contralateral, pineal, or suprasellar tumor

- **Phthisis Bulbi**
  - Key facts: End-stage condition of eye
    - Potential causes include trauma, infection, inflammation, chronic retinal detachment, and radiation
    - Pediatric causes include microphthalmia, retinopathy of prematurity, and Coats disease
    - Enucleation and prosthesis may be indicated for pain or cosmesis
  - Imaging: Shrunken crenated globe
    - Irregular coarse nodular calcification
    - Optic nerve atrophy common

- **Ocular Calcification, Miscellaneous**
  - Key facts: Nonspecific, degenerative
    - Increases with calcium disturbance
  - Imaging: Punctate hyperdensity
    - No soft tissue component
    - Preseptal sclera and pterygium
    - Trochlear sling of superior oblique

Helpful Clues for Rare Diagnoses
- **Osteoma, Choroidal**
  - Key facts: Benign osseous choristoma
    - Young adult women
    - Progressive vision loss
  - Imaging: Plate-like calcific plaque
    - Posterior pole, juxtapapillary location
    - Mild enhancement
    - Marrow space when large

Drusen

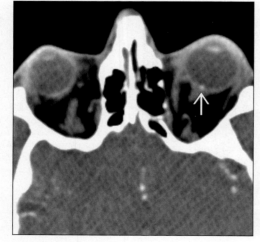

Axial CECT shows punctate calcification at the site of insertion of the left optic nerve ➡. When located at the optic nerve head, bulky drusen may mimic papilledema on funduscopy.

Drusen

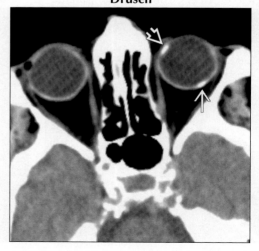

Axial NECT shows calcification near the posterior pole of the left eye ➡ in a patient with macular degeneration. Additional nonspecific degenerative calcification is seen anteriorly ➡.

Retinoblastoma
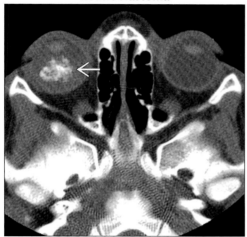

Retinoblastoma
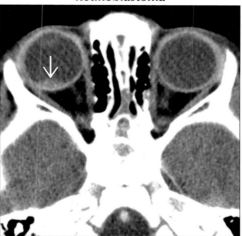

(Left) Axial bone CT shows dense flocculent calcification within an intraocular mass in the right eye of a child ➡. Calcification of large retinoblastomas may appear to be centered within the vitreous, despite the peripheral origin. (Right) Axial CECT shows a dense faintly calcified and plaque-like peripheral mass ➡ in the posterior aspect of the right globe in a child with leukocoria.

Phthisis Bulbi
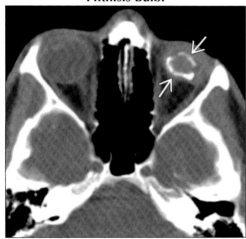

Phthisis Bulbi
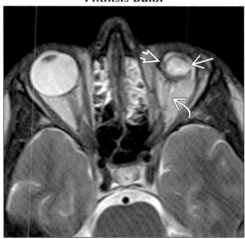

(Left) Axial NECT shows a small crenated left globe with irregular coarse peripheral calcification ➡. (Right) Axial T2WI MR in the same patient shows corresponding appearance of a small left globe ➡. Calcification is less obvious on MR, appearing as a peripheral signal void ➡. Note the severely atrophic left optic nerve ➡.

Ocular Calcification, Miscellaneous
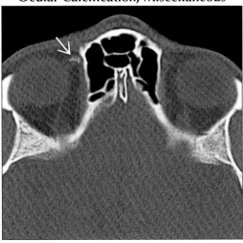

Osteoma, Choroidal
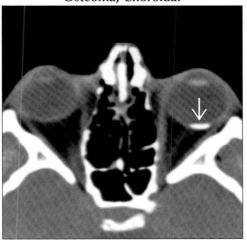

(Left) Axial bone CT shows irregular degenerative calcification adjacent to the right eye in the superomedial orbit anteriorly ➡, corresponding to the trochlea of the right superior oblique muscle. (Right) Axial NECT shows a densely calcified plaque-like mass at the posterior aspect of the globe ➡ in a young woman with monocular vision loss.

LEUKOCORIA

DIFFERENTIAL DIAGNOSIS

Common
- Retinoblastoma

Less Common
- Retinal Detachment
- Retinopathy of Prematurity
- Persistent Hyperplastic Primary Vitreous
- Coats Disease
- Coloboma
- Cataract, Congenital

Rare but Important
- Toxocariasis, Orbit
- Ocular Melanoma, Amelanotic
- Retinal Dysplasia

ESSENTIAL INFORMATION

Helpful Clues for Common Diagnoses
- **Retinoblastoma**
  - Key facts
    - Primary retinal malignancy, PNET type
    - Most common childhood ocular tumor
    - 60% sporadic; 40% inherited
    - RB1 gene mutation
  - Imaging
    - Punctate, speckled, or flocculent calcification in > 90%
    - Strong enhancement
    - Retinal detachment not unusual
    - Unilateral in 75%
    - Look for coincident contralateral, suprasellar, or pineal tumor in patients with inherited disease

Helpful Clues for Less Common Diagnoses
- **Retinal Detachment**
  - Key facts
    - Separation between inner sensory retina & outer pigmented epithelium
    - Myriad etiologies, including vascular, inflammatory, neoplastic, congenital, traumatic, & other processes
    - 3 mechanisms: Rhegmatogenous (tear), tractional (adhesions), and exudative (tumor or inflammation)
  - Imaging
    - Detached retina bulges toward vitreous, with underlying biconvex collection
    - Leaves of retina converge at optic disk, resulting in "V" contour

- Signal varies depending on content
- Often bloody or proteinaceous fluid
- Hyperdense on CT
- Hyperintense on most MR sequences

- **Retinopathy of Prematurity**
  - Key facts
    - Synonym: Retrolental fibroplasia
    - Fibrovascular proliferation of immature retina, presumably related to hyperoxia of extrauterine NICU environment
  - Imaging
    - Microphthalmia
    - Retinal detachment common, often with blood-fluid levels
    - Ca++ rare except in advanced stages

- **Persistent Hyperplastic Primary Vitreous**
  - Key facts
    - Primary vitreous = fetal ocular hyaloid vascular tissue
    - Normally regresses at 7 months gestation
    - Bilateral lesions typically syndromic, e.g., Norrie and Warburg syndromes
  - Imaging
    - Small globe
    - Hyperdense tissue in globe on CT
    - Hyperintense on T1WI & T2WI
    - Enhancing retrolental hyaloid remnant
    - Retinal detachment common

- **Coats Disease**
  - Key facts
    - Underlying lesion is retinal telangiectasia
    - Subretinal exudate causes retinitis and subsequent detachment
  - Imaging
    - Retinal detachment is *sine qua non*
    - Hyperdense exudate on CT
    - Hyperintense on T1WI and T2WI
    - Occasionally calcifies (~ 10%)

- **Coloboma**
  - Key facts
    - Defect of embryonic ocular cleft
    - Syndromic associations (e.g., CHARGE)
    - Morning glory anomaly is variation
    - Excavated defect on funduscopy
  - Imaging
    - May occur anywhere in eye; defects at disc are visible on imaging
    - Defect at optic nerve head with outpouching of vitreous
    - May be associated with microphthalmia &/or secondary cyst

LEUKOCORIA

- **Cataract, Congenital**
  - Key facts
    - Opacification of lens that presents from birth to 6 months of age
    - Bilateral cataracts often syndromic, including genetic, metabolic, infectious, gestational, and other processes
  - Imaging
    - Best seen with direct visualization
    - Shape & location of lesion indicate timing & etiology of insult
    - Often limited to central portion of lens

Helpful Clues for Rare Diagnoses

- **Toxocariasis, Orbit**
  - Key facts
    - *Toxocara canis/cati* (dog/cat roundworm)
    - Larvae migrate to eye from intestine
    - Sclerosing endophthalmitis with small eosinophilic abscess
  - Imaging
    - Uveoscleral thickening and nodularity
    - Subretinal exudate at site of larval infiltration, with variable hyperintensity
- **Ocular Melanoma, Amelanotic**
  - Key facts
    - Primary uveal tract malignancy
    - Most common adult ocular tumor
  - Imaging
    - US for initial evaluation and surveillance
    - MR or CT to assess retrobulbar invasion
    - Less intrinsic T1 signal when amelanotic
    - Moderate enhancement
    - Retinal detachment common

- **Retinal Dysplasia**
  - Key facts
    - Associated with congenital syndromes
  - Imaging
    - Retinal detachment, hyperintense fluid
    - Variably enhancing dysplastic tissue

Alternative Differential Approaches

- Calcification
  - Calcification present
    - Retinoblastoma (> 90%)
    - Late inflammatory or traumatic changes
  - Calcification absent
    - Persistent hyperplastic primary vitreous
    - Coats disease
    - Retinopathy of prematurity
    - Coloboma
    - Toxocariasis
- Globe size
  - Enlarged globe
    - Coloboma, except with microphthalmia
  - Normal globe size
    - Retinoblastoma, except bulky tumor
    - Retinal detachment
    - Coats disease
    - Toxocariasis
  - Small globe
    - Persistent hyperplastic primary vitreous
    - Retinopathy of prematurity
    - Coloboma, with microphthalmia

SELECTED REFERENCES

1. Kadom N et al: Radiological reasoning: leukocoria in a child. AJR Am J Roentgenol. 191(3 Suppl):S40-4, 2008

Retinoblastoma

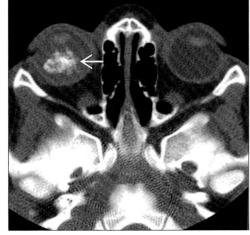

Axial NECT shows dense flocculent calcification ➡ centrally within an intraocular mass in the right eye of a child.

Retinoblastoma

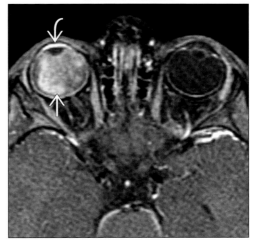

Axial T1WI FS MR reveals a bulky enhancing tumor ➡ that fills and slightly enlarges the right eye of a child. Enhancement in the anterior chamber ➡ is a poor prognostic sign.

Retinal Detachment

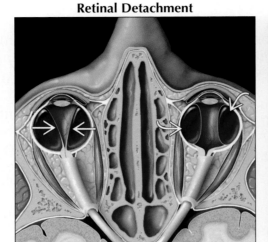

(Left) Graphic shows a detached retina in the right eye ➡. The retinal attachment at the optic nerve head results in the characteristic "V" shape. By comparison, choroidal detachment typically has a lenticular contour, as demonstrated in the left eye ➡. *(Right)* Axial T2WI MR shows a retinal detachment ➡ at the lateral aspect of the right eye. Detachment is often related to an underlying lesion, such as the ocular melanoma ➡ present in this patient.

Retinal Detachment

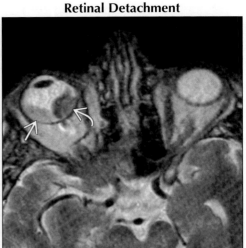

Retinopathy of Prematurity

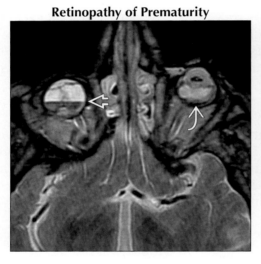

(Left) Axial T2WI FS MR shows bilateral small globes with a heterogeneous signal. Blood-fluid level is evident on the right ➡. Peripheral low signal on the left represents calcification ➡ due to advanced disease. *(Right)* Axial CECT shows enhancing tissue ➡ behind the lens of the left eye, representing persistent primary vitreous. A remnant of the hyaloid artery is seen as intense linear enhancement ➡.

Persistent Hyperplastic Primary Vitreous

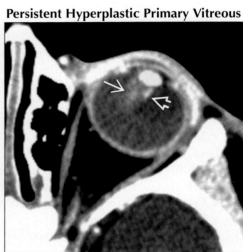

Persistent Hyperplastic Primary Vitreous

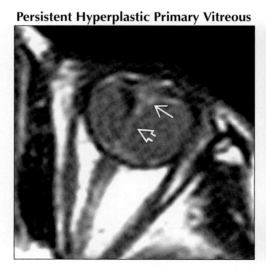

(Left) Axial T1 C+ MR shows triangular retrolental enhancing tissue ➡ and stalk-like hyaloid remnant ➡ representing failure of involution of embryonic fibrovascular tissue. The contour of this tissue has been described as resembling a "martini glass." *(Right)* Axial NECT shows ill-defined hyperdensity in the posterior aspect of the left globe ➡, representing subretinal exudate. A vague V-shaped contour of the vitreous ➡ is typical of retinal detachment.

Coats Disease

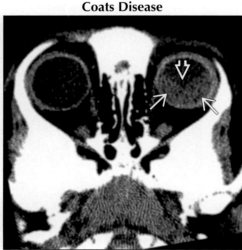

LEUKOCORIA

Coats Disease

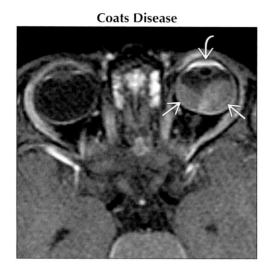

Coloboma

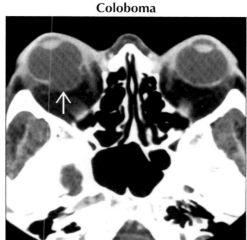

(Left) Axial T1 C+ FS MR shows moderately hyperintense subretinal exudates involving the left eye ➡. Anterior hyperintensity probably relates to anterior chamber cholesterolosis ➡. *(Right)* Axial NECT shows an optic disc coloboma ➡, seen as a dehiscence of the posterior globe through a broad defect centered at the location of the optic nerve head.

Cataract, Congenital

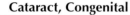
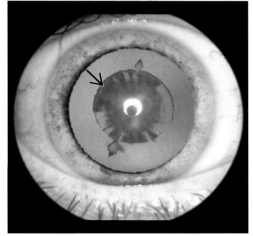

Toxocariasis, Orbit

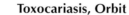
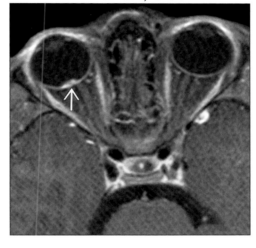

(Left) Clinical photograph shows opacity of the central portion of the lens corresponding to the fetal nucleus ➡, with relatively clear surrounding cortex. *(Right)* Axial T1 C+ FS MR shows ocular toxocariasis manifesting as uveoscleral nodularity in the posterior aspect of the right globe ➡. Hyperintensity is attributable to intrinsic signal of subretinal effusion and associated enhancement.

Ocular Melanoma, Amelanotic

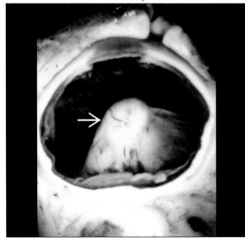

Retinal Dysplasia

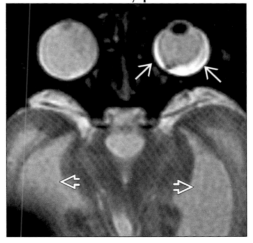

(Left) Gross pathology shows a large exophytic mass ➡ projecting into the vitreous from the posterior aspect of the eye. Melanoma was confirmed histologically, but the mass is largely without pigmentation. *(Right)* Axial T2WI MR in a newborn with Walker-Warburg syndrome shows peripheral T2 hyperintensity of the left globe ➡, indicating retinal dysplasia and associated subretinal hemorrhage. Note the presence of marked ventriculomegaly ➡.

DIFFERENTIAL DIAGNOSIS

Common
- Thyroid Ophthalmopathy
- Cavernous Malformation, Orbit
- Mucocele, Sinonasal
- Polyposis, Sinonasal

Less Common
- Lymphoproliferative Lesions, Orbit
- Metastasis, Orbit
- SCCa, Sinonasal
- Venous Varix, Orbit
- Meningioma, Skull Base
- Benign Mixed Tumor, Lacrimal

Rare but Important
- Esthesioneuroblastoma
- Idiopathic Orbital Inflammatory Disease (Pseudotumor)
- Lymphatic Malformation, Orbit
- Adenoid Cystic Carcinoma, Lacrimal

ESSENTIAL INFORMATION

Key Differential Diagnosis Issues
- Uni- or bilateral painless protrusion of globe
- Term "exophthalmos" reserved for proptosis due to endocrine dysfunction
- Bilateral: Measured clinically with Hertel exophthalmometer
- Unilateral: > 2 mm asymmetry of orbits
- Most common cause is thyroid ophthalmopathy (Graves ophthalmopathy)
- Remaining causes
  - Orbital mass lesion
  - Orbital wall lesion
  - Sinonasal disease
- Imaging strategy
  - CT typically 1st line study
    - > 2/3 of globe anterior to line drawn between lateral orbital rims
  - MR best for further characterization of mass & evaluation of soft tissues

Helpful Clues for Common Diagnoses
- **Thyroid Ophthalmopathy**
  - Key facts
    - Autoimmune inflammatory condition associated with thyroid dysfunction
    - Enlarged extraocular muscles (EOM) & proliferation of orbital fat
  - Imaging
    - Enlarged EOM sparing tendinous insertions
    - ↑ Orbital fat alone or enlarged large muscles
- **Cavernous Malformation, Orbit**
  - Key facts
    - Often called cavernous hemangioma
    - Endothelial-lined cavernous spaces
  - Imaging
    - Well circumscribed, avidly enhancing
    - Anywhere in orbit; intraconal most often
- **Mucocele, Sinonasal**
  - Key facts
    - Expansion of obstructed sinus/air cells
    - Ethmoid or frontal ⇒ proptosis
  - Imaging
    - Concentrated secretions result in variable imaging appearance
    - CT: Smoothly expanded, thinned bone contours, displaces adjacent structures; may be hyperdense
    - MR: Often T1 hyperintense, subtle rim enhancement
- **Polyposis, Sinonasal**
  - Key facts
    - Associated with asthma, allergy, cystic fibrosis, & aspirin insensitivity
  - Imaging
    - CT: Multiple lobulated masses, some sinuses obstructed; if severe, sinus expansion with bone thinning
    - MR: Heterogeneous signal with fungal infection

Helpful Clues for Less Common Diagnoses
- **Lymphoproliferative Lesions, Orbit**
  - Key facts
    - Wide spectrum of disease
    - Lymphoid hyperplasia ⇒ lymphoma
    - Intraconal, conal, extraconal (lacrimal)
  - Imaging
    - CT/MR: Solid, homogeneously enhancing
    - Most commonly extraconal
- **Metastasis, Orbit**
  - Key facts
    - Anywhere in orbit or orbit wall
    - Soft tissues/globe: Primary tumor from breast, lung, melanoma
    - Orbital walls: Primary tumor from prostate most often
    - May be painful if rapid growth

○ Imaging
- Single/multiple enhancing orbital mass(es) or destructive orbit wall mass
- **SCCa, Sinonasal**
  ○ Key facts
  - Most common sinonasal malignancy
  - Maxillary sinus > nasal cavity > ethmoid
  ○ Imaging
  - CT: Destruction of sinus & orbital walls
  - MR: Heterogeneous invasive tumor
- **Venous Varix, Orbit**
  ○ Key facts
  - Low-flow venous malformation
  - Most often retrobulbar and extraconal; frequently superolateral
  ○ Imaging
  - Variable contour from tubular to ovoid
  - Marked enhancement
  - Distends with Valsalva
- **Meningioma, Skull Base**
  ○ Key facts
  - Most common intracranial tumor
  - Meningioma of sphenoid wing may invade orbital wall
  ○ Imaging
  - CT: En plaque lesion often subtle
  - Sclerotic expanded lateral orbit wall
- **Benign Mixed Tumor, Lacrimal**
  ○ Key facts
  - Synonym: Pleomorphic adenoma
  - Progressive proptosis, lid swelling, ptosis
  ○ Imaging
  - CT: Diffusely enlarged gland with scalloped bone

- MR: Heterogeneously enhancing, T2 intense mass

Helpful Clues for Rare Diagnoses
- **Esthesioneuroblastoma**
  ○ Key facts
  - Malignant tumor of olfactory recess
  - Orbital & intracranial invasion frequent
  ○ Imaging
  - CT: Invasive homogeneous mass
  - MR: Homogeneous T2 mass with moderate enhancement
- **Idiopathic Orbital Inflammatory Disease (Pseudotumor)**
  ○ Key facts
  - Principal cause of *painful* proptosis
  - Previously treated disease with more fibrosis may have little/no pain
  ○ Imaging
  - Diffuse enhancing infiltrative or tumefactive process
- **Lymphatic Malformation, Orbit**
  ○ Key facts
  - Congenital malformation
  - Children or young adults
  ○ Imaging
  - Cystic mass with fluid-fluid levels
- **Adenoid Cystic Carcinoma, Lacrimal**
  ○ Key facts
  - Clinically painless or painful proptosis
  ○ Imaging
  - Diffusely enlarged enhancing gland
  - Erodes lateral wall of orbit

Thyroid Ophthalmopathy

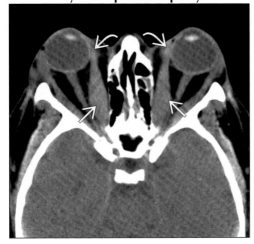

Axial NECT demonstrates symmetric proptosis with bilateral enlargement of medial rectus muscles ➥ and sparing of tendinous insertions at globe ➥. There is also a mild prominence of orbital fat.

Cavernous Malformation, Orbit

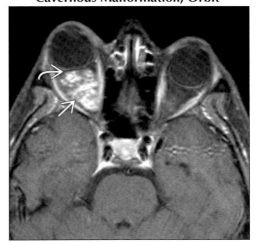

Axial T1 C+ FS MR shows a heterogeneously enhancing well-defined retrobulbar mass ➥ displacing the globe anteriorly and flattening its posterior margin ➥. This patient had slowly progressive proptosis.

Mucocele, Sinonasal

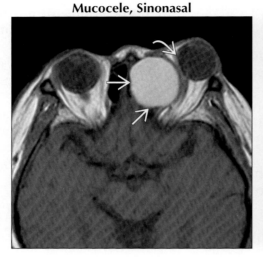

Polyposis, Sinonasal

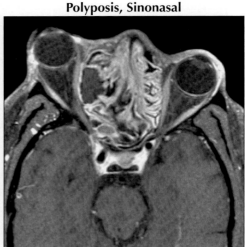

(Left) Axial T1WI MR shows left proptosis from an intrinsically hyperintense mass centered in the left ethmoid air cells ➡. This mucocele deforms the medial orbital wall and left globe ➡, displacing it anterolaterally. *(Right)* Axial T1 C+ MR demonstrates a heterogeneous mass expanding the ethmoids and deforming the right medial rectus. There is an infiltration of orbital fat. The smooth expansile contour of the ethmoid suggests chronic sinus disease.

Lymphoproliferative Lesions, Orbit

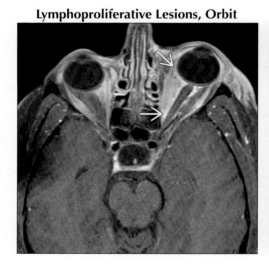

Metastasis, Orbit

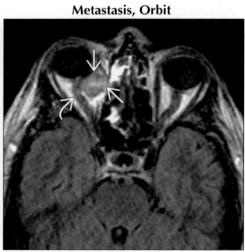

(Left) Axial T1 C+ FS MR reveals a left proptosis that had developed over 1 month secondary to infiltrative, predominantly intraconal enhancing soft tissue ➡. This was proven to be diffuse large B-cell lymphoma. *(Right)* Axial FLAIR MR demonstrates a mild right proptosis from an intraconal heterogeneous mass ➡ that abuts and displaces the right optic nerve ➡, which appears subtly hyperintense. Final pathologic diagnosis was melanoma metastasis.

SCCa, Sinonasal

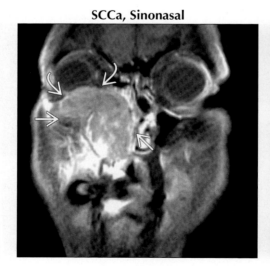

Venous Varix, Orbit

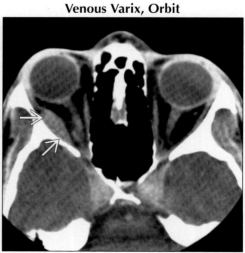

(Left) Coronal T1 C+ FS MR shows a large heterogeneously enhancing destructive mass ➡ arising from the right maxillary sinus, presenting with right proptosis. Orbit invasion ➡ necessitated surgical exenteration at time of maxillectomy. *(Right)* Axial CECT performed during Valsalva maneuver reveals an extraconal enhancing mass ➡ lateral to lateral rectus & mild proptosis. The lesion is virtually "invisible" without Valsalva (not shown), clinching diagnosis.

PAINLESS PROPTOSIS IN ADULT

Meningioma, Skull Base

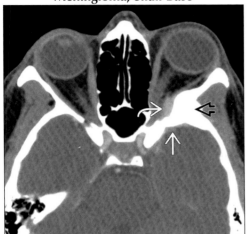

Benign Mixed Tumor, Lacrimal

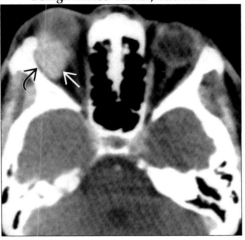

(Left) Axial CECT reveals left proptosis with a deformed thickened hyperostotic lateral orbital wall ⊳. Subtle enhancement of the middle cranial fossa ➡ and intraorbital tissues ➡ is another clue that this is meningioma. *(Right)* Axial CECT shows a well-marginated mass involving the orbital lobe of the lacrimal gland ➡, resulting in proptosis. Scalloped remodeling of the bony lacrimal fossa is evident even at soft tissue windows ⊳.

Esthesioneuroblastoma

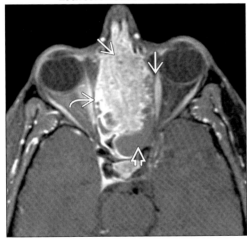

Idiopathic Orbital Inflammatory Disease (Pseudotumor)

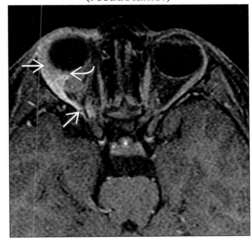

(Left) Axial T1 C+ FS MR reveals an enhancing mass ➡ involving the nasal vault and ethmoid air cells. There is lateral bowing ➡ of the right medial orbital wall but disruption of the orbital wall on the left with slight left proptosis. The mass obstructs the left sphenoid sinus ➡. *(Right)* Axial T1 C+ FS MR shows a diffusely enhancing mass in the right extraconal and intraconal orbit ➡ with mild proptosis. Note the involvement of the sclera ➡ in this patient with diffuse IOID.

Lymphatic Malformation, Orbit

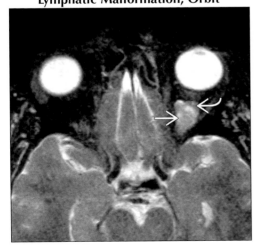

Adenoid Cystic Carcinoma, Lacrimal

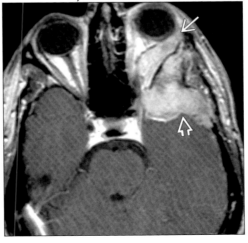

(Left) Axial STIR MR shows a left retrobulbar mass ➡ with heterogeneous signal and subtle layering of blood products within this multiloculated lesion ➡. The patient presented with acute proptosis. *(Right)* Axial T1 C+ MR shows an invasive lacrimal gland adenoid cystic carcinoma filling the lateral extraconal space ➡ of the left orbit. This tumor has invaded through the lateral orbital wall into the middle cranial fossa ➡.

PAINFUL PROPTOSIS IN ADULT

DIFFERENTIAL DIAGNOSIS

Common
- Idiopathic Orbital Inflammatory Disease
- Abscess, Subperiosteal, Orbit
- Cellulitis, Orbit
- Metastasis, Orbit

Less Common
- Lymphoproliferative Lesions, Orbit
- Thyroid Ophthalmopathy
- Sarcoidosis, Orbit
- Wegener Granulomatosis, Orbit

Rare but Important
- Carotid-Cavernous Fistula, Traumatic
- Thrombosis, Cavernous Sinus
- Orbital Malignancy, Other
  - Adenoid Cystic Carcinoma, Lacrimal
  - Adenocarcinoma, Lacrimal
  - Non-Hodgkin Lymphoma, Lacrimal

ESSENTIAL INFORMATION

Key Differential Diagnosis Issues
- Most common cause is pseudotumor
- Pathological processes fall into 4 groups
  - Inflammatory disease
  - Infection
  - Rapidly growing malignancies
  - Acute vascular disease
- Imaging strategies
  - CECT or MR may be 1st line study
  - CT best for acute infections
  - Always check for intracranial spread or vascular thrombosis

Helpful Clues for Common Diagnoses
- **Idiopathic Orbital Inflammatory Disease**
  - Key facts
    - Synonym: Orbital pseudotumor
    - Most common cause of painful proptosis
    - Nongranulomatous inflammatory process
    - Nonspecific infiltration of lymphocytes, plasma cells, neutrophils, & macrophages
    - No known local or systemic cause
  - Imaging
    - Diffuse enhancing, infiltrative, or tumefactive process
    - Anywhere in orbit
    - Does not distort or invade through sclera

- **Abscess, Subperiosteal, Orbit**
  - Key facts
    - Pus collection between orbit bony wall & periorbita, displacing muscles & globe
    - Mostly from ethmoid or frontal sinusitis
    - Abscess can rupture through septum to eyelids or through periorbita to postseptal fat
  - Imaging
    - CT: Rim-enhancing low density collection
    - MR: Hyperintense extraconal collection
- **Cellulitis, Orbit**
  - Key facts
    - Infection involves postseptal tissues
    - Distinct from periorbital preseptal cellulitis
    - Follows trauma, sinusitis, surgery, or extension of preseptal infection
  - Imaging
    - CT/MR: Postseptal fat infiltration
    - Look for cavernous sinus thrombosis
- **Metastasis, Orbit**
  - Key facts
    - Most common primaries: Breast, lung, melanoma
    - Rapid growth of bone or apex involvement → pain
  - Imaging
    - Diffuse, irregular, enhancing, often intraconal mass
    - Single/multiple enhancing orbital mass(es) or destructive orbit wall mass

Helpful Clues for Less Common Diagnoses
- **Lymphoproliferative Lesions, Orbit**
  - Key facts
    - Wide spectrum of disease from lymphoid hyperplasia to non-Hodgkin lymphoma
    - Intraconal, conal, extraconal (lacrimal)
    - Rapid growth &/or malignant lesions may produce pain
  - Imaging
    - Solid enhancing mass or infiltration anywhere in orbit
    - Most commonly extraconal
- **Thyroid Ophthalmopathy**
  - Key facts
    - Autoimmune inflammatory condition associated with thyroid dysfunction
    - Enlarged extraocular muscles (EOM) & proliferation of orbital fat

- Pain often perceived as retrobulbar or evoked on gaze maneuvers
  ○ Imaging
    ▪ Enlarged EOM sparing tendinous insertions
    ▪ Increased orbital fat or EOM alone
- **Sarcoidosis, Orbit**
  ○ Key facts
    ▪ Idiopathic systemic disease of noncaseating granulomas
    ▪ Orbital soft tissue or lacrimal disease in 20-25%; anterior uveitis up to 85%
    ▪ Pain is common, proptosis less common
  ○ Imaging
    ▪ Thickening and enhancement of uveal-scleral coat, intraorbital &/or chiasmatic optic nerve
- **Wegener Granulomatosis, Orbit**
  ○ Key facts
    ▪ Necrotizing granulomatous vasculitis affecting orbit
    ▪ Visual loss, pain, and less often proptosis
  ○ Imaging
    ▪ Irregular thickening and enhancement of sclera, often bilateral
    ▪ Frequently irregular ± enhancing soft tissue mass in orbit
    ▪ Majority have accompanying disease in paranasal sinus &/or nasal cavity

Helpful Clues for Rare Diagnoses
- **Carotid-Cavernous Fistula, Traumatic**
  ○ Key facts

- Arteriovenous fistula between ICA and cavernous sinus
- Proptosis, chemosis, pain, bruit
  ○ Imaging
    ▪ Proptosis, postseptal edema, and enlarged EOM
    ▪ Enlarged enhancing cavernous sinus and superior ophthalmic vein
- **Thrombosis, Cavernous Sinus**
  ○ Key facts
    ▪ Most often complication of sphenoethmoiditis
    ▪ May accompany orbital cellulitis
  ○ Imaging
    ▪ Enlarged heterogeneously enhancing cavernous sinus
    ▪ Enlargement &/or thrombosis of superior ophthalmic vein
    ▪ EOM may enlarge with venous engorgement
- **Adenoid Cystic Carcinoma, Lacrimal**
  ○ Key facts: May recur years later
  ○ Imaging: Enlarged enhancing gland; Ca++ uncommon
- **Adenocarcinoma, Lacrimal**
  ○ Key facts: Ductal type may be very aggressive
  ○ Imaging: Enlarged enhancing gland; Ca++ common
- **Non-Hodgkin Lymphoma, Lacrimal**
  ○ Key facts: Pain usually mild if present
  ○ Imaging: Enlarged enhancing gland; No Ca++
    ▪ MR: T2 signal often hypointense

Idiopathic Orbital Inflammatory Disease

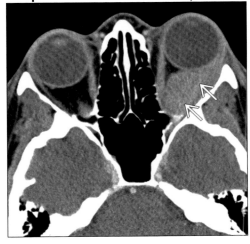

Axial CECT shows marked left proptosis with a moderately enhancing conal and intraconal orbital mass ➡. The mass is indistinguishable from lateral rectus muscle and encases optic nerve/sheath complex.

Idiopathic Orbital Inflammatory Disease

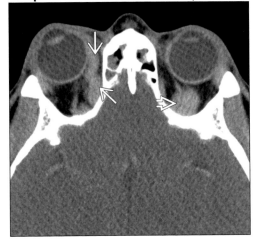

Axial CECT shows bilateral proptosis with enlarged enhancing medial rectus muscle ➡ and superior rectus muscle ➡ in a patient presenting with acute eye pain. This is a myositic form of pseudotumor.

(Left) Axial CECT in a child shows slight left proptosis & marked periorbital swelling ⇒ secondary to a rim-enhancing fluid collection ➡ along medial orbital wall, as well as a subperiosteal abscess secondary to ethmoid sinusitis ⇗. *(Right)* Axial T2WI FS MR demonstrates marked left proptosis with diffusely heterogeneous signal of intraconal ➡ & extraconal ⇒ postseptal fat. Opacification of ethmoid air cells ➡ is responsible for orbital spread of infection.

Abscess, Subperiosteal, Orbit

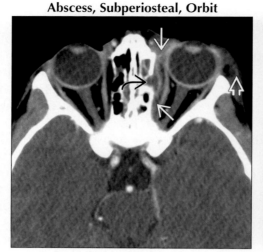

Cellulitis, Orbit

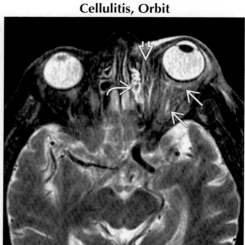

(Left) Axial T1 C+ FS MR shows bilateral enhancing soft tissue masses ➡ arising from sphenoid bone & sphenozygomatic sutures. There is marked distortion of right globe and proptosis. Intracranial extension is clearly evident ⇒. *(Right)* Axial T1WI MR demonstrates left proptosis with homogeneous soft tissue ➡ infiltrating left orbit intraconal fat around the optic nerve ⇗ & medial rectus muscle ⇒. This was found to be diffuse large B-cell lymphoma.

Metastasis, Orbit

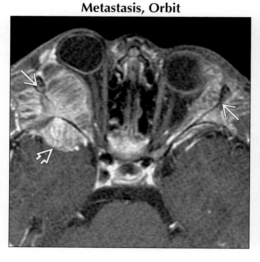

Lymphoproliferative Lesions, Orbit

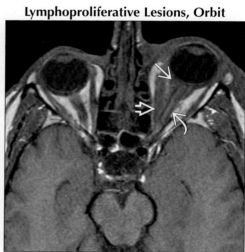

(Left) Axial NECT reveals bilateral marked enlargement of the medial rectus muscles ⇒ but sparing of tendinous insertions ➡. The lateral rectus muscles are relatively spared, and prominent retrobulbar fat also contributes to bilateral proptosis. *(Right)* Axial CECT demonstrates right proptosis with diffusely enlarged enhancing optic nerve sheath ⇒. Enlargement of the medial rectus ➡ is also noted, resulting in crowding at orbital apex ⇗.

Thyroid Ophthalmopathy

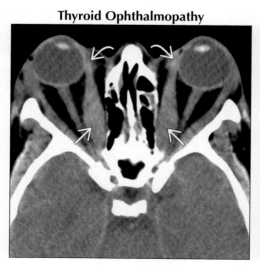

Sarcoidosis, Orbit

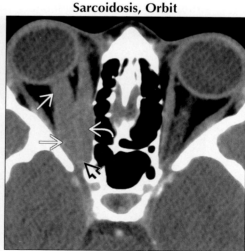

Wegener Granulomatosis, Orbit
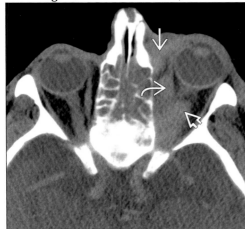

Carotid-Cavernous Fistula, Traumatic
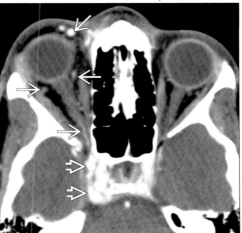

(Left) Axial CECT demonstrates extensive ethmoid sinus opacification adjacent to extensive solid enhancing soft tissue in the left orbit, resulting in mild proptosis. Orbital involvement is intraconal ➡, conal ➡, and extraconal ➡. *(Right)* Axial CECT demonstrates a distended enhancing right cavernous sinus ➡ in a patient with right proptosis. Prominent orbital veins ➡ are also noted, and there is subtle haziness of retrobulbar fat.

Thrombosis, Cavernous Sinus
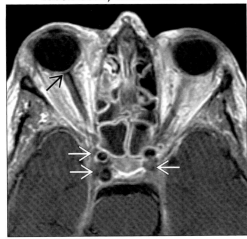

Adenoid Cystic Carcinoma, Lacrimal
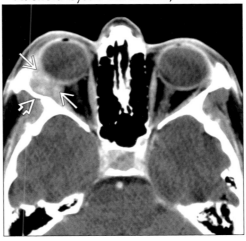

(Left) Axial T1 C+ MR in a patient with sphenoethmoidal sinusitis demonstrates heterogeneous enhancement of both cavernous sinuses with prominent bilateral filling defects ➡, indicating thrombosis. Note bilateral proptosis with subtle tenting of the right posterior globe ➡. *(Right)* Axial CECT shows an irregular noncalcified mass enlarging the lacrimal gland ➡. Scalloping of orbital wall and bone erosion is visible on soft tissue windows ➡.

Adenocarcinoma, Lacrimal
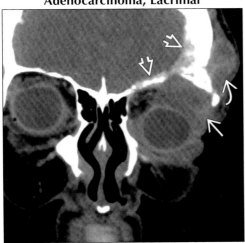

Non-Hodgkin Lymphoma, Lacrimal
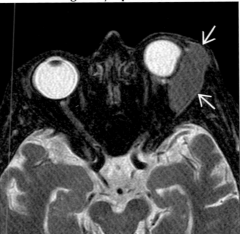

(Left) Coronal NECT shows an invasive lacrimal adenocarcinoma ➡ affecting the left lacrimal fossa with involvement of the orbital wall and calvarium ➡. Note that the tumor extends into the temporalis muscle ➡. *(Right)* Coronal NECT demonstrates a large hypointense soft tissue mass ➡ in the superolateral left orbit, replacing the lacrimal gland and displacing the globe anteromedially.

RAPIDLY DEVELOPING PROPTOSIS IN CHILD

DIFFERENTIAL DIAGNOSIS

Common
- Abscess, Subperiosteal, Orbit
- Infantile Hemangioma, Orbit
- Lymphatic Malformation, Orbit

Less Common
- Trauma, Orbit
- Idiopathic Orbital Inflammatory Disease (Pseudotumor)
- Rhabdomyosarcoma
- Neuroblastoma, Metastatic

Rare but Important
- Langerhans Histiocytosis
- Lymphoproliferative Lesions, Orbit
- Carotid-Cavernous Fistula, Traumatic

ESSENTIAL INFORMATION

Helpful Clues for Common Diagnoses
- **Abscess, Subperiosteal, Orbit**
  - Key facts
    - Pus between orbital wall & periosteum
    - Almost always associated with sinusitis
    - Anywhere in orbit, especially adjacent to ethmoid sinusitis
    - Brain MR if intracranial complication of sinusitis suspected
  - Imaging
    - Lentiform, rim-enhancing extraconal fluid collection (phlegmon or abscess)
    - ± Air-fluid level = drainable pus
    - Usually with preseptal cellulitis & deviation of extraocular muscle (EOM)
    - ± Edematous intraconal or extraconal fat, enlargement of EOMs (myositis)
- **Infantile Hemangioma, Orbit**
  - Key facts
    - Vascular neoplasm, NOT malformation
    - Not well seen at birth; more apparent within 1st few weeks of life
    - Proliferating phase: 1st year
    - Involuting phase: 1-5 years
    - Involuted phase: 5-7 years
    - GLUT-1: Specific immunohistochemical marker expressed in all 3 phases of infantile hemangioma
    - Congenital hemangioma: Rare variant, present at or before birth

- 2 subtypes of congenital hemangioma = rapidly involuting (RICH) & noninvoluting (NICH)
    - RICH shows involution by 8-14 months
  - Imaging
    - Proliferating phase: Solid, intensely enhancing mass with high-flow vessels
    - Involuting phase: Fat infiltration & ↓ size
    - May be part of PHACES syndrome: Posterior fossa abnormalities, hemangiomas, arterial anomalies, cardiovascular defects, eye abnormalities, sternal clefts
- **Lymphatic Malformation, Orbit**
  - Key facts
    - Congenital vascular malformation
    - Lymphatic channels of varying sizes
    - Present at birth, grows with child
    - Hemorrhage or respiratory infection causes sudden ↑ in size with resultant rapidly developing proptosis
    - Intracranial vascular anomalies present in ~ 2/3 of patients with periorbital lymphatic malformation
  - Imaging
    - Uni- or multilocular; macrocystic or microcystic
    - Intra- ± extraconal location
    - Only septations enhance, unless mixed venolymphatic malformation
    - Fluid-fluid levels best seen on MR

Helpful Clues for Less Common Diagnoses
- **Trauma, Orbit**
  - Key facts
    - Metallic foreign bodies (FB) most dense
    - Glass more dense than bone
    - Wood is very low density (~ air density)
    - Living plant material ~ soft tissue density
  - Imaging
    - FB, bone fragments, &/or adjacent hematoma ⇒ proptosis
    - ± Globe rupture, intraocular FB, intracranial injury
- **Idiopathic Orbital Inflammatory Disease (Pseudotumor)**
  - Key facts
    - Benign inflammatory process with fibrosis ⇒ painful proptosis
  - Imaging
    - Myositic: Most common subtype

- Diffuse enlargement & enhancement of EOMs, including tendinous insertions
- Lacrimal: Enlargement & enhancement
- Anterior: Thickening & enhancement of sclera ± choroid, ± involvement of retrobulbar fat, nerve, or sheath
- Diffuse: Intra- ± extraconal, may be mass-like, usually without globe deformity or bone erosion
- Apical: Enhancing orbital apex mass, extension through fissures

- **Rhabdomyosarcoma**
  - Key facts
    - H&N sites: Orbit, parameningeal (middle ear, paranasal sinus, nasopharynx), & all other H&N sites
  - Imaging
    - Soft tissue mass, variable enhancement
    - ± Bone erosion
    - ± Intracranial or sinus extension
- **Neuroblastoma, Metastatic**
  - Key facts
    - Most common malignant tumor in children < 1 year of age
    - Majority of primary tumors retroperitoneal adrenal origin
  - Imaging
    - Soft tissue mass + aggressive bone erosion & spiculated periosteal reaction
    - When bilateral, frequently involves lateral orbital walls
    - ± Intracranial extension

Helpful Clues for Rare Diagnoses
- **Langerhans Histiocytosis**
  - Key facts
    - In H&N: Orbit, maxilla, mandible, temporal bone, cervical spine, skull
  - Imaging
    - Enhancing soft tissue mass with smooth osseous erosion
- **Lymphoproliferative Lesions, Orbit**
  - Key facts
    - Includes NHL & lymphoid hyperplasia (benign polyclonal reactive hyperplasia & indeterminate atypical hyperplasia)
  - Imaging
    - Diffuse or focal masses
    - Homogeneous enhancing soft tissue mass anywhere in orbit
- **Carotid-Cavernous Fistula, Traumatic**
  - Key facts
    - Direct fistula between cavernous ICA & cavernous sinus
    - Secondary to trauma, venous thrombosis, or aneurysm
  - Imaging
    - Proptosis + large superior ophthalmic vein, cavernous sinus, & EOMs
    - "Dirty" orbital fat related to edema

SELECTED REFERENCES

1. Bisdorff A et al: Intracranial vascular anomalies in patients with periorbital lymphatic and lymphaticovenous malformations. AJNR Am J Neuroradiol. 28(2):335-41, 2007

Abscess, Subperiosteal, Orbit

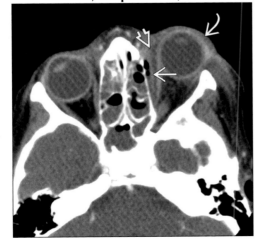

Axial CECT shows an elliptical subperiosteal abscess with air-fluid level ➡ in the medial left orbit with extraconal edema ➡, medial rectus muscle deviation, proptosis, & preseptal soft tissue edema ➡.

Abscess, Subperiosteal, Orbit

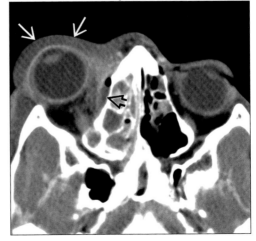

Axial CECT reveals significant right-sided ethmoid sinusitis, preseptal cellulitis ➡, proptosis, and small air-fluid level within a medial extraconal subperiosteal abscess ➡.

Infantile Hemangioma, Orbit

Infantile Hemangioma, Orbit

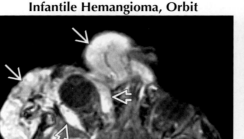

(Left) Axial T1 C+ FS MR shows a large, intensely enhancing infantile hemangioma ➡ involving the right orbit, face, and nose with postseptal extension ➡ resulting in proptosis. Solid, intensely enhancing mass with high-flow vessels indicates that the lesion is in the proliferating phase. *(Right)* Axial T1 C+ FS MR defines the preseptal ➡, postseptal intra- ➡ and extraconal ➡ extension of an infantile hemangioma. Note the resultant proptosis.

Lymphatic Malformation, Orbit

Lymphatic Malformation, Orbit

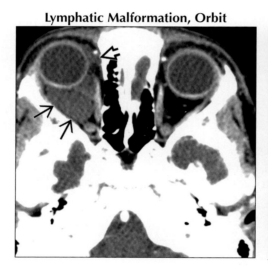
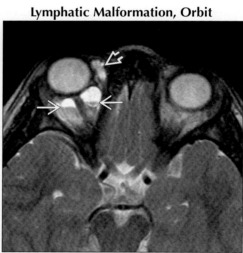

(Left) Axial CECT demonstrates a multilobular cystic-appearing intraconal right orbital lymphatic malformation ➡ with small anteromedial postseptal component ➡. *(Right)* Axial T2WI MR in the same patient better defines the mass as a large intraconal macrocystic lymphatic malformation with fluid-fluid levels ➡ secondary to intralesional hemorrhage. Note the smaller extraconal component anteromedially ➡. Acutely developing proptosis resulted.

Trauma, Orbit

Trauma, Orbit

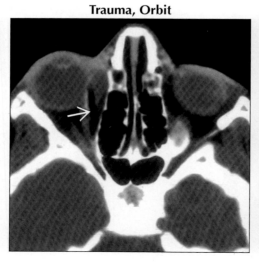
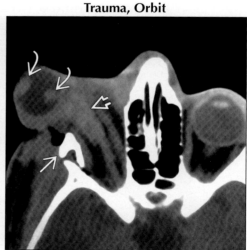

(Left) Axial NECT reveals mild right proptosis secondary to the penetration of the medial extraconal space by air that contains a twig ➡. Care must be taken not to confuse wood foreign body with air or fat. *(Right)* Axial NECT shows depressed lateral wall fracture fragments ➡ and orbital hemorrhage ➡, leading to severe proptosis and near complete traumatic enucleation of the small right globe with shattered fragments of lens ➡.

Idiopathic Orbital Inflammatory Disease (Pseudotumor)

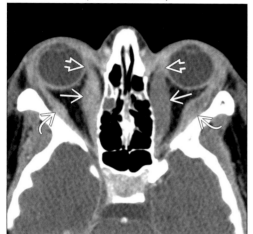

Idiopathic Orbital Inflammatory Disease (Pseudotumor)

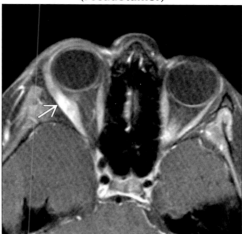

(Left) Axial CECT shows diffuse enlargement of bilateral medial ➡ & to a lesser extent lateral rectus muscles ➡, including involvement of the tendinous insertions ➡. This child presented with painful proptosis. Biopsy showed idiopathic orbital inflammatory disease. *(Right)* Axial T1 C+ FS MR reveals diffuse enlargement and increased enhancement of the lateral rectus muscle ➡. This child presented with mild pain and proptosis.

Rhabdomyosarcoma

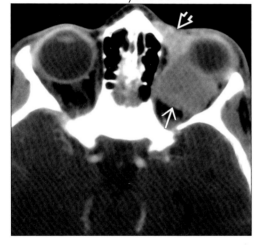

Langerhans Histiocytosis

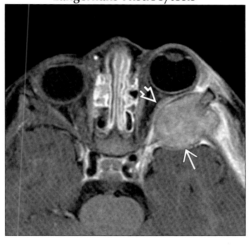

(Left) Axial CECT depicts an enhancing retrobulbar rhabdomyosarcoma ➡ that spreads into preseptal area medially ➡. Note the mild associated proptosis. *(Right)* Axial T1 C+ FS MR defines the cause of this child's left proptosis as a large, well-defined, moderately enhancing, expansile mass in the sphenoid wing with orbital ➡ and intracranial ➡ extension. Biopsy specimen showed Langerhans cell histiocytosis.

Lymphoproliferative Lesions, Orbit

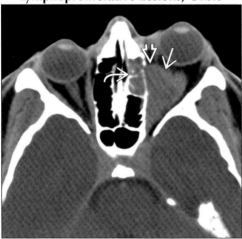

Carotid-Cavernous Fistula, Traumatic

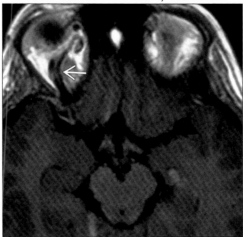

(Left) Axial CECT demonstrates an intraconal ➡ and extraconal ➡ left orbital mass with ethmoid extension ➡. This non-Hodgkin lymphoma explains this teenager's proptosis and periorbital ecchymosis. *(Right)* Axial T1 C+ MR reveals a large left superior ophthalmic vein ➡ in a child with post-traumatic carotid-cavernous fistula. This child's proptosis presented 2 years after skull base fractures.

INFECTIOUS & INFLAMMATORY ORBITAL LESIONS

DIFFERENTIAL DIAGNOSIS

Common
- Cellulitis, Orbit
- Abscess, Subperiosteal, Orbit
- Idiopathic Orbital Inflammatory Disease (Pseudotumor)
- Infection, Other Pathogen, Orbit

Less Common
- Sarcoidosis, Orbit
- Wegener Granulomatosis, Orbit
- Sjögren Syndrome, Orbit

Rare but Important
- Toxocariasis, Orbit
- Amyloidosis

ESSENTIAL INFORMATION

Helpful Clues for Common Diagnoses
- **Cellulitis, Orbit**
  - Key facts
    - Most common cause is sinusitis
    - Other causes = trauma or cutaneous, hematogenous, or iatrogenic infection
    - Chandler classification of orbital complications of sinusitis: Preseptal cellulitis, orbital cellulitis, subperiosteal abscess, orbital abscess, & cavernous sinus thrombophlebitis
    - Image brain if suspicion of intracranial complication (meningitis, extradural effusion or empyema, brain abscess)
  - Imaging
    - ↑ Density & enhancing periorbital soft tissue, lids, orbital septum
    - Postseptal extraconal ± intraconal fat infiltration
    - Intraconal disease may compromise optic nerve → requires surgical decompression
- **Abscess, Subperiosteal, Orbit**
  - Key facts: Subperiosteal collection of pus
  - Imaging
    - Lenticular rim-enhancing mass in extraconal orbit + displacement of adjacent extraocular muscles (EOMs)
    - Associated sinusitis common (ethmoid disease most common)
    - Look carefully for evidence of cavernous sinus thrombophlebitis (large superior ophthalmic vein + heterogeneous cavernous sinus enhancement)

- **Idiopathic Orbital Inflammatory Disease (Pseudotumor)**
  - Key facts: Benign inflammatory process of unknown etiology composed of lymphocytic infiltrates
  - Imaging: Space occupying infiltrative process
    - May involve any part of orbit: Classified into 5 types
    - Myositic: Most common; diffuse irregular enlargement & enhancement of EOMs; involves tendinous insertions
    - Diffuse: Infiltrative or tumefactive mass may involve retrobulbar, intraconal, & extraconal spaces; does not distort or invade globe; does not destroy bone
    - Apical: Irregular infiltration of orbital apex involving optic nerve & EOMs; results in orbital apex syndrome; Tolosa-Hunt = intracranial cavernous sinus involvement
    - Perineuritic (anterior): Ragged edematous enlargement of optic nerve sheath; may produce mild proptosis
    - Lacrimal (daycroadenitis): Diffuse, irregular enlargement of lacrimal gland
- **Infection, Other Pathogen, Orbit**
  - Key facts: Exogenous from surgery, penetrating injury
    - Endogenous from hematogenous route in diabetes, HIV, intravenous drug abuse, renal failure
  - Imaging
    - CT: Thickened, enhancing infiltrative sclera, preseptal/periorbital cellulitis
    - MR: Scleral-uveal enhancement; FLAIR may show intraocular lesions; restricted diffusion may reverse with treatment

Helpful Clues for Less Common Diagnoses
- **Sarcoidosis, Orbit**
  - Key facts: Idiopathic systemic disease
    - Noncaseating granulomas affecting orbit in ~ 25% of cases
  - Imaging
    - May involve any other part of orbit (fat, EOM, lacrimal gland) with thickening & enlargement
    - ± Thickening and enhancement of intraorbital ± chiasmatic optic nerve
    - ± Enhancement of optic nerve sheath (perineuritic)

- ± Infiltrative mass identical to IOID or lymphoma
- Rarely thickening, nodularity of sclera, uveal coat
- Look for intracranial involvement: Parenchymal, leptomeningeal, dural, or skull lesions
- **Wegener Granulomatosis, Orbit**
  - Key facts: Necrotizing granulomatous vasculitis affecting orbit present in ~ 20% cases
    - M:F = 3:2; ANCA antibody + in more than 90% of cases
  - Imaging
    - Most common: Irregular thickening & enhancement of sclera; often bilateral
    - Frequently presents as irregular soft tissue orbital mass ± enhancement adjacent to paranasal sinus with soft tissue/mucosal disease & bone erosion
    - Uncommon: Perineuritic form with enhancement of optic nerve sheath
    - Adjacent paranasal sinus & nasal involvement present in most cases
- **Sjögren Syndrome, Orbit**
  - Key facts: Autoimmune disease + lymphocytic infiltration of exocrine glands
    - Salivary and lacrimal most common
  - Imaging
    - Homogeneous enlargement ± enhancement of lacrimal glands (bilateral > unilateral)

- Look for enlargement of parotid glands with multiple cystic & solid intraparenchymal lesions & intraglandular calcifications

Helpful Clues for Rare Diagnoses
- **Toxocariasis, Orbit**
  - Key facts: Eosinophilic granuloma caused by nematode *Toxocara canis/cati* in infected soil
    - 90% have + ELISA test
  - Imaging
    - Thickened irregular & enhancing uveoscleral coat with no calcification
    - T2 hyperintense or isointense (cf. vitreous) or enhancing vitreal mass
    - Often associated with retinal detachment
- **Amyloidosis**
  - Key facts: Systemic or local disease with accumulation of amyloid fibrils
    - Orbital disease in 4% of local disease
  - Imaging
    - Homogeneous mass with Ca++ in extraconal orbit, most commonly involving lacrimal fossa or lacrimal gland
    - Remodeling, erosion, hyperostosis, or sclerosis of adjacent bone
    - Enlargement of EOMs with coarse or punctate Ca++

SELECTED REFERENCES

1. Chandler JR et al: The pathogenesis of orbital complications in acute sinusitis. Laryngoscope. 80(9):1414-28, 1970

Cellulitis, Orbit

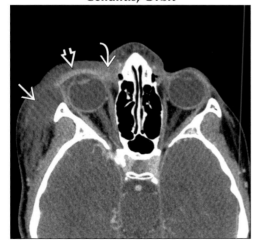

Axial CECT shows thickening & stranding of the subcutaneous periorbital soft tissues & temporalis muscle ➡, enhancement & thickening of lid ➡, and irregular thickening involving the orbital septum ➡.

Abscess, Subperiosteal, Orbit

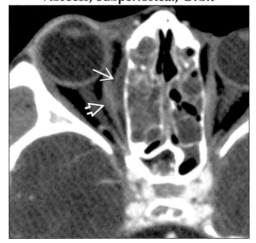

Axial CECT reveals a rim-enhancing medial extraconal abscess ➡ with mild displacement of medial rectus muscle ➡. Note the inflammatory opacification throughout the ethmoid complex.

Idiopathic Orbital Inflammatory Disease (Pseudotumor)

Idiopathic Orbital Inflammatory Disease (Pseudotumor)

(Left) Coronal CECT demonstrates enhancing tissue in the superior orbit, lacrimal fossa ➡, and sclera ➡. This is the diffuse form of idiopathic orbital inflammatory disease. *(Right)* Axial T1 C+ FS MR in the same patient shows diffuse homogeneous lateral rectus enhancement ➡, sclera ➡, and lid ➡. Note that the cortical signal of the lateral orbital wall is preserved.

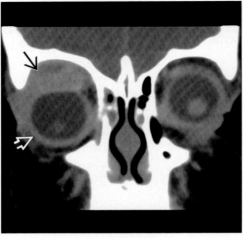

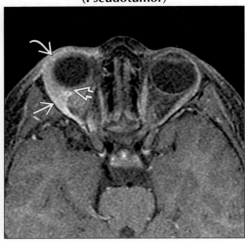

Idiopathic Orbital Inflammatory Disease (Pseudotumor)

Idiopathic Orbital Inflammatory Disease (Pseudotumor)

(Left) Coronal CECT reveals diffuse enlargement and enhancement of the right medial ➡ and inferior ➡ rectus, superior oblique ➡ and left superior rectus ➡ muscles in this 14 year old male patient with the myositic form of IOID. *(Right)* Axial T1 C+ MR in this patient with apical form of IOID shows abnormal enhancement in the right orbital apex and fissure ➡. Intracranial involvement in these cases may extend to the cavernous sinus ➡.

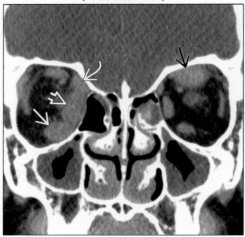

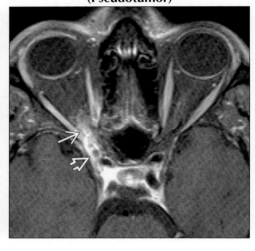

Idiopathic Orbital Inflammatory Disease (Pseudotumor)

Idiopathic Orbital Inflammatory Disease (Pseudotumor)

(Left) Axial CECT in this patient with the anterior perineuritis form of IOID demonstrates diffuse irregular enhancement of the left intraorbital optic nerve sheath ➡ and irregular thickening of the sclera ➡. *(Right)* Axial CECT in this patient with the lacrimal form of IOID shows diffuse enlargement and enhancement of the palpebral (eyelid) and orbital portions of the right lacrimal gland ➡ and thickening of the adjacent sclera ➡.

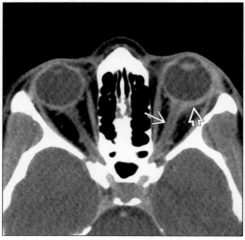

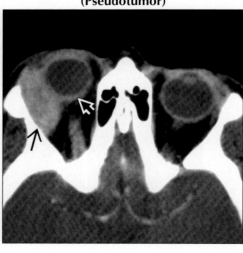

Infection, Other Pathogen, Orbit

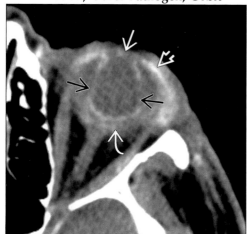

Sarcoidosis, Orbit

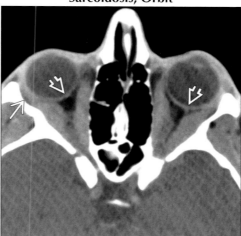

(Left) Axial CECT reveals endophthalmitis in a diabetic with corneal abrasion. Note corneal thinning ➡, orbital septum enhancement ➡, diffuse irregular scleral thickening ➡, & serous choroidal detachment ➡. *(Right)* Axial CECT shows irregular enlargement of the rectus muscles with subtle heterogeneous enhancement. The right lacrimal gland ➡ is enlarged, and the sclera is thickened with nodularity ➡. Scleral nodules help distinguish this from IOID.

Wegener Granulomatosis, Orbit

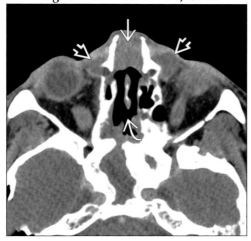

Sjögren Syndrome, Orbit

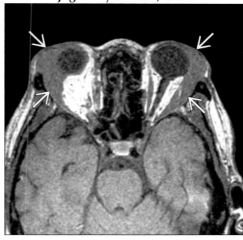

(Left) Axial CECT reveals enhancing tissue expanding the nasal cavity ➡, erosion of the septum ➡, and obstruction of both nasolacrimal ducts (dacryocystoceles) ➡ in this patient with severe Wegener granulomatosis. *(Right)* Axial T1WI MR shows diffuse bilateral enlargement of the palpebral (eyelid) & orbital portions of the lacrimal glands ➡ in a patient with Sjögren syndrome affecting the salivary glands.

Toxocariasis, Orbit

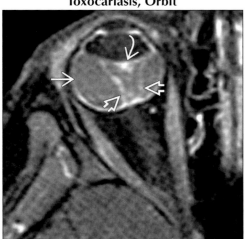

Amyloidosis

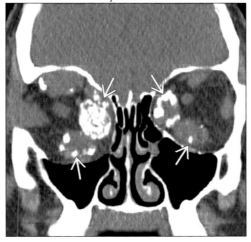

(Left) Axial T1WI FS MR shows diffuse hyperintensity and enhancement of the right vitreous ➡, retinal detachment ➡, and an enhancing vitreal mass located in the region of the ora serrata of the retina ➡. The relative anterior location of the retinal mass helps to distinguish this from retinoblastoma. *(Right)* Coronal NECT shows diffuse bilateral enlargement of the extraocular muscles with multiple coarse intramuscular calcifications ➡.

DIFFERENTIAL DIAGNOSIS

Common
- Abscess, Subperiosteal, Orbit
- Infantile Hemangioma, Orbit
- Lymphatic Malformation, Orbit
- Idiopathic Orbital Inflammatory Disease (Pseudotumor)

Less Common
- Neurofibromatosis Type 1, Orbit
- Glioma, Optic Pathway
- Lymphoproliferative Lesions, Orbit
- Rhabdomyosarcoma, Orbit
- Neuroblastoma, Metastatic
- Langerhans Histiocytosis, Orbit

Rare but Important
- Venous Malformation, Orbit
- Thyroid-Associated Orbitopathy
- Dermoid and Epidermoid, Orbit
- Sarcoidosis, Orbit

ESSENTIAL INFORMATION

Helpful Clues for Common Diagnoses
- **Abscess, Subperiosteal, Orbit**
  - Key facts: Pus between orbital wall & periosteum, secondary to sinusitis
  - Imaging
    - Lentiform rim-enhancing fluid collection (phlegmon or abscess)
    - ± Air-fluid level = drainable pus
    - ± Preseptal cellulitis, deviated extraocular muscle (EOM), edematous orbital fat, or large EOMs (myositis)
- **Infantile Hemangioma, Orbit**
  - Key facts
    - Vascular neoplasm, NOT malformation
    - Usually not well seen at birth, more apparent within 1st few weeks of life
    - 3 phases: Proliferating, involuting, & involuted; GLUT-1 positive
  - Imaging
    - Proliferating phase: Solid, intensely enhancing mass with high flow vessels
    - Involuting phase: Fat infiltration and ↓ size
    - ± Intracranial hemangiomas, cardiovascular anomalies, posterior fossa abnormalities, & eye abnormalities in children with PHACES syndrome
- **Lymphatic Malformation, Orbit**
  - Key facts: Congenital vascular malformation; grows with child; hemorrhage or infection ⇒ sudden size increase
  - Imaging
    - Uni- or multilocular; macro- or microcystic; intra- &/or extraconal
    - Only septations enhance, unless mixed venolymphatic malformation
    - Fluid-fluid levels best seen on MR
    - Intracranial vascular anomalies may be present in up to 2/3 of patients with periorbital lymphatic malformation
- **Idiopathic Orbital Inflammatory Disease (Pseudotumor)**
  - Key facts: Infiltration of inflammatory cells & fibrosis ⇒ painful masses
  - Imaging
    - Large, enhancing EOMs most common
    - ± Large, enhancing lacrimal gland
    - ± Thick, enhancing sclera &/or choroid, retrobulbar fat, nerve, or sheath
    - ± Intra- or extraconal enhancing mass; Tolosa-Hunt when in cavernous sinus

Helpful Clues for Less Common Diagnoses
- **Neurofibromatosis Type 1, Orbit**
  - Key facts
    - NF1; autosomal dominant; 50% new mutations, 17q11
    - Orbital involvement ⇒ pulsatile exophthalmos & buphthalmos
  - Imaging
    - Enhancing plexiform neurofibroma of orbit, face, infratemporal & middle cranial fossa
    - ± Sphenoid dysplasia = decalcification or remodeling of greater sphenoid wing + large middle fossa ⇒ herniation of intracranial contents into orbit
    - ± Enlarged globe secondary to glaucoma
    - ± Large optic nerve ± abnormal enhancement = optic pathway glioma
- **Glioma, Optic Pathway**
  - Key facts: Up to 60% of patients with optic nerve glioma (ONG) have NF1; up to 40% of children with NF1 have ONG
  - Imaging: Enlargement &/or enhancement of any segment of optic pathway ± cysts
- **Lymphoproliferative Lesions, Orbit**
  - Key facts: Includes lymphoma (usually non-Hodgkin) & lymphoid hyperplasia

○ Imaging: Homogeneous enhancing soft tissue mass anywhere in orbit
- **Rhabdomyosarcoma, Orbit**
  ○ Key facts: H&N sites = orbit, parameningeal (middle ear, paranasal sinus, nasopharynx), & all other H&N sites
  ○ Imaging: Soft tissue mass with variable enhancement ± bone erosion, intracranial or sinus extension
- **Neuroblastoma, Metastatic**
  ○ Key facts: Bilateral skull base metastases ⇒ periorbital ecchymosis (raccoon eyes)
  ○ Imaging: Soft tissue mass + aggressive bone erosion & spiculated periosteal reaction ± intracranial extension
- **Langerhans Histiocytosis, Orbit**
  ○ Key facts: H&N sites = orbit, maxilla, mandible, temporal bone, C-spine, skull
  ○ Imaging
    ▪ Enhancing soft tissue mass with smooth osseous erosion, lateral orbit most common
    ▪ ± Skull or temporal bone lesions
    ▪ ± Abnormal thickening and enhancement of pituitary infundibulum

Helpful Clues for Rare Diagnoses
- **Venous Malformation, Orbit**
  ○ Key facts: Vascular malformation, previously referred to as "cavernous hemangioma"
  ○ Imaging: Well-circumscribed enhancing "mass" of venous lakes, may "fill in" on delayed images ± phleboliths

- **Thyroid-Associated Orbitopathy**
  ○ Key facts: Autoimmune inflammation with thyroid dysfunction, usually hyper-, but may be hypo- or euthyroid
  ○ Imaging
    ▪ Exophthalmos with bilateral enlargement of EOM; inferior > medial > superior > lateral > oblique
    ▪ Spares tendinous insertion
    ▪ Increased orbital fat, ± lacrimal gland or superior ophthalmic vein enlargement
- **Dermoid and Epidermoid, Orbit**
  ○ Key facts: Congenital inclusion of epithelial + dermal elements = dermoid; epithelial elements only = epidermoid
  ○ Imaging
    ▪ Cystic mass adjacent to frontozygomatic or frontolacrimal suture; fat (dermoid) or fluid (dermoid or epidermoid) contents
    ▪ Smooth scalloped bony remodeling
- **Sarcoidosis, Orbit**
  ○ Key facts: Noncaseating granulomatous inflammation
  ○ Imaging: Lacrimal gland enlargement, EOM infiltration, optic nerve thickening & enhancement, or intraorbital mass

SELECTED REFERENCES

1. Chung EM et al: From the archives of the AFIP: Pediatric orbit tumors and tumorlike lesions: nonosseous lesions of the extraocular orbit. Radiographics. 27(6):1777-99, 2007

Abscess, Subperiosteal, Orbit

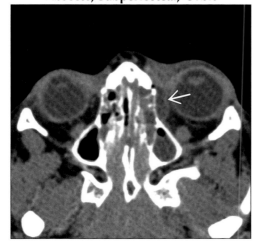

Axial CECT demonstrates a small rim-enhancing extraconal abscess ➡ in the medial left orbit, secondary to extensive ethmoid sinusitis.

Infantile Hemangioma, Orbit

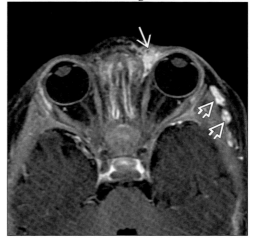

Axial T1 C+ FS MR shows intensely enhancing hemangiomas involving the left preseptal and postseptal orbit ➡ and in the left temporalis soft tissues ➡ of a 6 month old boy.

EXTRAOCULAR ORBITAL MASS IN CHILD

(Left) Axial CECT shows a primarily intraconal multiloculated macrocystic lymphatic malformation ➡ in the right orbit. *(Right)* Axial CECT reveals a large left lacrimal gland mass ➡. Notice the smooth bone remodeling, an uncommon finding in idiopathic orbital inflammatory disease.

Lymphatic Malformation, Orbit

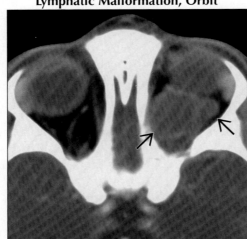

Idiopathic Orbital Inflammatory Disease (Pseudotumor)

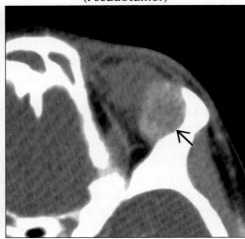

(Left) Axial T1 C+ FS MR demonstrates typical orbital features of neurofibromatosis type 1, including sphenoid wing dysplasia ➡, enhancing plexiform neurofibroma ➡, enlargement of the left middle cranial fossa, and resultant proptosis. *(Right)* Axial T1 C+ FS MR shows homogeneous enhancement of enlarged left optic nerve ➡ in a child with neurofibromatosis type 1. In this setting, the most likely diagnosis is optic pathway glioma.

Neurofibromatosis Type 1, Orbit

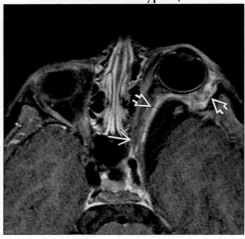

Glioma, Optic Pathway

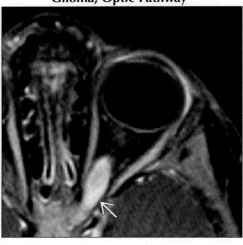

(Left) Axial T1 C+ FS MR in a patient with non-Hodgkin lymphoma reveals a moderately enhancing right preseptal orbital mass ➡ that mildly deforms the globe. *(Right)* Coronal CECT demonstrates a well-defined enhancing mass ➡ in the inferior left orbit, inseparable from the inferior rectus muscle, without bone erosion or globe deformity.

Lymphoproliferative Lesions, Orbit

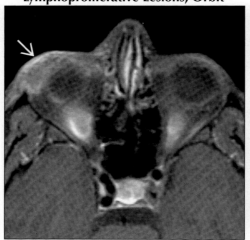

Rhabdomyosarcoma, Orbit

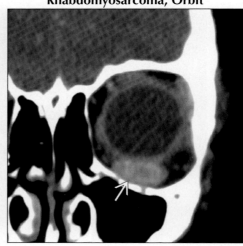

Neuroblastoma, Metastatic
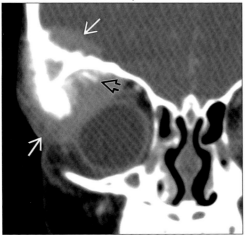

Langerhans Histiocytosis, Orbit
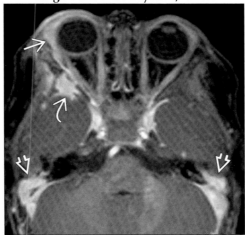

(Left) Coronal CECT shows a large enhancing mass in the right superolateral orbit ➡ with significant, aggressive periosteal reaction ➡. *(Right)* Axial T1 C+ FS MR shows a well-defined enhancing mass involving the right posterolateral orbit ➡ with extension into the right middle cranial fossa ➡, as well as bilateral enhancing temporal bone ➡ masses in a child who presented with diabetes insipidus.

Venous Malformation, Orbit
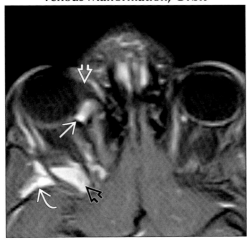

Thyroid-Associated Orbitopathy
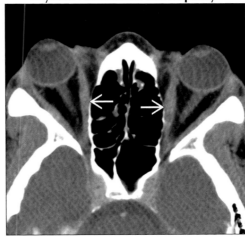

(Left) Axial T1 C+ FS MR reveals multiple enhancing venous malformations in the right orbit (intraconal ➡ and extraconal ➡), as well as the right sphenoid ➡. A small lymphatic component is also identified in the right medial postseptal orbit ➡. *(Right)* Axial CECT demonstrates subtle bilateral symmetric proptosis, enlarged medial rectus muscles ➡, and increased orbital fat in a patient with thyroid-associated orbitopathy.

Dermoid and Epidermoid, Orbit
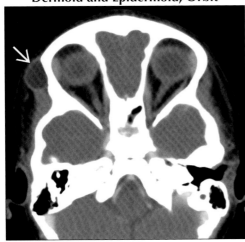

Sarcoidosis, Orbit
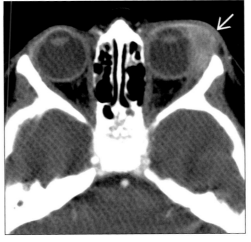

(Left) Axial CECT shows a well-defined cystic mass ➡ with smooth remodeling of the adjacent right lateral orbit. It may be difficult to distinguish epidermoid from dermoid unless fat or other complex elements are found within the mass (dermoid markers). *(Right)* Axial CECT depicts a heterogeneously enhancing focus of sarcoidosis in the preseptal and postseptal left orbit ➡, deforming the left globe.

SECTION 8
Temporal Bone

Anatomically Based Differentials

Generic Imaging Patterns

Clinically Based Differentials

EXTERNAL AUDITORY CANAL LESION

DIFFERENTIAL DIAGNOSIS

Common
- Atresia, EAC
- Cholesteatoma, EAC
- SCCa, EAC
- Osteoma, EAC

Less Common
- Medial Canal Fibrosis, EAC
- Exostoses, EAC
- Keratosis Obturans, EAC
- Necrotizing External Otitis

Rare but Important
- 1st Branchial Cleft Cyst
- Accessory Ossicle, EAC

ESSENTIAL INFORMATION

Key Differential Diagnosis Issues
- Clues for making external auditory canal (EAC) lesion diagnosis
  - Clinical examination of EAC often makes diagnosis; imaging needed to verify extent of lesion
  - Referring MD clinical information critical to differential diagnosis

Helpful Clues for Common Diagnoses
- **Atresia, EAC**
  - Key facts
    - Otoscopy: External ear microtia; EAC narrowed or absent
    - Degree of external ear deformity proportionate to severity of middle ear-ossicle malformation
  - CT imaging
    - Bony EAC stenotic or absent
    - Middle ear small; fused ossicles
    - Mastoid segment CN7 often ectopic
    - Oval ± round window atresia possible
    - Inner ear usually normal
- **Cholesteatoma, EAC**
  - Key facts
    - Otoscopy: Shows submucosal mass
    - Mucosa may be inflamed; mimic SCCa
  - CT imaging
    - EAC bony erosions present
    - Lesion matrix often shows bone fragments
- **SCCa, EAC**
  - Key facts

- Otoscopy: Mucosal lesion affects external ear structures ± external auditory canal
- SCCa of skin from sun exposure
  - CT imaging
    - Infiltrating mass ± EAC bony destruction
    - Middle ear spared; lesion stops at tympanic membrane
    - Note: SCCa EAC 1st order nodes in parotid space
- **Osteoma, EAC**
  - Key facts
    - Otoscopy: Hard submucosal mass; no mucosal lesion
  - CT imaging
    - Bony mass connects to EAC bony wall by broad base or stalk

Helpful Clues for Less Common Diagnoses
- **Medial Canal Fibrosis, EAC**
  - Key facts
    - Synonym: Idiopathic inflammatory medial meatal fibrosing otitis
    - Otoscopy: Medial IAC with fibrous plug ± medial mucosal inflammation
  - CT imaging
    - Variable thickness crescentic lesion abuts tympanic membrane
- **Exostoses, EAC**
  - Key facts
    - Synonym: Cold water ear
    - Otoscopy: Circumferential submucosal hard masses without mucosal abnormality
  - CT imaging
    - Circumferential bone encroachment on external auditory canal
- **Keratosis Obturans, EAC**
  - Key facts
    - Otoscopy: Unilateral or bilateral squamous plug in EAC(s)
    - May present with severe otalgia
  - CT imaging
    - Soft tissue plug in mildly enlarged EAC
    - No underlying bone erosion
- **Necrotizing External Otitis**
  - Key facts
    - Otoscopy: External ear and external auditory canal are swollen, inflamed with mucosal erosions
    - Found in diabetics and other immunocompromised patients
    - Age at presentation > 70 years

- Pseudomonas aeruginosa most common causal organism
  - CT imaging
    - Underlying bone destruction may vary from absent to severe depending on duration & severity of infection
    - Phlegmon ± abscess in subjacent suprahyoid neck spaces

Helpful Clues for Rare Diagnoses

- **1st Branchial Cleft Cyst**
  - Key facts
    - Otoscopy: Focal submucosal mass in lateral EAC
    - Variant 1st BCC within EAC lumen; usually in surrounding soft tissues
  - CT imaging
    - Cyst protrudes into EAC
    - Cyst "points" at bony-cartilaginous junction of EAC
- **Accessory Ossicle, EAC**
  - Key facts
    - Otoscopy: Normal or submucosal mass
  - CT imaging
    - Ovoid bony "ossicle" in vicinity of EAC

Alternative Differential Approaches

- Sort diagnoses by presence or absence of underlying bony destruction
  - EAC lesions with bony destruction
    - Cholesteatoma
    - SCCa
    - Necrotizing external otitis
  - EAC lesions without bone destruction
    - Atresia

- Keratosis obturans
- Medial canal fibrosis
- Exostoses
- 1st branchial cleft cyst
- Accessory ossicle
- Keratosis obturans
- Sort diagnoses by age at presentation
  - Congenital/pediatrics (< 20 years)
    - Atresia
    - 1st branchial cleft cyst
    - Accessory ossicle
  - Adults (20-70 years)
    - Cholesteatoma
    - SCCa
    - Osteoma
    - Exostoses
    - Medial canal fibrosis
  - Seniors (> 70 years)
    - SCCa
    - Medial canal fibrosis
    - Necrotizing external otitis

SELECTED REFERENCES

1. Lobo D et al: Squamous cell carcinoma of the external auditory canal. Skull Base. 18(3):167-72, 2008
2. Gassner EM et al: Preoperative evaluation of external auditory canal atresia on high-resolution CT. AJR Am J Roentgenol. 182(5):1305-12, 2004
3. Heilbrun ME et al: External auditory canal cholesteatoma: clinical and imaging spectrum. AJNR Am J Neuroradiol. 24(4):751-6, 2003
4. Hopsu E et al: Idiopathic inflammatory medial meatal fibrotizing otitis. Arch Otolaryngol Head Neck Surg. 128(11):1313-6, 2002
5. Grandis JR et al: Necrotizing (malignant) external otitis: prospective comparison of CT and MR imaging in diagnosis and follow-up. Radiology. 196(2):499-504, 1995

Atresia, EAC

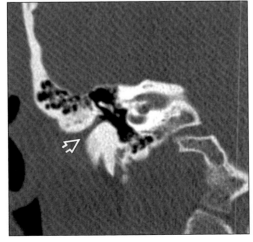

Coronal bone CT shows mild right EAC atresia as a stenotic bony external auditory canal with a membranous plug ➡. The middle ear cavity and ossicles are normal in this patient.

Atresia, EAC

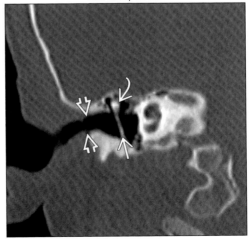

Coronal bone CT demonstrates a mild example of EAC atresia. Note the "ossified" tympanic membrane ➡, mildly narrowed EAC ➡, and ankylosis of the malleus to the tympanic membrane ➡.

EXTERNAL AUDITORY CANAL LESION

(Left) Coronal bone CT shows a typical EAC cholesteatoma as an erosive lesion on the inferior bony wall ➡. Notice the characteristic bony flecks within the lesion matrix ➡.
(Right) Coronal bone CT demonstrates EAC squamous cell carcinoma as soft tissue along the margins of the EAC itself ➡ and inferolateral osseous erosion with bone fragments ➡.

Cholesteatoma, EAC

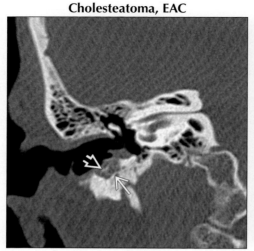

SCCa, EAC

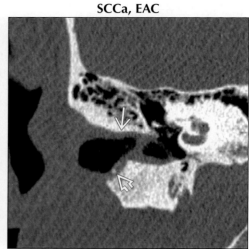

(Left) Axial bone CT shows an osteoma ➡ coming off the anterolateral wall of the bony external auditory canal.
(Right) Axial bone CT reveals a large intracanalicular EAC osteoma ➡. The hyperdense osteoma attaches to the anterior wall of the bony external auditory canal via a stalk ➡.

Osteoma, EAC

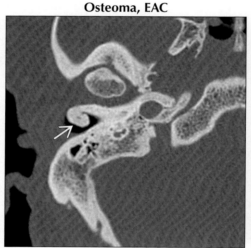

Osteoma, EAC

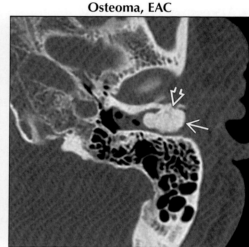

(Left) Coronal bone CT of the left ear shows medial canal fibrosis as benign-appearing soft tissue in the medial EAC with a convex crescentic margin ➡. Note absence of underlying bony erosion.
(Right) Axial bone CT reveals a variant case of mild medial canal fibrosis with associated calcification ➡.

Medial Canal Fibrosis, EAC

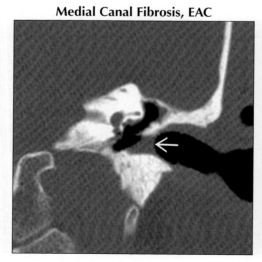

Medial Canal Fibrosis, EAC

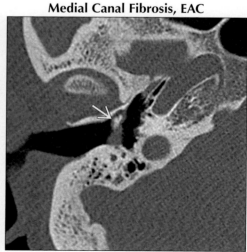

Exostoses, EAC

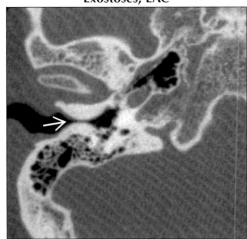

Exostoses, EAC

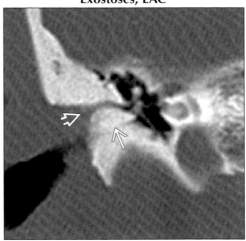

(Left) Axial bone CT of the right temporal bone reveals the classic appearance of EAC exostosis as a circumferential submucosal bony encroachment that narrows the lumen of the EAC ➡. *(Right)* Coronal bone CT of the right ear reveals an exostosis ➡ that occludes the external auditory canal ➡. Cold water exposure (surfer's ear) catalyzes this bony EAC reactive overgrowth.

Keratosis Obturans, EAC

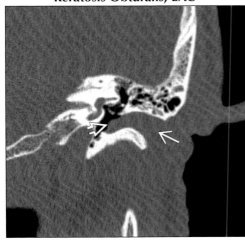

Necrotizing External Otitis

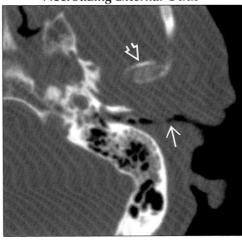

(Left) Coronal bone CT shows keratosis obturans as a benign-appearing mass ➡ filling the left EAC to level of the tympanic membrane ➡. Note the absence of EAC bony wall erosion. *(Right)* Axial bone CT shows the left EAC swollen shut ➡ by necrotizing external otitis in this patient with diabetes. Osteomyelitis of condylar head ➡ signals the presence of masticator space infection.

1st Branchial Cleft Cyst

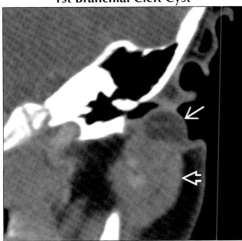

Accessory Ossicle, EAC

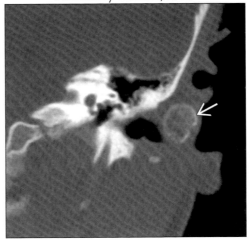

(Left) Coronal CECT demonstrates an unusual 1st branchial cleft cyst ➡ protruding from the upper parotid space ➡ into the lumen of the cartilaginous external auditory canal. *(Right)* Coronal bone CT demonstrates an ovoid bone with cortex and marrow space ➡ impinging on the superolateral portion of the cartilaginous EAC. Absence of stalk makes this an accessory ossicle.

DIFFERENTIAL DIAGNOSIS

Common
- Chronic Otitis Media
- Acquired Cholesteatoma, Pars Flaccida
- COM with Tympanosclerosis
- Cholesterol Granuloma, Middle Ear
- Paraganglioma, Glomus Tympanicum
- Paraganglioma, Glomus Jugulare

Less Common
- Jugular Bulb, Dehiscent
- Meningioma, T-Bone
- AOM with Coalescent Otomastoiditis
- Acquired Cholesteatoma, Pars Tensa
- Schwannoma, Middle Ear

Rare but Important
- Endolymphatic Sac Tumor
- Perineural Parotid Malignancy, T-Bone
- Aberrant Internal Carotid Artery
- Adenoma, Middle Ear

ESSENTIAL INFORMATION

Key Differential Diagnosis Issues
- Otoscopic findings provide clinician & imager critical information resulting in middle ear (ME) lesion pre-biopsy diagnosis
  - Is tympanic membrane (TM) ruptured? If so, which part? Is there cholesteatoma visible through rupture?
    - Pars flaccida & pars tensa cholesteatoma associated with TM rupture
    - Referring clinician often already knows cholesteatoma is present; wants to know about possible ME complications
  - Does retrotympanic lesion have a distinctive hue or location?

Helpful Clues for Common Diagnoses
- **Chronic Otitis Media**
  - Otoscopy: Thickened, retracted TM
  - CT: Linear, sporadic ME-mastoid tissue
    - Mastoid air cells underpneumatized
- **Acquired Cholesteatoma, Pars Flaccida**
  - Otoscopy: Pars flaccida portion of TM shows rupture or retraction pocket
  - CT: Nondependent soft tissue filling Prussak space & eroding ossicles ± middle ear walls ± scutum

- Dehiscence possible complications: Tegmen tympani, lateral semicircular canal, or facial nerve canal
- **COM with Tympanosclerosis**
  - Otoscopy: Opaque, thickened, calcified TM
  - CT: Post-inflammatory calcifications within TM or ME (ligaments, ossicles)
- **Cholesterol Granuloma, Middle Ear**
  - Otoscopy: Blue retrotympanic tissue
  - CT: Middle ear tissue with minimal bony or ossicular erosion
  - MR: High T1 & T2 signal
    - Old blood in lesion creates T1 shortening
- **Paraganglioma, Glomus Tympanicum**
  - Otoscopy: Red pulsatile mass behind anteroinferior TM quadrant
  - CT: Focal mass on cochlear promontory with intact ME bony floor
- **Paraganglioma, Glomus Jugulare**
  - Otoscopy: Red, pulsatile mass behind posteroinferior TM quadrant
  - CT: ME mass connects to jugular foramen through ME floor; invasive-destructive bone changes
  - MR: Enhancing mass spans jugular foramen into middle ear; high velocity flow voids ("pepper") on T1 images

Helpful Clues for Less Common Diagnoses
- **Jugular Bulb, Dehiscent**
  - Otoscopy: Blue lesion behind posteroinferior quadrant of TM
  - CT: Dehiscent sigmoid plate with jugular bulb "pseudopod" projecting into posteroinferior middle ear cavity
- **Meningioma, T-Bone**
  - Otoscopy: Pink retrotympanic mass
  - CT: Permeative-sclerotic or hyperostotic bone changes
  - MR: Enhancing middle ear mass extends from tegmen dura, jugular foramen, or IAC via inner ear
- **AOM with Coalescent Otomastoiditis**
  - Otoscopy: Thick, diffusely inflamed TM with retrotympanic pus
  - CT: ME & mastoid air cell opacification
    - Mastoid air cell trabecular breakdown indicate osteomyelitis is present
- **Acquired Cholesteatoma, Pars Tensa**
  - Otoscopy: Ruptured lower 2/3 TM (pars tensa) with marginal cholesteatoma visible

○ CT: Meso- and hypotympanic soft tissue mass often medial to ossicles; bone scalloping ± ossicle dehiscence
- **Schwannoma, Middle Ear**
  ○ Otoscopy: Tan-white retrotympanic mass
  ○ CT: ME mass pedunculating from CN7 or round window niche

Helpful Clues for Rare Diagnoses
- **Endolymphatic Sac Tumor**
  ○ Otoscopy: If enters middle ear, mixed hue retrotympanic mass
  ○ CT: Spiculated or coarse calcifications in tumor matrix; centered in vestibular aqueduct fovea on posterior T-bone wall
  ○ MR: High signal foci on T1 sequence from old blood trapped in tumor matrix
- **Perineural Parotid Malignancy, T-Bone**
  ○ Clinical: Parotid mass; CN7 paralysis
  ○ CT: Facial nerve canal enlarged variable distance; tumor may spill into ME cavity
  ○ MR: Invasive parotid neoplasm seen entering stylomastoid foramen; extends variable distance along facial nerve canal
- **Aberrant Internal Carotid Artery**
  ○ Otoscopy: Red tubular retrotympanic mass
  ○ CT: Tubular lesion passes through enlarged inferior tympanic canaliculus into posteroinferior middle ear cavity
    ▪ Lesion passes out ME cavity anteromedially by connecting to posterolateral horizontal petrous ICA
- **Adenoma, Middle Ear**
  ○ Otoscopy: Pink retrotympanic mass

○ CT: Middle ear soft tissue mass usually with no associated inflammatory changes
  ▪ Difficult to distinguish with bone CT from ME congenital cholesteatoma
○ MR: Enhancing middle ear mass
  ▪ Enhancement on MR differentiates from congenital cholesteatoma of middle ear

Alternative Differential Approaches
- Use hue and location of retrotympanic lesion, match with imaging findings
- White middle ear lesions
  ○ Acquired cholesteatoma, pars flaccida
    ▪ Upper 1/3 of TM retracted or ruptured; white cholesteatoma visible
  ○ Acquired cholesteatoma, pars tensa
    ▪ Rupture, lower 2/3 of TM; white lesion visible along rupture margin
  ○ Schwannoma, middle ear
    ▪ White mass behind mid- to upper TM
- Red middle ear lesions
  ○ Paraganglioma, glomus tympanicum
    ▪ Red mass behind anteroinferior TM
  ○ Paraganglioma, glomus jugulare
    ▪ Red mass behind posteroinferior TM
  ○ Aberrant internal carotid artery
    ▪ Red mass crosses behind lower TM
- Blue middle ear lesions
  ○ Cholesterol granuloma, middle ear
    ▪ Blue-black tissue behind entire TM
  ○ Chronic otitis media with hemorrhage
    ▪ Blue tissue behind entire TM
  ○ Jugular bulb, dehiscent
    ▪ Blue mass behind posteroinferior TM

Chronic Otitis Media

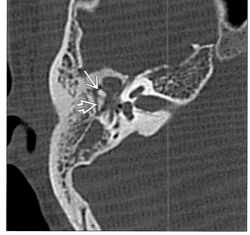

Axial bone CT shows opacification of epitympanum and mastoid antrum. Malleus head ➡ and short process of incus ▶ are both present within inflammatory tissue, making cholesteatoma unlikely.

Acquired Cholesteatoma, Pars Flaccida

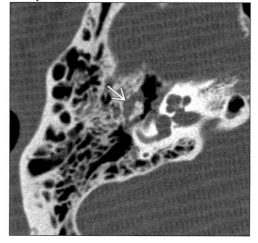

Axial bone CT through the epitympanum reveals cholesteatoma in lateral epitympanic recess ➡. On coronal images, the scutum was eroded, allowing cholesteatoma diagnosis to be made by CT.

(Left) Axial bone CT shows post-inflammatory ossification of manubrium of the malleus ➡. Tympanosclerosis involving an ossicle makes it appear larger with punctate high density on its margins. (Right) Axial T1WI MR reveals high signal within middle ear ➡ and mastoid air cells ➡. Mixed blood products within cholesterol granuloma create this appearance. Note basal turn of cochlea ➡.

COM with Tympanosclerosis

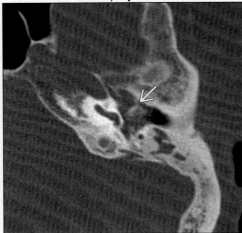

Cholesterol Granuloma, Middle Ear

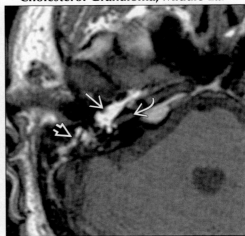

(Left) Coronal bone CT shows a small glomus tympanicum situated on the cochlear promontory ➡. Note the middle ear floor is intact ➡, excluding the diagnosis glomus jugulare paraganglioma. (Right) Coronal bone CT shows tumor spreading superolaterally through the floor of the middle ear ➡ into the middle ear cavity ➡ as well as superiorly to involve the floor of the IAC ➡.

Paraganglioma, Glomus Tympanicum

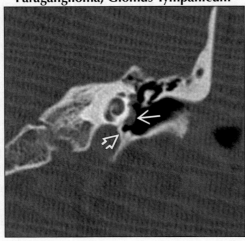

Paraganglioma, Glomus Jugulare

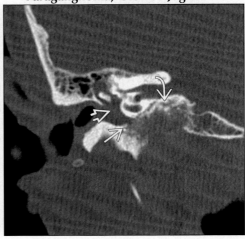

(Left) Axial bone CT shows a protrusion ➡ of the jugular bulb through a dehiscence of sigmoid plate ➡. A posteroinferior blue retrotympanic mass was visible at otoscopy. (Right) Coronal T1 C+ MR reveals en plaque meningioma along the tegmen tympani dura ➡. Notice the tumor spreads inferiorly into the middle ear cavity ➡ to surround the low signal ossicles.

Jugular Bulb, Dehiscent

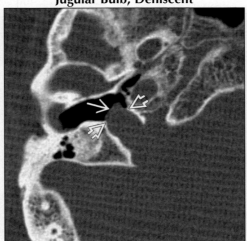

Meningioma, T-Bone

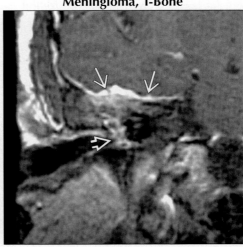

MIDDLE EAR LESION, ADULT

AOM with Coalescent Otomastoiditis

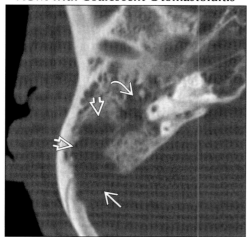

Acquired Cholesteatoma, Pars Tensa

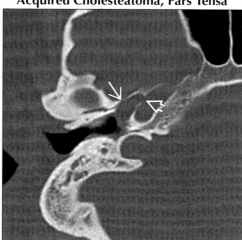

(Left) Axial bone CT shows acute otomastoiditis with coalescent mastoid air cells ⮊ and medial mastoid wall destruction ➡ resulting in meningitis. Note short process of incus destruction ⮊. (Right) Axial bone CT reveals pars tensa cholesteatoma that invades and enlarges the bony eustachian tube ➡. Note subtle focal erosion of horizontal petrous internal auditory canal bony wall ⮊.

Schwannoma, Middle Ear

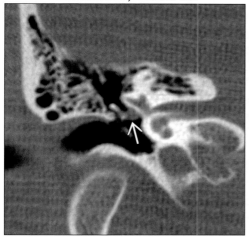

Endolymphatic Sac Tumor

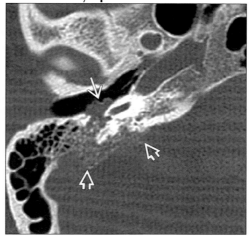

(Left) Coronal bone CT demonstrates a facial nerve schwannoma affecting the mid-tympanic segment of the facial nerve ➡. Lesion abuts ossicle and presents with conductive hearing loss. (Right) Axial bone CT reveals an invasive mass centered along the posterior wall of the T-bone ⮊ with punctate calcifications in its matrix. The lesion traverses the T-bone to enter the middle ear cavity ➡.

Perineural Parotid Malignancy, T-Bone

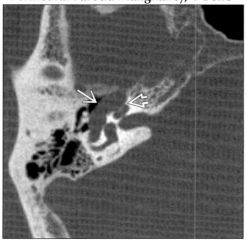

Aberrant Internal Carotid Artery

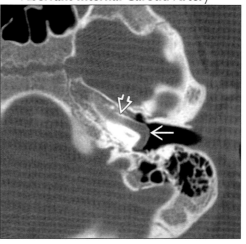

(Left) Axial bone CT shows an enlarged tympanic segment of the facial nerve canal ➡. An adenoid cystic carcinoma is present in the parotid gland (not shown). Note the erosion of the cochlea ⮊. (Right) Axial bone CT reveals the aberrant internal carotid artery crossing from posterior to anterior through the middle ear cavity ➡ and rejoining the normal horizontal petrous internal carotid artery ⮊.

DIFFERENTIAL DIAGNOSIS

Common
- Chronic Otitis Media
- Acquired Cholesteatoma, Pars Flaccida
- Congenital Cholesteatoma, Middle Ear

Less Common
- AOM with Coalescent Otomastoiditis
- Acquired Cholesteatoma, Pars Tensa
- Cholesterol Granuloma, Middle Ear
- COM with Tympanosclerosis
- COM with Ossicular Erosions

Rare but Important
- Rhabdomyosarcoma, Middle Ear
- Langerhans Histiocytosis, T-Bone
- Jugular Bulb, Dehiscent
- Aberrant Internal Carotid Artery

ESSENTIAL INFORMATION

Key Differential Diagnosis Issues
- Otoscopic findings often provide critical clues to precise diagnosis of middle ear lesion in child
  - Presence or absence of tympanic membrane (TM) rupture important
    - Pars tensa and flaccida acquired cholesteatoma have ruptured TM
  - Color and location of retrotympanic mass may be key to imaging diagnosis

Helpful Clues for Common Diagnoses
- **Chronic Otitis Media**
  - Otoscopy: Thickened tympanic membrane
  - Bone CT: Linear, sporadic middle ear-mastoid tissue; mastoid air cells may be under-pneumatized
- **Acquired Cholesteatoma, Pars Flaccida**
  - Otoscopy: Rupture or retraction pocket affecting pars flaccida portion of tympanic membrane
  - Bone CT: Nondependent soft tissue filling Prussak space with ossicle &/or bony wall erosions
    - Possible complications: Tegmen tympani, lateral semicircular canal, facial nerve canal dehiscence
- **Congenital Cholesteatoma, Middle Ear**
  - Otoscopy: White mass behind intact TM

- Bone CT: Smooth well-circumscribed soft tissue mass filling middle ear; often medial to ossicle chain
  - Ossicle erosion often absent
  - Mastoid pneumatization often normal

Helpful Clues for Less Common Diagnoses
- **AOM with Coalescent Otomastoiditis**
  - Otoscopy: Bulging, inflamed tympanic membrane
  - Bone CT: Complete middle ear-mastoid opacification with mastoid trabecular breakdown
    - **Hint:** Look on soft tissue windows for adjacent post-auricular abscess or epidural abscess
- **Acquired Cholesteatoma, Pars Tensa**
  - Otoscopy: Ruptured pars tensa portion of TM
  - Bone CT: Meso- and hypotympanic soft tissue mass often extending posteriorly or medially, ± ossicular erosion
- **Cholesterol Granuloma, Middle Ear**
  - Otoscopy: Blue-black material behind intact TM
  - Bone CT: Middle ear soft tissue mass with minimal bony erosion
  - MR: High T1 and high T2 signal of material in middle ear
    - **Hint:** Old blood in cholesterol granuloma creates T1 shortening
- **COM with Tympanosclerosis**
  - Otoscopy: Opaque, calcified tympanic membrane
  - Bone CT: Post-inflammatory calcifications may affect ossicles, ligaments or TM
- **COM with Ossicular Erosions**
  - Otoscopy: Thickened TM without normal ossicle impressions
  - Bone CT: Linear middle ear and mastoid air cell opacifications with partial ossicle absence
    - Long process of incus-lenticular process and stapes hub most commonly affected

Helpful Clues for Rare Diagnoses
- **Rhabdomyosarcoma, Middle Ear**
  - Otoscopy: EAC "polyp"
  - Bone CT: Destructive middle ear mass that often affects EAC, ossicles, surrounding bones, overlying dura
- **Langerhans Histiocytosis, T-Bone**
  - Otoscopy: Post-auricular mass common

8

MIDDLE EAR LESION, CHILD

○ Bone CT: Unilateral or bilateral (30%) destructive T-bone lesions affecting middle ear secondarily
  ▪ Mastoid air cell more commonly affected than petrous apex or inner ear
- **Jugular Bulb, Dehiscent**
  ○ Otoscopy: Blue lesion behind posteroinferior quadrant of TM
  ○ Bone CT: Dehiscent sigmoid plate projects jugular bulb into posteroinferior middle ear cavity
- **Aberrant Internal Carotid Artery**
  ○ Otoscopy: Reddish mass passes across inferior half of TM
  ○ Bone CT: Tubular lesion passes into posteroinferior middle ear cavity through enlarged inferior tympanic canaliculus
    ▪ Aberrant ICA passes out of middle ear cavity anteroinferiorly by accessing posterolateral margin of horizontal petrous ICA

Other Essential Information

- Best imaging tool for middle ear lesion in child: T-bone CT without contrast
  ○ Thin-section, fat-saturated MR only used for further evaluation of larger lesions involving inner ear, floor middle cranial fossa, or sigmoid sinus-posterior fossa
- Tumor or tumor-like lesions to consider in middle ear of child
  ○ Rhabdomyosarcoma & Langerhans cell histiocytosis
    ▪ May be difficult to distinguish

○ **Rhabdomyosarcoma, Middle Ear**
  ▪ Unilateral; centered in middle ear cavity; may present with EAC "polyp"
○ **Langerhans Histiocytosis, T-Bone**
  ▪ May be bilateral; centered around middle ear cavity, especially in mastoid; may present as post-auricular mass

Alternative Differential Approaches

- Otoscopic exam findings vs. diagnosis
  ○ White middle ear mass with associated ruptured or retracted pars flaccida TM
    ▪ Acquired cholesteatoma, pars flaccida
  ○ White middle ear mass with associated ruptured pars tensa TM
    ▪ Acquired cholesteatoma, pars tensa
  ○ White middle ear mass behind intact TM
    ▪ Congenital cholesteatoma, middle ear
  ○ Blue-black middle ear mass behind intact TM
    ▪ Cholesterol granuloma, middle ear
  ○ Red middle ear mass behind inferior half of intact TM
    ▪ Aberrant internal carotid artery
  ○ Blue middle ear mass behind posteroinferior intact TM
    ▪ Jugular bulb, dehiscent

Chronic Otitis Media

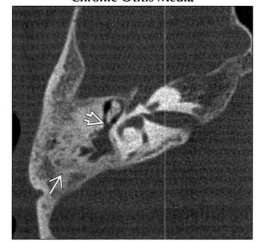

Axial bone CT shows inflammatory debris in posterior epitympanum ⊳ and mastoid antrum with under-pneumatization of the mastoid ➡, consistent with diagnosis of chronic otitis media.

Acquired Cholesteatoma, Pars Flaccida

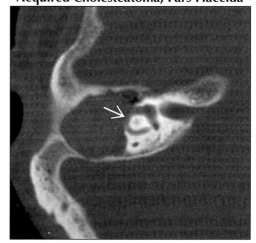

Axial bone CT shows large epitympanic & mastoid cholesteatoma causing dehiscence of lateral semicircular canal ➡. Notice scalloping enlargement of mastoid cavity and ossicle destruction.

MIDDLE EAR LESION, CHILD

(Left) Axial bone CT reveals a smooth soft tissue mass ➡ filling the anterior mesotympanum medial to ossicle chain. Subtle anterior bony wall erosion is associated ➡. (Right) Axial bone CT shows infection of mastoid has resulted in confluence of air cells ➡ and destruction of mastoid cortex ➡, resulting in TMJ infection with erosion of mandibular condyle ➡.

Congenital Cholesteatoma, Middle Ear

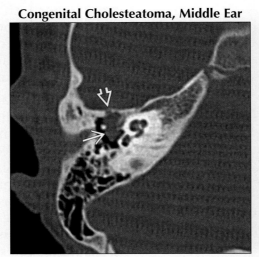

AOM with Coalescent Otomastoiditis

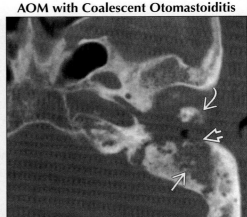

(Left) Axial bone CT shows middle ear soft tissue mass ➡ medial to ossicles with short process of incus erosion and sparing of Prussak space ➡. Otoscopy shows perforation in pars tensa TM. (Right) Axial T1WI MR shows high signal material in the middle ear ➡ and mastoid ➡ cavities. High T1 in cholesterol granuloma is due to a mixture of old blood and high protein.

Acquired Cholesteatoma, Pars Tensa

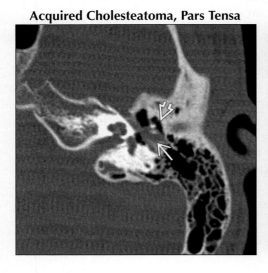

Cholesterol Granuloma, Middle Ear

(Left) Axial bone CT reveals multiple calcified foci ➡ in inflammatory debris surrounding the ossicles in the epitympanum. Under-pneumatized mastoid is a common finding of chronic otitis media. (Right) Axial bone CT shows absence of the distal incus-lenticular process as well as the hub of the stapes ➡. Notice also the linear stranding in the middle ear cavity from chronic otomastoiditis.

COM with Tympanosclerosis

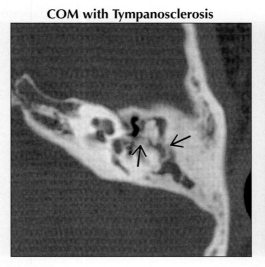

COM with Ossicular Erosions

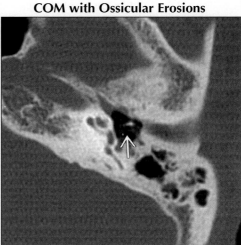

MIDDLE EAR LESION, CHILD

Rhabdomyosarcoma, Middle Ear

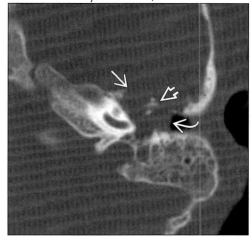

Langerhans Histiocytosis, T-Bone

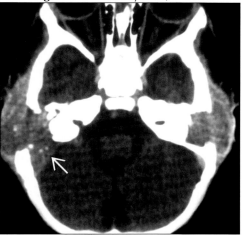

(Left) Axial bone CT demonstrates destructive mass in middle ear with loss of anterior bony wall ➡ and ossicular chain erosion ⇶. Otoscopic exam shows an EAC "polyp" ➡. *(Right)* Axial CECT shows bilateral enhancing masses in the middle ear, mastoids, and external ears. Note right temporal bone lesion has dehisced the sigmoid plate to involve the posterior fossa ➡.

Jugular Bulb, Dehiscent

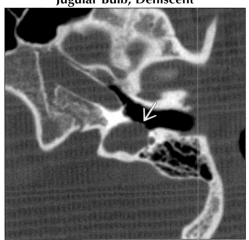

Jugular Bulb, Dehiscent

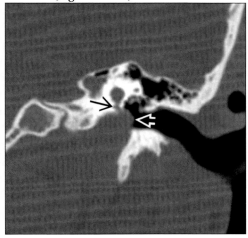

(Left) Axial bone CT reveals a large jugular bulb with a dehiscent lateral margin ➡. The protruding jugular bulb reaches the posteroinferior tympanic membrane where it is visible on otoscopy as a blue lesion. *(Right)* Coronal bone CT reveals dehiscent jugular bulb projecting superolateral into the middle ear cavity. Note it "leans" on the tympanic membrane ⇶ and fills the round window niche ➡.

Aberrant Internal Carotid Artery

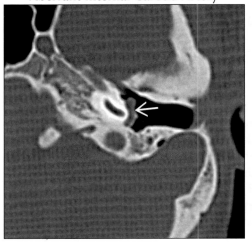

Aberrant Internal Carotid Artery

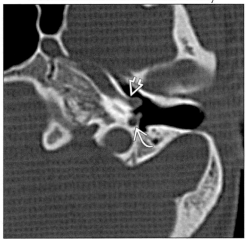

(Left) Axial bone CT demonstrates a tubular lesion ➡ on the cochlear promontory in the middle ear. Don't mistake the lesion for paraganglioma. The tubular appearance is the key. *(Right)* Axial bone CT shows an aberrant internal carotid artery entering middle ear via an enlarged inferior tympanic canaliculus ➡ and exiting through the horizontal petrous ICA canal ⇶.

INNER EAR LESION, ADULT

DIFFERENTIAL DIAGNOSIS

Common
- Semicircular Canal Dehiscence
- Fenestral Otosclerosis
- Labyrinthine Ossificans
- Jugular Bulb, High
- Jugular Bulb Diverticulum
- Fracture, T-Bone, Inner Ear

Less Common
- Large Endolymphatic Sac Anomaly (IP-2)
- Hemangioma, Facial Nerve, T-Bone
- Schwannoma, Facial Nerve, T-Bone
- Labyrinthitis
- Schwannoma, Intralabyrinthine

Rare but Important
- Cochlear Otosclerosis
- Intralabyrinthine Hemorrhage
- Endolymphatic Sac Tumor

ESSENTIAL INFORMATION

Key Differential Diagnosis Issues
- Differential encompasses all lesions, including normal variants, that may be found in inner ear region of an adult
- Inner ear region is temporal bone from medial wall of middle ear to lateral aspect of petrous apex

Helpful Clues for Common Diagnoses
- **Semicircular Canal Dehiscence**
  - Clinical clues: Tinnitus, dizziness, vertigo
    - Tullio phenomenon: Nystagmus caused by loud sound in affected ear
  - Focal dehiscence of superior semicircular canal causes "3rd" window in inner ear
  - CT: Superior semicircular canal roof is dehiscent into middle cranial fossa dura
    - Transverse oblique CT reformation best shows lesion
- **Fenestral Otosclerosis**
  - Clinical clues: Young adult develops gradual progressive conductive hearing loss
  - Begins at anterior margin of oval window (fissula antefenestrum)
  - CT: Lucent & sclerotic lesions along oval & round window margins
  - MR: Enhancing millimeter size lesions along margin of oval and round windows

- **Labyrinthine Ossificans**
  - Clinical clue: Profound sensorineural hearing loss following episode of meningitis
  - Healing of suppurative labyrinthitis may result in osteoneogenesis within inner ear fluid spaces
  - CT: Ossific plaques impinges on inner ear fluid spaces
  - MR: High-resolution T2 shows encroachment on membranous labyrinthine fluid spaces
- **Jugular Bulb, High**
  - Clinical clue: Asymptomatic normal variant
  - CT: Cephalad portion of jugular bulb projects to level of internal auditory canal
  - MR: On enhanced images may look like enhancing lesion posterior to IAC
- **Jugular Bulb Diverticulum**
  - Clinical clue: Asymptomatic normal variant
  - CT: Thumb-like projection off jugular bulb; usually projects cephalad but may project in any direction
  - MR: On enhanced images may look like focal enhancing lesion posterior to IAC
- **Fracture, T-Bone, Inner Ear**
  - CT: Transverse or longitudinal fracture line traverses inner ear structures; pneumolabyrinth possible
  - MR: T1 high signal (blood) within inner ear fluid spaces

Helpful Clues for Less Common Diagnoses
- **Large Endolymphatic Sac Anomaly (IP-2)**
  - Clinical clues: Bilateral congenital sensorineural hearing loss that appears in young adult with cascading hearing loss pattern
  - Most common congenital imaging abnormality in adult sensorineural hearing loss
  - CT: Enlarged bony vestibular aqueduct + mild cochlear dysplasia
  - MR: Enlarged endolymphatic sac + mild cochlear aplasia
- **Hemangioma, Facial Nerve, T-Bone**
  - Clinical clue: Facial nerve paralysis, often rapid, mimics Bell palsy
  - Location/morphology: Most commonly found in geniculate fossa; amorphous

- CT: ~ 50% show "honeycomb" ossific matrix
- MR: Amorphous enhancing geniculate ganglion area mass
- **Schwannoma, Facial Nerve, T-Bone**
  - Clinical clues: 50% present with hearing loss; facial nerve symptoms subtle or absent
  - Location/morphology: Most commonly found in geniculate fossa; smooth, tubular expanding lesion
  - CT: Focal or tubular enlargement of intratemporal facial nerve canal
  - MR: Enhancing mass follows intratemporal facial nerve
- **Labyrinthitis**
  - Clinical clue: Acute onset vertigo, hearing loss ± facial nerve paralysis
  - CT: Acute phase normal
  - MR: Often normal; if positive, diffuse enhancement of inner ear fluid spaces most common presentation
- **Schwannoma, Intralabyrinthine**
  - Clinical clue: Long history (10-20 years) of gradual sensorineural hearing loss
  - CT: Normal unless larger transmodiolar, transmacular, or transotic type present
  - MR: Focal area of enhancement within inner ear fluid space
    - Lesion name based on area of anatomic involvement

- Recommended descriptive terms include intracochlear, intravestibular, vestibulocochlear, transmodiolar, transmacular, and transotic options

Helpful Clues for Rare Diagnoses
- **Cochlear Otosclerosis**
  - Clinical clue: Bilateral "mixed" conductive and sensorineural hearing loss
  - CT: Lucent foci in bony labyrinth surrounding cochlea
  - MR: Punctate or linear foci of enhancing lesions in otic capsule
- **Intralabyrinthine Hemorrhage**
  - Clinical clue: May be idiopathic or post-traumatic
  - CT: Normal
  - MR: High T1 signal in inner ear fluid spaces
- **Endolymphatic Sac Tumor**
  - Clinical clues: Usually sporadic; von Hippel-Lindau disease associated in minority of cases
  - Location: Tumor centered along posterior wall of temporal bone in location of endolymphatic sac and duct
  - CT: Spiculated or coarse calcifications within tumor matrix; thin calcification seen along posterior margin
  - MR: T1 high signal foci from blood products trapped within tumor matrix

Semicircular Canal Dehiscence

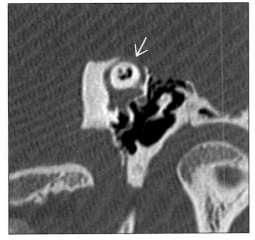

Transverse oblique reformation bone CT displays the dehiscent roof of the superior semicircular canal ➡ to best advantage by showing the entire extent of the dehiscence in a single image.

Fenestral Otosclerosis

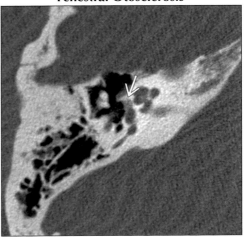

Axial bone CT demonstrates a subtle active otosclerotic plaque along the anterior margin of the oval window ➡ in the location of the fissula antefenestrum.

INNER EAR LESION, ADULT

(Left) Axial bone CT shows severe labyrinthine ossificans. Notice that the basal turn of the cochlea is ossified but still identifiable ➡, whereas the second turn is invisible ⏩. *(Right)* Axial bone CT shows a high jugular bulb ➡ visible at the level of the internal auditory canal ➡, abutting the bony vestibular aqueduct ⏩. Note that it does not enter the middle ear cavity.

Labyrinthine Ossificans

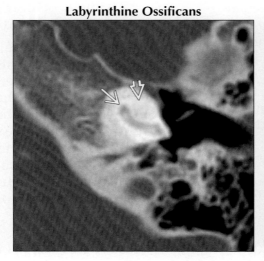

Jugular Bulb, High

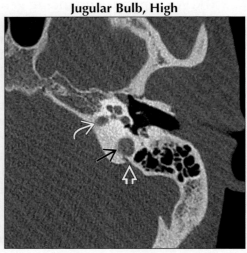

(Left) Coronal bone CT demonstrates the jugular bulb diverticulum as a superomedial projection off the top of the jugular bulb ➡. These lesions are asymptomatic. *(Right)* Axial bone CT reveals a transverse fracture traversing inner ear structures ➡. Notice the pneumolabyrinth ⏩ in the vestibule indicating perilymphatic fistula at the oval window level.

Jugular Bulb Diverticulum

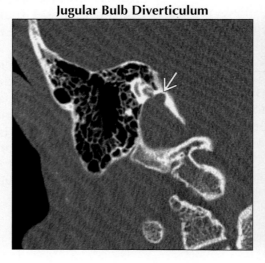

Fracture, T-Bone, Inner Ear

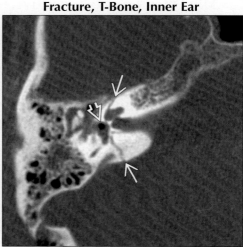

(Left) Axial T2WI MR shows a large endolymphatic sac ➡ along the posterior wall of the temporal bone. Note the associated cochlear dysplasia with modiolar deficiency and bulbous apical cochlear turn ⏩. *(Right)* Axial bone CT demonstrates a non-ossifying amorphous geniculate ganglion lesion ➡ pedunculating into the anterior epitympanic recess. The anterior tympanic segment of CN7 ⏩ is also shown.

Large Endolymphatic Sac Anomaly (IP-2)

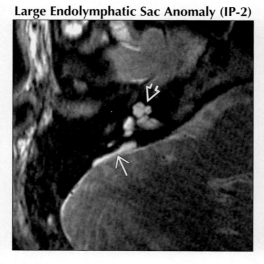

Hemangioma, Facial Nerve, T-Bone

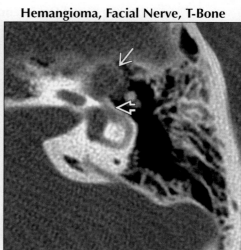

INNER EAR LESION, ADULT

Schwannoma, Facial Nerve, T-Bone

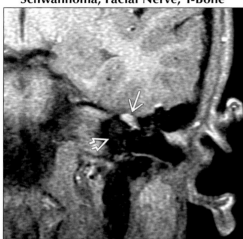

Labyrinthitis

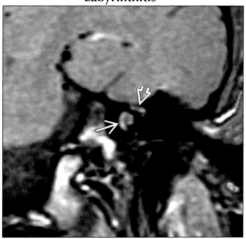

(Left) Coronal T1 C+ FS MR reveals an enhancing well-circumscribed lesion of the geniculate ganglion ➡. Notice this ovoid facial nerve schwannoma sits just superior to the cochlea ➡. (Right) Coronal T1 C+ MR shows a diffusely enhancing cochlea ➡ along with facial nerve enhancement in the geniculate ganglion area ➡. Clinical presentation was acute onset vertigo and sensorineural hearing loss.

Schwannoma, Intralabyrinthine

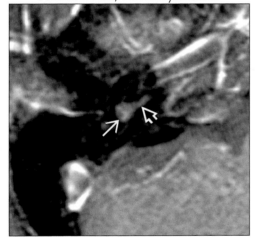

Cochlear Otosclerosis

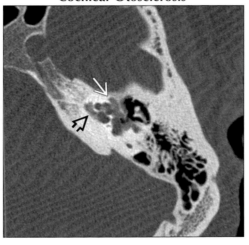

(Left) Axial T1 C+ FS MR shows a mildly enhancing schwannoma ➡ involving the posterolateral aspect of the basal turn of the cochlea ➡. Lesion protrudes into the middle ear cavity. (Right) Axial bone CT in a patient with severe cochlear ➡ and fenestral ➡ otosclerosis. The cochlear otospongiosis plaque at first appears to be a "third turn of the cochlea."

Intralabyrinthine Hemorrhage

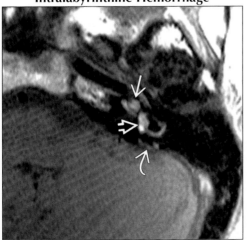

Endolymphatic Sac Tumor

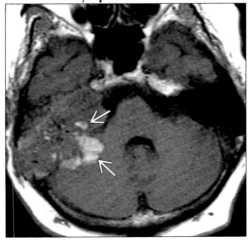

(Left) Axial T1WI MR reveals high signal intralabyrinthine hemorrhage involving the cochlea ➡, vestibule ➡, and endolymphatic sac ➡. (Right) Axial T1WI MR shows a very large right endolymphatic sac tumor. The high signal blood in the tumor matrix ➡ and broad involvement of posterior T-bone wall suggest this diagnosis.

8

PETROUS APEX LESION

DIFFERENTIAL DIAGNOSIS

Common
- Asymmetric Marrow, Petrous Apex
- Trapped Fluid, Petrous Apex
- Cholesterol Granuloma, Petrous Apex
- Metastasis, Petrous Apex

Less Common
- Cephalocele, Petrous Apex
- Meningioma, T-Bone
- Paget Disease, T-Bone
- Fibrous Dysplasia, T-Bone
- Schwannoma, Trigeminal, Skull Base
- Cholesteatoma, Petrous Apex
- Chondrosarcoma, Skull Base
- Plasmacytoma, Skull Base
- Langerhans Histiocytosis, Skull Base

Rare but Important
- Apical Petrositis
- Mucocele, Petrous Apex
- ICA Aneurysm, Petrous Apex

ESSENTIAL INFORMATION

Key Differential Diagnosis Issues
- Best imaging tool
  - CT and MR are complementary
    - Bone CT to evaluate petrous apex (PA) "bony" expansion or destruction
    - MR for lesion tissue analysis; characteristic signal per diagnosis
- Beware confusing high T1 MR signal in trapped fluid with PA cholesterol granuloma
  - When protein content is high, T1 signal may be high
  - In absence of bony expansion on CT, lesion should be considered trapped fluid

Helpful Clues for Common Diagnoses
- **Asymmetric Marrow, Petrous Apex**
  - Asymmetric pneumatization makes contralateral fatty marrow conspicuous
  - CT: Nonexpansile fat density PA
  - MR: High T1 normal fatty marrow
- **Trapped Fluid, Petrous Apex**
  - Remote otomastoiditis leaves behind PA air cell fluid of variable protein content
  - CT: Opacified air cells; trabeculae present
  - MR: Low T1, high T2 signal
- **Cholesterol Granuloma, Petrous Apex**
  - Chronic otitis media; pneumatized PA with recurrent hemorrhage
  - CT: Smooth, expansile margins; larger lesions affect clivus, jugular tubercle, ICA
  - MR: High T1 & T2 signal, expanded PA
- **Metastasis, Petrous Apex**
  - Spread from breast, lung, kidney, prostate, stomach cancer primaries most common
  - CT: Focal destructive PA lesion
  - MR: Intermediate T1 & T2 lesion, enhances on T1 C+ MR

Helpful Clues for Less Common Diagnoses
- **Cephalocele, Petrous Apex**
  - Incidental PA lesion where Meckel cave appears herniated into subjacent PA
  - CT: Expansile ovoid lesion
  - MR: Low T1, high T2 "pseudopod" from Meckel cave to PA; non-enhancing
- **Meningioma, T-Bone**
  - CT: Permeative, sclerotic, or hyperostotic bony changes
  - MR: Dural-based mass invades PA with avid contrast enhancement, dural tail
- **Paget Disease, T-Bone**
  - Bone dysplasia found in older males with excessive bony remodeling; alternating osteoblastic, & osteoclastic activity
    - Early phase: Bone demineralization
    - Intermediate: "Ground-glass" appearance
    - Late phase: Extreme bone thickening & otic capsule demineralization
  - CT: Disease phase dependent; bony expansion with "cotton wool" appearance
  - MR: Low T1 signal from fibrous tissue marrow replacement; T2 variable
- **Fibrous Dysplasia, T-Bone**
  - Bone disorder of younger women (< 30 years) with progressive replacement of normal marrow by mixture of fibrous tissue & disorganized trabeculae
    - Active phase: Cystic
    - Least active/burned out: Sclerotic
  - CT: Expansile bone lesion with mixed "ground-glass"/sclerotic & cystic components sparing otic capsule
  - MR: Low T1 & T2 signal; foci of enhancement common
- **Schwannoma, Trigeminal, Skull Base**
  - Larger trigeminal nerve schwannoma involves preganglionic segment as it passes into Meckel cave

- CT: Smooth PA remodeling of inferior porus trigeminus margin
- MR: Homogeneously enhancing tubular mass; intramural cysts when large
• **Cholesteatoma, Petrous Apex**
  ○ Congenital or acquired PA cholesteatoma
  ○ CT: Smooth, expansile low density lesion
  ○ MR: Low T1, high T2, nonenhancing PA lesion with restricted diffusion on DWI
• **Chondrosarcoma, Skull Base**
  ○ Originates from petrooccipital fissure
  ○ CT: Characteristic chondroid matrix in 50%, invasive bony changes
  ○ MR: T2 high signal; mixed enhancement
• **Plasmacytoma, Skull Base**
  ○ Intramedullary plasma cell tumor
  ○ CT: Intraosseous, lytic lesion with nonsclerotic margins
  ○ MR: Cellular lesion, T1 & T2 isointense to gray matter; homogeneous enhancement
• **Langerhans Histiocytosis, Skull Base**
  ○ Langerhans histiocytes proliferation forming lytic sites in skull & skull base
  ○ Peds: Onset 1 year; multifocal < 5 years
  ○ CT: Lytic lesion with beveled margins
  ○ MR: Avidly enhancing soft tissue mass

Helpful Clues for Rare Diagnoses
• **Apical Petrositis**
  ○ Fever, retro-orbital pain, diplopia, otorrhea
  ○ CT: Bony destructive changes
  ○ MR: Enhancing thick dura; PA pus does not enhance
• **Mucocele, Petrous Apex**
  ○ Mimics cholesteatoma; no DWI restriction
  ○ CT: Expansile, smooth margined lesion
  ○ MR: T1 low, T2 high signal fluid; no contrast enhancement
• **ICA Aneurysm, Petrous Apex**
  ○ Expansile, enhancing lesion most commonly involving horizontal segment of petrous ICA
  ○ CT: Focal expansion of petrous ICA canal
  ○ MR: Complex, heterogeneous T1 & T2 signal; flow void
    - MRA used to evaluate size, morphology & amount of clotted blood

Alternative Differential Approaches
• Destructive PA lesions: Metastasis, chondrosarcoma, plasmacytoma, apical periositis
• Nondestructive expansile PA lesions: Cholesteatoma, cholesterol granuloma, cephalocele, schwannoma, mucocele, aneurysm
• Nondestructive nonexpansile PA lesions: Trapped fluid, asymmetric bone marrow
• Enhancing PA lesions: Metastasis, meningioma, schwannoma, chondrosarcoma, plasmacytoma, Langerhans histiocytosis, apical petrositis
• Marked bone marrow expansion: Paget disease, fibrous dysplasia
• High T1 & T2 signal: Cholesterol granuloma, trapped fluid with high protein content

Asymmetric Marrow, Petrous Apex

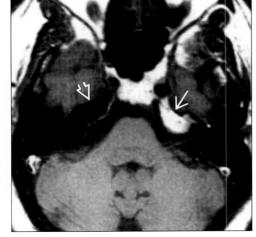

Axial T1WI MR shows high signal intensity fatty marrow in the left petrous apex ➡ without expansile or destructive changes. Contralateral aerated right petrous apex lacks signal ➡.

Trapped Fluid, Petrous Apex

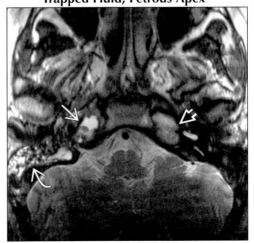

Axial T2WI MR shows high right petrous apex signal ➡, consistent with fluid. Signal in the left PA ➡ is fat intensity, similar to adjacent marrow. Right mastoid fluid is noted ➡.

PETROUS APEX LESION

Cholesterol Granuloma, Petrous Apex

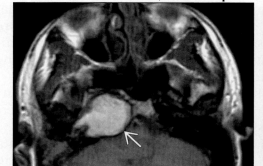

Metastasis, Petrous Apex

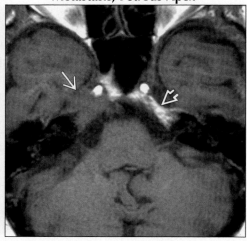

(Left) Axial T1WI MR shows a high signal expansile cholesterol granuloma of the petrous apex ➡. *(Right)* Axial T1WI MR demonstrates a low signal intensity invasive mass in the right petrous apex ➡. Compare to the normal high signal fatty marrow in the left petrous apex ➡.

Cephalocele, Petrous Apex

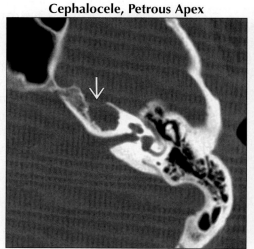

Meningioma, T-Bone

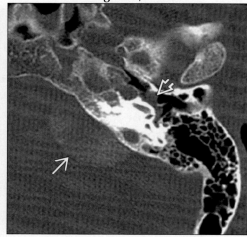

(Left) Axial bone CT reveals benign osseous expansion of the anterior left petrous apex ➡, posterior to the left Meckel cave, typical of petrous apex cephalocele. *(Right)* Axial bone CT shows a high attenuation dural-based mass in the CPA cistern ➡. Note the tumor passes through the petrous apex and inferior inner ear bone to access the middle ear ➡.

Paget Disease, T-Bone

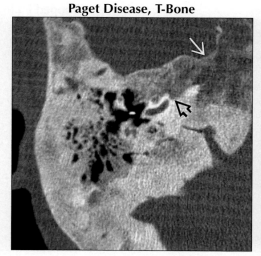

Fibrous Dysplasia, T-Bone

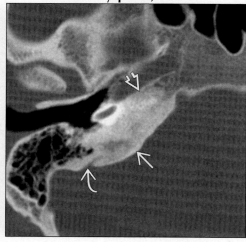

(Left) Axial bone CT shows diffuse enlargement and "cotton wool" appearance of petrous apex ➡ and mastoid bones with several areas of persistent demineralization. Note otic capsule involvement ➡. *(Right)* Axial bone CT demonstrates the characteristic expansile "ground-glass" appearance of the inner ear ➡ and petrous apex ➡ areas of the temporal bone. Vestibular aqueduct is engulfed ➡.

PETROUS APEX LESION

Schwannoma, Trigeminal, Skull Base

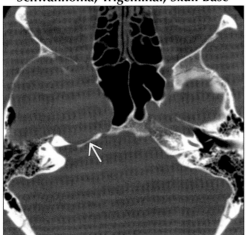

Cholesteatoma, Petrous Apex

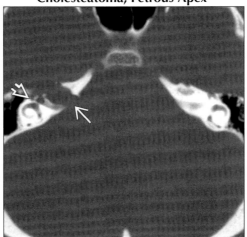

(Left) Axial bone CT reveals remodeling ➡ of inferior margin of porus trigeminus of Meckel cave from large trigeminal schwannoma affecting preganglionic segment and Meckel cave portion of CN5. *(Right)* Axial bone CT shows a smooth expansile lesion in the right petrous apex ➡ with bony erosion of the adjacent cochlea ⮞.

Chondrosarcoma, Skull Base

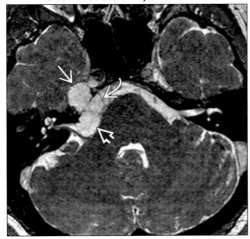

Langerhans Histiocytosis, Skull Base

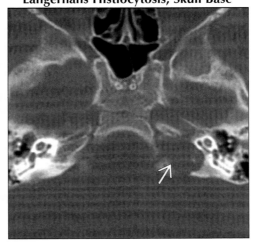

(Left) Axial T2WI MR 2 mm slice shows high signal chondrosarcoma extending up from petrooccipital fissure into the petrous apex ➡ and CPA cistern ⮞. CN6 is visible in the anterior CPA cistern ⮞. *(Right)* Axial bone CT shows a lytic lesion in the left petrous apex ➡ in a child. As rhabdomyosarcoma in this area is centered in the middle ear, Langerhans cell histiocytosis is first choice here.

Apical Petrositis

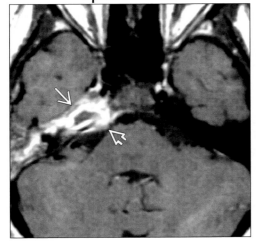

Mucocele, Petrous Apex

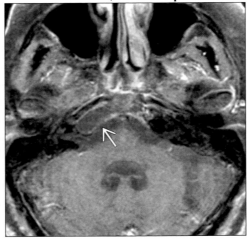

(Left) Axial T1 C+ MR reveals abnormal enhancement ➡ around a nonenhancing focus of pus in the petrous apex. Note associated dural enhancement and thickening ⮞. *(Right)* Axial T1 C+ FS MR image reveals the expansile right petrous apex mucocele ➡, which does not enhance. It lacks MR DWI restriction to distinguish it from cholesteatoma.

INNER EAR LESION, CHILD

DIFFERENTIAL DIAGNOSIS

Common
- Fracture, T-Bone
- Large Endolymphatic Sac Anomaly (IP-2)
- Labyrinthine Ossificans
- Subarcuate Artery Pseudolesion

Less Common
- Semicircular Canal Dysplasia, CHARGE Syndrome
- Labyrinthitis
- Intralabyrinthine Hemorrhage

Rare but Important
- Cystic Cochleovestibular Anomaly (IP-1)
- Aplasia-Hypoplasia, Cochlear Nerve Canal
- Common Cavity, Inner Ear
- Cochlear Aplasia, Inner Ear
- Osteogenesis Imperfecta, T-Bone
- Branchiootorenal Syndrome, Inner Ear
- X-Linked Mixed Hearing Loss Anomaly
- Labyrinthine Aplasia

ESSENTIAL INFORMATION

Key Differential Diagnosis Issues
- Congenital lesions in differential diagnosis
  - Congenital deafness has imaging diagnosis associated < 50%
  - If imaging diagnosis is found, large endolymphatic sac anomaly (incomplete partition type 2) is most common
  - All other inner ear congenital lesions that can be diagnosed by imaging are rare
- Imaging recommendations in childhood sensorineural hearing loss (SNHL)
  - Begin with T-bone CT
  - Add high-resolution T2 MR in axial & oblique sagittal plane when cochlear implant is under consideration
    - Define IAC size, integrity of cochlear nerve canal, presence of cochlear nerve

Helpful Clues for Common Diagnoses
- **Fracture, T-Bone**
  - Complex T-bone fractures may involve inner ear structures
  - T-bone CT: Fracture line crosses inner ear ± pneumolabyrinth
- **Large Endolymphatic Sac Anomaly (IP-2)**

- Clinical clues: Bilateral congenital SNHL that appears in child with cascading hearing loss pattern
  - Most common congenital imaging abnormality
  - CT: Enlarged bony vestibular aqueduct + mild cochlear dysplasia
  - MR: Enlarged endolymphatic sac + mild cochlear aplasia (modiolar deficiency, bulbous apical turn, scala vestibuli larger than scala tympani)
- **Labyrinthine Ossificans**
  - Clinical clues: Child develops profound SNHL after episode of meningitis or middle ear infection
  - Healing of suppurative labyrinthitis may result in osteoneogenesis within inner ear fluid spaces
  - CT: Ossific plaques impinges on inner ear fluid spaces
    - Define as cochlear and noncochlear for cochlear implant evaluation
  - MR: High-resolution T2 shows encroachment on membranous labyrinthine fluid spaces
- **Subarcuate Artery Pseudolesion**
  - Asymptomatic normal variant that disappears in 1st two years of life
  - CT: Prominent canal passes beneath superior semicircular canal arch
  - MR: Conspicuous high signal canal on T2 imaging underneath superior semicircular canal

Helpful Clues for Less Common Diagnoses
- **Semicircular Canal Dysplasia, CHARGE Syndrome**
  - Clinical clues: Colobomata, heart defects, choanal atresia, retardation, genitourinary problems, ear abnormalities
  - CT: Bilateral semicircular canal absence, small vestibules, oval window atresia, cochlear nerve canal atresia
  - MR: Cochlear nerve absence
- **Labyrinthitis**
  - Clinical clue: Acute onset vertigo, hearing loss ± facial nerve paralysis
  - CT: Acute phase normal
  - MR: Often normal; if positive, diffuse enhancement of inner ear fluid spaces most common presentation
- **Intralabyrinthine Hemorrhage**

○ Clinical clue: May be idiopathic or post-traumatic
○ CT: Normal unless associated with trauma
○ MR: High T1 signal in inner ear fluid

Helpful Clues for Rare Diagnoses
- **Cystic Cochleovestibular Anomaly (IP-1)**
  ○ Inner ear morphology: Inner ear looks like tilted "snowman" configuration on axial image
  ○ CT: Cochlea and vestibule cystic; bony vestibular aqueduct usually normal
  ○ MR: Both cochlea and vestibule are cystic; endolymphatic sac usually normal
- **Aplasia-Hypoplasia, Cochlear Nerve Canal**
  ○ CT: Complete or partial bony narrowing of base of cochlear nerve canal
  ○ MR: Fluid in cochlear nerve canal completely or partially replaced by low signal bone
    ▪ Cochlear nerve absent if aplasia of cochlear nerve canal
- **Common Cavity, Inner Ear**
  ○ Inner ear morphology: Inner ear looks like single cyst
  ○ CT: Single cyst with semicircular canals and vestibular aqueduct blended in
  ○ MR: Single inner ear fluid-filled cyst
- **Cochlear Aplasia, Inner Ear**
  ○ CT: Cochlea absent with variable deformity of vestibule, semicircular canals, and vestibular aqueduct
  ○ MR: Absent cochlea and cochlear nerve
- **Osteogenesis Imperfecta, T-Bone**
  ○ Clinical clues: Blue sclera; mild form develops deafness by age 40 years
  ○ Imaging same as cochlear otosclerosis
  ○ CT: Active disease shows lucent foci in otic capsule surrounding cochlea
  ○ MR: Active disease shows enhancing foci in otic capsule
- **Branchiootorenal Syndrome, Inner Ear**
  ○ Clinical clues: Auricular deformity, prehelical pits, mixed hearing loss, branchial fistulae, and renal abnormalities
  ○ Genetics: 40% with clinical manifestations have mutations of EYA1 gene on chromosome 8q13.3
  ○ CT: Hypoplastic apical turn of cochlea, medial deviation of facial nerve, funnel-shaped IAC, and patulous eustachian tube
- **X-Linked Mixed Hearing Loss Anomaly**
  ○ Clinical clues: Male child with bilateral mixed conductive and SNHL
    ▪ Open communication between IAC CSF pressure and cochlear fluid creates perilymphatic hydrops, with "gusher" resulting if stapes disturbed
  ○ CT: Cochlear nerve canal is enlarged with no modiolus
    ▪ Labyrinthine and anterior tympanic facial nerve canal may be enlarged
    ▪ Oval window atresia may be present
- **Labyrinthine Aplasia**
  ○ CT and MR: Inner ear structures and IAC absent

Fracture, T-Bone

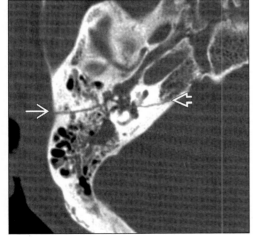

Axial bone CT shows a longitudinal fracture traversing the mastoid ➡, ossicles (note malleus head slightly separated from short process incus), oval window, and inner ear ➡.

Large Endolymphatic Sac Anomaly (IP-2)

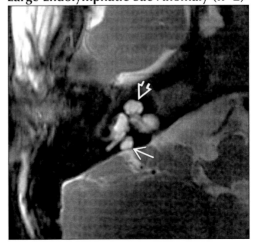

Axial T2WI MR reveals a large endolymphatic sac ➡ associated with significant cochlear dysplasia ➡ characterized by modiolar absence and cystic morphology.

INNER EAR LESION, CHILD

Labyrinthine Ossificans

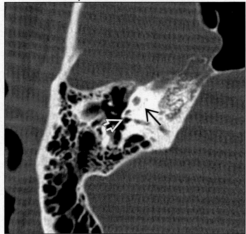

Subarcuate Artery Pseudolesion

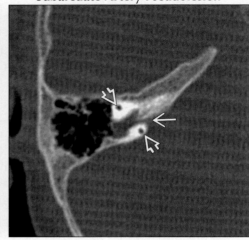

(Left) Axial bone CT reveals labyrinthine ossificans affecting the basal turn of the cochlea ➡. Notice the bony encroachment on the cochlear fluid space extends to the round window niche ➡. *(Right)* Axial bone CT shows a prominent but normal subarcuate artery canal and associated subarachnoid space ➡ passing under the superior semicircular canal arch ➡ prior to its involution.

Semicircular Canal Dysplasia, CHARGE Syndrome

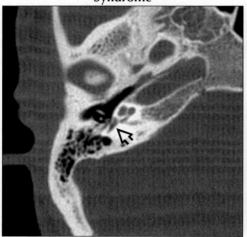

Labyrinthitis

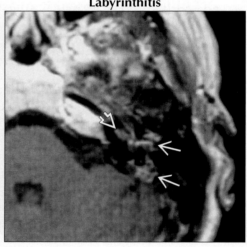

(Left) Axial bone CT shows CHARGE-related absent semicircular canals associated with oval window atresia. The "bare vestibule" has a characteristic small, slightly elongated shape ➡. *(Right)* Axial T1 C+ MR reveals acute otomastoiditis ➡ with secondary suppurative labyrinthitis. The cochlear membranous labyrinth enhances ➡ due to infection by middle ear pathogens.

Intralabyrinthine Hemorrhage

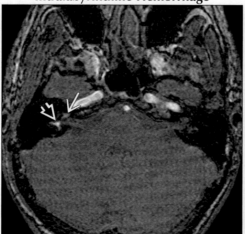

Cystic Cochleovestibular Anomaly (IP-1)

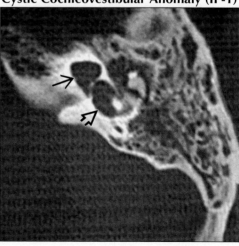

(Left) Axial MRA source image shows high signal blood in the ear vestibular ➡ and cochlear ➡ fluid space. Acute sensorineural hearing loss and vertigo heralded this intralabyrinthine bleed. *(Right)* Axial bone CT shows a grossly abnormal inner ear. Both the cochlea ➡ and the vestibule ➡ are cystic, hence the name cystic cochleovestibular anomaly.

INNER EAR LESION, CHILD

Aplasia-Hypoplasia, Cochlear Nerve Canal

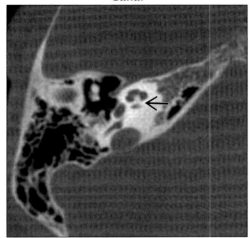

Common Cavity, Inner Ear

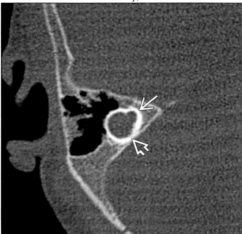

(Left) Axial bone CT demonstrates a bony bar ⇥ across the cochlea base separating it from the IAC fundus. Given the cochlear nerve canal is absent, no cochlear nerve is present in this lesion. *(Right)* Axial bone CT shows a multilobular inner common cavity with a large vestibular ⇥ and a small cochlear ⇥ component.

Cochlear Aplasia, Inner Ear

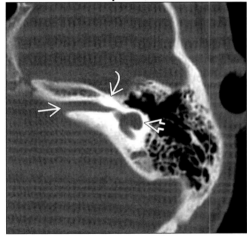

Osteogenesis Imperfecta, T-Bone

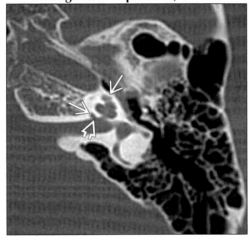

(Left) Axial bone CT reveals a small internal auditory canal ⇥, dysplastic vestibule-semicircular canals ⇥, and absent cochlea ⇥. Absent cochlea implies absent cochlear nerve. *(Right)* Axial bone CT shows multiple lucent foci ⇥ in the bony labyrinth. Notice that the active focus medial to the cochlea appears to communicate with the internal auditory canal ⇥.

Branchiootorenal Syndrome, Inner Ear

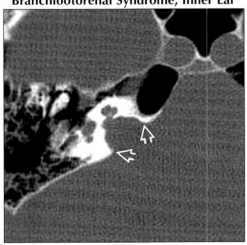

X-Linked Mixed Hearing Loss Anomaly

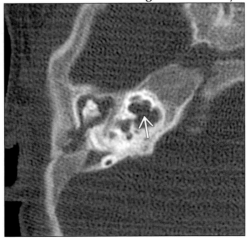

(Left) Axial bone CT shows a widely flared internal auditory canal ⇥, suggestive of branchiootorenal syndrome. A medialized labyrinthine segment of the facial nerve (not shown) is also seen in this lesion. *(Right)* Axial bone CT shows an enlarged cochlear nerve canal ⇥, which allows direct communication between the IAC and the cochlea. Note that the modiolus is absent.

DIFFERENTIAL DIAGNOSIS

Common
- Facial Nerve Enhancement, Intratemporal
- Bell Palsy
- Fracture, T-Bone, Involves CN7 Canal
- Perineural Parotid Malignancy, T-Bone
- Hemangioma, Facial Nerve, T-Bone
- Schwannoma, Facial Nerve, T-Bone

Less Common
- Oval Window Atresia, Ectopic CN7
- Atresia, EAC, Ectopic Facial Nerve

Rare but Important
- Prolapsing Facial Nerve, Middle Ear
- Ramsay Hunt Syndrome
- Lyme Borreliosis, Facial Nerve

ESSENTIAL INFORMATION

Key Differential Diagnosis Issues
- DDx contains lesions primary to intratemporal CN7 or lesions of T-bone where CN7 canal is routinely abnormal
- Routine acute onset Bell palsy NOT imaged
  - Image only "atypical Bell palsy"

Helpful Clues for Common Diagnoses
- **Facial Nerve Enhancement, Intratemporal**
  - Key facts
    - Normal finding; asymptomatic
    - More prominent on 3T MR
  - Imaging
    - T1 C+ MR: Area of geniculate ganglion, anterior tympanic segment, & posterior genu of CN7 normally enhances
- **Bell Palsy**
  - Key facts
    - Acute onset of unilateral peripheral facial nerve paralysis
    - > 90% recover & do not need imaging
    - MR imaging for "atypical Bell palsy"
  - Imaging
    - T-bone CT: Normal facial nerve canal
    - T1 C+ MR: Intratemporal CN7 enhances along entire course; IAC fundal "tuft" enhancement
- **Fracture, T-Bone, Involves CN7 Canal**
  - Key facts
    - Fracture line crosses facial nerve canal
    - Fracture line may be difficult to see; multiplanar reconstructions may help
  - Imaging
    - T-bone CT: Fracture may affect geniculate ganglion, tympanic or mastoid segment of CN7
    - Transverse fractures affect CN7 more commonly than longitudinal fractures do
- **Perineural Parotid Malignancy, T-Bone**
  - Key facts
    - If invasive parotid malignancy found on CT or MR, imaging of stylomastoid foramen & mastoid segment CN7 critical
    - Look for perineural malignancy on CN7
  - Imaging
    - T-bone CT: Enlarged mastoid CN7 canal; adjacent mastoid air cells may be opacified
    - T1 C+ MR: Invasive parotid mass affects stylomastoid foramen; climbs mastoid segment of CN7
- **Hemangioma, Facial Nerve, T-Bone**
  - Key facts
    - May be very subtle early in disease course
    - Any focal CN7 enhancement on MR should be investigated with T-bone CT
  - Imaging
    - Most common location: Geniculate fossa
    - T-bone CT: "Honeycomb" matrix (50%)
    - T1 C+ MR: Geniculate ganglion enhancing mass
- **Schwannoma, Facial Nerve, T-Bone**
  - Key facts
    - 50% present with hearing loss
    - Facial nerve symptoms may be delayed
  - Imaging
    - Most common location: Geniculate fossa
    - Often affects multiple contiguous segments of intratemporal CN7
    - T-bone CT: Expanded, tubular CN7 canal
    - T1 C+ MR: Enhancing mass along CN7

Helpful Clues for Less Common Diagnoses
- **Oval Window Atresia, Ectopic CN7**
  - Key facts
    - May be seen with external auditory canal atresia or as isolated lesion
    - Presents with conductive hearing loss with normal otoscopic exam
    - Key diagnosis to make, as CN7 ectopia may preclude surgery
  - Imaging

- T-bone CT: Oval window access narrowed with atresia plate covering window itself
- Tympanic segment CN7 moves medially from normal location under lateral semicircular canal
- Tympanic segment may be found on superior margin, within or on inferior margin of atresia plate
- **Atresia, EAC, Ectopic Facial Nerve**
  - Key facts
    - Severity of external ear microtia directly related to degree of EAC-middle ear dysplasia
    - Mastoid segment is most commonly ectopic
  - Imaging
    - T-bone CT: EAC atretic with mastoid segment CN7 anterior to normal location
    - EAC stenotic or absent; middle ear small with ossicle fusion mass ± oval window atresia

Helpful Clues for Rare Diagnoses
- **Prolapsing Facial Nerve, Middle Ear**
  - Key facts
    - Intratemporal facial nerve bordering middle ear cavity may have variable bone covering
    - If dehiscence of CN7 is accompanied by protrusion of nerve into middle ear, high risk of injury during surgery
  - Imaging

- T-bone CT: Tympanic segment CN7 dehiscent ± nerve hangs into middle ear cavity
- **Ramsay Hunt Syndrome**
  - Key facts
    - Herpes zoster oticus affects facial nerve ± vestibulocochlear nerve ± inner ear
    - External auditory canal vesicles usually precede CN7 symptoms
  - Imaging
    - T1 C+ MR: Enhancing CN7 in IAC & temporal bone
    - Enhancement of inner ear structures and CN8 variable
- **Lyme Borreliosis, Facial Nerve**
  - Key facts
    - Bacteria *Borrelia* is tick-borne systemic infection
    - May cause acute facial nerve paralysis
  - Imaging
    - T1 C+ MR: Holointratemporal CN7 enhancement

SELECTED REFERENCES
1. Chan EH et al: Facial palsy from temporal bone lesions. Ann Acad Med Singapore. 34(4):322-9, 2005
2. Kress B et al: Bell palsy: quantitative analysis of MR imaging data as a method of predicting outcome. Radiology. 230(2):504-9, 2004
3. Salzman KL et al: Dumbbell schwannomas of the internal auditory canal. AJNR Am J Neuroradiol. 22(7):1368-76, 2001
4. Gebarski SS et al: Enhancement along the normal facial nerve in the facial canal: MR imaging and anatomic correlation. Radiology. 183(2):391-4, 1992
5. Curtin HD et al: "Ossifying" hemangiomas of the temporal bone: evaluation with CT. Radiology. 164(3):831-5, 1987

Facial Nerve Enhancement, Intratemporal

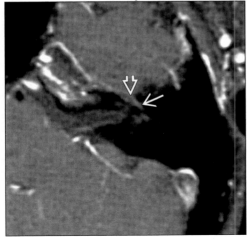

Axial T1 C+ FS MR shows normal enhancement of anterior tympanic segment ➡ and geniculate ganglion ⬧ portions of intratemporal facial nerve in this asymptomatic patient.

Facial Nerve Enhancement, Intratemporal

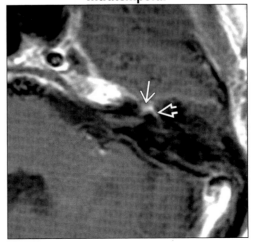

Axial T1 C+ MR reveals prominent but normal enhancement of the geniculate ganglion ➡ and anterior tympanic facial nerve ⬧.

FACIAL NERVE LESION, TEMPORAL BONE

(Left) Axial T1 C+ FS MR reveals an internal auditory canal fundal "tuft" of facial nerve enhancement ⇨ along with enhancement of the labyrinthine segment ⇨ and geniculate ganglion ⇨ in this patient with Bell palsy. *(Right)* Axial T1 C+ FS MR shows the mid-mastoid segment of facial nerve enhancing avidly ➡. A normal mastoid segment never enhances to this degree.

Bell Palsy

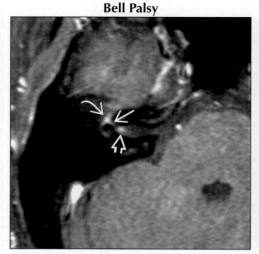

Bell Palsy

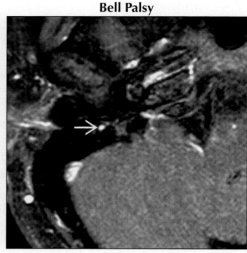

(Left) Axial bone CT demonstrates a transverse fracture through the inner ear. The fracture line ➡ passes anteriorly through the labyrinthine segment of the facial nerve canal ⇨. *(Right)* Coronal T1 C+ FS MR shows a small intraparotid adenoid cystic carcinoma ➡ centered below the stylomastoid foramen. Note mastoid segment facial nerve perineural tumor spread ➡.

Fracture, T-Bone, Involves CN7 Canal

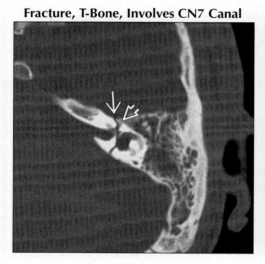

Perineural Parotid Malignancy, T-Bone

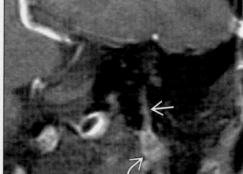

(Left) Axial bone CT shows a C-shaped hemangioma of the labyrinthine segment ⇨ and geniculate ganglion ➡ segments of the facial nerve. The anterior surface of the petrous apex ➡ is also involved. *(Right)* Axial bone CT demonstrates smooth enlargement of the geniculate fossa ➡ and the anterior tympanic segment of the facial nerve canal ⇨, typical of facial nerve schwannoma.

Hemangioma, Facial Nerve, T-Bone

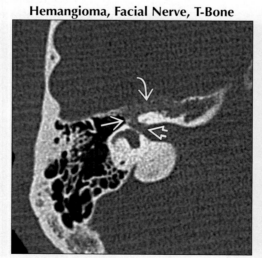

Schwannoma, Facial Nerve, T-Bone

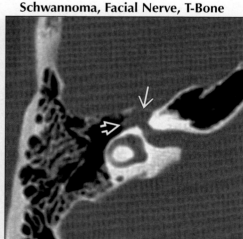

Oval Window Atresia, Ectopic CN7

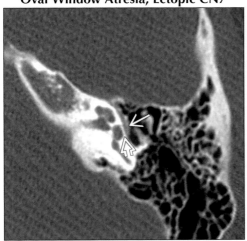

Oval Window Atresia, Ectopic CN7

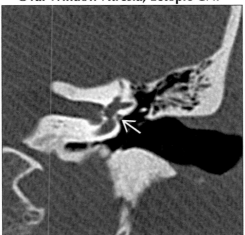

(Left) Axial bone CT demonstrates the tympanic segment of the facial nerve ➡ overlying the oval window, which has an atresia plate visible ➡. (Right) Coronal bone CT shows a typical case of oval window atresia with aberrant facial nerve ➡ overlying the site of the oval window. Any attempt to repair this atresia will result in injury to CN7.

Atresia, EAC, Ectopic Facial Nerve

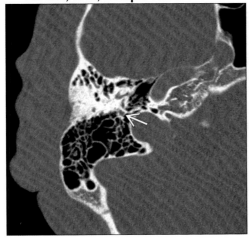

Prolapsing Facial Nerve, Middle Ear

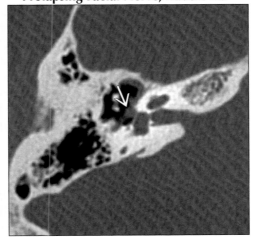

(Left) Axial bone CT demonstrates that the mastoid segment of the facial nerve is anterior to its normal location ➡ as a result of atresia of the EAC. (Right) Axial bone CT shows a typical case of mid-tympanic segment facial nerve prolapse into the middle ear cavity ➡. Facial nerve is sagging into oval window niche.

Ramsay Hunt Syndrome

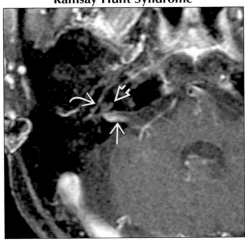

Lyme Borreliosis, Facial Nerve

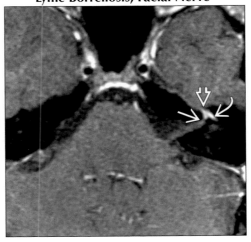

(Left) Axial T1 C+ FS MR reveals linear IAC ➡, cochlear ➡, and tympanic segments of the facial nerve ➡ enhancement. The patient had external ear vesicles at the time of imaging. (Right) Axial T1 C+ FS MR demonstrates intense enhancement of labyrinthine ➡, geniculate ➡, and anterior tympanic ➡ segments of the left intratemporal facial nerve.

ENHANCING MIDDLE EAR LESION

DIFFERENTIAL DIAGNOSIS

Common
- Paraganglioma, Glomus Tympanicum
- Paraganglioma, Glomus Jugulare
- Jugular Bulb, Dehiscent
- Acute Otitis Media

Less Common
- Hemangioma, Facial Nerve, T-Bone
- Schwannoma, Middle Ear
- Meningioma, T-Bone
- Metastasis, T-Bone
- Endolymphatic Sac Tumor
- Rhabdomyosarcoma, Middle Ear

Rare but Important
- Adenoma, Middle Ear
- Langerhans Histiocytosis, T-Bone
- Aberrant Internal Carotid Artery
- Schwannoma, Intralabyrinthine, Transotic

ESSENTIAL INFORMATION

Key Differential Diagnosis Issues
- DDx list includes all middle ear lesions that enhance on CT or MR
  - Lesions may arise in middle ear or access middle ear cavity from adjacent locations
  - Lesions arising in middle ear
    - Glomus tympanicum paraganglioma, acute otitis media, rhabdomyosarcoma, adenoma
  - Lesions arising in adjacent structures
    - Glomus jugulare paraganglioma, dehiscent jugular bulb, facial nerve hemangioma, schwannoma, meningioma, metastasis, endolymphatic sac tumor, Langerhans cell histiocytosis, aberrant ICA, and transotic schwannoma
- Remember that middle ear cholesterol granuloma does not enhance!
  - High signal on T1 MR prior to administration of contrast is responsible for high signal on enhanced T1 MR sequences

Helpful Clues for Common Diagnoses
- **Paraganglioma, Glomus Tympanicum**
  - Otoscopy: Reddish pulsatile retrotympanic mass similar to glomus jugulare paraganglioma

- Must differentiate tympanicum from jugulare paraganglioma as surgical issues are very different
  - Bone CT: Globular mass on cochlear promontory; middle ear bony floor intact
  - MR: Enhancing mass on cochlear promontory; no connection to jugular foramen
- **Paraganglioma, Glomus Jugulare**
  - Otoscopy: Reddish pulsatile retrotympanic mass similar to glomus tympanicum paraganglioma
  - Bone CT: Mass entering middle ear through inferomedial floor from jugular foramen; permeative destructive bone changes
  - MR: Enhancing jugular foramen-middle ear mass with high velocity flow voids; spreads superolaterally
- **Jugular Bulb, Dehiscent**
  - Otoscopy: Blue lesion behind posteroinferior quadrant of TM
  - Bone CT: Dehiscent sigmoid plate with jugular bulb "pseudopod" projecting into posteroinferior middle ear cavity
  - MR: Enhancing lobulation off of superolateral jugular bulb into middle ear
- **Acute Otitis Media**
  - Otoscopy: Bulging, inflamed tympanic membrane
  - Bone CT: Opacification of middle ear-mastoid without loss of ossicles or mastoid trabeculae; air-fluid level possible
  - MR: Enhancing middle ear-mastoid fluid

Helpful Clues for Less Common Diagnoses
- **Hemangioma, Facial Nerve, T-Bone**
  - Clinical clue: Atypical, non-resolving Bell palsy
  - Bone CT: Geniculate ganglion mass with "honeycomb" matrix calcification
  - MR: Enhancing lesion may extend along tympanic CN7 into middle ear
- **Schwannoma, Middle Ear**
  - Otoscopy: Tan-white retrotympanic mass
  - Bone CT: Middle ear mass pedunculating from facial nerve canal or round window niche
  - MR: Sharply marginated enhancing mass extends from facial nerve or round window niche
- **Meningioma, T-Bone**

ENHANCING MIDDLE EAR LESION

- ○ Otoscopy: Pink retrotympanic mass
- ○ Bone CT: Permeative-sclerotic or hyperostotic T-bone wall changes
- ○ MR: Enhancing middle ear mass extends from tegmen dura, jugular foramen, or IAC via inner ear
- • **Metastasis, T-Bone**
  - ○ Bone CT: Destructive middle ear mass
  - ○ MR: Enhancing, invasive middle ear mass
- • **Endolymphatic Sac Tumor**
  - ○ Otoscopy: If enters middle ear, mixed hue retrotympanic mass
  - ○ Bone CT: Spiculated or coarse calcifications in tumor matrix; centered in vestibular aqueduct fovea on posterior T-bone wall
  - ○ MR: High signal foci on T1 sequence from old blood trapped in tumor matrix; enhancing solid portions of tumor
- • **Rhabdomyosarcoma, Middle Ear**
  - ○ Otoscopy: EAC "polyp" in child or young adult; post-auricular mass also possible
  - ○ Bone CT: Destructive middle ear-mastoid mass that often affects EAC, ossicles, surrounding bones, overlying dura
  - ○ MR: Enhancing, invasive ear mass

Helpful Clues for Rare Diagnoses

- • **Adenoma, Middle Ear**
  - ○ Otoscopy: Pink retrotympanic mass
  - ○ Bone CT: Middle ear soft tissue mass usually with no associated inflammatory changes
    - ▪ Difficult to distinguish with bone CT from ME congenital cholesteatoma

- ○ MR: Enhancing middle ear mass
  - ▪ Enhancement on MR differentiates from congenital cholesteatoma of middle ear
- • **Langerhans Histiocytosis, T-Bone**
  - ○ Clinical clue: Post-auricular mass
  - ○ Bone CT: Unilateral or bilateral (30%) destructive T-bone lesions affecting middle ear secondarily
    - ▪ Mastoid air cells more commonly affected than petrous apex or inner ear
  - ○ MR: Avidly enhancing destructive lesion of middle ear & mastoid
- • **Aberrant Internal Carotid Artery**
  - ○ Otoscopy: Red-pink mass passes across inferior tympanic segment
  - ○ Bone CT: Tubular lesion passes into posteroinferior middle ear through enlarged inferior tympanic canaliculus
    - ▪ Passes out of middle ear anteroinferiorly by accessing horizontal petrous internal carotid artery
  - ○ MRA: Aberrant ICA swings more posterolateral than opposite normal petrous ICA
- • **Schwannoma, Intralabyrinthine, Transotic**
  - ○ Rarest form of intralabyrinthine schwannoma
  - ○ Schwannoma extends from CPA-IAC through inner ear to middle ear
  - ○ Bone CT: Middle ear remodeling
  - ○ MR: Enhancing mass from CPA-IAC to middle ear

Paraganglioma, Glomus Tympanicum

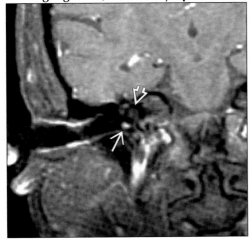

Coronal T1 C+ FS MR reveals a small enhancing mass ➡ sitting on the cochlear promontory without evidence for destruction of the floor of the middle ear cavity. Note cochlear fluid signal ➡.

Paraganglioma, Glomus Tympanicum

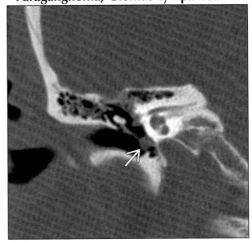

Coronal bone CT demonstrates this small glomus tympanicum paraganglioma as a round mass abutting the cochlear promontory ➡ with preservation of the middle ear bony floor.

ENHANCING MIDDLE EAR LESION

(Left) Coronal T1 C+ MR shows large glomus jugulare filling jugular foramen and nasopharyngeal carotid space, extending through the middle ear floor ➡ to reach the middle ear cavity and EAC ➡. (Right) Axial T1 C+ MR shows a large left jugular bulb ➡ with an anterolateral "tit" ➡ extending into the middle ear cavity. A posterolateral blue retrotympanic mass was visible on otoscopy.

Paraganglioma, Glomus Jugulare

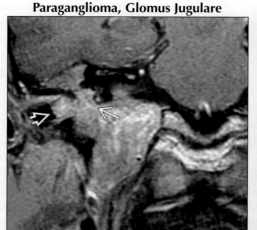

Jugular Bulb, Dehiscent

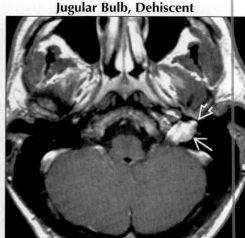

(Left) Axial bone CT reveals generalized mastoid air cell opacification ➡ and an air-fluid level in the petrous apex ➡ in this patient with ear pain, otorrhea, and fever. (Right) Axial T1 C+ MR shows a large enhancing facial nerve hemangioma ➡ of the geniculate fossa area with a tongue of the lesion extending around the cochlea into the middle ear cavity ➡.

Acute Otitis Media

Hemangioma, Facial Nerve, T-Bone

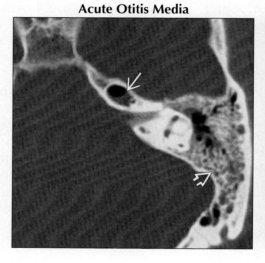

(Left) Axial T1 C+ MR reveals a large enhancing tubular schwannoma of the geniculate ganglion ➡ and tympanic segment ➡. An aditus ad antrum block has created enhancing mastoid fluid ➡. (Right) Axial T1 C+ MR demonstrates a large CPA meningioma ➡ extending through the temporal bone into the middle ear cavity ➡. This lesion can be seen behind an intact tympanic membrane.

Schwannoma, Middle Ear

Meningioma, T-Bone

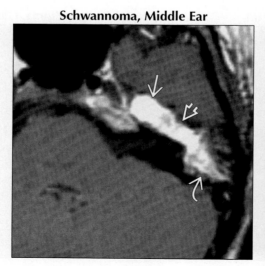

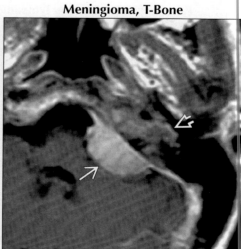

8

ENHANCING MIDDLE EAR LESION

Metastasis, T-Bone

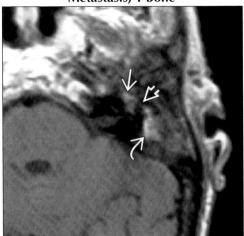

Endolymphatic Sac Tumor

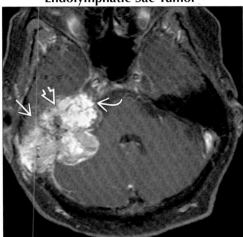

(Left) Axial T1 C+ MR demonstrates enhancing breast metastasis in the geniculate fossa ➡, from there tracking along the tympanic facial nerve ➡. Tumor in mastoid antrum ➡ is noted. *(Right)* Axial T1 C+ MR reveals a giant endolymphatic sac tumor involving the whole temporal bone including the middle ear and mastoid ➡, inner ear ➡, and petrous apex ➡.

Rhabdomyosarcoma, Middle Ear

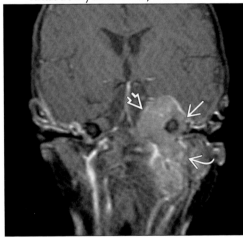

Adenoma, Middle Ear

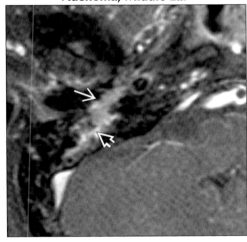

(Left) Coronal T1 C+ FS MR shows bilobed rhabdomyosarcoma involving the middle ear ➡, petrous apex ➡, and suprahyoid neck spaces ➡, including the parotid and parapharyngeal spaces. *(Right)* Axial T1 C+ MR reveals enhancing adenoma tissue in the middle ear ➡ and mastoid ➡. This rare lesion could be mistaken for glomus tympanicum paraganglioma on enhanced MR imaging.

Langerhans Histiocytosis, T-Bone

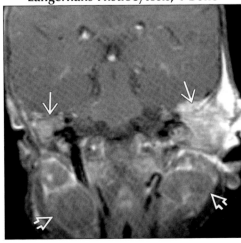

Aberrant Internal Carotid Artery

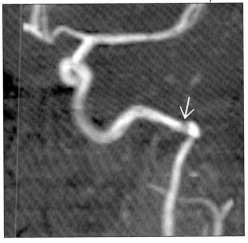

(Left) Coronal T1 C+ MR shows bilateral enhancing foci of Langerhans cell histiocytosis in the temporal bone ➡. Notice the associated neck adenopathy ➡. *(Right)* Anteroposterior MRA demonstrates the characteristic angular shape of the aberrant internal carotid artery. Note the stenosis ➡ seen where the lesion re-enters the horizontal petrous internal auditory canal.

EXPANSILE-DESTRUCTIVE PETROUS APEX LESION

DIFFERENTIAL DIAGNOSIS

Common
- Cholesterol Granuloma, Petrous Apex
- Cephalocele, Petrous Apex
- Metastasis, Petrous Apex

Less Common
- Apical Petrositis
- Cholesteatoma, Petrous Apex
- Aneurysm, ICA, T-Bone
- Chondrosarcoma, Skull Base

Rare but Important
- Plasmacytoma, Skull Base
- Mucocele, Petrous Apex
- Schwannoma, Petrous Apex

ESSENTIAL INFORMATION

Key Differential Diagnosis Issues
- Combining expansile and destructive petrous apex lesions allows discussion of wider range of diagnoses in petrous apex
- Benign congenital, inflammatory, and neoplastic lesions are expansile, while infection and malignant tumors are destructive

Helpful Clues for Common Diagnoses
- **Cholesterol Granuloma, Petrous Apex**
  - Key facts: Expansile "chocolate cyst" filled with old blood
    - Key imaging finding is high T1 signal on MR
  - Bone CT: Smooth expansile lesion with trabecular breakdown
  - MR: High T1 & T2 signal
    - No enhancement; high signal on T1 may fool observer
- **Cephalocele, Petrous Apex**
  - Key facts: Primarily "leave me alone" lesion of petrous apex
    - Rarely requires surgery if CSF leak into temporal bone air cells occurs
    - Key imaging finding is connection to Meckel cave
  - Bone CT: Enlarged inferior margin Meckel cave with expansile petrous apex lesion
  - MR: Low T1 & high T2 signal lesion extending from Meckel cave into petrous apex
    - No enhancement

- **Metastasis, Petrous Apex**
  - Key facts: Primary tumor usually known
  - Bone CT: Aggressive destructive margins
  - MR: Intermediate T1 & T2 signal lesion; enhances

Helpful Clues for Less Common Diagnoses
- **Apical Petrositis**
  - Key facts: Clinically very ill patient
    - May have all or part of Gradenigo syndrome (acute otomastoiditis, otalgia, CN6 palsy)
  - Bone CT: Petrous apex air cells coalesce; bony "destructive" changes
  - MR: Dural and air cell wall enhancement surrounds nonenhancing pus
- **Cholesteatoma, Petrous Apex**
  - Key facts: Congenital, rest of epithelium in petrous apex
    - Key imaging finding is restricted diffusion on DWI MR
  - Bone CT: Smooth expansile petrous apex lesion with trabecular breakdown
  - MR: Low T1 & high T2 signal; no enhancement
    - DWI: Restricted diffusion
- **Aneurysm, ICA, T-Bone**
  - Key facts: Post-traumatic or atherosclerotic
    - Key imaging finding is ovoid area of complex signal
  - Bone CT: Smooth ovoid expansion of petrous ICA canal; Ca++ in wall possible
  - MR: Complex signal (flow, Ca++, clot)
- **Chondrosarcoma, Skull Base**
  - Key facts: Involves petrous apex secondarily
  - Bone CT: 50% chondroid matrix; destructive bone changes
  - MR: Lesion centered in petrooccipital fissure
    - Low T1, high T2 signal; enhances

Helpful Clues for Rare Diagnoses
- **Plasmacytoma, Skull Base**
  - Key facts: Lesion seen as isolated tumor or part of multiple myeloma
  - Bone CT: Destructive lesion in petrous apex marrow
  - MR: Low T1, intermediate T2; enhances
- **Mucocele, Petrous Apex**
  - Key facts: Very rare location for mucocele
    - Requires petrous apex to be aerated to occur

EXPANSILE-DESTRUCTIVE PETROUS APEX LESION

- ○ Bone CT: Expansile petrous apex air cell lesion
- ○ MR: Low T1, high T2 petrous apex lesion; no enhancement
- **Schwannoma, Petrous Apex**
  - ○ Key facts: Nerve of origin uncertain
    - ▪ Key imaging finding is expansile and enhancing
  - ○ Bone CT: Remodeling, expansile bone changes
  - ○ MR: Intermediate T1, T2 signal; enhances

Alternative Differential Approaches

- Once lesion is identified in petrous apex, CT & MR imaging findings may identify its histopathology
- Organize thinking starting with bone CT feature of expansile versus destructive
- Then add T1, T2, DWI, and enhanced MR features
  - ○ Expansile lesions of petrous apex (bone CT)
    - ▪ Cholesterol granuloma: MR shows high T1, high T2
    - ▪ Cephalocele: MR shows low T1, high T2; no enhancement
    - ▪ Congenital cholesteatoma: MR shows low T1, high T2, high DWI; no enhancement
    - ▪ ICA aneurysm: MR shows complex signal from blood, calcium, & flow
    - ▪ Mucocele: MR shows low T1, high T2; no enhancement

- ▪ Schwannoma: MR shows intermediate T1 & T2; enhancement
- ○ Destructive lesions of petrous apex (bone CT)
  - ▪ Apical petrositis: MR shows heterogeneous T1 & T2 signal; dural enhancement surrounding pus
  - ▪ Metastasis: MR shows intermediate T1 & T2 signal; heterogeneous enhancement common
  - ▪ Chondrosarcoma: MR shows intermediate T1, high T2 signal; enhances
  - ▪ Plasmacytoma: MR signal intermediate T1, low T2 signal; enhances

SELECTED REFERENCES

1. Bonneville F et al: Unusual lesions of the cerebellopontine angle: a segmental approach. Radiographics. 21(2):419-38, 2001
2. Moore KR et al: Petrous apex cephaloceles. AJNR Am J Neuroradiol. 22(10):1867-71, 2001
3. Moore KR et al: 'Leave me alone' lesions of the petrous apex. AJNR Am J Neuroradiol. 19(4):733-8, 1998
4. Amedee RG et al: Petrous apex lesions. Skull Base Surg. 4(1):10-4, 1994
5. Lo WW et al: Cholesterol granuloma of the petrous apex: CT diagnosis. Radiology. 153(3):705-11, 1984

Cholesterol Granuloma, Petrous Apex

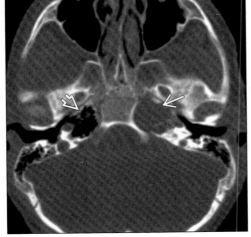

Axial bone CT reveals an expansile lesion of the left petrous apex ➡, which proved to be a cholesterol granuloma. Compare with the normally air-filled right petrous apex ➡.

Cholesterol Granuloma, Petrous Apex

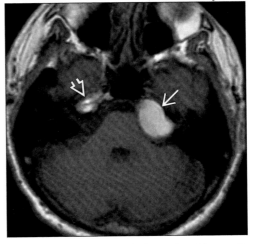

Axial T1WI MR shows a T1 high signal ovoid expansile mass in the left petrous apex ➡ of a different patient. Fatty marrow in right petrous apex ➡ is visible as a result of the absence of fat saturation.

EXPANSILE-DESTRUCTIVE PETROUS APEX LESION

(Left) Axial bone CT demonstrates bilateral petrous apex cephaloceles ➡ projecting into the petrous apex air cells. MR (not shown) demonstrates the cephaloceles connecting to the Meckel cave and following CSF-signal intensity on all sequences. *(Right)* Coronal T2WI MR in another patient shows bilateral "buds" off the inferomedial Meckel cave ➡ projecting into the petrous apices. Petrous apex cephaloceles maintain CSF signal on all MR sequences.

Cephalocele, Petrous Apex

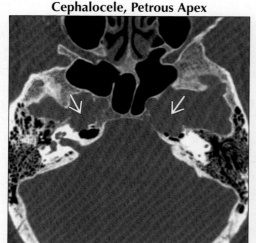

Cephalocele, Petrous Apex

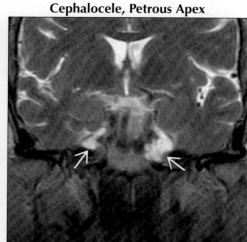

(Left) Axial T1 C+ FS MR demonstrates an irregular enhancing focus of metastatic breast carcinoma ➡ in the left petrous apex. PET/CT (not shown) revealed the lesion to be metabolically active. *(Right)* Axial T1 C+ MR shows pus in coalescent petrous apex air cells ➡ surrounded by dural enhancement. Notice the otomastoiditis ➡ visible as enhancing mastoid air cells.

Metastasis, Petrous Apex

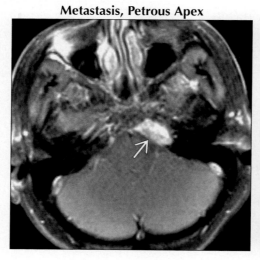

Apical Petrositis

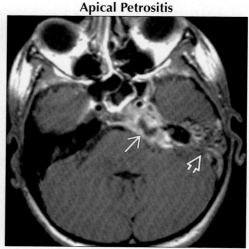

(Left) Axial bone CT shows an expansile congenital cholesteatoma of the lateral petrous apex ➡. Note connection with the enlarged geniculate fossa component ➡. *(Right)* Axial T2WI FS MR reveals a high signal congenital cholesteatoma in the lateral petrous apex ➡ that engulfs the superior semicircular canal ➡. Enhanced MR sequences (not shown) demonstrated no lesion enhancement.

Cholesteatoma, Petrous Apex

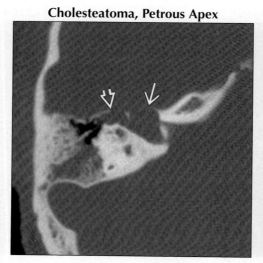

Cholesteatoma, Petrous Apex

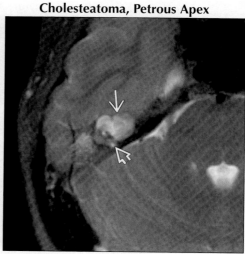

EXPANSILE-DESTRUCTIVE PETROUS APEX LESION

Aneurysm, ICA, T-Bone

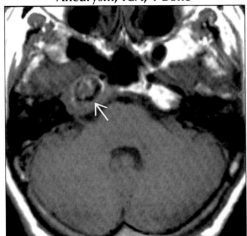

Aneurysm, ICA, T-Bone

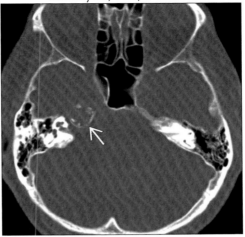

(Left) Axial T1WI MR demonstrates a complex signal ovoid mass ➡ in the petrous apex, found on angiography to be an aneurysm of the distal horizontal petrous internal carotid artery. *(Right)* Axial bone CT shows osseous expansion and destruction of the right petrous apex by an enlarging petrous internal carotid artery aneurysm. Note wall of aneurysm is marked by calcification ➡.

Chondrosarcoma, Skull Base

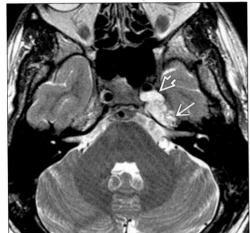

Plasmacytoma, Skull Base

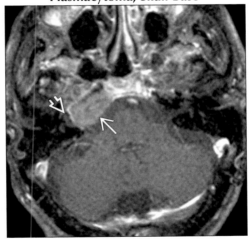

(Left) Axial T2WI MR shows a hyperintense chondrosarcoma of the petrooccipital fissure with its more cephalad component involving the petrous apex ➡ and cavernous internal carotid artery ➡. *(Right)* Axial T1 C+ FS MR shows an enhancing destructive plasmacytoma in the right petrous apex ➡ that is eroding the anteromedial aspect of the inner ear and internal auditory canal ➡.

Mucocele, Petrous Apex

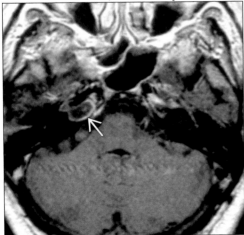

Schwannoma, Petrous Apex

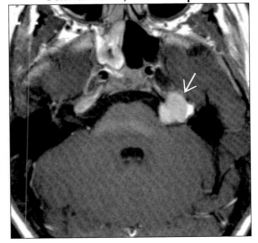

(Left) Axial T1 C+ MR reveals an oval low signal expansile mucocele in the petrous apex ➡ with minimal rim enhancement. DWI MR sequence will differentiate mucocele from epidermoid as needed. *(Right)* Axial T1 C+ MR shows an avidly enhancing schwannoma ➡ arising from the left petrous apex. All other lesions of the petrous apex that enhance are malignant (metastasis, chondrosarcoma, plasmacytoma) or infectious (apical petrositis).

8

BONY LESIONS OF THE TEMPORAL BONE

DIFFERENTIAL DIAGNOSIS

Common
- Fenestral Otosclerosis
- Cochlear Otosclerosis
- Chronic Otitis Media, Under-Pneumatized Mastoid
- Labyrinthine Ossificans
- Hemangioma, Facial Nerve, T-Bone

Less Common
- Fibrous Dysplasia, T-Bone
- Exostoses, EAC
- Osteoma, EAC
- Metastasis, T-Bone
- Meningioma, T-Bone

Rare but Important
- Paget Disease, T-Bone
- Osteopetrosis, T-Bone
- Endolymphatic Sac Tumor
- Osteogenesis Imperfecta, T-Bone

ESSENTIAL INFORMATION

Key Differential Diagnosis Issues
- "Bony" lesion defined as any lesion that affects the bony areas of T-bone and may have increased bone density as part of its imaging manifestation
- Best imaging tool: Temporal bone CT without contrast
  - Enhanced MR is complementary when tumor is suspected

Helpful Clues for Common Diagnoses
- **Fenestral Otosclerosis**
  - Clinical clue: Bilateral acquired conductive hearing loss (CHL)
  - Active disease: CT shows lucent foci along oval & round window margins
  - Chronic disease: CT shows sclerotic, thickened foci along oval & round window margins
- **Cochlear Otosclerosis**
  - Clinical clue: Bilateral mixed CHL and sensorineural hearing loss
  - Active disease: CT shows lucent foci of otic capsule surrounding cochlea
  - Chronic disease: CT shows sclerotic, thickened foci of otic capsule surrounding cochlea

- **Chronic Otitis Media, Under-Pneumatized Mastoid**
  - Clinical clue: Long history of ear infections
  - CT: Under-pneumatized mastoid in association with inflammatory changes of chronic otitis media
- **Labyrinthine Ossificans**
  - Clinical clue: History of meningitis as child; subsequent bilateral sensorineural hearing loss
  - Fibro-osseous material variably fills fluid spaces of inner ear including cochlea, vestibule, & semicircular canals
  - Mild: CT shows subtle increased density & size of modiolus
    - Subtle increased density with inner ear spaces
  - Severe: CT shows inner ear fluid spaces obliterated by bone density material
  - Remember to differentiate cochlear from non-cochlear sites of ossification
- **Hemangioma, Facial Nerve, T-Bone**
  - Clinical clue: Rapid onset facial nerve paralysis; does not resolve like typical Bell palsy
  - Geniculate fossa primary location > > IAC
  - CT: "Honeycomb bone" matrix (50%)
  - T1 C+ MR: Avidly enhancing amorphous mass

Helpful Clues for Less Common Diagnoses
- **Fibrous Dysplasia, T-Bone**
  - Clinical clue: Young patients generally under 30 years of age
  - CT: Typically expansile bony lesion with mixed ground-glass/sclerotic matrix and cystic components
    - Spares otic capsule
- **Exostoses, EAC**
  - Clinical clue: History of extensive scuba diving or other cold water exposure
  - CT: Circumferential bony encroachment on EAC
- **Osteoma, EAC**
  - CT: Bony lesion connected to EAC bony wall by broad base or stalk
- **Metastasis, T-Bone**
  - CT: Destructive bony lesion
    - Lytic or sclerotic appearance depends on primary tumor type
- **Meningioma, T-Bone**

- Meningioma arises from tegmen tympani, jugular foramen, or IAC
- CT: Hyperostotic or permeative-sclerotic bony changes
- T1 C+ MR: Enhancing meningioma of tegmen dura, jugular foramen, or IAC with adjacent bony invasion

Helpful Clues for Rare Diagnoses

- **Paget Disease, T-Bone**
  - Clinical clue: Older patients usually over 50 years in age
  - CT: Involved bone is enlarged with "cotton-wool" appearance
    - May involve otic capsule
- **Osteopetrosis, T-Bone**
  - Clinical clues: Progressive bilateral hearing loss in adult
  - CT: Diffuse increase in T-bone density
    - May involve ossicles
- **Endolymphatic Sac Tumor**
  - Clinical clues: Most are sporadic; von Hippel-Lindau disease present in minority of cases
  - Tumor centered in endolymphatic sac-duct area of posterior temporal bone wall
  - CT: Spiculated or coarse calcifications within tumor matrix with thin "eggshell" calcification along posterior tumor margin
  - MR: Multiple foci of T1 shortening (high signal) secondary to blood collections in interstices of tumor
- **Osteogenesis Imperfecta, T-Bone**

- Clinical clues: Blue sclera; patients with mild form develop deafness by age 40 years
- CT: Resembles cochlear otosclerosis with multiple lucent foci in otic capsule of inner ear

Alternative Differential Approaches

- Divide bony lesions of T-bone into focal and diffuse
  - Focal bony involvement can then further divided into tumors and other causes
  - Diffuse lesions
- Focal bony involvement of T-bone
  - Focal bony lesions: Tumor
    - Hemangioma, facial nerve, T-bone
    - Exostoses, EAC
    - Osteoma, EAC
    - Metastasis, T-bone
    - Meningioma, T-bone
    - Endolymphatic sac tumor
  - Focal bony lesions: Other causes
    - Fenestral otosclerosis
    - Cochlear otosclerosis
    - Chronic otitis media, under-pneumatized mastoid
    - Labyrinthine ossificans
    - Osteogenesis imperfecta, T-bone
- Diffuse bony involvement of T-bone
  - Fibrous dysplasia, T-bone
  - Metastasis, T-bone
  - Paget disease, T-bone
  - Osteopetrosis, T-bone

Fenestral Otosclerosis

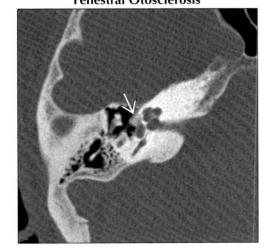

Axial bone CT shows fenestral otosclerosis as an active plaque involving the fissula ante fenestram ➡. The location and lucent-sclerotic density are characteristic.

Cochlear Otosclerosis

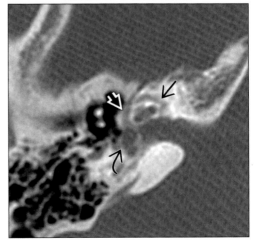

Axial bone CT reveals severe cochlear and fenestral otosclerosis. Note lucency around cochlea ➡, on cochlear promontory ➡, and across oval window margin ➡.

BONY LESIONS OF THE TEMPORAL BONE

Chronic Otitis Media, Under-Pneumatized Mastoid

Labyrinthine Ossificans

(Left) Axial bone CT shows under-pneumatized mastoid ➡ from pars tensa cholesteatoma ➡ with chronic otitis media. Middle ear aeration is required for normal mastoid pneumatization. *(Right)* Axial bone CT shows severe labyrinthine ossificans of the right inner ear. Notice the cochlear fluid space is encroached upon by bone ➡ and the ossific foci in the vestibule ➡.

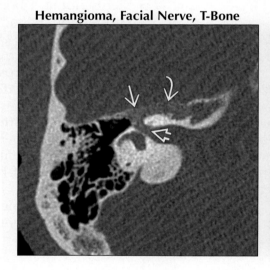
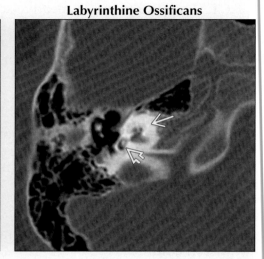

Hemangioma, Facial Nerve, T-Bone

Fibrous Dysplasia, T-Bone

(Left) Axial bone CT shows facial nerve hemangioma involving geniculate ganglion ➡, anteromedial T-bone ➡, and labyrinthine CN7 segment ➡. Subtle "honeycomb" ossification is present. *(Right)* Axial bone CT demonstrates enlarged ground-glass matrix lesion of the T-bone, typical of mature fibrous dysplasia. Mastoid aeration has been obliterated by the growth of this lesion.

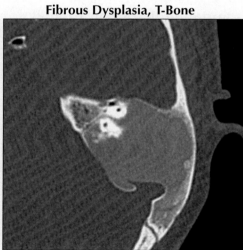

Exostoses, EAC

Osteoma, EAC

(Left) Axial bone CT demonstrates an EAC exostosis as a circumferential encroaching bony lesion ➡ causing narrowing of the bony external auditory canal ➡. *(Right)* Axial bone CT demonstrates a very large osteoma ➡ growing off the external cortex of the post-auricular temporal and occipital bones ➡.

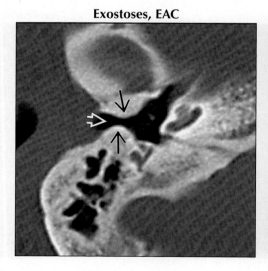
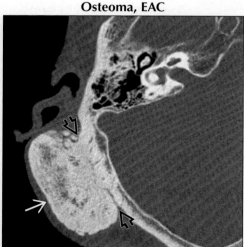

BONY LESIONS OF THE TEMPORAL BONE

Metastasis, T-Bone
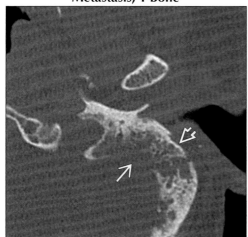

Meningioma, T-Bone
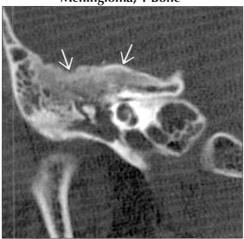

(Left) Axial bone CT shows metastatic tumor affecting the temporal bone. The tumor causes destruction of the medial mastoid cortex/sigmoid plate ➡ and marrow space invasion ➡. (Right) Coronal bone CT shows hyperostotic bone across the tegmen tympani ➡, signaling en plaque meningioma along the adjacent dura. MR (not shown) reveals enhancing meningioma across this area.

Paget Disease, T-Bone
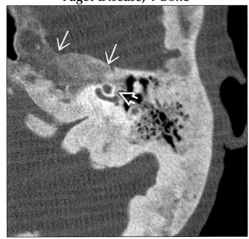

Osteopetrosis, T-Bone
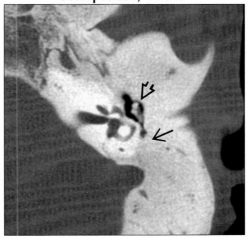

(Left) Axial bone CT shows late-phase Paget disease ➡ with some demineralization indicating acute/subacute phase. Notice the involvement of the bony labyrinth ➡. (Right) Axial bone CT shows severe type 1 autosomal recessive osteopetrosis. Notice generalized increase in bone density with absent mastoid air cells ➡ and encroachment on middle ear ➡.

Endolymphatic Sac Tumor
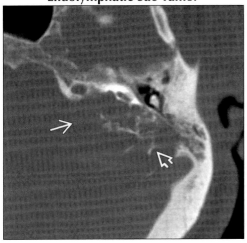

Osteogenesis Imperfecta, T-Bone
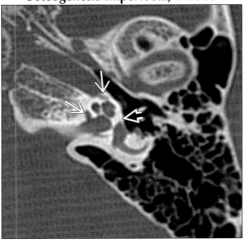

(Left) Axial bone CT reveals an endolymphatic sac tumor along the posterior wall of the T-Bone with both subtle posterior rim calcification ➡ and extensive stellate matrix calcification ➡. (Right) Axial bone CT shows osteogenesis imperfecta affecting the otic capsule of the inner ear as focal lucencies ➡ around the cochlea. Notice the fissula ante fenestram is normal ➡.

CONDUCTIVE HEARING LOSS

DIFFERENTIAL DIAGNOSIS

Common
- Acquired Cholesteatoma, Pars Flaccida
- Chronic Otitis Media
- Atresia, EAC
- Cholesteatoma, EAC
- Cholesterol Granuloma, Middle Ear
- Fenestral Otosclerosis
- Fracture, T-Bone, Ossicle Dislocation

Less Common
- Oval Window Atresia
- Congenital Cholesteatoma, Middle Ear
- COM with Tympanosclerosis
- Acquired Cholesteatoma, Pars Tensa
- Ossicular Fixation, Congenital
- Medial Canal Fibrosis, EAC

Rare but Important
- Osteoma, EAC
- COM with Ossicular Erosions
- Acquired Cholesteatoma, Mural
- Exostoses, EAC
- Keratosis Obturans, EAC

ESSENTIAL INFORMATION

Key Differential Diagnosis Issues
- Conductive hearing loss (CHL) results from disruption of sound conduction via external auditory canal, tympanic membrane (TM), ossicular chain, & oval window
  - Clinical (especially otoscopic) information critical to image interpretation
  - In addition to viewing CHL as a statistical list, this clinically based differential can be organized by lesion anatomic site

Helpful Clues for Common Diagnoses
- **Acquired Cholesteatoma, Pars Flaccida**
  - Otoscopy: Perforation in pars flaccida of tympanic membrane with visible cholesteatoma
  - CT: Prussak space tissue with scutum blunting
    - Ossicle, lateral semicircular canal or tegmen tympani erosion possible
- **Chronic Otitis Media**
  - Otoscopy: Thickened, reddish tympanic membrane ± perforation
  - CT: Linear middle ear-mastoid tissue

- If under-pneumatized mastoid present, COM longstanding
- **Atresia, EAC**
  - Ear examination: Deformed, microtic external ear with small or absent EAC
    - Severity of external ear deformity proportional to EAC-middle ear dysplasia
  - CT: EAC dysplasia and middle ear abnormalities variable
    - Middle ear cavity small with ossicle fusion common
    - CN7 mastoid segment often anterior
- **Cholesteatoma, EAC**
  - Otoscopy: Heaped up mucosa; if inflamed may mimic SCCa
  - CT: EAC mass + underlying bony erosion
    - Bony debris within lesion characteristic
- **Cholesterol Granuloma, Middle Ear**
  - Otoscopy: Blue-black material seen behind tympanic membrane
  - CT: Ossicle destruction ± tegmen or lateral semicircular canal dehiscence
    - Mimics acquired cholesteatoma on CT
  - MR: High T1 & T2 signal highly suggestive of this diagnosis
- **Fenestral Otosclerosis**
  - Otoscopy: If mild, normal; if severe, blue hue seen through TM (Schwartze sign)
  - CT: Lytic (otospongiotic) foci on anterior margin of oval window (fissula antefenestrum)
    - When diffuse disease present, margins of oval & round windows involved
- **Fracture, T-Bone, Ossicle Dislocation**
  - CT: Normal ossicle relationships disrupted by T-bone trauma
    - Incudo-stapedial articulation most commonly affected
    - Malleal-incudal articulation also affected; easily seen on axial CT

Helpful Clues for Less Common Diagnoses
- **Oval Window Atresia**
  - CT: Oval window niche is small or absent
    - Tympanic segment CN7 is in oval window niche, not under lateral semicircular canal
- **Congenital Cholesteatoma, Middle Ear**
  - Otoscopy: White mass behind intact TM
  - CT: Well-defined soft tissue lesion filling middle ear cavity; often medial to ossicles
- **COM with Tympanosclerosis**

- CT: Post-inflammatory calcific foci affect ossicles, ligament, TM
- **Acquired Cholesteatoma, Pars Tensa**
  - Otoscopy: Ruptured pars tensa with white mass in TM rent
  - CT: Meso- and hypotympanic soft tissue with ossicle, middle ear wall erosions
- **Ossicular Fixation, Congenital**
  - CT: Ossicle(s) ankylosed to middle ear wall
- **Medial Canal Fibrosis, EAC**
  - Otoscopy: Thickened TM with adjacent inflammation
  - CT: Crescentic medial EAC tissue

Helpful Clues for Rare Diagnoses
- **COM with Ossicular Erosions**
  - Mastoid shows air cell opacification with linear inflammatory debris in middle ear
  - All or part of ossicle(s) may be absent secondary to previous acute inflammation

Other Essential Information
- Best imaging tool for CHL: T-bone CT
- In cases of CHL, imaging is usually positive
  - Especially true with multislice CT at 0.4-0.6 mm slice thickness
  - Warning: If you cannot find lesion, keep looking!
- Of lesions in "Less Common" and "Rare" lists above, 3 are difficult imaging diagnoses
  - Oval window atresia, congenital ossicular fixation, and chronic otitis media with ossicular erosions can be missed unless specifically looked for in CHL patients

Alternative Differential Approaches
- Normal anatomic chain that permits conductive hearing loss includes EAC, tympanic membrane-ossicles, oval window
- Approaching CHL from anatomic perspective allows radiologist to inspect each of these areas looking for specific groups of diagnostic possibilities
  - Approach to image interrogation in setting of CHL is key to identifying subtle lesions such as oval window atresia
- EAC-related causes, CHL
  - Atresia, EAC
  - Cholesteatoma, EAC
  - Medial canal fibrosis, EAC
  - Osteoma, EAC
  - Exostoses, EAC
  - Keratosis obturans, EAC
- TM-ossicle related causes, CHL
  - Acquired cholesteatoma, pars flaccida
  - Chronic otitis media
  - Cholesterol granuloma, middle ear
  - Fracture, T-bone, ossicle dislocation
  - Congenital cholesteatoma, middle ear
  - COM with tympanosclerosis
  - Acquired cholesteatoma, pars tensa
  - Ossicular fixation, congenital
  - COM with ossicular erosions
  - Acquired cholesteatoma, mural
- Oval window related causes, CHL
  - Fenestral otosclerosis
  - Oval window atresia

Acquired Cholesteatoma, Pars Flaccida

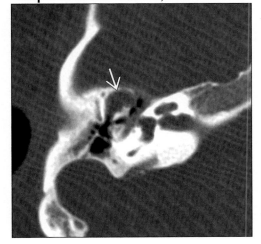

Axial bone CT shows a typical pars flaccida acquired cholesteatoma filling Prussak space ➡. Notice the medial displacement of the ossicles with subtle erosion along their lateral margin.

Acquired Cholesteatoma, Pars Flaccida

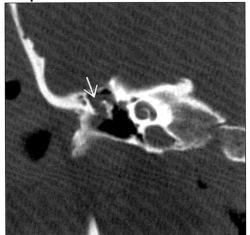

Coronal bone CT reveals typical case of cholesteatoma in Prussak space ➡ with ossicular erosion seen on the lateral surface of the malleus and minimal blunting of the scutum.

CONDUCTIVE HEARING LOSS

(Left) Axial bone CT shows chronic otitis media with linear middle ear inflammatory debris ⮑ and under-pneumatized mastoid ➡. Lack of mastoid aeration suggests this is a lifelong problem. *(Right)* Axial bone CT shows severe EAC atresia characterized by absent EAC ➡, small middle ear, and fused ossicles ⮑. Note the auricle is dysplastic ➡ and the inner ear is normal as is typically seen.

Chronic Otitis Media

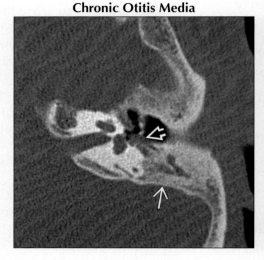

Atresia, EAC

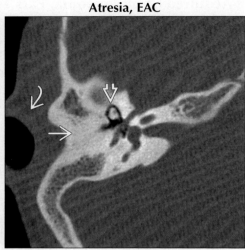

(Left) Axial bone CT shows EAC cholesteatoma eroding through posterior EAC wall ➡. Note the subtle bony flecks within cholesteatoma matrix ⮑, a radiologic marker for this lesion. *(Right)* Axial T1WI MR reveals middle ear cholesterol granuloma ➡ is high signal as expected. "Tympanogenic labyrinthine ossificans" obliterates cochlear ⮑ and vestibular ➡ fluid signal.

Cholesteatoma, EAC

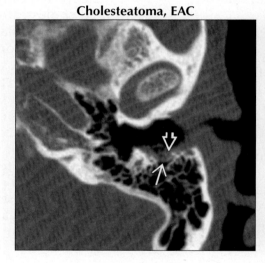

Cholesterol Granuloma, Middle Ear

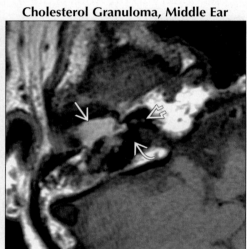

(Left) Axial bone CT shows a typical case of mild fenestral otosclerosis. Notice the small active otosclerotic plaque along the anterior oval window margin (fissula antefenestrum foci) ➡. *(Right)* Axial bone CT shows post-traumatic ossicular dislocation. Note disruption ➡ of "ice cream on a cone" relationship between head of malleus (ice cream) and short process of incus (cone).

Fenestral Otosclerosis

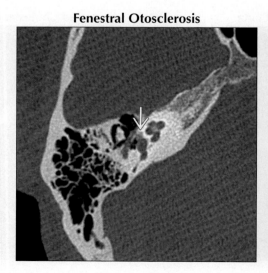

Fracture, T-Bone, Ossicle Dislocation

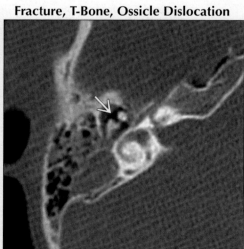

CONDUCTIVE HEARING LOSS

Oval Window Atresia
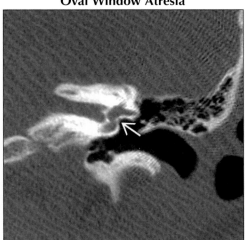

Congenital Cholesteatoma, Middle Ear
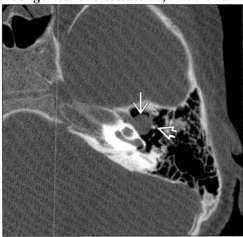

COM with Tympanosclerosis
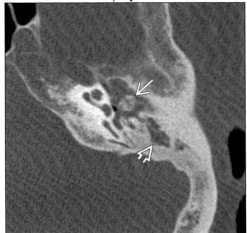

Acquired Cholesteatoma, Pars Tensa
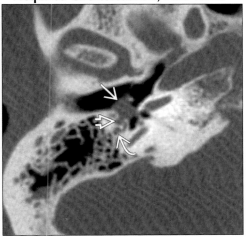

Ossicular Fixation, Congenital
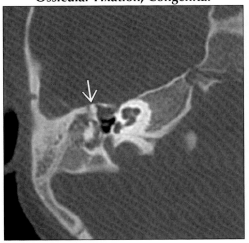

Medial Canal Fibrosis, EAC
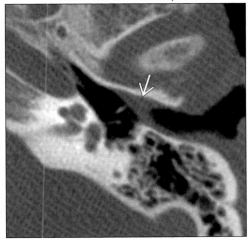

(Left) Coronal bone CT of oval window atresia shows thickened bony plate with tympanic segment of facial nerve along its inferior margin ➡. Surgical correction is not possible due to facial nerve position. *(Right)* Axial bone CT shows congenital middle ear cholesteatoma as an ovoid mass on the cochlear promontory ➡. Notice the displacement of the ossicles laterally ➡. Tympanic membrane is intact.

(Left) Axial bone CT of COM shows associated middle ear tympanosclerosis that looks like thickened ossicles with bony deposits along their margins ➡. Under-pneumatized mastoid is present ➡. *(Right)* Axial bone CT of acquired par tensa cholesteatoma shows posteroinferior cholesteatoma ➡ that involves the facial nerve recess ➡. Note mastoid segment of facial nerve ➡ is unaffected.

(Left) Axial bone CT of congenital ossicular fixation demonstrates bony ankylosis of the head of the malleus to the anterior wall of the middle ear ➡. *(Right)* Axial bone CT shows typical T-bone appearance of unilateral external auditory canal medial canal fibrosis. Note crescentic area of soft tissue abutting the tympanic membrane ➡.

DIFFERENTIAL DIAGNOSIS

Common
- Bell Palsy
- Fractures, Temporal Bone
- Metastases, CPA-IAC
- Acquired Cholesteatoma, Pars Flaccida

Less Common
- Schwannoma, Facial Nerve, T-Bone
- Hemangioma, Facial Nerve, T-Bone
- Paraganglioma, Glomus Jugulare
- Perineural Tumor, CN7, PS
- Meningioma, CPA-IAC
- Congenital Cholesteatoma, Middle Ear
- Acute Cerebral Ischemia-Infarction, Pons
- Meningioma, T-Bone
- Metastasis, T-Bone
- Multiple Sclerosis

Rare but Important
- Cavernous Malformation, Pons
- Adenoid Cystic Carcinoma, Parotid
- Mucoepidermoid Carcinoma, Parotid
- Sarcoidosis, CPA-IAC
- Langerhans Histiocytosis, T-Bone
- Rhabdomyosarcoma, Middle Ear
- Ramsay Hunt Syndrome
- Schwannoma, Facial Nerve, CPA-IAC

ESSENTIAL INFORMATION

Key Differential Diagnosis Issues
- Peripheral facial nerve paralysis
  - Definition: Unilateral CN7 injury with entire face including forehead involved
    - Motor: Facial expression muscles; stapedius muscles
    - Parasympathetic: Lacrimal gland
    - Special sensory: Anterior 2/3 tongue taste
- Imaging hints in searching for causes
  - Routine Bell palsy: Do not image
  - ATYPICAL Bell palsy best examined by thin-section enhanced (C+) MR
    - Subtle MR abnormalities: Imaged with T-bone CT to exclude CN7 hemangioma

Helpful Clues for Common Diagnoses
- **Bell Palsy**
  - Entire intratemporal CN7 enhances on MR without mass effect ± C+ fundal tuft
- **Fractures, Temporal Bone**
  - Tympanic segment CN7 most vulnerable

- **Metastases, CPA-IAC**
  - CPA-IAC mass with associated CN7 paralysis IS NOT vestibular schwannoma
  - Poorly marginated enhancing mass in CPA-IAC ± dural enhancement
- **Acquired Cholesteatoma, Pars Flaccida**
  - Nondependent soft tissue in middle ear filling Prussak space with ossicle + bone erosion ± involving CN7 canal

Helpful Clues for Less Common Diagnoses
- **Schwannoma, Facial Nerve, T-Bone**
  - Fusiform C+ mass along CN7 canal with expansile bone margins; geniculate fossa most common location
- **Hemangioma, Facial Nerve, T-Bone**
  - C+ mass with "honeycomb" matrix (50%); geniculate fossa most common location
- **Paraganglioma, Glomus Jugulare**
  - Jugular foramen C+ mass with high velocity flow voids (MR) projects superolateral through middle ear floor
- **Perineural Tumor, CN7, PS**
  - Parotid space cancer ascends through stylomastoid foramen to mastoid CN7
- **Meningioma, CPA-IAC**
  - Lobulated enhancing CPA mass with dural base; dural tails; hyperostosis (CT)
- **Congenital Cholesteatoma, Middle Ear**
  - Cholesteatomatous middle ear mass behind intact tympanic membrane
  - CT: Bony destruction usually minimal
- **Acute Cerebral Ischemia-Infarction, Pons**
  - DWI restricted diffusion/ADC low signal match signals pontine CVA (MR)
- **Meningioma, T-Bone**
  - Middle ear C+ tumor comes from tegmen tympani, jugular foramen, or transotic
- **Metastasis, T-Bone**
  - Destructive T-bone mass in patient with known malignancy
- **Multiple Sclerosis**
  - Young adult; supratentorial white matter disease
  - Pontine plaques may or may not be visible

Helpful Clues for Rare Diagnoses
- **Cavernous Malformation, Pons**
  - Pontine lesion with complex signal from blood products & calcifications
- **Adenoid Cystic Carcinoma, Parotid**
  - Flame-shaped enhancing parotid space invasive mass

PERIPHERAL FACIAL NERVE PARALYSIS

- **Mucoepidermoid Carcinoma, Parotid**
  - Ovoid invasive parotid space mass usually with complex matrix
- **Sarcoidosis, CPA-IAC**
  - Dural-based C+ meningioma mimic that may track along cistern-IAC CN7
- **Langerhans Histiocytosis, T-Bone**
  - Expansile lesion of T-bone in child
- **Rhabdomyosarcoma, Middle Ear**
  - Destructive lesion of T-bone in child
- **Schwannoma, Facial Nerve, CPA-IAC**
  - CPA-IAC enhancing vestibular schwannoma mimic that usually has "labyrinthine tail" off IAC fundus

Alternative Differential Approaches
- Another CN7 paralysis approach: Organize by ANATOMIC SEGMENT
  - Divide CN7 into its discrete segments
    - Intramedullary: 3 nuclei (motor & 2 sensory) tracts; motor fibers circle CN6 nucleus to create facial colliculus in floor of 4th ventricle
    - CPA-IAC cistern: Root exit zone of lateral brainstem to fundus of IAC
    - Intratemporal: Labyrinthine, tympanic, & mastoid intratemporal CN7
    - Extracranial: Stylomastoid foramen to functional endplates of CN7
  - By looking at CN7 injury from this vantage point you create a method for designing your imaging protocol
    - Scanning protocol must include pons, CPA-IAC cistern, T-bone, & parotid space

- Segmental anatomic approach to CN7 paralysis DDx
  - Intramedullary lesions
    - Cavernous malformation, pons
    - Multiple sclerosis
    - Cerebral ischemia-infarction, acute
  - CPA-IAC lesions
    - Metastases, CPA-IAC
    - Meningioma, CPA-IAC
    - Sarcoidosis, CPA-IAC
    - Ramsay Hunt syndrome
    - Schwannoma, facial nerve, CPA-IAC
  - T-bone lesions
    - Bell palsy
    - Fractures, temporal bone
    - Acquired cholesteatoma, pars flaccida
    - Schwannoma, facial nerve, T-bone
    - Hemangioma, facial nerve, T-bone
    - Paraganglioma, glomus jugulare
    - Congenital cholesteatoma, middle ear
    - Meningioma, T-bone
    - Metastasis, T-bone
    - Langerhans histiocytosis, T-bone
    - Rhabdomyosarcoma, middle ear
  - Parotid lesions
    - Perineural tumor, CN7
    - Adenoid cystic carcinoma
    - Mucoepidermoid carcinoma

SELECTED REFERENCES
1. Chan EH et al: Facial palsy from temporal bone lesions. Ann Acad Med Singapore. 34(4):322-9, 2005

Bell Palsy

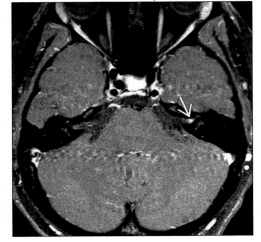

Axial T1 C+ FS MR shows a "tuft" sign ➡ in this patient with acute onset left peripheral CN7 paralysis. The enhancing fundal portion of the IAC CN7 often has this diffuse, less linear appearance.

Bell Palsy

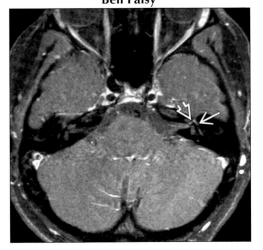

Axial T1 C+ FS MR demonstrates enhancement of the labyrinthine ➡ and tympanic ➡ segments of the intratemporal facial nerve. Mastoid segment enhancement was also present (not shown).

PERIPHERAL FACIAL NERVE PARALYSIS

(Left) Axial bone CT shows healing bone fragments in the lateral geniculate fossa ➡. This patient suffered temporal bone fracture with persistent facial nerve paralysis 6 weeks before this CT. *(Right)* Sagittal bone CT demonstrates disrupted ossicles in the attic ⇒ and healing bone in the lateral roof of the geniculate fossa ➡. 6 weeks after temporal bone fracture, persistent conductive hearing loss & facial nerve paralysis were still present.

Fractures, Temporal Bone

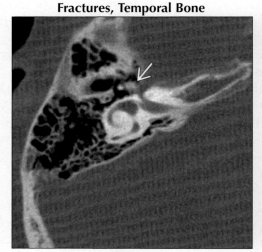

Fractures, Temporal Bone

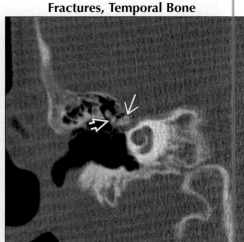

(Left) Axial T1 C+ MR shows breast carcinoma metastases in both internal auditory canals ➡. This type of linear enhancement is seen when the metastasis is in the pia-arachnoid of CN7 and CN8. *(Right)* Axial T2WI MR reveals bilateral internal auditory canal breast carcinoma metastases ➡ thickening the facial and vestibulocochlear nerve bundles. Pia-arachnoid metastasis has this "floating in CSF" appearance.

Metastases, CPA-IAC

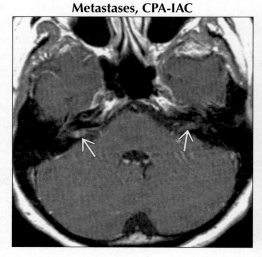

Metastases, CPA-IAC

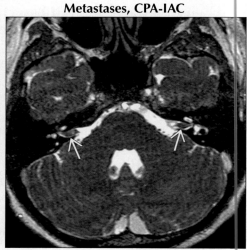

(Left) Axial bone CT demonstrates an epitympanic cholesteatoma that has eroded the anterior superior wall of the attic, shaved off the anterior head of the malleus ⇒, and dehisced the lateral bony wall of the anterior tympanic segment of the facial nerve canal ➡. *(Right)* Sagittal bone CT shows an anterior middle ear cholesteatoma that has both eroded the tegmen tympani ⇒ and dehisced the lateral bony wall of the geniculate fossa ➡.

Acquired Cholesteatoma, Pars Flaccida

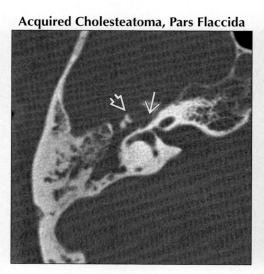

Acquired Cholesteatoma, Pars Flaccida

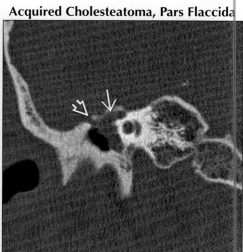

Schwannoma, Facial Nerve, T-Bone

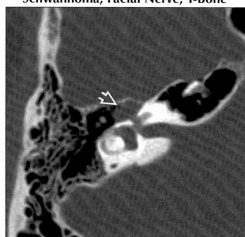

Hemangioma, Facial Nerve, T-Bone

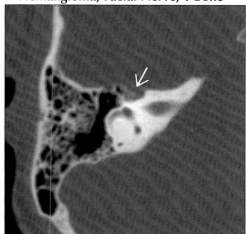

(Left) Axial bone CT shows smooth enlargement of the geniculate fossa ➡ by a facial nerve schwannoma. T1 enhanced MR (not shown) revealed enhancing tissue within the enlarged geniculate fossa. *(Right)* Axial bone CT reveals a hemangioma enlarging the geniculate fossa ➡. Note the central tumor matrix calcifications.

Paraganglioma, Glomus Jugulare

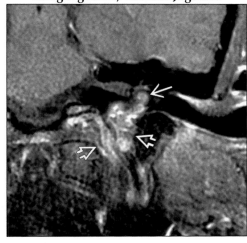

Perineural Tumor, CN7, PS

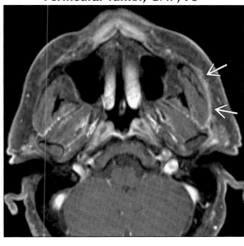

(Left) Coronal T1 C+ FS MR shows a glomus jugulare paraganglioma filling the jugular foramen ➡ and spreading superolaterally through middle ear floor to involve the tympanic segment of CN7 ➡. *(Right)* Axial T1 C+ FS MR demonstrates adenoid cystic carcinoma spreading along a branch of the extracranial facial nerve ➡. In cases where antegrade perineural tumor occurs from parotid distally along CN7, peripheral facial nerve paralysis may be only partial.

Meningioma, CPA-IAC

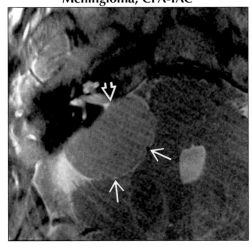

Congenital Cholesteatoma, Middle Ear

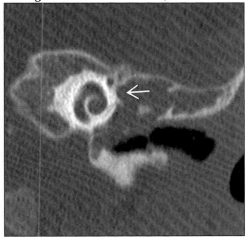

(Left) Axial T2WI FS MR reveals a lobulated dural-based meningioma with a CSF-vascular cleft ➡ and asymmetric relationship to the porus acusticus ➡. *(Right)* Coronal bone CT shows a large congential cholesteatoma of the middle ear that has eroded the lateral bony wall of the anterior tympanic segment of the facial nerve canal ➡. This child presented with a middle ear mass behind intact tympanic membrane and CN7 paresis.

PERIPHERAL FACIAL NERVE PARALYSIS

(Left) Axial T2WI MR demonstrates a subacute lateral pontine CVA ➡ on right. This patient presented with acute onset right facial nerve paralysis and facial numbness. (Right) Axial bone CT reveals the permeative-sclerotic bone changes of an anterior tegmen tympani meningioma ➡. Notice the lateral wall of the anterior tympanic segment of the facial nerve canal is affected by the meningioma ➡.

Acute Cerebral Ischemia-Infarction, Pons

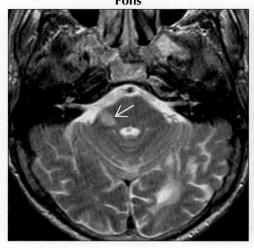

Meningioma, T-Bone

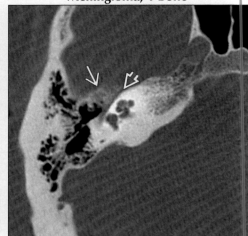

(Left) Axial bone CT shows a large floor of middle cranial fossa destructive metastasis eroding the anterior wall of the middle ear cavity ➡ and invading the geniculate fossa ➡. This patient with known colon cancer presented with acute onset facial nerve paralysis. (Right) Axial FLAIR MR demonstrates a large pontine multiple sclerosis plaque in this patient with florid supratentorial white matter disease (not shown).

Metastasis, T-Bone

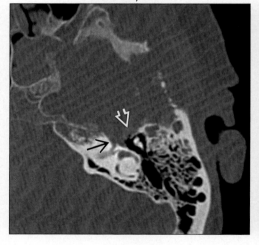

Multiple Sclerosis

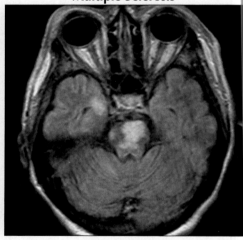

(Left) Coronal T2 GRE MR reveals a "blooming" cavernous malformation in the left pons ➡. T1 images (not shown) showed methemoglobin indicating that this lesion had recently bled. (Right) Axial CECT shows a poorly marginated adenoid cystic carcinoma ➡ of the parotid gland with deep invasion toward the stylomastoid foramen and proximal extracranial facial nerve ➡.*

Cavernous Malformation, Pons

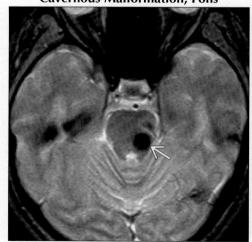

Adenoid Cystic Carcinoma, Parotid

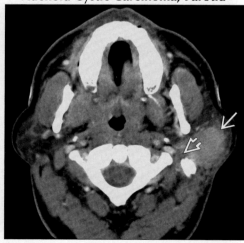

PERIPHERAL FACIAL NERVE PARALYSIS

Mucoepidermoid Carcinoma, Parotid

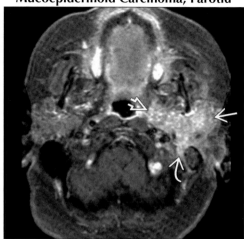

Sarcoidosis, CPA-IAC

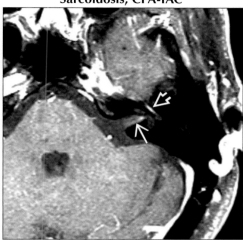

(Left) Axial T1 C+ FS MR shows an aggressive-appearing enhancing left parotid mucoepidermoid carcinoma that involves both the superficial ➡ and the deep ➡ lobes. Note the spread into the lower portion of the stylomastoid foramen ➡. (Right) Axial T1 C+ FS MR reveals a sarcoid affecting the 7th and 8th cranial nerves in the internal auditory canal ➡. Notice the tympanic segment of the facial nerve is also avidly enhancing ➡.

Langerhans Histiocytosis, T-Bone

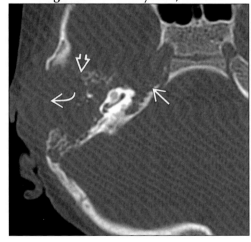

Rhabdomyosarcoma, Middle Ear

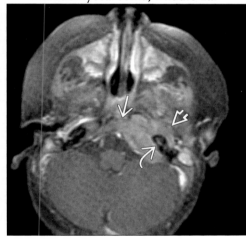

(Left) Axial bone CT demonstrates a lesion of the right temporal bone eroding the bones of the petrous apex ➡ and middle ear ➡. The lateral wall of the middle ear-mastoid is absent ➡ with periauricular soft tissue mass visible. (Right) Axial T1 C+ FS MR shows very large skull base ➡ and temporal bone ➡ rhabdomyosarcoma. The inner ear bony otic capsule is "floating" in the tumor ➡.

Ramsay Hunt Syndrome

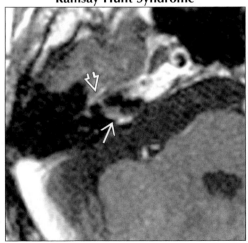

Schwannoma, Facial Nerve, CPA-IAC

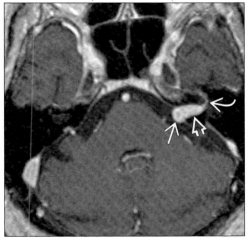

(Left) Axial T1 C+ MR reveals enhancement in the IAC ➡ and asymmetric enhancement of the intratemporal facial nerve ➡. This amount of enhancement is more than typically seen in Ramsay Hunt syndrome. (Right) Axial T1 C+ MR shows an enhancing tumor of the CPA ➡ and the IAC ➡. This tumor can be correctly identified as a facial nerve schwannoma because of the "labyrinthine tail" of enhancement of the facial nerve ➡.

VASCULAR RETROTYMPANIC MASS

DIFFERENTIAL DIAGNOSIS

Common
- Jugular Bulb, Dehiscent
- Paraganglioma, Glomus Tympanicum
- Paraganglioma, Glomus Jugulare

Less Common
- Cholesterol Granuloma, Middle Ear
- Lateralized Internal Carotid Artery
- Chronic Otitis with Hemorrhage
- Fenestral Otosclerosis

Rare but Important
- Persistent Stapedial Artery
- Aberrant Internal Carotid Artery

ESSENTIAL INFORMATION

Key Differential Diagnosis Issues
- Only 2 tumors on this whole list (paragangliomas)
- Caveat: Careful imaging diagnosis important in preventing biopsy or surgery on nonsurgical lesion!

Helpful Clues for Common Diagnoses
- **Jugular Bulb, Dehiscent**
  - Key facts: Congenital bulbous superolateral diverticulum protruding into posteromedial middle ear
  - Imaging: Focal dehiscence of sigmoid plate (CT); soft tissue density contiguous with jugular vein
    - Enhancement pattern on CECT or MR matches that of sigmoid sinus and jugular vein
- **Paraganglioma, Glomus Tympanicum**
  - Key facts: Typically small enhancing mass on cochlear promontory with normal middle ear (ME) bony floor
    - Tumor arises from glomus bodies of cochlear promontory
  - CT: Soft tissue mass on cochlear promontory, floor of ME intact
    - Medial wall of middle ear rarely demonstrates erosion
  - MR: T1 C+ avid enhancement; typically too small for high velocity flow voids
- **Paraganglioma, Glomus Jugulare**
  - Key facts: Vascular mass arises from jugular bulb

  - Vector of spread through inferomedial floor in superolateral direction
  - Imaging: Permeative-destructive changes to bone surrounding jugular foramen (CT)
    - T1/T2 MR: "Salt & pepper" high velocity flow voids
    - CECT/MR: Homogeneous enhancement

Helpful Clues for Less Common Diagnoses
- **Cholesterol Granuloma, Middle Ear**
  - Key facts: Post inflammatory granulation tissue from recurrent hemorrhage
  - Imaging: Expansile middle ear mass with ↑ T1 & T2 signal (MR)
    - No true enhancement of lesion; compare to pre-T1 (MR)
    - CT: Expansile soft tissue density, scalloping of surrounding bone if large, ± ossicular changes
- **Lateralized Internal Carotid Artery**
  - Key facts: Genu of vertical and horizontal petrous internal carotid artery congenitally displaced laterally
  - CT: Petrous ICA lateral wall dehiscence
    - Soft tissue density contiguous with carotid, adjacent to basal turn of cochlea
  - CECT: Enhancing internal carotid artery protrudes into medial middle ear
- **Chronic Otitis with Hemorrhage**
  - Key facts: Debris from chronic indolent infection with hemorrhage may appear dark blue on otoscopic exam
  - CT: Sclerotic, underdeveloped, or poorly aerated mastoid bone with soft tissue density in middle ear
    - Ossicular erosion may be present if infection-intense at one point; may mimic cholesteatoma
- **Fenestral Otosclerosis**
  - Key facts: Idiopathic spongiotic change in enchondral layer of labyrinth along margins of oval & round windows
    - If disease affects medial wall of middle ear widely, Schwartze sign results where clinically a vascular hue is seen through opaque tympanic membrane
  - CT: Subtle radiolucency at anterior margin of oval window (fissula ante fenestram) early
    - Late CT findings include sclerotic, heaped new bone
  - MR: T1 C+ punctate enhancing plaques

8

VASCULAR RETROTYMPANIC MASS

Helpful Clues for Rare Diagnoses

- **Persistent Stapedial Artery**
  - Key facts: Anomalous persistence of embryological remnant stapedial artery
    - Arises from petrous ICA; becomes middle meningeal artery
    - Passes through stapes footplate (not visible with imaging)
  - Imaging: Bone CT shows absent foramen spinosum
    - Anterior tympanic segment facial nerve canal enlarged or parallel canal present
- **Aberrant Internal Carotid Artery**
  - Key facts: Cervical internal carotid artery does not form
    - Collateral circuit via inferior tympanic artery reconnects to posterolateral horizontal petrous ICA
    - Absent vertical petrous carotid canal
  - Imaging: Bone CT reveals tubular lesion crossing cochlear promontory to rejoin horizontal petrous ICA at posterolateral margin
    - Enlarged inferior tympanic canaliculus present

Alternative Differential Approaches

- Otoscopic exam key
  - Contact referring MD for clinical/otoscopic impression before dictating case
- RED middle ear mass behind intact TM
  - Glomus tympanicum paraganglioma (GTP)

- Radiologist must distinguish GTP from GJP to guide appropriate surgical approach
  - Glomus jugulare paraganglioma (GJP)
  - Aberrant internal carotid artery
  - Lateralized internal carotid artery
  - Persistent stapedial artery
- BLUE middle ear mass behind intact TM
  - Jugular bulb, dehiscent
    - Dehiscent jugular bulb retrotympanic vascular mass is behind posteroinferior quadrant of tympanic membrane
  - Cholesterol granuloma, middle ear
    - Cholesterol granuloma usually fills entire middle ear
  - Fenestral otosclerosis
    - Vascular hue seen through tympanic membrane from large plaques involving middle ear bony wall is referred to as Schwartze sign
  - Chronic otitis media with hemorrhage

SELECTED REFERENCES

1. Koesling S et al: Vascular anomalies, sutures and small canals of the temporal bone on axial CT. Eur J Radiol. 54(3):335-43, 2005
2. Remley KB et al: Pulsatile tinnitus and the vascular tympanic membrane: CT, MR, and angiographic findings. Radiology. 174(2):383-9, 1990
3. Lo WW et al: High-resolution CT in the evaluation of glomus tumors of the temporal bone. Radiology. 150(3):737-42, 1984
4. Lo WW et al: High-resolution CT of the jugular foramen: anatomy and vascular variants and anomalies. Radiology. 150(3):743-7, 1984

Jugular Bulb, Dehiscent

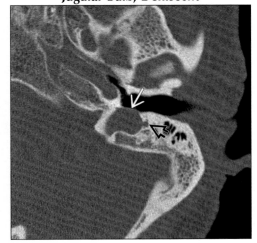

Axial bone CT demonstrates a dehiscent sigmoid plate ➡ with protrusion into the posterior mesotympanum just medial to the mastoid segment of the facial nerve ➡.

Jugular Bulb, Dehiscent

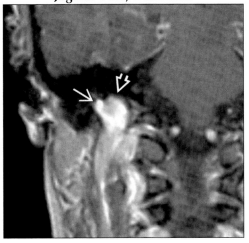

Coronal T1 C+ MR shows a jugular bulb ➡ with small diverticulum protruding superolaterally through the floor of the middle ear ➡, seen on otoscopy as a blue retrotympanic mass.

VASCULAR RETROTYMPANIC MASS

Paraganglioma, Glomus Tympanicum

(Left) Coronal bone CT reveals an ovoid soft tissue mass seated on the cochlear promontory ➡. Note floor of middle ear cavity is intact. Otoscopy showed a cherry red pulsatile retrotympanic mass. *(Right)* Coronal T1 C+ MR demonstrates an enhancing lesion filling the left middle ear ➡ that extends superiorly into the epitympanum ➡ and inferiorly to the middle ear floor ➡. Note absence of communication with inferomedial jugular bulb.

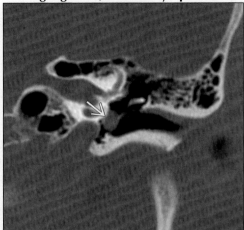

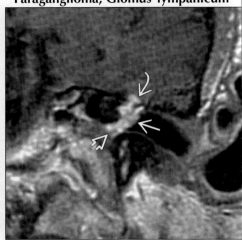

Paraganglioma, Glomus Jugulare

(Left) Coronal bone CT shows a tumor entering the middle ear cavity through the middle ear floor ➡. Permeative-destructive bone changes ➡ and superolateral vector of spread support the diagnosis. *(Right)* Coronal bone CT demonstrates a large glomus jugulare paraganglioma extending into the middle ear cavity ➡. Note the permeative-destructive bony changes affecting the lateral clivus ➡ and inferior temporal bone ➡.

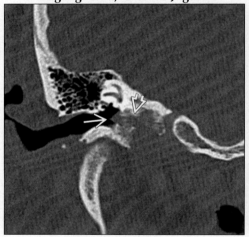

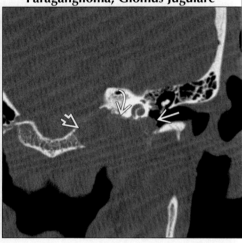

Cholesterol Granuloma, Middle Ear

(Left) Coronal T1WI MR reveals a hyperintense lesion filling the middle ear cavity ➡, representing a cholesterol granuloma. Note subtle bulge of tympanic membrane ➡. Otoscopy revealed a blue-black retrotympanic lesion. *(Right)* Axial T2WI MR shows a hyperintense left middle ear cholesterol granuloma ➡. Note the lesion extends into the eustachian tube ➡. The basal turn of the cochlea ➡ is also seen.

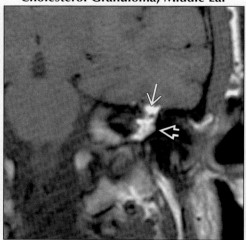

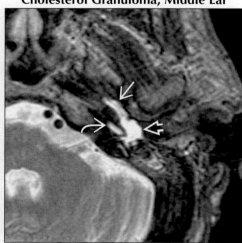

VASCULAR RETROTYMPANIC MASS

Lateralized Internal Carotid Artery

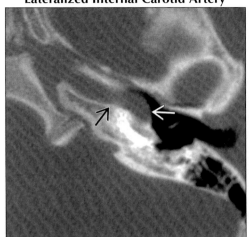

Chronic Otitis with Hemorrhage

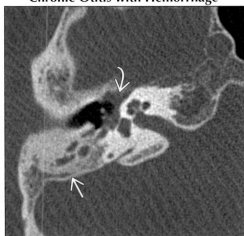

(Left) Axial bone CT of the left temporal bone reveals petrous left ICA ⇒ located slightly lateral to normal position. Note dehiscent lateral bony wall ➡. *(Right)* Axial bone CT shows under-pneumatized mastoid ⇒ associated with inflammatory debris in the mastoid antrum and middle ear ➡. Chronic otitis media may lead to build-up of fibrous debris with small foci of hemorrhage. In such cases, T1 MR shows high signal material in middle ear cavity.

Fenestral Otosclerosis

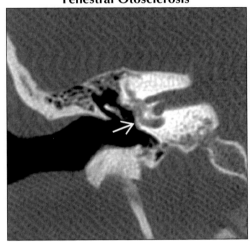

Persistent Stapedial Artery

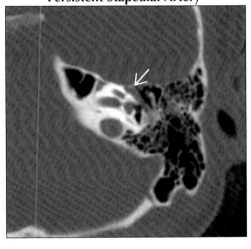

(Left) Coronal bone CT shows low-density bone around oval window extending inferiorly on upper cochlear promontory ➡. Schwartze sign, where a vascular hue is seen through opaque tympanic membrane, results. *(Right)* Axial bone CT reveals an enlarged anterior tympanic portion of the facial nerve canal ➡. In conjunction with ipsilateral absent foramen spinosum, diagnosis of persistent stapedial artery can be made.

Persistent Stapedial Artery

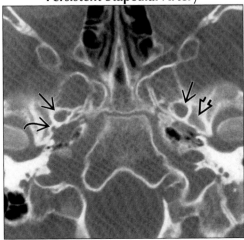

Aberrant Internal Carotid Artery

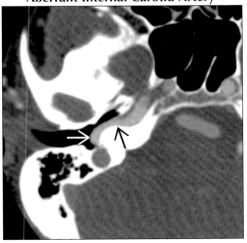

(Left) Axial bone CT shows normal bilateral foramen ovale ➡. Normal right foramen spinosum ➡ is identified. Absent left foramen spinosum ➡ is seen. Middle meningeal artery arises from persistent stapedial artery as a result. *(Right)* Axial CTA shows an aberrant internal carotid in right middle ear ➡. This lesion enters the middle ear through an enlarged tympanic canaliculus, with artery caliber change ➡ as carotid curves into horizontal petrous segment typical.

DIFFERENTIAL DIAGNOSIS

Common
- Intracranial Hypertension, Idiopathic
- Paraganglioma, Glomus Jugulare (GJP)
- Dural A-V Fistula, Skull Base

Less Common
- Paraganglioma, Glomus Tympanicum
- Jugular Bulb, Dehiscent
- Meningioma, T-Bone
- Carotid-Cavernous Fistula, Traumatic
- Arteriovenous Malformation
- Atherosclerosis, Carotid Artery, Neck
- Dissection, Carotid Artery, Neck

Rare but Important
- Cochlear Otosclerosis
- Dural Sinus Stenosis
- Diverticulum, Transverse-Sigmoid Sinus
- Aberrant Internal Carotid Artery (AbICA)

ESSENTIAL INFORMATION

Key Differential Diagnosis Issues
- Tinnitus, buzzing, or ringing in ear may be pulsatile or continuous (nonpulsatile)
- This differential diagnosis is focused on PULSATILE tinnitus (PT)
  - PT may be subjective (patient only hears) or objective (doctor hears)
  - PT suggests nonlaminar flow: Vascular anomaly, malformation, or vascular tumor
- Imaging recommendations
  - Enhanced MR with MRA-MRV best starting examination in setting of pulsatile tinnitus
  - If negative MR in setting of objective PT, angiography excludes small dural AVF

Helpful Clues for Common Diagnoses
- **Intracranial Hypertension, Idiopathic**
  - Key facts: Exclude underlying etiologies dural sinus stenosis, tumor, & SLE
    - CSF normal composition; opening pressure > 250 mm; obese females
  - Imaging: MR often normal; subtle signs may suggest diagnosis
    - Partially empty sella
    - Optic nerve sheath dilatation, tortuosity
    - Flattening of posterior sclera
- **Paraganglioma, Glomus Jugulare (GJP)**
  - Key facts: Originates in paraganglia of adventitia at jugular bulb

  - Imaging: Mass vector of spread from jugular foramen to hypotympanum through floor of middle ear
    - Bone CT: "Permeative-destructive" changes around jugular foramen
    - T1 MR: "Salt & pepper" appearance
    - T1 C+ fat saturation: Avidly enhancing
- **Dural A-V Fistula, Skull Base**
  - Key facts: Acquired, commonly secondary to trauma or thrombosis
    - Neoangiogenesis vessels converge on wall of thrombosed sinus
  - Imaging: MR normal if small lesion or slow flow; tortuous dural feeders
    - Higher grade lesions with enlarged cortical veins, retrograde flow
    - CTA/MRA/DSA: May show transosseous collaterals & enlarged external carotid artery branches
    - MR: Parenchymal edema, parenchymal hemorrhage if venous ischemia

Helpful Clues for Less Common Diagnoses
- **Paraganglioma, Glomus Tympanicum**
  - Key facts: Vascular pulsatile retrotympanic mass may mimic GJP when large
    - CAVEAT: Radiologist must differentiate glomus tympanicum paraganglioma from GJP to prevent incorrect surgery!
  - Imaging: Bone CT shows mass on cochlear promontory; middle ear (ME) floor intact
    - T1 C+ MR: Avid enhancement, noncontiguous with carotid
- **Jugular Bulb, Dehiscent**
  - Key facts: Focal sigmoid plate dehiscence
    - Otoscopy: Congenital blue retrotympanic posteroinferior mass
  - Imaging: Soft tissue projects from jugular bulb into ME cavity (CT)
    - MR variable: Complex signal always contiguous with jugular bulb
- **Meningioma, T-Bone**
  - Key facts: Typically ME extension of intracranial meningioma
    - Vector of spread to ME cavity typically via tegmen tympani or jugular foramen
  - Imaging: Permeative-sclerotic changes to temporal bone (CT)
    - MR C+ T1: Enhancing mass; dural tails
    - Jugular foramen lesion mimics glomus jugulare; no flow voids
- **Carotid-Cavernous Fistula, Traumatic**

PULSATILE TINNITUS

- ○ Key facts: Direct connection between cavernous carotid & cavernous sinus resulting in high velocity shunting
  - Pulsatile proptosis
  - Post-traumatic: From skull base fracture
  - Other causes: Rupture of cavernous carotid aneurysm or spontaneous
- ○ Imaging: Superior ophthalmic vein large; cavernous sinus lateral wall convexed (CECT/MR)
  - DSA: Direct communication visible
- • **Arteriovenous Malformation**
  - ○ Key facts: Tangle of arteries & veins
    - High flow shunting; no normal intervening brain or capillary bed
  - ○ Imaging (MR): Nidus of feeding arterial & draining venous flow voids; surrounding brain may reveal hemorrhage or gliosis
    - DSA: Evaluate for size, superficial vs. deep drainage, involvement of adjacent eloquent brain
- • **Atherosclerosis, Carotid Artery, Neck**
  - ○ Key facts: ICA above bifurcation narrowed
    - Turbulence, change in velocity causes PT
  - ○ Imaging: High velocity flow on ultrasound
    - CT: Ca++ plaque on CT
    - MR/MRA: Signal loss from plaque
- • **Dissection, Carotid Artery, Neck**
  - ○ Key facts: ICA intimal damage, false lumen
    - Spontaneous, 2° to trauma, hypertension, or vasculopathy
  - ○ Imaging: Intimal flap & false lumen may be present (CTA/MRA/DSA)
    - ICA smooth tapering; ends at skull base

- MR T1: Crescentic intramural ↑ signal

Helpful Clues for Rare Diagnoses
- • **Cochlear Otosclerosis**
  - ○ Key facts: Idiopathic primary lytic disease of enchondral layer of bony labyrinth
  - ○ Imaging: Pericochlear radiolucent foci (CT)
    - MR: T1 C+ foci enhance in active disease
- • **Dural Sinus Stenosis**
  - ○ Key facts: Stenosis → venous turbulence
    - Causes: Thrombosis, mass or idiopathic
  - ○ Imaging: MRV may be normal or demonstrate artifactual signal loss
    - Post-contrast MRV more sensitive
    - DSA: Modality of choice for imaging and grading pressure differential
- • **Diverticulum, Transverse-Sigmoid Sinus**
  - ○ Imaging (CTV): Sinus diverticulum extending into dehiscent mastoid bone
- • **Aberrant Internal Carotid Artery (AbICA)**
  - ○ Key facts: Rare but important diagnosis!
    - "Vascular-appearing" retrotympanic mass
    - Stenosis where AbICA rejoins horizontal petrous ICA is responsible for PT
  - ○ Imaging: Tubular mass traverses middle ear
    - Large inferior tympanic canaliculus

SELECTED REFERENCES

1. Krishnan A et al: CT arteriography and venography in pulsatile tinnitus: preliminary results. AJNR Am J Neuroradiol. 27(8):1635-8, 2006
2. Weissman JL et al: Imaging of tinnitus: a review. Radiology. 216(2):342-9, 2000
3. Remley KB et al: Pulsatile tinnitus and the vascular tympanic membrane: CT, MR, and angiographic findings. Radiology. 174(2):383-9, 1990

Intracranial Hypertension, Idiopathic

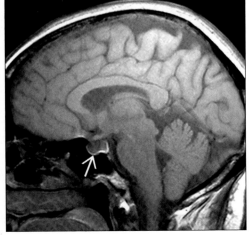

Sagittal T1WI MR shows enlarged, empty sella ➡. Enlarged, tortuous optic nerve sheaths are not shown. Both are seen as indirect clues to diagnosis of intracranial hypertension in < 50% of cases.

Paraganglioma, Glomus Jugulare (GJP)

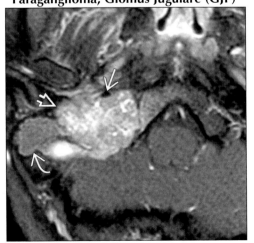

Axial T1 C+ FS MR reveals an enhancing glomus jugulare tumor spreading laterally into middle ear ➡, pushing internal carotid artery anteriorly ➡, and obstructing the mastoid air cells ➡.

(Left) Lateral angiography demonstrates findings of dural A-V fistula. In this selective internal carotid artery angiogram, a meningohypophyseal trunk ➡ is visible connecting to the transverse sinus ➡. **(Right)** Coronal bone CT reveals a glomus tympanicum paraganglioma arising along the cochlear promontory ➡ within the middle ear cavity. Note that otoscopy would show a vascular retrotympanic mass behind inferior tympanic membrane ➡.

Dural A-V Fistula, Skull Base
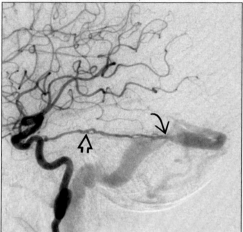

Paraganglioma, Glomus Tympanicum
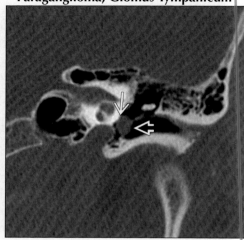

(Left) Coronal bone CT demonstrates a dehiscent jugular bulb ➡ protruding into the posterior middle ear cavity. Jugular bulb diverticulum ➡ is also incidentally present in this case. **(Right)** Coronal T1 C+ MR shows enhancing en plaque meningioma involving the tegmen tympani ➡ and spreading inferiorly into the middle ear cavity below ➡.

Jugular Bulb, Dehiscent
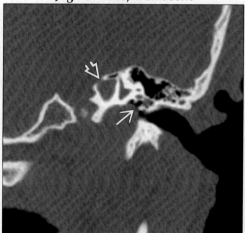

Meningioma, T-Bone
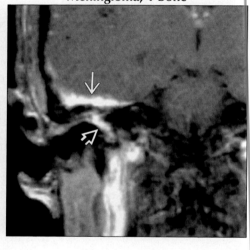

(Left) Anteroposterior angiography of left internal carotid injection reveals immediate filling of the contralateral cavernous sinus ➡ and high flow shunting into bilateral inferior petrosal sinuses ➡. **(Right)** Axial T2WI MR shows a medial temporal serpentine tangle of flow voids ➡ in the distribution of the right internal carotid artery. Notice the distended internal cerebral vein ➡.

Carotid-Cavernous Fistula, Traumatic
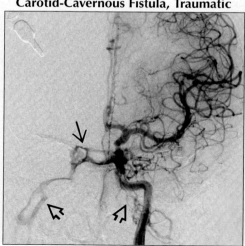

Arteriovenous Malformation
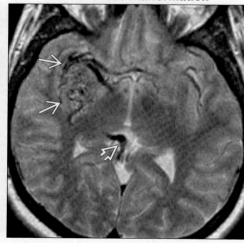

PULSATILE TINNITUS

Atherosclerosis, Carotid Artery, Neck

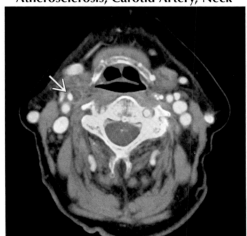

Dissection, Carotid Artery, Neck

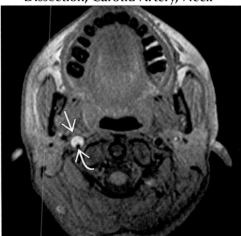

(Left) Axial CECT shows a high-grade stenosis ➔ of the proximal right cervical internal carotid artery. Jetting through such a stenosis may cause nonlaminar flow in the petrous internal carotid artery leading to pulsatile tinnitus. (Right) Axial T1WI FS MR reveals a crescentic focus of hyperintense signal ➔ representing dissection with subintimal hemorrhage surrounding an attenuated flow void ➔ (internal carotid artery lumen).

Cochlear Otosclerosis

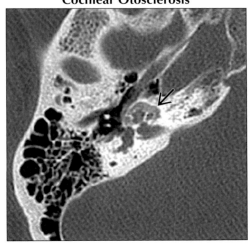

Dural Sinus Stenosis

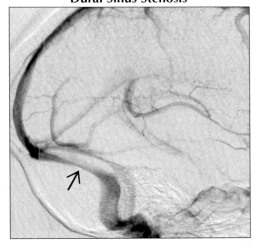

(Left) Axial NECT shows characteristic lytic "halo" ➔ surrounding the right cochlea, representing spongiform cochlear otosclerosis. (Right) Lateral angiography demonstrates the venous phase of contrast injection revealing a long segment smooth right transverse sinus stenosis ➔. Pressure transducer catheter (not pictured) revealed pre- and post-stenosis pressure differential of 35 mmHg.

Diverticulum, Transverse-Sigmoid Sinus

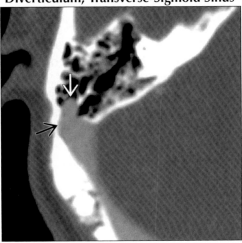

Aberrant Internal Carotid Artery (AbICA)

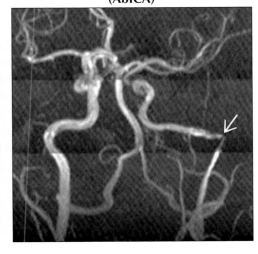

(Left) Axial CTV demonstrates dehiscence of the medial wall of the mastoid ➔ with projection of a right transverse-sigmoid sinus diverticulum ➔ into the posterior mastoid air cells. Turbulence in the diverticulum may be responsible for pulse synchronous sound. (Right) MRA demonstrates the characteristic "7-shaped" left aberrant internal carotid artery. Notice the abrupt change in caliber of the artery as it re-enters the horizontal petrous ICA ➔.

TRAUMATIC LESIONS OF THE TEMPORAL BONE

DIFFERENTIAL DIAGNOSIS

Common
- T-Bone Fractures, Longitudinal
- Ossicular Dislocation, Malleoincal
- T-Bone Fractures, Condylar Fossa
- T-Bone Fractures, Transverse
- T-Bone Fractures, Facial Nerve Injury

Less Common
- Ossicular Dislocation, Incudostapedial
- T-Bone Fractures, Mixed
- T-Bone Fractures, Tegmen Tympani, CSF Leak
- T-Bone Fractures, Pneumolabyrinth
- T-Bone Fractures, Dural Sinus Thrombosis

Rare but Important
- T-Bone Fractures, ICA Injury
- T-Bone Fractures, Tegmen Tympani, Cephalocele
- Ossicular Dislocation, Incus
- Ossicular Dislocation, Stapes
- T-Bone Fractures, Secondary Cholesteatoma

ESSENTIAL INFORMATION

Key Differential Diagnosis Issues
- Fractures (fx) classified by orientation relative to long axis of temporal bone
  - Longitudinal, transverse, & mixed
- Traumatic lesions of temporal bone (T-bone) affect multiple structures
  - Fractures of T-bone itself including bones of external auditory canal (EAC), middle ear (ME), inner ear (IE), condylar fossa
  - Dislocations of ossicles of ME
    - Malleoincal, incudostapedial, incus, stapes dislocations
    - Ossicle support from ligaments & tendons: Incus LEAST supported
    - Malleus support: Lateral & superior malleolar ligaments; tensor tympani tendon; embedded in tympanic membrane
    - Stapes support: Stapedius tendon (stapes hub); stapediovestibular articulation (stapes footplate & annular ligament)
  - Fx affecting neurovascular structures
    - Fx causing facial nerve injury
    - Fx causing sigmoid sinus thrombosis
    - Fx causing petrous ICA injury with secondary MCA stroke
    - Fx causing middle cranial fossa subdural or epidural hematoma
    - Fx causing temporal lobe contusion
  - Fx causing leptomeningeal injury
    - Tegmen tympani Fx causing cephalocele
    - Tegmen tympani Fx causing CSF leak

Helpful Clues for Common Diagnoses
- **T-Bone Fractures, Longitudinal**
  - Key facts: Extralabyrinthine
  - Imaging: Ossicle dislocation, tegmen tympani, & ICA injury
    - Less severe CN7 injury, typically at geniculate ganglia
- **Ossicular Dislocation, Malleoincal**
  - Key facts: True diarthrodial joint with joint capsule
  - Imaging: Best seen on axial CT
    - Malleus head ajar incus short process
- **T-Bone Fractures, Condylar Fossa**
  - Key facts: Transverse fx association
    - Condylar head driven into fossa
  - Imaging: Fx crosses glenoid fossa
- **T-Bone Fractures, Transverse**
  - Key facts: Crosses CN7 canal
    - CN7 may be severed
    - Perilymphatic fistula potential
  - Imaging: If medial, traverses IAC fundus with cochlear nerve transection
    - If lateral, traverses bony labyrinth; pneumolabyrinth, perilymphatic fistula into ME
- **T-Bone Fractures, Facial Nerve Injury**
  - Key facts: Immediate or delayed CN7 palsy
  - Imaging: Transverse fx, immediate, permanent CN7 paralysis (severed)
    - Longitudinal fx, delayed CN7 palsy
    - Bone fragment, displaced ossicle, or fx line may be responsible

Helpful Clues for Less Common Diagnoses
- **Ossicular Dislocation, Incudostapedial**
  - Key facts: Difficult to diagnose on CT
    - Use alternative plane views
  - Imaging: Anterior or posterior incus lenticular process relative to stapes head
- **T-Bone Fractures, Mixed**
  - Key facts: Longitudinal, oblique, & axial fractures mixed together
    - Severe fx with multiple complications
  - Imaging: Stellate fracture lines running in multiple directions

TRAUMATIC LESIONS OF THE TEMPORAL BONE

- **T-Bone Fractures, Tegmen Tympani, CSF Leak**
  - Key facts: Tegmen tympani fx with concomitant dural tear
    - CSF leaks into ME; CSF otorrhea if tympanic membrane ruptured
  - Imaging: Tegmen tympani fx; opacification of ME persists
- **T-Bone Fractures, Pneumolabyrinth**
  - Key facts: Usually associated with lateral type transverse fracture
  - Imaging: Transverse fracture through medial wall ME into bony labyrinth
    - Very common if fracture traverses round or oval window
    - Air seen in inner ear fluid spaces
- **T-Bone Fractures, Dural Sinus Thrombosis**
  - Key facts: Healing may result in dural A-V fistula
  - Imaging: Fx line crosses sigmoid plate of medial mastoid
    - CTA or MRA shows dural sinus thrombosis; often delayed appearance

Helpful Clues for Rare Diagnoses
- **T-Bone Fractures, ICA Injury**
  - Key facts: Usually longitudinal fx extending anteriorly through petrous internal carotid artery canal
  - Imaging: Fx line crosses petrous ICA canal
    - CTA: May show dissection or occlusion
    - DWI: May show restricted diffusion of middle cerebral artery stroke

- **T-Bone Fractures, Tegmen Tympani, Cephalocele**
  - Key facts: Tegmen tympani fx tears dura
  - Imaging: Delayed CSF pulsation driven enlargement of tegmen tympani fx
    - MR: Cephalocele with meninges ± brain
- **Ossicular Dislocation, Incus**
  - Key facts: Incus is least anchored ossicle
    - Both malleoincal and incudostapedial joints are disrupted
  - Imaging: Entire incus dissociates from malleus and incus
- **Ossicular Dislocation, Stapes**
  - Key facts: Stapes is anchored by stapedius tendon and stapediovestibular articulation (footplate and annular ligament)
    - Stapes fracture or dislocation rare and difficult to diagnose with CT because of very small size
    - Thin section (0.4-0.75 mm) MDCT may make this diagnosis more accessible
  - Imaging: Transverse fx line passes through oval window with stapes fragments visible
- **T-Bone Fractures, Secondary Cholesteatoma**
  - Key facts: Diastatic fx traps skin
    - Can be seen in EAC or lateral mastoid cavity
    - Delayed complication of serious temporal bone fx
  - Imaging: Enlarging scalloping soft tissue mass in site of fx

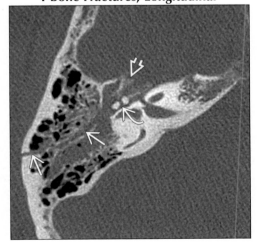

T-Bone Fractures, Longitudinal

Axial bone CT demonstrates a longitudinal temporal bone fracture ➡ with tegmen tympani fracture fragments ➡ and malleoincal dislocation ➡. Notice that the fracture does not involve the inner ear.

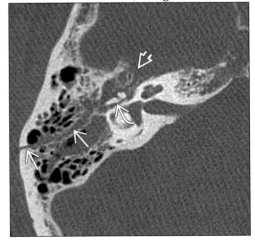

T-Bone Fractures, Longitudinal

Axial bone CT reveals a longitudinal temporal bone fracture ➡ with tegmen fracture debris ➡ pushing the short process of incus and malleus head against the lateral semicircular canal bone ➡.

TRAUMATIC LESIONS OF THE TEMPORAL BONE

(Left) Axial bone CT shows a longitudinal fracture passing through the mastoid air cells ➡. The malleoincal joint is widened, and the malleus head is tilted laterally ➡. *(Right)* Axial CECT reveals longitudinal fracture through mastoid air cells ➡ associated with malleoincal dislocation. Note head of malleus is no longer associated with short process ➡ of incus, which is itself posteriorly displaced ➡.

Ossicular Dislocation, Malleoincal

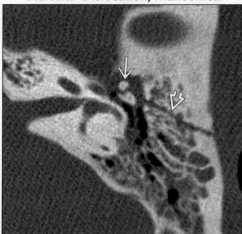

Ossicular Dislocation, Malleoincal

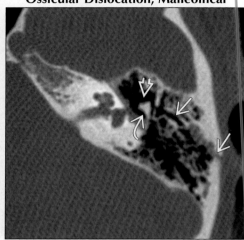

(Left) Axial bone CT demonstrates a transverse fracture that crosses through the inner ear ➡ and exits the oval window with pneumolabyrinth ➡. The fracture continues anteriorly through the condylar fossa ➡. *(Right)* Axial bone CT shows a transverse fracture crossing the posterior semicircular canal ➡, round window ➡, and the condylar fossa ➡. Such fractures usually present with acute onset of hearing loss.

T-Bone Fractures, Condylar Fossa

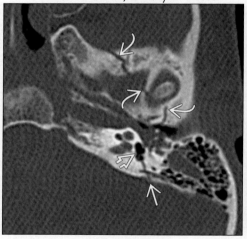

T-Bone Fractures, Condylar Fossa

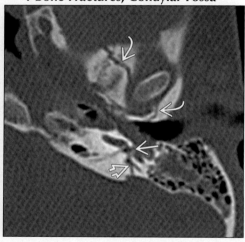

(Left) Axial bone CT depicts a transverse temporal bone fracture ➡ crossing the basal turn of the cochlea ➡. Perilymphatic fistula often occurs from a fracture with middle ear and mastoid opacification resulting. *(Right)* Axial bone CT at the level of the lateral semicircular canal shows a transverse fracture ➡ passing just deep to the vestibule. Notice the fracture line involving the labyrinthine segment of the facial nerve ➡.

T-Bone Fractures, Transverse

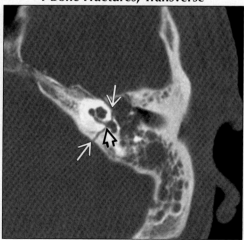

T-Bone Fractures, Transverse

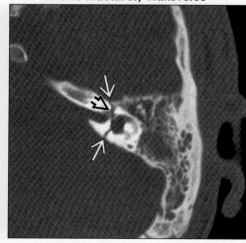

T-Bone Fractures, Facial Nerve Injury

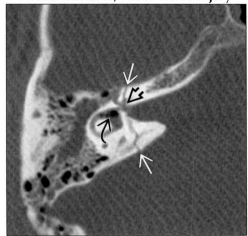

T-Bone Fractures, Facial Nerve Injury

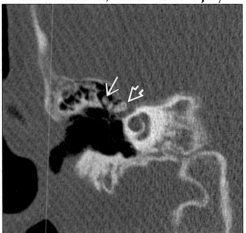

(Left) Axial bone CT demonstrates a transverse fracture ➡ through IAC fundus that crosses the base of the labyrinthine segment of CN7 ➡. A severed CN7 presents as acute CN7 paralysis. Pneumolabyrinth ➡ is seen. (Right) Coronal bone CT reveals complete disruption of ossicle chain with incus now in lateral epitympanum ➡ and the malleus protruding into the geniculate fossa ➡. Patient had acute onset of complete peripheral CN7 paralysis following trauma.

Ossicular Dislocation, Incudostapedial

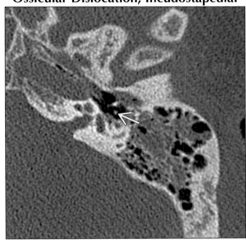

Ossicular Dislocation, Incudostapedial

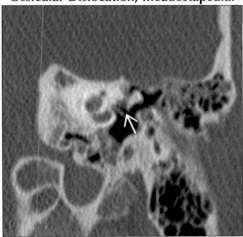

(Left) Axial bone CT at the level of the oval window shows inferior tip of long process of incus without a connection to the stapes ➡. Incudostapedial dislocation is difficult to diagnose with conventional CT planes. (Right) Coronal bone CT reveals an incudostapedial dislocation as a gap ➡ between the long process of the incus and the stapes head. Radiologists must look carefully for this type of dislocation or it will be missed.

T-Bone Fractures, Mixed

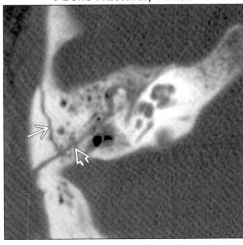

T-Bone Fractures, Tegmen Tympani, CSF Leak

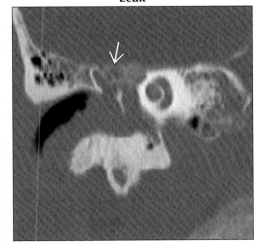

(Left) Axial bone CT demonstrates a mixed temporal bone fracture with lateral transverse ➡ and longitudinal ➡ fracture lines visible. More severe temporal bone trauma often creates mixed (complex) fracture patterns. (Right) Coronal bone CT at the level of cochlea depicts a comminuted tegmen tympani fracture with focal dehiscence ➡. Resulting CSF leaking into middle ear will present as otorrhea if the tympanic membrane is also ruptured.

8

63

TRAUMATIC LESIONS OF THE TEMPORAL BONE

T-Bone Fractures, Pneumolabyrinth

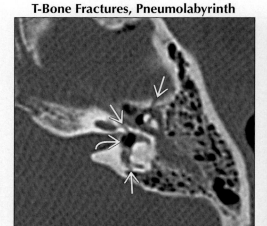

T-Bone Fractures, Pneumolabyrinth

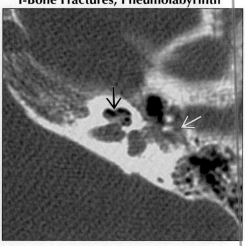

(Left) Axial bone CT at the level of the epitympanum reveals a zigzagging transverse fracture ➡ passing through the inner ear with associated air in the vestibule ➡ (pneumolabyrinth). *(Right)* Axial bone CT in a patient with hearing loss following minor trauma reveals pneumolabyrinth ➡ in the absence of fractures. Opacification around ossicles ➡ may be middle ear blood. Stapes disruption should be suspected.

T-Bone Fractures, Dural Sinus Thrombosis

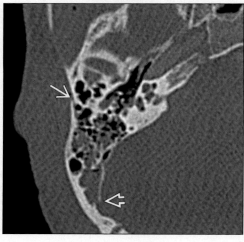

T-Bone Fractures, Dural Sinus Thrombosis

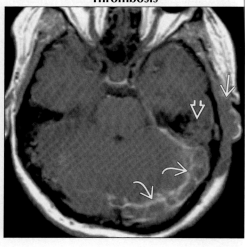

(Left) Axial bone CT shows an oblique temporal bone fracture through the mastoid sinus ➡ that involves the posterior medial wall at the sigmoid-transverse sinus junction ➡. Such fractures may result in sinus thrombosis and eventual dural A-V fistula. *(Right)* Axial T1 C+ MR demonstrates soft tissue swelling ➡ and middle ear fluid ➡ in this patient 1 week following head trauma. Persistent headache was explained by transverse sinus thrombosis ➡.

T-Bone Fractures, ICA Injury

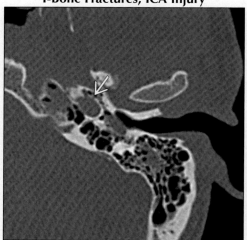

T-Bone Fractures, ICA Injury

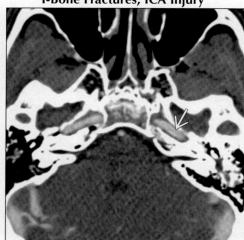

(Left) Axial bone CT shows a fracture through the vertical segment of the petrous internal carotid artery ➡. Middle ear and mastoid opacification is visible secondary to blood. Such patients are at risk for internal carotid artery dissection. *(Right)* Axial CTA shows a subtle "flap" of arterial intima ➡ in this patient with horizontal internal carotid artery dissection from temporal bone fracture.

8

TRAUMATIC LESIONS OF THE TEMPORAL BONE

T-Bone Fractures, Tegmen Tympani, Cephalocele

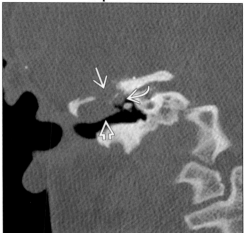

T-Bone Fractures, Tegmen Tympani, Cephalocele

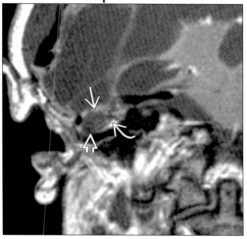

(Left) Coronal bone CT reveals a large tegmen tympani dehiscence ➡ with possible cephalocele in the roof of the external auditory canal ➡ and epitympanum ➡. MR imaging best evaluates for cephalocele in such circumstances. *(Right)* Coronal T1 C+ MR shows massive temporal lobe encephalomalacia with cephalocele passing through a large tegmen defect ➡ into the epitympanum ➡ and roof of the external auditory canal ➡.

Ossicular Dislocation, Incus

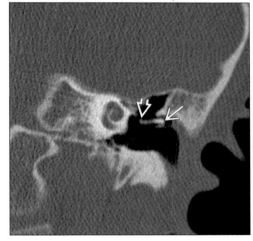

Ossicular Dislocation, Stapes

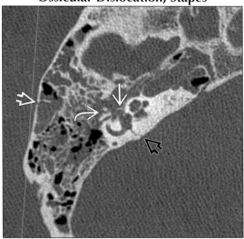

(Left) Coronal bone CT shows incus dislocation with projection through ruptured tympanic membrane into medial EAC ➡. Note lenticular process on medial end ➡. *(Right)* Axial bone CT reveals a transverse fracture zigzagging from outer cortex ➡ through middle & inner ear ➡. The anterior stapes crura is seen floating ➡ along the disrupted anterior margin of the oval window, while the malleus head & incus short process are posteriorly displaced ➡.

T-Bone Fractures, Secondary Cholesteatoma

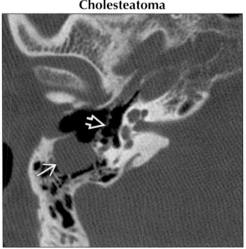

T-Bone Fractures, Secondary Cholesteatoma

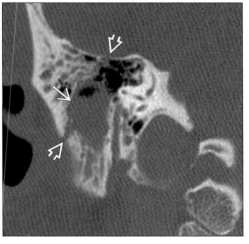

(Left) Axial bone CT demonstrates a scalloping post-traumatic cholesteatoma ➡ in the mastoid with dehiscence of posterior wall of middle ear in this patient 5 years following temporal bone fracture. Note thickened, healed tympanic membrane ➡. *(Right)* Coronal bone CT shows post-traumatic mastoid cholesteatoma ➡ in this patient with remote history of temporal bone fractures. Old oblique fracture line is still visible through mastoid air cells ➡.

SECONDARY (REFERRED) OTALGIA

DIFFERENTIAL DIAGNOSIS

Common
- Derangement, Articular Disc, TMJ
- Nasopharyngeal Carcinoma
- SCCa, Lingual Tonsil
- SCCa, Palatine Tonsil

Less Common
- Osteomyelitis, Mandible-Maxilla
- Rhinosinusitis, Chronic
- Suppurative Adenopathy, RPS
- Abscess, Palatine Tonsil
- SCCa, Hypopharynx
- Mucoepidermoid Carcinoma, Parotid
- Adenoid Cystic Carcinoma, Parotid

Rare but Important
- Parotitis, Acute
- Carotidynia, Acute Idiopathic
- SCCa, Nodal, RPS
- Thyroiditis, Chronic Lymphocytic (Hashimoto)
- Metastatic Node, Non-SCCa, RPS
- Rheumatoid Larynx
- Esophageal Carcinoma, Cervical

ESSENTIAL INFORMATION

Key Differential Diagnosis Issues
- Otalgia: Ear pain
  - Primary otalgia: Caused by ear disease
    - Otoscopy abnormal
  - Secondary (referred) otalgia: Caused by diseases remote from ear
    - Otoscopy normal
- Secondary otalgia: Structures & pathways that refer pain to ear
  - Trigeminal nerve (CN5): Referred along auriculotemporal nerve
    - Most frequent referred pain pathway
    - Structures innervated include nasopharynx, sinuses, teeth, major salivary glands (especially parotid)
  - Facial nerve (CN7): Referred along greater superficial petrosal nerve
    - Structures innervated by vidian nerve include nose, posterior ethmoid, sphenoid
  - Glossopharyngeal nerve (CN9): Referred along Jacobson nerve
    - Structures innervated include nasopharyngeal, oropharyngeal, & hypopharyngeal surface
  - Vagus nerve (CN10): Referred along Arnold nerve
    - Structures innervated include valleculae, pyriform sinuses, larynx, cervical trachea, & esophagus
- Imaging in otalgia
  - Primary: CT/MR focused to temporal bone
  - Secondary: C+ CT or MR must cover entire neck from skull base to clavicles
  - Scan review: Radiologist must review entire extracranial head and neck
    - CAVEAT: Remember to check TMJ, carotid wall (carotidynia), & cricoarytenoid areas

Helpful Clues for Common Diagnoses
- **Derangement, Articular Disc, TMJ**
  - Frequently overlooked cause of otalgia
  - Sagittal MR: Anteriorly dislocated & deformed TMJ meniscus
- **Nasopharyngeal Carcinoma**
  - Otalgia with fluid in ear
  - CT/MR: Nasopharyngeal mucosal space mass invades carotid, retropharyngeal, parapharyngeal spaces
    - Perivascular & perineural tumor spread
- **SCCa, Lingual Tonsil**
  - Often clinically silent until bulky; otalgia may be 1st symptom
  - CT/MR: Base of tongue invasive mass invades sublingual space
- **SCCa, Palatine Tonsil**
  - Clinically evident early
  - CT/MR: Enlarged palatine tonsil; invasion of parapharyngeal & masticator spaces

Helpful Clues for Less Common Diagnoses
- **Osteomyelitis, Mandible-Maxilla**
  - Dental infections of molars ± osteomyelitis frequent causes of otalgia
  - CT: Periapical lucency progresses to destructive osteomyelitis of mandible or maxilla in minority of cases
- **Rhinosinusitis, Chronic**
  - Longstanding sinus infections
  - CT: Partial sinus opacification & sinus wall thickening ± osteoneogenesis filling part of sinus lumen
- **Suppurative Adenopathy, RPS**
  - Pharyngitis "seeds" retropharyngeal nodes

- Oral antibiotics miss treatment goal
  - Reactive nodes suppurate
  - CT: Lateral retropharyngeal rim-enhancing node(s)
- **Abscess, Palatine Tonsil**
  - Sore throat & ear pain presentation
  - CT: Intrapalatine tonsil rim-enhancing low density lesion
    - If abscess extends to adjacent deep spaces, use term "peritonsillar abscess"
- **SCCa, Hypopharynx**
  - Sore throat, dysphagia, & otalgia
  - CT/MR: Pyriforms sinus invasive, enhancing mass ± malignant nodes
- **Mucoepidermoid Carcinoma, Parotid**
  - Most common parotid carcinoma
  - CT/MR: Invasive mass
- **Adenoid Cystic Carcinoma, Parotid**
  - 2nd most common carcinoma
  - CT/MR: Invasive; perineural tumor spread

Helpful Clues for Rare Diagnoses
- **Parotitis, Acute**
  - Viral gland infection vs. ductal obstruction
  - CT/MR: Enhancing, enlarged parotid
    - ± Large duct with stone or stenosis
- **Carotidynia, Acute Idiopathic**
  - Carotid bulb area pain & otalgia
  - CT/MR: C+, thickened carotid sheath
- **SCCa, Nodal, RPS**
  - Deep eye pain, occipital pain, otalgia
  - Primary sites: Nasopharynx, posterior wall oropharynx, & hypopharynx

- CT/MR: Enlarged, variably enhancing retropharyngeal space nodes
  - Primary site staged simultaneously
- **Thyroiditis, Chronic Lymphocytic (Hashimoto)**
  - Painful thyroid, angle of mandible & ear
  - CT/MR: Diffuse moderately enlarged lobular thyroid without calcifications or necrosis
- **Metastatic Node, Non-SCCa, RPS**
  - Deep eye pain, occipital pain, otalgia
  - Primary sites: Skin melanoma, thyroid carcinoma, lymphoma
  - CT/MR: Enlarged variably enhancing retropharyngeal space nodes
    - No visible primary tumor on scan
- **Rheumatoid Larynx**
  - Cricoarytenoid joint involvement causes otalgia
  - CT: Inflammatory cricoarytenoid mass may mimic SCCa
    - Cricoarytenoid erosions may be present
- **Esophageal Carcinoma, Cervical**
  - Throat pain, dysphagia, otalgia
  - CT/MR: Invasive mass centered behind trachea
    - Inferior images show distal esophageal wall thickening

SELECTED REFERENCES

1. Weissman JL: A pain in the ear: the radiology of otalgia. AJNR Am J Neuroradiol. 18(9):1641-51, 1997
2. Schellhas KP: Temporomandibular joint injuries. Radiology. 173(1):211-6, 1989

Derangement, Articular Disc, TMJ

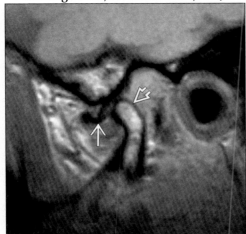

Sagittal T1WI MR shows open-mouthed view of a thickened, buckled TMJ meniscus ➾ dislocated anterior to the condylar head ➾. Chronic TMJ internal derangement of this kind can cause otalgia.

Derangement, Articular Disc, TMJ

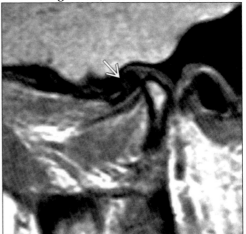

Sagittal T2WI MR reveals a closed-mouth view of a badly deformed TMJ meniscus ➾. In this case the disc is anteriorly dislocated and remains so in both closed and open (not shown) views.

(Left) Axial T1 C+ FS MR shows a large nasopharyngeal carcinoma ➡ filling the nasopharyngeal airway & extending posterolaterally toward the carotid space ⇨. Note the fluid in the left mastoid ➡. Primary & secondary otalgia are possible in this case. *(Right)* Coronal T1 C+ FS MR reveals a deeply invasive nasopharyngeal carcinoma ➡. Note left malignant retropharyngeal node ➡. Both the primary tumor or malignant retropharyngeal node can cause otalgia.

Nasopharyngeal Carcinoma

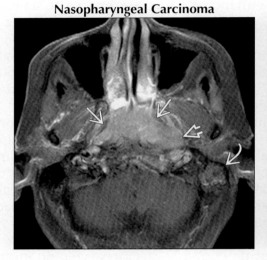

Nasopharyngeal Carcinoma

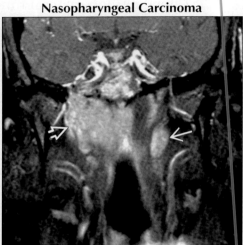

(Left) Axial CECT demonstrates a small right lingual tonsil squamous cell carcinoma primary ➡ with large malignant jugulodigastric lymph node ➡. *(Right)* Axial T1 C+ FS MR shows a large left palatine tonsil squamous cell carcinoma ➡. This lesion has invaded the deep masticator space and mandibular foramen-CNV3 ➡, parapharyngeal space, and deep portion of the parotid space ➡. Patient presented with jaw numbness and otalgia.

SCCa, Lingual Tonsil

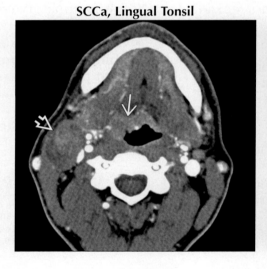

SCCa, Palatine Tonsil

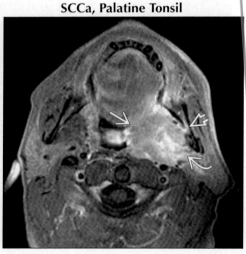

(Left) Coronal bone CT reveals periapical lucency/abscess ➡ associated with the root of the posterior mandibular molar. Notice the exuberant periosteal elevation ➡ indicating that osteomyelitis is also present. *(Right)* Sagittal 3D reconstruction in this patient with painful mandibular molar and otalgia shows a periapical abscess ➡, inframandibular sinus tract ➡, and periosteal reaction ➡, signaling concurrent mandibular osteomyelitis.

Osteomyelitis, Mandible-Maxilla

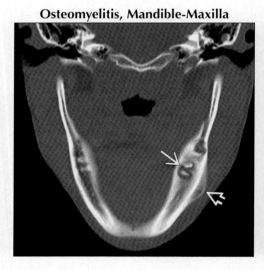

Osteomyelitis, Mandible-Maxilla

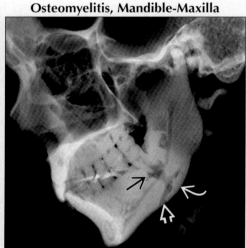

SECONDARY (REFERRED) OTALGIA

Rhinosinusitis, Chronic

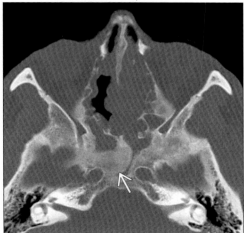

Rhinosinusitis, Chronic

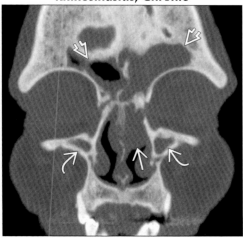

(Left) Axial bone CT shows a patient following FESS with continued significant ethmonasal opacification. Notice osteoneogenesis ➡ in the sphenoid sinus, indicating the patient's sinonasal inflammatory disease is chronic in nature. *(Right)* Coronal bone CT demonstrates intranasal inflammation ➡ along with frontal ➡ and maxillary ➡ sinus partial or complete opacification. These are typical CT findings of chronic rhinosinusitis.

Suppurative Adenopathy, RPS

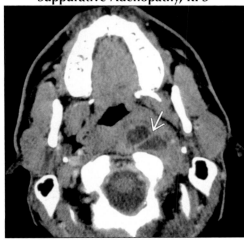

Abscess, Palatine Tonsil

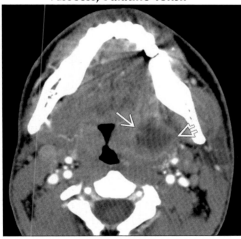

(Left) Axial CECT shows a left lateral retropharyngeal space suppurative nodal conglomerate ➡. If incompletely treated, this suppurative nodal group will evolve into frank retropharyngeal space abscess. *(Right)* Axial CECT reveals bilateral tonsillar enlargement with left palatine tonsil abscess ➡. The lateral wall of the abscess is "pointing" into the anterior parapharyngeal space ➡. If untreated, peritonsillar abscess will occur.

SCCa, Hypopharynx

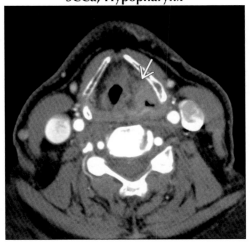

SCCa, Hypopharynx

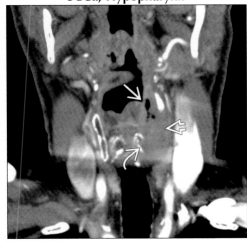

(Left) Axial CECT reveals an aggressive-appearing left pyriform sinus squamous cell carcinoma. This primary tumor has spread anteriorly into the supraglottic paraglottic space ➡. *(Right)* Coronal CECT demonstrates a left pyriform sinus squamous cell carcinoma ➡ that has spread anteriorly and inferiorly in the paraglottic space ➡ to destroy part of the cricoid cartilage ➡.

SECONDARY (REFERRED) OTALGIA

(Left) Axial T1 C+ FS MR shows a diffusely infiltrating left parotid mucoepidermoid carcinoma. Note the entire parotid is enhancing and poorly marginated. Tumor spreads anteriorly along a facial nerve branch ➡ *and posterosuperiorly into the bell of the stylomastoid foramen* ➡. *(Right) Axial CECT reveals an infiltrating mass in the deep right parotid space, invading the anterior tip of the sternocleidomastoid muscle* ➡ *and involving the deep lobe* ➡.

Mucoepidermoid Carcinoma, Parotid

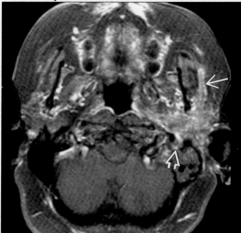

Adenoid Cystic Carcinoma, Parotid

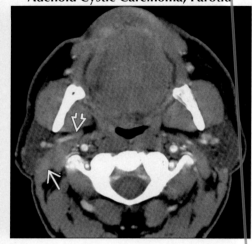

(Left) Coronal CECT shows left parotid enlargement with diffuse increase in enhancement in this patient with acute parotiditis. Within the gland are areas of low density ➡ *that may represent early abscess formation. (Right) Axial CECT demonstrates thickening of the left common carotid artery wall* ➡ *just below the bifurcation. This patient presented with a tender neck and left ear pain.*

Parotitis, Acute

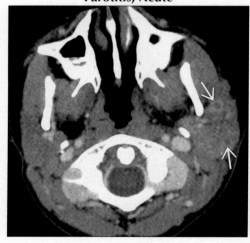

Carotidynia, Acute Idiopathic

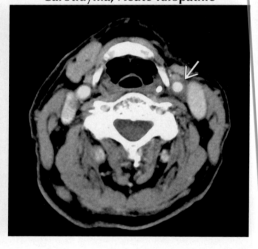

(Left) Axial T2WI FS MR shows a large left palatine tonsil squamous cell carcinoma ➡ *invading the parapharyngeal, masticator, and deep parotid spaces. Notice the left malignant retropharyngeal node* ➡. *(Right) Axial CECT reveals an enlarged and moderately enhancing thyroid gland* ➡, *typical of chronic lymphocytic thyroiditis. Calcifications and colloid cysts often seen in multinodular goiter are characteristically absent.*

SCCa, Nodal, RPS

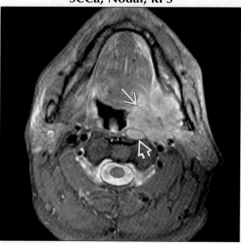

Thyroiditis, Chronic Lymphocytic (Hashimoto)

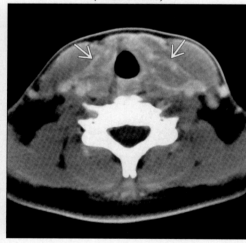

SECONDARY (REFERRED) OTALGIA

Metastatic Node, Non-SCCa, RPS

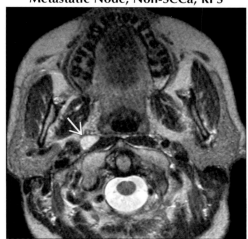

Metastatic Node, Non-SCCa, RPS

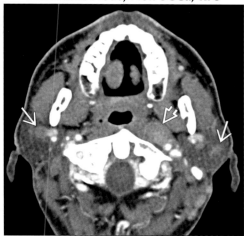

(Left) Axial T2WI MR reveals a malignant right lateral retropharyngeal node ➡ in a patient with a large bilobed nasal esthesioneuroblastoma. Other non-SCCa found in retropharyngeal nodes include non-Hodgkin lymphoma, melanoma, and differentiated thyroid carcinoma. *(Right)* Axial CECT demonstrates bilateral intraparotid lymph nodes ➡ in association with a large, non-necrotic left retropharyngeal lymph node ➡ in a patient with non-Hodgkin lymphoma.

Rheumatoid Larynx

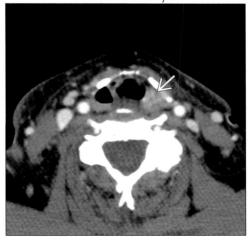

Rheumatoid Larynx

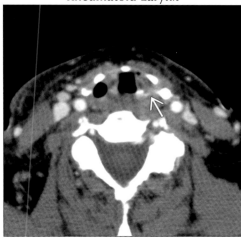

(Left) Axial CECT shows enhancement of an enlarged left aryepiglottic fold ➡ suspicious for squamous cell carcinoma of the supraglottis. The history of rheumatoid arthritis should suggest the alternative of rheumatoid larynx. *(Right)* Axial CECT reveals loss of soft tissue planes in the area of the left cricoarytenoid joint ➡. With this patient's history of longstanding rheumatoid arthritis, rheumatoid larynx should be the primary consideration.

Esophageal Carcinoma, Cervical

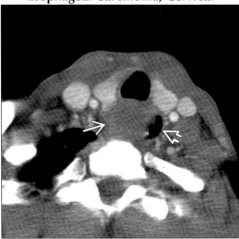

Esophageal Carcinoma, Cervical

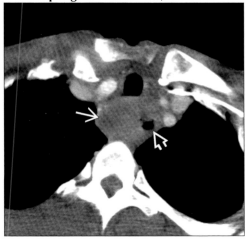

(Left) Axial CECT shows a bulbous mass ➡ behind the trachea involving the right lateral wall of the esophagus. Notice the air-filled lumen of the esophagus ➡ to the left of the mass. *(Right)* Axial CECT demonstrates the caudal end of a cervical esophageal carcinoma ➡. Despite the size of this lesion, the esophageal lumen is still visible to the left ➡. This lesion extended from the hypopharynx to the aortic arch.

SECTION 9
Skull Base

Anatomically Based Differentials

NORMAL SKULL BASE VENOUS VARIANTS

DIFFERENTIAL DIAGNOSIS

Common
- Jugular Foramen Asymmetry
- Jugular Bulb Pseudolesion
- Pterygoid Venous Plexus Asymmetry
- Emissary Vein, Transmastoid
- Posterior Condylar Canal, Asymmetric

Less Common
- High Jugular Bulb
- Jugular Bulb Diverticulum
- Dehiscent Jugular Bulb
- Sphenoidal Emissary Vein (of Vesalius), Asymmetric

Rare but Important
- Foramen Cecum
- Emissary Vein, Petrosquamosal

ESSENTIAL INFORMATION

Key Differential Diagnosis Issues
- Intracranial venous flow must exit through skull base foramina
- Normal structures may be asymmetric
- Normal variants may be uni- or bilateral
- Variants may be mistaken for masses, especially jugular foramen pseudolesion
  - MR pitfall results from variable signal intensity secondary to venous flow
  - Normal CECT ± normal bone CT clarifies
- Asymmetric or enlarged veins may be sign of pathology

Helpful Clues for Common Diagnoses
- **Jugular Foramen Asymmetry**
  - Key facts
    - Jugular veins usually asymmetric in size
    - Exaggerated asymmetry may result in larger side mimicking mass
    - More often MR pitfall
  - Imaging
    - MR: Unilateral high signal and enhancement
    - Look for ipsilateral enlarged transverse sinus
    - CECT: Normal jugular enhancement
    - Bone CT: Preservation of normal foraminal contours
- **Jugular Bulb Pseudolesion**
  - Key facts
    - Turbulent venous flow creates MR pitfall

- Asymmetric signal mimics pathology
  - Imaging
    - MR: Typically high signal intensity and avid enhancement
    - MRV or coronal T1 C+ usually clarify jugular bulb as normal
    - CECT: Normal jugular enhancement
    - Bone CT: Preservation of normal foraminal contours
- **Pterygoid Venous Plexus Asymmetry**
  - Key facts
    - Unilateral prominence of deep facial veins that drain from cavernous sinus
    - Often incidental finding
    - Asymmetry may be pathological: Increased venous flow with caroticocavernous fistula
  - Imaging
    - CT: Curvilinear enhancement in medial masticator &/or parapharyngeal space
    - MR: Enhancement or flow voids in deep face, but no mass effect
    - Normal signal intensity of adjacent masticator muscles
- **Emissary Vein, Transmastoid**
  - Key facts
    - Transverse sinus to posterior auricular or occipital veins
    - Large veins may be pathological
    - Skull base dysplasia with small jugular foramina (e.g., achondroplasia)
    - Emissary & suboccipital veins "replace" jugular veins and are surgical hazard
  - Imaging
    - CECT: Enhancement of veins traversing mastoid bone
    - Bone CT: Smooth well-corticated channels through bone
- **Posterior Condylar Canal, Asymmetric**
  - Key facts
    - Synonym: Condyloid canal
    - Posterolateral to hypoglossal canal
    - Important channel for venous flow with atretic jugular veins
    - Contents: Meningeal branch of ascending pharyngeal artery; emissary vein from sigmoid sinus to suboccipital veins
  - Imaging
    - Bone CT: Well-corticated venous channel
    - CECT/MR C+: Venous enhancement

NORMAL SKULL BASE VENOUS VARIANTS

Helpful Clues for Less Common Diagnoses
- **High Jugular Bulb**
  - Key facts
    - Usually incidental finding
    - May be associated with pulsatile tinnitus
  - Imaging
    - Axial bone CT: Bulb at level of cochlea
    - Coronal bone CT: Medial ± inferior to semicircular canals
    - MR: May be mistaken for unilateral mass because of high signal
    - MRV or coronal T1 C+ should clarify
- **Jugular Bulb Diverticulum**
  - Key facts
    - Normal variant, incidental finding
    - May be associated with pulsatile tinnitus
  - Imaging
    - Bone CT: Best evaluated in coronal plane
    - Small "pouch" projecting from superior aspect of jugular bulb
    - MR: May be mistaken for temporal bone mass because of high signal
    - MRV or coronal T1 C+ should clarify
- **Ddehiscent Jugular Bulb**
  - Key facts
    - Otoscopy: "Vascular" middle ear mass
    - May be associated with pulsatile tinnitus
    - Absence of bony covering between jugular bulb & middle ear cavity
  - Imaging
    - CT: Absence of bony plate over jugular bulb at posterior hypotympanum

- **Sphenoidal Emissary Vein (of Vesalius), Asymmetric**
  - Key facts
    - Synonym: Sphenoid emissary foramen
    - Transmits emissary vein from cavernous sinus to pterygoid venous plexus
    - Enlargement is pathological if ↑ venous flow from caroticocavernous fistula or tumor direct invasion
  - Imaging
    - May be partially assimilated with ovale or may be duplicated
    - Bone CT: Located medial to anterior aspect foramen ovale; usually < 2 mm

Helpful Clues for Rare Diagnoses
- **Foramen Cecum**
  - Key facts
    - Usually closes during embryogenesis
    - Contains vein from sup sagittal sinus
    - Large foramen can be pathological
    - Suspect anterior neuropore anomaly
  - Imaging
    - Bone CT: Midline anterior to crista galli
    - Usually < 2 mm
- **Emissary Vein, Petrosquamosal**
  - Key facts
    - Embryonic venous remnant
    - Connects transverse sinus & retromandibular vein
  - Imaging
    - Bone CT: Vertical channel, ≤ 4 mm
    - Posterior to TMJ, anterior to EAC

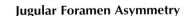

Jugular Foramen Asymmetry

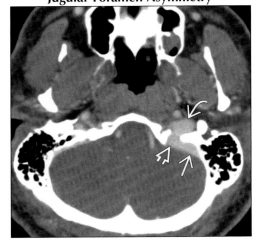

Axial CECT shows a normal left jugular foramen, though larger compared to the right. Note the left sigmoid sinus ➡, jugular foramen ⇒, and internal jugular vein ➡ are all significantly larger than the right.

Jugular Foramen Asymmetry

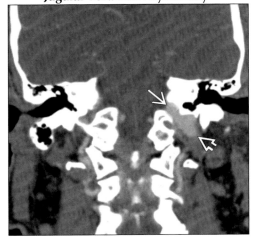

Coronal CECT in the same patient reveals the larger left jugular foramen ⇒ and internal jugular vein ⇒. Such asymmetry is normal and does not imply underlying pathology.

9

NORMAL SKULL BASE VENOUS VARIANTS

(Left) Axial T2WI FS MR performed during work-up of a possible metastatic disease reveals asymmetric hyperintensity in the right skull base ➡, which was intermediate intensity on T1 & enhanced with gadolinium (not shown). **(Right)** Axial CECT in the same patient reveals normal enhancement of right sigmoid sinus ➡ & jugular bulb ⇉ with normal foraminal contour. MR finding is attributed to turbulent venous flow in jugular foramen, not metastatic tumor.

Jugular Bulb Pseudolesion

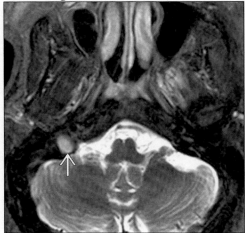

Jugular Bulb Pseudolesion

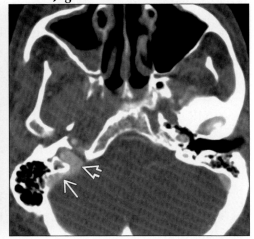

(Left) Axial CECT reveals curvilinear enhancement of the pterygoid venous plexus (PVP) bilaterally in deep face. The right PVP ➡ has several linear vessels while the left ➡ has a more prominent mass-like appearance. **(Right)** Coronal CECT in the same patient again shows asymmetry of the pterygoid plexus vessels ⇉ in deep face. It also better illustrates the curvilinear vascular appearance of the plexus, confirming that this is not a true mass.

Pterygoid Venous Plexus Asymmetry

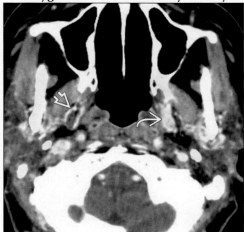

Pterygoid Venous Plexus Asymmetry

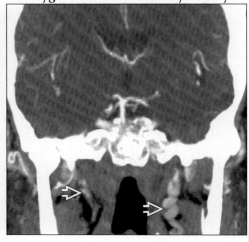

(Left) Axial bone CT demonstrates a right transmastoid emissary vein ➡ coursing from the transverse sinus through the bone adjacent to the occipital suture ➡. Portions of the left emissary vein are also evident ⇉. **(Right)** Sagittal bone CT reformat shows a well-corticated linear venous channel ➡ extending through the posterior mastoid bone, adjacent to occipital suture ➡.

Emissary Vein, Transmastoid

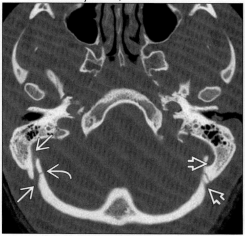

Emissary Vein, Transmastoid

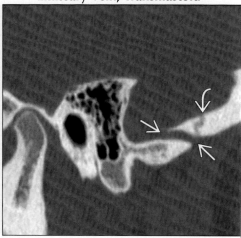

NORMAL SKULL BASE VENOUS VARIANTS

Posterior Condylar Canal, Asymmetric

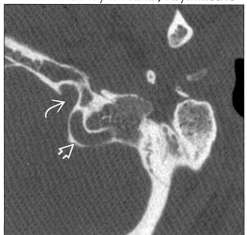

Posterior Condylar Canal, Asymmetric

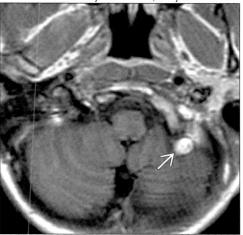

(Left) Axial bone CT through inferior temporal bone demonstrates a well-defined venous channel through the left skull base ➡ posterolateral to the left hypoglossal canal ➡, which is also known as the anterior condylar canal. *(Right)* Axial T1 C+ MR in a different patient shows asymmetric focal enhancement in the inferior skull base ➡, representing a normal but prominent left posterior condylar vein.

High Jugular Bulb

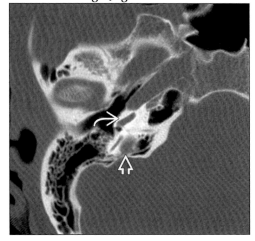

High Jugular Bulb

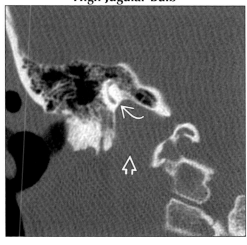

(Left) Axial bone CT through the temporal bone at the level of the basal turn of the cochlea ➡ demonstrates focal rounded lucency ➡ immediately medial to the posterior semicircular canal. *(Right)* Coronal bone CT in same patient reveals an enlarged right jugular foramen ➡ at this level. Large foramen is "scalloping" inferomedial margin of hyperdense otic capsule bone ➡ that contains membranous labyrinth.

Jugular Bulb Diverticulum

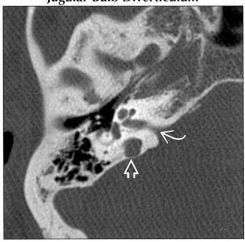

Jugular Bulb Diverticulum

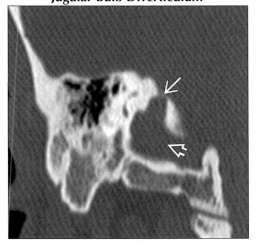

(Left) Axial bone CT demonstrates well-defined lucency ➡ in the posteromedial aspect of the right temporal bone at the level of the internal auditory canal ➡. *(Right)* Coronal bone CT reformat reveals this to be a focal diverticulum of the jugular bulb ➡, which extends superomedially from the normal-sized jugular foramen ➡. The overlying bone is intact.

NORMAL SKULL BASE VENOUS VARIANTS

(Left) Axial bone CT through the left temporal bone and external auditory canal ⮕ demonstrates a prominent jugular bulb without apparent bony covering to separate it from the middle ear cavity ⮕. *(Right)* Coronal bone CT through the external auditory canal ⮕ in the same patient again demonstrates the jugular bulb ⮕ "peeking" into the hypotympanum. The dehiscent jugular bulb can also be thought of as a lateral jugular bulb diverticulum.

Dehiscent Jugular Bulb

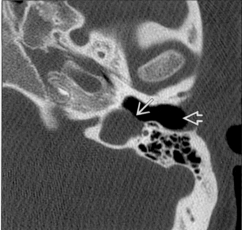

Dehiscent Jugular Bulb

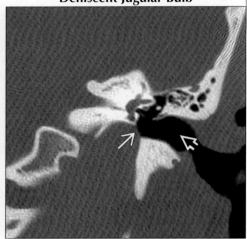

(Left) Axial bone CT demonstrates a very large right jugular bulb ⮕, which also appears to "herniate" into the hypotympanum ⮕. No overlying bony covering is evident; hence, the bulb is described as dehiscent. *(Right)* Coronal bone CT in the same patient reveals the bulb to have 2 diverticula: A lateral diverticulum into the middle ear ⮕ cavity and a medial superior jugular bulb diverticulum ⮕, which also creates a high jugular bulb.

Dehiscent Jugular Bulb

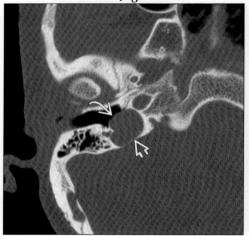

Dehiscent Jugular Bulb

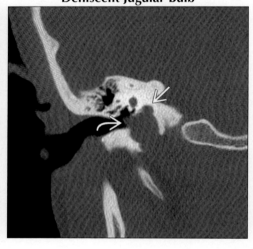

(Left) Axial bone CT through the skull base shows a small foramen of Vesalius ⮕ just medial to the foramen ovale ⮕. The foramen ovale and spinosum ⮕ are readily identified by searching for a "stiletto heel footprint." *(Right)* Axial T1 C+ FS MR shows normal enhancement of the foramen spinosum ⮕ (middle meningeal artery), foramen ovale ⮕, and foramen of Vesalius ⮕. The latter 2 carry emissary veins to the pterygoid venous plexus.

Sphenoidal Emissary Vein (of Vesalius), Asymmetric

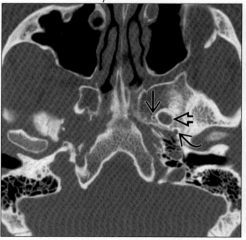

Sphenoidal Emissary Vein (of Vesalius), Asymmetric

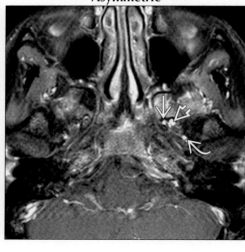

NORMAL SKULL BASE VENOUS VARIANTS

Sphenoidal Emissary Vein (of Vesalius), Asymmetric

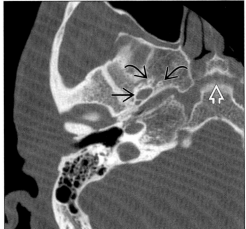

Sphenoidal Emissary Vein (of Vesalius), Asymmetric

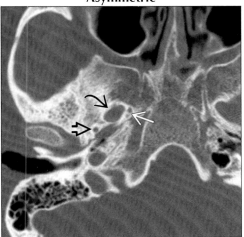

(Left) Axial bone CT through the right skull base in a child reveals 2 small foramina ➔ anteromedial to the foramen ovale ➔, indicating duplicated right foramina of Vesalius. Note the expected lack of fusion of the sphenooccipital synchondrosis ➔. *(Right)* Axial bone CT shows a normal-caliber foramen ovale ➔ and spinosum ➔. Notice the 2 small foramina of Vesalius ➔ just medial to the anterior margin of the foramen ovale.

Foramen Cecum

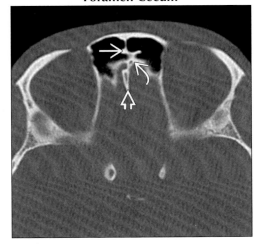

Foramen Cecum

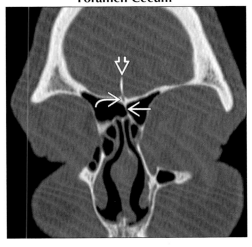

(Left) Axial bone CT in an adult patient demonstrates a small foramen cecum ➔ anterior to the crista galli ➔. This venous channel courses anteroinferiorly through the anterior skull base to the frontal intersinus septum ➔. *(Right)* Coronal reformat through the anterior fossa in the same patient shows the location of a small persistent foramen cecum ➔ at the anterior limit of the crista galli ➔ and coursing toward the intersinus septum ➔. The vein drains to the nasal cavity.

Emissary Vein, Petrosquamosal

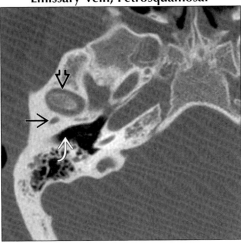

Emissary Vein, Petrosquamosal

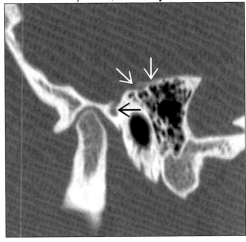

(Left) Axial bone CT shows the vertical component of the emissary vein ➔ as it descends through the temporal bone posterior to the TMJ ➔ and anterior to the external auditory canal ➔. *(Right)* Sagittal bone CT reformat reveals the distal course of the emissary vein ➔ posterior to TMJ as it exits down through the skull base. The more proximal aspect of the venous channel is also seen ➔ coursing through the lateral aspect of the petrous bone from the transverse sinus.

SKULL BASE FORAMINAL OR CANAL VARIANTS

DIFFERENTIAL DIAGNOSIS

Common
- Jugular Foramen Asymmetry
- Glossopharyngeal Canal

Less Common
- Petromastoid Canal
- Sphenoidal Emissary Vein (of Vesalius), Asymmetric
- Craniopharyngeal Canal, Persistent
- Medial Basal Canal (Basilaris Medianus)
- Internal Auditory Canal Hypoplasia
- Enlarged Emissary Vein, Transmastoid
- Posterior Condylar Vein, Asymmetric

Rare but Important
- Inferior Tympanic Canaliculus, Enlarged
- Absent Foramen Spinosum
- Innominate Canal
- Accessory Foramen Ovale

ESSENTIAL INFORMATION

Key Differential Diagnosis Issues
- Normal variants may be uni- or bilateral
- When normal structures are asymmetric, this may be normal variation or sign of pathology
- Many are incidental findings
- Imaging strategy
  ○ CT: Best defines or clarifies variants
  ○ MR: Often source of pitfalls

Helpful Clues for Common Diagnoses
- **Jugular Foramen Asymmetry**
  ○ Key facts
    ▪ Common developmental asymmetry of jugular foramen
  ○ Imaging
    ▪ CT: Smooth cortical bone surrounds enlarged jugular foramen
    ▪ MR: Various flow phenomena may result in misinterpretation of mass lesion
- **Glossopharyngeal Canal**
  ○ Key facts
    ▪ 30% have partial or complete canal
    ▪ Glossopharyngeal nerve (CN9) enters canal prior to jugular foramen
  ○ Imaging
    ▪ CT: Small funnel-shaped canal leading to anterior portion of jugular foramen (pars nervosa)

▪ MR: High-resolution T2 may show CN9

Helpful Clues for Less Common Diagnoses
- **Petromastoid Canal**
  ○ Key facts
    ▪ Synonyms: Subarcuate canaliculus
    ▪ From posterior CPA to mastoid air cells
    ▪ Canal passes between & below crura of superior semicircular canal
    ▪ Vestige of neonatal subarcuate fossa
    ▪ Contents: Subarcuate artery & vein; branch of AICA or labyrinthine artery
    ▪ In infant, subarcuate artery pseudolesion may confound radiologist
  ○ Imaging
    ▪ If seen in adult: ≤ 1 mm curvilinear canal below superior semicircular canal
    ▪ May be ≥ 2 mm in young children; subarachnoid space association may mimic lesion
- **Sphenoidal Emissary Vein (of Vesalius), Asymmetric**
  ○ Key facts
    ▪ Transmits emissary vein from cavernous sinus to pterygoid venous plexus
    ▪ May enlarge with ↑ venous flow from caroticocavernous fistula
  ○ Imaging
    ▪ Located medial to anterior aspect foramen ovale; usually < 2 mm
    ▪ May be partially assimilated with ovale or may be duplicated
- **Craniopharyngeal Canal, Persistent**
  ○ Key facts
    ▪ Synonym: Trans-sphenoidal canal; persistent hypophyseal canal
    ▪ Considered embryologic remnant of vascular channel
    ▪ Site of trans-sphenoidal cephalocele
  ○ Imaging
    ▪ Bone CT: Midline sphenoid, < 1.5 mm
    ▪ Anterior to sphenooccipital synchondrosis
- **Medial Basal Canal (Basilaris Medianus)**
  ○ Key facts
    ▪ Considered remnant of cephalic end of notochord
    ▪ Rarely enlarged to form basal cephalocele
  ○ Imaging
    ▪ Midline sphenoid; < 1.5 mm
    ▪ Posterior to sphenooccipital synchondrosis

SKULL BASE FORAMINAL OR CANAL VARIANTS

- **Internal Auditory Canal Hypoplasia**
  - Key facts
    - Contents: CN7 & CN8
    - Hypoplasia from congenital absence or deficiency of CN8
    - Associated with inner ear malformations
    - Normal canal diameter: 4-8 mm
  - Imaging
    - CT: Small caliber IAC, < 4 mm
    - MR: High resolution imaging may show deficient CN8
- **Enlarged Emissary Vein, Transmastoid**
  - Key facts
    - Connects transverse sinus to posterior auricular or occipital veins
    - Enlargement may be associated with small jugular foramen (JF)
  - Imaging
    - Horizontal canal through posteromedial mastoid bone adjacent to occipital suture
- **Posterior Condylar Vein, Asymmetric**
  - Key facts
    - Contents: Emissary vein from sigmoid sinus to suboccipital veins; meningeal branch of ascending pharyngeal artery
    - Enlargement associated with small JF
  - Imaging
    - Well-corticated curvilinear channel

Helpful Clues for Rare Diagnoses
- **Inferior Tympanic Canaliculus, Enlarged**
  - Key facts
    - Normally transmits Jacobsen nerve (inferior tympanic branch of CN9)

- Aberrant internal carotid artery (ICA) enters middle ear through this
  - Imaging
    - Aberrant ICA widens canaliculus to reach cochlear promontory
    - CTA or MRA to confirm aberrant ICA
- **Absent Foramen Spinosum**
  - Key facts
    - Normally transmits middle meningeal artery (MMA)
    - May be absent if MMA arises from ophthalmic artery or replaced by persistent stapedial artery (PSA)
    - Foramen rarely duplicated when MMA has anterior and posterior branches
  - Imaging
    - Foramen normally < 3 mm
    - Posterolateral to foramen ovale
    - Look for PSA and aberrant ICA
- **Innominate Canal**
  - Key facts
    - Synonym: Canal of Arnold
    - Contains lesser petrosal nerve
  - Imaging
    - Between foramen ovale and spinosum
    - Usually ≤ 2 mm
- **Accessory Foramen Ovale**
  - Key facts
    - Contains accessory meningeal artery
  - Imaging
    - Lateral to foramen ovale; < 2 mm
    - May be partially assimilated with ovale resulting in posterolateral groove

Jugular Foramen Asymmetry

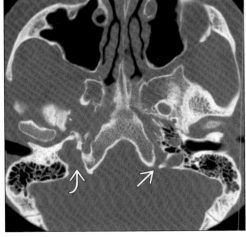

Axial bone CT through the low skull base demonstrates asymmetry of jugular foramina with the left foramen ➡ much smaller compared to the right ➘. This is a normal finding and does not indicate pathology.

Glossopharyngeal Canal

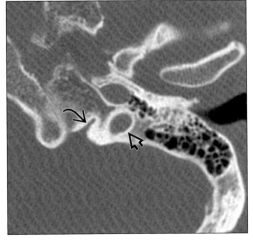

Axial bone CT demonstrates a funnel-shaped canal ➘ inferior to the level of the internal auditory canal. The canal connects inferiorly to the anterior portion of the jugular foramen ➘ (pars nervosa).

SKULL BASE FORAMINAL OR CANAL VARIANTS

Petromastoid Canal

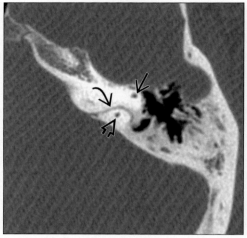

Petromastoid Canal

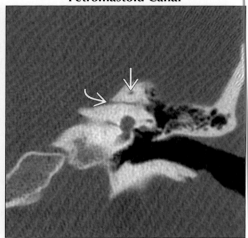

(Left) Axial bone CT in an adult patient demonstrates a curvilinear thin channel ⇗ coursing through the left petrous temporal bone between the posterior ⇗ and anterior ⇗ crura of the superior semicircular canal. (Right) Coronal bone CT reveals a petromastoid canal ⇗ coursing laterally from the posterior cerebellopontine angle to the mastoid air cells. The canal courses beneath the superior semicircular canal ⇗.

Sphenoidal Emissary Vein (of Vesalius), Asymmetric

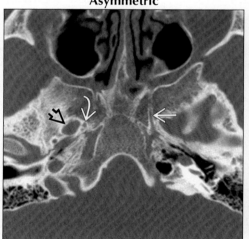

Craniopharyngeal Canal, Persistent

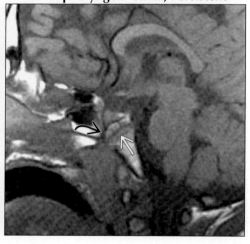

(Left) Axial bone CT shows 2 small foramina of Vesalius ⇗ at anteromedial margin of right foramen ovale ⇗. Left skull base shows anteromedial contour of the foramen ovale & vidian canal ⇗ but no accessory foramina. (Right) Sagittal T1WI MR in a child shows a small well-corticated canal ⇗ from inferior aspect of the sella to inferior aspect of the sphenoid bone. This craniopharyngeal canal is anterior to nonfused sphenooccipital synchondrosis ⇗.

Medial Basal Canal (Basilaris Medianus)

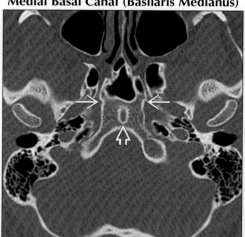

Internal Auditory Canal Hypoplasia

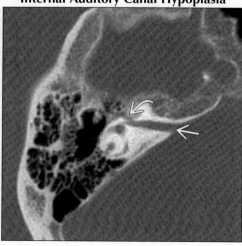

(Left) Axial bone CT demonstrates well-defined midline "keyhole"-shaped foramen ⇗ in posterior aspect of sphenoid (basisphenoid). This is posterior to the location of sella and posterior to site of fused sphenooccipital synchondrosis ⇗. (Right) Axial bone CT shows a small internal auditory canal ⇗ in an adult with history of congenital hearing loss. Even without measuring caliber, IAC is only slightly larger than caliber of labyrinthine segment of CN7 ⇗.

SKULL BASE FORAMINAL OR CANAL VARIANTS

Enlarged Emissary Vein, Transmastoid

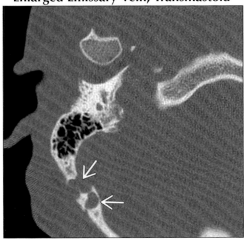

Posterior Condylar Vein, Asymmetric

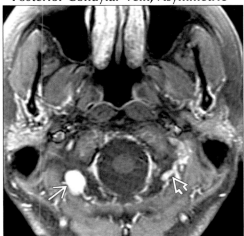

(Left) Axial NECT reveals multiple transmastoid emissary vein canals ➡ connecting the transverse sinus to the occipital veins. *(Right)* Axial T1 C+ FS MR demonstrates nodular enhancement just below the right skull base ➡ with more linear enhancement seen on the contralateral side ➡, which clearly appears vascular. Both are posterior condylar veins, and this asymmetry is a normal finding.

Inferior Tympanic Canaliculus, Enlarged

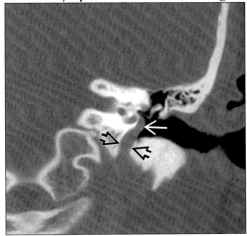

Absent Foramen Spinosum

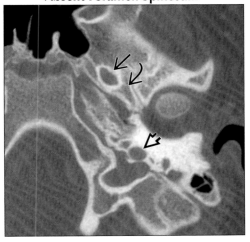

(Left) Coronal bone CT shows an enlarged inferior tympanic canaliculus ➡ secondary to an aberrant internal carotid artery ➡. *(Right)* Axial bone CT in the same patient shows an enlarged inferior tympanic canaliculus ➡. Note the additional finding of an absent ipsilateral foramen spinosum ➡ posterior to the foramen ovale ➡, indicating that a persistent stapedial artery is present.

Innominate Canal

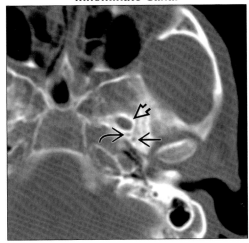

Accessory Foramen Ovale

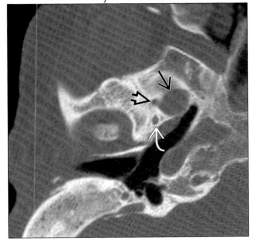

(Left) Axial bone CT demonstrates a tiny innominate canal ➡ anterior to the foramen spinosum ➡ and posterior to the foramen ovale ➡. This was an incidental unilateral variant. *(Right)* Axial bone CT shows an incidental unilateral small accessory foramen ➡ at the lateral margin of the foramen ovale ➡. The foramen spinosum containing the middle meningeal artery appears normal ➡.

CONGENITAL ANOMALIES OF THE SKULL BASE

DIFFERENTIAL DIAGNOSIS

Common
- Internal Jugular Vein, Asymmetry
- Jugular Bulb Diverticulum
- Chiari 1
- Chiari 2
- Neurofibromatosis Type 1

Less Common
- Aberrant Internal Carotid Artery
- Persistent Stapedial Artery
- Carotid Artery, Sphenoid Migration
- Agenesis Internal Carotid Artery

Rare but Important
- Craniostenoses
- 4th Occipital Sclerotome Anomalies
- Craniopharyngeal Canal, Persistent
- Medial Basal Canal (Basilaris Medianus)
- Chiari 3

ESSENTIAL INFORMATION

Helpful Clues for Common Diagnoses
- **Internal Jugular Vein, Asymmetry**
  - Key facts: Right internal jugular vein (IJV) dominant in 68-75%
    - Left IJV commonly smaller than right
    - IJV asymmetry < in larger cranial vault
  - Imaging
    - Most commonly seen normal asymmetry: Right sigmoid sinus, jugular bulb, & IJV larger than left
    - Increased signal of left IJV due to compression of left brachiocephalic vein during respiratory cycle
- **Jugular Bulb Diverticulum**
  - Key facts: Asymptomatic normal variant
  - Imaging
    - Coronal best: Bone CT, MRV, or T1 C+
    - "Pouch" projects from jugular bulb
    - High signal on MR may simulate mass
- **Chiari 1**
  - Key facts: Mismatch between posterior fossa size & cerebellar tissue
  - Imaging
    - Low-lying pointed (not rounded) "peg"-like cerebellar tonsils
    - Tonsils project below (≥ 5 mm) OR are impacted in foramen magnum
    - 4th occipital sclerotome anomalies in > 50% ⇒ small occipital enchondral skull

- **Chiari 2**
  - Key facts
    - 100% with neural tube closure defect
  - Imaging
    - Small bony posterior fossa
    - "Scalloped" petrous pyramid
    - "Notched" clivus
    - Low-lying tentorium/torcular
    - Large funnel-shaped foramen magnum
- **Neurofibromatosis Type 1**
  - Key facts: Neurocutaneous disorder
    - Characterized by diffuse neurofibromas, intracranial hamartomas, benign & malignant neoplasms
  - Imaging
    - Progressive sphenoid wing dysplasia
    - Enlarged optic foramina & fissures
    - Foramen magnum & skull base defects

Helpful Clues for Less Common Diagnoses
- **Aberrant Internal Carotid Artery**
  - Key facts: Displaced ICA courses through middle ear
  - Imaging
    - Enters posterior middle ear through enlarged inferior tympanic canaliculus
    - Courses anteriorly across cochlear promontory
    - Joins horizontal carotid canal through dehiscent carotid plate
    - Absent carotid foramen & vertical segment of petrous ICA
    - Look for associated persistent stapedial artery (PSA) in 30%
- **Persistent Stapedial Artery**
  - Key facts
    - Embryologic stapedial artery persists
    - PSA becomes middle meningeal artery
  - Imaging: Enlarged CN7 canal
    - Small canaliculus leaving carotid canal at genu of vertical & horizontal petrous ICA
    - Absent ipsilateral foramen spinosum
- **Carotid Artery, Sphenoid Migration**
  - Key facts: Seen in skull base syndromes involving enchondral bone
    - Achondroplasia, branchiootorenal syndrome, bicoronal synostoses (Apert, Pfeiffer, Crouzon)
  - Imaging
    - Medial migration of bony carotid artery walls at level of sphenoid
- **Agenesis Internal Carotid Artery**

CONGENITAL ANOMALIES OF THE SKULL BASE

○ Key facts
  ▪ Isolated or syndromic (PHACES, morning glory, Goldenhar, clefting syndromes)
○ Imaging
  ▪ Absent or hypoplastic vertical & horizontal petrous portions of ICA

Helpful Clues for Rare Diagnoses
• **Craniostenoses**
  ○ Key facts
    ▪ Syndromic (fibroblastic growth factor, TWIST, and MSX2 mutations) + nonsyndromic premature osseous obliteration of cranial sutures
  ○ Imaging
    ▪ Early fusion of occipital sutures surrounding foramen magnum
    ▪ Enchondral skull base: Achondroplasia, syndromic bicoronal synostoses, kleeblattschädel
• **4th Occipital Sclerotome Anomalies**
  ○ Synonym: Proatlas anomalies
  ○ Hypocentrum of 4th occipital sclerotome (OS) ⇒ anterior clival tubercle
  ○ Centrum of 4th OS ⇒ apical cap of dens & apical ligament
  ○ Ventral portion of neural component of 4th OS ⇒ anterior margin of foramen magnum & occipital condyle
  ○ Caudal portion of neural component of 4th OS ⇒ lateral atlantal masses & superior posterior arch of atlas
  ○ Imaging: 4th OSA finding
    ▪ Short clivus & atlas assimilation

  ▪ Craniovertebral bony anomalies
• **Craniopharyngeal Canal, Persistent**
  ○ Key facts
    ▪ Look for associated canal atresia or stenosis, moyamoya, coloboma
  ○ Imaging
    ▪ Small: Nonpituitary tissue containing remnant channel
    ▪ Large: Contains pituitary gland or frank encephalocele or artery
• **Medial Basal Canal (Basilaris Medianus)**
  ○ Key facts
    ▪ Notochord remnant cephalic terminus
  ○ Imaging: Midline clivus
    ▪ Posterior to sphenooccipital synchondrosis
    ▪ Currarino types A-F denote completeness and location of defect
    ▪ Tortuous canal may indent superior or inferior aspect of clivus
• **Chiari 3**
  ○ Key facts: Intracranial Chiari 2
    ▪ High cervical meningoencephalocele
  ○ Imaging: Occipital squama defect may involve upper cervical vertebrae
    ▪ Bony features of Chiari 2 in addition

SELECTED REFERENCES
1. Goodrich JT: Skull base growth in craniosynostosis. Childs Nerv Syst. 21(10):871-9, 2005
2. Jacquemin C et al: Canalis basilaris medianus: MRI. Neuroradiology. 42(2):121-3, 2000
3. Kjaer I et al: The craniopharyngeal canal indicating the presence of pharyngeal adenopituitary tissue. Eur J Radiol. 20(3):212-4, 1995

Internal Jugular Vein, Asymmetry

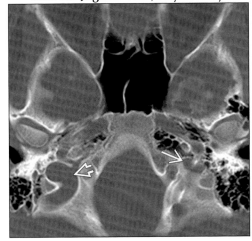

Axial bone CT demonstrates marked asymmetry with the jugular foramen on the right ⇒ larger than the small left jugular foramen ⇒.

Internal Jugular Vein, Asymmetry

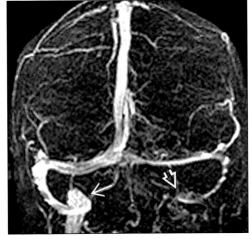

Coronal MRV in the same patient confirms marked asymmetry of the jugular veins. The left ⇒ tapers and is poorly visualized while the right ⇒ is normal in size.

CONGENITAL ANOMALIES OF THE SKULL BASE

(Left) Axial bone CT in a teenager with achondroplasia shows asymmetry of the jugular foramina ➡, both of which are stenosed. *(Right)* Sagittal MRV in a different patient with achondroplasia reveals severe restriction of the jugular vein ➡ at the level of the stenosed jugular foramina. There are excessive venous collaterals ➡ in the soft tissues of the neck.

Internal Jugular Vein, Asymmetry

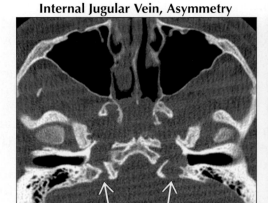

Internal Jugular Vein, Asymmetry

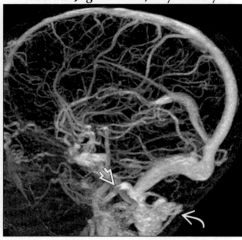

(Left) Coronal bone CT demonstrates a typical cephalad projecting jugular bulb diverticulum ➡. The diverticulum most commonly projects superiorly posterior to the internal auditory canal. *(Right)* Axial bone CT reveals the diverticulum ➡ to be located posterior to the internal auditory canal ➡. When the diverticulum is large, axial enhanced T1 MR imaging may appear to have an "enhancing lesion" in this location related to slow flow in the diverticulum.

Jugular Bulb Diverticulum

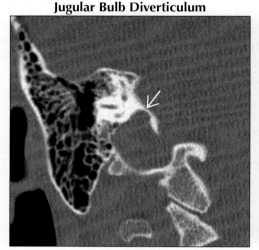

Jugular Bulb Diverticulum

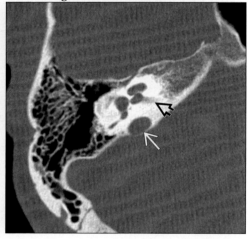

(Left) Sagittal T1WI MR shows marked herniation of the cerebellar tonsils ➡ behind the upper cervical spinal cord. There is an associated short scalloped clivus ➡. *(Right)* Sagittal T2WI MR reveals a typical enlarged foramen magnum, herniation of the uvula of the vermis, cascading cerebellar tissue ➡, and a notched clivus ➡. Note also the beaked tectum ➡ and the prominent massa intermedia ➡ associated with Chiari 2 malformation.

Chiari 1

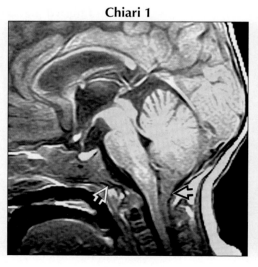

Chiari 2

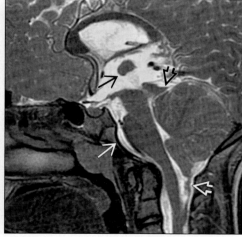

CONGENITAL ANOMALIES OF THE SKULL BASE

Neurofibromatosis Type 1

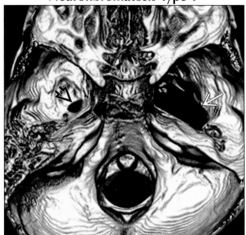

Neurofibromatosis Type 1

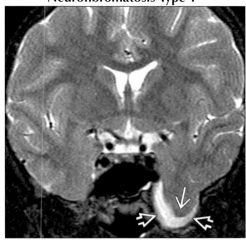

(Left) Axial bone CT 3D reconstruction shows a large defect ➡ of the left middle cranial fossa, centered on the foramen ovale. Note the normal-sized contralateral foramen ovale ➡. *(Right)* Coronal T2WI MR in the same child shows an encephalocele with herniation of the temporal lobe ➡ and hyperintense cerebral spinal fluid ➡ through the middle cranial floor defect.

Aberrant Internal Carotid Artery

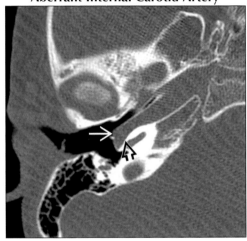

Aberrant Internal Carotid Artery

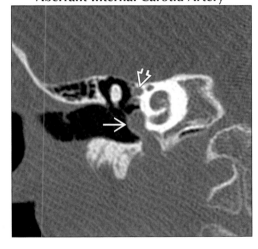

(Left) Axial bone CT demonstrates an aberrant internal carotid artery ➡ traversing the middle ear cavity over the cochlear promontory ➡. *(Right)* Coronal bone CT shows the aberrant internal carotid artery ➡ extending through the medial floor of the hypotympanum to overlie the cochlear promontory, inferior and lateral to the cochlea. The enlarged anterior tympanic CN7 canal ➡ suggests that the persistent stapedial artery is present.

Persistent Stapedial Artery

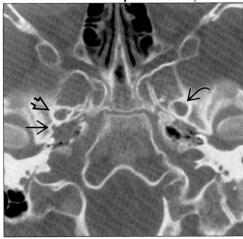

Persistent Stapedial Artery

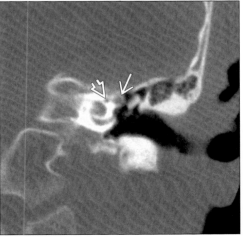

(Left) Axial bone CT shows a persistent stapedial artery in the absence of an aberrant internal carotid artery. Side-to-side comparison shows an absent left foramen spinosum with a normal left foramen ovale ➡. Note the normal right foramen ovale ➡ and foramen spinosum ➡. *(Right)* Coronal bone CT demonstrates an enlarged anterior tympanic segment of the facial nerve canal ➡ lateral to the normal labyrinthine segment ➡.

CONGENITAL ANOMALIES OF THE SKULL BASE

(Left) Axial bone CT in a child with achondroplasia shows marked medial deviation of the internal carotid arteries ➡. The bony covering remains, although indenting the posterior wall of the sphenoid sinus.
(Right) Axial bone CT reveals a normal-sized right horizontal petrous internal carotid artery canal ➡ and atretic left carotid canal ➡. Notice the prominent craniopharyngeal canal ➡ in this child with morning glory syndrome.

Carotid Artery, Sphenoid Migration

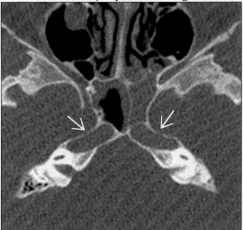

Agenesis Internal Carotid Artery

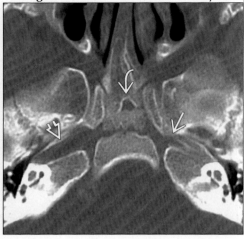

(Left) Axial bone CT 3D reconstruction in a newborn shows patency of the anterior ➡ and posterior ➡ intraoccipital sutures. The foramen ovale ➡ are symmetric. (Right) Axial bone CT 3D reconstruction in another newborn, this one with a disorder of enchondral cartilage, shows a deformed foramen magnum due to fusion of the sutures. There is hypertrophy of the internal occipital crest ➡. Note also the distortion of the left foramen ovale ➡.

Craniostenoses

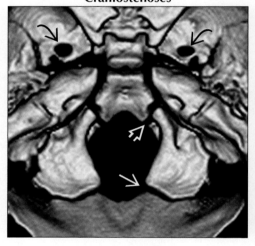

Craniostenoses

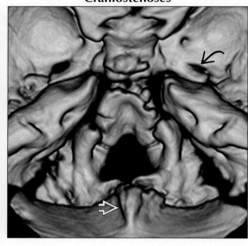

(Left) Axial CECT demonstrates absence of the clivus ➡ and an anomalous odontoid ➡ in an infant with severe anomalies of the skull base. (Right) Sagittal T1WI MR shows a pituitary gland ➡ "pointing" to a persistent craniopharyngeal canal ➡. Multiple midline anomalies are associated. The brainstem is thin, and the inferior 4th ventricle is open ➡. The anterior corpus callosum is thin ➡, and there is no anterior commissure.

4th Occipital Sclerotome Anomalies

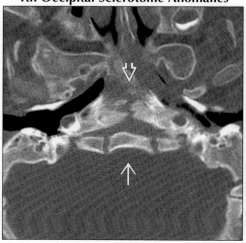

Craniopharyngeal Canal, Persistent

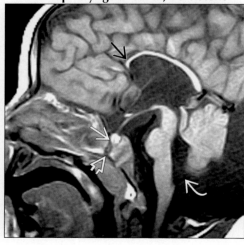

9

16

CONGENITAL ANOMALIES OF THE SKULL BASE

Craniopharyngeal Canal, Persistent

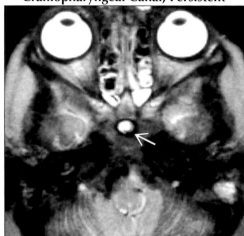

Craniopharyngeal Canal, Persistent

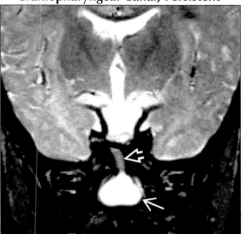

(Left) *Axial T2WI MR in a child with sphenoidal encephalocele reveals cerebrospinal fluid and pituitary tissue* ➡ *within the enlarged craniopharyngeal canal. This canal may contain fibrous tissue, CSF, pituitary tissue, and occasionally an artery.* *(Right)* *Coronal PD FSE FS MR shows a sphenoidal encephalocele* ➡ *projecting through a persistent craniopharyngeal canal* ⇥ *into pharynx. The pituitary gland is in the tissue signal within the canal.*

Medial Basal Canal (Basilaris Medianus)

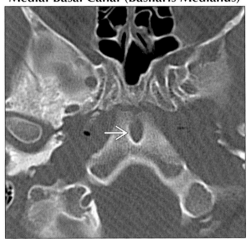

Medial Basal Canal (Basilaris Medianus)

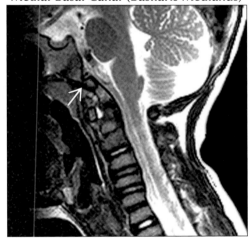

(Left) *Axial NECT demonstrates an incidental incomplete midline defect* ➡ *in the inferior aspect of the clivus.* *(Right)* *Sagittal T2WI MR in another child shows a complete defect* ➡ *traversing the clivus. Defects may be on the anterior or the posterior clival surface and may be through-and-through or incomplete.*

Chiari 3

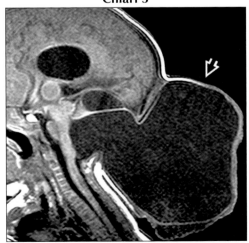

Chiari 3

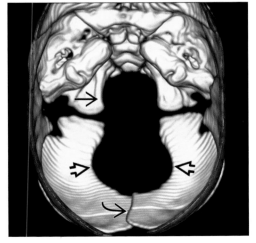

(Left) *Sagittal T1WI MR in a newborn shows a very large posterior encephalocele* ⇥ *involving the foramen magnum and supraoccipital bone. (Right)* *Axial bone CT 3D reconstruction in the same patient reveals a large bone defect* ⇥ *communicating with the foramen magnum* ➡. *There is an additional midline overlapping suture* ➢ *splitting the supraoccipital bone.*

DIFFERENTIAL DIAGNOSIS

Common
- Metastasis, Skull Base
- Fibrous Dysplasia, Skull Base
- Paget Disease, Skull Base
- Chordoma, Clivus
- Multiple Myeloma, Skull Base
- Plasmacytoma, Skull Base
- Chondrosarcoma, Skull Base
- Pneumatization Arrest, Sphenoid

Less Common
- Langerhans Histiocytosis, Skull Base
- Arachnoid Granulations, Dural Sinuses
- Osteomyelitis, Skull Base
- Meningioma, Skull Base

Rare but Important
- Giant Cell Tumor, Skull Base
- Cephalocele, Skull Base
- Ecchordosis Physaliphora
- Pseudotumor, Skull Base

ESSENTIAL INFORMATION

Key Differential Diagnosis Issues
- Lesion may be focal, diffuse, localized, or part of systemic disease
- Variable presentation of skull base lesion
  - Headache, cranial neuropathy
  - May be incidental imaging finding
- Imaging strategy
  - CT and MR often complementary
    - CT best demonstrates aggressive or benign bone features
    - MR may have characteristic signal intensity or enhancement

Helpful Clues for Common Diagnoses
- **Metastasis, Skull Base**
  - Key facts
    - Central skull base most frequent site
    - Most often prostate, breast, & lung carcinoma
  - Imaging
    - CT: Lytic, destructive, or sclerotic
    - MR: Variable signal, usually enhance
- **Fibrous Dysplasia, Skull Base**
  - Key facts
    - Benign expansile bone anomaly
    - Prone to enlarge during childhood
  - Imaging

- CT: Characteristic "ground-glass"; may narrow foramina and fissures
- MR: Heterogeneous, mass-like lesion
- T2: Ground-glass hypointense, lucent hyperintense, variable enhancement
- **Paget Disease, Skull Base**
  - Key facts
    - Chronic bone disorder with abnormal bone breakdown and formation
  - Imaging
    - CT: Sclerotic expansion of bone with "cotton wool" texture ± lytic areas
    - MR: T2 mainly low, lytic areas bright
- **Chordoma, Clivus**
  - Key facts
    - Benign but locally aggressive primary tumor of notochord remnants
    - From sphenooccipital synchondrosis
  - Imaging
    - CT: Lytic destructive midline sphenoid mass ± irregular bone spicules
    - MR: Characteristic high T2 signal, heterogeneous enhancement
- **Multiple Myeloma, Skull Base**
  - Key facts
    - Focal mass of malignant plasma cells
    - More frequently seen in calvarium
  - Imaging
    - CT: Multiple well-defined lytic lesions
- **Plasmacytoma, Skull Base**
  - Key facts
    - Isolated tumor of malignant plasma cells
  - Imaging
    - CT: Solitary lesion, bony lysis
    - MR: T2 intermediate signal; moderate enhancement
- **Chondrosarcoma, Skull Base**
  - Key facts
    - Malignant cartilaginous neoplasm
    - Arises from petroclival synchondrosis
  - Imaging
    - CT: Destructive mass at junction of sphenoid & temporal bones
    - "Arcs and whorls" of calcification
    - MR: T2 bright, intense enhancement
- **Pneumatization Arrest, Sphenoid**
  - Key facts
    - Incidental lesion of basisphenoid
  - Imaging
    - CT: Nonexpansile with sclerotic margin
    - Contains fat & curvilinear calcification

- MR: Heterogeneous, often focal T1 fat

Helpful Clues for Less Common Diagnoses

- **Langerhans Histiocytosis, Skull Base**
  - Key facts
    - Proliferation of bone marrow-derived Langerhans cells & eosinophils
    - Skull base involvement more often with multifocal or acute disseminated forms
  - Imaging
    - Nonspecific destructive soft tissue mass
- **Arachnoid Granulations, Dural Sinuses**
  - Key facts
    - Usually incidental imaging finding
  - Imaging
    - More numerous around dural sinuses
    - CT: Small well-defined "pits" in skull base
    - MR: Often subtle, focal T2 hyperintensity
- **Osteomyelitis, Skull Base**
  - Key facts
    - Primary bone infection, acute or chronic
  - Imaging
    - CT: Permeative lytic when acute; chronic may be lytic or lytic-sclerotic
    - MR: Marrow replacement, enhancement; often extensive involvement of dura
- **Meningioma, Skull Base**
  - Key facts
    - Dural-based, benign extraaxial tumor
    - May occur as intraosseous lesion
  - Imaging
    - CT: Bony changes may be hyperostosis, erosion, or permeative destruction
    - MR: Bone and thick dura enhance

Helpful Clues for Rare Diagnoses

- **Giant Cell Tumor, Skull Base**
  - Key facts
    - Benign long bone tumor
    - Skull base: Sphenoid & temporal bones
    - Can be locally aggressive &/or recur
  - Imaging
    - CT: Destructive mass with focally interrupted, thinned cortical shell
    - MR: Scant matrix, larger lesions more heterogeneous, marked enhancement
- **Cephalocele, Skull Base**
  - Key facts
    - Skull base defect with protrusion of meninges ± neural tissue
  - Imaging
    - CT: Focal bone defect
    - MR: Dura, CSF, ± neural elements
- **Ecchordosis Physaliphora**
  - Key facts
    - Notochordal remnant exophytic from dorsal aspect of clivus
  - Imaging
    - CT: Soft tissue density lesion
    - MR: T1 low, T2 high, no enhancement
- **Pseudotumor, Skull Base**
  - Key facts
    - Idiopathic inflammatory lesion
    - Inflammatory cells & variable fibrosis
  - Imaging
    - CT: Soft tissue mass, permeative bone
    - MR: Enhancing infiltrative process, T2 hypointense, T1 iso- to hypointense

Metastasis, Skull Base

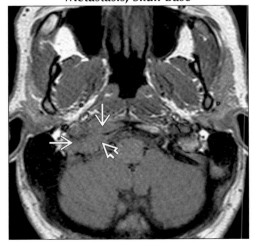

Axial T1WI MR in a patient with a history of lung cancer and new right CN12 palsy shows focal loss of bright marrow signal at the right skull base ➡, with abnormal tissue around the hypoglossal canal ➡.

Metastasis, Skull Base

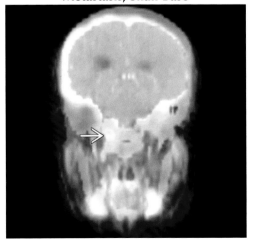

Coronal fused PET/CT image in the same patient shows markedly intense FDG uptake in the right skull base ➡, corresponding to metastasis. Multiple other bone and visceral metastases were also present.

INTRINSIC SKULL BASE LESION

(Left) *Axial T1 C+ FS MR reveals expansion of left greater sphenoid wing ➡, which is also heterogeneous but predominantly low in signal intensity. Note the focal ill-defined pools of enhancement demonstrated within substance of lesion ➡. **(Right)** Axial bone CT in the same patient clarifies cause. Most of the greater wing ➡ has characteristic "ground-glass" with areas of MR enhancement corresponding to regions of greater lucency ➡. Note narrowed vidian canal ➡.*

Fibrous Dysplasia, Skull Base

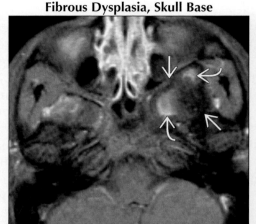

Fibrous Dysplasia, Skull Base

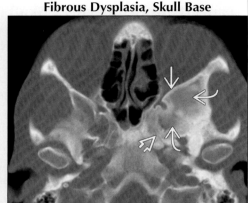

(Left) *Axial T1 C+ FS MR through skull base reveals intense heterogeneous enhancement of skull base ➡ & "fuzzy" heterogeneous expanded bones of skull base & calvarium ➡. **(Right)** Axial bone CT in the same patient shows diffuse "cotton wool" appearance of almost entire skull base with expansion of squamous temporal bone ➡, petrous apex ➡, & occipital bone ➡. Note also stapes prosthesis on the right ➡, placed for conductive hearing loss.*

Paget Disease, Skull Base

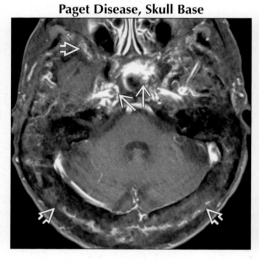

Paget Disease, Skull Base

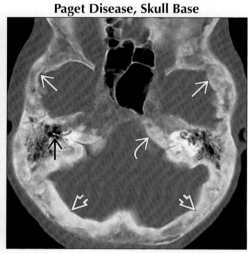

(Left) *Axial T2WI MR demonstrates an expansile, predominantly hyperintense mass ➡ arising in the clivus and eroding the posterior clival cortex ➡. Mass otherwise has more benign, rounded, well-defined contours as it extends anteriorly to involve longus capitis muscles and deform pharynx. **(Right)** Axial bone CT in the same patient reveals the lytic destructive nature of clival mass ➡. Only tiny spicules of residual bone ➡ are identified within soft tissue component.*

Chordoma, Clivus

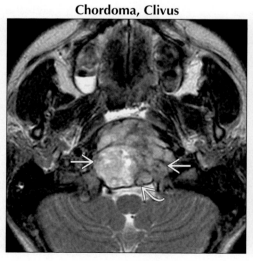

Chordoma, Clivus

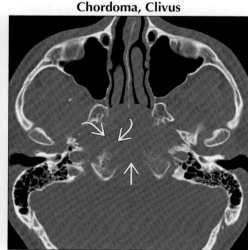

INTRINSIC SKULL BASE LESION

Multiple Myeloma, Skull Base

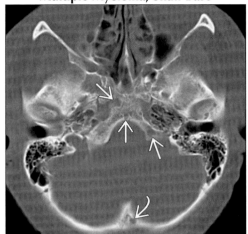

Multiple Myeloma, Skull Base

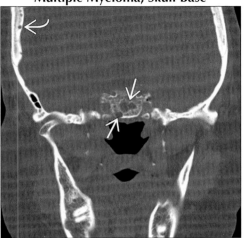

(Left) Axial bone CT shows multiple tiny lytic lesions ➡ in the skull base with sharply demarcated borders. Note the additional lesion in the occipital bone ➡. Lesions of this size are easily overlooked, especially without bone algorithm CT. (Right) Coronal bone CT in the same patient further demonstrates sharply contoured lytic lesions in the central skull base ➡ with a characteristic "punched out" appearance. Small right calvarial lesions ➡ are also noted.

Plasmacytoma, Skull Base

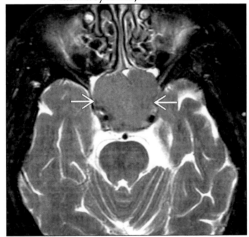

Plasmacytoma, Skull Base

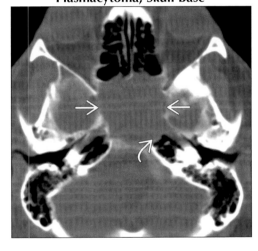

(Left) Axial T2WI FS MR reveals a large central skull base mass ➡, which expands bone and appears to extend laterally to the cavernous sinuses. The mass is homogeneous and has intermediate signal intensity. (Right) Axial bone CT in the same patient shows the sharply circumscribed nature of the lytic mass with narrow transition zone to normal bone. Note the complete loss of clival marrow ➡ and erosion of the left petrous apex ➡, without evidence of calcifications.

Chondrosarcoma, Skull Base

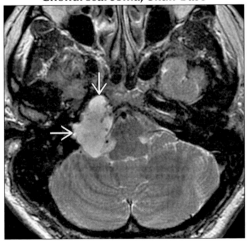

Chondrosarcoma, Skull Base

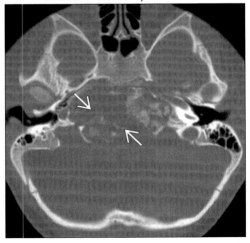

(Left) Axial T2WI MR through the skull base demonstrates a markedly high signal intensity tumor ➡ involving right petrous apex & extending into CPA cistern. Location suggests chondrosarcoma arising from petroclival synchondrosis. Such a tumor often has rounded contours, though aggressive malignancy. (Right) Axial bone CT in a different, younger patient shows large paramedian lytic lesion of right basiocciput & petrous bone with chondroid calcifications ➡.

INTRINSIC SKULL BASE LESION

(Left) Axial T1WI MR shows a soft-tissue-like mass of the right greater wing of the sphenoid ➡ with focal areas of intrinsic high signal intensity ➡. *(Right)* Axial bone CT in the same patient reveals the benign hyperdense appearance of the sphenoid body ➡ and greater wing ➡ mimicking fibrous dysplasia, but without the significant expansion seen with fibrous dysplasia.

Pneumatization Arrest, Sphenoid

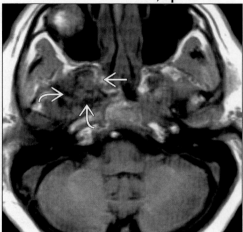

Pneumatization Arrest, Sphenoid

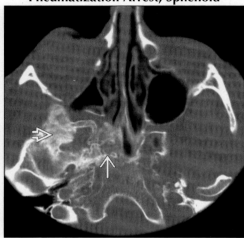

(Left) Axial CECT shows a nonspecific but destructive lesion ➡ of the central and anterior skull base with invasion to orbits ➡ bilaterally. The tumor surrounds carotid arteries ➡, indicating involvement of cavernous sinuses bilaterally also. Key to diagnosis is that this is a pediatric patient. *(Right)* Coronal bone CT shows a well-defined lytic lesion ➡ in the floor of the left middle fossa. Subtle lobulation of these well-defined lesions is typical, as is the location.

Langerhans Histiocytosis, Skull Base

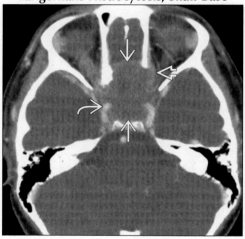

Arachnoid Granulations, Dural Sinuses

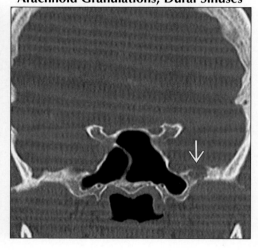

(Left) Axial T1 C+ FS MR in a patient with Gradenigo syndrome shows extensive enhancement of the petrous apex ➡ but also adjacent dural reflections. There is involvement of middle fossa dura ➡, dura of IAC ➡, and spasm of adjacent internal carotid artery ➡. *(Right)* Coronal T1 C+ MR demonstrates a homogeneously enhancing mass centered in sphenoid bone ➡. Key to diagnosis is the presence of overlying dural thickening and enhancement ➡.

Osteomyelitis, Skull Base

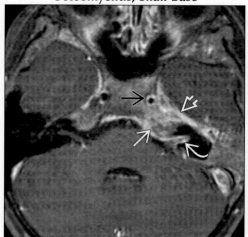

Meningioma, Skull Base

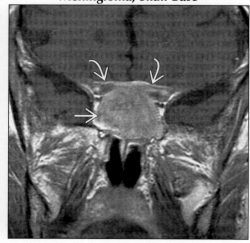

INTRINSIC SKULL BASE LESION

Giant Cell Tumor, Skull Base

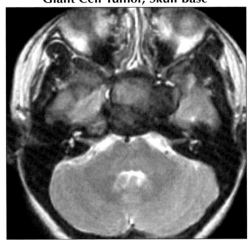

Giant Cell Tumor, Skull Base

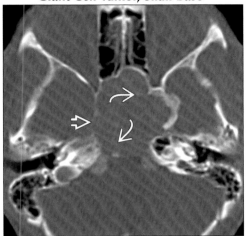

(Left) Axial T2WI MR shows a heterogeneous but predominantly low signal intensity expansile mass of the central skull base. T2 hypointensity is thought to reflect hemorrhage with hemosiderin deposition or calcification within lesion. (Right) Axial bone CT in the same patient reveals thin irregularly sclerotic "eggshell" of cortex. Expansile margins suggest a benign process. Focal areas of bone dehiscence ➡ and matrix calcifications are evident ➡.

Cephalocele, Skull Base

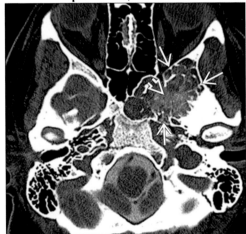

Ecchordosis Physaliphora

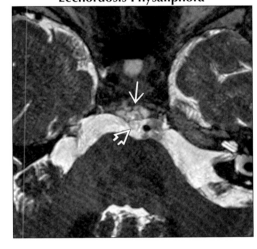

(Left) Axial CT cisternography reveals lobulated contour of large defect ➡ in left greater sphenoid wing, which has filled with contrast ➡, indicating communication with subarachnoid space. Note sphenoid wing is expanded in comparison to the right side. (Right) Axial T2WI MR demonstrates a subtle well-defined bilobed lesion ➡ arising from dorsal clivus and extending into the prepontine cistern ➡ although not causing any deformity of the pons.

Pseudotumor, Skull Base

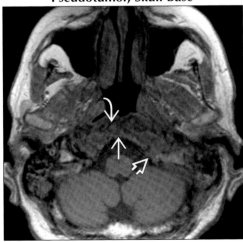

Pseudotumor, Skull Base

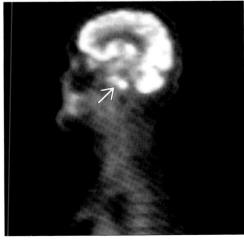

(Left) Axial T1WI MR shows symmetric low signal intensity of basiocciput ➡ but also infiltrating prevertebral muscles ➡ and hypoglossal canal ➡. This process could represent lymphoma, nasopharyngeal carcinoma, or metastases; here, it resolved on steroids following biopsies revealing inflammatory tissue only. (Right) Sagittal PET in the same patient prior to biopsies reveals intense uptake at base of skull ➡ in the site of soft tissue process identified on MR.

DIFFERENTIAL DIAGNOSIS

Common
- Meningioma, Skull Base
- Fibrous Dysplasia, Skull Base
- Mucocele, Sinonasal
- Esthesioneuroblastoma
- Osteoma, Sinonasal
- Metastasis, Skull Base

Less Common
- SCCa, Sinonasal
- Non-Hodgkin Lymphoma, Sinonasal
- Undifferentiated Carcinoma, Sinonasal
- Melanoma, Sinonasal
- Nerve Sheath Tumor, Sinonasal

Rare but Important
- Cephalocele, Frontoethmoidal
- Nasal Dermal Sinus
- Hemangiopericytoma

ESSENTIAL INFORMATION

Key Differential Diagnosis Issues
- Lesions here are intrinsic to skull base and arise in anterior fossa above skull base or from sinonasal cavities below skull base
- Characterization of bony changes aids in narrowing differential diagnosis

Helpful Clues for Common Diagnoses
- **Meningioma, Skull Base**
  - Key facts
    - Benign, extraaxial dural-based mass; ↑ incidence in older female patients
    - Classic locations: Olfactory groove and planum sphenoidale
  - Imaging
    - CT: Slightly hyperdense, ± Ca++ or hyperostosis of adjacent bone
    - MR: Isointense to brain on T1; ↓ T2, uniform and intense enhancement
- **Fibrous Dysplasia, Skull Base**
  - Key facts: Expansile lesion of bone development
  - Imaging
    - CT: Ground-glass appearance is classic; varies with amount of fibrous & ossified components
    - MR: ↓ T1, T2 signal with highly variable enhancement
- **Mucocele, Sinonasal**
  - Key facts
    - Expanded sinus from chronic obstruction; elevates anterior fossa floor
  - Imaging
    - CT: Airless, expanded sinus with bone remodeling
    - MR: Variable signal of secretions depending on age & protein:water ratio
- **Esthesioneuroblastoma**
  - Key facts
    - Vascular neoplasm of olfactory fibers with epicenter below floor of anterior fossa
    - ↑ Incidence of intracranial extension
    - Erosive skull base changes
  - Imaging
    - CT: Superior nasal cavity soft tissue mass
    - MR: Heterogeneous, avidly enhancing; characteristic cyst formation at brain-tumor interface
- **Osteoma, Sinonasal**
  - Key facts
    - Well-defined bony mass; most common in frontal & ethmoid sinuses
    - Elevates anterior fossa floor when large
  - Imaging
    - CT: Classically bone density lesion; often round or ovoid
    - MR: Hypointense on all sequences; may be mistaken for air in absence of obstructed secretions
- **Metastasis, Skull Base**
  - Key facts: History of primary malignancy is key; more common in older patients
  - Imaging: Bone destruction
    - May involve dura or brain parenchyma

Helpful Clues for Less Common Diagnoses
- **SCCa, Sinonasal**
  - Key facts
    - Most common sinonasal malignancy
    - Ethmoid sinus & nasal cavity primaries may involve anterior skull base
  - Imaging
    - Aggressive lesion with bony destruction; MR features are nonspecific
- **Non-Hodgkin Lymphoma, Sinonasal**
  - Key facts
    - Cephalad extension through skull base from nasal cavity
  - Imaging

- CT: Homogeneous, ↑ density on NECT, septal destruction, occasional bone remodeling
- MR: ↓ T2 signal (high nucleus:cytoplasm ratio); homogeneously enhancing
- **Undifferentiated Carcinoma, Sinonasal**
  - Key facts: Rare, highly aggressive sinonasal malignancy
  - Imaging
    - CT: Extensive bone destruction
    - MR: Mixed enhancement from tumoral necrosis; extranasal extension
- **Melanoma, Sinonasal**
  - Key facts
    - Highly malignant, pigmented neoplasm; often nasal cavity site of origin
  - Imaging
    - CT: Bone destruction > remodeling
    - MR: Characteristic ↑ T1 signal (paramagnetic properties of melanin), ↓ T2; avid enhancement 2° vascularity
- **Nerve Sheath Tumor, Sinonasal**
  - Key facts
    - Benign neoplasm from Schwann cells
  - Imaging
    - CT: Well-defined lesion with smooth remodeling; elevation of anterior skull base
    - MR: Enhancing, sharply marginated mass ± intramural cystic changes

Helpful Clues for Rare Diagnoses
- **Cephalocele, Frontoethmoidal**
  - Key facts

- Nasoethmoidal type involves anterior skull base
  - Imaging
    - Meninges ± brain parenchyma extend through skull base, defect into nasal cavity
- **Nasal Dermal Sinus**
  - Key facts
    - Midline developmental sinonasal/skull base lesion
    - May be associated with nasal pit or repetitive bouts of meningitis clinically
  - Imaging
    - CT & MR: Tract from nasal lesion to anterior fossa
    - Widened foramen cecum ± bifid crista galli or dermoid/epidermoid along tract
- **Hemangiopericytoma**
  - Key facts: Hypervascular lesion with aggressive growth pattern
  - Imaging: Dural-based mass ± flow voids; intensely enhancing

Other Essential Information
- Localization (center) of lesion suggests likely differential
  - Intrinsic to skull base: Fibrous dysplasia, metastasis
  - Dural-based: Meningioma, hemangiopericytoma, metastases
  - Elevation/destruction of floor of anterior fossa: Sinonasal lesion

Meningioma, Skull Base

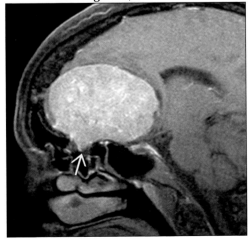

Sagittal T1 C+ FS MR shows an anterior fossa meningoma with extracranial extension into the ethmoid sinuses and upper nasal cavity ➡. Homogeneous intense enhancement is characteristic.

Fibrous Dysplasia, Skull Base

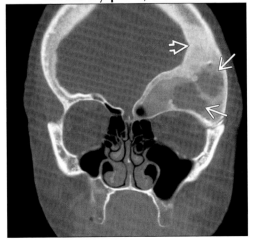

Coronal bone CT shows a mixed lucent ➡ and sclerotic ➡ or "Pagetoid" fibrous dysplasia affecting the orbital plate of the left frontal bone. Bone expansion is characteristic of this lesion.

ANTERIOR SKULL BASE LESION

(Left) Coronal CECT in a patient with sinonasal polyposis shows left anterior ethmoid mucocele ➡ formation due to chronic obstruction by polyps. There is diffuse opacification of all sinuses & osteitis, consistent with chronic inflammation. *(Right)* Coronal T1 C+ FS MR shows a "dumbbell" lesion of superior sinonasal cavity with extension into the anterior cranial fossa ➡. Note the destruction of the floor of the anterior fossa ➡ and bilateral orbital involvement ➡.

Mucocele, Sinonasal

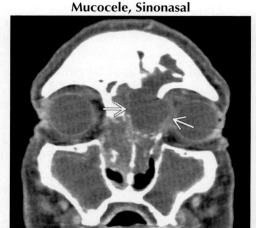

Esthesioneuroblastoma

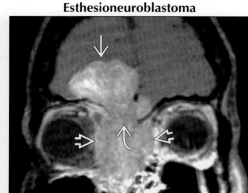

(Left) Coronal bone CT reveals a large osteoma involving both frontal sinuses. It is located centrally and extends into the anterior fossa ➡ over a broad region. This osteoma shows classic features including dense ossification and well-defined borders. *(Right)* Coronal T1 C+ FS MR shows anterior skull base metastases extending along the dura ➡, into the orbits ➡, and into the right temporalis fossa ➡. Marked bilateral proptosis was clinically apparent.

Osteoma, Sinonasal

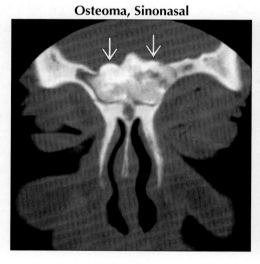

Metastasis, Skull Base

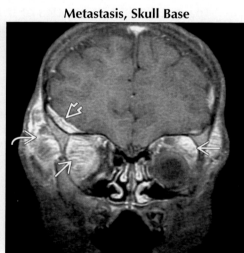

(Left) Coronal T1 C+ FS MR depicts a large aggressive sinonasal mass with extension into the skull base and infratemporal fossa ➡. The lesion involves the pterygopalatine fossa ➡ and dura along the floor of the anterior fossa ➡. *(Right)* Axial T1 C+ FS MR shows a large, homogeneously enhancing mass centered in the nasal cavity and ethmoid sinuses with invasion of the anterior skull base ➡ and orbits ➡. Note the obstructed secretions in the maxillary sinuses ➡.

SCCa, Sinonasal

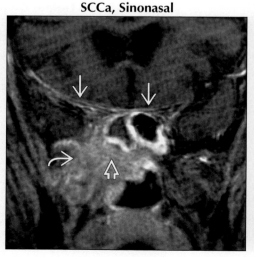

Non-Hodgkin Lymphoma, Sinonasal

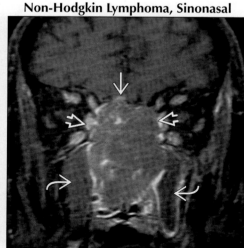

Undifferentiated Carcinoma, Sinonasal

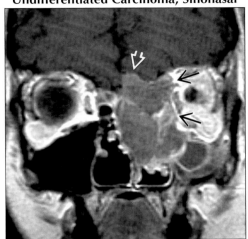

Melanoma, Sinonasal

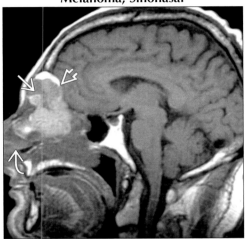

(Left) Coronal T1 C+ MR demonstrates an aggressive mass extending into the left orbit ➡ and anterior cranial fossa ⊳. The lesion shows moderate enhancement with no necrosis, a feature often seen in this rapidly growing malignancy. (Right) Sagittal T1WI MR reveals a characteristic high T1 signal mass with intracranial and orbital extension. The lesion arises in the anterior sinonasal cavity and extends into the nasal vestibule ➡, frontal sinus ➡, and cranial anterior fossa ⊳.

Nerve Sheath Tumor, Sinonasal

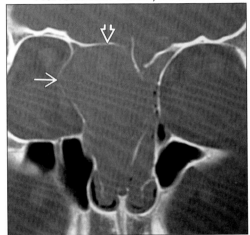

Cephalocele, Frontoethmoidal

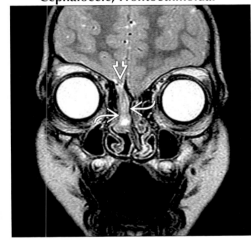

(Left) Coronal bone CT reveals a smooth, expansile right anterior ethmoidal lesion. Note the bowing of the medial orbital wall ➡ and upward remodeling of the fovea ethmoidalis ⊳. Differentiating schwannoma from mucocele requires contrast enhancement. (Right) Coronal T2WI MR shows a nasoethmoidal type of sincipital cephalocele extending through the anterior fossa cribriform plate ⊳. This mass in the nasal cavity ➡ is contiguous with the frontal lobe.

Nasal Dermal Sinus

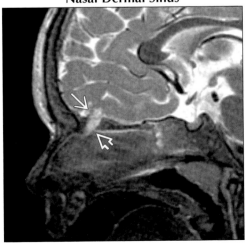

Hemangiopericytoma

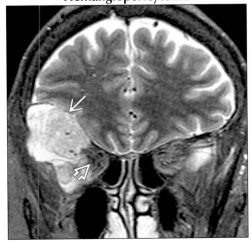

(Left) Sagittal T2WI MR shows a defect in the floor of the anterior fossa and a small intracranial mass at foramen cecum ⊳. A tract ⊳ extends into the nasal cavity, terminating at a small cutaneous bump on the nasal dorsum (not shown). (Right) Coronal T2WI FS MR shows an extraaxial mass ➡ that extends into the right orbit ⊳. The lesion enhances strongly and uniformly. Most hemangiopericytomas have flow voids on imaging; however, this one does not.

DIFFERENTIAL DIAGNOSIS

Common
- Meningioma, Skull Base
- Esthesioneuroblastoma
- SCCa, Sinonasal
- Fibrous Dysplasia, Skull Base
- Mucocele, Sinonasal
- Ossifying Fibroma, Sinus

Less Common
- Non-Hodgkin Lymphoma, Sinonasal
- Sarcoidosis, Sinonasal
- Melanoma, Sinonasal
- Undifferentiated Carcinoma, Sinonasal

Rare but Important
- Schwannoma, Olfactory
- Nasal Dermal Sinus
- Cephalocele, Frontoethmoidal

ESSENTIAL INFORMATION

Key Differential Diagnosis Issues
- Evaluation of integrity of cribriform plate (CP) is essential to narrow differential diagnosis
  - Sharply marginated dehiscence with distortion of bony anatomy suggests developmental lesion or benign neoplasm
  - Bone destruction implicates malignant lesions
  - Bone expansion with sclerosis suggests fibro-osseous lesions
  - Hyperostosis or bony sclerosis may be associated with anterior fossa meningioma

Helpful Clues for Common Diagnoses
- **Meningioma, Skull Base**
  - Arises in anterior fossa above CP (olfactory groove)
  - CT: Shows bone changes (hyperostosis, pneumosinus dilatans, erosion)
  - MR: Delineates tumor soft tissue extent
    - Marked enhancement & dural "tail" characteristic
- **Esthesioneuroblastoma**
  - Site of origin in superior nasal vault with cephalad extension through CP
  - CT: Ill-defined margins, intratumoral Ca++
  - MR: Heterogeneous, avid enhancement
    - Characteristic cyst formation at tumor-brain interface

- **SCCa, Sinonasal**
  - Nasal cavity, ethmoid sinus, or frontal sinus sites of origin ± extension through cribriform plate
  - CT: Aggressive bony destruction is classic
  - MR: Ill-defined mass with dural ± parenchymal invasion
- **Fibrous Dysplasia, Skull Base**
  - Slowly growing, expansile, intrinsic lesion of bone; monostotic and polyostotic forms
  - CT: Classic "ground-glass" density with bone expansion
    - Variable soft tissue (fibrous) & ossified components
  - MR: ↓ T1 and T2 signal with variable enhancement
- **Mucocele, Sinonasal**
  - Opacified, expanded sinus due to chronic obstruction; frontal & ethmoid lesions (most common) may involve CP
  - CT: Bony remodeling and expansion of involved sinus walls
  - MR: Variable signal of trapped secretions related to protein:water ratio
    - Mucosal enhancement at periphery
- **Ossifying Fibroma, Sinus**
  - Fibro-osseous lesion of facial skeleton
    - May mimic focal fibrous dysplasia
  - CT: Mixed soft tissue-osseous lesion of ethmoid or frontal sinus
    - Mass effect on CP
  - MR: Well-defined mass
    - Signal & contrast enhancement varies with fibrous:osseous ratio

Helpful Clues for Less Common Diagnoses
- **Non-Hodgkin Lymphoma, Sinonasal**
  - Origin most often in nasal cavity > paranasal sinuses
  - Solid & mass-like or superficially spreading
  - CT: Bone remodeling ± destruction
    - ↑ Attenuation on unenhanced images
  - MR: ↓ T2 signal, homogeneous enhancement
- **Sarcoidosis, Sinonasal**
  - Granulomatous disease with predilection for nasal cavity (septum & turbinate) > paranasal sinus involvement
    - Nonspecific sinonasal mucosal disease
    - Can result in bone destruction & extension into orbit or anterior fossa

CRIBRIFORM PLATE LESION

- Imaging features nonspecific & mimic rhinosinusitis
  - Clinical history is key
- CT/MR: Nodular soft tissue thickening with enhancement
  - May cause bone sclerosis or erosion
- **Melanoma, Sinonasal**
  - Highly malignant mucosal lesion
    - Nasal vault or ethmoid sinus origin
  - CT: May remodel or destroy bone
  - MR: Highly melanotic lesions show characteristic paramagnetic properties
    - ↑ T1, ↓ T2 signal
- **Undifferentiated Carcinoma, Sinonasal**
  - Aggressive malignancy with rapid growth
  - CT: Extensive bone destruction

Helpful Clues for Rare Diagnoses
- **Schwannoma, Olfactory**
  - Slowly growing benign neoplasm with bone remodeling
    - ↑ Incidence in neurofibromatosis type 1
  - CT: Remodeled cribriform plate
  - MR: Ovoid enhancing mass ± intramural cysts
    - Tumor ± extension through CP into superior nasal cavity
- **Nasal Dermal Sinus**
  - Sinus tract extends from nasal dorsum to foramen cecum through nasal septum
  - Dermoid or epidermoid may be found along sinus tract

- These associated lesions may be located from nasal dorsum to foramen cecum at skull base
- CT: Bony skull base defect & possible bifid crista galli
  - Epidermoid: Fluid attenuation lesion
  - Dermoid: May see fat, calcifications, fluid, or soft tissue density
- MR: Demonstrates entirety of tract
  - Epidermoid: Fluid signal on T1 & T2 with no enhancement; FLAIR & DWI differentiate from true cyst
  - Dermoid: ↑ T1 fat signal
- **Cephalocele, Frontoethmoidal**
  - Nasoethmoidal type presents as intranasal or sinus mass
  - CT: Smooth defect in CP
  - MR: Shows extent of cephalocele and contents of sac

Other Essential Information
- Based on anatomy
  - Lesions of CP can come from above (brain, meninges), within (skull base), and below (sinonasal)
  - Evaluation of bone changes may indicate vector of spread
    - Convex downward bone changes: Lesion arises above cribriform plate
    - Expansile bone changes: Lesion arises from anterior skull base
    - Convex upward bone changes: Lesion arises from upper sinonasal area

---

Meningioma, Skull Base

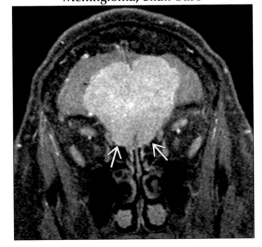

Coronal T1 C+ FS MR shows an anterior cranial fossa mass with extracranial extension into the ethmoid sinuses and upper nasal cavity. The enhancing lesion extends into the olfactory recess bilaterally ➡.

Esthesioneuroblastoma

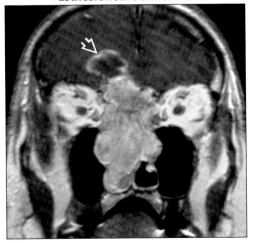

Coronal T1 C+ MR reveals a large mass originating in the superior sinonasal cavities with an extensive intracranial component and a classic cyst formation at the brain-tumor interface ➡.

CRIBRIFORM PLATE LESION

(Left) Coronal T1 C+ FS MR demonstrates an aggressive mass filling the left maxillary sinus, ethmoid sinus, and nose with extension through the cribriform plate into the anterior cranial fossa ➡. The left orbit is also invaded ➡. (Right) Axial bone CT shows diffuse expansion and "ground-glass" involving the facial bone and anterior skull base ➡. Note the sparing of the otic capsules ➡. This patient has fibrous dysplasia associated with McCune-Albright syndrome.

SCCa, Sinonasal

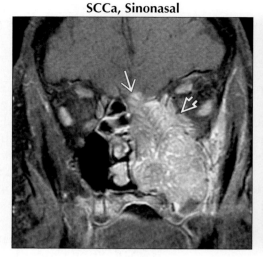

Fibrous Dysplasia, Skull Base

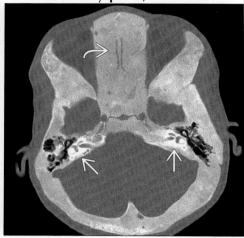

(Left) Sagittal T1WI MR shows a typical mucocele in the sphenoid sinus, an uncommon location. It contains a fluid-fluid level from the settling of varying elements ➡. The sinus is airless and expanded and elevates the floor of the anterior cranial fossa. (Right) Axial bone CT reveals a large ossifying fibroma centered in the ethmoid sinus involving the cribriform plate ➡, orbit ➡, and sphenoid sinus ➡.

Mucocele, Sinonasal

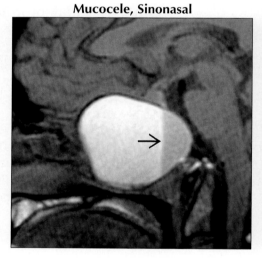

Ossifying Fibroma, Sinus

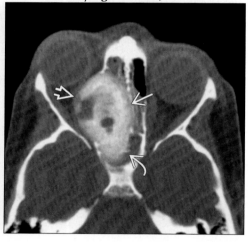

(Left) Coronal T1 C+ FS MR demonstrates a typical sinonasal lymphoma with a homogeneous enhancing mass that extends into the anterior fossa ➡ and involves the left lacrimal apparatus ➡. (Right) Coronal T1 C+ FS MR shows extensive sarcoid involvement of the sinonasal cavities ➡ and anterior cranial fossa ➡. The lesion involves the dura and adjacent frontal lobes.

Non-Hodgkin Lymphoma, Sinonasal

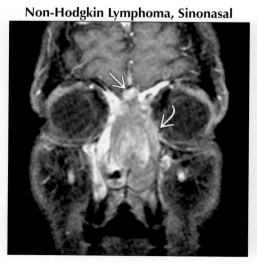

Sarcoidosis, Sinonasal

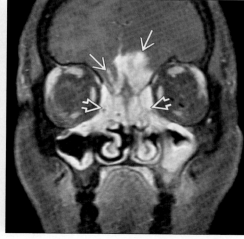

CRIBRIFORM PLATE LESION

Melanoma, Sinonasal
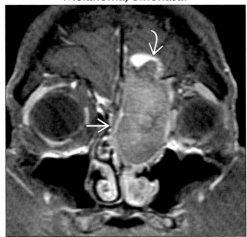

Undifferentiated Carcinoma, Sinonasal
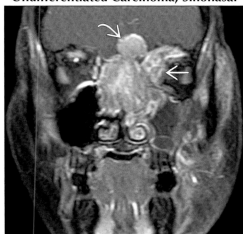

(Left) Coronal T1 C+ FS MR depicts the tendency of sinonasal melanoma to result in bone destruction as well as remodeling. The septum is smoothly displaced ➡ by the large nasal cavity/ethmoid mass that also invades the anterior cranial fossa through the cribriform plate ➡. *(Right)* Coronal T1 C+ FS MR reveals a typical large, aggressive sinonasal undifferentiated carcinoma (SNUC) with orbital ➡ and brain ➡ invasion through the cribriform plate.

Schwannoma, Olfactory
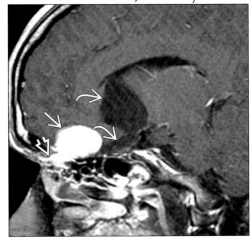

Nasal Dermal Sinus
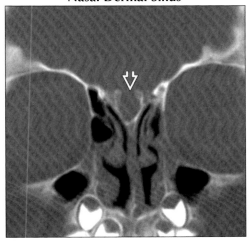

(Left) Sagittal T1 C+ MR shows a rare, avidly enhancing olfactory schwannoma ➡. Lesion extends through the anterior cribriform plate ➡. Fluid extends posterior to mass ➡ along anterior cranial fossa floor, leading to a deep frontal cyst that formed secondary to obstructed axonal flow. *(Right)* Coronal bone CT reveals the intracranial features of a nasal dermal sinus tract, with a "bifid" crista galli ➡ at the posterior aspect of foramen cecum defect.

Nasal Dermal Sinus
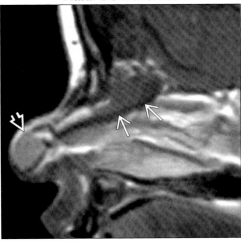

Cephalocele, Frontoethmoidal
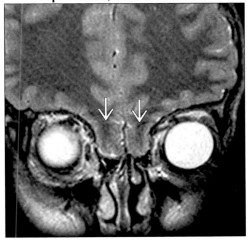

(Left) Sagittal T1 C+ MR shows a midline dermal sinus tract ➡ extending from the cribriform plate toward the nasal tip with associated dermoid cyst ➡ at the skin surface. *(Right)* Coronal T2WI MR shows a herniated frontal lobe parenchyma ➡ through a large defect in the anterior skull base. Note the normal appearance of the prolapsed cortex in this patient.

CENTRAL SKULL BASE LESION

DIFFERENTIAL DIAGNOSIS

Common
- Fibrous Dysplasia, Skull Base
- Metastasis, Skull Base
- Meningioma, Skull Base
- Multiple Myeloma, Skull Base
- Non-Hodgkin Lymphoma
- Pituitary Macroadenoma, Giant, Clivus
- Arachnoid Granulation, Skull Base

Less Common
- Langerhans Histiocytosis, Skull Base
- Chordoma, Clivus
- Paget Disease, Skull Base
- Chondrosarcoma, Skull Base

Rare but Important
- Cephalocele, Trans-sphenoidal (Craniopharyngeal Canal)
- Ecchordosis Physaliphora
- Aneurysm, ICA, T-Bone

ESSENTIAL INFORMATION

Key Differential Diagnosis Issues
- Diseases may secondarily involve central skull base by rising above or sinking below it
  - Disease intrinsic to central skull base must arise from its components
- Fibro-osseous lesions of central skull base are relatively common lesions
- Metastatic disease to central skull base is also common
  - Note: Clinical history of malignant disease is critical to correct radiologic report
- Characterization of matrix and eccentric origin can aid diagnosis of cartilaginous lesions
  - Bone CT superior for determination of calcified matrix

Helpful Clues for Common Diagnoses
- **Fibrous Dysplasia, Skull Base**
  - Key facts
    - Relatively common lesion of occiput and sphenoid
  - Imaging
    - Ground-glass matrix on CT is classic
    - Often hypointense on T2 MR; with intense T1 enhancement
- **Metastasis, Skull Base**
  - Key facts

- Patient with known malignant neoplasm
  - Imaging
    - Lytic, destructive lesion of skull base
    - May have associated soft tissue mass
    - Look for multiple lesions
- **Meningioma, Skull Base**
  - Key facts
    - Elderly female patient
  - Imaging
    - Uniform enhancement on CT or MR unless lesion significantly calcified
    - May see calcifications or intrinsic high density on CT
    - Bony changes may include hyperostosis, erosion, or permeative destruction
    - Isointense with brain on most sequences on MR
- **Multiple Myeloma, Skull Base**
  - Key facts
    - Multiple lesions; imaging identical to plasmacytoma
  - Imaging
    - Primarily osteolytic
- **Non-Hodgkin Lymphoma**
  - Key facts
    - May be primary bone disease, or originate from dura
  - Imaging
    - Wide range of appearances
    - Typically enhance uniformly
    - Dural-based disease is common
    - Can involve bone with destructive changes, extensive soft tissue mass
- **Pituitary Macroadenoma, Giant, Clivus**
  - Key facts
    - May occasionally extend inferior into clivus or sphenoid sinus
  - Imaging
    - Evaluation of sella is key; normal pituitary gland excludes this differential
    - Abnormal pituitary gland and sella characteristic
    - May see simultaneous suprasellar extension of macroadenoma
- **Arachnoid Granulation, Skull Base**
  - Key facts
    - Lesions found along dural sinuses, dural surface
    - When large may be tumefactive
  - Imaging
    - Well-defined, nonenhancing lytic lesions

Helpful Clues for Less Common Diagnoses
- **Langerhans Histiocytosis, Skull Base**
  - Key facts
    - May be multifocal disease
    - Evaluate pituitary area
    - Infundibular involvement possible
  - Imaging
    - CT: Destructive soft tissue mass
    - MR: Best to assess for sellar disease
- **Chordoma, Clivus**
  - Key facts
    - Patient may present with CN6 palsy
  - Imaging
    - CT: Destructive lesion of clivus with occasional bony spicules left behind by aggressive growth
    - MR: Characteristic T2 hyperintense signal may be seen
- **Paget Disease, Skull Base**
  - Key facts
    - Often asymptomatic; M:F = 2:1
    - Commonly isolated to skull base
  - Imaging
    - May be multifocal disease, with mixed lytic-sclerotic pattern
    - Expands bone and results in "cotton wool" appearance
- **Chondrosarcoma, Skull Base**
  - Key facts
    - Arises in skull base fissures, synchondroses
    - Petrooccipital fissure most common
  - Imaging

- CT: "Arcs and whorls" of calcification
- MR: Low signal intensity on T2, intense enhancement on post-contrast T1

Helpful Clues for Rare Diagnoses
- **Cephalocele, Trans-sphenoidal (Craniopharyngeal Canal)**
  - Key facts
    - Unusual cephalocele through sphenoid, into Meckel cave, or mid-face
  - Imaging
    - Contiguity of CSF spaces through bony defect, may contain neural tissue
- **Ecchordosis Physaliphora**
  - Key facts
    - Benign clival variant of chordoma
  - Imaging
    - MR: Hyperintense on T2, but lacks enhancement on post-contrast T1
- **Aneurysm, ICA, T-Bone**
  - Key facts
    - Rare location of internal carotid artery aneurysm; often in petrous apex
  - Imaging
    - MR: Flow-related enhancement or void

Other Essential Information
- Report of central skull base disease should include comments on integrity of internal carotid artery & cranial nerves 3-6
- Also report disease progression both intracranially and extracranially

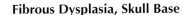

Fibrous Dysplasia, Skull Base

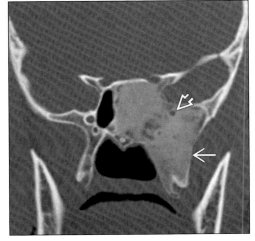

Coronal NECT shows expansion of the sphenoid bone. The foramen rotundum ⮞ is narrowed and laterally displaced. Expansion of the pterygoid process and pterygoid plates ⮞ is also visible.

Metastasis, Skull Base

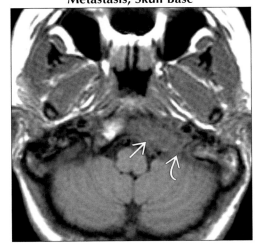

Axial T1WI MR shows a mass ⮞ of the basiocciput, which is of uniform low signal intensity, replacing normal marrow fatty signal. The mass extends laterally to involve the hypoglossal canal ⮞.

CENTRAL SKULL BASE LESION

(Left) Axial T1WI MR shows a dural-based mass ➔ with extensive skull base and middle ear involvement. The lesion extends inferiorly and anteriorly through the jugular foramen ➔ to involve the carotid space. *(Right)* Axial bone CT shows multiple myeloma of the skull base and calvarium, with multiple lytic lesions ➔ of the sphenoid and occipital bone. The lesions are well defined and without sclerotic margins.

Meningioma, Skull Base

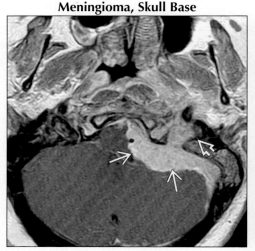

Multiple Myeloma, Skull Base

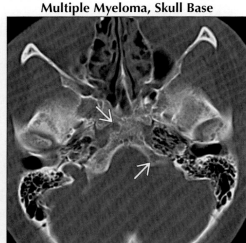

(Left) Axial CECT shows non-Hodgkin lymphoma involving the ethmoid ➔ and sphenoid ➔ sinuses with involvement at the extraconal orbit ➔. *(Right)* Axial bone CT shows a large mass that erodes the clivus and basisphenoid, extending laterally to involve the petrous ICAs ➔ and into the posterior fossa ➔. Coronal post-contrast MR is optimal to depict sellar, suprasellar, and juxtasellar disease.

Non-Hodgkin Lymphoma

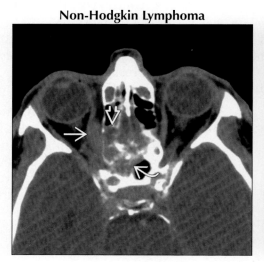

Pituitary Macroadenoma, Giant, Clivus

(Left) Axial bone CT shows central skull base arachnoid granulations ➔. An MR examination demonstrated multiple associated temporal lobe cephaloceles (not shown). *(Right)* Coronal bone CT shows a destructive mass centered in the basisphenoid ➔ that invades the posterior nasal cavity, medial orbit ➔, and planum sphenoidale ➔ to extend into the orbits and anterior fossa.

Arachnoid Granulation, Skull Base

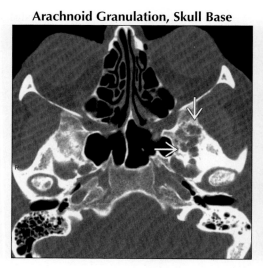

Langerhans Histiocytosis, Skull Base

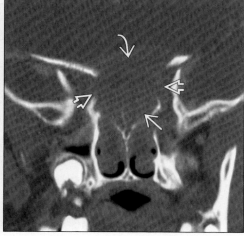

CENTRAL SKULL BASE LESION

Chordoma, Clivus

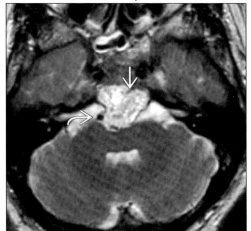

Paget Disease, Skull Base

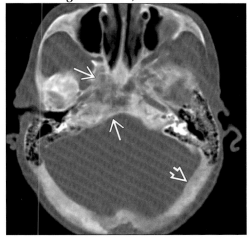

(Left) Axial T2WI MR shows a hyperintense mass ➔ with a peripheral hypointense rim involving the clivus, extending into the posterior fossa, and deforming the pons. The basilar artery ➔ is displaced by the mass. (Right) Axial bone CT reveals diffuse skull base Paget disease. Note the diffuse expansion and hyperdensity with "cotton wool" appearance ➔ and diffuse skull involvement ➔.

Chondrosarcoma, Skull Base

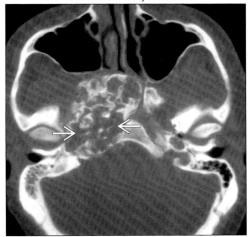

Cephalocele, Trans-sphenoidal (Craniopharyngeal Canal)

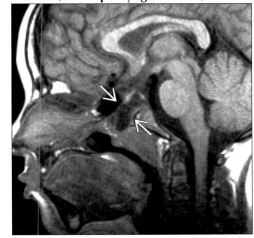

(Left) Axial bone CT shows a mass involving the petrooccipital fissure and demonstrating chondroid matrix calcification. Note the irregular ossification with "arcs and whorls" ➔ of calcification. (Right) Sagittal T1WI MR demonstrates a typical MR case of trans-sphenoidal cephalocele ➔ in the location of the craniopharyngeal canal. CSF extends through the defect into the roof of the nasopharynx.

Ecchordosis Physaliphora

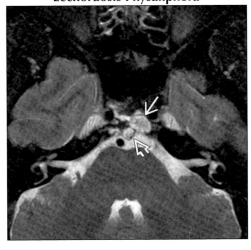

Aneurysm, ICA, T-Bone

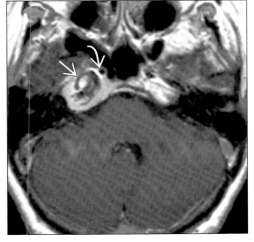

(Left) Axial T2WI FS MR shows a lesion of the clivus ➔ extending into prepontine cistern ➔, partially effacing the CSF within. The mass is well defined and hyperintense. Lack of significant enhancement is characteristic and distinguishes EP from chordoma. (Right) Axial T1 C+ MR reveals an ovoid aneurysm arising within the right petrous apex, with heterogeneous enhancement surrounding complex flow-related enhancement ➔ adjacent to the ICA ➔.

SELLAR/PARASELLAR MASS WITH SKULL BASE INVASION

DIFFERENTIAL DIAGNOSIS

Common
- Pituitary Macroadenoma
- Metastases

Less Common
- Lymphoma, Metastatic, Intracranial
- Myeloma
- Meningioma, Skull Base

Rare but Important
- Pseudotumor, Intracranial
- Langerhans Histiocytosis
- Hemangioma
- Thrombophlebitis, Cavernous Sinus
- Leukemia
- Erdheim-Chester Disease
- Chordoma, Extraosseous

ESSENTIAL INFORMATION

Key Differential Diagnosis Issues
- Pattern of skull base involvement
  - Included: Lesion(s) with permeative, infiltrative, destructive features
    - Invasive macroadenoma, metastases, lymphoma
  - Excluded: Lesion(s) with expansile, erosive pattern (e.g., trigeminal schwannoma)
- Anatomic origin
  - Included: Involvement from lesions mostly above or lateral to central skull base (BOS)
  - Excluded: Involvement from extending cephalad from structures below central BOS
    - Sphenoid sinus (e.g., aggressive polyposis, invasive fungal sinusitis)
    - Nasopharynx (carcinomas with direct or perineural extension)
- Specific origin of mass helpful
  - Pituitary gland
    - Macroadenoma
    - Less commonly lymphoma, metastasis
  - Cavernous sinus/dura
    - Metastasis, lymphoma, meningioma, myeloma
    - Less commonly hemangioma, thrombophlebitis, histiocytoses
- Key imaging findings help
  - Look for pituitary gland separate from mass!

- Can't find it? Mass probably of pituitary origin (gland = mass)
  - Adult: Macroadenoma > metastasis, lymphoma, pseudotumor
  - Child: Histiocytosis > macroadenoma, leukemia
- Intracranial dural involvement
  - Adult: Metastasis, meningioma, lymphoma, invasive pseudotumor
  - Child: Histiocytosis, leukemia
- Multiple enhancing cranial nerves
  - Adult: Metastases, lymphoma
  - Child: Leukemia

Helpful Clues for Common Diagnoses
- **Pituitary Macroadenoma**
  - Pituitary gland = mass
  - Most commonly invades upward through diaphragma sellae
  - Less common = inferior extension
  - Rare but important = invasion, destruction of central BOS
  - Adult male with invasive, destructive central BOS mass? Check prolactin prior to surgery, biopsy!
- **Metastases**
  - Can involve, infiltrate pituitary gland/stalk
  - Extend into central BOS, cavernous sinus(es)
  - Look for other lesions (e.g., calvarium, brain)

Helpful Clues for Less Common Diagnoses
- **Lymphoma, Metastatic, Intracranial**
  - Metastatic > primary lymphoma in/around central BOS, sella/cavernous sinuses (CS)
  - Uni- > bilateral CS involvement
  - May infiltrate pituitary gland, stalk, cranial nerves
  - Isointense, avidly enhancing
  - Look for dural involvement, other lesions
- **Myeloma**
  - Multifocal or solitary (plasmacytoma)
  - Central BOS > > pituitary, CS
  - Bilateral > unilateral CS
  - Usually elevates, displaces pituitary gland but occasionally invades gland, stalk
- **Meningioma, Skull Base**
  - Most common = suprasellar mass extending into CS
  - Unilateral, asymmetric > bilateral involvement

SELLAR/PARASELLAR MASS WITH SKULL BASE INVASION

○ Look for pituitary gland separate from mass
- Pituitary usually displaced inferiorly, laterally
- Occasionally can be elevated

○ Beware: Meningiomas occasionally appear aggressive, invade adjacent skull (mimic metastasis, lymphoma, etc.)

Helpful Clues for Rare Diagnoses

• **Pseudotumor, Intracranial**
○ 90% of intracranial pseudotumors occur without orbital disease
- Originates in CS, dura
- Smooth > "lumpy-bumpy" dural thickening, enhancement
- Typically ↓ following steroids

○ Less common: Posterior extension from orbit
- Tolosa-Hunt syndrome (painful ophthalmoplegia) = CS involved
- Uni- > bilateral disease
- Look for associated meningeal thickening (can be extensive)

○ Rare variant = idiopathic invasive pseudotumor
- Can invade, destroy bone, mimic neoplasm or aggressive infection

• **Langerhans Histiocytosis**
○ Child > > adult
○ Osteolysis ± soft tissue mass
- Varies from small "punched out" lesion to widespread, diffuse involvement

○ Variable brain lesions (pituitary stalk/gland, meninges > parenchyma, choroid plexus)

• **Hemangioma**
○ True vasoformative neoplasm of CS, dura
○ May mimic meningioma
- Child without NF2, lesion that looks like meningioma? Consider hemangioma

○ If large, may involve adjacent bone

• **Thrombophlebitis, Cavernous Sinus**
○ Usually secondary to paranasal sinus infection
○ Look for dural thickening, filling defects in CS
○ Osteolysis central BOS rare

• **Leukemia**
○ Paranasal sinus/orbit involvement typical
○ May extend into 1 or both cavernous sinuses, pituitary gland/stalk

• **Erdheim-Chester Disease**
○ Rare non-Langerhans cell histiocytosis
○ Disseminated xanthogranulomatous infiltrative disease
○ Adults > children
○ Long bones > brain, CS, orbits (rare)

• **Chordoma, Extraosseous**
○ Typical chordoma originates in clivus
- Destructive midline mass

○ Rare: Extraosseous origin
- Laterally located mass in CS, Meckel cave
- Osseous invasion secondary
- Typically hyperintense on T2WI, strong uniform enhancement

Pituitary Macroadenoma

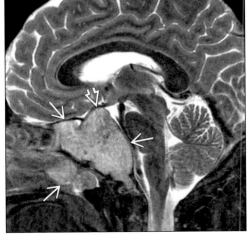

Sagittal T2WI MR shows a hyperintense extensively invasive mass ➡. Pituitary gland ➡ cannot be identified separately from the lesion in this male patient with elevated prolactin and an invasive macroadenoma.

Metastases

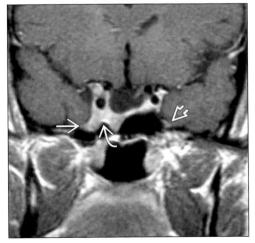

Coronal T1 C+ MR shows a mass in the right cavernous sinus ➡ extending into the foramen rotundum ➡ in a patient with ovarian cancer and right facial numbness. Compare to the normal left side ➡.

SELLAR/PARASELLAR MASS WITH SKULL BASE INVASION

(Left) Sagittal T1 C+ MR demonstrates an enhancing mass invading the pituitary gland, stalk ➡, central skull base, and nasopharynx. Note the dural involvement ➡. (Right) Sagittal T1WI MR in a patient with myeloma reveals an infiltrative destructive lesion with involvement of the cavernous sinus, sphenoid sinus, clivus, and dura. The pituitary gland ➡ is identifiable as separate from the mass ➡.

Lymphoma, Metastatic, Intracranial

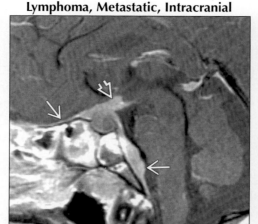

Myeloma

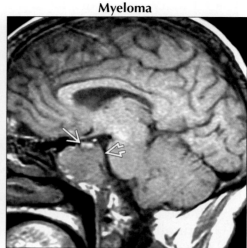

(Left) Coronal T1 C+ MR shows a large enhancing mass that elevates and displaces the pituitary gland ➡. Note the bone erosion ➡. A trans-sphenoidal biopsy specimen disclosed a typical meningioma. (Right) Coronal T1 C+ MR in a patient with multiple left-sided cranial neuropathies shows an enhancing left cavernous sinus mass ➡ extending into the skull base & nasopharynx ➡. Note dural involvement ➡. Symptoms resolved completely with steroids.

Meningioma, Skull Base

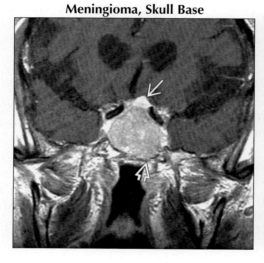

Pseudotumor, Intracranial

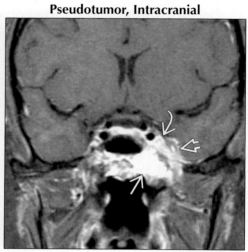

(Left) Sagittal T1 C+ MR demonstrates an extensive enhancing mass ➡ involving the pituitary gland and stalk ➡, central skull base, and nasopharynx. This patient was a 6 year old with a history of sinus treatment and new onset right vision loss. (Right) Coronal T1 C+ FS MR in the same patient shows an extensive destructive central mass that erodes the skull base and infiltrates the pituitary gland and cavernous sinuses.

Langerhans Histiocytosis

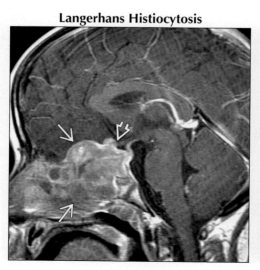

Langerhans Histiocytosis

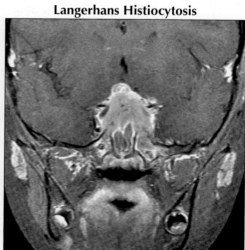

SELLAR/PARASELLAR MASS WITH SKULL BASE INVASION

Hemangioma

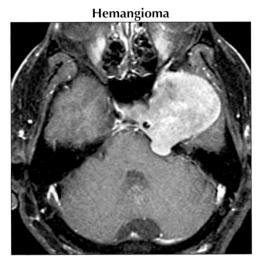

Hemangioma

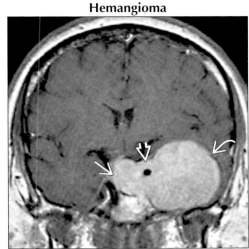

(Left) Axial T1 C+ MR in a 13 year old shows an enormous left cavernous invasive enhancing mass. An initial trigeminal schwannoma or meningioma differential diagnosis gave way to surgical pathologic diagnosis of hemangioma. (Right) Coronal T1 C+ MR in the same patient reveals that the hemangioma involves the sella ➡, cavernous sinus ➡, and floor of the middle cranial fossa ➡.

Thrombophlebitis, Cavernous Sinus

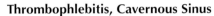
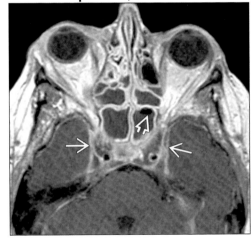

Leukemia

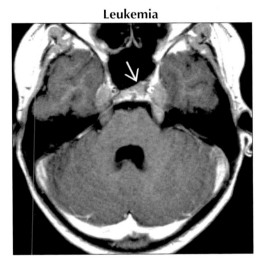

(Left) Axial T1 C+ MR shows bilateral nonenhancing areas in the cavernous sinuses ➡ occurring as a complication of acute chronic sinusitis. Note the opacified sinuses with an air-fluid level in the sphenoid sinus ➡. (Right) Axial T1 C+ MR in a patient with acute lymphoblastic leukemia and multiple cranial neuropathies shows cavernous sinuses and trigeminal nerves. Note the involvement of the adjacent sphenoid ➡.

Erdheim-Chester Disease

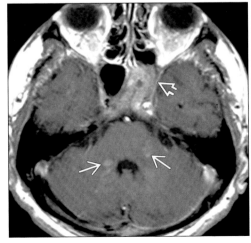

Chordoma, Extraosseous

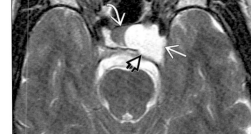

(Left) Axial T1 C+ MR reveals large bilateral cavernous sinuses and a mass that invades the skull base ➡ with multifocal parenchymal lesions ➡. (Courtesy M. Warmuth-Metz, MD.) (Right) Axial T2WI MR reveals a very hyperintense mass that originates in the left cavernous sinus ➡ with bone destruction ➡. Note the displacement of the pituitary gland ➡.

UNILATERAL CAVERNOUS SINUS MASS

DIFFERENTIAL DIAGNOSIS

Common
- Pituitary Macroadenoma
- Meningioma
- Schwannoma
- Metastases, Skull and Meningeal
- Lymphoma, Metastatic, Intracranial
- Nasopharyngeal Carcinoma

Less Common
- Saccular Aneurysm
- Carotid-Cavernous Fistula, Traumatic
- Thrombosis, Cavernous Sinus
- Dermoid Cyst
- Epidermoid Cyst
- Neurosarcoid
- Pseudotumor, Intracranial
- Hemangioma

Rare but Important
- Plexiform Neurofibroma
- Chordoma
- Tuberculosis
- Iatrogenic

ESSENTIAL INFORMATION

Key Differential Diagnosis Issues
- Lateral dural walls of cavernous sinuses (CSs) should be flat or concave on axial/coronal imaging
  - Convex outer margin indicates abnormality
  - Lateral dural wall thick, easy to see; medial = thin, difficult to delineate
- CSs are septated (not single pool of venous blood in venous spaces)
- CSs enhance strongly but contain normal filling "defects" (Meckel cave, cranial nerves, ICA)
- If mass present, is it intrinsic or extrinsic to cavernous sinus?
- Where does mass originate?
  - Sella: Pituitary macroadenoma
  - Sphenoid sinus/central skull base: Metastasis, nasopharyngeal carcinoma
  - Dura: Meningioma, hemangioma, pseudotumor
- Does it contain "flow voids"?
  - Aneurysm
  - Dural AVF

Helpful Clues for Common Diagnoses
- **Pituitary Macroadenoma**
  - Cavernous sinus invasion common with macroadenoma
  - Difficult to determine unless florid
  - Mass, gland indistinguishable (gland IS mass)
- **Meningioma**
  - Diffusely infiltrates sinus, thickens dura
  - Lateral dural wall can sometimes be identified within thickened, intensely enhancing CS mass
  - Look for dural "tail" along clivus, tentorium
  - Look for other meningiomas (multiple meningioma syndrome, neurofibromatosis type 2)
- **Schwannoma**
  - Most common = trigeminal, in Meckel cave
  - Typically well marginated
  - Usually hyperintense on T2WI
  - Solitary > multiple (neurofibromatosis type 2)
- **Metastases, Skull and Meningeal**
  - 3 patterns
    - Hematogenous (direct or extension from skull base)
    - Perineural along cranial nerve (usually from nasopharyngeal or sinus tumor)
    - Direct geographic invasion (squamous cell, minor salivary gland tumors most common primaries)
- **Lymphoma, Metastatic, Intracranial**
  - Primary CS rare; usually history of disease elsewhere
- **Nasopharyngeal Carcinoma**
  - 2 patterns
    - Direct cephalad extension into central skull base, CS
    - Perineural extension into cavernous sinus(es) along CNV2

Helpful Clues for Less Common Diagnoses
- **Saccular Aneurysm**
  - Can be spontaneous, post-traumatic (pseudoaneurysm)
  - Can be patent or partially thrombosed
  - Prominent "flow void," pulsation (phase) artifact
- **Carotid-Cavernous Fistula, Traumatic**
  - Superior ophthalmic vein enlarged

UNILATERAL CAVERNOUS SINUS MASS

- ○ ± Basilar skull fracture
- ○ Usually at junction of vertical, horizontal ICA segments
- **Thrombosis, Cavernous Sinus**
  - ○ Nonenhancing thrombus, thickened enhancing dural walls
  - ○ May be secondary to sinusitis (thrombophlebitis)
  - ○ Superior ophthalmic vein(s) often enlarged
  - ○ Proptosis common
- **Dermoid Cyst**
  - ○ Typically in Meckel cave, not CS proper
  - ○ Fat density/signal intensity
- **Epidermoid Cyst**
  - ○ Typically in Meckel cave, not CS proper
  - ○ CSF density/signal intensity
  - ○ Usually occurs as extension from CPA lesion
- **Neurosarcoid**
  - ○ Can be uni- or bilateral
  - ○ Look for thickened infundibular stalk, dural masses
- **Pseudotumor, Intracranial**
  - ○ Uni- > bilateral
  - ○ Typically extends posteriorly from orbital apex into CS
  - ○ Extensive dural enhancement along middle fossa can be present
  - ○ Occasionally can be invasive, destructive; mimics neoplasm or aggressive infection
- **Hemangioma**
  - ○ True vasoformative neoplasm in CS, dura
  - ○ May mimic meningioma

Helpful Clues for Rare Diagnoses
- **Plexiform Neurofibroma**
  - ○ Occurs only in neurofibromatosis type 1
  - ○ Involves cutaneous, orbital branches of CN5
  - ○ Infiltrative, unencapsulated mass
  - ○ Look for
    - Scalp neurofibromas
    - Sphenoid wing dysplasia
- **Chordoma**
  - ○ Destructive mass, midline > lateral
  - ○ Occasionally can originate in CS or extend asymmetrically from clivus into CS
  - ○ Most are very hyperintense on T2WI
- **Tuberculosis**
  - ○ History of pulmonary TB
  - ○ Dura-arachnoid thickening from basilar meningitis
- **Iatrogenic**
  - ○ Post-operative packing after trans-sphenoidal macroadenoma resection
  - ○ Look for surgical defect in sellar floor
  - ○ Caused by overpacking of defect
  - ○ May appear very bizarre
  - ○ Fat-suppression sequence helpful

Pituitary Macroadenoma

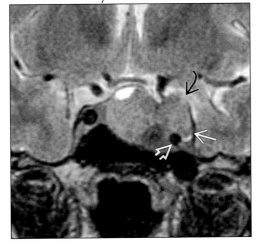

Coronal T2WI MR shows macroadenoma that extends into the left cavernous sinus ⮕, displacing and encasing the cavernous internal carotid artery ⮕. The tumor lateral to the ICA ⮕ confirms CS invasion.

Meningioma

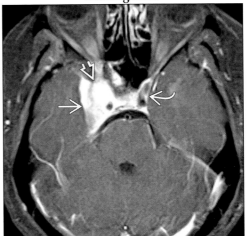

Axial T1 C+ FS MR shows meningioma of the right cavernous sinus ⮕ with thickening along both sides of the lateral dural wall ⮕ and effacement of the internal architecture compared to the normal left side ⮕.

9

41

UNILATERAL CAVERNOUS SINUS MASS

(Left) Axial T1 C+ MR shows a classic trigeminal schwannoma in the right Meckel cave ▷. Compare with the normal left side ➔. Schwannomas are typically hyperintense on T2WI, enhancing strongly. (Right) Coronal T1 C+ FS MR shows a unilateral cavernous sinus metastasis ▷.

Schwannoma

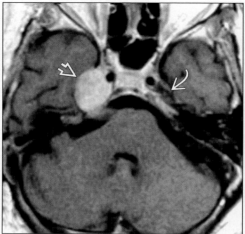

Metastases, Skull and Meningeal

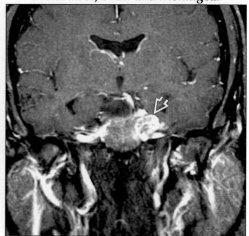

(Left) Axial T1 C+ FS MR in patient with non-Hodgkin lymphoma who presented with left-sided facial weakness shows an enhancing mass along the maxillary division of CN5 in the cavernous sinus ➔, extending into the apex of the pterygopalatine fossa ▷. (Right) Axial T1 C+ FS MR shows nasopharyngeal carcinoma spreading into the clivus ➔, the left cavernous sinus/Meckel cave ▷, and intracavernous carotid artery wall ▷.

Lymphoma, Metastatic, Intracranial

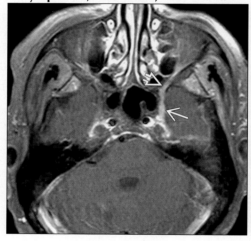

Nasopharyngeal Carcinoma

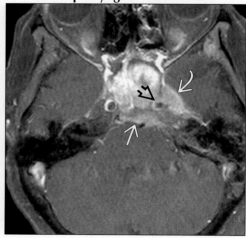

(Left) Axial CTA in a man with a headache and a remote history of MVA shows a partially calcified right cavernous carotid artery pseudoaneurysm ➔. (Right) Axial CECT shows prominent orbital vessels ➔ and a markedly enlarged right superior ophthalmic vein ➔ in a patient with trauma and right-sided proptosis. The right cavernous sinus is also distended, showing abnormal enhancement ➔.

Saccular Aneurysm

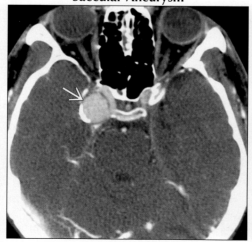

Carotid-Cavernous Fistula, Traumatic

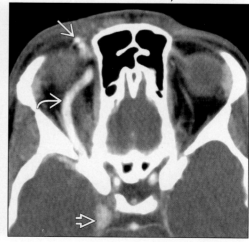

UNILATERAL CAVERNOUS SINUS MASS

Thrombosis, Cavernous Sinus

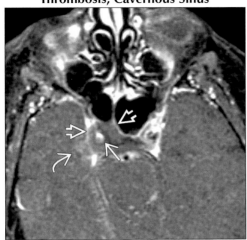

Dermoid Cyst

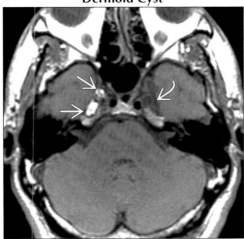

(Left) Axial T1 C+ FS MR in a patient with acute sphenoid sinusitis shows a unilateral nonenhancing clot in the right cavernous sinus ➡, a thrombosed cavernous ICA ➡, and early cerebritis in the adjacent brain ➡. *(Right)* Axial T1WI MR shows a dermoid cyst in the right Meckel cave and cavernous sinus ➡. Compare to the normal CSF-filled left Meckel cave ➡.

Epidermoid Cyst

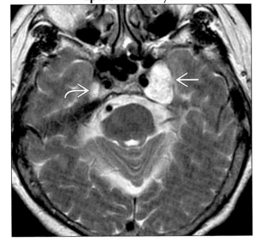

Neurosarcoid

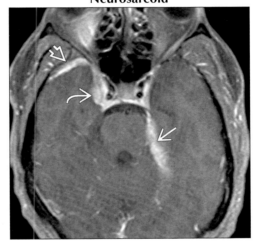

(Left) Axial T2WI MR shows an epidermoid cyst originating in the left Meckel cave ➡. Note that the epidermoid-filled Meckel cave is slightly more hyperintense than the normal right CSF-filled left Meckel cave ➡. *(Right)* Axial T1 C+ FS MR shows sarcoidosis infiltrating the right cavernous sinus ➡ and extending along the dura of the tentorium ➡ and the right middle cranial fossa ➡.

Pseudotumor, Intracranial

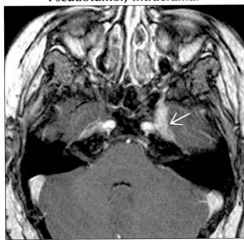

Chordoma

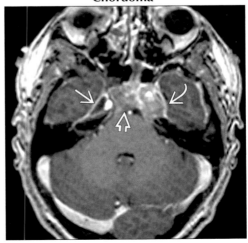

(Left) Axial T1 C+ MR in woman with headache, nausea, and vomiting shows thickened dura along the left cavernous sinus ➡. Symptoms and findings resolved quickly after the administration of IV steroids. *(Right)* Axial T1 C+ MR shows a clival chordoma ➡ with extension into the left cavernous sinus ➡. The right cavernous sinus, including the Meckel cave ➡, is normal.

BILATERAL CAVERNOUS SINUS MASS

DIFFERENTIAL DIAGNOSIS

Common
- Pituitary Macroadenoma
- Meningioma
- Metastasis, Skull Base
- Lymphoma, Metastatic, Intracranial

Less Common
- Neurofibromatosis Type 2
- Carotid-Cavernous Fistula
- Thrombosis, Cavernous Sinus
- Chordoma, Clivus
- Plasmacytoma
- Neurosarcoid
- Langerhans Histiocytosis, Skull Base

Rare but Important
- Pseudotumor, Intracranial
- Leukemia
- Extramedullary Hematopoiesis
- Germ Cell Neoplasms
- Erdheim-Chester Disease
- Benign Nonmeningothelial Tumors

ESSENTIAL INFORMATION

Key Differential Diagnosis Issues
- Is lesion intrinsic to cavernous sinus (CS)?
- Does it arise from skull base or extracranial tissues?
- Is it destructive?

Helpful Clues for Common Diagnoses
- **Pituitary Macroadenoma**
  - Pituitary gland indistinguishable from mass (gland IS mass)
    - Enlarged, "figure 8" mass
    - Extends laterally through thin medial dural wall into CS
    - May surround, encase ICAs but rarely occludes
    - Mass typically isointense with brain; avid, uniform enhancement
  - Dynamic MR shows mass enhances more slowly than CS
  - If symptoms of pituitary apoplexy, hemorrhage common
    - Sphenoid sinusitis often present
- **Meningioma**
  - Unilateral > bilateral involvement
  - Thick, uniformly enhancing dura along lateral walls

- Variable extension into CS proper
  - Look for dural "tail" (thickening along tentorium, middle fossa)
  - Look for obliteration of CSF in Meckel caves
  - May extend inferiorly along clivus
- **Metastasis, Skull Base**
  - Permeative, destructive mass
    - Hematogenous spread from extracranial primary common (e.g., breast)
    - Most commonly centered in central skull base (BOS), secondary extension into CS
    - May also be direct geographic extension from nasopharyngeal carcinoma
  - CS involvement can be uni-, bilateral; symmetric or asymmetric
  - Sagittal T1, coronal T1 C+ FS scans useful
- **Lymphoma, Metastatic, Intracranial**
  - Primary central BOS lymphoma rare
  - Unilateral > bilateral involvement
  - Isointense, avidly enhancing
  - Associated cranial nerve, meningeal (dural) lesions common
  - Tumor often surrounds, encases but does not occlude cavernous ICAs

Helpful Clues for Less Common Diagnoses
- **Neurofibromatosis Type 2**
  - Multiple schwannomas, meningiomas
    - Most common CS schwannoma = trigeminal (Meckel cave)
    - Look for meningiomas of CS, optic nerve sheath, tentorium
  - Look for bilateral vestibular schwannomas (VS, diagnostic of neurofibromatosis type 2), evidence for prior CPA/temporal bone surgery
    - 1 VS + other schwannoma, meningioma highly suggestive
- **Carotid-Cavernous Fistula**
  - Uni- > bilateral carotid-cavernous fistulas
  - Look for CS "flow voids" in addition to ICAs
  - Look for ↑ superior ophthalmic vein(s) (SOV) caliber
    - CTA helpful screening study
    - DSA delineates fistula site(s)
- **Thrombosis, Cavernous Sinus**
  - Can be spontaneous, sterile, or septic (thrombophlebitis)
    - Look for infection in paranasal sinuses, orbits

- Nonenhancing areas within intensely enhancing CS
  - Lateral dural wall, CS septations enhance, thrombus does not
  - Look for ↑ SOVs caliber
- **Chordoma, Clivus**
  - Destructive T2 hyperintense mass centered in clivus
  - Large lesions may invade CS
    - Displace but rarely occlude ICAs
  - Chondrosarcoma may mimic
    - Usually unilateral, arises from petrooccipital fissure
- **Plasmacytoma**
  - Solitary destructive mass of central BOS
    - Centered in sphenoid sinus, clivus
    - Isointense, strongly enhancing mass
    - Bi- > unilateral
- **Neurosarcoid**
  - CS rare site
  - Look for other lesions
    - Pituitary, infundibular stalk lesion
    - Cranial nerve involvement
    - Dural-based masses
  - Infiltrating CS mass(es)
    - Lesions enhance strongly, uniformly
    - Bone destruction rare
- **Langerhans Histiocytosis, Skull Base**
  - Osteolysis with sharply defined scalloped margins ± soft tissue mass
  - Varies from small "punched out" lesion to widespread diffuse bony involvement
    - May destroy almost entire BOS
  - Homogeneous enhancement

Helpful Clues for Rare Diagnoses
- **Pseudotumor, Intracranial**
  - 90% of intracranial pseudotumors occur without orbital disease
  - Tolosa-Hunt syndrome (painful ophthalmoplegia) when CS involved
    - Uni- > bilateral
    - Look for associated meningeal thickening (can be extensive)
    - Bone invasion, destruction may occur
- **Leukemia**
  - Paranasal sinus/orbit involvement typical
  - Bilateral CS involvement rare
- **Extramedullary Hematopoiesis**
  - CS involvement rare
  - Look for associated dural-based masses (calvarium, spine)
- **Germ Cell Neoplasms**
  - Rare; typically involve pituitary gland/stalk
- **Erdheim-Chester Disease**
  - Rare non-Langerhans cell histiocytosis
  - Disseminated xanthogranulomatous infiltrative disease of unknown origin
  - Adults > children
  - Long bones > brain, CS, orbits (rare)
- **Benign Nonmeningothelial Tumors**
  - Benign cartilaginous tumors may arise from central BOS
  - If large, extend intracranially into CS

Pituitary Macroadenoma

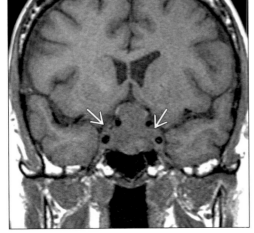

Coronal T1WI MR shows a large macroadenoma with the "figure 8" configuration and extension into the suprasellar cistern and both cavernous sinuses ➡.

Meningioma

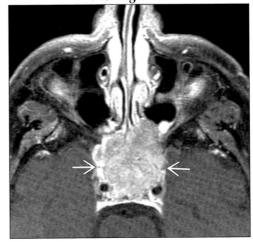

Axial T1 C+ FS MR shows a strongly enhancing central skull base mass extending laterally into both cavernous sinuses ➡. A histologically typical meningioma was found at surgery.

BILATERAL CAVERNOUS SINUS MASS

(Left) Axial T1 C+ FS MR shows a classic case of nasopharyngeal carcinoma extending superiorly into the sphenoid sinus, clivus, and cavernous sinuses ➡. The left Meckel cave is involved while the right ➡ is spared. *(Right)* Axial T1 C+ MR shows an extensive, destructive central skull base mass that infiltrates the sphenoid sinus and both cavernous sinuses ➡. The mass encases both cavernous carotid arteries ➡.

Metastasis, Skull Base

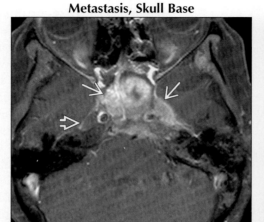

Lymphoma, Metastatic, Intracranial

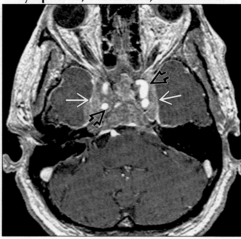

(Left) Coronal T1 C+ FS MR shows schwannomas in both Meckel caves ➡. Bilateral vagal schwannomas are also present ➡. *(Right)* Axial T2WI MR shows numerous abnormal "flow voids," predominately in the left ➡ but also the right ➡ cavernous sinuses, in this patient with red eye and proptosis 2 weeks following head trauma.

Neurofibromatosis Type 2

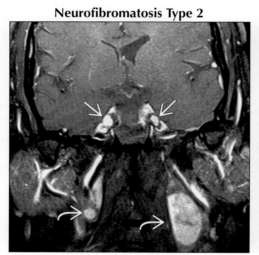

Carotid-Cavernous Fistula

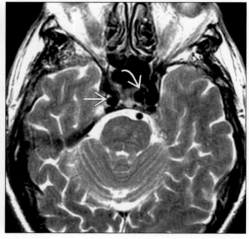

(Left) Axial T1 C+ MR shows bilateral cavernous sinus thrombosis, resulting as a complication of acute sinusitis. Note the nonenhancing areas within the cavernous sinus ➡, thickened enhancing dura of the tentorium ➡, and sphenoid wings ➡. *(Right)* Coronal T2WI MR shows a large clival chordoma with bilateral cavernous sinus invasion ➡.

Thrombosis, Cavernous Sinus

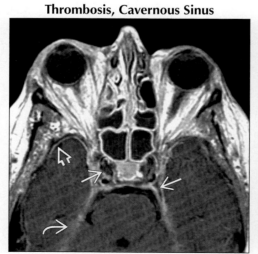

Chordoma, Clivus

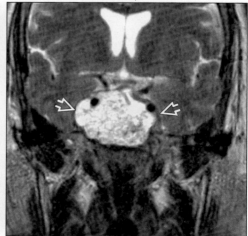

BILATERAL CAVERNOUS SINUS MASS

Plasmacytoma

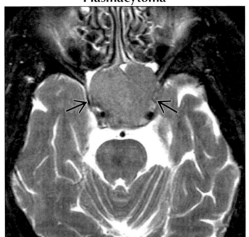

Neurosarcoid

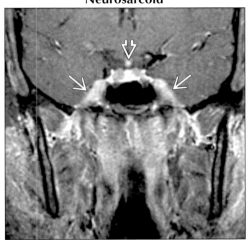

(Left) Axial T2WI FS MR shows an isointense central skull base mass that extends superiorly into the sella turcica and both cavernous sinuses →. *(Right)* Coronal T1 C+ FS MR shows both Meckel caves filled with strongly enhancing tissue →. Note that the infundibular stalk → and pituitary gland appear normal.

Langerhans Histiocytosis, Skull Base

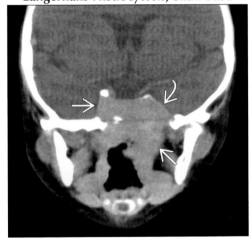

Pseudotumor, Intracranial

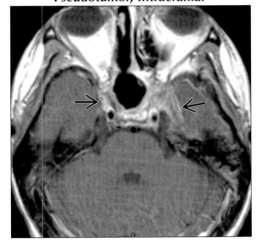

(Left) Coronal CECT shows a central skull base lytic lesion with sharply defined margins. A large soft tissue component invading the skull base, both cavernous sinuses →, and nasopharynx → enhances strongly and uniformly. *(Right)* Axial T1 C+ MR shows bilateral cavernous sinus enhancement →, left more striking than right, in a patient with left-sided cranial neuropathies. Symptoms resolved with the administration of steroids.

Leukemia

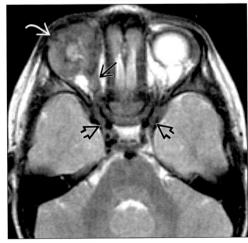

Germ Cell Neoplasms

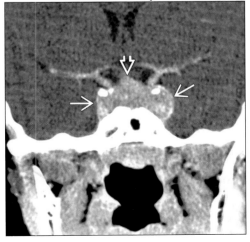

(Left) Axial T2WI MR shows a leukemic mass in the right orbit → infiltrating the lacrimal gland and the superior rectus muscle →. Note the isointense tissue in both cavernous sinuses →, suggesting extension of leukemic infiltrate. *(Right)* Coronal CECT shows an enhancing mass infiltrating the pituitary gland → and both cavernous sinuses →.

9

MECKEL CAVE LESION

DIFFERENTIAL DIAGNOSIS

Common
- Schwannoma, Trigeminal, Intracranial
- Meningioma
- Metastasis, Skull Base

Less Common
- Metastasis, CSF/Meningeal
- Metastasis, Perineural CNV3
- Meningitis
- Neurosarcoid
- Neurofibroma
- Pseudotumor, Intracranial
- Pituitary Macroadenoma

Rare but Important
- Metastasis, Perineural CNV2
- Trigeminal Herpetic Neuritis
- Lipoma
- Epidermoid Cyst
- Dermoid Cyst
- Neurocysticercosis
- Chronic Thrombosis, Dural Sinus

ESSENTIAL INFORMATION

Key Differential Diagnosis Issues
- Normal Meckel cave (MC)
  - Anatomy
    - CSF-filled, dura-arachnoid lined invagination into cavernous sinus (CS)
    - Contains CN5 fascicles, semilunar ganglion
    - Communicates directly, freely with prepontine/cerebellopontine cisterns
  - Normal imaging
    - Ovoid, smooth, CSF-filled cisterns on axial, coronal scans resemble "open eyes"
    - Bilaterally symmetric hypointensity on T1WI
    - Bilaterally symmetric hyperintensity on T2WI
- Abnormal Meckel cave
  - "Winking" Meckel cave sign
    - 1 MC filled with soft tissue, not CSF
    - 1 MC therefore NOT = CSF density/intensity
    - Asymmetric appearance = "winking" Meckel cave (1 "eye" appears closed)
  - Look for CN5 motor denervation secondary to MC mass
    - May be only sign of subtle lesion

- Acute → hyperintensity, enhancement of muscles of mastication
- Chronic → atrophy, fatty infiltration of muscles of mastication

Helpful Clues for Common Diagnoses
- **Schwannoma, Trigeminal, Intracranial**
  - Variable configuration
    - "Dumbbell" tumor with CPA component, constriction of tumor at entrance to Meckel cave, Meckel cave mass
    - May involve MC only
    - ± Extracranial extension along V1, V2, &/or V3
  - Unilateral unless NF2
  - Hyperintense on T2WI, avid enhancement on T1 C+
  - May result in atrophy of muscles of mastication
- **Meningioma**
  - Uni- > bilateral involvement
  - Dural thickening along cavernous sinus, tentorium (dural "tail" sign)
  - ± Ipsilateral denervation, atrophy of muscles of mastication
- **Metastasis, Skull Base**
  - Metastases to Meckel cave can be hematogenous, direct geographic extension, perineural, or CSF spread
    - Hematogenous spread to central skull base (BOS) with secondary involvement of cavernous sinus
    - Direct extension from extracranial primary (e.g., nasopharyngeal squamous cell carcinoma) into central BOS
    - Uni- > bilateral involvement
  - Sagittal T1WI helpful
    - Look for replacement of normal fatty clival marrow ± cortical destruction

Helpful Clues for Less Common Diagnoses
- **Metastasis, CSF/Meningeal**
  - Pia-arachnoid tumor spread may extend into MCs
  - ± Enhancement along cisternal CN5
- **Metastasis, Perineural CNV3**
  - Retrograde tumor spread along mandibular nerve
  - Look for mass in retromolar trigone, masticator space
  - Adenoid cystic carcinoma, squamous cell carcinoma most common

- CNV3 appears thick, enhancing ± erosion of foramen ovale
- **Meningitis**
  - Any etiology (e.g., pyogenic, TB)
  - Dura-arachnoid disease can extend into MC
  - Look for basal cistern enhancement
- **Neurosarcoid**
  - Pituitary gland, infundibular stalk, dural masses common
  - Uni- or bilateral involvement
- **Neurofibroma**
  - Orbit/scalp/lid plexiform in NF1
  - May extend posteriorly through superior orbital fissure, infiltrate V1 branches → MC
- **Pseudotumor, Intracranial**
  - Typically originates in/around orbit
  - Extends through SOF into CS, MC
  - Variable dura-arachnoid thickening, enhancement
  - Idiopathic invasive subtype
    - May erode bone, mimic aggressive infection, neoplasm
- **Pituitary Macroadenoma**
  - Can extend into 1 or both CSs, MCs
  - Pituitary gland generally cannot be distinguished from mass
    - Gland IS mass
  - Aggressive invasive type may destroy central skull base, clivus
    - Pituitary adenoma > > > carcinoma
    - Can mimic malignant disease, so do endocrine workup

Helpful Clues for Rare Diagnoses
- **Metastasis, Perineural CNV2**
  - Often skin carcinomas (basal, squamous cell)
  - Infiltrates along inferior orbital canal
  - May enlarge/erode foramen rotundum
  - Thickened, enhancing maxillary nerve
- **Trigeminal Herpetic Neuritis**
  - Herpes zoster oticus > trigeminal neuritis
  - Edematous, enhancing CN5
    - Ophthalmic division most commonly involved
- **Lipoma**
  - MC is rare site
  - Uni- > bilateral
- **Epidermoid Cyst**
  - May originate in MC or as extension from CPA epidermoid
  - Does not suppress on FLAIR; restricts on DWI
- **Dermoid Cyst**
  - Looks like fat in MC, not CSF
  - May occur ± rupture, CSF fatty droplets
- **Neurocysticercosis**
  - Cysts in basal cisterns may extend into 1 or both MCs
- **Chronic Thrombosis, Dural Sinus**
  - Chronically occluded dural sinus(es)
  - Dural thickening, enhancement secondary to collateral venous drainage
  - May involve 1 or both MCs

Schwannoma, Trigeminal, Intracranial

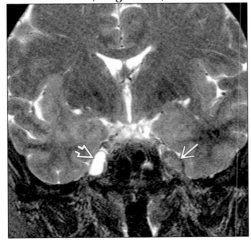

Coronal T2WI MR shows a classic "winking" Meckel cave sign. The normal (right) Meckel cave is CSF-filled and hyperintense ➡. The left side is filled with a mass that is hypointense and expands the Meckel cave ➡.

Schwannoma, Trigeminal, Intracranial

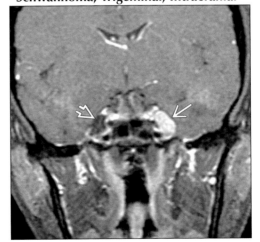

Coronal T1 C+ MR in the same patient shows that the normal Meckel (right) is CSF-filled and hypointense ➡ on this sequence. Contrast this with the enhancing mass that fills the left Meckel cave ➡.

MECKEL CAVE LESION

(Left) Coronal T1 C+ MR shows a meningioma expanding the right Meckel cave ➡. The left Meckel cave is filled with CSF ➡ as is normal. *(Right)* Axial T1 C+ MR shows a metastasis to the left petrous apex that extends into the clivus and the left Meckel cave ➡. The right Meckel cave ➡ is normal and CSF filled.

Meningioma

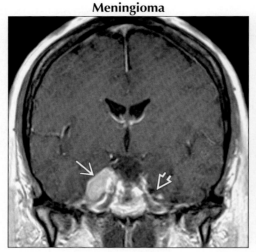

Metastasis, Skull Base

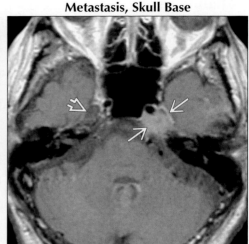

(Left) Axial T1 C+ FS MR in patient with diffuse CSF spread of glioblastoma multiforme shows pial metastases covering the cerebellum ➡. The tumor has spread into the left Meckel cave ➡. Note the normal CSF in the right Meckel cave ➡. *(Right)* Coronal T1 C+ FS MR shows perineural tumor extension of squamous cell carcinoma from the masticator space ➡ through an enlarged foramen ovale ➡ into the left cavernous sinus and Meckel cave ➡.

Metastasis, CSF/Meningeal

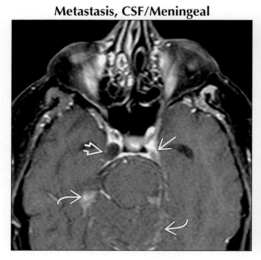

Metastasis, Perineural CNV3

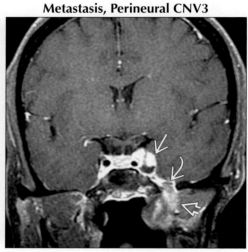

(Left) Coronal T1 C+ MR shows basilar and cisternal meningitis ➡ with thickened, enhancing meninges and extension into the right Meckel cave ➡. *(Right)* Coronal T1 C+ FS MR shows a sarcoid infiltrating the pituitary gland ➡ as well as both Meckel caves ➡.

Meningitis

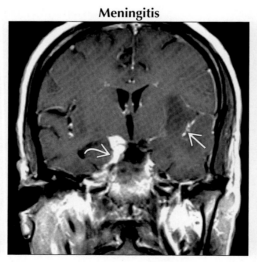

Neurosarcoid

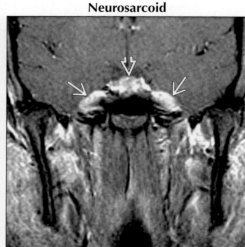

MECKEL CAVE LESION

Pseudotumor, Intracranial

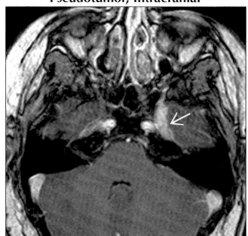

Metastasis, Perineural CNV2

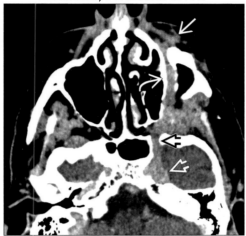

(Left) Axial T1 C+ MR shows an enhancing lesion in left cavernous sinus & Meckel cave ➡. Thickened dura, enhancing pituitary gland, & infundibulum were also present. Symptoms/findings resolved after steroids. *(Right)* Axial CECT with curved reformatted image shows cheek melanoma ➡ spreading along left CNV2 from infraorbital foramen through inferior orbital canal ➡ & foramen rotundum ➡ into Meckel cave ➡. (Courtesy S. van der Westhuizen, MD.)

Trigeminal Herpetic Neuritis

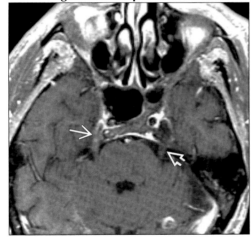

Epidermoid Cyst

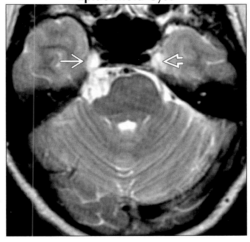

(Left) Axial T1 C+ MR shows an enhancing right CN5 ➡ extending into the Meckel cave. The left trigeminal nerve ➡ and Meckel cave appear normal. *(Right)* Axial T2WI MR shows an epidermoid in the upper CPA cistern wrapped around CN5, extending into the right Meckel cave ➡. The epidermoid cyst is slightly hyperintense to CSF in the normal left Meckel cave ➡.

Dermoid Cyst

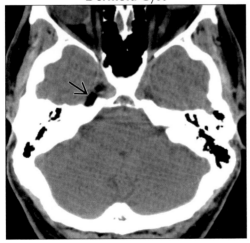

Chronic Thrombosis, Dural Sinus

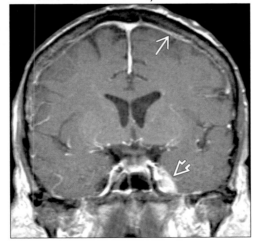

(Left) Axial NECT shows a fat-density lesion in the right Meckel cave ➡, found incidentally in a patient with a headache after trauma. MR disclosed a ruptured dermoid cyst with multiple fat droplets in the CSF cisterns (not shown). *(Right)* Coronal T1 C+ MR in a patient with multiple chronically occluded venous sinuses shows dural ➡ and Meckel cave ➡ engorgement caused by collateral venous drainage pathways. (Courtesy M. Castillo, MD.)

9

POSTERIOR SKULL BASE LESION

DIFFERENTIAL DIAGNOSIS

Common
- Meningioma, Skull Base
- Metastasis, Skull Base
- Paraganglioma, Glomus Jugulare
- Schwannoma, Jugular Foramen
- Meningioma, Jugular Foramen
- Arachnoid Granulations, Dural Sinuses

Less Common
- Dural Sinus Thrombosis, Skull Base
- Chordoma, Clivus
- Schwannoma, Hypoglossal Nerve
- Dural A-V Fistula, Skull Base

Rare but Important
- Chondrosarcoma, Skull Base
- Plasmacytoma, Skull Base
- Giant Cell Tumor, Skull Base

ESSENTIAL INFORMATION

Key Differential Diagnosis Issues
- Most lesions arise from
  - Bone: Basiocciput and lower clivus; occipital condyles and jugular tubercles; squamous occipital bone
  - Apertures and canals: Foramen magnum, hypoglossal canal, condylar foramen, jugular foramen (JF)
- Imaging strategy
  - MR and CT provide complementary information and may both be required for diagnosis

Helpful Clues for Common Diagnoses
- **Meningioma, Skull Base**
  - Key facts
    - Extraaxial, dural-based mass
  - Imaging
    - CT: 75% hyperdense on NECT; 25% intralesional Ca++; permeative/sclerotic/hyperostotic bone changes
    - MR: Dural "tails" extend from periphery; Ca++ hypointense; avid enhancement
- **Metastasis, Skull Base**
  - Key facts
    - Primary neoplasm often known at presentation
  - Imaging

- CT: Irregular bone destruction, centered in marrow space
- MR: Intermediate or ↓ T1 & ↑ T2 with variable enhancement; may involve dura, brain, or extracranial soft tissues

- **Paraganglioma, Glomus Jugulare**
  - Key facts: Benign neoplasm arising from glomus bodies
  - Imaging
    - CT: Permeative destructive bone change; jugular spine erosion common
    - MR: "Salt & pepper" appearance; flow voids and avid enhancement
- **Schwannoma, Jugular Foramen**
  - Key facts
    - Benign tumor arising from CN9-11
    - Clinical presentation may mimic vestibular schwannoma
  - Imaging
    - CT: Smooth remodeling and enlargement of JF; amputation of lateral jugular tubercle ("bird's beak")
    - MR: ↑ T2 signal and homogeneous enhancement; intratumoral cysts & heterogeneity in larger lesions
- **Meningioma, Jugular Foramen**
  - Key facts
    - Arises from arachnoid cap cells in jugular foramen
    - Centrifugal pattern of growth
  - Imaging
    - CT: ↑ density on NECT; permeative-sclerotic bone change; matrix Ca++ uncommon
    - MR: T1 hypo- to isointense mass to muscle; absence of flow voids with avid enhancement
- **Arachnoid Granulations, Dural Sinuses**
  - Key facts
    - Enlarged arachnoid villi projecting into venous sinus or subarachnoid space
  - Imaging
    - CT: Isodense to CSF; scalloping of inner table (calvarial pits); round/ovoid filling defect in sinus on CECT or CTV
    - MR: Isointense to CSF on T1; ↑ T2 surrounded by venous flow void; nonenhancing

Helpful Clues for Less Common Diagnoses
- **Dural Sinus Thrombosis, Skull Base**
  - Key facts

POSTERIOR SKULL BASE LESION

- Clot formation in transverse or sigmoid sinus
  - Imaging
    - Note absence of normal sinus contrast enhancement or flow void
    - Evaluate for parenchymal venous infarction ± hemorrhage
    - CT: High density on NECT; lack of enhancement on CECT ("empty delta" sign) or CTV
    - MR: Clot signal varies with age
- **Chordoma, Clivus**
  - Key facts
    - Malignant tumor arising from remnants of primitive notochord
  - Imaging
    - CT: Destructive midline clival mass; high attenuation foci in tumor matrix (50%)
    - MR: Characteristic ↑ T2; foci of ↑ T1 signal = hemorrhage or mucoid material; moderate to marked enhancement
- **Schwannoma, Hypoglossal Nerve**
  - Key facts
    - Benign tumor in hypoglossal canal
    - Results in ipsilateral tongue denervation
  - Imaging
    - CT: Smooth scalloped margins & enlargement of hypoglossal canal
    - MR: ↑ T2 signal, "dumbbell"-shaped mass; fatty infiltration of ipsilateral tongue on T1 MR
- **Dural A-V Fistula, Skull Base**
  - Key facts
    - A-V shunting within dura

- Adult type: Network of tiny, "crack"-like vessels in wall of thrombosed dural venous sinus
  - Imaging
    - CT: NECT usually normal; tortuous dural feeders and enlarged cortical draining veins on CTA/V
    - MR: Thrombosed sinus with small flow voids

Helpful Clues for Rare Diagnoses
- **Chondrosarcoma, Skull Base**
  - Key facts
    - Off-midline lesion of skull base centered at petrooccipital fissure
  - Imaging
    - CT: "Arcs and whorls" of Ca++ in chondroid matrix
    - MR: Heterogeneous enhancement with ↑ T2 signal
- **Plasmacytoma, Skull Base**
  - Key facts
    - Solitary form: Absence of multiple myeloma (MM)
    - Malignant form: Patient has MM
  - Imaging
    - CT: Lytic with nonsclerotic scalloped margins; usually homogeneous
    - MR: ↑ T2 with variable enhancement
- **Giant Cell Tumor, Skull Base**
  - Key facts: Benign intraosseous neoplasm of multinucleated giant cells
  - Imaging: Expansile mass with cortical thinning and avid enhancement

Meningioma, Skull Base

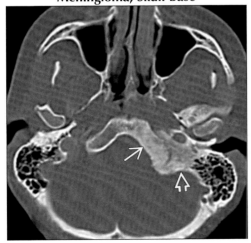

Axial bone CT reveals an extensive meningioma involving the lower clivus ➡ and inferomedial temporal bone ➡. Note the hyperostotic bony changes, signaling the presence of meningioma.

Metastasis, Skull Base

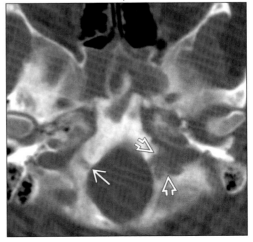

Axial T1WI MR shows destructive bony metastasis in the condylar occipital bone ➡. The lesion involves the hypoglossal canal. Note the opposite normal hypoglossal canal ➡.

POSTERIOR SKULL BASE LESION

Paraganglioma, Glomus Jugulare

(Left) Axial bone CT shows a permeative destructive pattern of bone destruction around the left jugular foramen ➡, characteristic of a paraganglioma in this location. *(Right)* Axial T1 C+ MR shows the classic appearance of a paraganglioma ➡ of the jugular foramen. The lesion has ill-defined margins, shows internal flow voids, and avidly enhances.

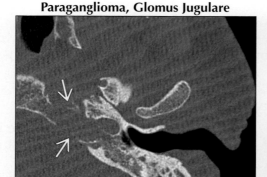

Paraganglioma, Glomus Jugulare

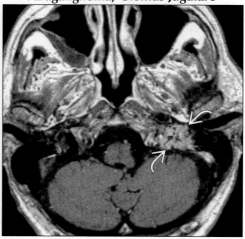

Schwannoma, Jugular Foramen

(Left) Coronal bone CT reveals the characteristic bony changes of a jugular foramen schwannoma. There is smooth lobulated expansion of the foramen ➡ with a sharp transition between the mass and the adjacent bone. *(Right)* Axial T1 C+ FS MR shows a well-defined enhancing schwannoma within the left jugular foramen ➡ and nasopharyngeal carotid space ➡. The internal carotid artery ➡ is pushed anteriorly by the tumor.

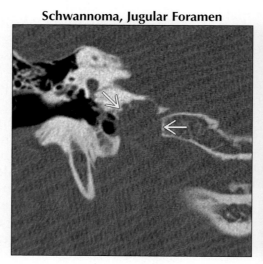

Schwannoma, Jugular Foramen

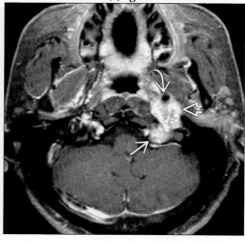

Meningioma, Jugular Foramen

(Left) Axial T1 C+ MR demonstrates an enhancing mass centered in the jugular foramen with a component extending into the posterior fossa ➡. This component has a broad dural base with "tails" extending laterally and medially ➡. *(Right)* Axial T2WI MR shows posterior fossa arachnoid granulations as sharply marginated, rounded foci of CSF signal intensity ➡ in the occipital bone. They are located near the transverse sinuses.

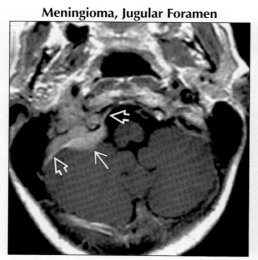

Arachnoid Granulations, Dural Sinuses

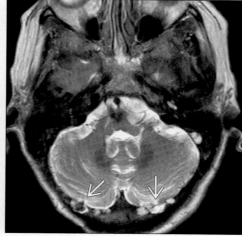

POSTERIOR SKULL BASE LESION

Dural Sinus Thrombosis, Skull Base

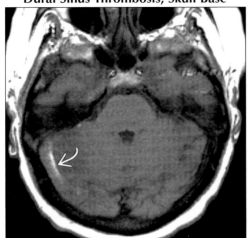

Chordoma, Clivus

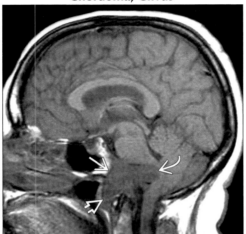

(Left) Axial T1WI MR illustrates a venous sinus thrombosis involving the right transverse sinus ⮕, secondary to oral contraceptive use. T1 shortening is noted within the thrombus on this unenhanced image. *(Right)* Sagittal T1WI MR shows a destructive chordoma of the lower clivus ⮕, extending anteroinferiorly into the nasopharynx ⮕ and posteriorly ⮕ to "thumb" the lower pons and medulla.

Schwannoma, Hypoglossal Nerve

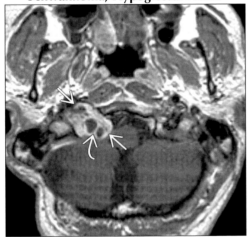

Dural A-V Fistula, Skull Base

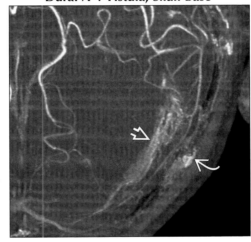

(Left) Axial T1 C+ MR shows a smoothly marginated, heterogeneously enhancing mass ⮕ extending through an expanded right hypoglossal canal. Larger schwannomas may demonstrate intratumoral cystic change ⮕. *(Right)* Axial MRA shows a transverse sinus dural arteriovenous fistula. Transosseous collateral vessels are seen in the bone. Note the distal occipital artery ⮕ and partially recanalized transverse sinus ⮕.

Chondrosarcoma, Skull Base

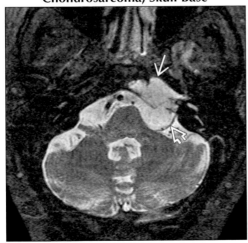

Plasmacytoma, Skull Base

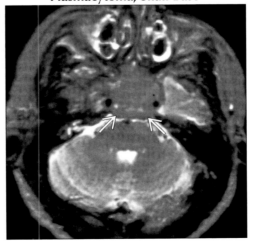

(Left) Axial T2WI FS MR shows an aggressive high signal mass ⮕ centered in the petrooccipital fissure. The lesion extends into the prepontine cistern with displacement of the vestibulocochlear nerve ⮕. *(Right)* Axial T2WI MR shows a plasmacytoma of the skull base in a patient with multiple myeloma. There is posterior extension from the clivus into the prepontine cistern ⮕. Homogeneous signal is characteristic of this lesion.

CLIVAL LESION

DIFFERENTIAL DIAGNOSIS

Common
- Fibrous Dysplasia, Skull Base
- Metastasis, Skull Base
- Non-Hodgkin Lymphoma
- Plasmacytoma, Skull Base
- Nasopharyngeal Carcinoma
- Chordoma, Clivus
- Pituitary Macroadenoma, Giant, Clivus

Less Common
- Meningioma, Clivus
- Pneumatization Arrest, Sphenoid
- Paget Disease, Skull Base
- Langerhans Histiocytosis, Skull Base
- Chondrosarcoma, Skull Base
- Giant Cell Tumor, Skull Base
- Rhabdomyosarcoma

Rare but Important
- Cephalocele, Skull Base
- Osteomyelitis, Skull Base
- Osteosarcoma, Skull Base

ESSENTIAL INFORMATION

Key Differential Diagnosis Issues
- Clival lesion may present with headache, cranial neuropathies, especially CN6
  - May be incidental imaging finding
- MR best modality to detect and characterize
  - Sagittal T1 is key MR sequence
    - Lesion seen as loss of bright fatty marrow
    - Does lesion invade from nasopharynx? If so, think nasopharyngeal carcinoma, lymphoma
    - Does lesion arise from pituitary? If so, think pituitary macroadenoma
  - MR T2 high signal intensity? Consider chordoma & chondrosarcoma
- CT complementary to MR but often best for primary bone lesions
  - Clarifies bone lesions such as Paget disease, fibrous dysplasia, bone tumors, sinus pneumatization arrest

Helpful Clues for Common Diagnoses
- **Fibrous Dysplasia, Skull Base**
  - Key facts
    - Be careful to distinguish from arrested pneumatization of sphenoid
  - Imaging
    - CT: Diagnosis suggested by ground-glass appearance; cranial foraminal narrowing
    - MR: Frequently heterogeneous; low T2 signal intensity unless cystic
- **Metastasis, Skull Base**
  - Imaging
    - CT: Lytic, sclerotic, or mixed; variable
    - MR: Signal varies; best on T1 or T1 C+ FS
    - DWI: May detect subtle lesions
- **Non-Hodgkin Lymphoma**
  - Key facts
    - Clival metastasis or invasion of clivus from adjacent mass
  - Imaging
    - CT: Most commonly lytic, may be sclerotic or mixed
    - MR: Best seen on T1 or T1 C+ FS
- **Plasmacytoma, Skull Base**
  - Key facts
    - Solitary or part of multiple myeloma
  - Imaging
    - Permeative and destructive mass with variable soft tissue component
- **Nasopharyngeal Carcinoma**
  - Key facts
    - Clival invasion from nasopharyngeal primary; denotes T3 disease
  - Imaging
    - CT: Cortex erosion; marrow invasion subtle
    - MR: Best for marrow infiltration
- **Chordoma, Clivus**
  - Key facts
    - 2nd most common site after sacrum
  - Imaging
    - CT: Destructive ± residual bone flecks
    - MR: Characteristic high T2 signal
- **Pituitary Macroadenoma, Giant, Clivus**
  - Key facts
    - Most often nonsecreting adenoma, but any type may extend into skull base
  - Imaging
    - CT: Expanded sella characteristic
    - MR: Shows pituitary origin

Helpful Clues for Less Common Diagnoses
- **Meningioma, Clivus**
  - Key facts
    - More common in females
  - Imaging
    - CT: Look for clival hyperostosis

- MR: Dural-based mass, extension along dural surfaces, marked C+
- **Pneumatization Arrest, Sphenoid**
  - Key facts
    - Incidental imaging finding
    - Asymptomatic
  - Imaging
    - CT: Nonexpansile, osteosclerotic border, internal fat, curvilinear calcifications
    - MR: Heterogeneous, fatty signal ± C+
- **Paget Disease, Skull Base**
  - Key facts
    - Incidental finding or cranial nerve foraminal narrowing
  - Imaging
    - Sclerotic, expanded bone
- **Langerhans Histiocytosis, Skull Base**
  - Key facts
    - Skull is most common bone site
  - Imaging
    - CT: Destructive lesion
    - MR: ± pituitary & infundibular enlargement & contrast enhancement
- **Chondrosarcoma, Skull Base**
  - Key facts
    - Usually cranial neuropathies (CN5-6)
    - Arises in petroclival synchondrosis
  - Imaging
  - CT: Destructive mass; may see "arcs and whorls" of calcium
  - MR: High signal on T2 like chordoma
    - Centered along lateral clivus
- **Giant Cell Tumor, Skull Base**
  - Key facts

- Benign tumor; uncommon location
  - Imaging
    - CT: Expansile mass, thin cortical shell
    - MR: Marked contrast enhancement
- **Rhabdomyosarcoma**
  - Key facts
    - Most commonly extension from nasopharynx, sinuses, or orbit
    - Many present with intracranial disease
  - Imaging
    - CT: Aggressive, rapid destruction
    - MR: Solid mass with heterogeneous C+

Helpful Clues for Rare Diagnoses
- **Cephalocele, Skull Base**
  - Key facts
    - Frequently secondary to trauma
  - Imaging
    - CT: Multiplanar reconstructions helpful, very useful with cisternography
    - MR: High T2 CSF ± neural elements
- **Osteomyelitis, Skull Base**
  - Key facts
    - May be secondary to sphenoid sinusitis, petrous apicitis
  - Imaging
    - CT: Permeative lytic bone changes
    - MR: Heterogeneous high T2 and C+; occasional depiction of abscess
- **Osteosarcoma, Skull Base**
  - Key facts
    - Rare site; difficult imaging diagnosis
  - Imaging
    - CT: Destructive lesion ± osteoid matrix

Fibrous Dysplasia, Skull Base

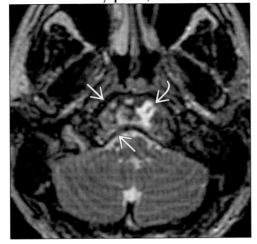

Axial T2WI MR shows an expanded clivus with heterogeneous signal intensity. Although predominantly low signal, focal areas of high signal ➡ are noted, but the low intensity cortex ➡ is preserved.

Fibrous Dysplasia, Skull Base

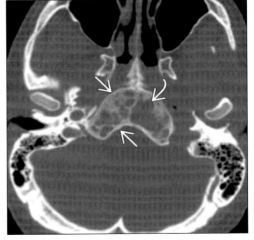

Axial NECT clarifies that the lesion is fibrous dysplasia with marked expansion of sphenoid bone and preservation of cortex ➡. Higher signal areas on T2 MR correspond to low or less dense regions ➡ on CT.

CLIVAL LESION

(Left) Sagittal T1WI MR demonstrates focal loss of normal bright fatty marrow at the inferior lateral aspect of the clivus ➡. Loss of clival T1 signal should be evaluated further in every patient. (Right) Axial T1 C+ FS MR reveals heterogeneous enhancement of a metastatic lesion ➡, extending laterally toward the jugular foramen. There is also expansion of the inferior clivus and irregular dural enhancement ➡.

Metastasis, Skull Base

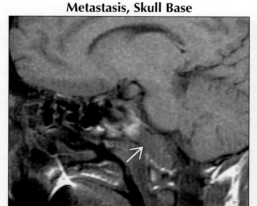

Metastasis, Skull Base

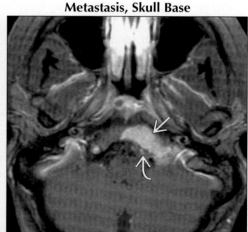

(Left) Sagittal T1WI MR shows diffuse replacement of normal bright marrow with low signal intensity ➡ that also extends to the dorsal clivus ➡. The contour of the sella floor is preserved, suggesting that this did not arise in the pituitary fossa. (Right) Axial T2WI FS MR in the same patient reveals subtle expansion of clivus ➡, with replacement of marrow by a process with diffusely low signal intensity. This suggests a tumor with high nuclear:cytoplasmic ratio such as NHL.

Non-Hodgkin Lymphoma

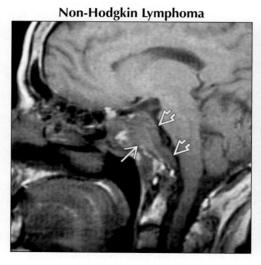

Non-Hodgkin Lymphoma

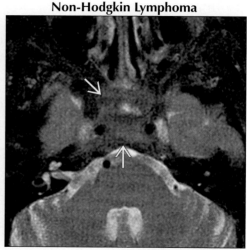

(Left) Sagittal T1WI MR shows a soft tissue mass ➡ replacing marrow & expanding clivus. Normal pituitary gland ➡ is elevated by mass, excluding invasive pituitary macroadenoma as differential consideration. Clival lymphoma, metastasis, & plasmacytoma are often not differentiated by imaging. (Right) Axial T2WI FS MR reveals mass ➡ to be isointense to brain and not as bright as chordoma. Mass bulges into the prepontine cistern, abutting the basilar artery ➡.

Plasmacytoma, Skull Base

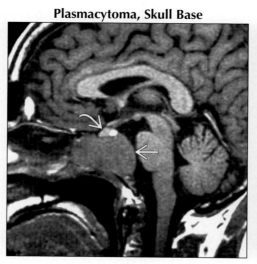

Plasmacytoma, Skull Base

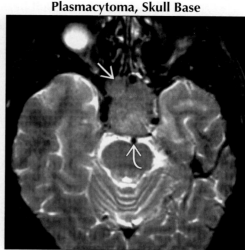

CLIVAL LESION

Nasopharyngeal Carcinoma

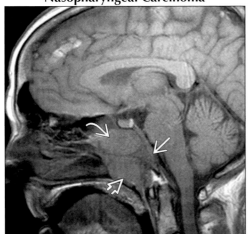

Nasopharyngeal Carcinoma

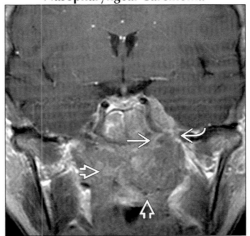

(Left) Sagittal T1WI MR through midline reveals loss of clival fatty marrow ➡ but also a nasopharyngeal soft tissue mass ➡ abutting the skull base, the origin of the infiltrating tumor. Superior extension to the sphenoid sinus ➡ is also seen. (Right) Coronal T1 C+ FS MR in the same patient best shows a bulky nasopharyngeal tumor ➡ with superior extension to the sphenoid sinus as well as invasion through foramen lacerum ➡ and through foramen ovale ➡ to Meckel cave.

Chordoma, Clivus

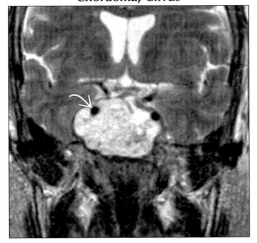

Chordoma, Clivus

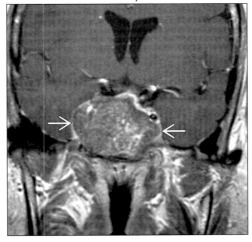

(Left) Coronal T2WI MR shows homogeneous T2 hyperintensity, typically seen with chordoma. Mass engulfs clivus & cavernous sinuses & surrounds right ICA ➡, explaining cranial neuropathy presentation. (Right) Coronal T1 C+ MR in the same patient reveals "honeycomb" pattern of enhancement often seen with chordoma. T2 hyperintensity in midline expansile clival mass ➡ with irregular but solid enhancement is highly suggestive of chordoma.

Pituitary Macroadenoma, Giant, Clivus

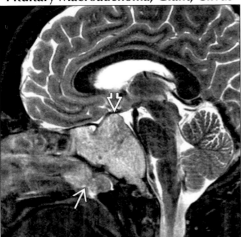

Pituitary Macroadenoma, Giant, Clivus

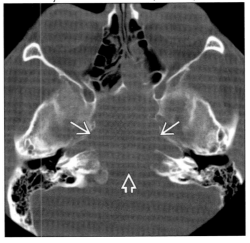

(Left) Sagittal T2WI FS MR shows a large intermediate signal intensity mass replacing & expanding the clivus. Note the tumor also involves the posterior nose and nasopharynx ➡. Key to the pituitary origin of the tumor is the absence of a definable pituitary gland ➡. (Right) Axial bone CT reveals marked remodeling of the central skull base with erosion ➡ of the dorsal clivus ➡ and medial aspects of the petrous ICA canals.

(Left) Sagittal T1 C+ MR demonstrates uniformly enhancing tissue that arises from the dorsal aspect of the clivus ⮕ and extends into the suprasellar cistern and sella ⮕, with filling of the prepontine cistern. (Right) Coronal T1 C+ MR in a different patient shows a moderately enhancing mass filling the sphenoid ⮕. Although this is nonspecific in appearance, dural involvement of the planum ⮕ is a clue to tumor origin.

Meningioma, Clivus

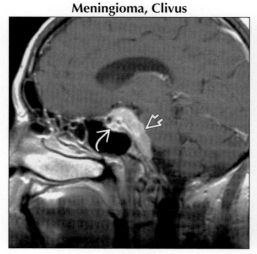

Meningioma, Clivus

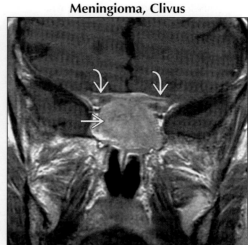

(Left) Axial bone CT through the skull base in a patient with headache reveals a heterogeneous right sphenoid body & greater wing with areas of sclerotic ⮕ & lucent ⮕ expansion. Lesion is heterogeneous on MR (not shown); hence, it may be mistaken for tumor. (Right) Axial bone CT shows diffuse expansion and hyperdensity of skull base with "fluffy" appearance of thickened bone. Process also extends to involve petrous apices of temporal bones ⮕ up to otic capsules ⮕.

Pneumatization Arrest, Sphenoid

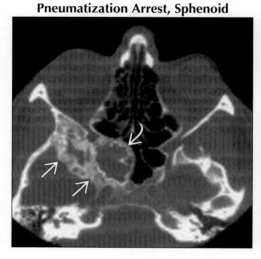

Paget Disease, Skull Base

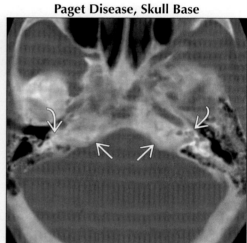

(Left) Sagittal T1 C+ MR in a child shows a large mass ⮕ extending into the sella with displacement of the infundibulum ⮕ posteriorly. Anteriorly the mass ⮕ elevates the inferior frontal lobes. The lesion exhibits moderate heterogeneous enhancement. (Right) Axial T2WI MR shows a markedly hyperintense lesion centered at the lateral aspect of clivus at petroclival fissure ⮕. The lesion involves the petrous apex and extends to the proximal petrous ICA ⮕ and into the CPA cistern ⮕.

Langerhans Histiocytosis, Skull Base

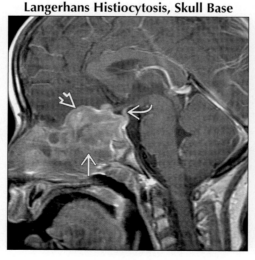

Chondrosarcoma, Skull Base

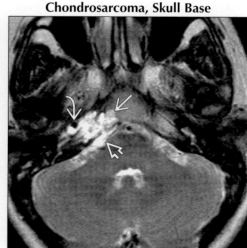

Giant Cell Tumor, Skull Base

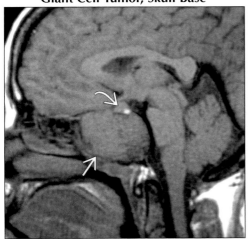

Giant Cell Tumor, Skull Base

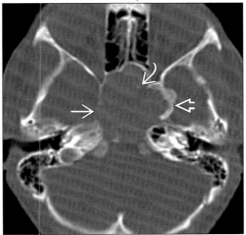

(Left) Sagittal T1WI MR demonstrates a large expansile skull base mass centered in the clivus & obliterating the sphenoid sinus ➡. Note the pituitary gland ➡ is elevated by the mass & clearly distinct from it. (Right) Axial bone CT demonstrates expansile nature of clival mass. Areas of markedly thin cortex ➡ and other more irregularly sclerotic cortex ➡ are seen. Focal areas of bone dehiscence and more subtle matrix calcifications ➡ are also evident.

Rhabdomyosarcoma

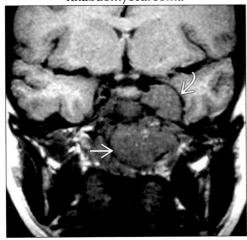

Cephalocele, Skull Base

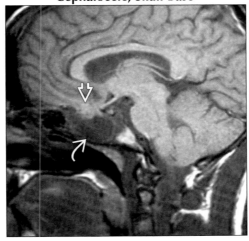

(Left) Coronal T1WI MR in a child shows a large heterogeneous nasopharyngeal mass ➡ invading the clivus and extending through the skull base to distend the left cavernous sinus ➡. (Right) Sagittal T1WI MR in a patient with a proven CSF-leak and a history of trauma shows the cystic collection distending the sphenoid sinus ➡. Inferior prolapse of frontal gyri ➡ into the collection and absence of low intensity linear sinus roof suggests the diagnosis.

Osteomyelitis, Skull Base

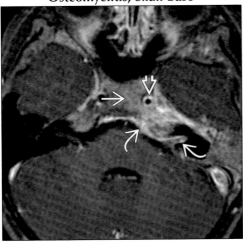

Osteosarcoma, Skull Base

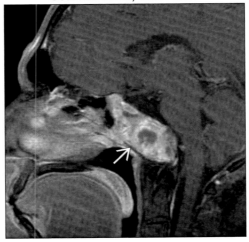

(Left) Axial T1 C+ FS MR shows a typical case of apical petrositis with involvement of the clivus. Extensive enhancement of petrous apex, clivus ➡, & dura ➡ is evident. Inflammation results in ICA narrowing ➡. (Right) Sagittal T1 C+ MR shows a large lesion replacing normal marrow & expanding the clivus. Note heterogeneous enhancement in the lesion ➡. Absence of bony matrix makes it difficult to characterize this as primary osteosarcoma.

JUGULAR FORAMEN LESION

DIFFERENTIAL DIAGNOSIS

Common
- Paraganglioma, Glomus Jugulare
- Schwannoma, Jugular Foramen
- Meningioma, Jugular Foramen
- Jugular Foramen Asymmetry
- Jugular Bulb Pseudolesion
- Jugular Bulb, High
- Metastasis, Skull Base

Less Common
- Jugular Bulb, Dehiscent
- Jugular Bulb Diverticulum
- Chondrosarcoma, Skull Base
- Plasmacytoma, Skull Base

Rare but Important
- Dural Sinus Thrombosis, Skull Base
- Dural A-V Fistula, Skull Base
- Langerhans Histiocytosis, Skull Base

ESSENTIAL INFORMATION

Key Differential Diagnosis Issues
- Lesions arise primarily within jugular foramen (JF) or secondarily invade it
  - Primary lesions centered in JF
  - Secondary invasion from lesions arising in petrous apex & petrooccipital fissure
- Asymmetry of normal JF is rule
- Bony margins of JF lesions yield clues to diagnosis
  - Irregular destruction: Think glomus jugulare paraganglioma (GJP), metastasis, other malignant neoplasm
  - Smooth cortical remodeling/expansion: Think normal variants, schwannoma
- Do not mistake turbulent flow (pseudolesion) of JF for neoplasm

Helpful Clues for Common Diagnoses
- **Paraganglioma, Glomus Jugulare**
  - CT: Permeative-destructive bony margins of JF
  - MR: "Salt & pepper" appearance in lesions > 2 cm on T2 and T1 C+ sequences
    - Salt = parenchyma; pepper = flow voids
  - Vector of spread: Superolaterally into middle ear cavity
- **Schwannoma, Jugular Foramen**
  - CT: Soft tissue density mass with sharp, smoothly expanded margins of JF

- MR: Fusiform enhancing mass usually without flow voids, ± intramural cysts
  - Small number may be hypervascular & exhibit flow voids ("puddling" of angiographic contrast seen in this type)
- Vector of spread: Superomedially toward retro-olivary sulcus of lateral medulla
- **Meningioma, Jugular Foramen**
  - CT: High density mass ± intralesional Ca++
    - Hyperostotic or permeative-sclerotic adjacent bone
  - MR: ↓ T2, isointense to brain on T1
    - Uniform enhancement, unless calcified
    - May see enhancing dural "tail"
  - Vector of spread: Centrifugal (away from center) along dural surfaces
- **Jugular Foramen Asymmetry**
  - Asymmetry in size of JF & associated dural sinuses is rule
  - Typically right > left
- **Jugular Bulb Pseudolesion**
  - MR: Turbulent flow produces heterogeneous bulb signal on some, but not all MR sequences
    - JF schwannoma or thrombosis mimic
  - CT: Normal bony margins
  - CTV or MRV show normal venous flow
- **Jugular Bulb, High**
  - Limited clinical relevance (patients may have tinnitus)
  - CT or MR: Roof of jugular bulb extending cephalad to level of IAC is diagnostic
- **Metastasis, Skull Base**
  - Hematogenous spread to adjacent skull base with secondary involvement of JF
  - CT: Invasive/destructive bony margins
  - MR: Typically ↓ T1 signal with enhancement; features primary dependent

Helpful Clues for Less Common Diagnoses
- **Jugular Bulb, Dehiscent**
  - Bluish mass ("vascular tympanic membrane") visible on otoscopy
  - Absence of normal bony jugular plate with prolapse into middle ear cavity
  - CT: Diagnostic with absence of bone between bulb & middle ear cavity
  - MR: Bulb "ear" extends into middle ear
- **Jugular Bulb Diverticulum**
  - Asymptomatic; normal variant
  - CT: Outpouching from jugular bulb into temporal bone

9

JUGULAR FORAMEN LESION

- Most commonly projects superiorly posterior to IAC
- May extend in any direction
- Well-corticated; "finger"-like or broad based
- **Chondrosarcoma, Skull Base**
  - Centered on petrooccipital fissure with secondary JF invasion
  - CT: Sharply marginated with nonsclerotic bony margins
    - 50% with chondroid matrix
  - MR: ↑ T2 signal; chondroid matrix poorly visualized compared to CT
- **Plasmacytoma, Skull Base**
  - Involves adjacent bone with secondary JF involvement; multiple lesions usually present (check calvarium)
  - CT: Osteolytic with nonsclerotic margins
    - Biconvex expansion of bone

Helpful Clues for Rare Diagnoses
- **Dural Sinus Thrombosis, Skull Base**
  - Usually result of dehydration, otomastoiditis, trauma, blood dyscrasia
  - CT: Hyperdense sinus/JF
  - MR: Abnormal signal in sinus/JF
    - ↑ T1 on nonenhanced images
- **Dural A-V Fistula, Skull Base**
  - Arterialized flow in dural venous sinuses
  - CTA: May suggest diagnosis
  - MR: MRA source images may show transosseous collaterals
    - Flow voids on MRA
  - Angiography confirms diagnosis

- **Langerhans Histiocytosis, Skull Base**
  - Presents in 1st decade; M > F
  - CT: Lytic lesion with sharply defined, "punched out" margins
  - MR: Heterogeneous enhancement

Other Essential Information
- Imaging findings can be very helpful in differentiating JF lesions
  - Bone CT imaging
    - GJP: Permeative-destructive
    - Schwannoma: Sharp, smooth margins with JF expansion
    - Meningioma: Permeative-sclerotic or hyperostotic
    - Metastasis: Destructive/invasive margins
  - MR imaging
    - GJP: High velocity flow voids ("pepper")
    - Schwannoma: No high velocity flow voids; intramural cysts
    - Meningioma: Hypointense foci from Ca++; dural "tail" sign
    - Metastasis: Invasive margins
  - Lesion vector of spread
    - GJP: Superolateral into middle ear
    - Schwannoma: Superomedial toward brainstem
    - Meningioma: Centrifugal along dural surfaces

SELECTED REFERENCES

1. Caldemeyer KS et al: The jugular foramen: a review of anatomy, masses, and imaging characteristics. Radiographics. 17(5):1123-39, 1997

Paraganglioma, Glomus Jugulare

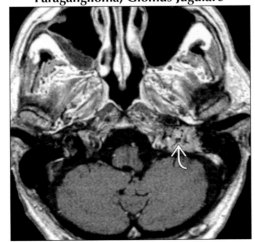

Axial T1 C+ MR shows serpiginous flow voids ⮞ within the mass, consistent with arterial feeders. These flow voids within the parenchyma give paragangliomas their classic "salt & pepper" appearance.

Schwannoma, Jugular Foramen

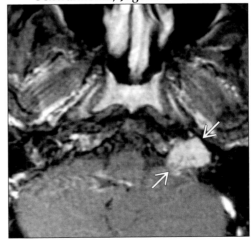

Axial T1 C+ FS MR shows a well-defined enhancing mass ➡ within the left jugular foramen with no appreciable flow voids in the lesion. Intact cortical margins would be better seen on CT.

(Left) Axial T1 C+ MR shows a large dural-based mass ➡ within the right posterior fossa. This en plaque lesion involves the jugular foramen with extensive surrounding infiltration of the skull base and extension into the carotid space ➡. (Right) Axial CTV shows a normal variation in the size of the jugular foramina. The right jugular bulb ➡ is larger than the left ➡. Asymmetry in the size of the jugular bulbs is the rule rather than the exception.

Meningioma, Jugular Foramen

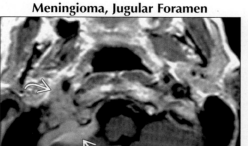

Jugular Foramen Asymmetry

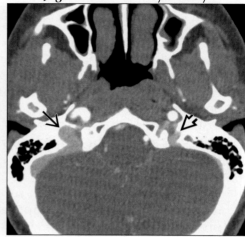

(Left) Axial T1 C+ MR demonstrates heterogeneous enhancement of a large right jugular bulb ➡ with lower signal toward the center. The adjacent sigmoid sinus also has a central lower signal stripe ➡. The MRV in this patient was normal, excluding sinus and bulb thrombosis. (Right) Coronal bone CT shows cephalad extension of the left jugular bulb ➡. By definition, the bulb reaches the level of the internal auditory canal (not shown on this image).

Jugular Bulb Pseudolesion

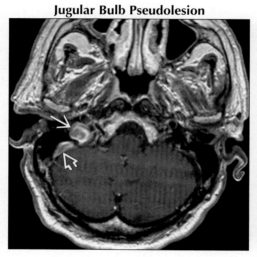

Jugular Bulb, High

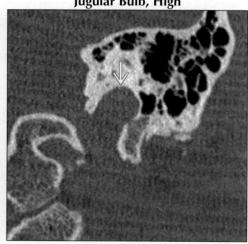

(Left) Axial CECT shows metastatic medullary thyroid carcinoma to the skull base extending into the jugular foramen ➡, cerebellopontine angle cistern ➡, and the middle ear ➡. On this CT image, the metastasis is difficult to distinguish from a paraganglioma. (Right) Axial bone CT shows a dehiscent jugular bulb ➡ bulging into the posteroinferior aspect of middle ear cavity. Note intact, smooth cortical bone at the remaining margins of the jugular foramen.

Metastasis, Skull Base

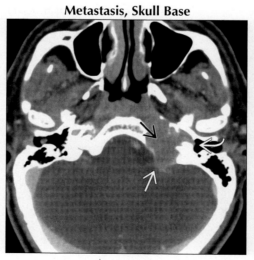

Jugular Bulb, Dehiscent

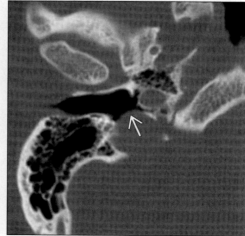

JUGULAR FORAMEN LESION

Jugular Bulb Diverticulum

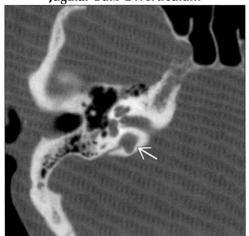

Chondrosarcoma, Skull Base

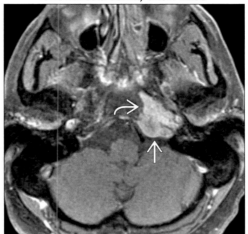

(Left) Axial bone CT shows a typical jugular bulb diverticulum ➡ rising into a location posterior to the internal auditory canal. *(Right)* Axial T1 C+ MR demonstrates a skull base chondrosarcoma with homogeneous enhancement centered in the left petrooccipital fissure ➡ and extending laterally to involve the jugular foramen ➡.

Plasmacytoma, Skull Base

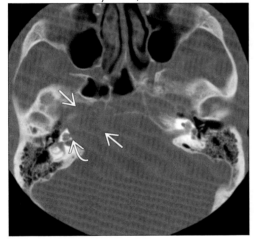

Dural Sinus Thrombosis, Skull Base

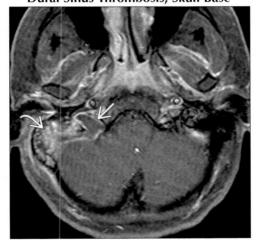

(Left) Axial bone CT shows a plasmacytoma ➡ involving the petrous apex, jugular foramen, inner ear, and clivus. This lytic lesion erodes into the cochlea ➡ and ICA. The margins of this mass are sharply defined but noncorticated. *(Right)* Axial T1 C+ FS MR shows dural sinus thrombosis as a complication of suppurative otomastoiditis. Note lack of enhancement in the thrombosed jugular bulb ➡ and enhancement within the inflamed mastoid air cells ➡.

Dural A-V Fistula, Skull Base

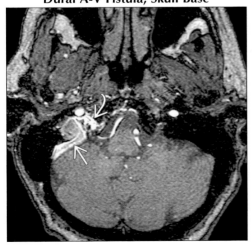

Langerhans Histiocytosis, Skull Base

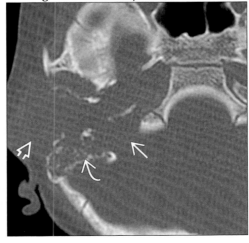

(Left) Axial MRA source image reveals a dural A-V fistula of the jugular foramen and skull base. Note the multiple extra vessels visible as flow-related enhancement ➡. High velocity flow is also noted in the adjacent sigmoid sinus ➡. *(Right)* Axial bone CT in a child with Langerhans cell histiocytosis demonstrates a unilateral destructive lesion involving the external ear ➡, temporal bone ➡, and jugular foramen ➡.

DURAL SINUS LESION, GENERAL

DIFFERENTIAL DIAGNOSIS

Common
- Arachnoid Granulations, Dural Sinuses
- Dural Sinus Hypoplasia-Aplasia
- Thrombosis, Dural Sinus
- Dural A-V Fistula

Less Common
- Meningioma
- Metastasis
- Lymphoma
- Depressed Skull Fracture
- Intracranial Hypotension

Rare but Important
- Dural Venous Sinus Stenosis
- Thrombophlebitis
- Polycythemia
- Hemangioma
- Leukemia
- Rosai-Dorfman Disease
- Extramedullary Hematopoiesis
- Lipoma
- Masson Vegetant Intravascular Hemangioendothelioma

ESSENTIAL INFORMATION

Key Differential Diagnosis Issues
- Includes generic lesions affecting ALL dural venous sinuses
  - Cavernous sinus (CS) unique because of contents, proximity to skull base
  - CS diagnoses (e.g., perineural metastasis, aneurysm, schwannoma) do not typically affect other sinuses
- Imaging challenge: Differentiate dural sinus thrombosis (DST) from stenosis, anatomic variants
  - CTV best
  - MRV shows anatomical narrowing/occlusion
  - T2* (GRE/SWI) shows thrombus

Helpful Clues for Common Diagnoses
- **Arachnoid Granulations, Dural Sinuses**
  - Can be large (> 1 cm), remodel calvarium
    - May narrow but not occlude sinus
  - Round/ovoid, well circumscribed
  - CSF density/signal intensity
- **Dural Sinus Hypoplasia-Aplasia**
  - Seen in up to 1/3 of normal scans

- Transverse sinus (TS) most common site
  - "Flow gaps" on MRV can mimic DST
    - Confirm "flow gaps" on source data
    - No "blooming" thrombus on T2*
    - If MRV is unclear, CTV helpful
- **Thrombosis, Dural Sinus**
  - Symptoms vary with extent of thrombus, collaterals, cortical vein involvement
  - NECT
    - Hyperdense clot in sinus
    - Cortical/subcortical hemorrhages (bilateral parasagittal if superior sagittal sinus or temporal lobe if vein of Labbe)
    - ± Edema (vasogenic > cytotoxic)
  - CECT shows "empty delta" sign
  - MR
    - Loss of normal "flow void"
    - Clot elongated, fills sinus, shows susceptibility on T2*
    - Confirm with MRV
  - Chronic thrombosis difficult diagnosis
    - Progressive recanalization &/or granulation tissue forms
    - Chronic thrombus enhances, mimicking patent dural sinus
    - Dura also thickens, enhances; bizarre-appearing collaterals may mimic vascular malformation
    - May have clinical, imaging findings of intracranial hypertension (pseudotumor cerebri)
- **Dural A-V Fistula**
  - Most acquired; clinical manifestations vary
    - Pulsatile tinnitus, exophthalmos
    - Less common = progressive encephalopathy (dementia), diffuse white matter hyperintensity from chronic venous hypertension
  - Imaging
    - Flow voids within wall of thrombosed dural sinus common
    - High-grade lesions prone to intracranial (usually parenchymal) hemorrhage
    - Small web of vessels on collapsed MRA images may suggest diagnosis
    - DSA gold standard for diagnosis

Helpful Clues for Less Common Diagnoses
- **Meningioma**
  - Enhancing dural-based mass ± "tail"
  - May invade, occlude, or compress dural sinuses

○ Bony hyperostosis variable
- **Metastasis**
  ○ Systemic primaries may compress or invade dural sinuses
  ○ Usually arise from calvarium with secondary dural sinus involvement
- **Lymphoma**
  ○ Dural-based mass(es) common in metastatic lymphoma
- **Depressed Skull Fracture**
  ○ May lacerate/compress/occlude dural sinus
  ○ ± Venous epidural hematoma (EDH)
  ○ Venous EDH develops slowly, presents late!
- **Intracranial Hypotension**
  ○ Dural venous engorgement, enhancement
  ○ Slumping midbrain, tonsillar descent, subdural hematomas

Helpful Clues for Rare Diagnoses
- **Dural Venous Sinus Stenosis**
  ○ Focal short segmental narrowing on CTV, MRV, or DSA (venous phase)
  ○ May cause intractable headaches (intracranial hypertension)
  ○ Patients with suspected symptomatic venous outflow restriction, pressure gradient at venography may improve after stent
- **Thrombophlebitis**
  ○ Complication of infection (meningitis, rhinosinusitis, or mastoiditis)
  ○ Infection spreads easily due to valveless nature of intracranial venous system

○ May cause septic venous thrombosis
- **Polycythemia**
  ○ High hematocrit → "dense" dural sinus
- **Hemangioma**
  ○ Capillary/cavernous vasoformative neoplasm
  ○ Convex dura or venous sinus (CS most common)
  ○ May present with mass effect or intracranial hypertension
- **Leukemia**
  ○ Dural-based enhancing masses
  ○ May compress/invade dural sinuses
- **Rosai-Dorfman Disease**
  ○ Younger patients
  ○ Lymphadenopathy > paranasal sinus disease
  ○ Lymphadenopathy usually coexists if CNS disease is present
  ○ Solitary/multiple dural-based enhancing masses
- **Extramedullary Hematopoiesis**
  ○ Dural-based enhancing masses
  ○ Dural sinus compression/invasion rare
- **Lipoma**
  ○ Fat in dural sinus rare; CS most common
- **Masson Vegetant Intravascular Hemangioendothelioma**
  ○ Rare benign tumor of young patients
  ○ Papillary endothelial hyperplasia
  ○ Can cause stenosis, hypertension
  ○ Can mimic meningioma

Arachnoid Granulations, Dural Sinuses

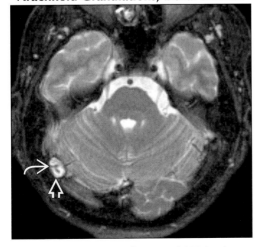

Axial T2WI FS MR shows a large ovoid CSF-signal mass ⬌ in the right transverse sinus with an internal flow void ⬀, probably representing a vein.

Arachnoid Granulations, Dural Sinuses

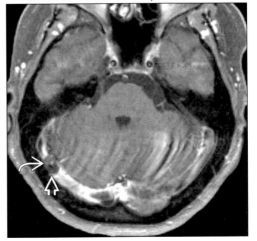

Axial T1 C+ FS MR in the same patient shows that the lesion ⬌ does not enhance and is the same signal as CSF. The vein ⬀ enhances. This was an incidental finding in an asymptomatic patient.

9

DURAL SINUS LESION, GENERAL

(Left) Axial CECT shows a hypodense CSF-like lobulated filling defect in the right transverse sinus ➡. Note the adjacent calvarial scalloping ⇨. *(Right)* Axial bone CT in the same patient shows smooth, well-delineated erosion ➔ of the calvarium caused by arachnoid granulation.

Arachnoid Granulations, Dural Sinuses

Arachnoid Granulations, Dural Sinuses

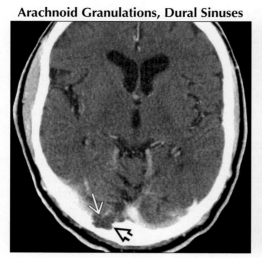
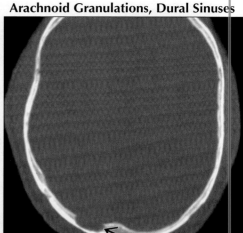

(Left) Sagittal T1WI MR shows a round, fluid signal, cystic lesion within the superior sagittal sinus ➡ that followed CSF on all sequences. This is a variant appearance because of the atypical size and location of the lesion. *(Right)* Coronal oblique angiography shows a large filling defect ➡ in the superior sagittal sinus caused by giant arachnoid granulation.

Arachnoid Granulations, Dural Sinuses

Arachnoid Granulations, Dural Sinuses

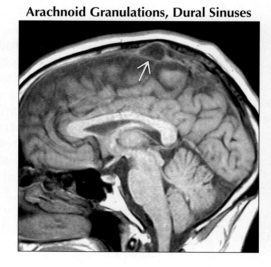

(Left) Axial T2WI MR with video inversion shows a cluster of sharply marginated CSF-like cysts ⇨ remodeling the inner calvarium. *(Right)* Axial T2WI MR shows an arachnoid granulation that appears to communicate directly with the adjacent subarachnoid space via a defect in its inner margin along the inner table of the calvarium ➔. It also contains a hypointense "knuckle" of tissue ⇨ that forms an intraosseous meningoencephalocele.

Arachnoid Granulations, Dural Sinuses

Arachnoid Granulations, Dural Sinuses

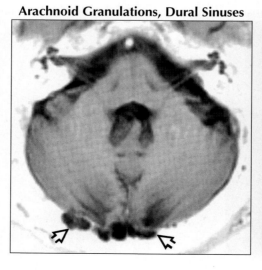

DURAL SINUS LESION, GENERAL

Dural Sinus Hypoplasia-Aplasia

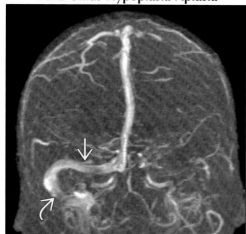

Dural Sinus Hypoplasia-Aplasia

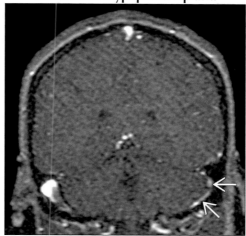

(Left) Coronal MRV shows no flow-related signal within the left transverse or sigmoid sinuses on the MRV MIP projection. Compare this to the normal dominant right transverse ➡ and sigmoid ➡ sinuses. *(Right)* Coronal MRV shows flow-related signal within an asymmetrically smaller left transverse sinus ➡; it is important to review the source images before concluding that lack of flow on MIPs is genuine.

Thrombosis, Dural Sinus

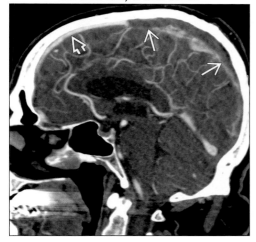

Thrombosis, Dural Sinus

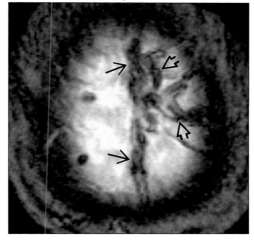

(Left) Sagittal CTA shows that the anterior 1/3 of the superior sagittal sinus is patent ➡. The posterior 2/3 are filled with nonenhancing clot ➡. *(Right)* Axial T2* GRE MR in the same patient shows "blooming" of the clot in the superior sagittal sinus ➡. Note the extension into the adjacent cortical veins ➡.

Thrombosis, Dural Sinus

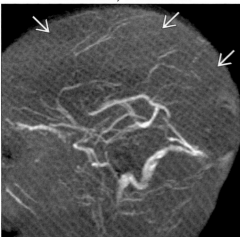

Thrombosis, Dural Sinus

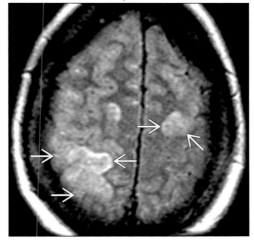

(Left) Lateral MRV shows lack of flow-related enhancement in the expected location of the superior sagittal sinus ➡, consistent with acute thrombosis. *(Right)* Axial T2WI MR shows bilateral parenchymal foci of swelling and high T2 signal in areas of associated cortical venous ischemia ➡ in the same patient as the prior image. These findings are due to associated cortical venous occlusion.

DURAL SINUS LESION, GENERAL

(Left) Lateral angiography shows thrombosis at the junction of the transverse sigmoid sinus ⊳ with retrograde filling of the transverse & contralateral dural sinuses. Several enlarged transosseous perforating branches from occipital artery supply dAVF ➡. **(Right)** Axial T2WI MR shows a normal right "flow void" ⊳. The left side is hyperintense and contains numerous tiny "flow voids" ➡. Dural AVF developed in chronically occluded left transverse sinus (not shown).

Dural A-V Fistula

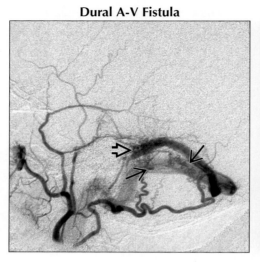

Dural A-V Fistula

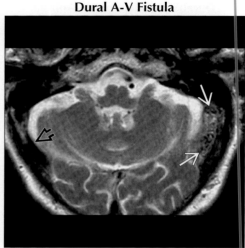

(Left) Axial NECT shows a densely calcified meningioma that originated within and mildly expands the superior sagittal sinus ➡. **(Right)** Coronal T1 C+ MR shows dural-based metastasis ➡ on both sides of the superior sagittal sinus, which is invaded and thrombosed by the tumor ➡.

Meningioma

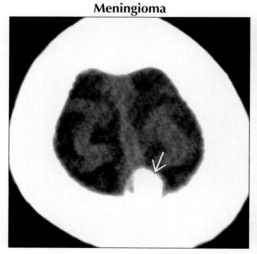

Metastasis

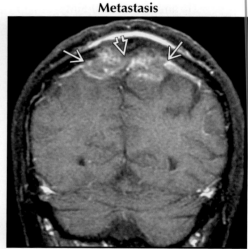

(Left) Sagittal T1 C+ MR shows an enhancing dural-based mass ➡ in the region of the cisterna magna that is encroaching into the region of the torcular herophili ⊳ in a patient with systemic lymphoma. **(Right)** Axial NECT shows a large acute epidural hematoma ➡ due to a depressed skull fracture through the torcular and transverse sinus (not shown), resulting in dural sinus laceration and bleeding.

Lymphoma

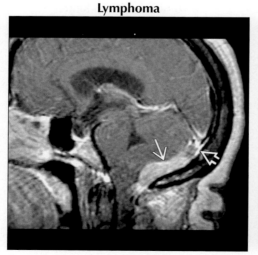

Depressed Skull Fracture

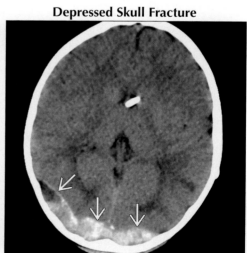

DURAL SINUS LESION, GENERAL

Intracranial Hypotension

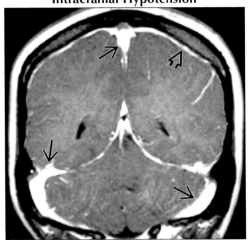

Dural Venous Sinus Stenosis

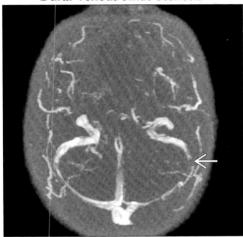

(Left) Coronal T1 C+ MR in this patient with intracranial hypotension shows engorged dural venous sinuses ⇥ and thickened enhancing dura ⇥. The pituitary gland (not shown) also appeared enlarged. *(Right)* Axial MRV shows small caliber of both transverse-sigmoid sinus junctions, with focal stenosis in the left transverse sinus ⇥ in a patient with papilledema and headaches.

Thrombophlebitis

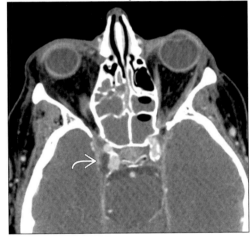

Polycythemia

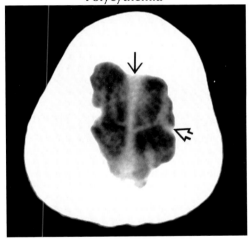

(Left) Axial CECT shows bilateral proptosis. The cavernous sinuses are enlarged with a lack of contrast opacification due to thrombosis ⇥. Mucosal disease and fluid levels consistent with acute rhinosinusitis can be seen in multiple sinuses. *(Right)* Axial NECT shows hyperdense superior sagittal sinus ⇥ and cortical veins ⇥ and mimics CECT in this 22 year old patient with chronic right-to-left cardiac shunt and a hematocrit of 67.

Hemangioma

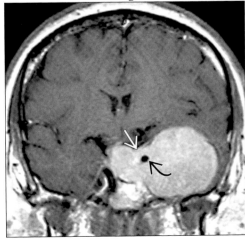

Leukemia

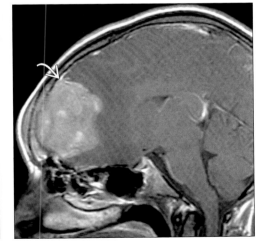

(Left) Coronal T1 C+ MR in this 13 year old shows a strongly enhancing ⇥ left cavernous sinus lesion encasing the left internal carotid artery ⇥, extending into the sella and middle cranial fossa. *(Right)* Sagittal T1 C+ MR in another 13 year old with frontal soft tissue swelling shows a dural, calvarial, enhancing mass that occludes the anterior superior sagittal sinus ⇥. Acute lymphoblastic leukemia was found.

DIFFERENTIAL DIAGNOSIS

Common
- Acquired Tonsillar Herniation
- Chiari 1
- Chiari 2
- Meningioma, Clivus
- Rheumatoid Arthritis, Adult
- Schwannoma, Jugular Foramen

Less Common
- Chordoma, Clivus
- Ependymoma
- Chondrosarcoma, Skull Base
- Retro-Odontoid Pseudopannus
- Hemangioblastoma
- CPPD
- Metastasis, Skull Base

Rare but Important
- Fusiform Aneurysm, ASVD
- Fusiform Aneurysm, Non-ASVD
- Brainstem Glioma, Pediatric
- Epidermoid Cyst
- Neurenteric Cyst

ESSENTIAL INFORMATION

Key Differential Diagnosis Issues
- Foramen magnum (FM): Posterior skull base aperture in occipital bone
  - Transmits medulla oblongata, vertebral arteries, & CN11
- Lesions of FM can be intraaxial, extraaxial, & bony skull base in origin
- Cisternal magna: Skull base cistern between medulla anteriorly & occiput posteriorly

Helpful Clues for Common Diagnoses
- **Acquired Tonsillar Herniation**
  - Key facts: Secondary to posterior fossa mass effect or severe hydrocephalus
  - Imaging: Cerebellar tonsils ⇒ into FM
    - Cisterna magna obliterated
    - 4th ventricle obstructs ⇒ hydrocephalus
- **Chiari 1**
  - Key facts: May be incidental
  - Imaging: Small posterior fossa
    - Low-lying "pegged" tonsils
    - Tonsils > 5 mm below FM
- **Chiari 2**
  - Key facts: Complex hindbrain malformation + lumbar myelomeningocele

- "Beaked" tectum, "towering" cerebellum, dysgenic corpus callosum
  - Imaging: Tonsillar ectopia
    - "Straw"-like 4th ventricle; hydrocephalus
- **Meningioma, Clivus**
  - Key facts: Older, female patients
    - Tends to encase & narrow vessels
  - Imaging: Enhancing dural-based mass with "tails"; extends through FM when clivial
    - CT: High density lesion ± Ca++
    - MR: Low signal on T2 MR
- **Rheumatoid Arthritis, Adult**
  - Key facts: Inflammatory pannus in retro-odontoid soft tissues
  - Imaging: Odontoid erosions common
    - CT: Cranial settling in severe cases
    - MR: Markedly hypointense on T2; T1 variable; enhances
- **Schwannoma, Jugular Foramen**
  - Key facts: Arises from CN9-11
    - Cisternal component may involve FM
    - May arise primarily within FM
  - Imaging: Fusiform jugular foramen mass
    - CT: Smooth enlargement of JF
    - MR: Enhances, high T2 signal; intramural cysts

Helpful Clues for Less Common Diagnoses
- **Chordoma, Clivus**
  - Key facts: Midline mass; exophytic
    - Extension into prepontine cistern "thumbs" pons
  - Imaging: Lower clival location ⇒ FM
    - CT: Irregular destructive mass lesion within clivus
    - MR: Characteristic high T2 signal; intensely enhancing
- **Ependymoma**
  - Key facts: Soft tumor, "squeezes out" 4th ventricle foramina
    - 2/3 infratentorial, 4th ventricle
  - Imaging: Heterogeneously enhancing 4th ventricle mass
    - Inferiorly extending tumor in FM
- **Chondrosarcoma, Skull Base**
  - Key facts: Chondroid malignancy; petrooccipital fissure most common
  - Imaging: 50% chondroid Ca++ (CT)
    - MR: Destructive enhancing T2 hyperintense tumor
    - When large, affects FM
- **Retro-Odontoid Pseudopannus**

- Key facts: Calcific debris arising posterosuperior to C1-2
  - Associated with degenerative arthritis, gout, CPPD
- Imaging: Look for medullary or cervical cord compression
  - CT: Calcifications of ligaments & within joint capsule
  - MR: Low signal intensity mass behind odontoid
- **Hemangioblastoma**
  - Key facts: Associated with von Hippel Lindau
    - 80% cerebellar hemispheres, 15% vermis, 5% medulla, 4th ventricle
  - Imaging: Cystic cerebellar mass + enhancing mural nodule (60%)
    - 40% solid mass
- **CPPD**
  - Key facts: Calcium pyrophosphate dihydrate deposition disease
  - Imaging: Retro-odontoid mass may cause instability ± cervical cord compression
- **Metastasis, Skull Base**
  - Key facts: Involvement of occiput by bony metastatic lesion
  - Imaging: Irregular bone destruction ± soft tissue mass
    - When large, compresses brainstem

Helpful Clues for Rare Diagnoses
- **Fusiform Aneurysm, ASVD**
  - Key facts: Aneurysm of distal vertebral artery or proximal basilar artery

- Imaging
  - CT: Lamellated layers of calcific & noncalcific thrombus; residual lumen
  - MR: Flow-related changes of lumen, with varying age thrombus in wall, phase artifact from aneurysm pulsation
  - MRA: Shows residual lumen
- **Fusiform Aneurysm, Non-ASVD**
  - Key facts: Associated with collagen vascular diseases, other vasculopathies
  - Imaging
    - CT: Shows fusiform enlargement of vessel involved
    - MR: Layered thrombus or enlarged vessel
- **Brainstem Glioma, Pediatric**
  - Key facts: Infiltrative glioma, typically low grade, involving medulla & pons
  - Imaging: Enlarged brainstem
    - Usually no enhancement
    - High T2 & FLAIR signal
- **Epidermoid Cyst**
  - Key facts: Ectodermal rest in cistern
    - CPA 40-50%, 4th ventricle 15-20%
  - Imaging: CSF-like, lobular, extraaxial
    - Insinuates into cisterns, encases nerves/vessels
- **Neurenteric Cyst**
  - Key facts: Developmental lesion resulting in intradural midline cystic mass
  - Imaging: Smooth extraaxial mass at skull base, ventral to brainstem
    - Iso- to hyperintense to CSF on T1
    - High T2 signal; conspicuous on FLAIR

Acquired Tonsillar Herniation

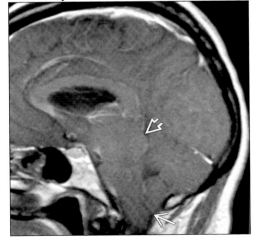

Sagittal T1WI MR reveals acquired tonsillar herniation ➡ as a result of intracranial hypotension with the "slumping midbrain" ⇨ squeezing the pons inferiorly.

Acquired Tonsillar Herniation

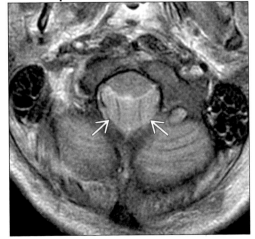

Axial T2WI MR demonstrates tonsils herniated into the foramen magnum ➡, secondary to a large supratentorial stroke (not shown).

(Left) *Sagittal T1WI MR shows a Chiari 1 malformation demonstrating tonsillar herniation. The tonsils ⇨ protrude the through foramen magnum, below an imaginary line drawn between the basion ⇨ and opisthion ⇨. **(Right)** Sagittal T2WI MR reveals pegged cerebellar tonsils ⇨ protruding inferiorly. Additionally, a focal cavity is seen in the upper cervical cord ⇨, representing focal syringohydromyelia in this Chiari 1 patient.*

Chiari 1

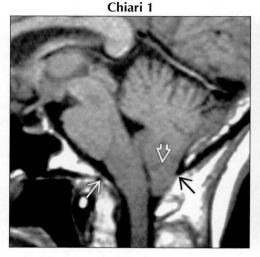

Chiari 1

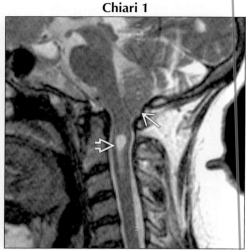

(Left) *Sagittal T1WI MR shows caudal descent of the cerebellar tissue and 4th ventricle ⇨ associated with callosal dysgenesis ⇨. Abnormal tectum, or beaking ⇨, is an important associated finding. **(Right)** Sagittal T2WI MR in a patient with Chiari 2 malformation reveals corpus callosum dysgenesis ⇨, "beaked" tectum ⇨, and downward shift of the pons, 4th ventricle, and cerebellum ⇨.*

Chiari 2

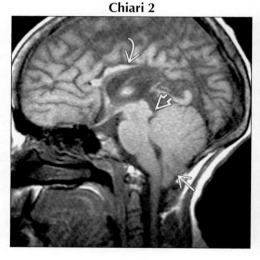

Chiari 2

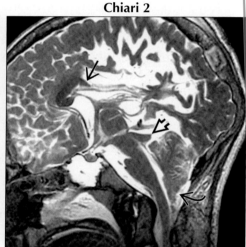

(Left) *Sagittal T1 C+ MR demonstrates a homogeneously enhancing meningioma with conspicuous dural "tails" ⇨ along the anterior margin of the foramen magnum. **(Right)** Sagittal T1 C+ MR shows a dural-based meningioma ⇨ protruding into the posterior fossa. Avid enhancement is noted, and thickening of the adjacent dura is obvious ⇨. The lesion extends into the anterior foramen magnum.*

Meningioma, Clivus

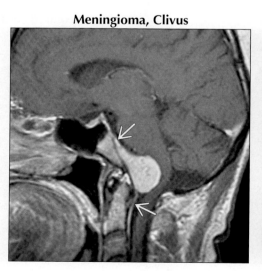

Meningioma, Clivus

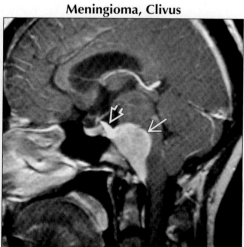

FORAMEN MAGNUM MASS

Rheumatoid Arthritis, Adult

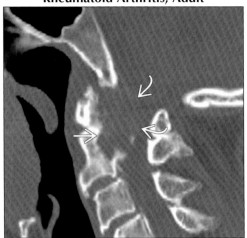

Rheumatoid Arthritis, Adult

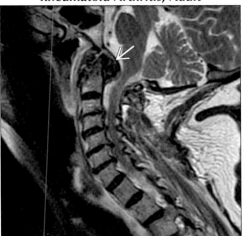

(Left) Sagittal bone CT shows craniocervical rheumatoid arthritis with extensive odontoid & C2 body erosions ➡. Note the associated large pannus that contains a "pseudotumor" ➡ severely compressing the upper cervical canal and foramen magnum. (Right) Sagittal T2WI MR reveals a large amount of rheumatoid pannus ➡ with effacement of the spinal canal and posterior displacement of the lower medulla. The odontoid process is abnormally "pointed" and eroded.

Schwannoma, Jugular Foramen

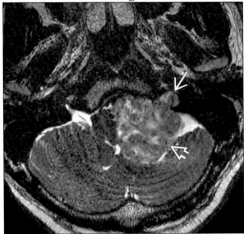

Schwannoma, Jugular Foramen

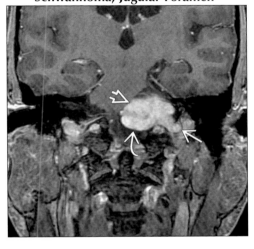

(Left) Axial T2WI MR shows a jugular foramen schwannoma with a very large cisternal component ➡ displacing the medulla and filling the basal cistern. Note that the left jugular foramen is filled by schwannoma ➡. (Right) Coronal T1 C+ MR reveals a schwannoma beginning in the left jugular foramen ➡, extending to compress the inferolateral pons ➡, and projecting into the upper foramen magnum ➡.

Chordoma, Clivus

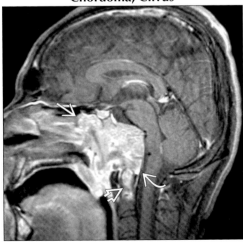

Chordoma, Clivus

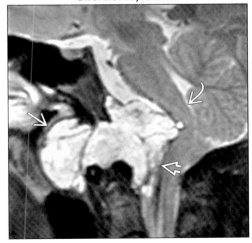

(Left) Sagittal T1 C+ MR shows a very large enhancing chordoma of the clivus with involvement of the sphenoid sinus ➡ and C2 vertebra ➡ with extension into the posterior fossa and foramen magnum ➡. (Right) Sagittal T1WI FS MR reveals a hyperintense midline chordoma arising from the inferior clivus, projecting anteriorly into the nasopharynx ➡ and posteriorly into the foramen magnum ➡. Note the medullary compression ➡.

Ependymoma

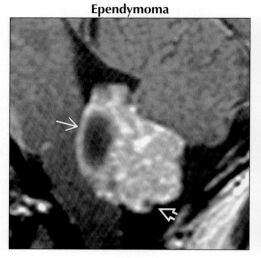

Chondrosarcoma, Skull Base

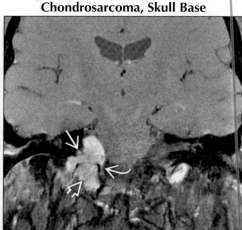

(Left) Sagittal T1 C+ MR shows an enhancing ependymoma ➡ projecting from the inferior 4th ventricle into the superior foramen magnum ➡. (Right) Coronal T1 C+ FS MR demonstrates an enhancing petrooccipital fissure chondrosarcoma ➡ extending into the occipital condyle ➡ and lateral foramen magnum ➡.

Retro-Odontoid Pseudopannus

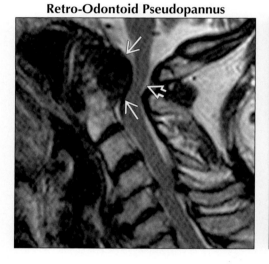

Hemangioblastoma

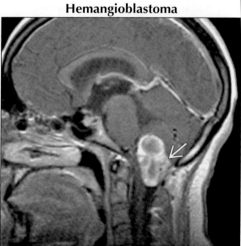

(Left) Sagittal T2WI MR shows gouty involvement of the upper cervical spine with an associated low signal mass ➡ compressing the lower medulla ➡. Pseudopannus is nonspecific with differential diagnoses that include gout, degenerative arthritis, and CPPD. (Right) Sagittal T1 C+ MR reveals a solid and cystic hemangioblastoma centered in the posterior foramen magnum ➡.

CPPD

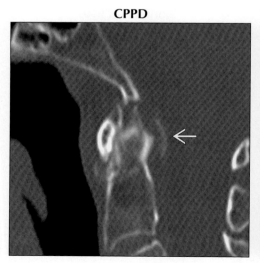

Metastasis, Skull Base

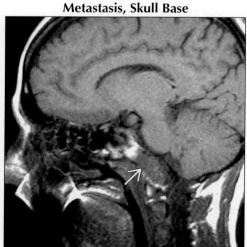

(Left) Sagittal bone CT shows calcifications of the retrodental soft tissues ➡ resulting in a mass at the foramen magnum with some mild canal stenosis. (Right) Sagittal T1WI MR shows metastasis to the basioccipital aspect of the central skull base at the anterior and lateral aspect of the foramen magnum ➡. The low signal intensity of the mass replaces the normal fatty marrow of the basiocciput.

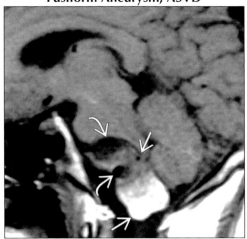
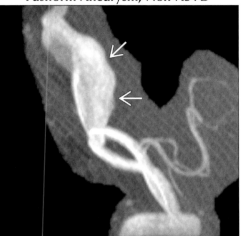
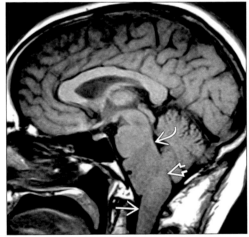
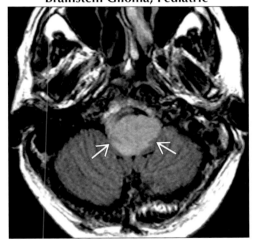
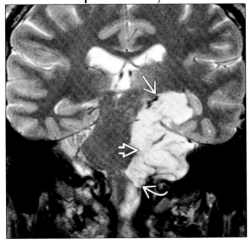
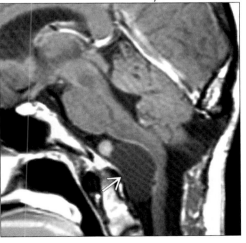

Fusiform Aneurysm, ASVD

Fusiform Aneurysm, Non-ASVD

Brainstem Glioma, Pediatric

Brainstem Glioma, Pediatric

Epidermoid Cyst

Neurenteric Cyst

(Left) Sagittal T1WI MR shows a mixed signal intensity extraaxial mass ➡. An extraaxial lesion with evidence of flow and thrombosis is strongly suggestive of aneurysm. Only small residual "flow voids" are seen on this sagittal image ➡. *(Right)* Sagittal MRA depicts a fusiform nonatherosclerotic aneurysm of the basilar artery in a young adolescent male. The vessel wall is somewhat irregular ➡ but without stenosis.

(Left) Sagittal T1WI MR shows a markedly expanded upper cervical cord ➡, medulla ➡, and inferior pons ➡ resulting from an infiltrative mass isointense to the brainstem. Brainstem gliomas often smoothly enlarge the brainstem. *(Right)* Axial T2WI MR in the same patient demonstrates diffuse medullary gliomas ➡ with increased signal compared to normal brain.

(Left) Coronal T2WI MR shows a very hyperintense lobulated epidermoid cyst that extends from the ambient cistern ➡ above to the cerebellopontine angle cistern ➡ and foramen magnum ➡ below. *(Right)* Sagittal T1 C+ MR shows an extraaxial mass ➡ in the anterior foramen magnum elevating and displacing the medulla. This neurenteric cyst is slightly hyperintense compared to CSF and was conspicuous on FLAIR (not shown).

SECTION 10
CPA-IAC & Posterior Fossa

Anatomically Based Differentials

Generic Imaging Patterns

Clinically Based Differentials

CPA MASS, ADULT

DIFFERENTIAL DIAGNOSIS

Common
- Vestibular Schwannoma

Less Common
- Meningioma, CPA-IAC
- Epidermoid Cyst, CPA-IAC
- Aneurysm, CPA-IAC
- Arachnoid Cyst, CPA-IAC
- Metastases, CPA-IAC

Rare but Important
- Neurofibromatosis Type 2, CPA-IAC
- Sarcoidosis, CPA-IAC
- Choroid Plexus Papilloma, CPA
- Lipoma, CPA-IAC
- Ependymoma, CPA
- Pseudotumor, Intracranial
- Schwannoma, Facial Nerve, CPA-IAC
- Schwannoma, Jugular Foramen
- Hemangioma, IAC
- Neurenteric Cyst

ESSENTIAL INFORMATION

Key Differential Diagnosis Issues
- Idealized imaging protocol in evaluating CPA mass lesions
  - T1 C+ fat-saturated MR is gold standard
    - Fat saturation differentiates lipoma from vestibular schwannoma
    - Add DWI for possible epidermoid
    - Add GRE for aneurysm wall clot & calcification; tumor calcifications
  - T2 thin-section, high-resolution MR gives more surgical data when vestibular schwannoma diagnosed
    - Amount of CSF cap in lateral IAC
    - Assessment of relationship to cochlear nerve canal
    - If small schwannoma, nerve of origin
- Knowledge of relative incidence of lesions key in cerebellopontine angle
  - Vestibular schwannoma: ~ 90% all CPA-IAC masses
  - Meningioma, epidermoid cyst, aneurysm, arachnoid cyst together represent ~ 8% all CPA-IAC masses
  - All other diagnoses in differential list ~ 2% of CPA-IAC masses

Helpful Clues for Common Diagnoses
- **Vestibular Schwannoma**
  - Morphology: Ovoid intracanalicular mass (IAC); "ice cream on cone" shape (CPA-IAC)
  - T1 C+ MR: Enhancing ± intramural cysts

Helpful Clues for Less Common Diagnoses
- **Meningioma, CPA-IAC**
  - Morphology: "Mushroom" dural-based mass capping IAC asymmetrically
  - T1 C+ MR: Enhancing ± dural "tails" ± CSF-vascular cleft if CPA component is larger
    - 25% of CPA meningiomas have extension/dural tail into IAC
- **Epidermoid Cyst, CPA-IAC**
  - Morphology: Insinuating ± scalloping brainstem margin
  - T1 C+ MR: Nonenhancing; may be difficult to see
  - DWI: Restricted diffusion (high signal) makes diagnosis
- **Aneurysm, CPA-IAC**
  - Morphology: Ovoid or fusiform; rarely IAC
  - T1 & T1 C+ MR: Complex signal mass from wall calcification, clot, & flow
  - MRA, CTA, or angiography sort out diagnosis
- **Arachnoid Cyst, CPA-IAC**
  - Morphology: Fills cistern with rounded margins
  - T1 C+ MR: No enhancement
    - MR: FLAIR attenuates; DWI: No restricted diffusion
- **Metastases, CPA-IAC**
  - Morphology: Irregular invasive margins
  - T1 C+ MR: Single or multiple enhancing masses in CPA area
    - 4 sites primarily involved: Flocculus, choroid plexus, arachnoid-dura, or pia

Helpful Clues for Rare Diagnoses
- **Neurofibromatosis Type 2, CPA-IAC**
  - Morphology: Bilateral ovoid IAC or "ice cream on cone" CPA-IAC masses
  - T1 C+ MR: Bilateral enhancing CPA-IAC masses
    - Other schwannomas & meningiomas may be present
- **Sarcoidosis, CPA-IAC**

- Laboratory: CSF lymphocytosis; ↑ blood angiotensin converting enzyme (ACE)
- Morphology: En plaque or nodular dural lesion(s)
- T1 C+ MR: Enhancing multifocal dural-based lesions
- **Choroid Plexus Papilloma, CPA**
  - Morphology: "Dumbbell" shape with 4th ventricle and CPA cistern components
    - Pear-shaped if begins in foramen of Luschka
  - T1 C+ MR: Avidly enhancing mass in 4th ventricle projecting through foramen of Luschka into CPA cistern
- **Lipoma, CPA-IAC**
  - Morphology: Ovoid if IAC; CPA lesion may be broad-based against brainstem
  - CT: Fat-density lesion of CPA ± IAC ± inner ear
  - T1 MR: High signal lesion, suppresses with fat-saturation
  - Caveat: If T1 C+ without fat saturation, may be mistaken for vestibular schwannoma
- **Ependymoma, CPA**
  - Morphology: Irregular soft tumor squeezes out through 4th ventricle foramen of Luschka into CPA cistern
    - Tumor margins amorphous
  - CT: Calcifications in 50%
  - T1 C+ MR: Heterogeneous enhancement of solid tumor components
    - Marginal enhancement of tumor cyst wall

- **Pseudotumor, Intracranial**
  - Morphology: En plaque
  - T1 C+ MR: Thickened, enhancing dura
  - Caveat: May mimic meningioma, sarcoidosis, or metastatic disease
- **Schwannoma, Facial Nerve, CPA-IAC**
  - Morphology: CPA-IAC mass with "labyrinthine tail"
  - CT: Labyrinthine segment CN7 may be enlarged
  - T1 C+ MR: Enhancing tubular mass in CPA-IAC and labyrinthine segment CN7
  - Caveat: If no labyrinthine segment CN7 involvement, cannot differentiate from vestibular schwannoma
- **Schwannoma, Jugular Foramen**
  - T1 C+ MR: Enhancing mass arising from jugular foramen
    - Mass projects cephalad into CPA cistern
- **Hemangioma, IAC**
  - Morphology: Ovoid IAC mass with punctate calcifications
  - CT: Punctate calcifications in IAC mass
  - T1 C+ MR: Enhancing IAC mass with focal low signal foci (calcifications)
- **Neurenteric Cyst**
  - Morphology: Rounded ovoid mass in prepontine cistern
  - MR: Intermediate to high signal T1 prepontine mass
  - Caveat: T1 increased signal differentiates from epidermoid cyst

Vestibular Schwannoma

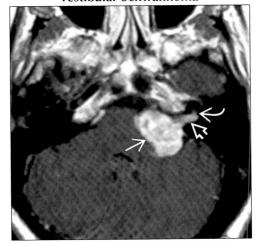

Axial T1 C+ MR reveals enhancing mass filling the CPA ➡ and internal auditory canal ➡. Note that the cochlear nerve canal is involved ➡, making resection with hearing preservation difficult.

Meningioma, CPA-IAC

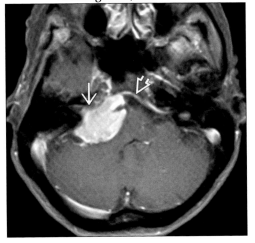

Axial T1 C+ FS MR reveals an enhancing dural-based mass centered over the IAC but with minimal IAC involvement ➡. The shape and the associated dural tail ➡ make meningioma the diagnosis.

CPA MASS, ADULT

(Left) Axial T1WI MR shows a low signal mass in the right CPA cistern that insinuates and enlarges the foramen of Luschka ⮕ and scallops the ventral cerebellar hemisphere ⮕. *(Right)* Axial T1 C+ MR demonstrates a large enhancing distal vertebral artery aneurysm ⮕ projecting up into the CPA cistern and compressing the area where CN7 and CN8 exit the brainstem ⮕.

Epidermoid Cyst, CPA-IAC

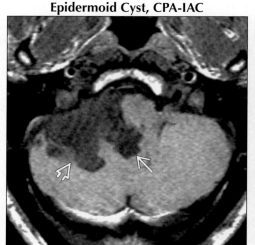

Aneurysm, CPA-IAC

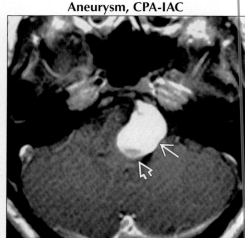

(Left) Axial T2WI FS MR shows high signal lesion ⮕ in low CPA cistern. Note the anterior displacement of proximal CN8 by arachnoid cyst ⮕. The high signal results from absence of CSF flow. *(Right)* Axial T1 C+ FS MR reveals an inhomogeneously enhancing metastatic focus arising from the dura along the prepontine cistern. This metastasis reaches the anterior margin of the porus acusticus ⮕.

Arachnoid Cyst, CPA-IAC

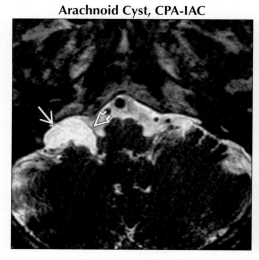

Metastases, CPA-IAC

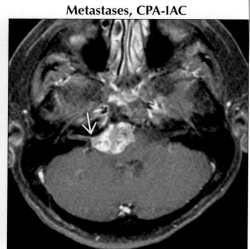

(Left) Axial T1 C+ MR shows bilateral enhancing CPA-IAC schwannomas ⮕. The left schwannoma involves the intratemporal facial nerve ⮕, indicating it is most likely a facial nerve schwannoma. *(Right)* Axial T1 C+ MR shows heaped-up dural-based sarcoid deposit in the right CPA ⮕ that enters the internal auditory canal ⮕. Meckel cave is also affected ⮕. This lesion mimics meningioma.

Neurofibromatosis Type 2, CPA-IAC

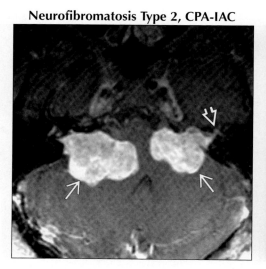

Sarcoidosis, CPA-IAC

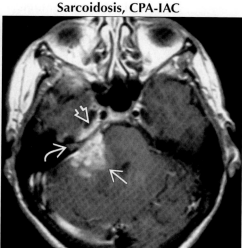

Choroid Plexus Papilloma, CPA

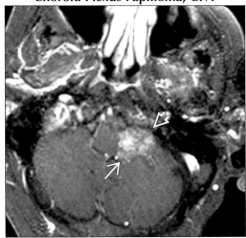

Lipoma, CPA-IAC

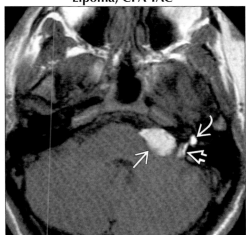

(Left) Axial T1 C+ MR reveals a pear-shaped inhomogeneously enhancing papilloma ➡ projecting from the lateral recess of the 4th ventricle through the foramen of Luschka into the low CPA cistern ➡. *(Right)* Axial T1WI MR shows a variant three-part lipoma affecting the CPA cistern ➡, high anterior jugular foramen ➡, and the vestibule of the inner ear ➡. Surgical resection is not performed for these lesions.

Ependymoma, CPA

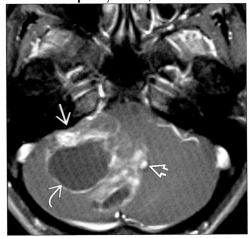

Pseudotumor, Intracranial

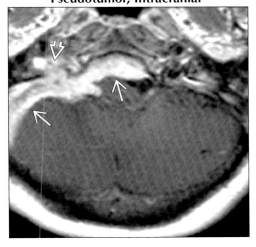

(Left) Axial T1 C+ MR demonstrates an aggressive mixed cystic-solid enhancing ependymoma of the right CPA cistern ➡, 4th ventricle ➡, and cerebellar hemisphere ➡. *(Right)* Axial T1 C+ MR demonstrates an extensive area of enhancing dural thickening ➡ along the right low CPA cistern. The intracranial pseudotumor also involves the subjacent jugular foramen ➡.

Schwannoma, Facial Nerve, CPA-IAC

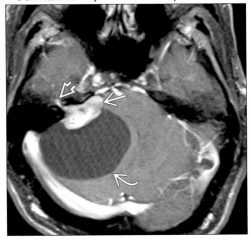

Schwannoma, Jugular Foramen

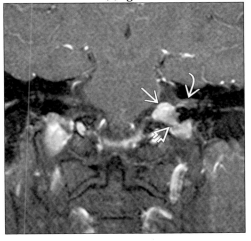

(Left) Axial T1 C+ MR shows a variant facial nerve schwannoma with enhancing CPA-IAC component ➡ extending into the geniculate ganglion ➡. Note associated arachnoid cyst ➡. *(Right)* Coronal T1 C+ FS MR reveals a schwannoma ➡ projecting cephalad from the jugular foramen ➡ into the CPA cistern. Note the normal IAC ➡ is at the level of upper margin of the tumor.

DIFFERENTIAL DIAGNOSIS

Common
- CSF Flow Artifact
- Dolichoectasia (Vertebrobasilar)
- Fusiform Aneurysm, ASVD
- Meningioma
- Metastases, Skull and Meningeal

Less Common
- Epidermoid Cyst
- Chiari 2 ("Creeping Cerebellum")
- Exophytic Brainstem Glioma, Pediatric
- Pituitary Macroadenoma (Giant)
- Neurocysticercosis
- Intracranial Hypotension

Rare but Important
- Inflammatory Mass
  - Tuberculosis
  - Fungal Diseases
  - Neurosarcoid
- Clival Neoplasms
  - Chordoma, Clivus
  - Chondrosarcoma, Skull Base
  - Plasmacytoma, Skull Base
  - Nasopharyngeal Tumor (Invading Clivus)
- Schwannoma
- Arachnoid Cyst
- Craniopharyngioma
- Neurenteric Cyst
- Ecchordosis Physaliphora

ESSENTIAL INFORMATION

Key Differential Diagnosis Issues
- Anatomy
  - Extensive CSF space along ventral & lateral pons, dorsal to clivus (a.k.a. pontine cistern)
  - Bounded superiorly by interpeduncular cistern, inferiorly by subarachnoid space of spinal cord, & continuous about medulla with cerebellomedullary cistern
- Many abnormalities, often from transpatial processes

Helpful Clues for Common Diagnoses
- **CSF Flow Artifact**
  - MR artifacts divided into 2 categories: Time-of-flight effects & turbulent flow
  - Worsens with thinner slices, longer TE, and imaging perpendicular to flow
  - Assess real vs. artifact in other planes
  - Minimize TOF losses: Use short TE, image parallel to flow, acquire thicker slices
- **Dolichoectasia (Vertebrobasilar)**
  - Older patients, ± ASVD in other vessels
  - Ectasia often extends into branches
  - May have significant mass effect on pons
- **Fusiform Aneurysm, ASVD**
  - Long segment fusiform arterial dilatation
  - Involves long nonbranching segments
  - Calcifications common
  - Lumen enhances strongly, clot does not
- **Meningioma**
  - Clival dural-based enhancing mass
  - Infratentorial (8-10%): CPA most common
  - Causes cranial neuropathies or ataxia
- **Metastases, Skull and Meningeal**
  - Enhancing lesion(s) with skull/meningeal destruction/infiltration
  - Manifestations: Smooth thickening, nodularity, loculation, fungating masses
  - Image entire neuraxis!

Helpful Clues for Less Common Diagnoses
- **Epidermoid Cyst**
  - Usually extends medially from CPA cistern
  - Lobulated, insinuating CSF-like mass
  - Doesn't completely suppress on FLAIR; restricts on DWI
- **Chiari 2 ("Creeping Cerebellum")**
  - Small posterior fossa with low torcular herophili
  - Cerebellar hemispheres/tonsils herniate anteriorly → "creeping"
  - Pons, cranial nerve roots often elongated
- **Exophytic Brainstem Glioma, Pediatric**
  - Nonenhancing mass markedly expanding pons; may engulf basilar artery
  - Infiltrative have poor survival
  - Focal are uncommon, better prognosis
- **Pituitary Macroadenoma (Giant)**
  - No distinct pituitary gland
  - Bone CT shows benign bony margins
  - Early intense but heterogeneous CTST+
  - Dural "tail" may mimic meningioma
- **Neurocysticercosis**
  - Cisterns > parenchyma > ventricles
  - Basal cistern cysts may be racemose
  - Cysts variable, typically 1 cm, range from 5-20 mm, contain a 1-4 mm scolex
  - Most are isointense to CSF
- **Intracranial Hypotension**

PREPONTINE CISTERN MASS

- ○ Sagittal shows brain descent in 40-50%
- ○ Pons may be compressed against clivus
- ○ Diffusely, avidly enhancing dura in 85%
- ○ Bilateral subdural fluid collections in 15%

Helpful Clues for Rare Diagnoses
- **Inflammatory Mass**
  - ○ **Tuberculosis**
    - ▪ Basilar meningitis, pulmonary TB
    - ▪ Thick basilar exudate ± tuberculomas/abscesses
  - ○ **Fungal Diseases**
    - ▪ Blastomycosis, coccidiomycosis, histoplasmosis, candidiasis
    - ▪ Meningeal enhancement, multiple enhancing brain lesions
  - ○ **Neurosarcoid**
    - ▪ Classically infiltrates dura, leptomeninges, basal cisterns
    - ▪ Solitary or multifocal CNS mass(es) ± abnormal CXR
- **Clival Neoplasms**
  - ○ **Chordoma, Clivus**
    - ▪ Destructive midline mass centered in clivus with high T2 signal intensity
    - ▪ Sagittal images show tumor "thumb" indenting anterior pons
  - ○ **Chondrosarcoma, Skull Base**
    - ▪ Arises from petrooccipital fissure
    - ▪ ± Extend posterior into prepontine cistern
    - ▪ Hyperintense on T2WI, enhances strongly but heterogeneously
    - ▪ Chondroid mineralization on CT (50%)

- ○ **Plasmacytoma, Skull Base**
  - ▪ Solitary intraosseous osteolytic soft tissue mass with non-sclerotic margins
  - ▪ Peripherally displaced osseous expansion/fragmentation may be seen
- ○ **Nasopharyngeal Tumor (Invading Clivus)**
  - ▪ Often squamous cell carcinoma arising from nasopharyngeal mucosal space
  - ▪ Multiplanar MR images best show invasion of clivus
- **Schwannoma**
  - ○ T2 hyperintense, enhance
- **Arachnoid Cyst**
  - ○ Extra-axial cyst follows CSF attenuation/signal
  - ○ Complete FLAIR suppression; no DWI restriction
- **Craniopharyngioma**
  - ○ 90% Ca++, 90% cystic, 90% enhance
  - ○ May extend behind sella into posterior fossa
- **Neurenteric Cyst**
  - ○ Round/lobulated, nonenhancing, slightly hyperintense to CSF mass
  - ○ Benign malformative endodermal CNS cyst
- **Ecchordosis Physaliphora**
  - ○ Notochord remnant
  - ○ Extends from clivus into prepontine cistern
  - ○ Hyperintense on T2WI

CSF Flow Artifact

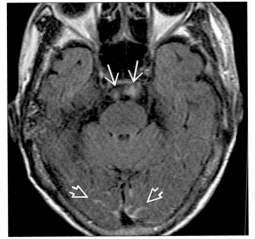

Axial FLAIR MR reveals a hyperintense artifact ➡ due to CSF turbulent flow. Also note sulcal hyperintensity from subarachnoid hemorrhage ➡.

Dolichoectasia (Vertebrobasilar)

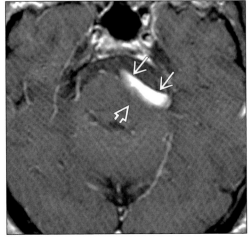

Axial T1 C+ MR demonstrates luminal enhancement of a dolichoectatic basilar artery ➡ with associated deformation of the pons ➡.

10

PREPONTINE CISTERN MASS

(Left) Sagittal T1WI MR shows a large mass anterior to the pons and medulla ➡. Note mixed hyper-, isointense signal caused by slow flow and laminated clot in this classic ASVD fusiform aneurysm. *(Right)* Sagittal T1 C+ MR demonstrates avid meningioma enhancement ➡ as well as enhancing dural tails ➡.

Fusiform Aneurysm, ASVD

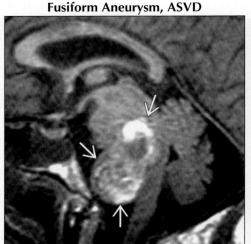

Meningioma

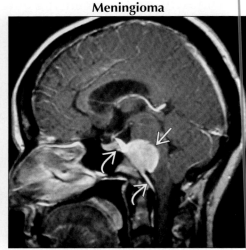

(Left) Axial T1 C+ MR demonstrates extensive renal cell metastatic disease involving the clivus and overlying dura ➡, effacing the prepontine cistern ➡. *(Right)* Axial T1 C+ MR shows a typical MR appearance of leptomeningeal seeding of carcinoma along the folia of the cerebellum and the brainstem ➡, as well as within bilateral Meckel cave ➡.

Metastases, Skull and Meningeal

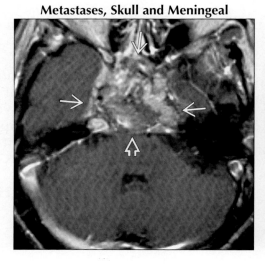

Metastases, Skull and Meningeal

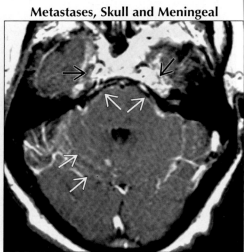

(Left) Sagittal T1WI MR depicts a nearly CSF isointense nonenhancing multilobulated epidermoid within prepontine ➡, interpeduncular, and quadrigeminal cisterns. Note flattening of the pons ➡. *(Right)* Axial T2WI MR shows cerebellar hemispheres herniating or "creeping" ➡ anteriorly due to a congenitally small posterior fossa of Chiari 2.

Epidermoid Cyst

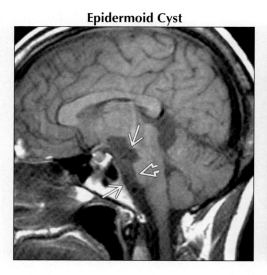

Chiari 2 ("Creeping Cerebellum")

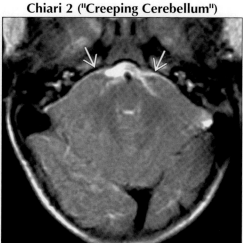

Exophytic Brainstem Glioma, Pediatric

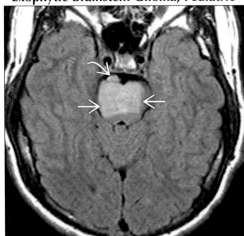

Pituitary Macroadenoma (Giant)

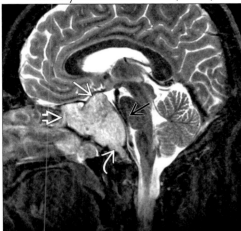

(Left) Axial FLAIR MR shows a diffuse brainstem glioma asymmetrically involving the pons ➜ with a small anterior exophytic component extending into the right prepontine cistern ➔. (Right) Sagittal T2WI MR shows a giant macroadenoma with suprasellar extension ➔, invading anteriorly into basisphenoid ➔ and posteriorly into basi-occiput ➔. Pons and basilar are flattened ➡.

Neurocysticercosis

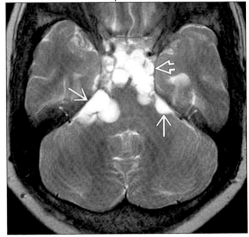

Intracranial Hypotension

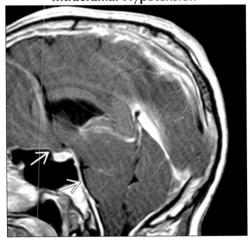

(Left) Axial T2WI MR shows multiple racemose cysts in the subarachnoid spaces including the CPA and quadrigeminal and prepontine cisterns ➔. Also note cysts within suprasellar cistern ➔. (Right) Sagittal T1 C+ MR demonstrates obliteration of the suprasellar and prepontine cisterns ➔ with a sagging midbrain, pontine flattening against the clivus, dural enhancement, and tonsillar descent.

Tuberculosis

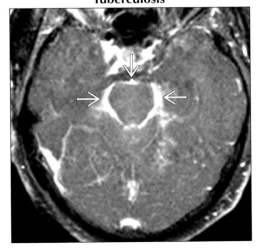

Tuberculosis

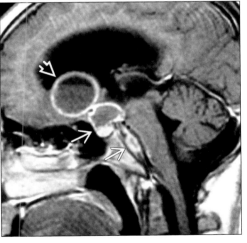

(Left) Axial T1 C+ MR demonstrates typical tuberculosis enhancing exudative meningitis filling the basilar cisterns ➔. (Right) Sagittal T1 C+ MR shows tuberculosis abscesses within the basal and prepontine cisterns ➔ as well as 3rd ventricle ➔.

PREPONTINE CISTERN MASS

(Left) *Axial T1 C+ MR shows thick enhancement in the subarachnoid space and along the pia filling the prepontine cistern* ➡️ *and extending into the left IAC* ➡️. *Diagnosis: Cocci meningitis.* *(Right)* *Axial T1 C+ MR demonstrates fine linear enhancement along the pia* ➡️ *from candida meningitis.*

Fungal Diseases

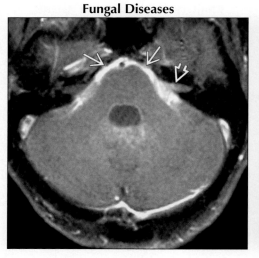

Fungal Diseases

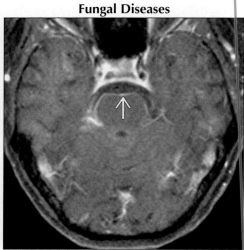

(Left) *Sagittal T1 C+ MR demonstrates a typical neurosarcoid appearance and location with marked multifocal dural-based enhancement* ➡️. *Sella/parasellar and basal cisternal location is classic.* *(Right)* *Sagittal T1 C+ MR shows a "honeycomb" pattern of enhancement with replacement of the clivus* ➡️, *"thumbing" of the pons posteriorly* ➡️, *and anterior extension into the sphenoid sinus* ➡️.

Neurosarcoid

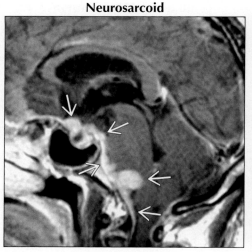

Chordoma, Clivus

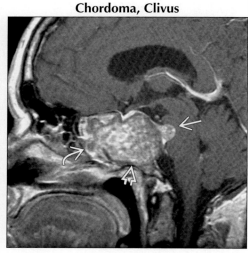

(Left) *Axial T1 C+ MR reveals chondrosarcoma* ➡️ *originating from petrooccipital fissure, extending posterosuperiorly into Meckel cave* ➡️, *prepontine, and cerebellopontine angle cisterns.* *(Right)* *Sagittal T1WI MR demonstrates plasmacytoma* ➡️ *expanding the clivus and elevating the pituitary gland* ➡️.

Chondrosarcoma, Skull Base

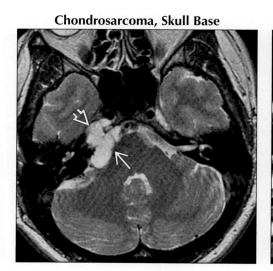

Plasmacytoma, Skull Base

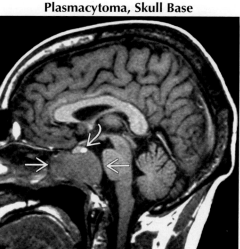

PREPONTINE CISTERN MASS

Nasopharyngeal Tumor (Invading Clivus)

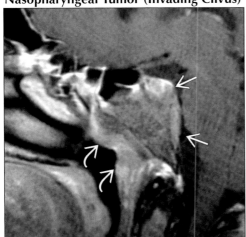

Schwannoma

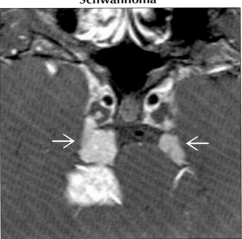

(Left) Sagittal T1 C+ MR demonstrates nasopharyngeal carcinoma infiltration of the pharyngeal mucosal space ➡, as well as abnormal marrow signal and cortical destruction involving an expanded clivus ➡. *(Right)* Axial T1 C+ MR demonstrates bilateral trigeminal ➡ schwannomas in a patient with neurofibromatosis type 2.

Arachnoid Cyst

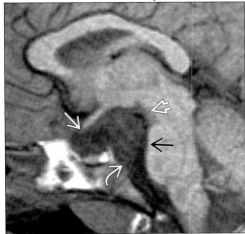

Craniopharyngioma

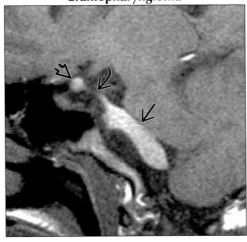

(Left) Sagittal T1WI MR demonstrates a primarily suprasellar cistern arachnoid cyst ➡ extending into the interpeduncular ➡ and prepontine cisterns ➡. Note flattening of the pons ➡. *(Right)* Sagittal T1WI MR demonstrates hyperintense mass in prepontine cistern ➡ that is connected to suprasellar mass ➡ by a thin stalk ➡. Craniopharyngioma was found at surgery. Predominance of tumor mass in posterior fossa is unusual.

Neurenteric Cyst

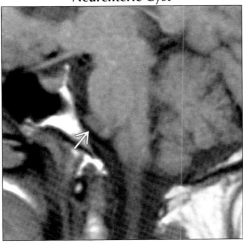

Ecchordosis Physaliphora

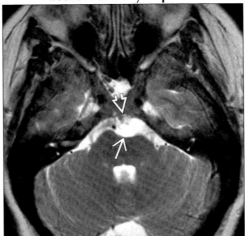

(Left) Sagittal T1WI MR reveals a well-delineated, slightly ovoid, lobulated mass ➡ that was hyperintense to CSF on all sequences. *(Right)* Axial T2WI FS MR shows a lobulated mass in prepontine cistern that indents pons ➡ and is hyperintense to CSF. Note subtle dehiscence of clivus ➡, from which lesion arose.

10

DIFFERENTIAL DIAGNOSIS

Common
- Herniation Syndromes, Intracranial
- Chiari 1
- Chiari 2
- Dandy-Walker Continuum (DWC)

Less Common
- Arachnoid Cyst
- Ependymoma
- Meningioma
- Metastasis
- Intracranial Hypotension

Rare but Important
- Subependymoma
- Epidermoid Cyst
- Dermoid Cyst
- Hemangioblastoma
- Neurenteric Cyst

ESSENTIAL INFORMATION

Key Differential Diagnosis Issues
- Cisterna magna (CM) between medulla (anterior), occiput (posterior) (a.k.a. cerebellomedullary cistern)
  - Below/behind inferior vermis
  - Large medullary cistern masses may extend laterally, posteriorly into CM
- Most common adult lesions are tonsillar associated
  - Indirect (secondary effect on tonsil) > direct (lesion in tonsil)
- MR and clinical information helps DDx

Helpful Clues for Common Diagnoses
- **Herniation Syndromes, Intracranial**
  - Most often 2° to posterior fossa (PF) mass effect
  - Tonsils pushed down into CM
  - "Peg-like" configuration of tonsils
  - Tonsil folia usually oriented horizontally → become vertically oriented when herniated
  - 4th ventricle may obstruct, cause obstructive hydrocephalus
- **Chiari 1**
  - Pointed cerebellar tonsils ≥ 5 mm below foramen magnum
  - Posterior fossa (PF) usually normal size
  - Age-related tonsil descent below "opisthion-basion line" common

- Treatment aim = restore normal CSF flow at foramen magnum (FM)
- **Chiari 2**
  - Small PF → contents shift ↓
  - "Cascade" of tissue (vermis, not tonsil) herniates ↓ through FM
  - ~ 100% associated myelomeningocele
- **Dandy-Walker Continuum (DWC)**
  - DWC a broad spectrum of cystic posterior fossa (PF) malformations
  - DW malformation: Large posterior fossa and large CSF cyst, normal 4th ventricle absent, lambdoid-torcular inversion
  - DW variant: Failure of "closure" of 4th ventricle, vermian hypoplasia
  - Mega cisterna magna: Communicates freely with 4th ventricle, basal subarachnoid spaces
  - 2/3 have associated CNS &/or extracranial anomalies

Helpful Clues for Less Common Diagnoses
- **Arachnoid Cyst**
  - Sharply demarcated extra-axial cyst that follows CSF attenuation/signal
  - FLAIR suppresses; no diffusion restriction
  - Size varies from a few mms to giant
  - Often asymptomatic, found incidentally
  - CPA location > CM
- **Ependymoma**
  - Cellular ependymomas more common in children
  - Soft or "plastic" tumor squeezes out of 4th ventricle foramina into cisterns
  - Ca++ common (50%); ± cysts, hemorrhage
  - Sagittal imaging can distinguish origin as roof vs. floor of 4th ventricle (subependymoma)
  - Heterogeneous T1/T2 signal with mild to moderate enhancement
- **Meningioma**
  - CM rare PF location (CPA, medullary cisterns more common)
  - CM meningiomas usually arise from occipital squamosa
  - Well-demarcated, lobulated/rounded enhancing mass with dural attachment
  - Hyperostosis, tumoral calcifications, ↑ vascular markings
- **Metastasis**
  - Linear or nodular meningeal enhancement

10

CISTERNA MAGNA MASS

- MR CSF flow may be helpful establishing location and degree of CSF obstruction
- Primary tumors include breast, lung, melanoma, prostate
- Lymphoproliferative malignancy = lymphoma and leukemia
- Primary CNS tumor seed basal cisterns (drop metastases)
- Image entire neuroaxis!
- **Intracranial Hypotension**
  - Sagittal shows brain descent in 40-50%
  - Caudal displacement of tonsils in 25-75%
  - Diffusely intensely enhancing dura in 85%
  - Bilateral subdural fluid collections in 15%
  - Frequently misdiagnosed syndrome of headache caused by ↓ intracranial CSF pressure from spontaneous spinal CSF leak

Helpful Clues for Rare Diagnoses
- **Subependymoma**
  - T2 hyperintense lobular, nonenhancing intraventricular mass
  - Arises from 4th ventricle floor, may extend posteroinferiorly into cisterna magna
  - More common in middle-aged, older adults
  - 0.7% of intracranial neoplasms
- **Epidermoid Cyst**
  - Lobulated, irregular, CSF-like mass, "fronds" insinuates cistern
  - FLAIR usually doesn't completely null; diffusion yields high signal restriction
  - 0.2-1.8% of all primary intracranial tumors

- Congenital inclusion cysts; rare malignant degeneration into SCCa
- **Dermoid Cyst**
  - Fat appearance: Use fat-suppression sequence to confirm
  - With rupture find fat droplets in cisterns, sulci, ventricles with extensive MR enhancement possible from chemical meningitis
  - < 0.5% of primary intracranial tumors
  - Rupture can cause significant morbidity/mortality
  - Rare malignant degeneration into squamous cell carcinoma
- **Hemangioblastoma**
  - Intra-axial posterior fossa mass with cyst, enhancing mural nodule abutting pia
  - Classified as meningeal tumor of uncertain histogenesis
  - Familial = von Hippel-Lindau
  - 7-10% of posterior fossa tumors
- **Neurenteric Cyst**
  - Round/lobulated nonenhancing, slightly hyperintense to CSF mass
  - Most intracranial neurenteric cysts found in posterior fossa
  - Benign malformative endodermal CNS cyst
  - Part of split spinal cord malformation spectrum; persistent neurenteric canal
  - Location
    - Thoracic (42%), cervical (32%)
    - Others: Lumbar spine, basilar cisterns, brain parenchyma
    - Anterior medullary, CPA cisterns > CM

Herniation Syndromes, Intracranial

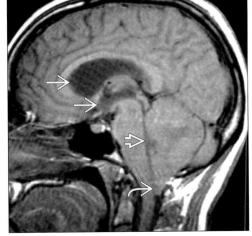

Sagittal T1WI MR shows cerebellar tonsillar herniation ➡ from a large left posterior fossa mass. Note compression of 4th ventricle ➡. Supratentorial ventricles are enlarged ➡.

Chiari 1

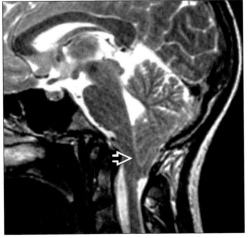

Sagittal T2WI MR shows a classic case of Chiari 1 with pointed cerebellar tonsils ➡ protruding through the foramen magnum and effacing the cisterna magna.

CISTERNA MAGNA MASS

(Left) Sagittal T1WI MR shows caudal descent of cerebellar vermian tissue ⇒ and elongated 4th ventricle ⇒, as well as callosal dysgenesis ⇒ and a small posterior fossa. *(Right)* Sagittal T1WI MR demonstrates markedly enlarged posterior fossa with huge cisterna magna cyst ⇒ in continuity with 4th ventricle. Note upwardly rotated superior vermian remnant ⇒.

Chiari 2
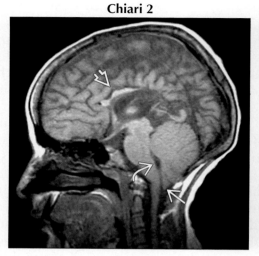

Dandy-Walker Continuum (DWC)
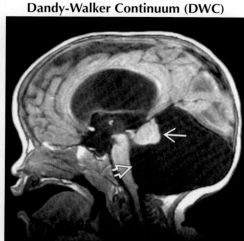

(Left) Sagittal T1WI MR shows a CSF isointense arachnoid cyst ⇒ filling the cisterna magna, flattening the cervicomedullary junction ⇒, and extending caudally into the upper cervical canal. *(Right)* Sagittal T1 C+ MR shows enhancing tissue extruding through the foramen of Magendie, filling cisterna magna ⇒, and causing enlarged cerebral aqueduct ⇒ and a dilated 3rd ventricle ⇒.

Arachnoid Cyst
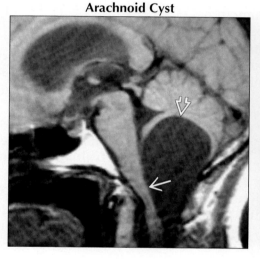

Ependymoma
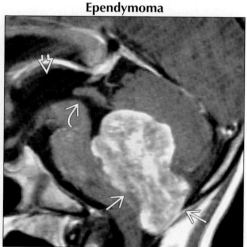

(Left) Sagittal T1WI MR demonstrates dural-based tumor ⇒ with significant mass effect compressing and displacing the cerebellum. Note the trapped CSF clefts ⇒ indicating extra-axial lesion. The tumor encroaches on cisterna magna. *(Right)* Axial T1 C+ MR shows a typical case of primary CNS lymphoma with subependymal tumor spread. Note a posterior fossa mass near the foramen of Luschka ⇒, as well as a 2nd dural-based mass ⇒.

Meningioma
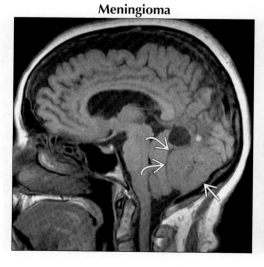

Metastasis
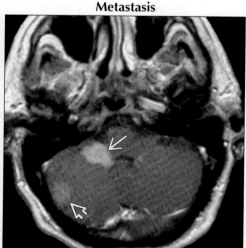

Intracranial Hypotension

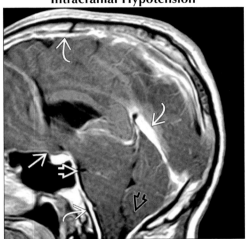

Subependymoma

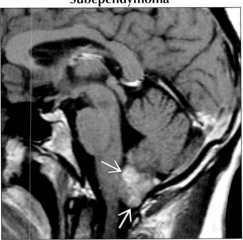

(Left) Sagittal T1 C+ MR shows obliteration of the suprasellar cistern ➡, sagging/fat midbrain with a closed angle between the peduncles and the pons ➡, dural enhancement ➡, and tonsillar descent ➡. *(Right)* Sagittal T1 C+ MR in a 40 year old man shows an enhancing mass at the bottom of the 4th ventricle ➡ filling the cisterna magna.

Epidermoid Cyst

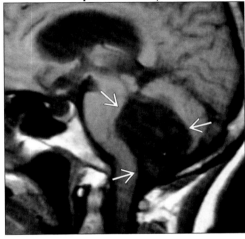

Dermoid Cyst

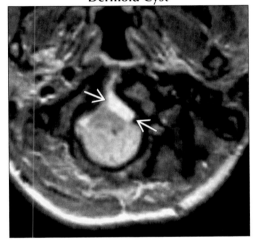

(Left) Sagittal T1WI MR shows a typical case of a large 4th ventricular epidermoid cyst ➡, which follows CSF intensity but is often slightly brighter and mildly heterogeneous in signal. *(Right)* Axial T2WI MR demonstrates a T2 hyperintense mass ➡ encroaching laterally upon the cisterna magna. There was evidence of rupture (not shown) causing recurrent meningitis.

Hemangioblastoma

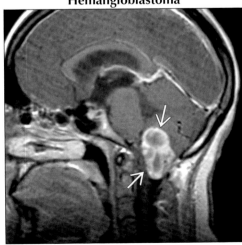

Neurenteric Cyst

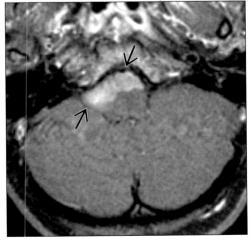

(Left) Sagittal T1 C+ MR demonstrates a mostly solid hemangioblastoma ➡ involving the cerebellar tonsils and effacing the cisterna magna. *(Right)* Axial T1 C+ MR shows a neurenteric cyst encroaching upon the cisterna magna ➡. Although most often these are located anteriorly, when large they may extend posteriorly as in this case.

10

15

DIFFERENTIAL DIAGNOSIS

Common
- Vestibular Schwannoma

Less Common
- Meningioma, CPA-IAC
- Metastases, CPA-IAC
- Metastases, Parenchymal
- Hemangioblastoma
- Other Schwannomas
  - Schwannoma, Trigeminal, Intracranial
  - Schwannoma, Facial Nerve, CPA-IAC
  - Schwannoma, Jugular Foramen
  - Schwannoma, Hypoglossal Nerve
- Subependymoma
- Choroid Plexus Papilloma

Rare but Important
- Astrocytomas
  - Glioblastoma Multiforme (GBM)
  - Anaplastic Astrocytoma
  - Diffuse Astrocytoma, Low-Grade
  - Pilocytic Astrocytoma
- Paraganglioma, Glomus Jugulare
- Dysplastic Cerebellar Gangliocytoma (Lhermitte-Duclos)
- Medulloblastoma (Desmoplastic Variant)
- Hemangiopericytoma
- Lymphoma
- Ecchordosis Physaliphora
- Rosette-Forming Glioneuronal Tumor of the Fourth Ventricle
- Cerebellar Liponeurocytoma

ESSENTIAL INFORMATION

Key Differential Diagnosis Issues
- With exception of vestibular schwannoma, posterior fossa (PF) neoplasms rare in adults
- Most important question: Is lesion intra- or extra-axial?
- Extra-axial
  - Most adult PF neoplasms are extra-axial
  - By far most common is vestibular schwannoma
  - Meningioma > metastasis > other schwannomas > glomus jugulare paraganglioma
- Intra-axial: Parenchymal or intraventricular?
  - Adult parenchymal neoplasms all uncommon/rare
    - Overall most common = metastasis

- Hemangioblastoma most common primary, PF neoplasm
- Astrocytomas, most common supratentorial tumors, rare in PF
  - 4th ventricle
    - Subependymoma > choroid plexus papilloma (CPP)
    - Subependymoma in inferior fourth ventricle (obex)
    - CPP in body/lateral recess, CPA

Helpful Clues for Common Diagnoses
- **Vestibular Schwannoma**
  - By far most common adult posterior fossa neoplasm; all others less common or rare!
  - 90% of all CPA-IAC masses
  - Looks like "ice cream on cone" (CPA-IAC)
  - Extra-axial enhances strongly
  - ± Intra- or extratumoral cysts

Helpful Clues for Less Common Diagnoses
- **Meningioma, CPA-IAC**
  - "Mushroom-shaped," extra-axial mass caps IAC
  - Flat base towards dural surface
  - ± Hyperostosis, dural tail sign
  - 25% show IAC involvement!
- **Metastases, CPA-IAC**
  - CPA metastases can arise in 4 locations
    - Dura-arachnoid
    - Cranial nerves (7, 8 most common)
    - Flocculus
    - Choroid plexus (foramen of Luschka)
  - Irregular, invasive margins
- **Metastases, Parenchymal**
  - 2nd only to vestibular schwannoma as adult PF neoplasm
  - Most common parenchymal PF tumor
  - Rarely solitary brain metastasis!
- **Hemangioblastoma**
  - 95% posterior fossa (hemispheres > > vermis > brainstem, 4th ventricle)
  - < 50% of patients have VHL (look for multiple lesions, visceral cysts, etc.)
  - Imaging
    - 60% nonenhancing cyst + strongly enhancing mural nodule abutting pia
    - 40% solid, ± blood products
- **Other Schwannomas**
  - **Schwannoma, Trigeminal, Intracranial**
    - Upper CPA mass
    - Look for "dumbbell" shape (CPA + Meckel cave components)

- ○ **Schwannoma, Facial Nerve, CPA-IAC**
  - ▪ CPA-IAC mass with "labyrinthine tail"
  - ▪ Look for labyrinthine segment tumor (if absent, can't distinguish from VS)
  - ○ **Schwannoma, Jugular Foramen**
  - ▪ Enhancing mass arising from jugular foramen
  - ▪ Smooth remodeling of bony margins
  - ▪ Projects cephalad into CPA cistern
  - ○ **Schwannoma, Hypoglossal Nerve**
  - ▪ Smooth remodeling of hypoglossal canal
  - ▪ Look for ipsilateral tongue atrophy
- • **Subependymoma**
  - ○ Middle-aged/elderly adult patients
  - ○ Small, asymptomatic nonenhancing mass
  - ○ T2 hyperintense lobulated mass in inferior 4th ventricle (obex)
  - ○ May have cysts, Ca++; hemorrhage rare
- • **Choroid Plexus Papilloma**
  - ○ 40% of CPPs occur in 4th ventricle, CPA
  - ○ Most common CPP location in adults
  - ○ Cauliflower- or frond-like excrescences
  - ○ Avid, relatively uniform enhancement

Helpful Clues for Rare Diagnoses
- • **Astrocytomas**
  - ○ **Glioblastoma Multiforme (GBM)**
  - ▪ Infratentorial GBMs rare
  - ▪ Typically necrotic, ring-enhancing
  - ○ **Anaplastic Astrocytoma**
  - ▪ Also rare; infiltrative, variable enhancement
  - ○ **Diffuse Astrocytoma, Low-Grade**
  - ▪ Young adults

- ○ **Pilocytic Astrocytoma**
  - ▪ Rare in adults
- • **Paraganglioma, Glomus Jugulare**
  - ○ Superolateral into middle ear >> CPA
  - ○ Look for "salt & pepper" "flow voids"
  - ○ Erosive, destructive, infiltrative
- • **Dysplastic Cerebellar Gangliocytoma (Lhermitte-Duclos)**
  - ○ Widened, irregular cerebellar folia with layered/laminated "striped" appearance
  - ○ May cause significant mass effect
  - ○ Typically doesn't enhance (rarely may)
- • **Medulloblastoma (Desmoplastic Variant)**
  - ○ "Desmoplastic" variant more common in 2nd, 3rd decades
  - ▪ Off-midline (lateral cerebellar hemisphere) location
  - ▪ Enhances; CSF spread less common
- • **Ecchordosis Physaliphora**
  - ○ Small, gelatinous tissue mass considered ectopic notochordal remnant
  - ○ Midline of craniospinal axis from dorsum sellae to sacrococcygeal region
  - ○ Clival/retroclival in posterior fossa
  - ○ Found in 2% of autopsies
  - ○ Typically asymptomatic
  - ○ Hypointense on T1WI, hyperintense on T2WI; nonenhancing
  - ○ May involve/erode clivus, ± stalk-like connection to mass

Vestibular Schwannoma

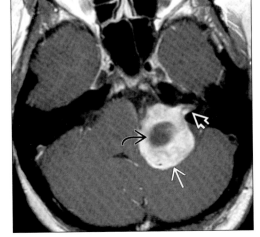

Axial T1 C+ MR shows a large extra-axial enhancing mass ➡ displacing/rotating the pons to the right. Note the extension into IAC ➡ and a central intratumoral cyst ➡.

Meningioma, CPA-IAC

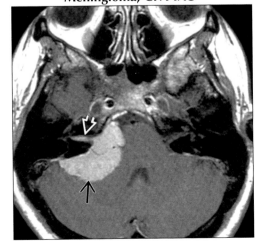

Axial T1 C+ MR shows a large, mushroom-shaped, enhancing mass ➡ in the right CPA cistern. The mass has a broad base towards the dural surface. Note dural tail sign ➡ of reactive meningeal thickening in IAC.

10

Metastases, CPA-IAC

Metastases, Parenchymal

(Left) Axial T2WI MR in a female with breast carcinoma shows a lobulated extra-axial mass in the right flocculus ➡ with associated parenchymal edema ➡. Normal flocculus on left ➡. *(Right)* Coronal T1 C+ MR shows enhancing nodule ➡ with rim-enhancing cyst ➡. This was the only lesion in a patient with known systemic cancer. Lesion resembles a hemangioblastoma (HGB), but the cyst wall in most HGBs is nonneoplastic (nonenhancing compressed cerebellum).

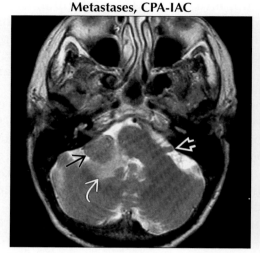
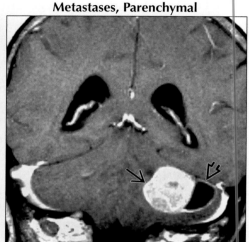

Hemangioblastoma

Schwannoma, Jugular Foramen

(Left) Axial T1 C+ FS MR shows classic hemangioblastoma with solid tumor nodule ➡ abutting pial surface of cerebellum. Associated cyst ➡ does not enhance because wall is a compressed, nonneoplastic cerebellum. *(Right)* Axial T1 C+ MR shows a large solid intensely enhancing extra-axial mass extending into enlarged, smoothly remodeled jugular foramen ➡. Intratumoral cysts, not present in this case, are common in posterior fossa schwannomas.

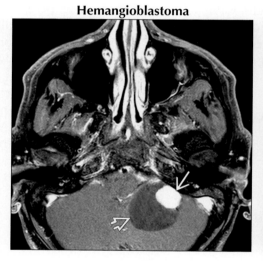
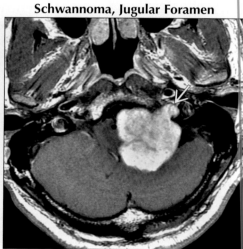

Subependymoma

Choroid Plexus Papilloma

(Left) Sagittal T2WI MR shows a small, mildly hyperintense mass ➡ in the inferior fourth ventricle, found incidentally in this 43 year old male with headache and trigeminal neuralgia. No hydrocephalus was identified. Presumed subependymoma. *(Right)* Coronal T1 C+ MR in a 43 year old female with headaches shows a "speckled" or "bubbly" strongly but heterogeneously enhancing mass in the fourth ventricle ➡ with extension into the lateral recess ➡.

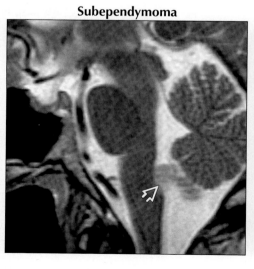
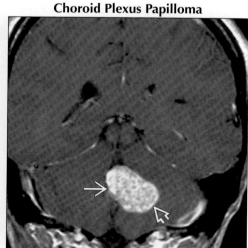

POSTERIOR FOSSA NEOPLASM, ADULT

Anaplastic Astrocytoma
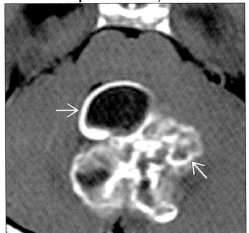

Diffuse Astrocytoma, Low-Grade
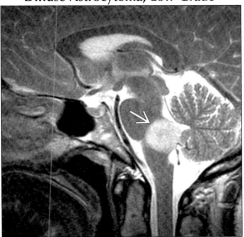

(Left) Axial T1 C+ MR in an older teenager with nausea & vomiting shows inhomogeneously enhancing vermian mass ➡ with cystic, solid components. Preoperative diagnosis was malignant astrocytoma. WHO grade II tumor was found at biopsy, possibly secondary to sampling as this tumor looks nasty! (Right) Sagittal T2WI MR in 25 year old female with lower cranial nerve palsies shows dorsally exophytic pontomedullary mass ➡. Biopsy-proven WHO grade II astrocytoma.

Dysplastic Cerebellar Gangliocytoma (Lhermitte-Duclos)
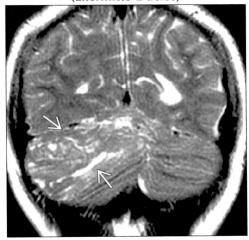

Medulloblastoma (Desmoplastic Variant)
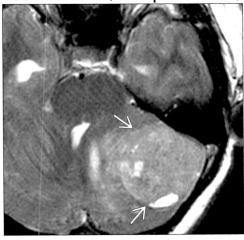

(Left) Coronal T2WI MR shows enlarged, dysplastic-appearing cerebellar folia with striated, mixed hyper-/isointense mass in right cerebellum ➡. (Right) Axial T2WI MR in a 26 year old male shows inhomogeneously hyperintense mass in lateral cerebellum ➡. Mass enhanced heterogeneously. Desmoplastic medulloblastoma is most likely etiology; were this a child, atypical teratoid-rhabdoid tumor would be a consideration.

Hemangiopericytoma
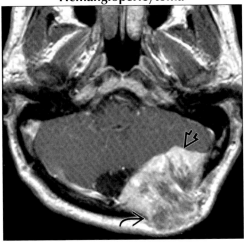

Ecchordosis Physaliphora
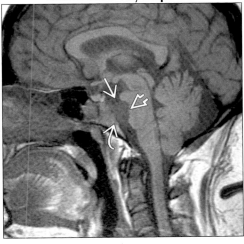

(Left) Axial T1 C+ MR shows a large, inhomogeneously enhancing, destructive, transcalvarial mass with both intracranial ➡ and extracranial ➡ components. (Right) Sagittal T1WI MR shows a midline mass ➡ in front of and indenting the pons ➡. Note the loss of cortical margin in the clivus ➡ from which the mass originates. The mass was extremely hyperintense on T2WI (not shown), consistent with its notochordal remnant origin.

DIFFERENTIAL DIAGNOSIS

Common
- Pilocytic Astrocytoma
- Medulloblastoma (PNET-MB)
- Ependymoma
- Brainstem Glioma, Pediatric

Less Common
- Ganglioglioma
- Schwannoma
- Meningioma, CPA-IAC
- Hemangioblastoma
- Choroid Plexus Papilloma

Rare but Important
- Anaplastic Astrocytoma
- Atypical Teratoid-Rhabdoid Tumor
- Choroid Plexus Carcinoma
- Medulloblastoma Variants
- Medulloepithelioma
- Dysplastic Cerebellar Gangliocytoma

ESSENTIAL INFORMATION

Key Differential Diagnosis Issues
- Most common pediatric posterior fossa (PF) tumors
  - Astrocytomas
    - Pilocytic astrocytoma (PA)
    - Infiltrating "glioma" (astrocytoma, WHO grade II)
  - Medulloblastoma (PNET-MB)
  - Ependymoma
- Imaging
  - Findings on conventional MR overlap
  - Location helpful in differential diagnosis
    - Tectum, cerebellum: PA
    - Pons: Diffusely infiltrating astrocytomas
    - Midline (vermis, 4th ventricle): PNET-MB, PA
    - 4th ventricle + lateral recess/CPA mass: Ependymoma
  - DWI, MRS (normalized to water)
    - Can discriminate between pediatric PF tumors
    - PNET-MB, atypical teratoid-rhabdoid tumor (ATRT) show DWI restriction
  - Examine **entire** neuraxis in child with PF tumor prior to surgery!
    - T1 C+ essential (look for CSF spread)
- History, physical examination (e.g., cutaneous markers) important

Helpful Clues for Common Diagnoses
- **Pilocytic Astrocytoma**
  - Cystic cerebellar mass + mural nodule
  - Solid component low density NECT, high signal T2
- **Medulloblastoma (PNET-MB)**
  - Early childhood: Solid vermis mass extends into, fills, &/or obstructs 4th ventricle
  - Later onset: Lateral cerebellar mass
  - Hypercellular: ↑ Density on NECT, ↓ T2
  - DWI: Restricts
  - 2-5% have nevoid basal cell carcinoma (Gorlin) syndrome (BCCS)
    - Typically seen with desmoplastic variant
    - Look for jaw cysts, bifid ribs, etc.
    - XRT can lead to induced basal cell carcinomas, other intracranial neoplasms within irradiated field
- **Ependymoma**
  - Extrudes through 4th ventricle outlet foramina into cisterns
  - Coarse calcifications
  - Diffusion restriction uncommon, may predict anaplastic behavior
- **Brainstem Glioma, Pediatric**
  - Tectal plate glioma
    - NECT: Increased density progresses to Ca++
    - CECT/MR: Faint or no enhancement
  - Pontine glioma
    - Enlarged pons engulfs basilar artery
    - Enhances late in course, rarely at diagnosis
  - Dorsal exophytic glioma
    - Tumor protrudes into 4th ventricle
    - If large, may be difficult to differentiate from PA
    - Look for FLAIR signal change in dorsal brainstem or peduncles

Helpful Clues for Less Common Diagnoses
- **Ganglioglioma**
  - Brainstem most common PF site
  - Look for expansion of nucleus cuneatus/gracilis
- **Schwannoma**
  - Vestibular schwannoma (ICA/CPA) looks like "ice cream on cone"
  - T2 hyperintensity helps differentiate from meningioma
  - Multiple in NF2
- **Meningioma, CPA-IAC**

○ Broad dural base, covers IAC
○ Variable signal, but T2 hypointensity common
○ Hyperostosis, tumoral calcifications
○ May have intra- or juxtatumoral cyst(s)
• **Hemangioblastoma**
○ Late teen or adult
○ Intra-axial (cerebellum > medulla, cord)
  ▪ Cyst + enhancing nodule > solid
  ▪ Solid component shows flow voids, enhances avidly
  ▪ Multiple lesions diagnostic of von Hippel-Lindau (VHL)
○ Avidly enhancing mural nodule abuts pia
○ Look for visceral cysts of VHL in any child/young adult with hemangioblastoma
• **Choroid Plexus Papilloma**
○ Frond-like 4th ventricle or CPA tumor
○ Avidly enhancing, lobulated mass
○ Hydrocephalus common

Helpful Clues for Rare Diagnoses
• **Anaplastic Astrocytoma**
○ Infiltrating mass involves predominantly white matter
○ Enhancement none to sparse or patchy
○ Ring enhancement suggests progression to GBM
• **Atypical Teratoid-Rhabdoid Tumor**
○ Imaging similar to PNET-MB plus
  ▪ ATRT patients generally younger
  ▪ Cysts, hemorrhage more common
  ▪ CPA involvement more common
  ▪ Frequent metastases at diagnosis

○ Both ATRT, PNET-MB show diffusion restriction
• **Choroid Plexus Carcinoma**
○ Similar to CPP plus
  ▪ Cysts, necrosis, hemorrhage
  ▪ CSF/ependymal/parenchymal spread
• **Medulloblastoma Variants**
○ Desmoplastic medulloblastoma (MB)
  ▪ 5-25% of all medulloblastomas
  ▪ 55-60% of PNET-MBs in children < 3 yo
  ▪ PNET-MB in older children, young adults often desmoplastic variant
  ▪ Desmoplastic subtype of MB in children < 2 is major diagnostic criterion for basal cell nevus syndrome (Gorlin syndrome)
  ▪ Nodular collections of neurocytic cells bounded by desmoplastic zones
  ▪ Lateral (cerebellar) location
○ MB with extensive nodularity (MBEN)
  ▪ Formerly called "cerebellar neuroblastoma"
  ▪ Usually occurs in infants
  ▪ Gyriform or "grape-like" appearance
  ▪ May mature → better prognosis
• **Medulloepithelioma**
○ Rare embryonal brain &/or ocular tumor
○ Inhomogeneous signal, enhancement
• **Dysplastic Cerebellar Gangliocytoma**
○ Diffuse or focal hemispheric mass
○ Thick cerebellar folia with "striated" appearance
○ Evaluate for Cowden syndrome

Pilocytic Astrocytoma

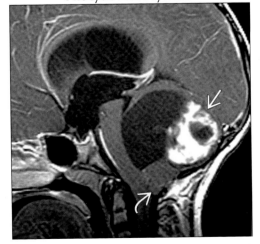

Sagittal T1 C+ MR shows a typical tumor cyst with enhancing mural nodule ➡. There is hydrocephalus and protrusion of the cerebellar tonsils ➡ through the foramen magnum (acquired Chiari 1).

Pilocytic Astrocytoma

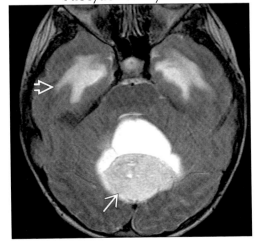

Axial T2WI MR shows increased signal of the solid component ➡ of the mass. Interstitial edema ➡ is present in the temporal lobes.

POSTERIOR FOSSA NEOPLASM, PEDIATRIC

(Left) Sagittal T2WI MR shows a hyperintense mass ➡ filling and expanding the 4th ventricle. The tumor does not extend through the 4th ventricular outlet foramina. There is hydrocephalus with acquired tonsillar herniation ➡. **(Right)** Coronal T1 C+ MR shows heterogeneous enhancement ➡ of the 4th ventricular PNET-MB. Note enlargement of lateral ventricles.

Medulloblastoma (PNET-MB)

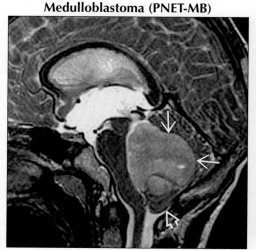

Medulloblastoma (PNET-MB)

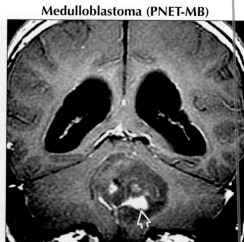

(Left) Sagittal T1WI MR shows a large tumor filling the 4th ventricle ➡ and extruding ➡ through the obex into the upper spinal canal. **(Right)** Axial T2WI MR shows a heterogeneous tumor expanding and extruding through the right foramen of Luschka ➡. There are a few coarse calcific foci ➡ within the tumor.

Ependymoma

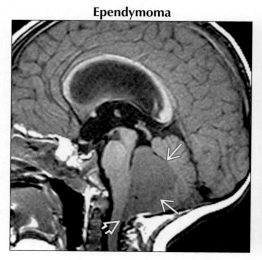

Ependymoma

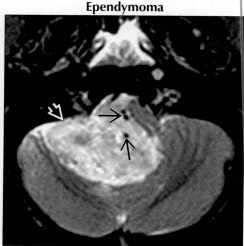

(Left) Sagittal T2WI MR in an infant with a tectal plate glioma shows marked hydrocephalus involving the 3rd and lateral ventricles. The corpus callosum ➡ is stretched thin. The tectal plate ➡ is bulbous and slightly increased in signal intensity. The aqueduct of Sylvius is obstructed ➡. **(Right)** Sagittal T2WI MR in this child with a diffusely infiltrating pontine glioma shows homogeneous high signal intensity of the expanded pons ➡.

Brainstem Glioma, Pediatric

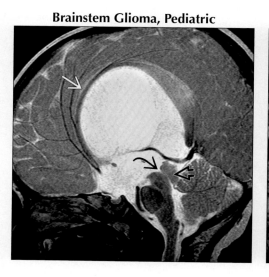

Brainstem Glioma, Pediatric

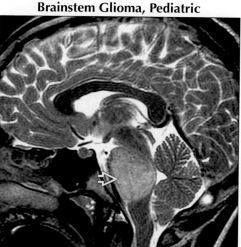

POSTERIOR FOSSA NEOPLASM, PEDIATRIC

Brainstem Glioma, Pediatric

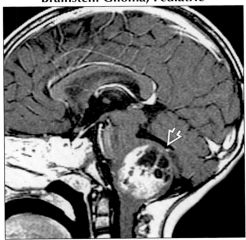

Ganglioglioma

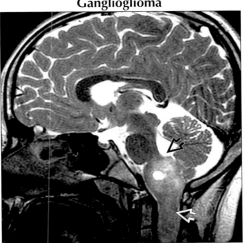

(Left) Sagittal T1 C+ MR shows marked expansion of the medulla ⇉ by a complex mass with intralesional cystic areas and avid, but heterogeneous, enhancement in this child with dorsal exophytic brainstem glioma. The inferior 4th ventricle is deformed by the protruding mass. (Right) Sagittal T2WI MR shows marked expansion of the medulla and upper cervical spinal cord ⇉. The inferior 4th ventricle is deformed ⇉ by the dorsally protruding mass.

Schwannoma

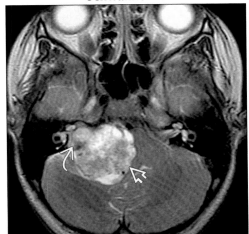

Schwannoma

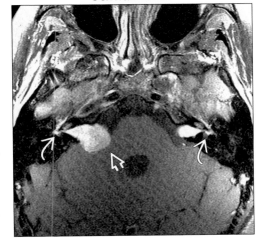

(Left) Axial T2WI MR shows a bulky heterogeneous right cerebellopontine angle mass ⇉, which crosses the midline. There is also extensive remodeling of the right internal auditory canal ⇉ by this schwannoma. (Right) Axial T1 C+ MR in another child shows small bilateral vestibular schwannomas. The right lesion ⇉ assumes the appearance of "ice cream on a cone." Both demonstrate intralabyrinthine extension ⇉.

Meningioma, CPA-IAC

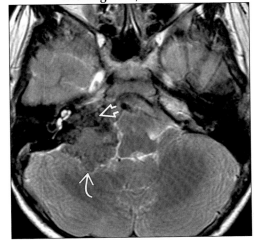

Meningioma, CPA-IAC

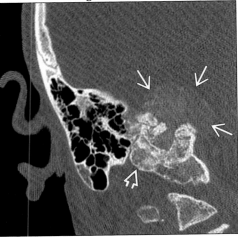

(Left) Axial T2WI MR shows a low signal, lobular cerebellopontine angle mass ⇉ with hyperostosis ⇉ of the adjacent petrous apex. There is mild rotation of the medulla due to mass effect. (Right) Coronal NECT shows diffuse hyperostosis ⇉ adjacent to the meningioma ⇉.

10

23

(Left) Sagittal T2WI MR shows a solid component with multiple flow voids ⇨, a cyst →, and edema of the medulla and upper cervical cord ⇨. *(Right)* Sagittal T1 C+ MR shows the cyst ⇨ to better advantage than the prior T2WI image. Here, the cyst's contents have slightly increased signal.

Hemangioblastoma

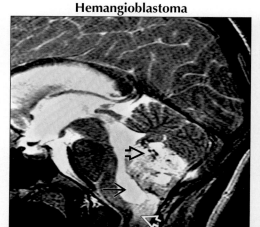

Hemangioblastoma

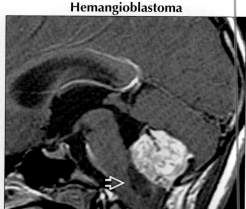

(Left) Axial T2WI MR shows multiple foci of abnormal signal intensity in the peripheral right cerebellar hemisphere and in the cerebellar white matter ➡ adjacent to the lateral recess of the 4th ventricle. *(Right)* Axial T1 C+ MR shows enhancement ➡ following gadolinium administration. The lesion adjacent to the 4th ventricle lateral recess has ill-defined margins.

Anaplastic Astrocytoma

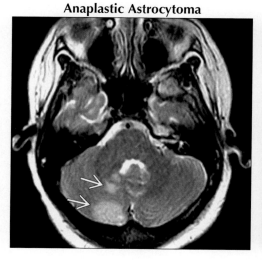

Anaplastic Astrocytoma

(Left) Sagittal T2WI MR shows extensive posterior fossa ⇨, pineal region →, and intraventricular ⇨ low signal intensity masses. Multifocal deposits of tumor at diagnosis are strongly suggestive of an atypical teratoid-rhabdoid tumor. *(Right)* Sagittal T1 C+ MR shows quite variable enhancement of the posterior fossa ⇨, pineal region ➡, and intraventricular ⇨ tumor deposits. There is marked hydrocephalus.

Atypical Teratoid-Rhabdoid Tumor

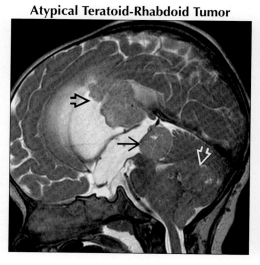

Atypical Teratoid-Rhabdoid Tumor

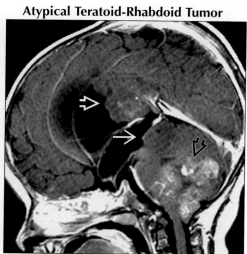

Choroid Plexus Carcinoma

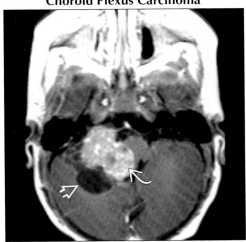

Choroid Plexus Carcinoma

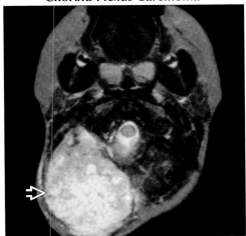

(Left) Axial T1 C+ MR shows a slightly heterogeneous, but avidly enhancing, mass within the right foramen of Luschka ➡. There is an associated cyst ⇒. *(Right)* Axial T2WI MR in a different child undergoing treatment for choroid plexus carcinoma shows a large skull base metastatic deposit ⇒.

Medulloepithelioma

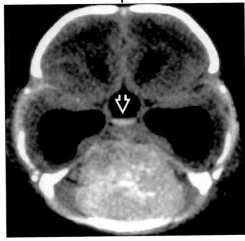

Medulloepithelioma

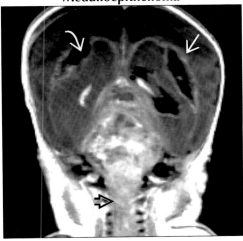

(Left) Axial NECT in a one day old infant shows a dense lobular mass filling the posterior fossa. Foci of increased density superimposed in the mass are due to hemorrhage. Note the blood-CSF level in the dilated infundibular recess ⇒. *(Right)* Coronal T1 C+ MR in the same infant following biopsy shows extension into the spinal canal ⇒. Gas ➡ in the ventricular system follows neurosurgical intervention. There is extensive ependymal seeding ➡.

Dysplastic Cerebellar Gangliocytoma

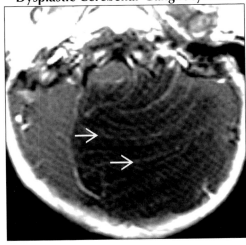

Dysplastic Cerebellar Gangliocytoma

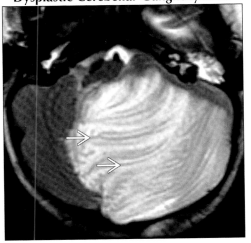

(Left) Axial T1 C+ MR shows a large nonenhancing mass involving the left cerebellar hemisphere. Preservation of the cerebellar folia pattern, or "striated cerebellum" ➡, is characteristic for dysplastic cerebellar gangliocytoma (Lhermitte-Duclos). This disease has a strong association with Cowden syndrome. *(Right)* Axial T2WI MR again shows the pattern of a "striated cerebellum" ➡.

DIFFERENTIAL DIAGNOSIS

Common
- Epidermoid Cyst, CPA-IAC
- Arachnoid Cyst, CPA-IAC

Less Common
- Vestibular Schwannoma with Intramural Cyst(s)
- Neurocysticercosis, CPA
- Hemangioblastoma
- Large Endolymphatic Sac Anomaly (IP-2)

Rare but Important
- Vestibular Schwannoma with Arachnoid Cyst
- Schwannoma, Facial Nerve, CPA-IAC with Cyst
- Neurenteric Cyst
- Schwannoma, Jugular Foramen with Intramural Cyst

ESSENTIAL INFORMATION

Key Differential Diagnosis Issues
- This differential diagnosis is constructed around lesions of CPA that may have cystic manifestation
  - Lesions that are characteristically cystic include epidermoid cyst, arachnoid cyst, neurocysticercosis, large endolymphatic sac anomaly, & neurenteric cyst
  - Many of solid CPA tumors may have either intramural cysts, necrosis, or extramural cysts as normal or variant MR imaging manifestation
    - Schwannoma: Vestibular, facial nerve, or jugular foramen schwannoma with intramural or extramural/arachnoid cyst can all be found in CPA area
    - Cystic meningioma
    - Hemangioblastoma
- Idealized imaging protocol in evaluating cystic CPA mass lesions
  - T1 C+ fat-saturated MR is gold standard
    - Contrast helps differentiate solid from cystic components of tumors such as vestibular or facial nerve schwannoma, meningioma, & hemangioblastoma
    - Use DWI sequence for possible epidermoid (restricted diffusion)
  - T2 thin-section high-resolution MR

- Also sorts out solid and cystic components of lesions
- May help with associated cranial nerve and arterial anatomy

Helpful Clues for Common Diagnoses
- **Epidermoid Cyst, CPA-IAC**
  - Key facts
    - Congenital rest of epithelial tissue in CPA
  - Imaging
    - Insinuating ± scalloping brainstem margin
    - T1 C+ MR: Nonenhancing, cystic appearing; may be difficult to see
    - DWI: Restricted diffusion (high signal) makes diagnosis
- **Arachnoid Cyst, CPA-IAC**
  - Key facts
    - Congenital lesion resulting from failure of embryonic meninges to merge with cyst between split in arachnoid membrane
  - Imaging: Fills cistern with rounded margins
    - T1 C+ MR: No enhancement
    - Other MR: FLAIR attenuates; DWI: No restricted diffusion

Helpful Clues for Less Common Diagnoses
- **Vestibular Schwannoma with Intramural Cyst(s)**
  - Key facts
    - Vestibular schwannoma may have either intramural or extramural (arachnoid cyst) cysts
  - Imaging
    - Solid CPA-IAC mass with intramural cysts
    - T1 C+ MR: Enhancing solid tumor component ± intramural cysts (common) ± arachnoid cyst (rare)
- **Neurocysticercosis, CPA**
  - Key facts
    - Intracranial infection caused by pork tapeworm (*Taenia solium*)
  - Imaging
    - Cysts with "dots" inside
    - Appearance varies with stage
    - T1 C+ MR: Cysts with enhancing thin or thick wall
- **Hemangioblastoma**
  - Key facts

CYSTIC CPA MASS

- Adult with intra-axial posterior fossa mass abutting pia
  - Imaging
    - Cerebellar cystic & solid tumor
    - T1 C+ MR: 60% of tumors with solid enhancing & cystic components (40% solid only)
- **Large Endolymphatic Sac Anomaly (IP-2)**
  - Key facts
    - Bilateral congenital sensorineural hearing loss that appears in child with cascading hearing loss pattern
    - Most common congenital imaging abnormality
  - Imaging
    - CT: Enlarged bony vestibular aqueduct
    - T2 high-resolution MR: Enlarged endolymphatic sac + mild cochlear aplasia (modiolar deficiency, bulbous apical turn, scalar chamber asymmetry)

Helpful Clues for Rare Diagnoses

- **Vestibular Schwannoma with Arachnoid Cyst**
  - Key facts
    - Vestibular schwannoma with extramural (arachnoid cyst) cyst
    - Neuro-otologists refer to as "herald cyst"
  - Imaging
    - CPA-IAC mass with extramural cyst
    - T1 C+ MR: Enhancing solid tumor component rare ± arachnoid cyst
- **Schwannoma, Facial Nerve, CPA-IAC with Cyst**
  - Key facts
    - Rare CPA-IAC mass with "labyrinthine tail" involving labyrinthine segment of facial nerve canal
    - Often present with hearing loss before facial nerve symptoms
  - Imaging
    - CT: Labyrinthine segment CN7 may be enlarged
    - T1 C+ MR: Enhancing tubular mass in CPA-IAC & labyrinthine segment of facial nerve; intramural or extramural cyst visible
- **Neurenteric Cyst**
  - Key facts
    - Incidental rounded to ovoid mass in prepontine cistern
  - Imaging
    - MR shows intermediate to high signal T1 prepontine mass
- **Schwannoma, Jugular Foramen with Intramural Cyst**
  - Key facts
    - Presents with some mixture of 9-12 cranial neuropathy
  - Imaging
    - Bone CT: Enlarged sharply marginated jugular foramen
    - T1 C+ MR shows enhancing mass with intramural cysts arising from jugular foramen & projecting superomedially into CPA cistern, often with brainstem compression

Epidermoid Cyst, CPA-IAC

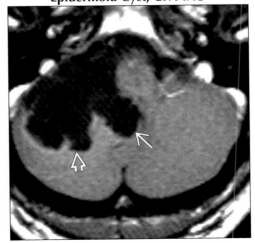

Axial T1 C+ MR reveals a low signal epidermoid cyst that insinuates into foramen of Luschka ➡ and cerebellar hemisphere ➡. DWI MR sequence would show restricted diffusion.

Arachnoid Cyst, CPA-IAC

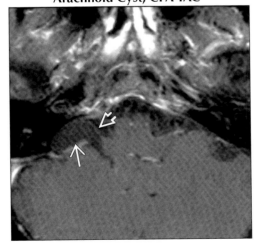

Axial T1 C+ FS MR demonstrates a right CPA cistern arachnoid cyst ➡ displacing the proximal facial and vestibulocochlear nerves anteriorly ➡.

CYSTIC CPA MASS

Vestibular Schwannoma with Intramural Cyst(s)

Vestibular Schwannoma with Intramural Cyst(s)

(Left) Axial T1 C+ MR shows a large enhancing vestibular schwannoma projecting from the IAC ➡ into the CPA. The tumor has a large intramural cyst ⬂ and compresses the brainstem and cerebellum. *(Right)* Axial T1 C+ MR reveals the inferior aspect of a large enhancing vestibular schwannoma in the left CPA cistern. An unusually prominent intramural cyst ⬂ is present.

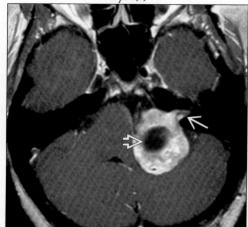
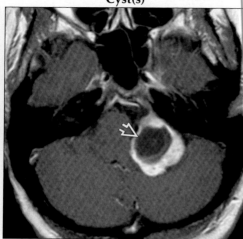

Neurocysticercosis, CPA

Neurocysticercosis, CPA

(Left) Axial T1 C+ FS MR demonstrates a cystic mass in the right cerebellopontine angle cistern with an enhancing wall ➡. Adjacent enhancing thickened meninges ⬂ also seen. *(Right)* Coronal T1 C+ FS MR shows multiple cysts in the right cerebellopontine angle cistern ➡ causing mass effect on the brainstem. Secondary hydrocephalus is present.

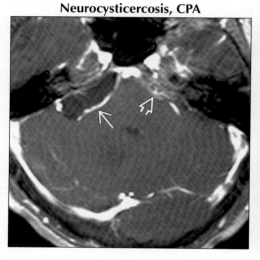
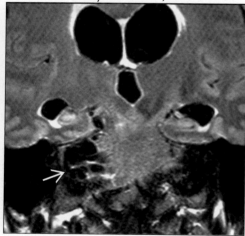

Hemangioblastoma

Hemangioblastoma

(Left) Axial T1 C+ FS MR shows an intracerebellar mixed cystic-solid hemangioblastoma projecting into the left cerebellopontine angle cistern area. The solid nodule is avidly enhancing ➡. *(Right)* Axial T2WI MR reveals an intracerebellar high signal hemangioblastoma projecting into the cerebellopontine angle cistern area. Contrast is required to define enhancing nodule if present.

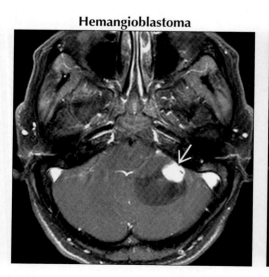

CYSTIC CPA MASS

Large Endolymphatic Sac Anomaly (IP-2)

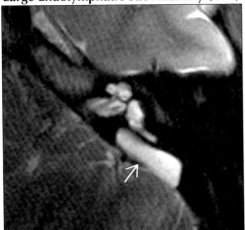

Vestibular Schwannoma with Arachnoid Cyst

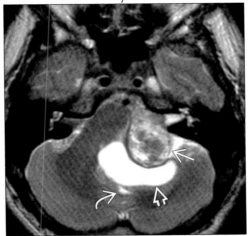

(Left) Axial T2WI MR shows a large endolymphatic sac ➡ within the posterior wall of the temporal bone. CT would reveal a large bony vestibular aqueduct in this patient with large endolymphatic sac anomaly. *(Right)* Axial T2WI MR shows a vestibular schwannoma ➡ projecting from the IAC into the CPA cistern. An associated arachnoid cyst is visible ➡ compressing the brainstem and 4th ventricle ➡.

Schwannoma, Facial Nerve, CPA-IAC with Cyst

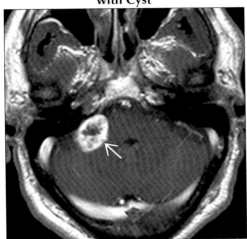

Neurenteric Cyst

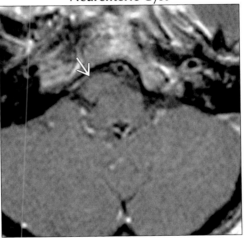

(Left) Axial T1 C+ MR reveals a cerebellopontine angle enhancing tumor ➡ with prominent intramural cysts. The lesion did project into the IAC but did not involve the labyrinthine facial nerve. *(Right)* Axial T1WI MR shows a small mass anterior to the pontomedullary junction ➡. The neurenteric cyst is well delineated and does not enhance significantly.

Schwannoma, Jugular Foramen with Intramural Cyst

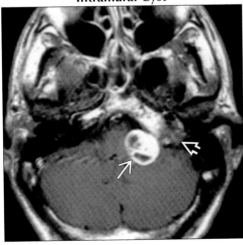

Schwannoma, Jugular Foramen with Intramural Cyst

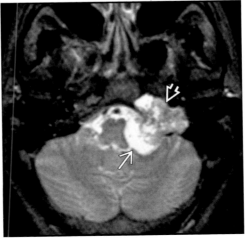

(Left) Axial T1 C+ MR demonstrates an ovoid enhancing mass in low CPA cistern ➡. Multiple intramural cysts suggest the diagnosis of schwannoma. Extension into jugular foramen is evident ➡. *(Right)* Axial T2WI FS MR reveals a large sharply marginated lesion in the jugular foramen ➡. The high signal mass projects medially into the low CPA cistern where it compresses the brainstem ➡.

DIFFERENTIAL DIAGNOSIS

Common
• Vascular Loop Syndrome, CPA-IAC

Less Common
• Epidermoid Cyst, CPA-IAC
• Meningioma, CPA-IAC
• Aneurysm, CPA-IAC
• Schwannoma, Facial Nerve, CPA-IAC
• Schwannoma, Facial Nerve, T-Bone
• Perineural Tumor, CN7, Parotid Space
• Hemangioma, Facial Nerve, T-Bone

Rare but Important
• Multiple Sclerosis
• Arteriovenous Malformation
• Cerebral Ischemia-Infarction, Acute
• Hemangioma, IAC

ESSENTIAL INFORMATION

Key Differential Diagnosis Issues
• Overall statistics
  ○ > 95% of the time, arterial vascular loop is cause of hemifacial spasm
  ○ All other causes listed above (< 5%)
• Hemifacial spasm (HFS)
  ○ HFS definition: Segmental myoclonus of muscles of the face innervated by facial nerve
  ○ HFS presentation: 50-80 year olds, unilateral; begins around eye, spreading gradually to other facial muscles
  ○ Principal symptom: Rhythmic involuntary myoclonic facial muscle contractions
  ○ Pathophysiology: Irritation of facial nerve or facial nucleus
• Vascular loop syndrome, facial nerve
  ○ By far most common cause of HFS
    ▪ Aberrant or ectatic vessels in cistern (AICA, VA, PICA, SCA)
  ○ Anterior inferior cerebellar artery most common offending artery (40-50%)
  ○ Vertebral artery alone or in combination with posterior inferior cerebellar artery less commonly responsible
  ○ High-resolution MR-MRA can now identify compressive aberrant or ectatic arteries routinely

Helpful Clues for Common Diagnoses
• **Vascular Loop Syndrome, CPA-IAC**
  ○ Negative high-resolution MR exam does not preclude surgery for smaller vascular loop causing HFS
  ○ MR-MRA: Asymmetric looping artery impinges on CN7 root exit zone in CPA
  ○ AICA, VA, PICA, SCA all possible culprits

Helpful Clues for Less Common Diagnoses
• **Epidermoid Cyst, CPA-IAC**
  ○ Morphology: Assumes shape of cistern it occupies; insinuating margins
  ○ MR: Near CSF intensity makes difficult to see on T1, T2, & FLAIR sequences
    ▪ DWI shows restricted diffusion
• **Meningioma, CPA-IAC**
  ○ Morphology: Dural-based sessile mass
  ○ Bone CT: Bony hyperostosis possible
  ○ MR: Enhancing mass with dural tail(s)
• **Aneurysm, CPA-IAC**
  ○ Morphology: Ovoid or fusiform shape
  ○ MR: Complex lesion signal from wall calcification, clot, and flow
• **Schwannoma, Facial Nerve, CPA-IAC**
  ○ Morphology: CPA-IAC "ice cream on cone" and labyrinthine segment tail
  ○ Bone CT: Labyrinthine segment CN7 enlarged
  ○ MR: Enhancing tubular mass with tail; may have intramural cysts
• **Schwannoma, Facial Nerve, T-Bone**
  ○ Morphology: Tubular mass within enlarged facial nerve canal may pedunculate into middle ear cavity (tympanic segment CN7) or mastoid air cells (mastoid segment CN7)
  ○ Bone CT: Obvious enlargement of CN7 canal
    ▪ Geniculate ganglion most commonly affected
  ○ MR: Enhancing mass enlarges bony facial nerve canal
• **Perineural Tumor, CN7, Parotid Space**
  ○ Morphology: Enlargement of intratemporal CN7 connected through stylomastoid foramen with invasive parotid malignancy
  ○ Bone CT: Enlargement of bony CN7 canal
    ▪ Mastoid segment most common
  ○ MR: Enhancing minimally enlarged intratemporal CN7
    ▪ Mastoid segment 1st involved
• **Hemangioma, Facial Nerve, T-Bone**

- Morphology: Amorphous geniculate ganglion area mass
- Bone CT: "Honeycomb bone" matrix (50%)
- MR: Avidly enhancing mass with low signal foci

Helpful Clues for Rare Diagnoses

- **Multiple Sclerosis**
  - Hemifacial spasm is rare presentation of multiple sclerosis
  - MR: T2/FLAIR ↑ signal supratentorial white matter plaques
    - Plaques in vicinity of facial nerve nucleus in floor of 4th ventricle may not be seen
- **Arteriovenous Malformation**
  - More commonly supratentorial
  - MR: Large ectatic arterial flow voids
    - Enhancing nidus on T1 C+ fat-saturated sequence
    - Large draining veins
- **Cerebral Ischemia-Infarction, Acute**
  - Acute onset brainstem-related symptoms
    - Pontine CVA secondary to basilar artery perforator injury
  - MR: DWI shows restricted diffusion in pons with ADC map mirrored low signal
- **Hemangioma, IAC**
  - Morphology: Distal intracanalicular (IAC) ovoid to round mass
  - Bone CT: Tumor matrix with punctate calcifications
  - MR: Enhancing IAC lesion with focal low signal areas (calcifications)

Alternative Differential Approaches

- Radiologist generally searches for cause of cranial neuropathy by following cranial nerve from origin to functional endplate
  - Such an anatomic approach permits segmentation of potential causes into anatomic groups
- Anatomic delineation of HFS causes
  - Three general anatomic sites where facial nerve may be injured causing hemifacial spasm
    - Intra-axial (nuclear)
    - Cisternal (CPA or IAC cistern)
    - Intratemporal (intratemporal facial nerve canal)
- Intra-axial (nuclear)
  - Arteriovenous malformation
  - Cerebral ischemia-infarction, acute
  - Multiple sclerosis
- Cisternal (CPA or IAC cistern)
  - Vascular loop syndrome, CPA-IAC
  - Epidermoid cyst, CPA-IAC
  - Meningioma, CPA-IAC
  - Aneurysm, CPA-IAC
  - Schwannoma, facial nerve, CPA-IAC
  - Hemangioma, IAC
- Intratemporal (intratemporal CN7 canal)
  - Schwannoma, facial nerve, T-bone
  - Hemangioma, facial nerve, T-bone
  - Perineural parotid malignancy, T-bone

Vascular Loop Syndrome, CPA-IAC

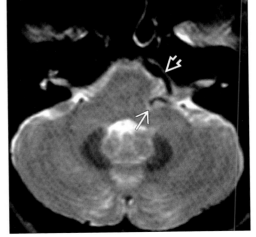

Axial T2WI MR shows a markedly asymmetric left vertebral artery ➡ lifting the posterior inferior cerebellar artery ➡ into the medial aspect of the CPA cistern in the CN7 root exit zone vicinity.

Vascular Loop Syndrome, CPA-IAC

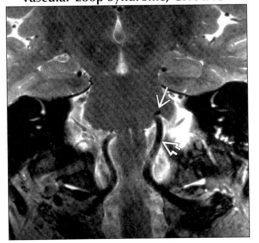

Coronal T2WI MR shows an ectatic vertebral artery ➡ "lifting" the posterior inferior cerebellar artery into the root exit zone of the facial nerve ➡. Note compression of lateral pons.

HEMIFACIAL SPASM

(Left) Axial T2WI MR shows right CPA cistern epidermoid cyst ➥ scalloping the cerebellar contour and bowing the cisternal facial nerve anteriorly ➥. The root exit zone is also affected ➥. (Right) Axial T2WI MR demonstrates right CPA cistern epidermoid cyst with penetration of porus acusticus ➥ and lobulated mass effect on the lateral margin of the brachium pontis ➥.

Epidermoid Cyst, CPA-IAC

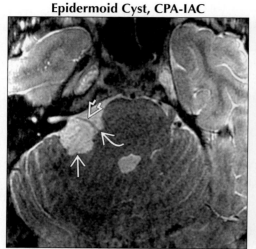

Epidermoid Cyst, CPA-IAC

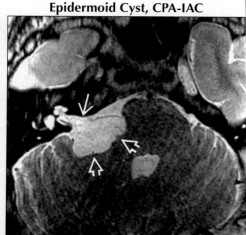

(Left) Axial T2WI MR reveals a dural-based CPA mass with IAC penetration ➥ with a "CSF-vascular cleft" ➥ between it and the adjacent brachium pontis-pons. Note the normal root exit zone CN7 ➥. (Right) Axial T1WI MR shows a complex signal associated with a vertebral artery aneurysm ➥. The aneurysm is wedged into the medial CPA cistern in the immediate vicinity of the CN7 root exit zone.

Meningioma, CPA-IAC

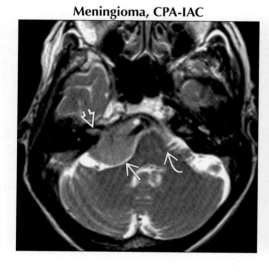

Aneurysm, CPA-IAC

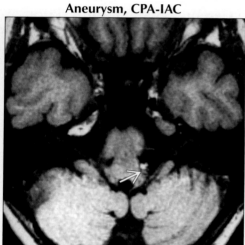

(Left) Axial T1 C+ MR shows a small facial nerve schwannoma of the lateral internal auditory canal ➥, labyrinthine segment ➥, and geniculate ganglion ➥ portions of the facial nerve. (Right) Axial T1 C+ MR demonstrates a mastoid segment facial nerve schwannoma ➥. Notice the enhancing tumor has dehisced the posterior wall of the external auditory canal ➥.

Schwannoma, Facial Nerve, CPA-IAC

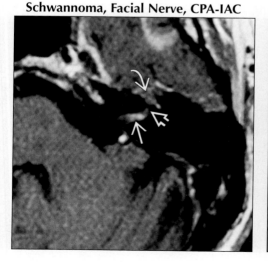

Schwannoma, Facial Nerve, T-Bone

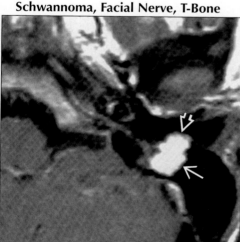

HEMIFACIAL SPASM

Perineural Tumor, CN7, Parotid Space

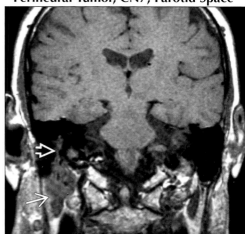

Hemangioma, Facial Nerve, T-Bone

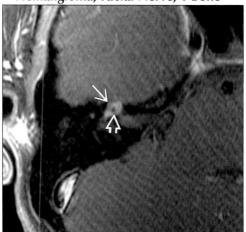

(Left) Coronal T1WI MR shows invasive parotid space malignancy ➡ with perineural tumor spread cephalad through the stylomastoid foramen to involve the mastoid segment of the facial nerve ➡. *(Right)* Axial T1 C+ FS MR shows an enhancing lesion ➡ within enlarged geniculate fossa. Note the black central dot of calcification ➡ suggesting the diagnosis of facial nerve hemangioma.

Multiple Sclerosis

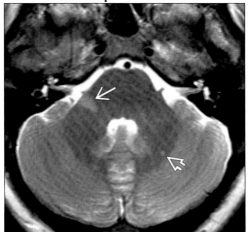

Arteriovenous Malformation

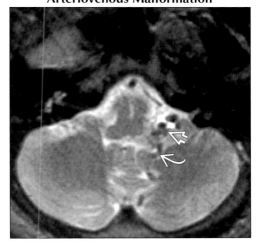

(Left) Axial T2WI MR shows a multiple sclerosis plaque ➡ situated in the lateral pons near the root exit zone of the facial nerve. Note a 2nd more subtle plaque cerebellar lesion ➡. *(Right)* Axial T2WI MR shows a left cerebellopontine cistern arteriovenous malformation nidus ➡ with a large posterior draining vein ➡.

Cerebral Ischemia-Infarction, Acute

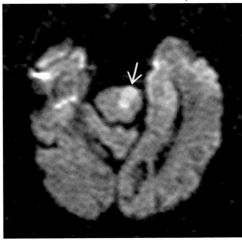

Hemangioma, IAC

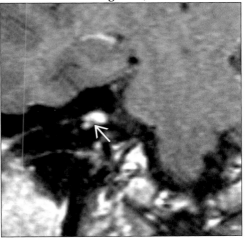

(Left) Axial DWI MR shows left pontine acute CVA ➡ as a high signal area of restricted diffusion. Patients with brainstem strokes may develop hemifacial spasm in the subacute to chronic phase. *(Right)* Coronal T1 C+ MR reveals a calcified internal auditory canal hemangioma as a lateral IAC enhancing mass with subtle evidence of intratumoral calcification ➡.

SENSORINEURAL HEARING LOSS IN ADULT

DIFFERENTIAL DIAGNOSIS

Common
- Vestibular Schwannoma
- Meningioma, CPA-IAC
- Epidermoid Cyst, CPA-IAC
- Aneurysm, CPA-IAC
- Fracture, T-Bone

Less Common
- Cochlear Otosclerosis
- Metastases, CPA-IAC
- Schwannoma, Facial Nerve, CPA-IAC
- Lipoma, CPA-IAC
- Large Endolymphatic Sac Anomaly (IP-2)
- Schwannoma, Intralabyrinthine
- Labyrinthitis
- Neuritis, Vestibulocochlear
- Paget Disease, T-Bone
- Fibrous Dysplasia, T-Bone

Rare but Important
- Endolymphatic Sac Tumor
- Sarcoidosis, CPA-IAC
- Superficial Siderosis, CPA-IAC
- Hemangioma, IAC
- Ramsay Hunt Syndrome

ESSENTIAL INFORMATION

Key Differential Diagnosis Issues
- Many diagnoses may cause sensorineural hearing loss (SNHL)
- Important to know relative statistical incidence of major diagnoses in this list
  - Vestibular schwannoma: 90% of all lesions causing SNHL
  - CPA meningioma, epidermoid cyst, aneurysm: 5% of all lesions causing SNHL
  - All other diagnoses in SNHL differential diagnosis list: 5%
- Best imaging tool
  - MR best for SNHL patients
    - High-resolution, thin slice (< 1 mm) T2: Best for surgical anatomy, nerve of origin, and fundal CSF cap (vestibular schwannoma)
    - Enhanced T1 fat-saturated: Helps make labyrinthitis, vestibular neuritis, Ramsay Hunt syndrome diagnoses

Helpful Clues for Common Diagnoses
- **Vestibular Schwannoma**
  - Morphology: "Ice cream on cone"-shaped mass aligned with CPA-IAC
  - T1 C+ MR: Enhancing lesion ± intramural cysts
- **Meningioma, CPA-IAC**
  - Morphology: Dural-based sessile mass often asymmetric to porus acusticus
  - T1 C+ MR: Enhancing mass ± dural tails ± CSF-vascular cleft between mass and brainstem
- **Epidermoid Cyst, CPA-IAC**
  - Morphology: Insinuating with brainstem margin "scalloping"
  - T1 C+ MR: Nonenhancing mass may be difficult to see
  - Diffusion weighted imaging: Restricted diffusion (high signal) makes diagnosis
- **Aneurysm, CPA-IAC**
  - Morphology: Ovoid or fusiform CPA mass; rarely IAC
  - T1 and T1 C+ MR: Complex signal mass from wall calcification, clot, and flow
  - MRA, CTA, or angiography can confirm diagnosis
- **Fracture, T-Bone**
  - T-bone CT essential
  - Transverse or longitudinal fracture crosses inner ear structures
  - Pneumolabyrinth may be associated

Helpful Clues for Less Common Diagnoses
- **Cochlear Otosclerosis**
  - CT: Radiolucent foci in bony labyrinth
  - T1 C+ MR: Multiple enhancing foci in bony labyrinth
- **Metastases, CPA-IAC**
  - T1 C+ MR: Multiple enhancing lesions involving flocculus, choroid plexus, arachnoid-dura, or pia
- **Schwannoma, Facial Nerve, CPA-IAC**
  - CT: Labyrinthine segment facial nerve canal enlarged
  - T1 C+ MR: Enhancing tubular mass affects CPA-IAC and labyrinthine segment of facial nerve
- **Lipoma, CPA-IAC**
  - CT: Fatty lesion of CPA, IAC ± inner ear
  - T1 MR: High signal lesion as above; fat saturation makes lesion disappear
- **Large Endolymphatic Sac Anomaly (IP-2)**
  - CT: Large bony vestibular aqueduct + mild cochlear dysplasia

SENSORINEURAL HEARING LOSS IN ADULT

- ○ MR: Large endolymphatic sac and duct
- **Schwannoma, Intralabyrinthine**
  - ○ T1 C+ MR: Intralabyrinthine enhancing lesion
    - Intracochlear, intralabyrinthine, vestibulocochlear, transmodiolar, transmacular, and transotic types
- **Labyrinthitis**
  - ○ T1 C+ MR: Diffuse (less commonly focal) enhancement of labyrinth
    - Facial or vestibulocochlear nerves may also enhance
- **Neuritis, Vestibulocochlear**
  - ○ T1 C+ MR: Linear enhancement in CPA-IAC cisterns
- **Paget Disease, T-Bone**
  - ○ Clinical: Patient over 50 years of age
  - ○ CT: Expansile bony lesion with "cotton-wool" appearance; may involve otic capsule
  - ○ T1 C+ MR: Heterogeneous enhancement within expanded T-bone, skull base, and calvarium
- **Fibrous Dysplasia, T-Bone**
  - ○ Clinical: Patient under 30 years of age
  - ○ CT: Expansile lesion with mixed ground-glass/sclerotic and cystic components; spares otic capsule
  - ○ MR: Expansile lesion with low signal components on most sequences
    - T1 C+ MR: Heterogeneous mixture of avid enhancement mixed with areas of minimal to no enhancement

Helpful Clues for Rare Diagnoses

- **Endolymphatic Sac Tumor**
  - ○ Tumor centered in endolymphatic duct or sac area of posterior T-bone
  - ○ CT: Spiculated or coarse calcifications within tumor matrix with thin posterior marginal calcification
  - ○ T1 MR: Multifocal high signal tumor foci (blood products in tumor matrix)
- **Sarcoidosis, CPA-IAC**
  - ○ Laboratory: CSF lymphocystosis; increased blood angiotensin converting enzyme (ACE)
  - ○ Morphology: En plaque, nodular, or linear masses
  - ○ T1 C+ MR: Multifocal dural-based enhancing lesions
- **Superficial Siderosis, CPA-IAC**
  - ○ Clinical: Bilateral SNHL with ataxia
  - ○ T* GRE MR: Blooming dark signal (hemosiderin) along surface of cerebellum and cranial nerves
  - ○ MR: May identify site of chronic oozing: Surgical site, aneurysm, tumor, or AVM
- **Hemangioma, IAC**
  - ○ CT: Punctate calcification in IAC lesion
  - ○ T1 C+ MR: Enhancing lesion in IAC with focal low signal areas (calcifications)
- **Ramsay Hunt Syndrome**
  - ○ Clinical: External ear vesicles characteristic ± CN7 or CN8 neuropathy
  - ○ T1 C+ MR: Linear enhancing foci in IAC

Vestibular Schwannoma

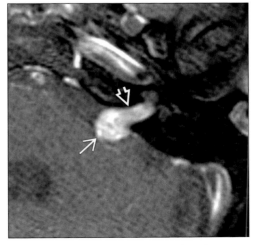

Axial T1 C+ FS MR shows typical mid-sized CPA-IAC vestibular schwannoma. "Ice cream" (CPA component) ➡ "on cone" (IAC component) ⊃ morphology is highly suggestive of this diagnosis.

Meningioma, CPA-IAC

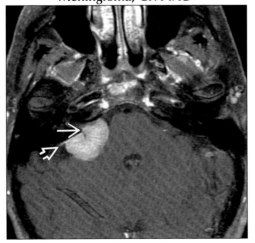

Axial T1 C+ FS MR shows the sessile morphology of meningioma as it "sits" on the posterior T-bone wall. Note the characteristic dural tail ⊃ and dural artery ➡ feeding the tumor center.

SENSORINEURAL HEARING LOSS IN ADULT

Epidermoid Cyst, CPA-IAC

(Left) Axial DWI MR shows a CPA epidermoid identified by its restricted diffusion ➥. CPA epidermoids often are not directly over the porus acusticus, as in this case. *(Right)* Axial T2WI MR shows vertebral artery aneurysm as an ovoid mass ➡ with complex signal in the cerebellopontine angle cistern bowing the vestibulocochlear nerve ▷ posterolaterally.

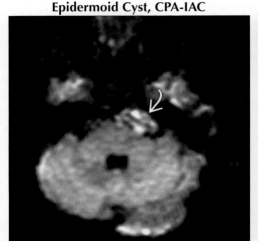

Aneurysm, CPA-IAC

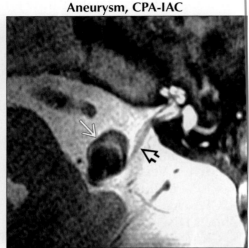

Fracture, T-Bone

(Left) Axial bone CT shows an oblique T-bone fracture ➡ traversing the oval window and extending to the IAC area ➡. Notice the air bubble (pneumolabyrinth) along the anterior margin of vestibule ➡. *(Right)* Axial bone CT shows severe otosclerosis as radiolucent foci along the medial middle ear wall ➡ (fenestral otosclerosis) and within the bony labyrinth ➡ (cochlear otosclerosis).

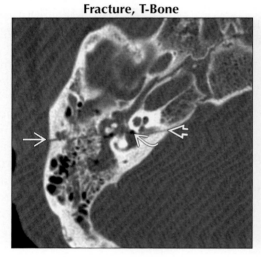

Cochlear Otosclerosis

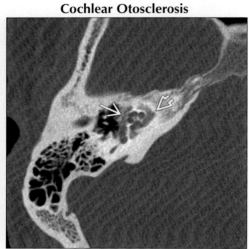

Metastases, CPA-IAC

(Left) Axial T2WI MR demonstrates a right floccular metastasis ➡ with associated high signal cerebellar and brachium pontis edema. Normal left flocculus ➡ is also seen. *(Right)* Axial T1 C+ FS MR reveals an enhancing facial nerve schwannoma traversing CPA ➡ and IAC ➡ into facial nerve labyrinthine segment ➡. The "labyrinthine tail" ➡ is characteristic.

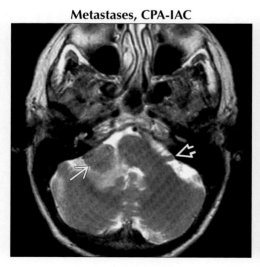

Schwannoma, Facial Nerve, CPA-IAC

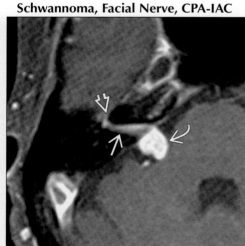

SENSORINEURAL HEARING LOSS IN ADULT

Lipoma, CPA-IAC

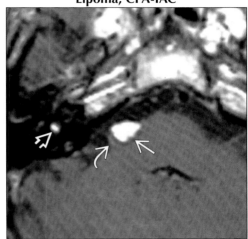

Large Endolymphatic Sac Anomaly (IP-2)

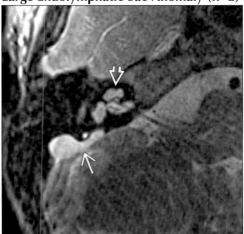

(Left) Axial T1WI MR demonstrates CPA ➡ and intravestibular ⧁ lipoma. Notice the CPA lipoma effaces the most proximal vestibulocochlear nerve bundle ➡. These lesions are left alone. (Right) Axial T2WI FS MR shows a large endolymphatic sac ➡ along the posterior wall of the temporal bone associated with a dysplastic cochlea (modiolar deficiency and bulbous apical turn) ➡.

Schwannoma, Intralabyrinthine

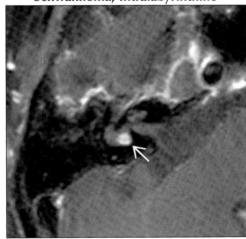

Labyrinthitis

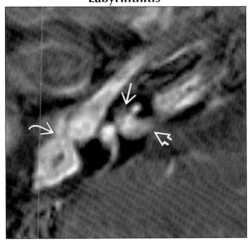

(Left) Axial T1 C+ FS MR demonstrates a nodule of enhancing tissue in the vestibule ➡ of the inner ear secondary to intralabyrinthine schwannoma. CT of the temporal bone was normal. (Right) Axial T1 C+ FS MR shows enhancement of the middle ear ➡, inner ear membranous labyrinth ➡, and internal auditory canal ⧁ in this pediatric patient with acute actinomycosis.

Neuritis, Vestibulocochlear

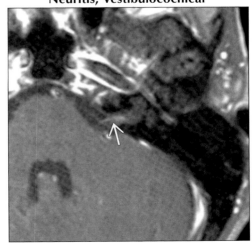

Paget Disease, T-Bone

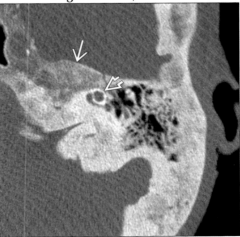

(Left) Axial T1 C+ FS MR shows typical 3T MR case of vestibulocochlear neuritis in this patient with rapid onset of sensorineural hearing loss. Note area of linear enhancement in the proximal IAC ➡. (Right) Axial bone CT shows late-phase Paget disease with diffuse bony expansion with areas of demineralization ➡. Notice that the bony labyrinth along anterior cochlear surface is involved ➡.

SENSORINEURAL HEARING LOSS IN CHILD

DIFFERENTIAL DIAGNOSIS

Common
- Large Endolymphatic Sac Anomaly (IP-2)
- Fractures, Temporal Bone
- Semicircular Canal Dysplasia
- Labyrinthine Ossificans

Less Common
- Labyrinthitis
- Cochlear Nerve Deficiency
- Cystic Cochleovestibular Anomaly (IP-1)
- Lipoma, CPA-IAC

Rare but Important
- Common Cavity, Inner Ear
- Cochlear Aplasia, Inner Ear
- Labyrinthine Aplasia
- Neurofibromatosis 2, CPA-IAC
- Schwannoma, Facial Nerve, CPA-IAC

ESSENTIAL INFORMATION

Key Differential Diagnosis Issues
- History is important
  - In setting of fluctuating or "cascading" sensorineural hearing loss in child who could hear at birth (without history of meningitis)
    - Look for large vestibular aqueduct ± cochlear dysplasia & modiolar deficiency on CT
    - Look for enlarged endolymphatic sac & duct with cochlear dysplasia & modiolar deficiency on MR
  - Trauma: Look for fracture involving inner ear structures ± pneumolabyrinth on CT
  - Genetic disorders: In CHARGE, Alagille, Waardenburg, Crouzon or Apert syndrome, look for semicircular canal (SCC) dysplasia
  - Prior meningitis
    - Look for labyrinthine ossificans on CT
    - Look for enhancement or replacement of high T2 intensity with low T2 intensity within structures of the membranous labyrinth on MR (depends on timing of imaging)
- Best imaging tool
  - Thin-section T-bone CT identifies many congenital inner ear anomalies

- High-resolution T2 MR imaging identifies large endolymphatic sac, cochlear dysplasia, best to show cochlear nerve aplasia/hypoplasia
- Contrast MR best evaluates schwannoma, acute labyrinthitis, & lipoma

Helpful Clues for Common Diagnoses
- **Large Endolymphatic Sac Anomaly (IP-2)**
  - Most common congenital anomaly of inner ear found by imaging
  - Vestibular aqueduct on CT ≥ 1.5 mm bony transverse dimension
    - Newer literature suggests ≥ 2 mm at operculum or ≥ 1 mm at midpoint
  - Look for associated cochlear dysplasia, modiolar deficiency, vestibule, &/or SCC dysplasia
  - Additional diagnosis information
    - Avoidance of contact sports or other activities that may lead to head trauma is recommended in children with IP-2 anomaly
    - Genetic testing for Pendred syndrome is becoming increasingly recommended in children with IP-2 anomaly
    - Up to 15% of all patients with IP-2 will have Pendrin gene = Pendred syndrome, with severe profound bilateral SNHL; 50% with goiter and 50% of those with goiter will be hypothyroid
- **Fractures, Temporal Bone**
  - Thin-section T-bone CT (0.625-1 mm)
  - Transverse or longitudinal fracture may cross inner ear structures, ± pneumolabyrinth
- **Semicircular Canal Dysplasia**
  - Spectrum of abnormalities: One or more of SCC dysmorphic, hypoplastic, or aplastic
  - Unilateral or bilateral: Bilateral more common in syndromic form
  - Most common is short, dilated lateral SCC & vestibule forming single cavity
  - Look for associated cochlear dysplasia, oval window atresia, & ossicular anomalies
  - CHARGE syndrome
    - Bilateral absence of all SCCs
    - Associated anomalies: Small vestibule, absent cochlear nerve aperture ("isolated cochlea"), oval window atresia (± overlying tympanic segment of CN7), choanal atresia, coloboma

SENSORINEURAL HEARING LOSS IN CHILD

Labyrinthitis

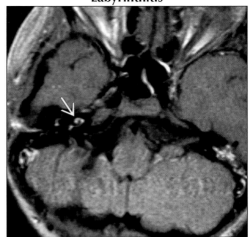

Labyrinthitis

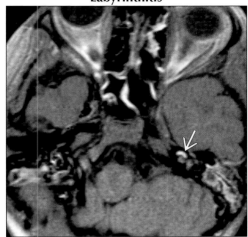

(Left) Axial T1 C+ FS MR shows abnormal enhancement of the right cochlea ➡ in this patient with Cogan syndrome. (Right) Axial T1 C+ FS MR in the same patient demonstrates abnormal enhancement of the left cochlea ➡.

Labyrinthitis

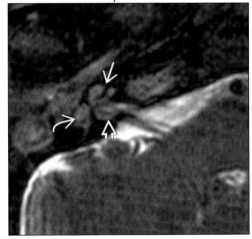

Labyrinthitis

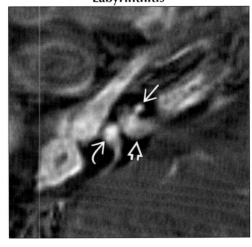

(Left) Axial T2WI FS MR shows corresponding loss of hyperintense T2 signal in the cochlea ➡, vestibule ➡, and internal auditory canal ➡. (Right) Axial T1 C+ FS MR shows abnormal contrast enhancement in the middle ear, mastoid, cochlea ➡, vestibule ➡, and internal auditory canal ➡, secondary to actinomycosis labyrinthitis.

Cochlear Nerve Deficiency

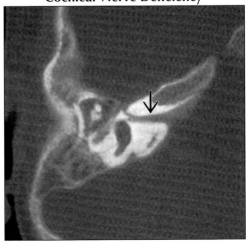

Cochlear Nerve Deficiency

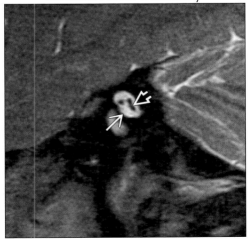

(Left) Axial bone CT reveals hypoplastic right IAC ➡ related to right cochlear nerve deficiency. (Right) Sagittal oblique T2WI MR shows an absent cochlear nerve on the left ➡ in association with a small internal auditory canal. The superior and inferior vestibular nerves are connected ➡.

SENSORINEURAL HEARING LOSS IN CHILD

(Left) Axial T2WI MR shows a tiny left IAC ➡ and nonvisualization of the cochlear nerve. *(Right)* Sagittal oblique T2WI MR shows nonvisualization of the cochlear nerve ➡ in association with a small internal auditory canal. CN8 and CN7 formation in the IAC area provides the IAC formation stimulation.

Cochlear Nerve Deficiency

Cochlear Nerve Deficiency

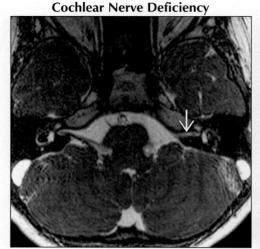
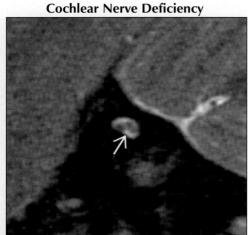

(Left) Axial bone CT shows typical CT appearance of cystic cochleovestibular anomaly. The vestibule is enlarged ➡. *(Right)* Axial bone CT in the same patient reveals a featureless cochlea ➡ without a definable modiolus.

Cystic Cochleovestibular Anomaly (IP-1)

Cystic Cochleovestibular Anomaly (IP-1)

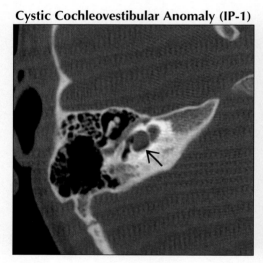

(Left) Axial NECT shows typical CT appearance of a small lipoma in the left CPA cistern ➡. Low-density focus of tissue is diagnostic of CPA lipoma. *(Right)* Coronal T1WI MR shows hyperintense T1 lipoma in the left CPA cistern ➡.

Lipoma, CPA-IAC

Lipoma, CPA-IAC

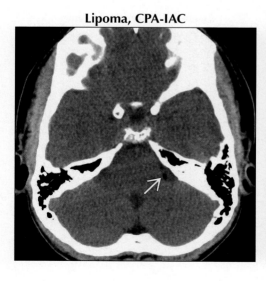

SENSORINEURAL HEARING LOSS IN CHILD

- ○ Lateral SCC last to form embryologically; therefore if posterior & superior SCC are normal, lateral should be normal
  - Except if obliterated by labyrinthine ossificans or hypoplastic in Waardenburg and Alagille syndrome
- **Labyrinthine Ossificans**
  - ○ Synonyms: Labyrinthitis ossificans, labyrinthine ossification, chronic labyrinthitis, ossifying labyrinthitis
  - ○ Acute inflammatory response results in fibrous and then osseous replacement of membranous labyrinth
    - May involve cochlea ± vestibule ± semicircular canals
  - ○ Bilateral in meningogenic form (meningitis), and in hematogenic form (blood-borne infections)
    - Unilateral in tympanogenic form (middle ear infection)
  - ○ T-bone CT: High-attenuation bone deposition in formerly fluid-filled membranous labyrinth
  - ○ T2 MR: Focal or diffuse low intensity replaces high intensity fluid, with apparent "enlargement" of modiolus if cochlea is involved
  - ○ T1 C+: Enhancement of involved membranous labyrinth structures in early stage, may persist into ossifying stages

Helpful Clues for Less Common Diagnoses
- **Labyrinthitis**
  - ○ Subacute inflammation of fluid-filled inner ear structures
  - ○ T-bone CT: Normal in early phases, may progress to labyrinthine ossificans
  - ○ T2 MR: Low intensity replaces normal fluid signal within membranous labyrinth structures
  - ○ T1 C+: Mild to moderate enhancement
- **Cochlear Nerve Deficiency**
  - ○ Very small or absent cochlear nerve with small IAC
- **Cystic Cochleovestibular Anomaly (IP-1)**
  - ○ Cochlea & vestibule form bilobed cyst
- **Lipoma, CPA-IAC**
  - ○ Fatty lesion of CPA, IAC ± inner ear

Helpful Clues for Rare Diagnoses
- **Common Cavity, Inner Ear**
  - ○ Cystic cochlea & vestibule form a common cavity ± SCC absence or dysplasia
- **Cochlear Aplasia, Inner Ear**
  - ○ Absent cochlea
- **Labyrinthine Aplasia**
  - ○ Absent membranous labyrinth
- **Neurofibromatosis 2, CPA-IAC**
  - ○ Bilateral hearing loss in 1st decade
  - ○ T1 C+ MR: Bilateral CPA-IAC CN7 ± CN8 enhancing schwannomas
- **Schwannoma, Facial Nerve, CPA-IAC**
  - ○ Enlarged labyrinthine segment CN7 canal with enhancing tubular mass in CPA-IAC & labyrinthine segment of CN7
  - ○ Rare in children

Large Endolymphatic Sac Anomaly (IP-2)

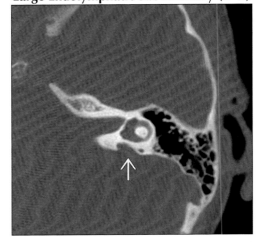

Axial bone CT demonstrates enlargement of the left bony vestibular aqueduct ➜.

Large Endolymphatic Sac Anomaly (IP-2)

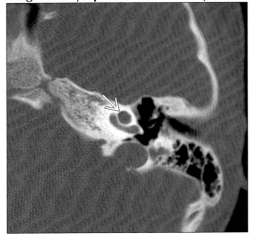

Axial bone CT in the same patient shows associated incomplete partitioning of the left cochlea ➜.

SENSORINEURAL HEARING LOSS IN CHILD

Fractures, Temporal Bone

Fractures, Temporal Bone

(Left) Axial bone CT shows longitudinal temporal bone fracture ➡ with associated pneumolabyrinth ➘. *(Right)* Coronal oblique bone CT shows transverse temporal bone fracture ➡ with associated pneumolabyrinth and gas in the vestibule ⊟ and lateral semicircular canal.

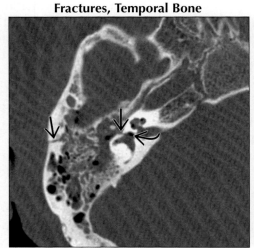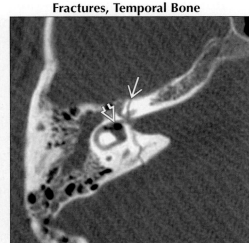

Semicircular Canal Dysplasia

Semicircular Canal Dysplasia

(Left) Axial bone CT shows severe hypoplasia of the right IAC ➡ and hypoplasia of the vestibule and semicircular canals with only a small remnant ⊟. *(Right)* Axial bone CT shows lack of the normal right cochlear aperture ➡ and severe hypoplasia of the vestibule and SCCs ➡ in a patient with CHARGE syndrome.

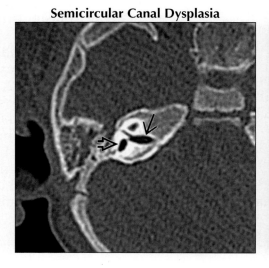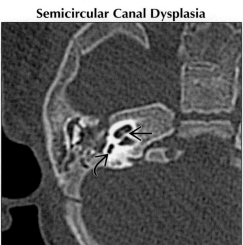

Labyrinthine Ossificans

Labyrinthine Ossificans

(Left) Axial bone CT shows osseous replacement of the vestibule and right lateral semicircular canals ➡. *(Right)* Axial bone CT shows complete osseous replacement of the right cochlea ➡. Notice the presence of the normal right cochlear promontory, convex laterally ➡.

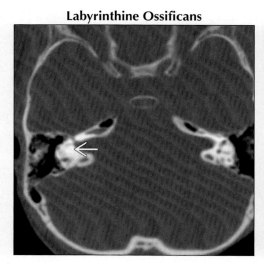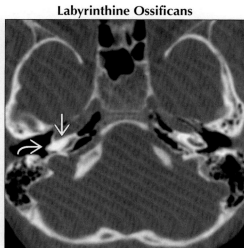

SENSORINEURAL HEARING LOSS IN CHILD

Cochlear Aplasia, Inner Ear

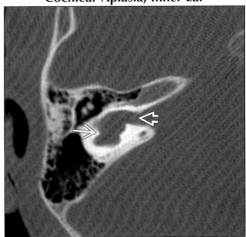

Labyrinthine Aplasia

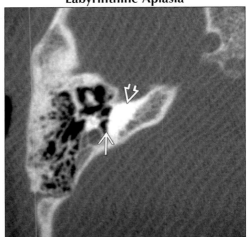

(Left) Axial bone CT demonstrates a dysplastic vestibule ➡ that communicates with a small IAC through a broad gap at the IAC fundus ➡. There is no cochlea anterior to the vestibule. (Right) Axial bone CT shows a featureless otic capsule ➡ without definable labyrinthine structures. The lateral wall is flat ➡, indicating congenital absence rather than acquired ossificans.

Neurofibromatosis 2, CPA-IAC

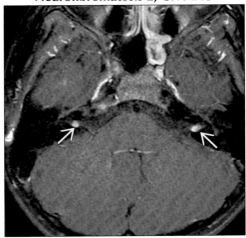

Neurofibromatosis 2, CPA-IAC

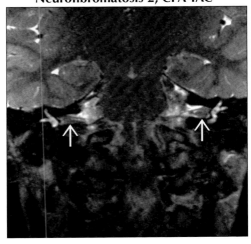

(Left) Axial T1 C+ FS MR shows enhancement of small bilateral vestibular schwannomas ➡. (Right) Coronal T2WI MR in a patient with known neurofibromatosis type 2 demonstrates hypointense masses ➡ in the inferior aspect of the IACs, consistent with vestibular schwannomas.

Schwannoma, Facial Nerve, CPA-IAC

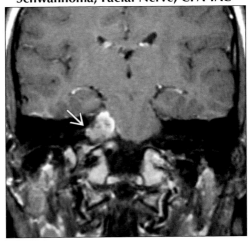

Schwannoma, Facial Nerve, CPA-IAC

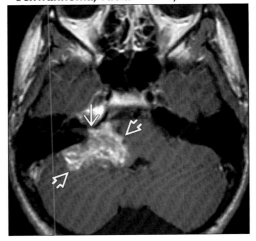

(Left) Coronal T1 C+ MR shows a large heterogeneously enhancing mass in the CPA cistern and proximal internal auditory canal ➡. (Right) Axial T1 C+ MR shows variant appearance of a heterogeneously enhancing extra-axial mass ➡ in the right CPA with extension into the porous acusticus of the right IAC ➡.

SECTION 11
Cranial Nerve & Brainstem

DIFFERENTIAL DIAGNOSIS

Common
- Cerebral Ischemia-Infarction, Acute
- Trauma (Diffuse Axonal Injury, Contusion)
- Demyelinating Disease (MS, ADEM)
- Metastasis
- Cavernous Malformation
- Enlarged Perivascular Spaces
- Wallerian Degeneration

Less Common
- Aqueductal Stenosis
- Brainstem Tumor
  - Tectal Glioma
  - Low-Grade Neoplasm
    - JPA, Diffuse Fibrillary Astrocytoma
  - High-Grade Neoplasm
    - Anaplastic Astrocytoma, GBM, PNET
- Wernicke Encephalopathy
- Mitochondrial Cytopathy

Rare but Important
- Infection
  - Progressive Multifocal Leukoencephalopathy (PML)
  - Abscess, Encephalitis
- Vasculitis
- Intracranial Hypotension
- Progressive Supranuclear Palsy (PSP)
- Parkinson Disease
- Amyotrophic Lateral Sclerosis (ALS)
- Drug Toxicity

ESSENTIAL INFORMATION

Key Differential Diagnosis Issues
- Most common midbrain lesions are ischemic, traumatic, demyelinating, vascular, or neoplastic
- Hemorrhage usually due to trauma, vascular malformation, or hemorrhagic metastasis; hypertensive hemorrhage rare in midbrain

Helpful Clues for Common Diagnoses
- **Cerebral Ischemia-Infarction, Acute**
  - Acute onset of clinical symptoms, often hemiparesis (corticospinal tracts), cranial neuropathy (nuclei of 3, 4; a nucleus of 5), &/or ataxia (red nucleus)
  - Presence of reduced diffusion: High SI on DWI, low SI on ADC map
    - Often accompanied by lesion of basilar artery, so consider MRA or CTA
- **Trauma (Diffuse Axonal Injury, Contusion)**
  - Appropriate clinical history; FLAIR, DWI particularly helpful to assess for edema (cytotoxic &/or vasogenic); GRE to assess for hemorrhage
  - Brainstem DAI typically dorsolateral, usually seen with hemispheric & callosal involvement; check for additional sites of injury
- **Demyelinating Disease (MS, ADEM)**
  - T2 bright lesions typically without reduced diffusion or GRE abnormality, often enhance post-gadolinium
  - Assess rest of brain for additional white matter (WM) lesions
  - Consider MR of optic nerves, spinal cord
- **Metastasis**
  - Typically enhance, associated with vasogenic edema; additional lesions often present in brain, meninges, or bone
  - May be hemorrhagic
- **Cavernous Malformation**
  - Often bright T1 & T2WI; hemosiderin rim "popcorn wall" morphology; ↓ SI on GRE
  - Associated developmental venous anomaly (DVA) may be present
- **Enlarged Perivascular Spaces**
  - Usually seen at base of cerebral peduncles
  - Follow CSF on all MR sequences
- **Wallerian Degeneration**
  - Acute: Variable ↓ diffusion and ↑ SI on T2
  - Chronic: Volume loss; variable T2 SI

Helpful Clues for Less Common Diagnoses
- **Aqueductal Stenosis**
  - Cause of "congenital" hydrocephalus: May be due to a web or adhesion; often post-inflammatory or post-intraventricular hemorrhage
  - Assess tectum carefully on axial T2 & FLAIR to exclude subtle nonenhancing tectal glioma
- **Brainstem Tumor**
  - Multiple histologies can affect midbrain & other parts of brainstem
  - Imaging varies with tumor histology
  - "Tectal gliomas": Typically confined to tectum, nonenhancing, present with chronic hydrocephalus

- - Generally better prognosis then other brainstem tumors; associated with NF1
- **Wernicke Encephalopathy**
  - Thiamine deficiency; most commonly seen in alcoholics; also malnutrition, malabsorption, HIV/AIDS
  - Classic clinical triad: Ataxia, encephalopathy, oculomotor dysfunction
  - Symmetrical ↑ T2 SI variably involves periaqueductal gray matter, dorsomedial thalami, mamillary bodies
  - ↓ Diffusion, post-gad enhancement variably present acutely
- **Mitochondrial Cytopathy**
  - Typically affects deep gray nuclei of cerebrum &/or gray matter structures of brainstem in symmetrical fashion
  - ↓ Diffusion, ↑ T2 SI typically present with acute flare of disease
  - ↑ Lactate peak may be seen with MR spectroscopy

Helpful Clues for Rare Diagnoses
- **Infection**
  - **Progressive Multifocal Leukoencephalopathy (PML)**
    - Usually severely immunocompromised patients (AIDS, organ transplant, chemotherapy)
    - Classic: WM lesions without enhancement or mass effect
    - May cause pattern of "small dots" in WM or brainstem that eventually coalesces into more typical geographic lesions

- - Abscess, Encephalitis
    - Central ↓ diffusion; also ring enhancement, vasogenic edema
- **Vasculitis**
  - Nonspecific ↑ SI on T2WI; often ↓ diffusion
- **Intracranial Hypotension**
  - Downward displacement of midbrain, loss of cisterns; "folding" if severe
- **Progressive Supranuclear Palsy (PSP)**
  - Atypical Parkinsonian syndrome
    - Supranuclear ophthalmoplegia, pseudobulbar palsy, dysarthria, postural instability, frontotemporal dementia
  - Neuropathological hallmark: Midbrain atrophy; tau + aggregates
  - MR: Midbrain atrophy; variable midbrain T2 hyperintensity
- **Parkinson Disease**
  - Imaging findings typically subtle; possible ↓ volume of substantia nigra, ↓ hypointensity of lateral margin of substantia nigra
- **Amyotrophic Lateral Sclerosis (ALS)**
  - Degenerative disease of upper and lower motor neurons in the motor cortex, brainstem, and spinal cord
  - Imaging hallmark: ↑ T2 SI of corticospinal tracts; no mass effect, enhancement
- **Drug Toxicity**
  - Notably metronidazole; symmetrical ↑ T2 SI, variable ↓ diffusion
  - Dentate nuclei usually involved

Cerebral Ischemia-Infarction, Acute

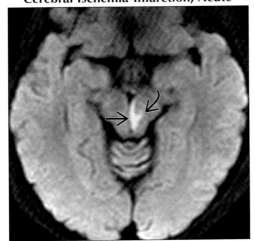

Axial DWI MR in a 71 year old shows high signal intensity representing reduced diffusion in the midbrain ➔. This lesion sharply respects midline ➔. An ADC map confirmed true reduced diffusion.

Trauma (Diffuse Axonal Injury, Contusion)

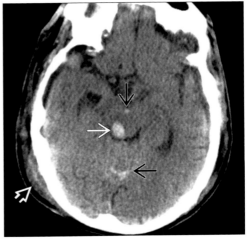

Axial NECT shows a shear hemorrhage ➔ in the right dorsolateral midbrain. This patient with severe head trauma has evidence of scalp injury ➔ and post-traumatic SAH ➔, among other injuries.

11

MIDBRAIN LESION

(Left) Axial FLAIR MR shows a focal lesion in the right midbrain ➘, consistent with an MS plaque. This lesion enhanced and was symptomatically acute. Periventricular white matter lesions ➾ are also present in this young woman with MS. (Right) Axial NECT shows a focal hemorrhage in the right midbrain with surrounding edema ➘. Additional hemorrhagic lesions are present in the temporal lobe ➾. This patient had metastatic melanoma.

Demyelinating Disease (MS, ADEM)

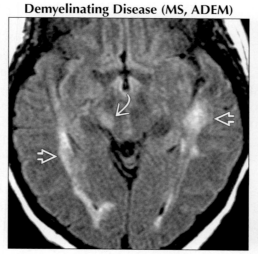

Metastasis

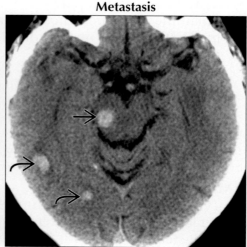

(Left) Axial T2WI MR shows a well-circumscribed lesion ➘ with a hemosiderin rim & heterogeneous internal signal due to blood products. The trunk of a large associated DVA that drains brainstem and cerebellum ➾ is also seen. (Right) Axial T2WI MR shows bilateral linear T2 bright structures at the base of the cerebral peduncles bilaterally ➘. These followed CSF on all sequences. Small perivascular or Virchow-Robin spaces are common in this location.

Cavernous Malformation

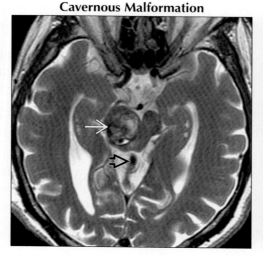

Enlarged Perivascular Spaces

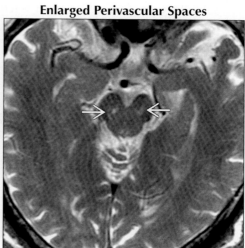

(Left) Axial T2WI MR shows a hyperintense and mildly atrophic left cerebral peduncle ➘. This patient had a prior left MCA stroke, and left temporal atrophy is present. (Right) Sagittal T2WI MR shows a funnel-shaped aqueduct of Sylvius ➘, normal 4th ventricle ➚, thinned & stretched corpus callosum ➘, & downward displacement of the floor of the 3rd ventricle ➘. The aqueductal obstruction is due to a web or adhesion, and no mass is present.

Wallerian Degeneration

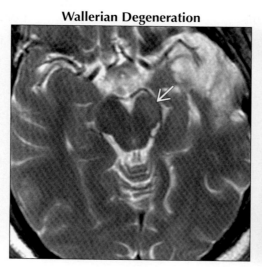

Aqueductal Stenosis

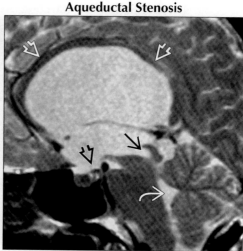

MIDBRAIN LESION

Tectal Glioma

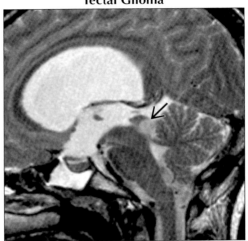

Low-Grade Neoplasm

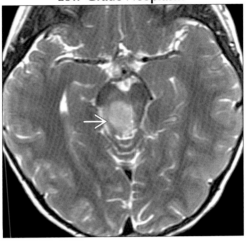

(Left) Sagittal T2WI MR shows a high signal intensity mass ⇨ confined to the tectum, causing severe obstructive hydrocephalus. There was no associated enhancement or surrounding edema. *(Right)* Axial T2WI MR shows an expansile mass of the midbrain ⇨ that extends well beyond the tectum. There is no associated edema. Surprisingly, no hydrocephalus is present. The mass enhanced intensely & homogeneously. Pathology confirmed JPA.

High-Grade Neoplasm

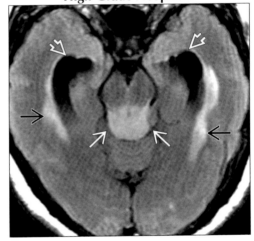

Wernicke Encephalopathy

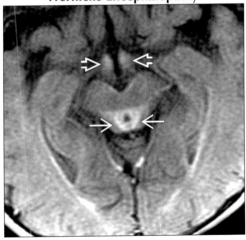

(Left) Axial FLAIR MR shows an expansile lesion involving the dorsal midbrain ⇨. The lesion has an ill-defined interface with normal midbrain. Severe obstructive hydrocephalus is present ⇨ with transependymal flow of CSF ⇨. *(Right)* Axial FLAIR MR shows symmetrical ↑ SI of the dorsal midbrain & periaqueductal gray matter ⇨, as well as ↑ SI of the mamillary bodies ⇨. This patient was severely malnourished & responded to thiamine treatment.

Mitochondrial Cytopathy

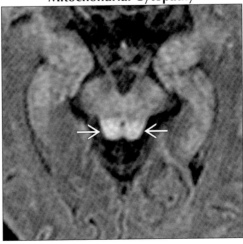

Progressive Multifocal Leukoencephalopathy (PML)

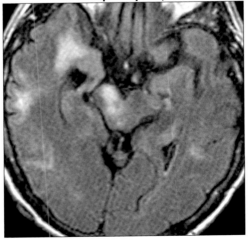

(Left) Axial FLAIR MR shows symmetrical ↑ SI of the dorsal midbrain & periaqueductal gray matter ⇨ in a 2 year old. The lesion demonstrated ↓ diffusion & no enhancement. Additional symmetrical lesions were present in the putamina. *(Right)* Axial FLAIR MR shows patchy ↑ T2 SI in right midbrain & cerebral peduncle, associated with mild volume loss. Additional multifocal peripheral/subcortical WM lesions are present in the right temporal lobe.

PONTINE LESION

DIFFERENTIAL DIAGNOSIS

Common
- Arteriolosclerosis (Ischemic Rarefaction)
- Cerebral Ischemia-Infarction, Acute
- Hypertensive Intracranial Hemorrhage
- Brainstem Tumor
- Vascular Lesion
  - Capillary Telangiectasia, Cavernous Malformation, AVM

Less Common
- Demyelinating Disease (MS, ADEM)
- Malignant Neoplasm
  - Metastasis, High-Grade Tumor, Lymphoma
- Pilocytic Astrocytoma
- Wallerian Degeneration
- Acute Hypertensive Encephalopathy, PRES
- Focal or Multifocal Infection
  - Pyogenic Abscess, Tuberculoma, PML
- Osmotic Demyelination Syndrome
- Neurofibromatosis Type 1

Rare but Important
- Brainstem Encephalitis
- Vasculitis
- Multiple System Atrophy
- Radiation Necrosis
- Mitochondrial Disorder
- Maple Syrup Urine Disease
- Infiltrative Disorder
  - Langerhans Cell Histiocytosis; Neurosarcoid; Whipple Disease

ESSENTIAL INFORMATION

Key Differential Diagnosis Issues
- Pontine lesions that present acutely are typically ischemic or hemorrhagic
- Diffuse astrocytomas present in a more insidious fashion

Helpful Clues for Common Diagnoses
- **Arteriolosclerosis (Ischemic Rarefaction)**
  - Ischemic rarefaction of pons very common in older patients with ASVD risk factors
  - Mild diffuse ↑ SI on T2WI without mass effect, enhancement, or ↓ diffusion
- **Cerebral Ischemia-Infarction, Acute**
  - Pontine infarct typically respects the midline & shows reduced diffusion
    - Consider CTA or MRA to assess vertebrobasilar circulation

- **Hypertensive Intracranial Hemorrhage**
  - Hypertensive hemorrhages usually central
  - Acute pontine hemorrhage usually hypertensive, but may be due to cavernoma or AVM
  - CTA or MR/MRA to look for AVM
- **Brainstem Tumor**
  - Massive expansion of pons, "engulfing" basilar artery, often nonenhancing
  - Typically diffuse fibrillary astrocytoma
- **Vascular Lesion**
  - Capillary telangiectasia: Small, asymptomatic; "brush-like" enhancement; signal loss on GRE; common in pons

Helpful Clues for Less Common Diagnoses
- **Demyelinating Disease (MS, ADEM)**
  - Often involvement of middle cerebellar peduncles; incomplete ring enhancement
  - Additional lesions in corpus callosum, hemispheric white matter (WM), spinal cord, optic nerves
- **Malignant Neoplasm**
  - High-grade tumor (GBM, PNET) often accompanied by edema, irregular enhancement, increased CBV
  - Metastases to pons associated with edema, often other enhancing lesions of brain parenchyma, dura, bone
  - Lymphoma usually homogeneously enhances, may show mildly ↓ diffusion
- **Pilocytic Astrocytoma**
  - Focal enhancing lesion without edema
- **Wallerian Degeneration**
  - Acute: Variable ↓ diffusion and ↑ SI on T2
  - Chronic: Volume loss; variable T2 SI
- **Acute Hypertensive Encephalopathy, PRES**
  - Most commonly involves parietooccipital subcortical WM
  - Infratentorial T2 hyperintensity often present in pons, cerebellum
  - Best appreciated on FLAIR; usually no enhancement or DWI abnormality
- **Focal or Multifocal Infection**
  - Pyogenic abscess will typically restrict diffusion, whereas tuberculoma may not
  - PML often causes multiple small dots of T2 hyperintensity in the brainstem
- **Osmotic Demyelination Syndrome**
  - Commonly involves central pons, spares corticospinal tracts, may show ↓ diffusion

PONTINE LESION

- **Neurofibromatosis Type 1**
  - Common in dorsal pons, due to dysmyelination/myelin vacuolization
  - No mass effect, enhancement

Helpful Clues for Rare Diagnoses
- **Brainstem Encephalitis**
  - Multiple causative agents including listeria monocytogenes, West Nile, HSV 1
  - Acute presentation, swelling, irregular enhancement, variable ↓ diffusion
- **Vasculitis**
  - May mimic demyelinating lesions; look for reduced diffusion, vascular irregularity, irregular enhancement
- **Multiple System Atrophy**
  - Sporadic neurodegenerative disorder encompasses olivopontocerebellar atrophy, striatonigral degeneration, & Shy-Drager
  - When Parkinsonism predominates, MSA-P; when cerebellar signs predominate, MSA-C
  - Imaging may show putaminal volume loss, "slit-like" lateral putaminal T2 hyperintensity (MSA-P), or "hot cross bun" appearance, atrophy of pons/middle cerebellar peduncles (MSA-C)
- **Radiation Necrosis**
  - Correlate with history; look for evidence of port (fatty marrow in skull base)
  - May occur many years after radiation
- **Mitochondrial Disorder**
  - May be congenital or acquired (e.g., perinatal exposure to zidovudine)
  - Symmetrical T2 hyperintensity that often involves hemispheric WM, deep gray nuclei, & pons
  - Often ↓ diffusion acutely; volume loss in chronic phase
- **Maple Syrup Urine Disease**
  - Neonate: Cerebellar WM, brainstem > supratentorial edema
- **Infiltrative Disorder**
  - Enhancing lesions typical

Other Essential Information
- MR is study of choice for pontine pathology
- Parallel imaging techniques may be helpful to reduce susceptibility artifacts that can obscure pontine pathology

Alternative Differential Approaches
- Pontine lesion in child: Demyelination (ADEM), brainstem encephalitis, or diffuse astrocytoma; metabolic or mitochondrial disorder
- Pontine lesion in adult: Likely to be ischemic or hemorrhagic
  - Hypertensive hemorrhage in older adult
  - Vascular malformation (AVM, cavernoma) in young adult
- Enlargement of pons: Diffuse astrocytoma; brainstem encephalitis; severe ADEM, PRES
- Atrophy of pons: Prior injury (ischemic, hemorrhagic, infectious, metabolic); wallerian degeneration; MSA; other neurodegenerative disorder

Arteriolosclerosis (Ischemic Rarefaction)

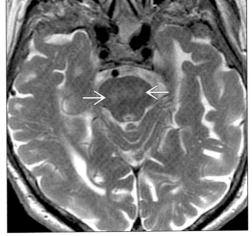

Axial T2WI MR shows ill-defined central pontine T2 high signal ➡ in an elderly man. Cerebrum demonstrated volume loss as well as periventricular and subcortical white matter T2 hyperintensities.

Cerebral Ischemia-Infarction, Acute

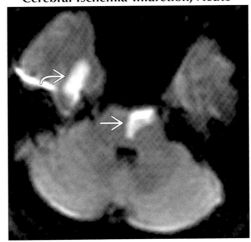

Axial DWI MR shows reduced diffusion in the left pons that respects the midline ➡ in a patient with acute onset right hemiparesis. A 2nd area of acute infarct ➡ is seen in the temporal lobe.

11

PONTINE LESION

(Left) Axial NECT shows central pontine high density ⬌, consistent with acute hemorrhage. This hypertensive patient had an abrupt onset of headache followed by loss of consciousness. *(Right)* Axial FLAIR MR shows massive expansion of the pons ➡ in a young girl with gradual onset difficulty walking & cranial neuropathy. The pons is diffusely bright, and the basilar artery ➡ appears to be "engulfed" by tumor. The lesion did not enhance or restrict diffusion.

Hypertensive Intracranial Hemorrhage

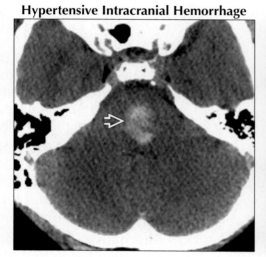

Brainstem Tumor

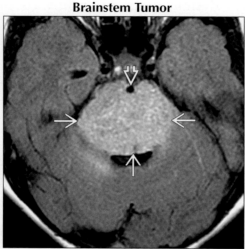

(Left) Axial T2WI MR shows a central "popcorn ball" high signal lesion with a dark rim of hemosiderin ➡. This appearance is classic for a cavernous malformation. A developmental venous anomaly is often seen post-gadolinium. *(Right)* Axial T1 C+ MR shows a central pontine lesion with "brush-like" enhancement. The T2 was normal, and the GRE image (not shown) showed signal loss in this region. This constellation of findings is typical of capillary telangiectasia.

Vascular Lesion

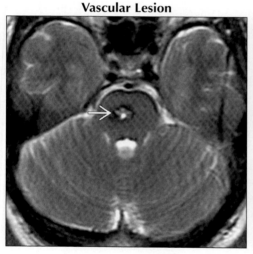

Vascular Lesion

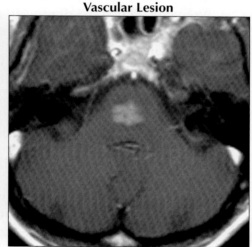

(Left) Axial T2WI MR shows numerous well-defined T2 bright lesions in the pons & middle cerebellar peduncles in a patient with known multiple sclerosis. These lesions showed no enhancement or reduced diffusion. *(Right)* Axial T2WI MR shows multiple large, bright, somewhat ill-defined lesions in the pons and middle cerebellar peduncles. Several of the lesions showed mild enhancement but no reduced diffusion. This child was subsequently diagnosed with ADEM.

Demyelinating Disease (MS, ADEM)

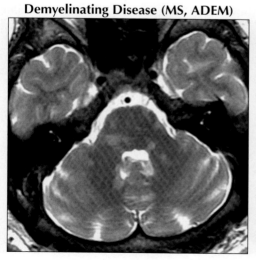

Demyelinating Disease (MS, ADEM)

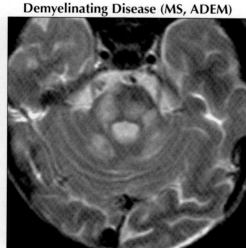

PONTINE LESION

Malignant Neoplasm

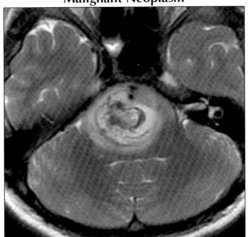

Pilocytic Astrocytoma

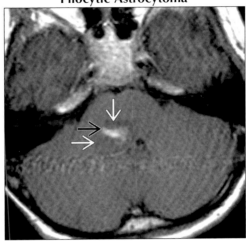

(Left) Axial T2WI MR shows a centrally hemorrhagic lesion with a low signal intensity rim and surrounding vasogenic edema. The pons is moderately expanded in this 15 year old. Biopsy confirmed GBM. *(Right)* Axial T1 C+ MR shows a fairly well-circumscribed low SI lesion in the dorsal pons ➡ with central enhancement ➡. The lesion was T2 bright, and there was no associated edema. Biopsy showed juvenile pilocytic astrocytoma in this young boy.

Focal or Multifocal Infection

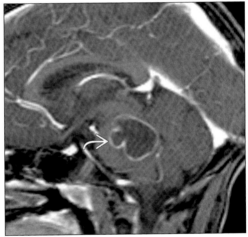

Osmotic Demyelination Syndrome

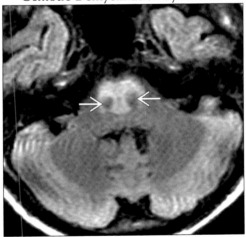

(Left) Sagittal T1 C+ MR shows a large rim-enhancing lesion in the dorsal pons. A "daughter" lesion ➡ is beginning to form. There was associated vasogenic edema & central reduced diffusion. Pyogenic abscess. *(Right)* Axial FLAIR MR shows central pontine high signal intensity, with sparing of a thin peripheral rim of pontine tissue as well as the descending corticospinal tracts ➡. There was reduced diffusion & no enhancement in the lesion. CPM.

Multiple System Atrophy

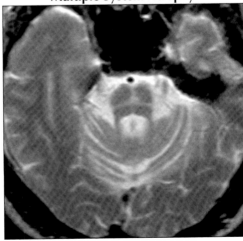

Infiltrative Disorder

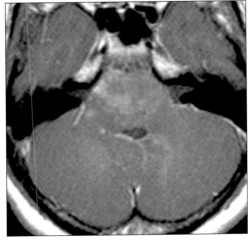

(Left) Axial T2WI MR shows marked atrophy of the pons & visualized cerebellum. The pons shows a "hot cross bun" appearance due to selective loss of myelinated transverse pontocerebellar fibers & neurons in the pontine raphe. Corticospinal tracts are preserved. *(Right)* Axial T1 C+ MR shows irregular linear & nodular enhancement throughout the pons, extending to middle cerebellar peduncles & cerebellum. High signal on T2 was present. Neurosarcoidosis.

11

MEDULLA LESION

DIFFERENTIAL DIAGNOSIS

Common
- Lateral Medullary Infarct
- Wallerian Degeneration
- Demyelinating Lesion (MS, ADEM)
- Vascular Lesion
  - Cavernous Malformation; AVM
- Brainstem Glioma, Pediatric
  - Diffuse Fibrillary Astrocytoma
  - Exophytic Cervicomedullary Glioma

Less Common
- Brainstem Neoplasm, Adult
  - Glioma, High or Low Grade
  - Hemangioblastoma
  - Metastasis, Lymphoma
- Vasculitis
- Medial Medullary Infarct
- Infection (Abscess, Tuberculoma, PML)
- Syringobulbia

Rare but Important
- Hypertrophic Olivary Degeneration
- Infiltrative Disorders (Langerhans Cell Histiocytosis, Neurosarcoid)
- Mitochondrial Disorder
- Viral Encephalitis

ESSENTIAL INFORMATION

Key Differential Diagnosis Issues
- Acute onset of cranial nerve deficits and Horner syndrome in older patient suggests medullary infarction
  - CT suboptimal for evaluation of medulla; MR with diffusion is indicated
  - Posterior circulation should be assessed intra- & extracranially with CTA or MRA
  - Vertebral artery dissection a consideration in younger patient
    - Add axial T1 with fat saturation
- Reduced diffusion in focal medullary lesion usually due to acute medullary infarction
- Volume loss of medullary pyramid(s) usually due to wallerian degeneration
  - Look for remote infarct
- Expanded medulla? Neoplasm > infarction, demyelination, infection

Helpful Clues for Common Diagnoses
- **Lateral Medullary Infarct**
  - Reduced diffusion; often subtle T2 bright abnormality in acute phase
  - Typically dorsolateral, due to occlusion of vertebral artery or PICA; check CTA or MRA
  - Wallenberg syndrome: Deficits in pain/temperature sense, dysphagia, hoarseness, vertigo, diplopia, Horner syndrome
- **Wallerian Degeneration**
  - Acute wallerian degeneration may lead to medullary pyramid T2 hyperintensity, mildly reduced diffusion
  - Chronic infarction along corticospinal tract leads to volume loss of medullary pyramid; variable T2 signal
- **Demyelinating Lesion (MS, ADEM)**
  - Usually associated with WM lesions in other parts of brain, may enhance, diffusion typically not reduced
- **Vascular Lesion**
  - Cavernous malformation may be associated with developmental venous anomaly; GRE hypointense
  - CTA or MRA may help to evaluate for high flow vascular malformation
- **Brainstem Glioma, Pediatric**
  - Diffuse infiltrative astrocytoma: Medullary expansion, ↑ T2 SI, usually nonenhancing
  - Pediatric astrocytoma may also be exophytic from cervicomedullary junction
    - Dorsal or ventral; often enhancing

Helpful Clues for Less Common Diagnoses
- **Brainstem Neoplasm, Adult**
  - Medullary expansion, areas of irregular enhancement likely high grade glioma
  - Hemangioblastoma presents as enhancing nodule ± cyst
    - Usually in setting of von Hippel-Lindau; look for other lesions in cerebellum, spinal cord
  - Focal enhancing lesion + associated edema: Consider metastasis, lymphoma
- **Vasculitis**
  - Multifocal T2 lesions, variable ↓ DWI
  - CTA or MRA may show vascular irregularity, but catheter angiography generally indicated
  - Often associated with systemic symptoms, abnormal CSF
- **Medial Medullary Infarct**

MEDULLA LESION

- Less common vertebrobasilar stroke syndrome
- Classic: Ipsilateral hypoglossal palsy, contralateral hemiparesis, contralateral lemniscal sensory loss
- **Infection (Abscess, Tuberculoma, PML)**
  - Medullary pyogenic abscess rare; reduced diffusion, peripheral enhancement
  - Tuberculoma: Ring or nodular enhancement, central T2 hypointensity, diffusion variable
  - PML: Multifocal T2 abnormality, no mass effect, immunocompromised patient
- **Syringobulbia**
  - Cervical syrinx may extend cephalad into medulla
  - Assess for Chiari 1 malformation, spinal cord tumor, other obstruction to CSF flow

Helpful Clues for Rare Diagnoses
- **Hypertrophic Olivary Degeneration**
  - Insult to dentato-rubro-olivary pathway
  - Classic symptom: Palatal tremor
  - Uni- or bilateral enlargement, T2 hyperintensity of inferior olivary nucleus
  - No reduced diffusion, no post-gad enhancement
  - Chronic phase: Possible volume loss
- **Infiltrative Disorders (Langerhans Cell Histiocytosis, Neurosarcoid)**
  - T2 abnormality, irregular linear and nodular enhancement
  - Diffusion typically not reduced, vascular imaging studies normal

- **Mitochondrial Disorder**
  - Symmetrical ↑ T2 SI, often ↓ diffusion
  - May mimic medullary encephalitis, or vice versa
- **Viral Encephalitis**
  - Typically symmetrical, nonspecific ↑ SI on T2WI; variably ↓ diffusion
  - Specific diagnosis usually made with CSF analysis

Other Essential Information
- MR is always the imaging study of choice for medullary pathology

Alternative Differential Approaches
- Medullary lesion with reduced diffusion
  - Typically medullary infarct; assess vertebrobasilar circulation
  - Occasionally seen with demyelination: Look elsewhere for typical lesions
  - May occur with mitochondrial disease or brainstem encephalitis (more diffuse, symmetrical)
- Medullary lesion with GRE hypointensity
  - Typically cavernous malformation; give gadolinium to look for DVA
  - Other possibilities: Hemorrhage due to AVM, neoplasm, infection, prior trauma
- Medullary lesion with gadolinium enhancement
  - Neoplasm, infection, demyelination
- Medullary expansion
  - Usually seen with diffuse infiltrative astrocytoma in child or young adult

Lateral Medullary Infarct

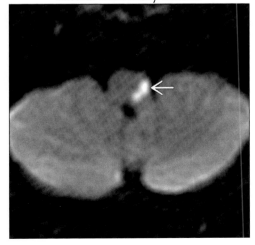

Axial DWI MR shows high signal intensity ➡, consistent with reduced diffusion in the left lateral medulla of a young man with acute onset of dysphagia and left vocal cord paralysis.

Lateral Medullary Infarct

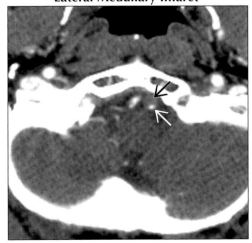

Axial CTA shows narrowing of the contrast-enhanced lumen of the left vertebral artery ➡ as well as intermediate density intramural hematoma ➡, consistent with arterial dissection.

MEDULLA LESION

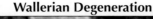

Wallerian Degeneration

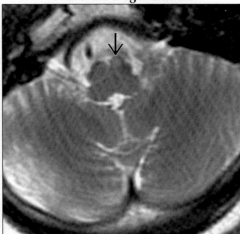

(Left) Axial T2WI MR shows a small, mildly hyperintense medullary pyramid →. This patient had a left MCA stroke with right hemiparesis 1 year earlier. *(Right)* Axial T2WI MR shows extensive high signal in the central medulla → and the right medullary pyramid →. The lesion does not respect the midline or usual vascular boundaries. This patient had known MS and presented with subacute onset of left-sided weakness and lower cranial neuropathies.

Demyelinating Lesion (MS, ADEM)

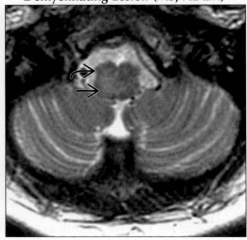

Cavernous Malformation; AVM

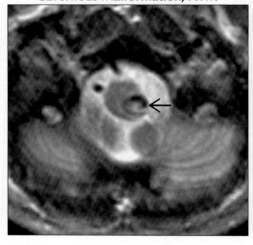

(Left) Axial T2WI MR shows a well-circumscribed lesion in the dorsolateral medulla with peripheral hemosiderin rim →. There is central hyperintensity and subtle surrounding edema. The patient was acutely symptomatic and had bled into this cavernous malformation. *(Right)* Axial T2WI MR shows diffuse but asymmetrical medullary expansion and T2 hyperintensity → in a 7 year old. This medullary astrocytoma did not enhance.

Diffuse Fibrillary Astrocytoma

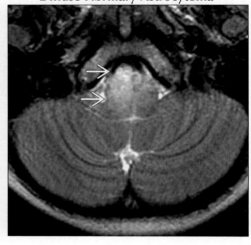

Exophytic Cervicomedullary Glioma

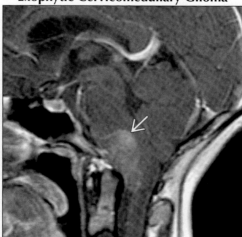

(Left) Sagittal T1 C+ MR shows a lobulated, ventrally exophytic, moderately enhancing mass arising from the medulla → of a child. The pons and upper spinal cord were not involved by tumor. *(Right)* Axial T1 C+ MR shows an irregular peripherally enhancing mass → with central necrosis involving the medulla in a 39 year old man. The patient had no symptoms of infection, and diffusion was not reduced in the lesion. Pathology confirmed glioblastoma.

Glioma, High or Low Grade

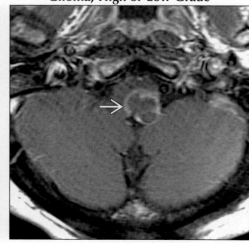

MEDULLA LESION

Hemangioblastoma

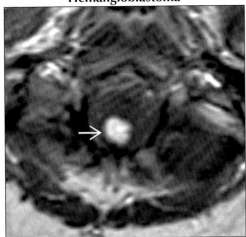

Medial Medullary Infarct

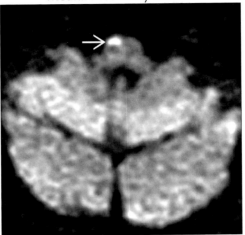

(Left) Axial T1 C+ MR shows a well-circumscribed intensely enhancing nodule ➡ in the dorsal medulla. Additional enhancing nodules were present in the cerebellum in this von Hippel-Lindau disease patient with multiple hemangioblastomas. *(Right)* Axial DWI MR shows focal high signal intensity, consistent with reduced diffusion in the medullary pyramid ➡ in an elderly patient with acute onset of left hemiparesis and right vertebral artery occlusion.

Infection (Abscess, Tuberculoma, PML)

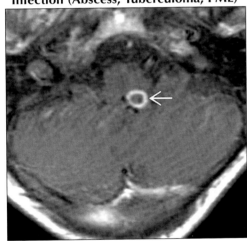

Infection (Abscess, Tuberculoma, PML)

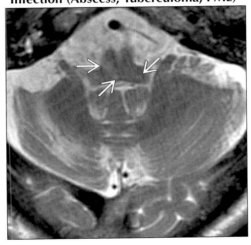

(Left) Axial T1 C+ MR shows a well-defined peripherally enhancing lesion with a thin regular rim ➡ involving the left dorsal medulla. The lesion was intermediate on T2WI. This patient also had lung nodules and epididymo-orchitis. Tuberculosis. *(Right)* Axial T2WI MR shows multiple small T2 hyperintense lesions ➡ scattered in the medulla. There was no associated enhancement or reduced diffusion. This patient had AIDS & progressive neurological decline. PML.

Syringobulbia

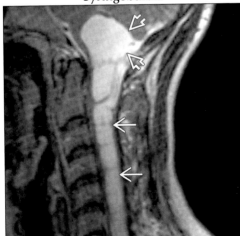

Hypertrophic Olivary Degeneration

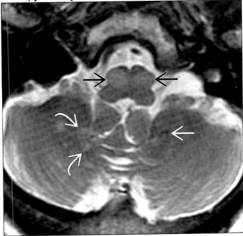

(Left) Sagittal T2WI MR shows an extensive cervical spinal cord syrinx ➡ with extension cephalad to the medulla ➡. This syrinx was secondary to hemangioblastoma. *(Right)* Axial T2WI MR shows enlargement & hyperintensity of the medullary olives ➡, R > L, in a patient with prior hemorrhage into a brainstem cavernoma. An additional cavernoma is present in the left cerebellum ➡, & branches of a large DVA are faintly seen in the right cerebellum ➡.

MONOCULAR VISION LOSS

DIFFERENTIAL DIAGNOSIS

Common
- Trauma, Orbit
- Ocular Hemorrhage
- Retinal Detachment
- Optic Neuritis
- Meningioma, Optic Nerve Sheath
- Glioma, Optic Pathway
- Intracranial Hypertension, Idiopathic
- Meningioma, Parasellar

Less Common
- Persistent Hyperplastic Primary Vitreous
- Retinoblastoma
- Coloboma
- Melanoma, Ocular
- Optic Perineuritis
- Endophthalmitis
- Ocular Toxocariasis/Sclerosing Endophthalmitis

Rare but Important
- Coats Disease
- Metastasis, Orbital or Ocular
- Pituitary Apoplexy

ESSENTIAL INFORMATION

Key Differential Diagnosis Issues
- Scotoma is focal area of visual field loss
- Unilateral (monocular) loss of vision due to lesion anywhere from globe ⇒ optic nerve ⇒ chiasm
  - Unilateral central scotoma = optic nerve lesion
- Bilateral loss of vision uncommon, unless pathology involves chiasm or intracranial hypertension is present

Helpful Clues for Common Diagnoses
- **Trauma, Orbit**
  - Many different manifestations
    - Dislocated lens, traumatic cataract, ruptured globe, retrobulbar hematoma, tented globe, avulsion of optic nerve
  - CT is typically first-line study
- **Ocular Hemorrhage**
  - Collection in vitreous, subretinal, or subchoroidal space
  - Imaging: Hyperdense fluid level on CT
    - MR: Signal depends on sequence & stage of blood products over time

- **Retinal Detachment**
  - Subretinal fluid collection
  - Imaging: Characteristically V-shaped
    - Apex at optic disc with distal ends at ciliary body
  - Compare choroidal detachment: Fluid collection with parallel or unilateral biconvex choroidal leaves
    - Ciliary bodies to posterior sclera
- **Optic Neuritis**
  - May be isolated or associated with MS or Devic neuromyelitis optica
  - Imaging: MR is modality of choice
    - CN2 may be slightly enlarged, T2 hyperintense, focal or diffuse enhancement
- **Meningioma, Optic Nerve Sheath**
  - Calcifying, enhancing mass surrounding and extending along optic nerve
  - Imaging: Coronal MR best demonstrates perineural location
- **Glioma, Optic Pathway**
  - Up to 40% of patients develop optic glioma with NF1
    - Bilateral gliomas almost pathognomonic of NF1
  - Imaging: Variably enhancing, noncalcifying fusiform mass involving intraorbital CN2 or chiasm
    - Cannot distinguish optic nerve from mass
- **Intracranial Hypertension, Idiopathic**
  - Clinical: Middle-aged obese female with headache, papilledema, visual loss, diplopia
    - Visual loss typically binocular, but may be monocular acutely
  - Imaging: Flattening of posterior sclera, enlarged subarachnoid space in optic nerve sheath, empty sella
- **Meningioma, Parasellar**
  - Imaging: Avidly enhancing dural-based mass ± adjacent bony hyperostosis
    - MR T1 C+ fat-saturated sequences best delineate extension along optic canal

Helpful Clues for Less Common Diagnoses
- **Persistent Hyperplastic Primary Vitreous**
  - Developmental disorder of vitreous with persistent Cloquet canal for hyaloid artery
    - Usually unilateral with microphthalmia

- Imaging: Small globe with hyperdense vitreous & without calcification (CT)
  - MR: Retrolental mass, hemorrhage fluid levels, linear structure from optic nerve to lens = Cloquet canal
- **Retinoblastoma**
  - Malignant retinal tumor arising < 3 years
    - Frequently presents as leukocoria
  - Imaging: Calcified, enhancing intraocular mass in normal or large globe
    - ~ 70% unilateral
    - May extend into vitreous, subretinal space, or optic nerve
- **Coloboma**
  - Isolated or feature of CHARGE syndrome
  - Imaging: Focal defect in posterior scleral wall at optic nerve-head with outpouching of vitreous
    - Bilateral > > unilateral
- **Melanoma, Ocular**
  - Most common intraocular tumor in adults
  - Imaging: Dome-shaped posterior segment mass with broad choroidal base
    - MR: T1 variably hyperintense & moderately enhancing; T2 hypointense
- **Optic Perineuritis**
  - Form of orbital pseudotumor with primary involvement of intraorbital optic nerve
    - Less common than myositic or lacrimal pseudotumor
  - Imaging: Ragged edematous enlargement of optic nerve sheath
    - Apical form has infiltration of orbital apex & optic nerve

- **Endophthalmitis**
  - From intraocular surgery, penetrating orbital injury, diabetes, intravenous drug abuse, renal failure
  - Imaging: Thickened, enhancing infiltrative sclera, preseptal/periorbital cellulitis (CT)
    - MR: Scleral-uveal enhancement; FLAIR may show intraocular lesions
- **Ocular Toxocariasis/Sclerosing Endophthalmitis**
  - Eosinophilic granuloma caused by infection of nematode toxocara canis/cati
  - Imaging: Thickened, irregular, enhancing uveoscleral coat; no calcification (CT)
    - MR: Retinal mass may also be evident

Helpful Clues for Rare Diagnoses
- **Coats Disease**
  - Idiopathic retinal telangiectasia with exudative detachment
    - Typically young males, unilateral
  - Imaging: No calcifications (CT)
    - MR: Thickened retinal leaves, subretinal effusion, retinal detachment, no enhancing mass
- **Metastasis, Orbital or Ocular**
  - Commonly from breast, prostate, lung
  - Imaging: Diffuse C+ intraconal mass
- **Pituitary Apoplexy**
  - Severe retro-orbital headache ± vision loss
  - Imaging: Heterogeneous sella mass extending superiorly to suprasellar cistern

Trauma, Orbit

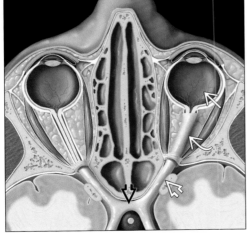

Axial graphic shows potential sites of traumatic monocular vision loss: Globe ➡, intraorbital ➡ segment, and canalicular ➡ segment of the optic nerve. Chiasm ➡ injury results in bilateral vision loss.

Trauma, Orbit

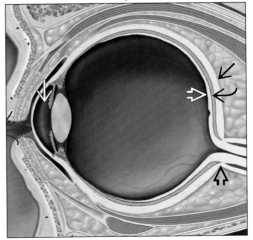

Sagittal graphic shows globe components that may be injured: Anterior chamber ➡, posterior segment vitreous & lined by retina ➡, choroid ➡, & sclera ➡. CN2 joins globe at optic nerve head ➡.

(Left) Axial NECT shows the normal position and contour of right lens ➡, but the dislocated left lens is deformed and lies in dependent portion of globe ⮰. There are also old fractures of the left medial orbital wall ➡. *(Right)* Axial NECT of traumatic cataract shows normal position of right lens; however, there is asymmetric loss of density in lateral aspect ➡ following penetrating injury. Note adjacent preseptal soft tissue swelling ➡.

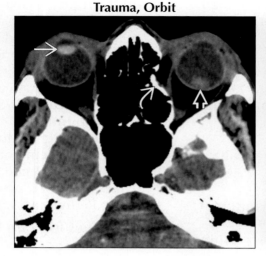

Trauma, Orbit

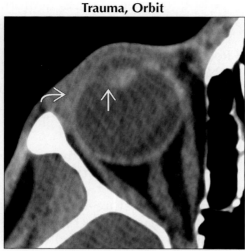

Trauma, Orbit

(Left) Axial NECT of orbital foreign body shows high-density shrapnel in right vitreous ➡ with streak artifact and adjacent subtle scleral laceration seen as abnormal outer contour of globe. Absence of increased vitreous density suggests that no significant hemorrhage occurred. *(Right)* Axial NECT shows unilateral traumatic globe rupture. The right globe is misshapen and dense with internal hemorrhage. There is dislocated lens and periocular hematoma ⮰.

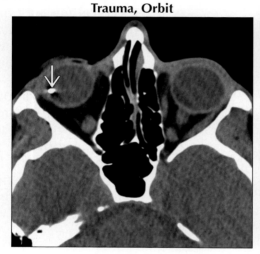

Trauma, Orbit

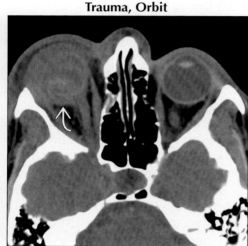

Trauma, Orbit

(Left) Axial NECT shows a retrobulbar hematoma in a patient following a motor vehicle crash. Globe & optic nerve ➡ are of normal contour, but there is abnormal density in retrobulbar fat at optic nerve head ➡. *(Right)* Axial NECT of tented globe in trauma patient shows a relatively acute angle of posterior sclera at the optic nerve head ➡, measuring approximately 125°. Angles < 120° require emergent decompression to prevent permanent vision loss.

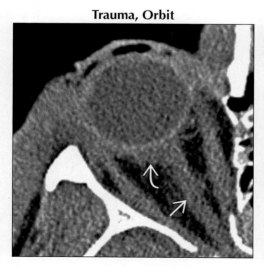

Trauma, Orbit

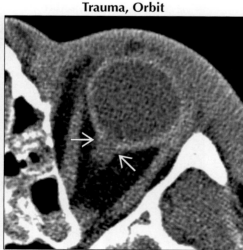

Trauma, Orbit

MONOCULAR VISION LOSS

Ocular Hemorrhage

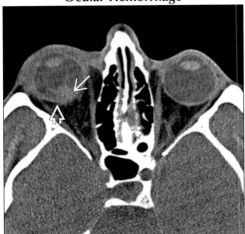

Retinal Detachment

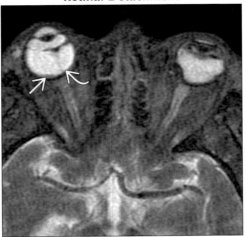

(Left) Axial NECT shows hyperdense hemorrhage posteriorly in vitreous body ➡ in this patient with unilateral right globe trauma. Note also the thickened adjacent sclera ➡. (Right) Axial T2WI FS MR performed in a patient with diabetic retinopathy and blindness reveals slightly hypointense retinal leaves with their apex at retina ➡. There is also subtle adjacent hyaloid detachment ➡. Contralateral globe has total retinal detachment.

Optic Neuritis

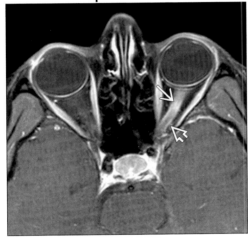

Meningioma, Optic Nerve Sheath

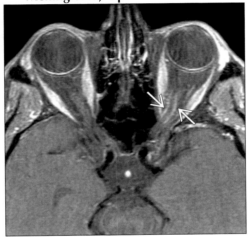

(Left) Axial T1 C+ FS MR shows focal enhancement of distal left optic nerve ➡, but also subtle enhancement of nerve sheath ➡, which may accompany inflammatory disease of nerve. Left globe appears subtly proptotic in this patient with MS. (Right) Axial T1 C+ FS MR reveals subtle left proptosis and linear enhancement of left optic nerve sheath, outlining the optic nerve ➡. This appearance is referred to as "tram track" enhancement.

Glioma, Optic Pathway

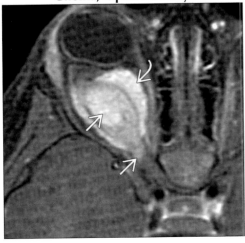

Intracranial Hypertension, Idiopathic

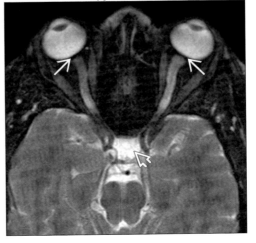

(Left) Axial T1 C+ FS MR shows fusiform-enhancing mass of intraorbital right optic nerve ➡. This distorts proptotic globe and is also associated with enhancement and enlargement of surrounding nerve sheath ➡. (Right) Axial T2WI MR shows prominent bilateral optic nerve sheaths, more apparent on the left. There is also a more subtle finding of flattened posterior sclerae ➡, which correlates with clinical papilledema. Patient has empty sella ➡.

11

MONOCULAR VISION LOSS

(Left) Sagittal oblique T1 C+ FS MR shows an extra-axial mass ➔ over the posterior roof of orbit that also involves anterior clinoid process. This meningioma extends anteriorly along canalicular optic nerve ➔. Patient had vision loss and diplopia. **(Right)** Axial STIR MR shows small right globe with hemorrhagic fluid levels in vitreous ➔. The central linear structure ➔ traversing vitreous from optic nerve head to posterior aspect of lens is Cloquet canal.

Meningioma, Parasellar

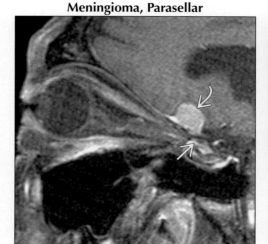

Persistent Hyperplastic Primary Vitreous

(Left) Axial NECT in a 2 year old shows a large unilateral densely calcified mass ➔ in posterior aspect of slightly enlarged left globe. No contralateral mass is seen. **(Right)** Axial T2WI MR shows large mass ➔ within left globe with very low T2 signal. Calcification is often very difficult to appreciate on MR; however, MR is important for staging, notably to determine extraocular spread through sclera to retrobulbar fat or along optic nerve and intracranially.

Retinoblastoma

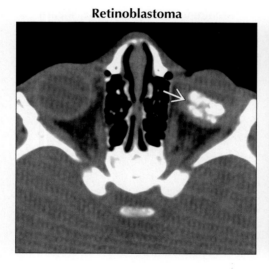

Retinoblastoma

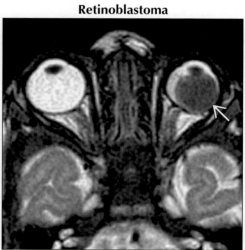

(Left) Axial NECT shows optic nerve head defect ➔ with outpouching of vitreous ➔ in typical posterior location. Size of coloboma will determine extent of loss of visual field. **(Right)** Axial T1WI MR reveals well-defined intrinsically T1 hyperintense mass ➔ in globe. The hyperintense signal on T1 is typical. Most ocular melanomas are dome-shaped early but acquire mushroom configuration with a "waist" ➔ after breaking through Bruch membrane.

Coloboma

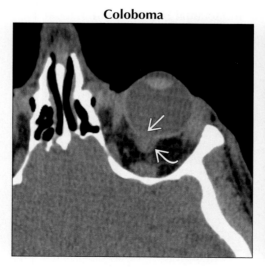

Melanoma, Ocular

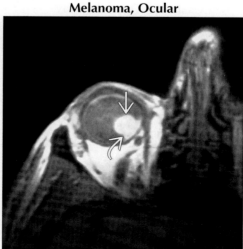

MONOCULAR VISION LOSS

Optic Perineuritis

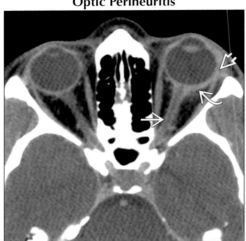

Endophthalmitis

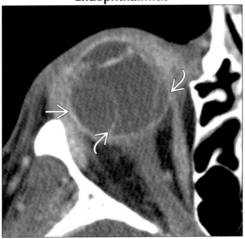

(Left) Axial NECT shows diffuse irregular thickening of optic nerve sheath ➡, irregular thickening of posterior sclera ➡, and preseptal cellulitis, seen as thickening of Tenon capsule at insertion of lateral rectus ➡. This is a form of orbital pseudotumor. (Right) Axial CECT in a patient with vision loss shows enhancing and irregular sclera ➡ with serous choroidal detachment ➡. This proved to be pseudomonas scleritis.

Ocular Toxocariasis/Sclerosing Endophthalmitis

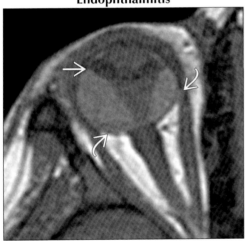

Coats Disease

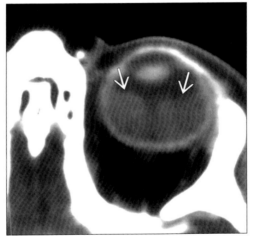

(Left) Axial T1WI MR shows diffuse increased signal in vitreous, retinal detachments ➡, and subtle nodularity of sclera ➡. This proved to be a toxocariasis infection in a 6 year old with 2 month history of painful "red" eye and no vision or light perception on examination. (Right) Axial NECT shows subtle posterior chamber hyperdensity from subretinal/subhyaloid detachment ➡. Lack of Cloquet canal or scleral findings distinguishes this from PHPV and toxocariasis.

Metastasis, Orbital or Ocular

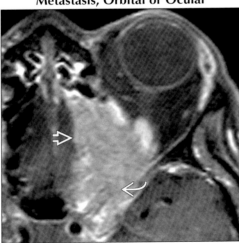

Pituitary Apoplexy

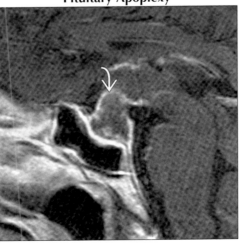

(Left) Axial T1 C+ FS MR shows a large enhancing intraconal & extraconal mass that encases intraorbital optic nerve ➡ & extends through medial orbital wall ➡. This unusual tumor was proven to be metastatic prostate carcinoma. (Right) Sagittal T1 C+ FS MR shows an irregular peripherally enhancing mass ➡ arising from sella, but with significant suprasellar extension. Patient had known pituitary macroadenoma & presented with sudden vision loss.

BITEMPORAL HETERONYMOUS HEMIANOPSIA

DIFFERENTIAL DIAGNOSIS

Common
- Pituitary Macroadenoma
- Craniopharyngioma
- Meningioma, Parasellar
- Saccular Aneurysm

Less Common
- Neoplastic
  - Pilocytic Astrocytoma, Chiasm
  - Germinoma
- Congenital
  - Tuber Cinereum Hamartoma, Hypothalamus
  - Rathke Cleft Cyst
- Inflammatory/Infectious
  - Lymphocytic Hypophysitis
  - Neurosarcoid
  - Tuberculosis
- Vascular
  - Pituitary Apoplexy
- Other
  - Langerhans Cell Histiocytosis

Rare but Important
- Pituicytoma
- Metastases, Intracranial, Other
- Abscess, Pituitary

ESSENTIAL INFORMATION

Key Differential Diagnosis Issues
- Loss of vision in temporal crescents of both eyes produce "tunnel vision" caused by lesions involving optic chiasm
- Key questions
  - Pediatric or adult patient?
  - History of head trauma?
  - Mass extra- or intra-pituitary?
- Best tool to investigate BHH: T1 C+ MR
- Rule out vascular (aneurysm or apoplexy) vs. all other causes
  - Ruptured aneurysm or acute apoplexy symptoms need emergent treatment

Helpful Clues for Common Diagnoses
- **Pituitary Macroadenoma**
  - Key facts: Intrasellar mass > 10 mm
    - Cannot be separated from pituitary
  - Imaging: Isointense to gray matter
    - Suprasellar extension through diaphragma sella → "snowman" shape

- Intense early but heterogeneous C+
- **Craniopharyngioma**
  - Key facts: Cystic, solid ± Ca++ components
    - Children: Cystic & Ca++, adamantinomatous histology
    - Adults: Solid/papillary histology
  - Imaging: Suprasellar location
    - CT: Mixed iso- & hypodense mass with nodular or eggshell Ca++; C+ rim & solid components
    - MR: ↑ Signal intensity on T1 with high protein content in cyst; solid parts iso- to hyperintense, T1 & T2
- **Meningioma, Parasellar**
  - Key facts: Uncommonly prechiasmatic
  - Imaging: Dural-based mass
    - CT: Ca++, hyperostosis adjacent bone
    - MR: Dural "tail," avid C+
- **Saccular Aneurysm**
  - Key facts: Basilar tip, cavernous sinus ICA
  - Imaging: Complex ovoid mass
    - CT: Wall calcification possible
    - MR: Complex signal from wall clot, Ca++, & phase artifact

Helpful Clues for Less Common Diagnoses
- **Pilocytic Astrocytoma, Chiasm**
  - Key facts: WHO grade I astrocytoma; child
    - Neurofibromatosis type 1 association
  - Imaging: Chiasmal enlargement, often has retrochiasmatic extension
    - T1 C+: Variably enhancing enlarged optic nerve/chiasm/tract
    - Isointense T1WI, slightly hyperintense T2WI, variable enhancement
- **Germinoma**
  - Key facts: Pediatric population
    - Suprasellar lesions, girls > boys
  - Imaging: Suprasellar hyperdense non-Ca++ mass (CT)
    - MR: Iso- to hyperintense T2 signal, restricted diffusion (DWI)
    - ± Synchronous pineal lesion, CSF seeding
- **Tuber Cinereum Hamartoma, Hypothalamus**
  - Key facts: Child with precocious puberty ± gelastic seizures
  - Imaging: Tuber cinereum, mammillary bodies of hypothalamus
    - T1 isointense, ↑ T2, nonenhancing
- **Rathke Cleft Cyst**

BITEMPORAL HETERONYMOUS HEMIANOPSIA

- Imaging: Intrasellar → suprasellar extension
  - Nonenhancing intracystic nodule
- **Lymphocytic Hypophysitis**
  - Key facts: Peripartum female
  - Imaging: Thickened, enhancing pituitary stalk with suprasellar extension
    - May mimic pituitary adenoma
- **Neurosarcoid**
  - Key facts: Uveitis, SNHL
    - Multifocal or solitary dural, leptomeningeal, or parenchymal lesions
  - Imaging: T1 C+ plaque-like or nodular masses; optic chiasm ± optic nerve
- **Tuberculosis**
  - Key facts: Basilar meningitis ± parenchymal tuberculomas
    - Isolated optic pathway involvement rare
  - Imaging: T1 C+ nodular masses involving optic chiasm, may involve optic nerves
- **Pituitary Apoplexy**
  - Key facts: Severe bifrontal/retro-orbital HA
    - Laboratory evidence of hypopituitarism
  - Imaging: Hemorrhage or infarction into preexisting pituitary adenoma
    - CT: Hyperdense large pituitary
    - MR: Heterogeneous ↑ T1 pituitary
- **Langerhans Cell Histiocytosis**
  - Key facts: Panhypopituitarism
  - Imaging: T1 C+ thick pituitary stalk
    - May mimic chiasmal glioma

Helpful Clues for Rare Diagnoses
- **Pituicytoma**

- Key facts: Diabetes insipidus
  - Peak incidence 5th decade
- Imaging: Neurohypophysis or stalk mass
  - Well-defined hyperdense or enhancing
- **Metastasis, Intracranial, Other**
  - Key facts: Breast, lung, prostate, gastric
  - Imaging: T1 C+ supra or intrasellar mass
    - ± Pituitary gland involvement; may involve or encase optic chiasm
- **Abscess, Pituitary**
  - Key facts: Preexisting pituitary adenoma
    - ± Clinical signs of infection
  - Imaging: T1 C+ intrasellar mass

Alternative Differential Approaches
- Imaging findings & BHH presentation
- Hyperdense suprasellar mass (CT)
  - Craniopharyngioma: Parenchyma Ca++
  - Aneurysm: ± Peripheral calcification
  - Germinoma: No calcification
  - Pilocytic astrocytoma: No calcification
- Enhancing intrasellar mass
  - Pituitary macroadenoma: Mass is one with pituitary gland
  - Pituitary apoplexy: Look for hemorrhagic components or diffusion restriction
- Nonenhancing intrasellar-suprasellar mass
  - Rathke cleft cyst
  - Hypothalamic hamartoma
- Lesions centered at chiasm
  - Chiasmatic glioma: Retrochiasmatic
  - Neurosarcoid: Multicentric
  - TB: Multicentric ± basilar meningitis
  - Langerhans cell histiocytosis

Pituitary Macroadenoma

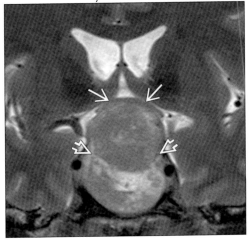

Coronal T2WI MR of a 53 year old male with BHH. The heterogeneous intrasellar mass extends through the diaphragma sella ➡ and displaces and compresses the optic chiasm ➡ upward.

Pituitary Macroadenoma

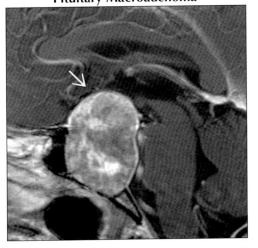

Sagittal T1 C+ MR demonstrates a heterogeneously enhancing pituitary macroadenoma that extends to the level of the infundibular recess and mamillary body, compressing the chiasm from below ➡.

BITEMPORAL HETERONYMOUS HEMIANOPSIA

(Left) Coronal T1 C+ MR in a 10 year old girl shows a minimally enhancing mixed cystic and solid mass ➡. It extends to the pituitary fossa ➯ and displaces the optic chiasm ➡ to the chiasmatic recess of the 3rd ventricle. *(Right)* Axial T2WI MR reveals a large cystic suprasellar epicenter of a sellar craniopharyngioma with mixed solid and calcified components ➡. This lesion showed adamantinomatous histology.

Craniopharyngioma

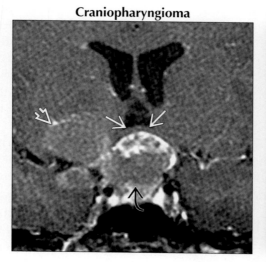

Craniopharyngioma

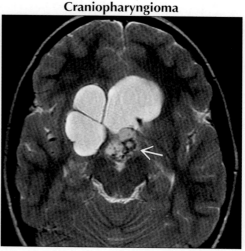

(Left) Sagittal T1 C+ MR shows enhancing suprasellar mass extending into the pituitary fossa ➡ and displacing the pituitary gland ➡. Note the dural tail ➯ and thickened hyperostotic planum sphenoidale ➡. *(Right)* Sagittal T1 C+ MR reveals an enhancing suprasellar meningioma that bows diaphragma sellae inferiorly ➯. Note the anterior and posterior margin dural tails ➡ and the normal pituitary gland below the diaphragma sellae ➡.

Meningioma, Parasellar

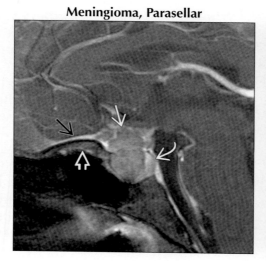

Meningioma, Parasellar

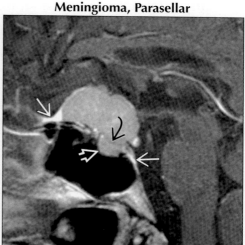

(Left) Sagittal T1WI MR shows a basilar tip aneurysm ➡ extending anteriorly and superiorly in the interpeduncular aspect of the suprasellar cistern. A flow void is present in its most anterior aspect ➡. Note that the mass is clearly separate from the pituitary gland. *(Right)* Axial T1 C+ MR reveals a large enhancing pilocytic astrocytoma enlarging the optic chiasm ➡ and extending along the canalicular and intraorbital optic nerve ➡.

Saccular Aneurysm

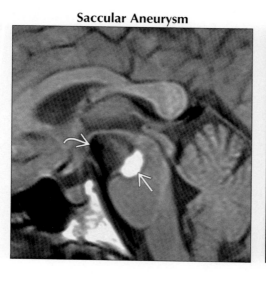

Pilocytic Astrocytoma, Chiasm

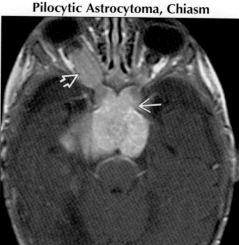

BITEMPORAL HETERONYMOUS HEMIANOPSIA

Germinoma

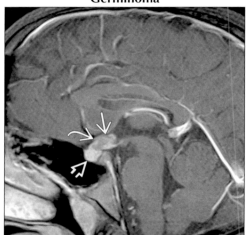

Germinoma

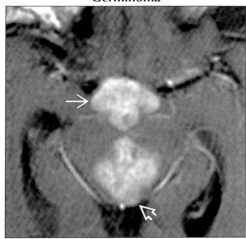

(Left) Sagittal T1 C+ MR demonstrates an enhancing suprasellar germinoma ➡ with sellar involvement and extension to chiasm ➡. Note normal anterior pituitary gland with avid homogeneous enhancement ➡ compared to the less enhancing tumor. *(Right)* Axial T1 C+ MR shows optic chiasm involvement with germinoma ➡ with a 2nd focus of this tumor that emanates from the pineal region ➡ and spreads to involve the subjacent midbrain.

Tuber Cinereum Hamartoma, Hypothalamus

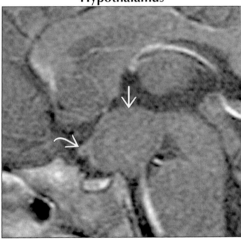

Tuber Cinereum Hamartoma, Hypothalamus

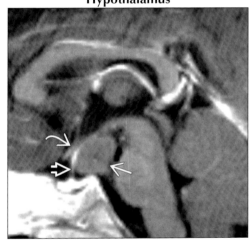

(Left) Sagittal T1 C+ MR shows a large T1 isointense nonenhancing suprasellar mass ➡ extending from the hypothalamus and impinging upon the optic chiasm ➡. This 20 month old girl presented with precocious puberty. *(Right)* Sagittal T1 C+ MR reveals an ovoid nonenhancing mass ➡ hanging from the tuber cinereum just posterior to the infundibulum ➡. Notice the optic chiasm ➡ pushed cephalad by this hamartoma.

Rathke Cleft Cyst

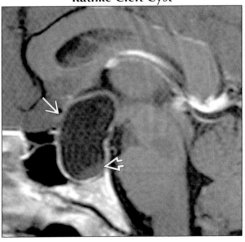

Rathke Cleft Cyst

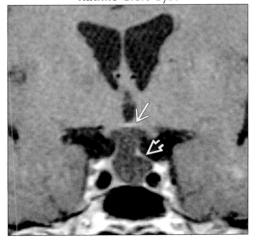

(Left) Sagittal T1 C+ MR reveals a lobulated nonenhancing cystic mass arising from the sella and extending into the suprasellar cistern, where it elevates and compresses the optic chiasm ➡. Note the isointense layer of debris in the floor ➡. *(Right)* Coronal T1 C+ MR demonstrates an intra- and suprasellar Rathke cleft cyst extending cephalad to bow the optic chiasm superiorly ➡. Note that the infundibular stalk ➡ forms a "claw" around the lesion.

BITEMPORAL HETERONYMOUS HEMIANOPSIA

(Left) Coronal T1 C+ MR shows a homogeneous avidly enhancing intrasellar mass with suprasellar extension and compression of the optic chiasm ➡ in a postpartum woman. The differential for this lesion includes pituitary macroadenoma. *(Right)* Coronal T2WI MR shows a slightly hyperintense pituitary mass ➡ that elevated the optic chiasm ➡. Preoperative diagnosis was pituitary macroadenoma. Lymphocytic hypophysitis was found at surgery.

Lymphocytic Hypophysitis

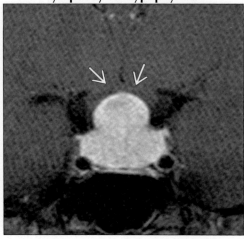

Lymphocytic Hypophysitis

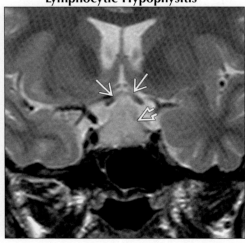

(Left) Sagittal T1 C+ FS MR shows multiple enhancing "fluffy" or nodular masses involving subependymal lateral and 3rd ventricles ➡ and diffuse enlargement of the optic chiasm ➡. *(Right)* Axial CECT reveals an irregular, ring-shaped hyperdense mass in the suprasellar cistern ➡ with adjacent pial enhancement extending around the suprasellar cistern and into the sylvian fissure ➡.

Neurosarcoid

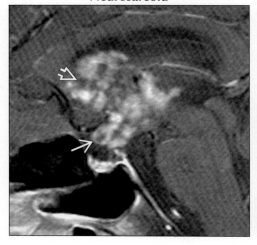

Tuberculosis

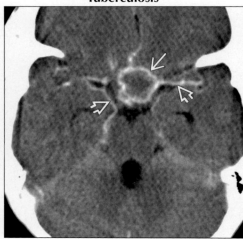

(Left) Sagittal T1 C+ MR shows a patchy enhancing intrasellar mass with suprasellar extension to chiasm ➡. GRE images showed suprasellar hemorrhage. Patient had a known macroadenoma & presented acutely with headache & BHH. *(Right)* Sagittal T1WI MR shows moderate-sized, high signal intrasellar mass ➡ that projects superiorly into suprasellar cistern & abuts optic chiasm ➡. Necrotic hemorrhagic macroadenoma was found at surgery.

Pituitary Apoplexy

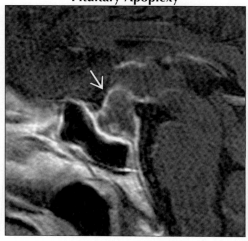

Pituitary Apoplexy

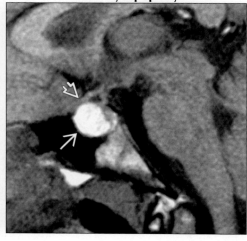

BITEMPORAL HETERONYMOUS HEMIANOPSIA

Langerhans Cell Histiocytosis

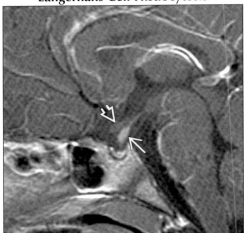

Langerhans Cell Histiocytosis

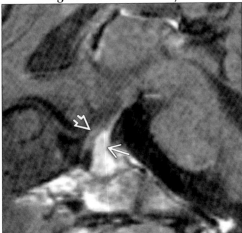

(Left) Sagittal T1 C+ FS MR demonstrates an irregular thickening and enhancement of the pituitary stalk ➡ with extension to the chiasm ➡ in a 5 year old patient with diabetes insipidus. *(Right)* Sagittal T1WI MR shows a thick pituitary stalk ➡ from Langerhans cell histiocytosis. The optic chiasm is upwardly bowed ➡ by the enlarged pituitary stalk.

Pituicytoma

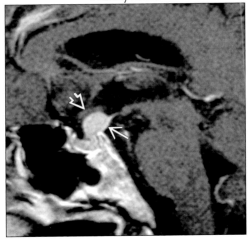

Pituicytoma

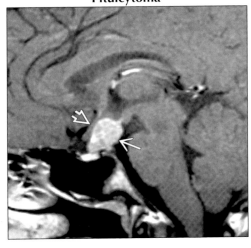

(Left) Sagittal T1 C+ MR reveals a well-defined enhancing suprasellar pituicytoma arising from the infundibulum ➡ and compressing the optic chiasm ➡. *(Right)* Sagittal T1 C+ MR demonstrates a pituicytoma ➡ in a patient with hypopituitarism. Mild mass effect upon the optic chiasm by the lesion is visible ➡.

Metastases, Intracranial, Other

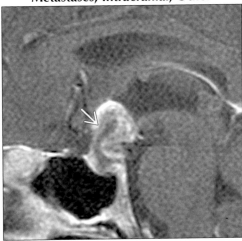

Abscess, Pituitary

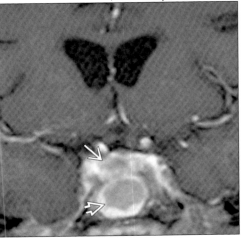

(Left) Sagittal T1 C+ FS MR reveals a heterogeneously enhancing invasive metastatic melanoma with both sellar and suprasellar components. Notice that the optic chiasm is encased ➡ by this metastasis. *(Right)* Coronal T1 C+ MR shows an irregular enhancing mass in the pituitary fossa ➡ in a patient who presented acutely with fever, visual loss, and ophthalmoplegia. Note the adjacent sphenoid sinusitis ➡.

11

Cranial Nerve & Brainstem

DIFFERENTIAL DIAGNOSIS

Common
- Posterior Cerebral Artery Ischemia
- CNS Neoplasm in Temporal-Occipital Region or Retrochiasmatic Optic Pathway
  - Glioblastoma Multiforme
- Demyelinating Diseases
  - Multiple Sclerosis
  - ADEM
- CNS Trauma Affecting Temporal-Occipital Region or Retrochiasmatic Optic Pathway
  - Subdural Hematoma, Acute
  - Cerebral Contusion

Less Common
- Fusiform Aneurysm, ASVD, PCA, or MCA
- Abscess, Temporal-Occipital Brain
- Cavernous Malformation, Temporal-Occipital Brain

Rare but Important
- Opportunistic Infection, AIDS, PML
- Creutzfeldt-Jakob Disease, Heidenhain Variant

ESSENTIAL INFORMATION

Key Differential Diagnosis Issues
- Type of hemianopsia pinpoints relative location along visual pathway
  - Incongruous homonymous hemianopsia (HH) with afferent pupillary defect and bow-tie atrophy = optic tract
  - Homonymous sectoranopia = lateral geniculate nucleus (LGN)
  - Incongruous homonymous hemianopsia is same as lateral geniculate nucleus
  - Homonymous upper quadrant defect ("pie in the sky") = temporal lobe
  - Homonymous defect, denser more inferiorly = parietal lobe
  - Complete homonymous hemianopsia = temporoparietal ± occipital
  - Homonymous upper quadrantanopsia with macular sparing = lower bank of occipital lobe
  - Homonymous lower quadrantanopsia, macular sparing = upper bank of occipital lobe
  - Isolated homonymous defect (macular sparing) without other neurological findings = occipital lobe

Helpful Clues for Common Diagnoses
- **Posterior Cerebral Artery Ischemia**
  - Key facts: PCA distribution infarct is most common cause of HH (40-90%)
    - Significant association with hypertension, diabetes, & renal impairment
  - MR findings
    - Acute PCA CVA: Diffusion restriction & ADC map correlate in PCA territory
    - Subacute: Wedge-shaped area in PCA distribution with edema on T1, T2, FLAIR; gyral enhancement T1 C+; ↑ diffusion restriction, ↓ ADC with reversal through subacute stage
    - Chronic: Nonenhancing, hypodense, or CSF isointense area with gliosis along margin; no diffusion restriction
- **Glioblastoma Multiforme**
  - Key facts
    - Many primary and metastatic CNS neoplasms affect temporal-occipital brain or retrochiasmatic optic pathway
    - Most are gliomas; most of gliomas are glioblastoma multiforme
    - Pilocytic astrocytoma: ± enhancing & enlarged optic chiasm or optic tract; pediatric population; ~ 30% neurofibromatosis type 1
    - Parenchymal metastasis: Often multiple C+ masses at gray-white junction
  - MR findings
    - Temporal, parietal, or occipital focal or diffuse C- or C+ white matter or cortical mass involving retrochiasmatic optic pathway or optic radiations
    - Diffusion tensor imaging: FA maps ± fiber tracts may show infiltration or compression of optic radiation ± inferior occipitofrontal fasciculus
    - Look for lack of diffusion restriction to differentiate from ischemia/infarction
- **Multiple Sclerosis**
  - Key facts: Polyphasic illness
  - MR findings: Look for additional lesions involving callpososeptal interface; optic neuritis
- **ADEM**
  - Key facts: Monophasic illness
  - MR findings: Multifocal ± enhancing white matter, basal ganglia lesions

11

- Typically does not involve callososeptal interface
- **Subdural Hematoma, Acute**
  - Key facts: Mass effect may affect temporal-occipital region or retrochiasmatic optic pathway
    - Specific visual field testing usually not performed in emergent or acute setting
  - CT findings: Shows hyper- to hypodense extra-axial fluid collection
    - Enhancement of bridging veins
    - Compression & displacement of underlying brain
- **Cerebral Contusion**
  - Key facts: May affect temporal-occipital region or retrochiasmatic optic pathway
    - Has reported association with encephalomalacia following traumatic subdural hematoma
  - CT findings: Look for multiple patchy ill-defined punctate or linear areas of gyral hemorrhage
    - Look for subarachnoid hemorrhage & associated skull fracture

Helpful Clues for Less Common Diagnoses
- **Fusiform Aneurysm, ASVD, PCA, or MCA**
  - Key facts: Chronically enlarging posterior or middle cerebral artery fusiform aneurysm cause HH from mass effect
  - MR findings: Fusiform mass with complex signal
- **Abscess, Temporal-Occipital Brain**
  - Key facts: Systemically ill patient with decreased consciousness
  - MR findings: Hemispheric parenchymal ring-enhancing mass with restricted diffusion
- **Cavernous Malformation, Temporal-Occipital Brain**
  - Key facts: Benign vascular hamartoma prone to intralesional hemorrhage
  - MR findings: Mixed signal lesion with GRE blooming

Helpful Clues for Rare Diagnoses
- **Opportunistic Infection, AIDS, PML**
  - Key facts: Occurs in immunocompromised patients due to JC polyomavirus
    - Majority of patients present with HH
  - MR findings: Frontal & parietal-occipital subcortical white matter patchy high T2 signal without enhancement
    - Peripherally located lesions in contrast to periventricular lesions in MS
- **Creutzfeldt-Jakob Disease, Heidenhain Variant**
  - Key facts: Rapidly progressive dementia cause by prion
    - Heidenhain variant: Isolated visual symptoms from predominantly occipital lobe degeneration
  - MR findings: T2 & FLAIR high signal in occipital lobe white matter tracts with associated encephalomalacia

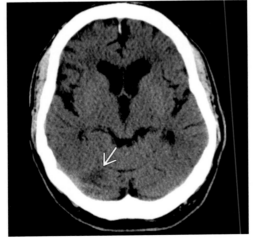

Posterior Cerebral Artery Ischemia

Axial NECT of a patient with an acute onset of left binocular visual field defect shows a hypodense area in the right occipital lobe ➡.

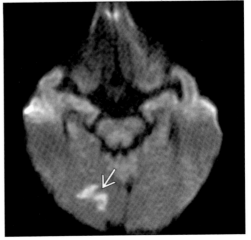

Posterior Cerebral Artery Ischemia

Axial DWI MR shows ↑ DW signal ➡ in the right occipital lobe, which showed restricted diffusion on ADC maps. On examination, the patient had a left superior homonymous quadrantanopsia.

HOMONYMOUS HEMIANOPSIA

Glioblastoma Multiforme

Multiple Sclerosis

(Left) Axial FLAIR MR reveals extensive confluent hyperintensity involving the white matter of the right temporal lobe ➡ and thalamus ➡. *(Right)* Axial T1 C+ MR demonstrates peripherally enhancing ➡ tumefactive multiple sclerosis plaque in the region of the left optic radiations.

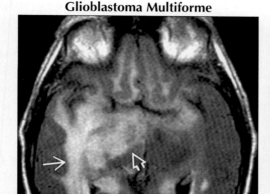
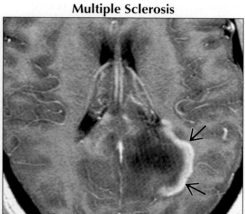

ADEM

Subdural Hematoma, Acute

(Left) Axial T2WI MR shows confluent regions of high signal in the white matter of the cerebral hemispheres ➡ in this patient with acute disseminated encephalomyelitis. Note the additional regions of T2 hyperintense signal seen in the thalami ➡. *(Right)* Axial NECT shows crescentic hyperdense extra-axial hemorrhage along right occipital lobe ➡ & temporal lobe ➡. Acute onset homonymous hemianopsia with severe headache were the presenting symptoms.

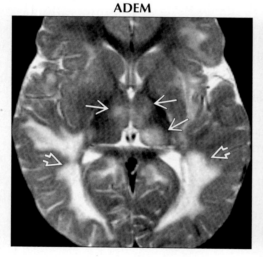
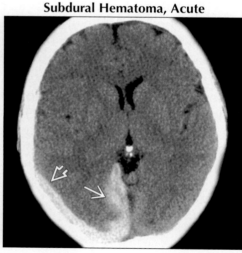

Cerebral Contusion

Fusiform Aneurysm, ASVD, PCA, or MCA

(Left) Axial NECT shows traumatic contrecoup hemorrhagic contusion of the right temporal lobe ➡. Also notice the subdural blood layering along the tentorium ➡. A large left subcutaneous hematoma ➡ is also noted. *(Right)* Axial MRA reveals a partially thrombosed fusiform aneurysm of the middle cerebral artery. Contrast-enhanced MRA source image delineates the residual lumen ➡ and rim-enhancing clot.

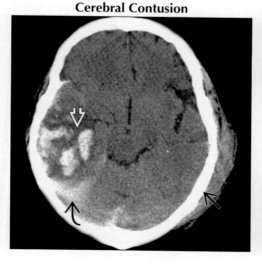
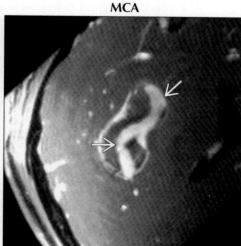

Abscess, Temporal-Occipital Brain

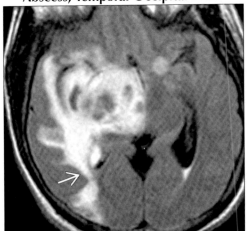

Cavernous Malformation, Temporal-Occipital Brain

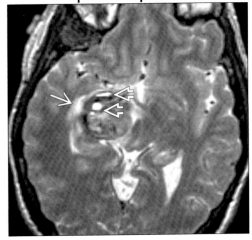

(Left) Axial FLAIR MR shows extensive confluent high signal intensity in the temporal lobe, midbrain, basal ganglia, and deep white matter. Note involvement of the retrochiasmatic pathway ➡. (Right) Axial T2WI MR demonstrates classic "popcorn" mixed attenuation with multiple fluid-fluid levels ➡ contained within a low signal hemosiderin ring. Edema is present in the temporal lobe adjacent to the malformation ➡.

Cavernous Malformation, Temporal-Occipital Brain

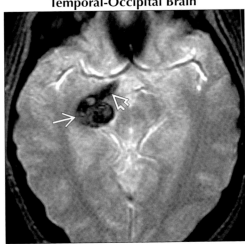

Opportunistic Infection, AIDS, PML

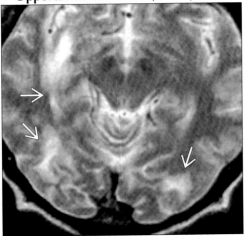

(Left) Axial T2 GRE MR reveals blooming ➡ blood products from a previous hemorrhage in a medial temporal lobe cavernous malformation. Note the extension of the blooming blood products anteromedially along the optic tract ➡. (Right) Axial T2WI MR reveals the typical appearance of PML with patchy increased signal in the white matter bilaterally ➡. PML typically causes a subacute demyelination.*

Creutzfeldt-Jakob Disease, Heidenhain Variant

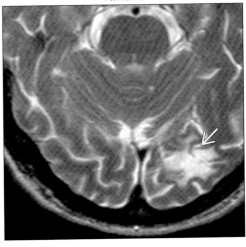

Creutzfeldt-Jakob Disease, Heidenhain Variant

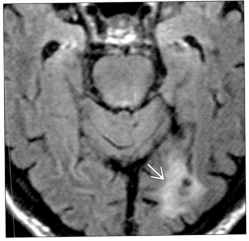

(Left) Axial T2WI MR shows occipital lobe white matter confluent high signal ➡ without mass effect. The Heidenhain variant of Creutzfeldt-Jakob disease is characterized by early isolated visual symptoms and signs. (Right) Axial FLAIR MR demonstrates a confluent high signal abnormality in the left occipital lobe ➡ with the appearance of encephalomalacia.

OCULOMOTOR, TROCHLEAR, OR ABDUCENS NEUROPATHY

DIFFERENTIAL DIAGNOSIS

Common
- Microvascular Infarction (CN3,4,6)
- Saccular Aneurysm, Posterior Communicating Artery (CN3)
- Multiple Sclerosis
- Cerebral Ischemia-Infarction, Acute
- Meningioma, Cavernous Sinus (CS)
- Metastases, Intracranial, Cavernous Sinus
- Schwannoma, Cavernous Sinus (CN3,4,6)
- Metastases, Parenchymal, Brainstem
- Thrombosis, Cavernous Sinus

Less Common
- Idiopathic Orbital Inflammatory Disease
- Pseudotumor, Intracranial
- Carotid-Cavernous Fistula, Traumatic
- Saccular Aneurysm, Cavernous ICA
- Lymphoproliferative Lesions, Orbit

Rare but Important
- Metastasis, Orbit
- Pituitary Macroadenoma
- Cavernous Malformation
- Schwannoma, Cisternal (CN3,4,6)

ESSENTIAL INFORMATION

Key Differential Diagnosis Issues
- CN3,4,6 supply 6 extraocular muscles
  - CN3: All muscles but superior oblique (CN4) & lateral rectus (CN6)
- All 3 CN's have brainstem, cisternal, cavernous sinus, & orbital components
- CN3 anatomy
  - Nucleus in dorsal midbrain at level superior colliculus
  - Cisternal CN3 parallels posterior communicating artery
  - Midbrain → interpeduncular cistern → oculomotor cistern → cavernous sinus → superior orbital fissure (SOF) → orbit
  - Arterial supply to CN3 feeds nerve core
  - Parasympathetic fibers (pupillary sphincter) in superficial CN3
- CN3 neuropathy in patient > 40 years of age
  - Patient old enough to suffer from vasculopathic oculomotor neuropathy
  - Pupillary sparing often followed clinically
- CN3 neuropathy in patient < 40 years of age or any complete CN3 neuropathy

- Posterior communicating artery aneurysm must be excluded!
  - CTA or MR/MRA followed by angio if unanswered questions
- CN4 anatomy
  - Midbrain nucleus → dorsal decussation → free margin tentorium → cavernous sinus → superior orbital fissure → orbit
- CN6 anatomy
  - Pontine tegmentum nucleus → exits at ventral pontomedullary junction → prepontine cistern → Dorello canal → cavernous sinus → SOF → orbit

Helpful Clues for Common Diagnoses
- **Microvascular Infarction (CN3,4,6)**
  - Key facts: Acute onset CN3,4,6 neuropathy
    - CN3: Usually pupil-sparing
    - Diabetics ± hypertension
  - Imaging: Enhancing CN3, 4, or 6 rare
- **Saccular Aneurysm, Posterior Communicating Artery (CN3)**
  - Key facts: Complete CN3 neuropathy
  - Imaging: CTA, MRA, angiography
    - CTA: Ovoid contrast collection with Ca++ in wall
    - MR/MRA: Complex signal from flow, clot, & Ca++ in wall
- **Multiple Sclerosis**
  - Key facts: CN3,4,6 symptoms in younger patient, suspect MS
  - Imaging: White matter plaques
    - Lesions in midbrain may not be visible
- **Cerebral Ischemia-Infarction, Acute**
  - Key facts: Acute onset CN3 symptoms
  - Imaging: DWI shows restricted diffusion in midbrain with low signal ADC
- **Meningioma, Cavernous Sinus (CS)**
  - Key facts: From dural margin of CS
  - Imaging: Extra-axial, "dural tails"
- **Metastases, Intracranial, Cavernous Sinus**
  - Imaging: Enlarged, irregular C+ CS
- **Schwannoma, Cavernous Sinus (CN3,4,6)**
  - Key facts: May be asymptomatic
  - Imaging: Smoothly C+, enlarged CS
- **Metastases, Parenchymal, Brainstem**
  - Imaging: Enhancing brainstem lesion often with significant associated edema
- **Thrombosis, Cavernous Sinus**
  - Key facts: Septic patient
  - Imaging: Nonenhancing clot in enlarged CS ± large superior orbital veins

OCULOMOTOR, TROCHLEAR, OR ABDUCENS NEUROPATHY

Helpful Clues for Less Common Diagnoses

- **Idiopathic Orbital Inflammatory Disease**
  - Key facts: Painful limited eye movement
  - Imaging: May involve any part of orbit
- **Pseudotumor, Intracranial**
  - Imaging: Thickened, enhancing meninges of cavernous sinus wall
    - Low T2 signal often
    - May have "dural tails" like meningioma
- **Carotid-Cavernous Fistula, Traumatic**
  - Key facts: Post-traumatic red eye
  - Imaging: Enlarge CS & superior ophthalmic vein
- **Saccular Aneurysm, Cavernous ICA**
  - Imaging: Unilateral CS enlargement
    - Complex signal from clot, flow, & Ca++
- **Lymphoproliferative Lesions, Orbit**
  - Imaging: Invasive mass anywhere in orbit

Helpful Clues for Rare Diagnoses

- **Metastasis, Orbit**
  - Key facts: Breast, prostate, lung
  - Imaging: Variable; diffuse enhancing intraconal mass
- **Pituitary Macroadenoma**
  - Key facts: > 10 mm; suprasellar ± CS
  - Imaging: Large pituitary with suprasellar ± cavernous sinus involvement
- **Cavernous Malformation**
  - Key facts: Solitary or multiple (familial)
  - MR: Lesion blood products & "popcorn" calcifications bloom on GRE
- **Schwannoma, Cisternal (CN3,4,6)**
  - Key facts: May be incidental

  - Imaging: Enhancing fusiform mass extending along cranial nerve course

Alternative Differential Approaches

- Segmental anatomic approach
  - For CN3,4,6 includes brainstem, cistern, cavernous sinus, & orbit
- Segment approach to oculomotor neuropathy differential diagnosis
  - Midbrain (CN3, CN4) & pons (CN6)
    - Multiple sclerosis
    - Cerebral ischemia-infarction, acute
    - Metastases, parenchymal, brainstem
    - Cavernous malformation
  - Cistern
    - Microvascular infarction (CN3,4,6)
    - Saccular aneurysm, posterior communicating artery (CN3)
    - Pituitary macroadenoma
    - Schwannoma, cisternal (CN3,4,6)
  - Cavernous sinus
    - Saccular aneurysm, cavernous ICA
    - Thrombosis, cavernous sinus
    - Meningioma, cavernous sinus
    - Metastases, intracranial, cavernous sinus
    - Carotid-cavernous fistula, traumatic
    - Schwannoma, cavernous sinus (CN3,4,6)
  - Orbit
    - Idiopathic orbital inflammatory disease
    - Pseudotumor, intracranial
    - Lymphoproliferative lesions, orbit
    - Metastasis, orbit

Saccular Aneurysm, Posterior Communicating Artery (CN3)

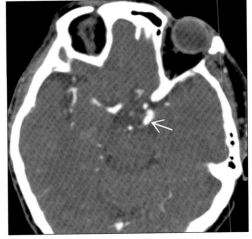

Axial CTA reveals a left posterior communicating artery aneurysm ➡ in this patient presenting with a complete CN3 palsy including pupillary reflex absence.

Saccular Aneurysm, Posterior Communicating Artery (CN3)

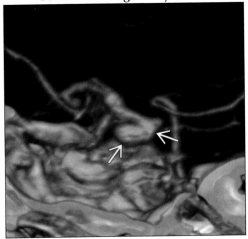

Sagittal 3D CTA reconstruction shows a large posterior communicating artery aneurysm ➡ with a complex shape. This patient presented with a complete CN3 palsy on the side of the aneurysm.

OCULOMOTOR, TROCHLEAR, OR ABDUCENS NEUROPATHY

Multiple Sclerosis

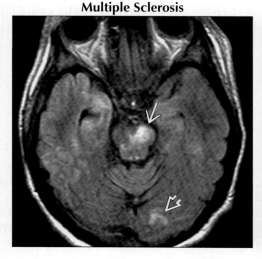

Multiple Sclerosis

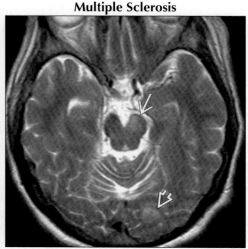

(Left) Axial FLAIR MR demonstrates a large amorphous multiple sclerosis plaque ➡ in left midbrain. CN3 fibers pass through this lesion on their way ventrally to exit the midbrain in the interpeduncular cistern. 2nd lesion is seen in the occipital lobe white matter ➡.
(Right) Axial T2WI MR shows a left midbrain extensive multiple sclerosis lesion ➡ in a patient with known MS & new onset left CN3 palsy. Note 2nd occipital white matter lesion ➡.

Cerebral Ischemia-Infarction, Acute

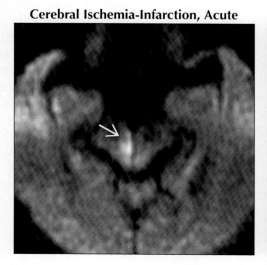

Cerebral Ischemia-Infarction, Acute

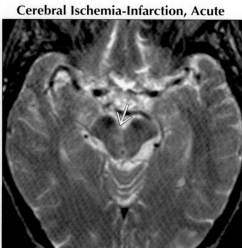

(Left) Axial DWI MR shows restricted diffusion ➡ in the ventromedial midbrain in a patient with acute onset of a right CN3 palsy. This midbrain infarction involves the area of CN3 fibers coursing from the dorsal CN3 nucleus to exit the midbrain in the interpeduncular cistern.
(Right) Axial T2WI MR demonstrates a subtle area of high signal in the right ventral midbrain ➡ in a patient with acute onset of right CN3 palsy.

Meningioma, Cavernous Sinus (CS)

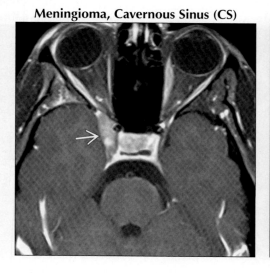

Meningioma, Cavernous Sinus (CS)

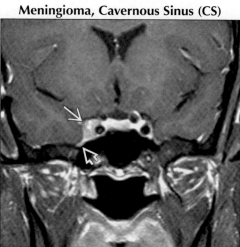

(Left) Axial T1 C+ MR reveals an enhancing dural-based mass involving the right cavernous sinus ➡. Intracranial pseudotumor and cavernous sinus schwannoma were both considered along with cavernous sinus meningioma in the differential diagnosis.
(Right) Coronal T1WI MR shows convexed right cavernous sinus wall from meningioma involvement ➡. Lesion extends to abut the right maxillary division of the trigeminal nerve in foramen rotundum ➡.

11

Metastases, Intracranial, Cavernous Sinus

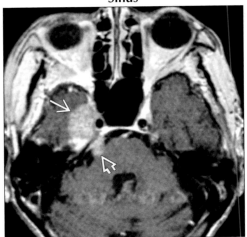

Metastases, Intracranial, Cavernous Sinus

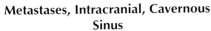
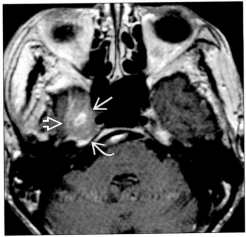

(Left) Axial T1 C+ MR demonstrates a large cavernous sinus metastasis ➡ in this patient with known breast cancer and acute onset of right CN3, CN4, and CN6 palsies. Note perineural spread ➡ along preganglionic segment of the trigeminal nerve. *(Right)* Axial T1 C+ MR shows a large right cavernous sinus metastatic deposit of breast carcinoma ➡. Note the tumor spreads laterally along the middle cranial fossa floor ➡ and involves the petrous apex ➡.

Schwannoma, Cavernous Sinus (CN3,4,6)

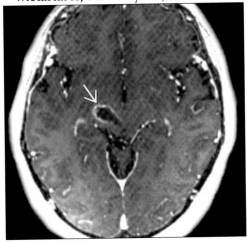

Schwannoma, Cavernous Sinus (CN3,4,6)

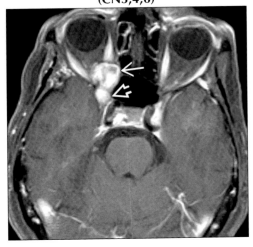
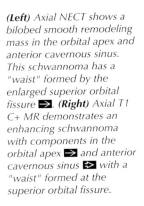

(Left) Axial NECT shows a bilobed smooth remodeling mass in the orbital apex and anterior cavernous sinus. This schwannoma has a "waist" formed by the enlarged superior orbital fissure ➡. *(Right)* Axial T1 C+ MR demonstrates an enhancing schwannoma with components in the orbital apex ➡ and anterior cavernous sinus ➡ with a "waist" formed at the superior orbital fissure.

Metastases, Parenchymal, Brainstem

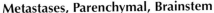

Metastases, Parenchymal, Brainstem

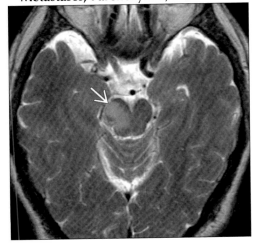

(Left) Coronal T1 C+ MR reveals a necrotic right midbrain lung carcinoma metastasis ➡ crossing the plane of the oculomotor nerve fibers as they track ventrally to exit the interpeduncular cistern. *(Right)* Axial T2WI MR demonstrates midbrain edema ➡ associated with a lung carcinoma metastasis. Left body weakness accompanied oculomotor palsy in this patient.

11

33

(Left) Axial T1 C+ FS MR shows sphenoid sinusitis ➡ causing cavernous sinus thrombosis ➡ and cavernous ICA spasm and possible occlusion ➡. Patient presented with right CN3, CN4, and CN6 palsies. (Right) Coronal T1 C+ FS MR reveals right cavernous sinus septic thrombosis with ICA spasm ➡. The cavernous sinus clot is seen as low signal nonenhancing material around the cavernous carotid artery. Right sphenoid sinus is infected ➡.

Thrombosis, Cavernous Sinus

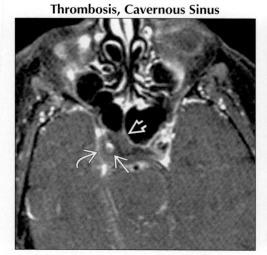

Thrombosis, Cavernous Sinus

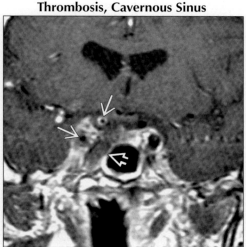

(Left) Axial T1 C+ MR shows apical subtype of idiopathic orbital inflammatory disease, involving the orbital apex ➡ and superior orbital fissure ➡, with resultant optic and oculomotor nerve involvement. (Right) Coronal T1 C+ MR demonstrates idiopathic orbital inflammatory disease in the orbital apex ➡. Notice the adjacent enhancement of the meninges just superomedial to the orbital apex disease ➡. Such proximal intracranial disease is not uncommon.

Idiopathic Orbital Inflammatory Disease

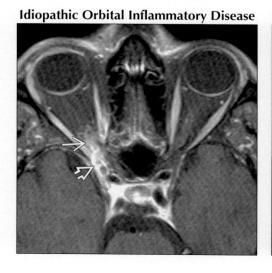

Idiopathic Orbital Inflammatory Disease

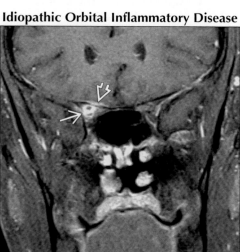

(Left) Axial T1 C+ MR reveals intracranial pseudotumor involving the left cavernous sinus ➡ and tentorium cerebelli ➡. Cavernous ICA is narrowed ➡. Distinguishing this lesion from meningioma with imaging may be extremely difficult. (Right) Axial T1WI MR shows large left cavernous sinus ➡ filled with multiple high velocity flow voids. This patient had severe head trauma and returned for evaluation of left pulsatile exophthalmos and palsies of CN3 and CN6.

Pseudotumor, Intracranial

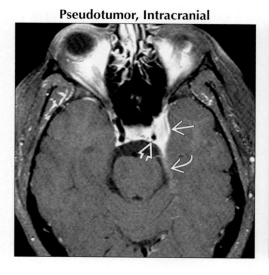

Carotid-Cavernous Fistula, Traumatic

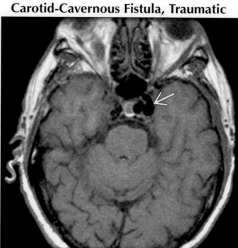

11

34

OCULOMOTOR, TROCHLEAR, OR ABDUCENS NEUROPATHY

Saccular Aneurysm, Cavernous ICA

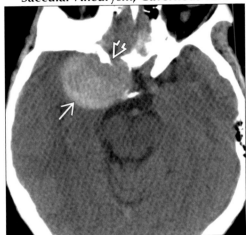

Lymphoproliferative Lesions, Orbit

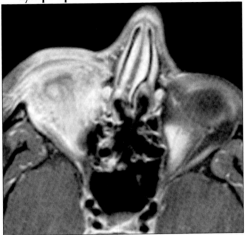

(Left) Axial NECT demonstrates a giant thrombosed internal carotid artery aneurysm extending from the cavernous sinus into the right middle cranial fossa ➡. The aneurysm erodes the tip of the anterior clinoid ➡. MR (not shown) showed complex aneurysm signal with luminal flow void. (Right) Axial T1 C+ FS MR shows infiltrating avidly enhancing lymphoma of the right orbit involving the extraconal, conal, intraconal, and preseptal areas.

Metastasis, Orbit

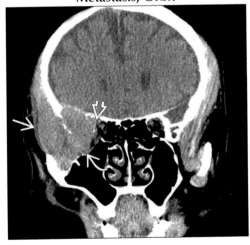

Pituitary Macroadenoma

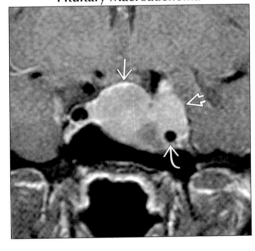

(Left) Coronal NECT reveals a large destructive right lateral orbital wall metastasis that involves the suprazygomatic masticator space ➡, orbital apex ➡, and retromaxillary fat pad ➡. (Right) Coronal T1 C+ MR shows a pituitary macroadenoma ➡ that invades the left cavernous sinus ➡. Notice the cavernous internal carotid artery on the left is completely surrounded by adenoma ➡.

Cavernous Malformation

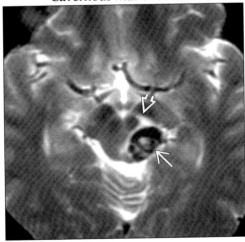

Schwannoma, Cisternal (CN3,4,6)

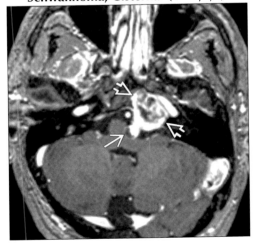

(Left) Axial T2WI MR shows a hemorrhagic midbrain cavernous malformation ➡ with low signal associated with matrix blood products. Note the associated midbrain high signal edema tracks ➡. (Right) Axial T1 C+ FS MR reveals an abducens nerve schwannoma as an enhancing mass "pointing" inferomedially toward the pontomedullary junction ➡. The lesion remodels the clivus-petrous apex area ➡. Intramural cysts are present.

11

TRIGEMINAL NEUROPATHY

DIFFERENTIAL DIAGNOSIS

Common
- Perineural Tumor, CNV2, Sinus-Nose
- Perineural Tumor, CNV3, MS
- Vascular Loop Syndrome, CN5
- Schwannoma, Trigeminal, Skull Base
- Meningioma, CPA-IAC

Less Common
- Metastases, CPA-IAC
- Neurofibromatosis 2, CPA-IAC
- Schwannoma, CNV3, MS
- Metastasis, Skull Base
- Sarcoidosis, CPA-IAC
- Perineural Tumor, CNV1

Rare but Important
- Multiple Sclerosis
- Cavernous Malformation, Pontine
- Cerebral Ischemia-Infarction, Acute
- Chondrosarcoma, Skull Base

ESSENTIAL INFORMATION

Key Differential Diagnosis Issues
- NEUROPATHY vs. NEURALGIA
  - Trigeminal neuropathy is ANY dysfunction of CN5, sensory or motor
    - Facial pain or numbness, weakness of masticator muscles or trismus
  - Trigeminal neuralgia (tic douloureux) is specific disorder with episodic severe pain in distribution of branch(es) of CN5
    - Vascular loop compressing CN5 at root entry zone (REZ) most common cause
- Best imaging tool for trigeminal neuropathy
  - MR is modality of choice
    - T2 for brainstem & cisternal segment
    - Thin-slice heavily T2-weighted most helpful for detecting vascular loop
    - T1: For skull base & main nerve branches in deep face
    - T1 C+ fat-sat: Perineural tumor search
  - Look for denervation changes in masticator muscles
    - Acute: T1 normal, bright T2, may enhance, muscles enlarged
    - Subacute: Bright T1 & T2, usually enhances, muscles normal volume
    - Chronic: Bright T1, T2 normal, variable enhancement, muscles atrophic
- Perineural tumor (PNT) of V1, V2, V3

  - Appears as focal or segmental thickening of CN5 or branch or abnormal nerve C+
    - Cisternal segment PNT best seen as abnormal enhancement on MR
    - Deep face PNT best seen on T1 C+ MR as thick "cord" displacing normal fat

Helpful Clues for Common Diagnoses
- **Perineural Tumor, CNV2, Sinus-Nose**
  - Key facts: Maxillary division, CN5 PNT
    - CNV2: Sensory only to cheek, palate, maxillary teeth
    - CNV2 exits skull base through foramen rotundum to pterygopalatine fossa, then along inferior orbital canal to cheek
    - Primary (SCCa, adenoid cystic carcinoma) in palate, maxillary gingiva, sinus, & skin of cheek
  - CT/MR: Enhancing enlarged nerve projects from primary tumor along CNV2
    - PNT may involve inferior orbital nerve → pterygopalatine fossa → foramen rotundum → cavernous sinus → Meckel cave → preganglionic CN5
- **Perineural Tumor, CNV3, MS**
  - Key facts: Mandibular division, CN5 PNT
    - CNV3: 2 motor & 4 sensory branches
    - Sensory: Chin, anterior tongue, floor of mouth and jaw
    - Motor: Muscles of mastication, anterior belly of digastric, mylohyoid, tensor tympani, tensor veli palatini
    - CNV3 exits skull base through foramen ovale to masticator space (MS), then along inferior alveolar canal of mandible
    - Primary tumor (SCCa, melanoma) in floor of mouth, tongue mandibular gingiva, skin of chin; MS sarcoma
  - CT/MR: Enhancing enlarged nerve projects from primary tumor along CNV3
    - PNT may involve inferior alveolar nerve → masticator nerve → foramen ovale → Meckel cave → preganglionic CN5
- **Vascular Loop Syndrome, CN5**
  - Key facts: Arterial loop abuts CN5 at REZ
    - Presentation: Trigeminal neuralgia
    - Superior cerebellar artery > AICA > vertebrobasilar dolichoectasia
    - CN5 atrophy may be associated
  - MR/MRA: Deforming arterial loop in REZ
- **Schwannoma, Trigeminal, Skull Base**
  - Key facts: NF2 or isolated

- CT/MR: Bilobed Meckel cave → superior CPA cistern mass
  - Avid enhancement ± intramural cysts
  - If bilobed, isthmus of mass created by constriction at entrance to Meckel cave
  - If Meckel cave only, large medial middle cranial fossa mass
- **Meningioma, CPA-IAC**
  - Key facts: From dura of dorsal clivus, petrous bone, petroclival ligament, tentorium
  - CT/MR: C+ mass with dural base
    - When extends to Meckel cave, mimics trigeminal schwannoma
    - Look for DURAL TAILS to make diagnosis

Helpful Clues for Less Common Diagnoses
- **Metastases, CPA-IAC**
  - CT/MR: Invasive mass along course of CN5
- **Neurofibromatosis 2, CPA-IAC**
  - CT/MR: Bilateral CPA-IAC schwannomas with trigeminal schwannoma possible
- **Schwannoma, CNV3, MS**
  - CT/MR: Fusiform enhancing CNV3 mass
    - Large foramen ovale possible
- **Metastasis, Skull Base**
  - CT/MR: Destructive mass in bones of skull base affects foramen ovale (CNV3), foramen rotundum (CNV2), or superior orbital fissure (CNV1)
- **Sarcoidosis, CPA-IAC**
  - CT/MR: Dural-based enhancing lesion may affect CN5 directly or occur in proximity, including Meckel cave or cavernous sinus

- **Perineural Tumor, CNV1**
  - Key facts: Malignant primary tumor of forehead, skin, or orbit
  - CT/MR: Enlarged, enhancing CN1 may extend from tumor → orbit → superior orbital fissure → cavernous sinus → Meckel cave → preganglionic CN5

Helpful Clues for Rare Diagnoses
- **Multiple Sclerosis**
  - Key facts: CN5 symptoms in younger patient, suspect MS
  - MR: Supratentorial white matter plaques
    - Lesions in pons may not be visible
    - Enhancing preganglionic CN5 reported
- **Cavernous Malformation, Pontine**
  - Key facts: Solitary or multiple (familial)
  - MR: Lesion blood products & calcifications bloom on GRE
- **Cerebral Ischemia-Infarction, Acute**
  - MR: DWI restricted diffusion signals pontine CVA presence
- **Chondrosarcoma, Skull Base**
  - CT/MR: Petro-occipital fissure invasive mass involves Meckel cave-CN5 early

SELECTED REFERENCES

1. Woolfall P et al: Pictorial review: Trigeminal nerve: anatomy and pathology. Br J Radiol. 74(881):458-67, 2001
2. Caldemeyer KS et al: Imaging features and clinical significance of perineural spread or extension of head and neck tumors. Radiographics. 18(1):97-110; quiz 147, 1998
3. Majoie CB et al: Trigeminal neuropathy: evaluation with MR imaging. Radiographics. 15(4):795-811, 1995

Perineural Tumor, CNV2, Sinus-Nose

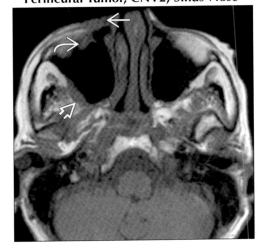

Axial T1WI MR image shows right cheek subcutaneous thickening ➡ and a cord of tumor extending along the infraorbital nerve ➡ to the retromaxillary fat ➡.

Perineural Tumor, CNV3, MS

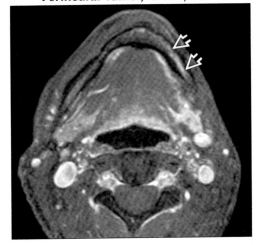

Axial T1 C+ FS MR shows abnormal thickening and enhancement of the left inferior alveolar nerve ➡ due to perineural adenoid cystic carcinoma.

11

TRIGEMINAL NEUROPATHY

(Left) Axial T2WI MR shows a dark flow void of the superior cerebellar artery ⇒ medial to the most proximal cisternal segment of the right trigeminal nerve ⇒, known as the root entry zone.
(Right) Axial T1 C+ FS MR shows an enhancing bilobed schwannoma of the cisternal segment of the right trigeminal nerve ⇒, extending into the Meckel cave ⇒.

Vascular Loop Syndrome, CN5

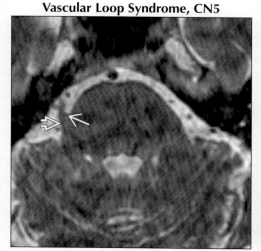

Schwannoma, Trigeminal, Skull Base

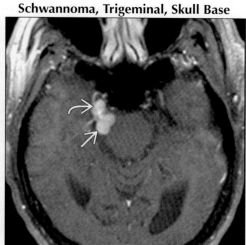

(Left) Axial T1 C+ MR shows a dural-based mass ⇒ in the left CPA extending into the left Meckel cave ⇒. Dural tail ⇒ is key to distinguishing from trigeminal schwannoma.
(Right) Coronal T1 C+ MR shows left IAC ⇒ enhancement from leptomeningeal adenocarcinoma metastases, with additional involvement of the left trigeminal nerve cisternal segment ⇒.

Meningioma, CPA-IAC

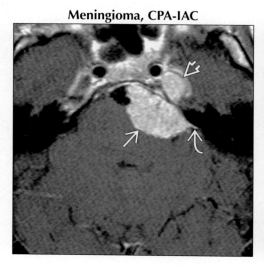

Metastases, CPA-IAC

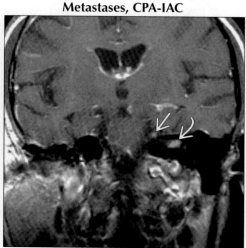

(Left) Axial T1 C+ MR shows bilateral enhancing IAC lesions ⇒, suggesting schwannomas and neurofibromatosis type 2, and an enhancing mass in the left Meckel cave ⇒ at the trigeminal ganglion.
(Right) Coronal T1WI FS MR shows a large enhancing mass ⇒ centered on and enlarging the foramen ovale. The mass extends inferiorly to the masticator space ⇒ along the course of V3.

Neurofibromatosis 2, CPA-IAC

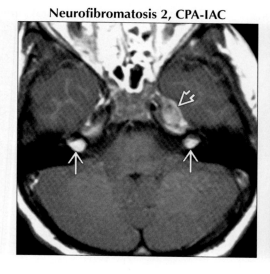

Schwannoma, CNV3, MS

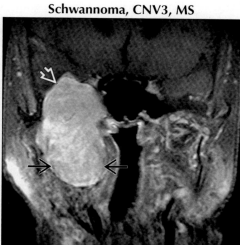

TRIGEMINAL NEUROPATHY

Metastasis, Skull Base

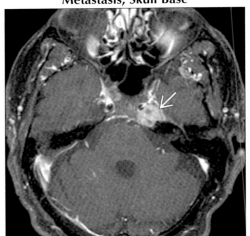

Sarcoidosis, CPA-IAC

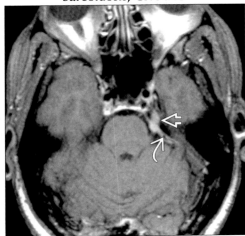

(Left) Axial T1 C+ FS MR shows heterogeneously enhancing metastatic disease ➡ to the left petrous apex and encroaching on the Meckel cave, to affect the trigeminal ganglion. *(Right)* Axial T1 C+ MR shows dural thickening along the course of the preganglionic segment of the left trigeminal nerve ⇨ toward the Meckel cave and also along the left petroclival ligament ➡.

Perineural Tumor, CNV1

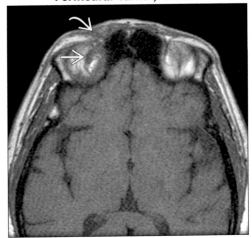

Multiple Sclerosis

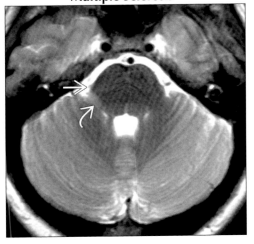

(Left) Axial T1WI MR shows subcutaneous thickening ➡ at the site of the previous SCCa resection, but also an asymmetrically thickened right supraorbital nerve ➡ indicating perineural tumor. *(Right)* Axial T2WI MR shows abnormal T2 signal in the right lateral pons ➡ at the level of the root entry zone of the 5th nerve ➡, explaining the patient's history of paresthesias.

Cavernous Malformation, Pontine

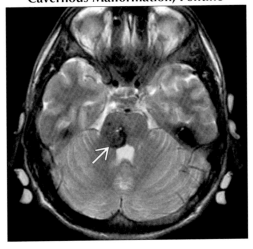

Cerebral Ischemia-Infarction, Acute

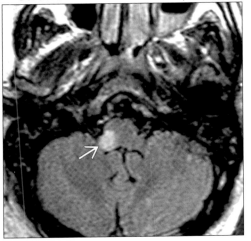

(Left) Axial T2WI MR shows an expansile heterogeneous cavernous hemangioma in the right mid-pons ➡ with peripheral low T2 signal intensity suggesting hemorrhage. *(Right)* Axial FLAIR MR shows high signal in the right lateral medulla ➡. This affects the nucleus of the spinal tract of the trigeminal nerve, which is responsible for facial pain and temperature.

11

TRIGEMINAL NEURALGIA

DIFFERENTIAL DIAGNOSIS

Common
- Vascular Loop Syndrome, CN5

Less Common
- Epidermoid Cyst, CPA-IAC
- Meningioma, CPA-IAC
- Multiple Sclerosis, Pons
- Aneurysm, CPA-IAC
- Schwannoma, Trigeminal, Skull Base

Rare but Important
- Perineural Tumor, CNV3, MS
- Perineural Tumor, CNV2, SN
- Cavernous Malformation, Pons
- Arteriovenous Malformation, Posterior Fossa
- Cerebral Ischemia-Infarction, Acute

ESSENTIAL INFORMATION

Key Differential Diagnosis Issues
- Overall statistics
  - \> 90% of the time, arterial vascular loop in root exit zone CN5 causes trigeminal neuralgia
  - All other causes listed above (< 10%)
- Trigeminal neuralgia (tic douloureux)
  - Presentation: > 60 years old, unilateral paroxysmal facial pain
  - Principal symptom: Unilateral stabbing facial pain typically radiating in maxillary (CNV2) or mandibular (CNV3) areas
  - Pathophysiology: Irritation of root entry zone of CN5
  - Treatments options
    - Medical: Carbamazepine
    - Radiation treatment: Gamma knife stereotactic radiosurgery
    - Surgical treatment: Microvascular decompression
  - Best imaging study
    - MR with MRA
    - Focused MR imaging must include pons, cavernous sinus, face to level of inferior mandible (distal CNV3)

Helpful Clues for Common Diagnoses
- **Vascular Loop Syndrome, CN5**
  - Key facts: Aberrant or ectatic vessels in CPA cistern
    - High-resolution MR-MRA can now identify compressive artery routinely

  - Imaging: Asymmetric looping artery impinges on CN5 root entry zone
    - Superior cerebellar artery > AICA > PICA > vertebral artery

Helpful Clues for Less Common Diagnoses
- **Epidermoid Cyst, CPA-IAC**
  - Key facts: Congenital squamous rest grows slowly, presents in adulthood
  - Imaging
    - Lesion assumes shape of CPA cistern; insinuating margins
    - MR: Near CSF intensity lesion; DWI shows restricted diffusion
- **Meningioma, CPA-IAC**
  - Key facts: Arises from arachnoid cap cells
  - Imaging
    - Dural-based sessile mass
    - MR: Enhancing mass with dural tail(s)
    - CT: Underlying bony hyperostosis or permeative sclerosis possible
- **Multiple Sclerosis, Pons**
  - Key facts: Trigeminal neuralgia in younger patient, suspect multiple sclerosis
  - Imaging: Supratentorial white matter plaques
    - Lesions in area of root entry zone of CN5 may or may not be seen
- **Aneurysm, CPA-IAC**
  - Key facts: May present with sensorineural hearing loss & trigeminal neuralgia
  - Imaging: MR shows complex signal ovoid to fusiform-shaped mass
    - Complex signal due to wall calcification & clot plus luminal flow
- **Schwannoma, Trigeminal, Skull Base**
  - Key facts: Often in setting of neurofibromatosis type 2
  - Imaging: MR shows "dumbbell" schwannoma extending from Meckel cave to root entry zone CN5
    - Intramural cysts (cystic degeneration) common along with avid enhancement

Helpful Clues for Rare Diagnoses
- **Perineural Tumor, CNV3, MS**
  - Key facts: Malignant tumor arises from jaw skin, oral cavity, masticator space
  - Imaging: MR shows enlarged, enhancing CNV3

TRIGEMINAL NEURALGIA

- Inferior alveolar nerve, masticator nerve, foramen ovale, Meckel cave, preganglionic segment, & lateral pons may all be involved
- **Perineural Tumor, CNV2, SN**
  - Key facts: Malignant tumor arises in cheek skin, sinus, or nose
  - Imaging: MR shows enlarged, enhancing CNV2
    - Infraorbital nerve, pterygopalatine fossa, foramen rotundum, cavernous sinus, Meckel cave, preganglionic segment, & lateral pons may all be involved
- **Cavernous Malformation, Pons**
  - Key facts: Solitary or multiple (familial)
  - Imaging: GRE MR shows blooming lesion(s) in pons
- **Arteriovenous Malformation, Posterior Fossa**
  - Key facts: Posterior fossa location uncommon
  - Imaging: CTA/MRA shows large, ectatic arteries
    - Enhancing nidus & large draining veins
- **Cerebral Ischemia-Infarction, Acute**
  - Key facts: Pontine > upper medullary stroke
    - Pontine CVA secondary to basilar artery perforator occlusion
    - Vertebral dissection or atherosclerosis
  - Imaging: DWI MR with restricted diffusion in pons with ADC map mirrored low signal

Alternative Differential Approaches

- Intra-axial
  - Multiple sclerosis, pons
  - Cavernous malformation, pons
  - Arteriovenous malformation, posterior fossa
  - Cerebral ischemia-infarction, acute
- Cisternal (CPA cistern)
  - Vascular loop syndrome, CN5
  - Epidermoid cyst, CPA-IAC
  - Meningioma, CPA-IAC
  - Aneurysm, CPA-IAC
  - Schwannoma, trigeminal, skull base
- Distal cranial nerve 5 branches (CNV2, CNV3)
  - Perineural tumor, CNV2
  - Perineural tumor, CNV3, MS

SELECTED REFERENCES

1. Yoshino N et al: Trigeminal neuralgia: evaluation of neuralgic manifestation and site of neurovascular compression with 3D CISS MR imaging and MR angiography. Radiology. 228(2):539-45, 2003
2. Ueda F et al: In vivo anatomical analysis of arterial contact with trigeminal nerve: detection with three-dimensional spoiled grass imaging. Br J Radiol. 72(861):838-45, 1999
3. Majoie CB et al: Symptoms and signs related to the trigeminal nerve: diagnostic yield of MR imaging. Radiology. 209(2):557-62, 1998
4. Majoie CB et al: Trigeminal neuropathy: evaluation with MR imaging. Radiographics. 15(4):795-811, 1995
5. Meaney JF et al: Association between trigeminal neuralgia and multiple sclerosis: role of magnetic resonance imaging. J Neurol Neurosurg Psychiatry. 59(3):253-9, 1995
6. Hutchins LG et al: Trigeminal neuralgia (tic douloureux): MR imaging assessment. Radiology. 175(3):837-41, 1990

Vascular Loop Syndrome, CN5

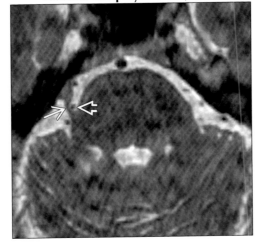

Axial T2WI MR reveals the preganglionic segment of the trigeminal nerve is laterally convex ➡ as a result of a loop of the superior cerebellar artery ➡. Right trigeminal neuralgia results.

Vascular Loop Syndrome, CN5

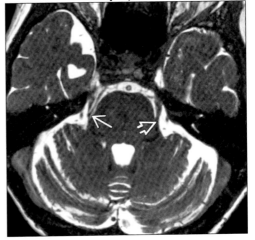

Axial T2WI MR shows 3T MR image of superior cerebellar artery impinging on right root entry zone of the trigeminal nerve preganglionic segment ➡. Note normal root entry zone on the left ➡.

TRIGEMINAL NEURALGIA

(Left) Axial T2WI MR reveals an epidermoid cyst ⬧ of the right superior aspect of the CPA cistern with scalloping of the lateral pons ⬧ and impingement on the root entry zone of the trigeminal nerve ⬧. *(Right)* Axial DWI MR demonstrates a high CPA epidermoid cyst in the superior aspect of the CPA cistern ⬧ that stretches the preganglionic segment of the trigeminal nerve and abuts the root entry zone ⬧.

Epidermoid Cyst, CPA-IAC

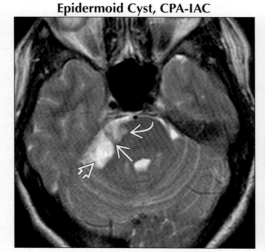

Epidermoid Cyst, CPA-IAC

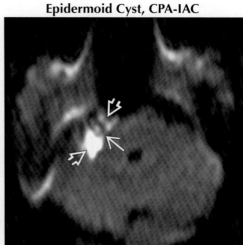

(Left) Axial T1 C+ FS MR shows a meningioma involving the left cavernous sinus ⬧, Meckel cave ⬧, and prepontine cistern ⬧. The area of the root entry zone ⬧ is normal on the right side. *(Right)* Coronal T1 C+ MR reveals a tentorial meningioma ⬧ projecting into the left lateral prepontine cistern in this patient presenting with trigeminal neuralgia. The preganglionic segment of the trigeminal nerve ⬧ is normal on the right side.

Meningioma, CPA-IAC

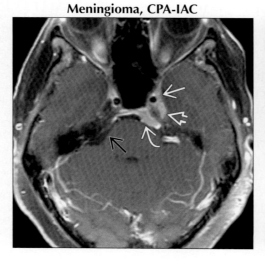

Meningioma, CPA-IAC

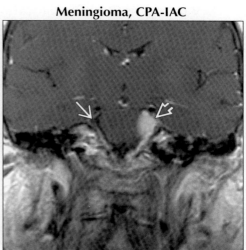

(Left) Axial FLAIR MR demonstrates multiple sclerosis plaques involving the pons. Notice the single largest lesion ⬧ is just deep to the root entry zone ⬧ of the trigeminal nerve. *(Right)* Axial T1WI MR shows a large, fusiform, partially thrombosed basilar artery aneurysm ⬧. The basilar artery is on the left lateral margin of the aneurysm ⬧, while the trigeminal nerve root entry zone impingement ⬧ is on the right.

Multiple Sclerosis, Pons

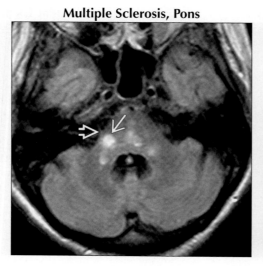

Aneurysm, CPA-IAC

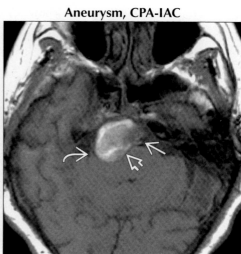

TRIGEMINAL NEURALGIA

Schwannoma, Trigeminal, Skull Base

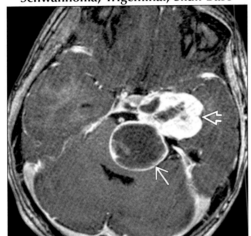

Perineural Tumor, CNV3, MS

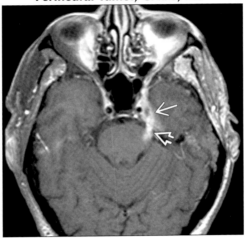

(Left) Axial T1 C+ MR reveals a bilobed trigeminal schwannoma with a cystic prepontine cistern component ➡ and Meckel cave component ⮞ mostly solid and enhancing. The area of the trigeminal nerve root entry zone is significantly compressed. *(Right)* Axial T1 C+ MR shows Meckel cave ➡ & preganglionic segment ⮞ CN5 perineural tumor. This primary retromolar trigone SCCa invaded the masticator space & ascended on CNV3 through the foramen ovale.

Perineural Tumor, CNV2, SN

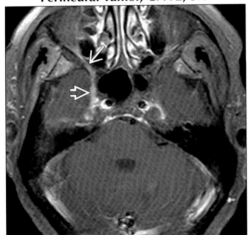

Cavernous Malformation, Pons

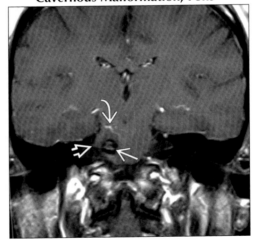

(Left) Axial T1 C+ FS MR demonstrates perineural non-Hodgkin lymphoma extending from the pterygopalatine fossa ➡ along CNV2 in foramen rotundum ⮞. *(Right)* Coronal T1 C+ MR shows right pontine cavernous malformation ➡ just deep to the root entry zone ⮞ of the trigeminal nerve. Notice the associated developmental venous anomaly ➡.

Arteriovenous Malformation, Posterior Fossa

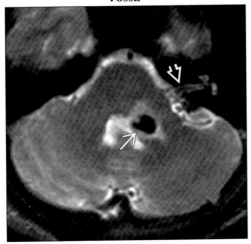

Cerebral Ischemia-Infarction, Acute

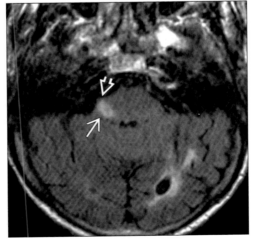

(Left) Axial T2WI MR reveals arteriovenous malformation hemorrhage ➡ with surrounding high signal edema along with large looping anterior inferior cerebellar artery ⮞ in the CPA-IAC cistern. *(Right)* Axial FLAIR MR demonstrates an acute lateral pontine stroke ➡ in this patient with vertebral dissection. Notice this focal CVA is just beneath the root entry zone ⮞ of the preganglionic segment of the trigeminal nerve.

COMPLEX CRANIAL NERVE 9-12 NEUROPATHY

DIFFERENTIAL DIAGNOSIS

Common
- Paraganglioma, Glomus Jugulare
- Nasopharyngeal Carcinoma
- SCCa, Nodes, Internal Jugular
- Cerebral Ischemia-Infarction, Acute, PICA
- Metastasis, Skull Base
- Brainstem Glioma, Pediatric

Less Common
- SCCa, Palatine Tonsil
- Schwannoma, Jugular Foramen
- Cavernous Malformation, Medulla
- Metastases, Meningeal
- Dissection, Carotid Artery, Neck
- Paraganglioma, Glomus Vagale
- Schwannoma, Carotid Space

Rare but Important
- Ependymoma, Basal Cistern
- Multiple Sclerosis, Medulla
- Meningioma, Jugular Foramen
- Chondrosarcoma, Skull Base
- Schwannoma, Hypoglossal Nerve

ESSENTIAL INFORMATION

Key Differential Diagnosis Issues
- Lesions causing injury to CN9-12 are found anywhere along nerve's course from medulla to mid-oropharynx
  - CN9 & CN12 remain suprahyoid
  - CN10 & CN11 course infrahyoid
    - CN10 in carotid space (CS); CN11 in posterior cervical space
- Proximal CN9-12 course together
  - Intracranial course: Medullary nuclei, basal cisterns
  - Skull base: Jugular foramen (CN9-11), hypoglossal canal (CN12)
  - Extracranial: Naso- & oropharyngeal CS
- Imaging approach
  - Enhanced MR: Medulla to hyoid bone
  - Bone CT: Evaluate bones if MR positive

Helpful Clues for Common Diagnoses
- **Paraganglioma, Glomus Jugulare**
  - Benign tumor arises from paraganglia cells along margin of jugular foramen (JF)
  - Centered along superolateral margin of JF; superolateral vector of spread

- CT: Permeative-destructive appearing bone changes; middle ear floor not seen
- MR: Flow voids; avidly enhancing
- **Nasopharyngeal Carcinoma**
  - Tumor usually invasive at presentation
  - CT/MR: Invasion from nasopharynx ⇒ CS
- **SCCa, Nodes, Internal Jugular**
  - Internal jugular chain metastases
    - Primary tumor from nasopharynx or oropharynx
  - CT/MR: Extranodal extension affects CS
- **Cerebral Ischemia-Infarction, Acute, PICA**
  - PICA infarct affects lateral medulla & inferior cerebellar hemisphere
  - MR: DWI ↑ signal, ADC ↓ signal
- **Metastasis, Skull Base**
  - CT: Invasive/destructive bony margins
  - MR: T1 ↓ signal in fatty skull base; enhances
- **Brainstem Glioma, Pediatric**
  - MR: High T2 & FLAIR signal in brainstem
    - Variable, often subtle enhancement

Helpful Clues for Less Common Diagnoses
- **SCCa, Palatine Tonsil**
  - Deeply invasive SCCa
  - Large palatine tonsil with posterolateral invasive margin reaching CS
- **Schwannoma, Jugular Foramen**
  - Bone CT: Smooth, expansion of JF
  - MR: Tubular enhancing mass centered in JF; "points" toward lateral medulla
- **Cavernous Malformation, Medulla**
  - CT: Punctate Ca++; high-density blood
  - MR: GRE blooming ± developmental venous anomaly
- **Metastases, Meningeal**
  - Synonym: Meningeal carcinomatosis
  - MR: Enhancing, thickened meninges
    - Sometimes nodular in appearance
- **Dissection, Carotid Artery, Neck**
  - Ipsilateral Horner syndrome; history of previous trauma or vasculopathy
  - CTA/MRA: Carotid lumen narrowing
    - Suprabifurcation location; terminates at carotid canal of skull base
    - High-density/intensity mural thrombus
- **Paraganglioma, Glomus Vagale**
  - Arises in vagal nodose ganglion of CS
  - CT/MR: Centered ~ 2 cm below skull base
    - Intense enhancement
    - High velocity flow voids (MR)

COMPLEX CRANIAL NERVE 9-12 NEUROPATHY

- **Schwannoma, Carotid Space**
  - CT: Tubular enhancing CS mass; displaces carotid anteriorly
  - MR: Enhancing mass ± intramural cysts

Helpful Clues for Rare Diagnoses
- **Ependymoma, Basal Cistern**
  - Childhood tumor; 4th ventricle origin often; spreads to basal cisterns
  - CT: ~ 50% shows some Ca++
  - MR: Complex signal 4th ventricle-basal cistern tumor
    - Ca++, hemorrhage, cystic changes all possible
- **Multiple Sclerosis, Medulla**
  - MR: High signal lesions in suprasellar white matter
    - Medullary lesions not always visible
- **Meningioma, Jugular Foramen**
  - Bone CT: Permeative-sclerotic hyperostotic changes in bones around jugular foramen
  - MR: "Centrifugal" spreading tumor along dural surfaces
    - Enhancing lesion; "dural tails"
- **Chondrosarcoma, Skull Base**
  - Bone CT: 50% chondroid matrix; centered on petro-occipital fissure most commonly
  - MR: ↑ T2 signal; enhances avidly
- **Schwannoma, Hypoglossal Nerve**
  - Bone CT: Benign expansion hypoglossal canal
  - MR: Tubular enhancing lesion ± intramural cysts

Alternative Differential Approaches
- CN9-12 neuropathy via **segmental anatomic approach**
  - Anatomic segments
    - Intramedullary: Nuclei-tracts
    - Cisternal: Nerves in basal cistern
    - Skull base: Jugular foramen (CN9-11); hypoglossal canal (CN12)
    - Naso- & oropharyngeal CS: CN9-12
- Segmental approach complex CN9-12 neuropathy DDx
  - Medulla
    - Cerebral ischemia-infarction, acute
    - Brainstem glioma, pediatric
    - Cavernous malformation, medulla
    - Multiple sclerosis, medulla
  - Basal cistern
    - Ependymoma, basal cistern
    - Metastases, meningeal
  - Skull base around jugular foramen
    - Paraganglioma, glomus Jugulare
    - Metastasis, skull base
    - Schwannoma, jugular foramen
    - Meningioma, jugular foramen
    - Chondrosarcoma, skull base
    - Schwannoma, hypoglossal nerve
  - Carotid space, naso- & oropharynx
    - Paraganglioma, glomus vagale
    - SCCa, nodes
    - Nasopharyngeal carcinoma
    - SCCa, palatine tonsil
    - Dissection, carotid artery, neck
    - Schwannoma, carotid space

Paraganglioma, Glomus Jugulare

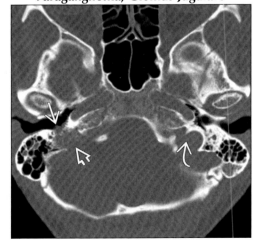

Axial bone CT reveals a jugular foramen permeative-destructive lesion ➡ with soft tissue evident in the middle ear cavity ➡. Note opposite normal corticated jugular foramen bony margins ➡.

Paraganglioma, Glomus Jugulare

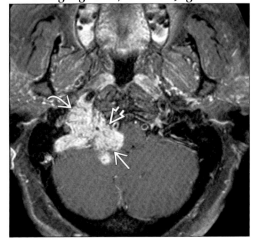

Coronal T1 C+ FS MR shows the inferior portion of a large glomus jugulare paraganglioma involving the basal cistern ➡, area of hypoglossal canal ➡, and nasopharyngeal carotid space ➡.

COMPLEX CRANIAL NERVE 9-12 NEUROPATHY

Nasopharyngeal Carcinoma

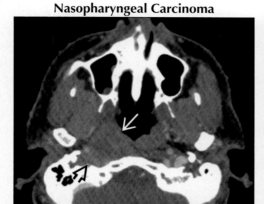

Nasopharyngeal Carcinoma

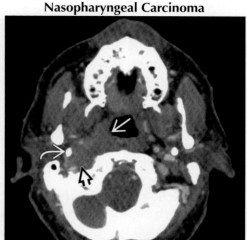

(Left) Axial CECT shows an invasive carcinoma in the right lateral nasopharyngeal recess ➡. Notice that the carotid space (containing CN9-12 at this level) has lost its distinct soft tissue planes ⇨ as a result of tumor invasion. *(Right)* Axial CECT in the same patient demonstrates the inferior aspect of the nasopharyngeal carcinoma ➡ with invasion of the carotid space ⇨ deep to the styloid process ➡.

SCCa, Nodes, Internal Jugular

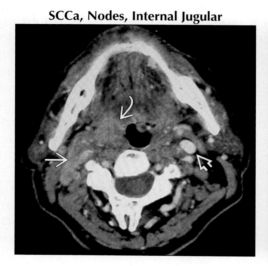

SCCa, Nodes, Internal Jugular

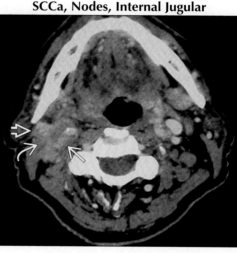

(Left) Axial CECT reveals a right tonsillar mass extending anteriorly into the tongue base ➡. Internal jugular nodes ➡ appear infiltrating and extranodal as they invade the carotid space. Note the normal carotid space on the left, deep to the posterior belly of digastric muscle ⇨. *(Right)* Axial CECT in the same patient shows extranodal tumor invading the deep parotid space ⇨, sternocleidomastoid muscle ➡, and the carotid space ➡.

Cerebral Ischemia-Infarction, Acute, PICA

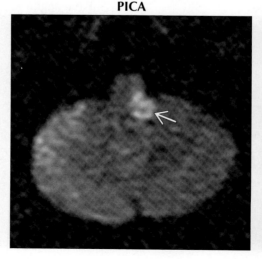

Cerebral Ischemia-Infarction, Acute, PICA

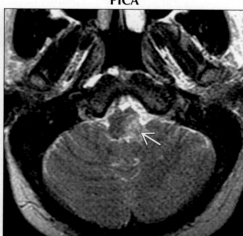

(Left) Axial DWI MR shows high signal (restricted diffusion) ➡ of the left lateral medulla in the area of the lower cranial nerve nuclei. An ADC map image (not shown) revealed a matching low signal, indicating that this brainstem stroke is acute to subacute. *(Right)* Axial T2WI MR in the same patient reveals a medullary high signal area ➡ that is from a subacute stroke based on T2 signal presence and DWI restricted diffusion, as seen on the previous image.

COMPLEX CRANIAL NERVE 9-12 NEUROPATHY

Metastasis, Skull Base

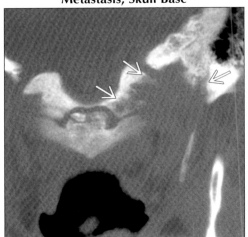

Metastasis, Skull Base

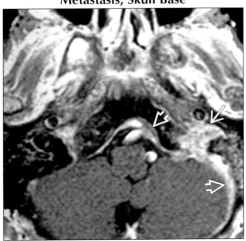

(Left) Coronal bone CT demonstrates abnormal lucent areas ➡ along the margin of the jugular foramen, indicating a widely invasive lesion. Metastatic tumor was the final tissue diagnosis. *(Right)* Axial T1 C+ MR in the same patient shows the left jugular foramen is filled with metastatic carcinoma ➡. Notice the metastatic tumor also involves the meninges along the adjacent posterior fossa ➡.

Brainstem Glioma, Pediatric

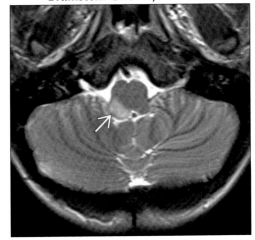

Brainstem Glioma, Pediatric

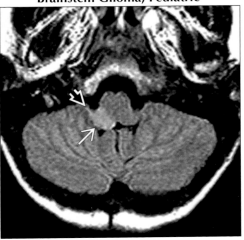

(Left) Axial T2WI MR reveals a small high signal posterolateral medullary glioma ➡ affecting the area of cranial nerve nuclei 9-12. *(Right)* Axial FLAIR MR in the same patient reveals a high signal brainstem glioma ➡. Notice the thickened high signal proximal CN9-11 cranial nerve bundle ➡.

SCCa, Palatine Tonsil

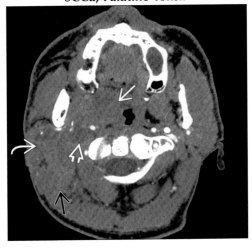

SCCa, Palatine Tonsil

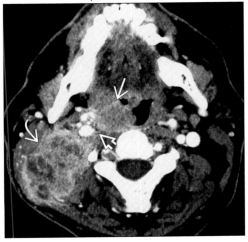

(Left) Axial CECT demonstrates an invasive right palatine tonsil SCCa primary ➡ with extensive extranodal disease in the right carotid space ➡, parotid space ➡, and perivertebral space ➡. *(Right)* Axial CECT shows a right palatine tonsil SCCa primary tumor ➡ spreading posterolaterally into the oropharyngeal carotid space ➡ where cranial nerves 9-12 reside. Note also the massive extranodal SCCa in the right posterior cervical space ➡.

COMPLEX CRANIAL NERVE 9-12 NEUROPATHY

(Left) Axial T1 C+ FS MR in a patient with left vocal cord paralysis shows a well-circumscribed enhancing schwannoma ➡️ emerging from the left jugular foramen ⏩. *(Right)* Axial T2WI MR in the same patient reveals the schwannoma ➡️. Notice that the vector of spread of the lesion is along the CN9-11 bundle ⏩ toward the lateral medulla. It is impossible to predict which nerve this lesion arises from based on imaging alone.

Schwannoma, Jugular Foramen

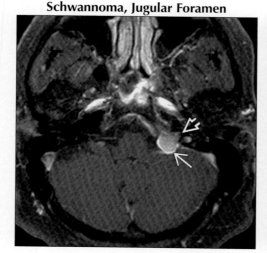

Schwannoma, Jugular Foramen

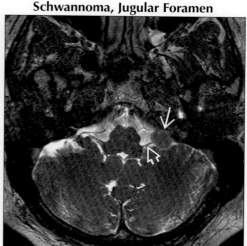

(Left) Axial T1 C+ FS MR demonstrates a partially enhancing left medullary cavernous malformation ➡️ with associated developmental venous anomaly ⏩. A GRE image (not shown) revealed significant blooming of the lesion, indicating previous hemorrhage. *(Right)* Coronal T1 C+ MR shows extensive carcinomatosis of the posterior fossa meninges ➡️. Note the metastatic tumor has entered the internal auditory canals ➡️.

Cavernous Malformation, Medulla

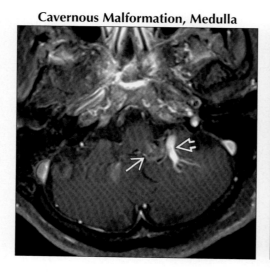

Metastases, Meningeal

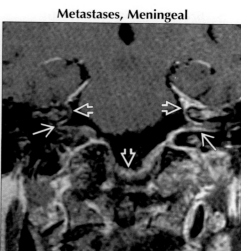

(Left) Axial MRA source image shows residual lumen of internal carotid artery dissection ➡️ in association with a pseudoaneurysm ⏩. *(Right)* Coronal T1 C+ FS MR reveals an ovoid, avidly enhancing carotid space mass ➡️ with a few sporadic high velocity flow voids ⏩ visible. Note the lesion is centered above the carotid bifurcation and does not reach the skull base (jugular foramen) as is characteristic of glomus vagale paraganglioma.

Dissection, Carotid Artery, Neck

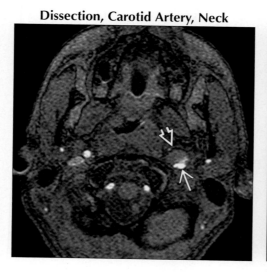

Paraganglioma, Glomus Vagale

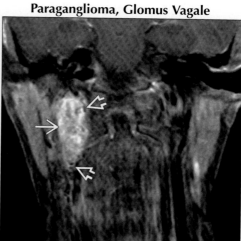

Schwannoma, Carotid Space

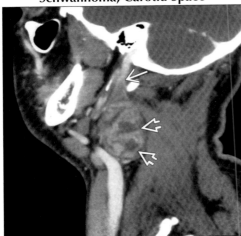

Ependymoma, Basal Cistern

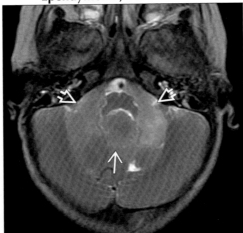

(Left) Sagittal CECT demonstrates a lenticular-shaped schwannoma with multiple intramural cysts ➡. The superior margin "points" ➡ toward the jugular foramen. *(Right)* Axial T2WI MR reveals a 4th ventricular ependymoma ➡ that has spread through both foramina of Luschka into the basal cisterns ➡.

Multiple Sclerosis, Medulla

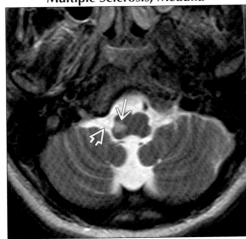

Meningioma, Jugular Foramen

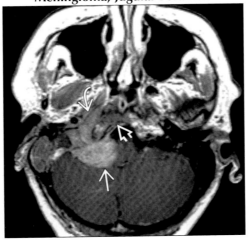

(Left) Coronal T2WI MR shows a lateral medullary focus ➡ of multiple sclerosis. The CN9-11 bundle ➡ emerging from the post-olivary sulcus is just visible within the basal cistern high signal CSF. *(Right)* Axial T1 C+ MR reveals a jugular foramen meningioma projecting into the basal cistern ➡, involving both the lateral clival bone marrow ➡ and the nasopharyngeal carotid space ➡.

Chondrosarcoma, Skull Base

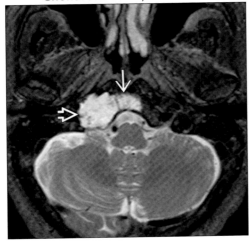

Schwannoma, Hypoglossal Nerve

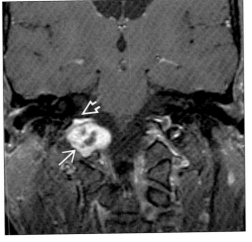

(Left) Axial T2WI FS MR demonstrates the inferior portion of a high signal petro-occipital fissure chondrosarcoma. Note the tumor invasion of the clival marrow space ➡ and the jugular foramen ➡. *(Right)* Coronal T1 C+ FS MR shows an enhancing hypoglossal schwannoma ➡ within an enlarged hypoglossal canal. The tumor encroaches upon the superolateral jugular foramen ➡. Multiple intramural cysts are present within the tumor.

HYPOGLOSSAL NEUROPATHY

DIFFERENTIAL DIAGNOSIS

Common
- Skull Base Metastasis
- Glomus Jugulare Paraganglioma
- Jugular Foramen Meningioma
- Nasopharyngeal Carcinoma
- Hypoglossal Nerve Schwannoma
- Carotid Artery Dissection, Neck

Less Common
- Trauma, Hypoglossal Nerve
- Radiation Changes, Chronic
- Skull Base Fracture
- Chordoma, Clivus
- Skull Base Chondrosarcoma
- Skull Base Plasmacytoma
- Meningioma, Clivus

Rare but Important
- Perineural Tumor Spread, CN12
- Pseudotumor, Skull Base
- Syringomyelia

ESSENTIAL INFORMATION

Key Differential Diagnosis Issues
- Hypoglossal nerve = CN12
- Each nerve innervates 1/2 of tongue
- Nerve injury produces recognizable patterns of denervation
  - Acute: Edematous enhancing muscles
  - Later: Less edema, ongoing enhancement
  - Chronic: Fatty atrophy, variable enhancement
- Key imaging points
  - MR signal/CT enhancement
    - Can be confusing depending on denervation phase
    - Do not mistake enhancing/enlarged tongue for tumor
    - Unilateral tongue abnormal *to midline* = ipsilateral CN12 denervation
  - FDG PET: No uptake in denervated side
- Imaging strategies
  - Once neuropathy is recognized, follow CN12 course in suprahyoid neck
    - Hypoglossal canal → carotid sheath to hyoid → tongue

Helpful Clues for Common Diagnoses
- **Skull Base Metastasis**
  - Key facts

- Most often: Lung, breast, prostate
  - Imaging
    - CT: Destructive hypoglossal canal lesion
    - MR: Loss of normal fat T1 signal
- **Glomus Jugulare Paraganglioma**
  - Key facts
    - Hypervascular neuroendocrine tumor of jugular foramen (JF)
  - Imaging
    - CT: Permeative lytic destructive lesion
    - MR: Infiltrative mass, large flow voids
    - T1 hemorrhage, marked enhancement
- **Jugular Foramen Meningioma**
  - Key facts
    - Benign tumor of arachnoid cap cells
  - Imaging
    - Bone CT: Permeative-sclerotic JF margins
    - MR: Enhancing JF mass, ± dural tail
- **Nasopharyngeal Carcinoma**
  - Key facts
    - Malignancy associated with EBV
    - Originates in lateral pharyngeal recess
    - Infiltrates skull base; nodal metastases
  - Imaging
    - CT: Nasopharynx mass; wide CN12 canal
    - MR: Tumor infiltration at CN12 canal
- **Hypoglossal Nerve Schwannoma**
  - Key facts
    - Benign nerve sheath tumor of CN12
  - Imaging
    - CECT/MR: CN12 canal enhancing lesion
    - May be suprahyoid carotid space lesion
    - Bone CT: Smoothly enlarged CN12 canal
- **Carotid Artery Dissection, Neck**
  - Key facts
    - Spontaneous or following trauma
    - Lower cranial nerve palsies in 10-20%
  - Imaging
    - CECT: Difficult diagnosis without CTA
    - MR T1 FS: Hyperintense crescentic ICA rim

Helpful Clues for Less Common Diagnoses
- **Trauma, Hypoglossal Nerve**
  - Key facts
    - Necessary CN12 surgical sacrifice
    - May be from operative misadventure
  - Imaging
    - 1/2 of tongue is flaccid & edematous
    - Operative changes along ipsilateral carotid sheath or tongue base
- **Radiation Changes, Chronic**

- Key facts
  - Probably microvascular radiation effect
- Imaging: Diagnosis of exclusion
  - Must exclude CN12 tumor
- **Skull Base Fracture**
  - Key facts
    - Acute: Fracture through CN12 canal
    - Late: Canal stenotic as callus forms
  - Imaging
    - Bone CT: Lucency through canal
- **Chordoma, Clivus**
  - Key facts
    - Benign infiltrative notochordal tumor arising within midline clivus
  - Imaging
    - CT: Expansile and destructive
    - MR: T2 hyperintense, heterogeneous enhancement
- **Skull Base Chondrosarcoma**
  - Key facts
    - Chondroid tumor of petroclival fissure
  - Imaging
    - T2 MR: Characteristically hyperintense
    - CT: Destructive mass; 50% chondroid calcifications
- **Skull Base Plasmacytoma**
  - Key facts
    - Malignant mass of plasma cells without systemic multiple myeloma
  - Imaging
    - Nonspecific enhancing clival mass
- **Meningioma, Clivus**
  - Key facts
    - Benign meningothelial tumor

- Imaging
  - CT: Permeative sclerotic bone changes
  - MR: Dural-based enhancing mass

Helpful Clues for Rare Diagnoses

- **Perineural Tumor Spread, CN12**
  - Key facts
    - Most often tumor of tongue base invades neurovascular bundle
    - Tumor spreads along endoneurium/perineurium
    - Or direct spread to CN12 canal by nasopharynx mass: Nasopharyngeal cancer, lymphoma
  - Imaging
    - May be difficult to find unless extending to CN12 canal
    - CT: May see widened CN12 canal
    - MR: Enlarged enhancing nerve
- **Pseudotumor, Skull Base**
  - Key facts
    - Nonspecific inflammatory infiltrate
    - Responds to steroid treatment
  - Imaging
    - Submucosal mildly enhancing infiltrate
    - MR: Tends to be low signal T2
- **Syringomyelia**
  - Key facts
    - Cystic glial-lined spinal cord cavity
    - Usually other neurologic symptoms
  - Imaging
    - MR: CSF-intensity eccentric cord lesion extends to medulla
    - Mild cord expansion

Skull Base Metastasis

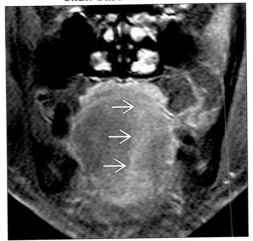

Coronal T1 C+ FS MR shows asymmetric tongue enhancement extending up toward midline to a defined line ➡. This unilateral enhancement is a key finding indicating hypoglossal palsy rather than tongue tumor.

Skull Base Metastasis

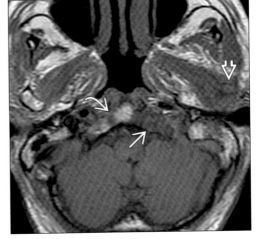

Axial T1WI MR reveals loss of fat marrow hyperintensity ➡ in left basiocciput at hypoglossal canal. Note additional tiny right occipital ➡ and left mandibular ➡ metastases from known prostatic cancer.

HYPOGLOSSAL NEUROPATHY

(Left) Axial T1WI MR shows a hyperintense signal within the left half of the tongue. Note signal has a sharply defined medial margin ➡, suggesting denervation & fat replacement. (Right) Axial T1 C+ FS MR in the same patient shows an avidly enhancing mass ➡ arising in the right jugular foramen & infiltrating much of the left posterior skull base, including hypoglossal canal. Notice normal right canal ➡. Large flow voids ➡ are evident within lesion. (Courtesy W. Smoker, MD.)

Glomus Jugulare Paraganglioma

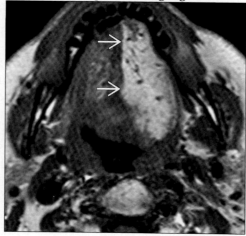

Glomus Jugulare Paraganglioma

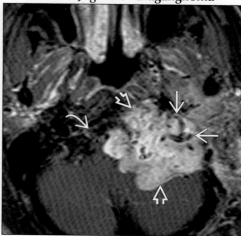

(Left) Axial CECT in a patient with longstanding left vagal (CN10) and spinal accessory (CN11) neuropathy shows fatty atrophy in left tongue with sharply defined medial contour ➡, indicating left CN12 neuropathy. (Right) Axial CECT shows an enhancing destructive mass ➡ of the left skull base with small fragments of residual bone ➡ evident. This is a recurrent glomus tumor, which extends medially to involve the left hypoglossal canal ➡, resulting in CN12 neuropathy.

Glomus Jugulare Paraganglioma

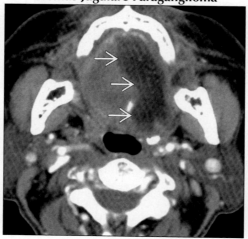

Glomus Jugulare Paraganglioma

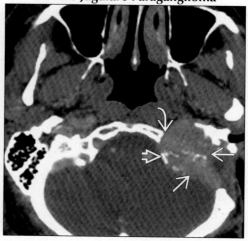

(Left) Coronal T1 C+ FS MR shows an avidly enhancing mass engulfing the left basiocciput ➡ & occipital condyle ➡, filling the left jugular foramen ➡ and hypoglossal canal. The mass has a smooth dural surface. (Courtesy W. Smoker, MD.) (Right) Axial bone CT in a different patient shows a partially calcified mass ➡ below the skull base at the inferior aspect of the left jugular foramen and also within the left hypoglossal canal ➡. (Courtesy W. Smoker, MD.)

Jugular Foramen Meningioma

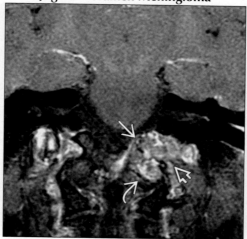

Jugular Foramen Meningioma

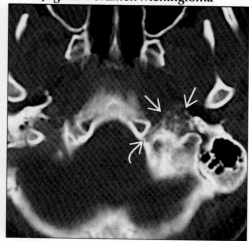

HYPOGLOSSAL NEUROPATHY

Nasopharyngeal Carcinoma

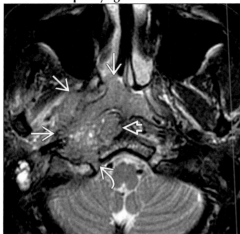

Nasopharyngeal Carcinoma

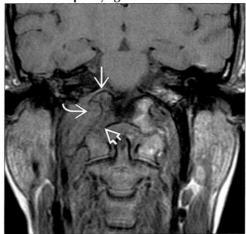

(Left) Axial T2WI FS MR shows a large heterogeneous right nasopharyngeal mass ➡, which extends posteriorly through right prevertebral muscle ➡ and fills right hypoglossal canal ➡. (Right) Coronal T1WI MR in the same patient demonstrates replacement of fatty marrow of right basiocciput ➡ & occipital condyle ➡ with tumor, which also fills right hypoglossal canal ➡. Involvement of cranial nerves indicates T4 nasopharyngeal carcinoma.

Hypoglossal Nerve Schwannoma

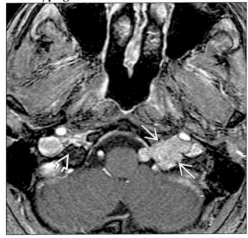

Hypoglossal Nerve Schwannoma

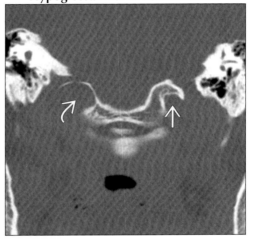

(Left) Axial T1 C+ FS MR shows well-defined lobulated mass ➡ expanding left hypoglossal canal. Note normal right hypoglossal canal ➡. Hypoglossal schwannoma may be found in suprahyoid carotid space as well but typically does not have CN12 symptoms preoperatively. (Right) Coronal bone CT demonstrates smooth scalloping & enlargement of right hypoglossal canal ➡ compared to normal left contour ➡, suggesting schwannoma.

Carotid Artery Dissection, Neck

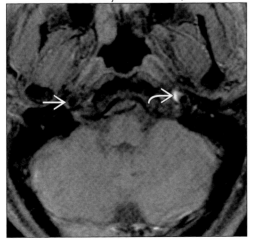

Carotid Artery Dissection, Neck

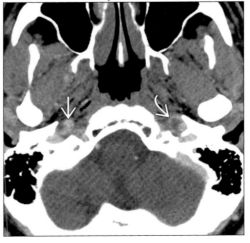

(Left) Axial T1WI FS MR shows a crescentic area of signal hyperintensity ➡ at the medial rim of enlarged left internal carotid artery at skull base. Note the normal flow void of right internal carotid artery ➡. (Right) Axial CECT in the same patient shows dissection to be a subtle rim of low density at anteromedial margin of ICA below skull base ➡. Enlarged caliber of ICA indicates pseudoaneurysm formation. Normal enhancement of right ICA is noted ➡.

HYPOGLOSSAL NEUROPATHY

(Left) Axial CECT in a patient with acute CN12 neuropathy demonstrates an edematous & flaccid left half of tongue ➡ deforming oropharynx contour, often mistaken for tongue mass. Note small focus of air in neck ➡ from left carotid endarterectomy. (Right) Axial T1 C+ FS MR shows a flaccid right tongue ➡ deforming oropharynx contour in a patient with prior neck radiation for laryngeal carcinoma. Note extensive radiation changes in the neck with no evidence of tumor recurrence.

Trauma, Hypoglossal Nerve

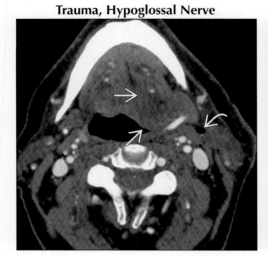

Radiation Changes, Chronic

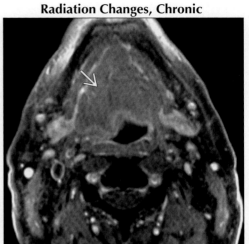

(Left) Axial bone CT shows a sharp lucent fracture line through the right skull base ➡, extending through the right hypoglossal canal. Note the normal left hypoglossal canal ➡. (Right) Axial T2WI MR shows a lobulated hyperintense expansile mass arising from the inferior clivus ➡. The mass involves both hypoglossal canals and extends anteriorly to displace the prevertebral muscles ➡ without altering their signal.

Skull Base Fracture

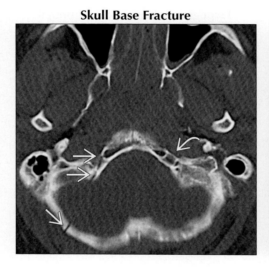

Chordoma, Clivus

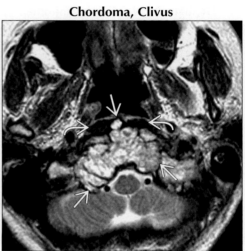

(Left) Axial T2WI MR reveals a uniformly high signal lesion ➡ centered in the right petroclival fissure and involving the lateral clivus. Lesion signal intensity appears brighter than CSF, which is typical of chondroid neoplasms. (Right) Coronal T1 C+ FS MR in the same patient shows a right skull base mass ➡ that homogeneously enhances and engulfs the right hypoglossal canal ➡ and jugular foramen ➡.

Skull Base Chondrosarcoma

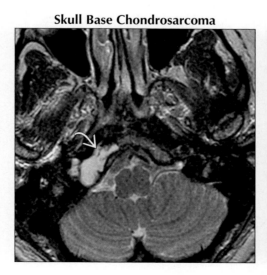

Skull Base Chondrosarcoma

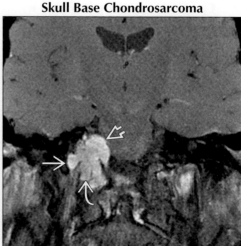

Skull Base Plasmacytoma

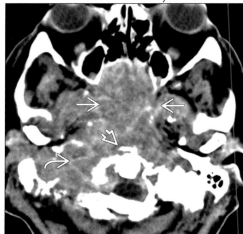

Meningioma, Clivus

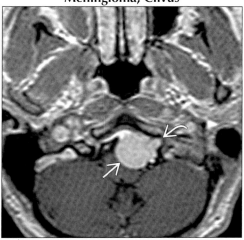

(Left) Axial CECT shows a large destructive central skull base mass ➡, which posteriorly involves the basiocciput, occipital condyles, and anterior arch C1 ➡. This heterogeneous mass infiltrates the right jugular foramen ➡ as well. (Right) Axial T1 C+ MR reveals a well-defined homogeneously enhancing extra-axial mass ➡ in the inferior aspect of the posterior fossa, deforming the medulla. Meningioma extends into the left hypoglossal canal ➡.

Perineural Tumor Spread, CN12

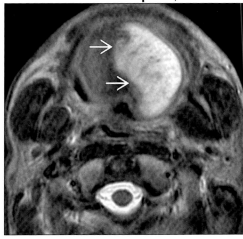

Perineural Tumor Spread, CN12

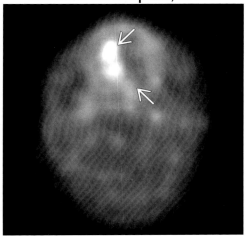

(Left) Axial T2WI MR shows left base of tongue SCCa & ipsilateral residual adenopathy following chemoradiation. The denervation of left tongue is seen as enlarged edematous tissue ➡ from tumor infiltration of left CN12. (Right) Axial PET in the same patient demonstrates FDG uptake in right half of tongue only, due to denervation of left half. This should not be mistaken for a right tongue neoplasm. Again, medial well-defined margin ➡ suggests denervation.

Pseudotumor, Skull Base

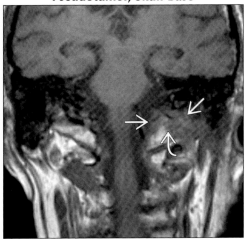

Syringomyelia

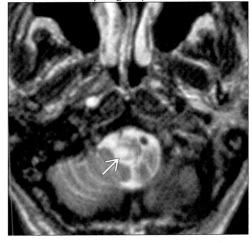

(Left) Coronal T1WI MR shows a subtle infiltrative mass ➡ of left basiocciput with signal loss around the hypoglossal canal ➡. Patient had left CN12 neuropathy & marked improvement after steroid treatment following multiple biopsies negative for tumor. (Right) Axial T2WI MR shows a focal cyst ➡ within the right upper cervical cord extending into medulla. This brainstem involvement indicates syringobulbia in addition to syringomyelia. No enhancement was seen.

11

HORNER SYNDROME

DIFFERENTIAL DIAGNOSIS

Common
- Dissection, Carotid Artery, Neck
- Nasopharyngeal Carcinoma
- Thrombosis, Cavernous Sinus
- Paraganglioma, Glomus Jugulare
- Fibromuscular Dysplasia, Carotid, Neck
- Pancoast Tumor
- Brachial Plexus Traction Injury
- Lymphoproliferative Lesions, Orbit

Less Common
- Metastases, Cavernous Sinus
- Paraganglioma, Carotid Body
- Metastasis, Orbit
- Pseudoaneurysm, Carotid Artery, Neck
- Anaplastic Carcinoma, Thyroid
- Paraganglioma, Glomus Vagale

Rare but Important
- Schwannoma, Sympathetic
- Aneurysm, Subclavian Artery
- Aneurysm, ICA, T-Bone
- Neuroblastoma, Primary Cervical

ESSENTIAL INFORMATION

Key Differential Diagnosis Issues
- Horner syndrome (HS): Occurs when oculosympathetic pathway is interrupted
- DDx focuses on peripheral preganglionic-postganglionic HS differential
- Oculosympathetic pathway (OSP)
  - Supplies sympathetic innervation to sweat glands, dilator muscles of eye, & retractor muscles of upper & lower eyelids
  - 1st order neuron (FON)
    - In posterolateral aspect of hypothalamus
    - Postganglionic fibers from FON descend in reticular formation to cervical spinal cord & proximal thoracic spinal cord
    - Synapse with 2nd order neurons in ciliospinal center C8-T2 spinal cord
  - 2nd order neuron (SON)
    - In ciliospinal center C8-T2 spinal cord
    - Postganglionic fibers exit spine in ventral spinal roots (C8, T1, T2)
    - Fibers pass through inferior cervical (stellate) & middle cervical ganglion
    - Synapse in superior cervical ganglion
  - 3rd order neuron (TON)

- Superior cervical ganglion (located at C2-3 level posteromedial to carotid space)
- Postganglionic fibers ascend in ICA adventitia (carotid plexus) to cavernous sinus
- Fibers follow CN6 to ophthalmic nerve (CN5 ophthalmic branch) to long ciliary nerve branch, entering orbit through superior orbital fissure
- HS clinical presentation
  - Ptosis (drop of upper eyelid)
  - Miosis (↓ pupil size)
  - Anhydrosis (absence of sweat)
- Preganglionic HS: 1st & 2nd order neuron Horner syndrome
  - Segment of OSP proximal to superior cervical (stellate) ganglion
    - Central (FON) subsegment OSP between hypothalamus & C8-T2 ciliospinal center
    - Peripheral (SON) subsegment OSP between C8-T2 ciliospinal center & superior cervical ganglion
- Postganglionic HS: 3rd order neuron HS
  - Segment of OSP between superior cervical ganglion & eye
- Imaging of postganglionic and peripheral preganglionic HS
  - Both present with all 3 symptoms of HS
  - Imaging area of interest: T2 to orbit
    - CECT with CTA most efficient approach
    - Radiologist must interrogate proximal brachial plexus, carotid space (CS), longus colli muscle, carotid canal in skull base, cavernous sinus, & orbit

Helpful Clues for Common Diagnoses
- **Dissection, Carotid Artery, Neck**
  - Key facts: Periorbital pain, ipsilateral visual loss, headache ± HS following trauma
  - Imaging: ICA lumen narrowed with subintimal hematoma
    - CTA: Supra-bifurcation ICA stenosis
    - T1 MR: ↑ signal subintimal hematoma
- **Nasopharyngeal Carcinoma**
  - Imaging: Invasive nasopharyngeal SCCa with CS involvement
- **Thrombosis, Cavernous Sinus**
  - Imaging: Nonenhancing clot in enlarged CS ± large superior ophthalmic vein
- **Paraganglioma, Glomus Jugulare**

- Imaging: Enhancing jugular foramen tumor with high velocity flow voids
  - Spreads into middle ear through floor
- **Fibromuscular Dysplasia, Carotid, Neck**
  - Key facts: Medium-large artery wall dysplasia in younger women
  - Imaging: Multifocal stenosis, long tubular stenosis, & single wall outpouching
- **Pancoast Tumor**
  - Imaging: Apical lung carcinoma invades cervical-thoracic inlet
- **Brachial Plexus Traction Injury**
  - Key facts: Severe shoulder injury
  - Imaging: 1 or multiple brachial plexus roots avulsed
- **Lymphoproliferative Lesions, Orbit**
  - Key facts: Most non-Hodgkin lymphoma
  - Imaging: Enhancing, solid mass involving any area of orbit

Helpful Clues for Less Common Diagnoses
- **Metastases, Cavernous Sinus**
  - Imaging: Enlarged, enhancing cavernous sinus with convex border
- **Paraganglioma, Carotid Body**
  - Key facts: Pulsatile mass, angle of mandible
  - Imaging: Carotid bifurcation location
    - Ovoid enhancing mass; splays ICA from ECA; high velocity flow voids
- **Metastasis, Orbit**
  - Imaging: Invasive, enhancing mass anywhere in orbit
- **Pseudoaneurysm, Carotid Artery, Neck**
  - Key facts: Complication of dissection

- Imaging: Focal arterial enlargement with variable residual lumen; wall thrombus
- **Anaplastic Carcinoma, Thyroid**
  - Imaging: Rapidly enlarging invasive thyroid tumor ± metastatic nodes
- **Paraganglioma, Glomus Vagale**
  - Key facts: Vagal nodose ganglion origin
  - Imaging: Nasopharyngeal carotid space
    - Enhancing mass with flow voids

Helpful Clues for Rare Diagnoses
- **Schwannoma, Sympathetic**
  - Key facts: Asymptomatic neck mass ± HS
  - Imaging: Enhancing, fusiform mass posteromedial to CS; ± intramural cysts
- **Aneurysm, Subclavian Artery**
  - Imaging: Focal subclavian artery enlargement
    - Variable residual lumen size with thrombotic material in wall
- **Aneurysm, ICA, T-Bone**
  - Imaging: Focal ICA enlargement with variable residual lumen; wall thrombus
- **Neuroblastoma, Primary Cervical**
  - Key facts: Presents in 1st 3 years of life
    - Neural crest lesion
  - Imaging: Calcifications in 90% (CT)
    - MR: Enhancing mass in or adjacent to CS; in sympathetic ganglia

SELECTED REFERENCES

1. Digre KB et al: Selective MR imaging approach for evaluation of patients with Horner's syndrome. AJNR Am J Neuroradiol. 13(1):223-7, 1992

Dissection, Carotid Artery, Neck

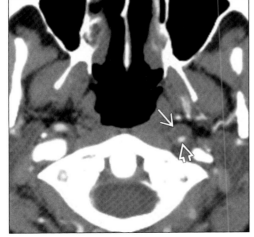

Axial CECT reveals a left internal carotid artery dissection with subintimal hematoma seen as low-density material ➡ surrounding the high-density stenotic residual lumen ➡.

Dissection, Carotid Artery, Neck

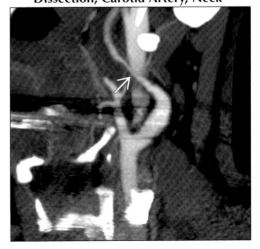

Sagittal oblique CTA demonstrates tapered narrowing ➡ of the internal carotid artery above the carotid bifurcation, secondary to dissection.

HORNER SYNDROME

(Left) Axial T1 C+ FS MR shows a nasopharyngeal carcinoma spreading cephalad through nasopharynx roof into the cavernous sinus ➡ with encasement of the left cavernous internal carotid artery ➡. (Right) Axial T1 C+ FS MR in the same patient demonstrates a large nasopharyngeal carcinoma filling pharyngeal mucosal space. Notice posterolateral left tumor extension into the nasopharyngeal carotid space ➡ with encasement of the left ICA ➡.

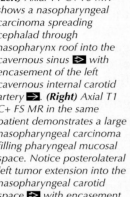

Nasopharyngeal Carcinoma

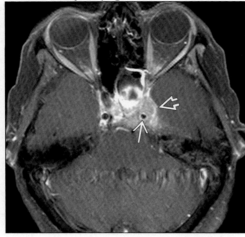

Nasopharyngeal Carcinoma

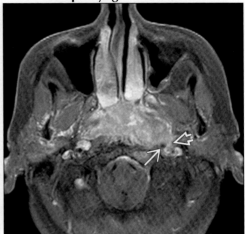

(Left) Axial T1 C+ MR shows bilateral cavernous sinus thrombosis that developed as a complication of acute pansinusitis. Note patchy contrast enhancement within the cavernous sinuses with areas of low signal intensity thrombus ➡. (Right) Coronal T1 C+ MR demonstrates bilateral cavernous sinus fullness, secondary to thrombosis. The multiple low signal areas within the enhancing cavernous sinuses represent clots ➡.

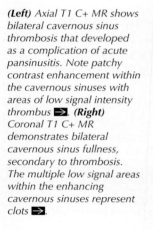

Thrombosis, Cavernous Sinus

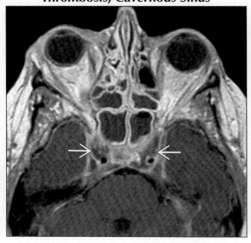

Thrombosis, Cavernous Sinus

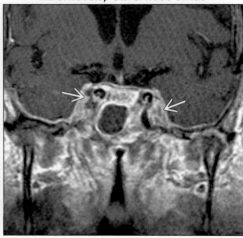

(Left) Axial T1 C+ FS MR shows a large right glomus jugulare paraganglioma as an enhancing jugular foramen ➡, basal cistern ➡, and intrasigmoid sinus ➡ mass with multiple intralesional flow voids. (Right) Coronal T1 C+ FS MR reveals a greatly enlarged jugular foramen filled with an avidly enhancing mass ➡ with flow voids. Note the projection of the paraganglioma into the middle ear cavity ➡.

Paraganglioma, Glomus Jugulare

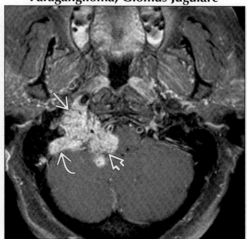

Paraganglioma, Glomus Jugulare

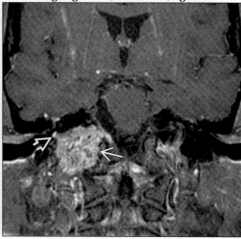

HORNER SYNDROME

Fibromuscular Dysplasia, Carotid, Neck

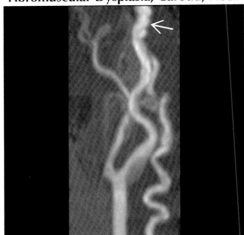

Fibromuscular Dysplasia, Carotid, Neck

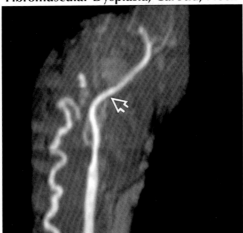

(Left) Sagittal extracranial MRA right shows an abnormal internal carotid artery with a "string of beads" appearance in the distal extracranial ICA ➡, allowing diagnosis of fibromuscular dysplasia. *(Right)* Anteroposterior MRA of opposite carotid system in the same patient reveals the external carotid artery ➡ with complete occlusion of the ICA. Dissected fibromuscular dysplasia vessel with occlusion was suspected based on FMD in opposite ICA.

Pancoast Tumor

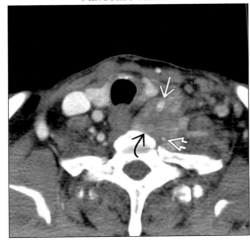

Pancoast Tumor

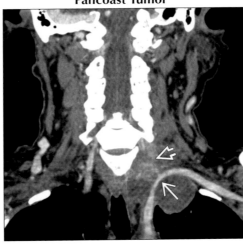

(Left) Axial CECT demonstrates invasive lung carcinoma spreading superiorly to encase the left common carotid artery ➡ and vertebral artery ➡ and invading the longus colli muscle ➡. *(Right)* Coronal CECT shows apical lung carcinoma encasing the left subclavian artery ➡ and spreading into the prevertebral soft tissues ➡.

Brachial Plexus Traction Injury

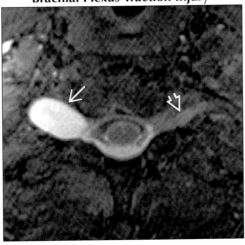

Brachial Plexus Traction Injury

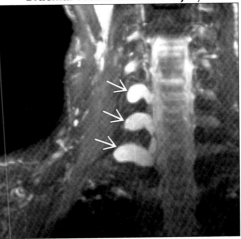

(Left) Axial STIR MR through C7 roots shows pseudomeningocele ➡ with lack of internal neural elements within the right C7 root. The normal left C7 root complex ➡ serves for comparison. *(Right)* Coronal STIR MR reveals multiple avulsion pseudomeningoceles of the right C6, C7, and C8 roots ➡ in this patient with severe brachial plexus traction injury.

(Left) Axial CECT demonstrates an amorphous, mildly enhancing intraorbital focus of non-Hodgkin lymphoma primarily involving the rectus muscles. *(Right)* Coronal CECT in the same patient shows the orbital non-Hodgkin lymphoma involving the superior ➡ and lateral ➡ rectus muscles.

Lymphoproliferative Lesions, Orbit

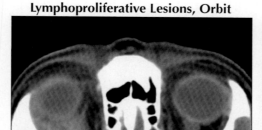

Lymphoproliferative Lesions, Orbit

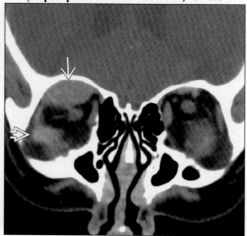

(Left) Axial CECT shows an enlarged, enhancing left cavernous sinus ➡ due to perineural spread of invasive skin squamous cell carcinoma of the left cheek. *(Right)* Coronal CECT depicts a large right carotid body paraganglioma ➡. The extensive peritumoral arterial feeders ➡ are highly suggestive of paraganglioma.

Metastases, Cavernous Sinus

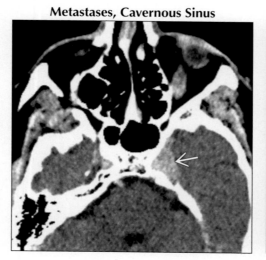

Paraganglioma, Carotid Body

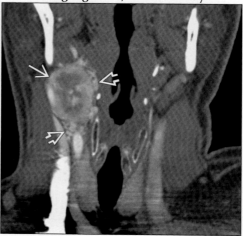

(Left) Coronal T1 C+ FS MR reveals bilateral lateral orbital wall metastases ➡ with significant extraosseous soft tissue spread. On the left, dural involvement is present ➡. Extensive conal and extraconal tumor is also present on the left ➡. *(Right)* Axial CECT shows a large, complex, carotid artery pseudoaneurysm arising from the distal right common carotid artery ➡. Note irregular filling of the patent pseudoaneurysm lumen ➡.

Metastasis, Orbit

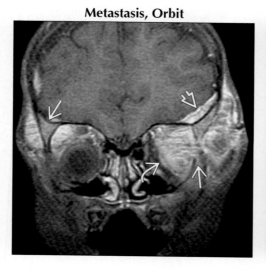

Pseudoaneurysm, Carotid Artery, Neck

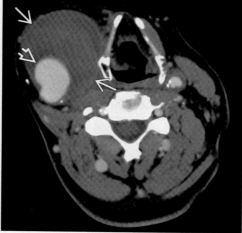

11

Anaplastic Carcinoma, Thyroid

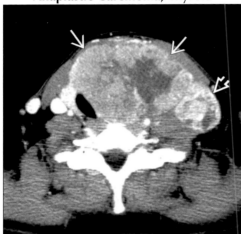

Paraganglioma, Glomus Vagale

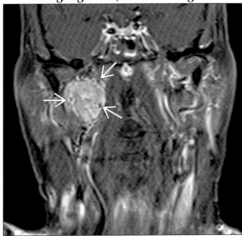

(Left) Axial CECT demonstrates a very large, inhomogeneously enhancing left thyroid mass ➡ associated with malignant-appearing adenopathy ➡. *(Right)* Coronal T1 C+ FS MR reveals an ovoid enhancing tumor 1-2 cm below the skull base with associated high velocity flow voids ➡, identifying the tumor as a glomus vagale paraganglioma.

Schwannoma, Sympathetic

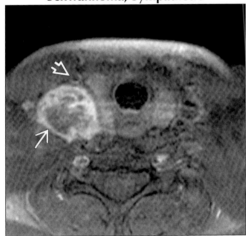

Aneurysm, Subclavian Artery

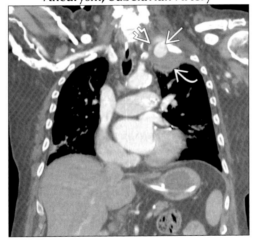

(Left) Axial T1 C+ FS MR shows an infrahyoid neck enhancing tumor at the level of the middle cervical ganglion ➡. Note that the common carotid artery is displaced anteriorly by the lesion ➡. *(Right)* Coronal CECT shows a mycotic subclavian artery aneurysm affecting the proximal left subclavian artery. The eccentric aneurysm lumen ➡, its thrombosed inferior component ➡, and its origin from the subclavian artery ➡ are all visible.

Aneurysm, ICA, T-Bone

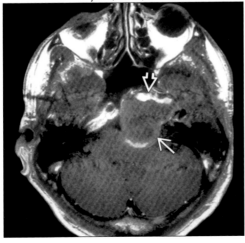

Neuroblastoma, Primary Cervical

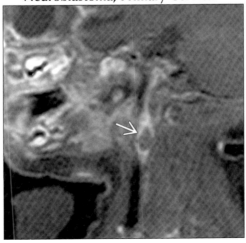

(Left) Axial T1 C+ MR reveals a petrous internal carotid aneurysm with residual arterial lumen seen anteriorly ➡ and a large clot within the aneurysm ➡. *(Right)* Sagittal T1 C+ FS MR in a 9 month old child with Horner syndrome shows a small rim-enhancing cervical neuroblastoma ➡ in the oropharyngeal carotid space.

DIFFERENTIAL DIAGNOSIS

Common
- Metastases
- Neurofibromatosis Type 2
- Neurofibromatosis Type 1
  - Plexiform Neurofibroma
  - Optic Nerve Glioma
- Multiple Sclerosis
  - Optic Neuritis

Less Common
- Viral, Post-Viral Neuritis
  - Bell Palsy
  - Herpes Zoster
  - ADEM
- Lyme Disease
- Lymphoma
- Neurosarcoid
- Opportunistic Infection, AIDS
- Leukemia

Rare but Important
- Ischemia
  - Diabetes
  - Arteriolosclerosis (Microvascular Disease)
- Langerhans Cell Histiocytosis
- Chronic Inflammatory Demyelinating Polyneuropathy

ESSENTIAL INFORMATION

Key Differential Diagnosis Issues
- Enhancement of cisternal, cavernous sinus CN segments always abnormal
- Which cranial nerve(s) affected?
  - Optic nerve: MS, NF1 (optic glioma), viral/post-viral
  - CN3, 6: Often ischemia (diabetes, arteriolosclerosis)
  - CN7: Bell palsy, Herpes zoster (Ramsay Hunt)
  - CN8: Schwannoma (sporadic or NF2 associated), metastasis
- If multiple nerves involved, consider
  - Metastases, lymphoma, leukemia
  - NF2
  - Lyme disease
  - CIDP (especially if nerves massively enlarged)
- History important
  - Optic neuritis (majority have or develop MS)

  - Known neoplasm
  - Flu-like illness (ADEM, viral neuritis)

Helpful Clues for Common Diagnoses
- **Metastases**
  - Most common: CSF spread
    - Involves pia, CNs, may extend along perivascular spaces
    - Multiple thickened nerves > solitary involvement
    - Fundus of CPA/IAC most common site
  - Less common: Perineural tumor extension from extracranial primary
    - Extension into cisternal CN uncommon
    - Squamous cell, adenoid cystic carcinoma (CN5,7 involvement most common)
- **Neurofibromatosis Type 2**
  - Multiple schwannomas
  - Bilateral acoustic schwannomas diagnostic
  - Acoustic schwannoma plus schwannoma of one other CN highly suggestive
  - Schwannoma of "small" CN (e.g., CN3,4) should raise consideration of NF2
- **Neurofibromatosis Type 1**
  - **Plexiform Neurofibroma**
    - Intracranial involvement less common than scalp, orbit, face (e.g., parotid gland)
    - Plexiform neurofibromas of CN3 or CN5 may extend intracranially, involve cavernous sinus
  - **Optic Nerve Glioma**
    - Most are typical pilocytic astrocytomas (PAs)
    - 15-20% of NF1 patients develop pilocytic astrocytoma (most commonly in optic pathway)
    - Up to 1/3 of patients with optic pathway PA have NF1
    - Enhancement varies from none to avid
    - May be uni- or bilateral, extend to/from orbit, involve nerves/chiasm/hypothalamus
- **Multiple Sclerosis**
  - Optic nerve most commonly affected
  - 50-60% of patients with optic neuritis ultimately develop MS
  - Imaging
    - Mildly enlarged, enhancing optic nerve
    - 40% extend to intracanalicular, prechiasmatic/chiasmatic segments

- Other CNs (e.g., trigeminal nerve) less commonly affected
  - Non-MS associated optic neuropathy
    - Infectious (viral)
    - Anterior ischemic optic neuropathy

Helpful Clues for Less Common Diagnoses
- **Viral, Post-Viral Neuritis**
  - **Bell Palsy**
    - Enhancement of intratemporal facial nerve
    - "Tuft" of enhancement in IAC less common
  - **Herpes Zoster**
    - Ramsay Hunt syndrome (Herpes zoster oticus) = vesicular rash of pinna, involvement of CN7,8 in IAC, cochlea
    - Other CNs (e.g., 5) less common
  - **ADEM**
    - Rare manifestation of post-viral demyelination
    - Affected nerve minimally enlarged, enhances transiently
- **Lyme Disease**
  - Most common = MS-like lesions in patient with skin rash, flu-like illness following deer tick bite
  - Can involve multiple CNs (CN7 most common)
- **Lymphoma, Leukemia**
  - Diffuse pial tumor spread → multiple CNs
- **Neurosarcoid**
  - Most common intracranial involvement = optic nerve/chiasm/hypothalamus

- Other CNs rare
- **Opportunistic Infection, AIDS**
  - Tuberculous meningitis, CMV neuritis (retina, optic nerve)

Helpful Clues for Rare Diagnoses
- **Ischemia**
  - Diabetes, microvascular disease
    - CN3,6 most commonly affected
    - Optic nerve (anterior ischemic optic neuropathy) less common
  - Transient enhancement, then atrophy
- **Langerhans Cell Histiocytosis**
  - Usually children
  - Optic nerve/chiasm/hypothalamus/infundibular stalk most common
    - Infiltrated, thickened structures enhance strongly, uniformly
  - Disseminated intracranial Langerhans cell histiocytosis rare
    - Sulcal/cisternal enhancement
    - Multiple enhancing CNs
- **Chronic Inflammatory Demyelinating Polyneuropathy**
  - Typical setting = chronic MS
  - Serial demyelination, remyelination → "onion bulb" thickening of affected nerves
  - Massive enlargement, enhancement of spinal, cranial nerves (spinal > > CNs)

Metastases

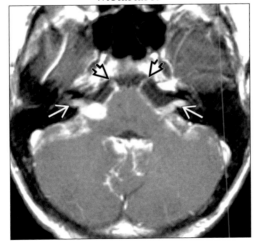

Axial T1 C+ MR in a patient with disseminated malignant glial neoplasm shows diffuse enhancing metastases covering the brain, CPA/IACs ➡, and both abducens nerves ▷.

Metastases

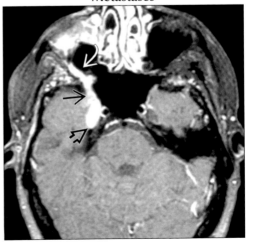

Axial T1 C+ FS MR shows thickened, enhancing V2 in a patient with adenoid cystic carcinoma with perineural tumor spread in pterygopalatine fossa ➘, extending along foramen rotundum ➡ into Meckel cave ▷.

ENHANCING CRANIAL NERVE(S)

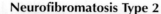

(Left) Axial T1 C+ MR shows bilateral acoustic schwannomas with classic "ice cream on cone" appearance ➡. Note arachnoid cyst associated with left lesion ➡. *(Right)* Coronal T1 C+ FS MR in a patient with known NF2 shows trigeminal schwannomas in both Meckel caves ➡, as well as multiple schwannomas involving cervical spinal nerve roots ➡.

Neurofibromatosis Type 2
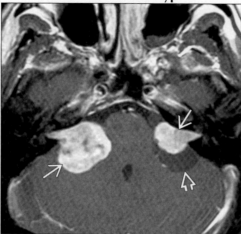

Neurofibromatosis Type 2
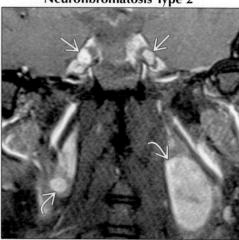

(Left) Axial T1 C+ FS MR in a patient with NF1 shows unusually extensive plexiform neurofibroma of CN3 branches, extending from orbit through markedly enlarged orbital fissure into expanded cavernous sinus ➡. Note scalp plexiform neurofibroma ➡. *(Courtesy M. Martin, MD.)* *(Right)* Axial CECT in a child with NF1 shows bilateral optic nerve gliomas extending through optic canals to chiasm ➡. The right optic nerve is noticeably enlarged and enhancing ➡.

Plexiform Neurofibroma
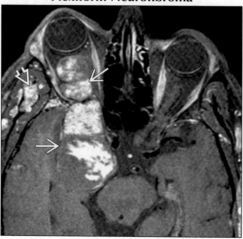

Optic Nerve Glioma
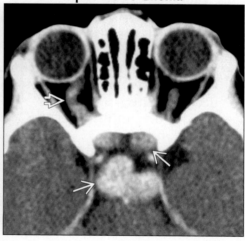

(Left) Axial T1 C+ FS MR shows enhancement of almost the entire length of the left optic nerve ➡, including segment within optic canal ➡. *(Right)* Coronal T1 C+ FS MR in a patient with multiple sclerosis and left trigeminal neuralgia shows enhancing left CN5 ➡. Compare to normal nonenhancing right side ➡.

Multiple Sclerosis
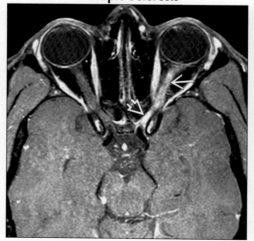

Multiple Sclerosis
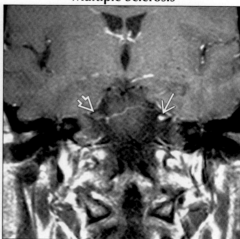

Bell Palsy

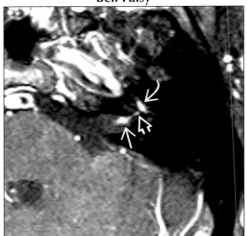

Lyme Disease

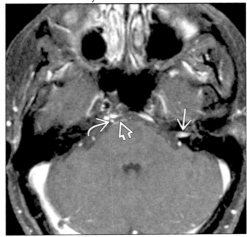

(Left) Axial T1 C+ FS MR with magnified view shows variant case with enhancing "fundal tuft" in IAC ➡, with enhancing labyrinthine segment ➡ leading to geniculate ganglion ➡. (Right) Axial T1 C+ FS MR shows enhancement in left IAC involving both CN7 and CN8 ➡. Note pial enhancement along pons ➡ extending along CN6 from its brainstem exit to Dorello canal ➡.

Lymphoma

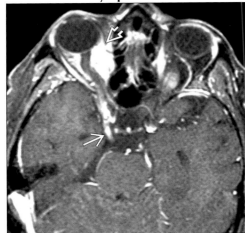

Neurosarcoid

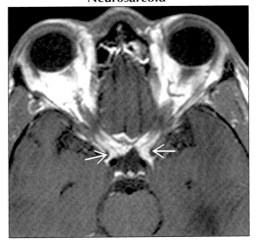

(Left) Axial T1 C+ FS MR in a patient with known systemic lymphoma and right 3rd nerve palsy shows thickened, enhancing right oculomotor nerve ➡, intraconal retrobulbar enhancing tumor ➡. (Right) Axial T1 C+ MR shows enhancement of both thickened optic nerves extending from optic canal to optic chiasm ➡.

Opportunistic Infection, AIDS

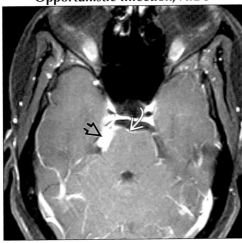

Chronic Inflammatory Demyelinating Polyneuropathy

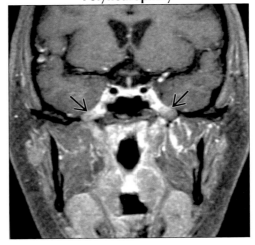

(Left) Axial T1 C+ MR in a patient with HIV/AIDS who presented with confusion and seizures shows tubercular meningitis ➡ that thickens and encases the right trigeminal nerve ➡. (Right) Coronal T1 C+ FS MR in a 39 year old woman with longstanding MS and left facial pain shows both trigeminal nerves are thickened and enhancing ➡.

INDEX

A

INDEX

INDEX

INDEX

C

INDEX

INDEX

INDEX

INDEX

INDEX

F

INDEX

INDEX

INDEX

INDEX

INDEX

INDEX

INDEX

INDEX

INDEX

INDEX

INDEX

INDEX

INDEX

INDEX

INDEX

INDEX

INDEX

INDEX

INDEX

INDEX

INDEX

INDEX